MW00837330

SECOND EDITION

PRIMARY CARE *of* WOMEN

Edited by

BARBARA K. HACKLEY, PHD, CNM

Clinical Director of Women's Health Services
Director of Resiliency Initiative
South Bronx Health Center
Bronx, New York

JAN M. KRIEBS, MSN, CNM, FACNM

Clinical Assistant Professor
Department of Obstetrics, Gynecology, and Reproductive Sciences
University of Maryland, Baltimore
Baltimore, Maryland

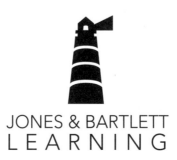

JONES & BARTLETT
LEARNING

World Headquarters
Jones & Bartlett Learning
5 Wall Street
Burlington, MA 01803
978-443-5000
info@jblearning.com
www.jblearning.com

Jones & Bartlett Learning books and products are available through most bookstores and online booksellers. To contact Jones & Bartlett Learning directly, call 800-832-0034, fax 978-443-8000, or visit our website, www.jblearning.com.

Substantial discounts on bulk quantities of Jones & Bartlett Learning publications are available to corporations, professional associations, and other qualified organizations. For details and specific discount information, contact the special sales department at Jones & Bartlett Learning via the above contact information or send an email to specialsales@jblearning.com.

Production Credits

VP, Executive Publisher: David D. Cella
Executive Editor: Amanda Martin
Acquisitions Editor: Teresa Reilly
Editorial Assistant: Emma Huggard
Senior Production Editor: Amanda Clerkin
Marketing Communications Manager: Katie Hennessy
Product Fulfillment Manager: Wendy Kilborn

Composition: S4Carlisle Publishing Services
Cover Design: Scott Moden
Rights & Media Specialist: Wes DeShano
Media Development Editor: Troy Liston
Cover Image: © Gregor Buir/Shutterstock
Printing and Binding: Edwards Brothers Malloy
Cover Printing: Edwards Brothers Malloy

Library of Congress Cataloging-in-Publication Data
Names: Hackley, Barbara, editor. | Kriebs, Jan M., editor.
Title: Primary care of women/edited by Barbara K. Hackley and Jan M. Kriebs.
Description: Second edition. | Burlington, Massachusetts: Jones & Bartlett
    Learning, [2017] | Includes bibliographical references.
Identifiers: LCCN 2016014028 | ISBN 9781284045970
Subjects: | MESH: Primary Health Care | Women's Health | Midwifery | Nurse
    Midwives | Nurse's Role | United States
Classification: LCC RG950 | NLM W 84.6 AA1 | DDC 618.2/0233—dc23
LC record available at https://lccn.loc.gov/2016014028

6048

Printed in the United States of America
20 19 18 17 16   10 9 8 7 6 5 4 3 2 1

Contents

Preface

Primary care is first-contact care; it is care across health and disease; it is care across a lifetime. Midwives and other women's health providers are often a woman's most frequent source for care. Whether we expected to be in the role or not, we become primary care clinicians and need resources that will provide a holistic approach. As clinicians, we have sought information that focused on women. As educators, we have searched for materials that addressed the learning needs of our students.

With this *Second Edition*, the authors offer a text that is designed for students of women's health, as well as for practicing midwives and women's health practitioners. In order to meet the primary health-care needs of women, we require knowledge about health promotion, screenings, immunizations, and environmental health as well as lifestyle changes needed to prevent long-term health problems. The clinician must also be able to manage a wide range of infections and mild presentations of chronic conditions, and have an understanding of when, where, and to whom to refer women with more complicated clinical presentations. This text addresses all of these issues. Primary care material is presented in a manner that is appropriate to the clinical scope of practice.

Because many midwives and women's health practitioners care predominantly for younger reproductive-aged women, they have the unique opportunity to help women adopt healthier lifestyle behaviors early enough to prevent chronic conditions such as cardiovascular disease, diabetes, and cancer, which are leading causes of death and disability in women. They also have the skills and ability to help women with already established health conditions better manage their care. Our goal is that this text will help us, as professionals, more effectively "be with women across the life span."

Acknowledgment

This work is our thank you to all the women who have entrusted their health to us over the years, believing that we will care as much about their general well-being as we do their reproductive health.

Contributors

Janet R. Beardsley, MSN, ANP-C, CNM
Adult Nurse Practitioner/Certified
 Nurse-Midwife
Central Maine Pulmonary and Sleep Medicine
Lewiston, ME

Diane Berry, PhD, ANP-BC, FAANP, FAAN
Associate Professor
School of Nursing
The University of North Carolina at Chapel Hill
Chapel Hill, NC

Carolynn Spera Bruno, APRN PhD, CNS, FNP-C
Assistant Professor of Nursing
Specialty Coordinator, Adult-Gerontological
 Primary Care and Family
 Nurse Practitioner Programs
Yale School of Nursing
Orange, CT

Melanie Cheung MBBS, MRCS
Senior House Officer
Surgical Department
South West Acute Hospital
Enniskillen Fermanagh,
Northern Ireland

Matija Daniel, PhD, FRCS
Otorhinolaryngology
Nottingham University Hospitals
NIHR Nottingham
Hearing Biomedical Research Unit
 and Otology & Hearing Group
The University of Nottingham
Nottingham, UK

Deborah S. Finnell, DNS, PMHNP-BC, CARN-AP, FAAN
Associate Professor
Director of Master's and DNP Programs
School of Nursing
Johns Hopkins University
Baltimore, MD

Barbara W. Graves, CNM, MN, MPH, FACNM
Staff Nurse-Midwife
Baystate Medical Center
Springfield, MA

Barbara K. Hackley, PhD, CNM
Clinical Director of Women's Health Services
Director of Resiliency Initiative
South Bronx Health Center
Bronx, NY

Deborah A. Hall, PhD, BSc
Director
National Institute for Health Research
Nottingham Hearing Biomedical Research Unit
The Ropewalk, Nottingham
Nottingham, UK

Jennifer G. Hensley, EdD, CNM, WHNP-BC, LCCE
Assistant Professor, Nurse-Midwifery Option
 Coordinator
College of Nursing
Anschutz Medical Campus
University of Colorado
Aurora, CO

Derek Hoare, MRes, PhD
Senior Research Fellow
NIHR Nottingham Hearing Biomedical
    Research Unit
Nottingham, UK

Katie Huffling, MS, RN, CNM
Director of Programs
Alliance of Nurses for Healthy Environments
Mount Rainier, MD

Jan M. Kriebs, MSN, CNM, FACNM
Clinical Assistant Professor
Department of Obstetrics, Gynecology,
    and Reproductive Sciences
University of Maryland at Baltimore
Baltimore, MD

Julia Lange Kessler, CM, DNP, FACNM
Program Director, Nurse Midwifery/
    WHNP Program
Assistant Professor
Georgetown University
Washington, DC

Elaine A. Leigh, DNP, FNP-BC
Nurse Practitioner
Mercy Health
Muskegon, MI

Jenna A. LoGiudice, PhD, CNM
Assistant Professor
The Marion Peckham Egan School of Nursing
    and Health Studies
Fairfield University
Fairfield, CT

Kathryn Niemeyer, PhD, MSc, MSN, FNP-BC
Assistant Professor Ferris State University
    School/College of Nursing
Integrative Practitioner, Radicle Wellness
Research Associate, Mederi Foundation
Big Rapids, MI

Megan Sapp Madsen, CNM, FNP, MSN
Women's Healthcare Associates, LLC
Portland, OR

Christine L. Savage, RN, PhD, CARN, FAAN
Professor
John Hopkins University School of Nursing
Baltimore, MD

Deborah L. Schofield, DNP, CRNP, FAANP
Clinical Program Manager and Lead NP for
    Specialty Areas
Director, Postgraduate Nurse Practitioner
    Residency Program
University of Maryland Medical Center
Baltimore, MD

Lynn C. Simko, RN, PhD, CCRN
Clinical Associate Professor
School of Nursing
Duquesne University
Pittsburgh, PA

Karen A. Stemler, MS, RN, APRN, FNP-BC
Nurse Practitioner
Quinnipiac Medical Group, LLC
Branford, CT

Holly Thomas, Audiology BSc
National Institute for Health Research
Nottingham Hearing Biomedical
    Research Unit
The Ropewalk, Nottingham
Nottingham, UK

Allison A. Vorderstrasse, DNSc, APRN, FAAN
Associate Professor
School of Nursing
Duke University
Durham, NC

Penny Wortman, DNP, CNM
Instructor
Frontier Nursing University
Hyden, KY

Susan M. Yount, PhD, CNM, WHNP-BC, FACNM
Associate Professor
Frontier Nursing University
Hyden, KY

CHAPTER 1

DEFINING PRIMARY CARE

Jan M. Kriebs

Primary care has been described in many ways: by provider type, by specialty, and by care provided. In 1978, the World Health Organization described primary care as "first level contact. . . . address[ing] the main health problems in the community" and with a variety of clinicians including midwives "suitably trained socially and technically to work as a team."[1] One commonly accepted definition was developed by the Institute of Medicine's (IOM) Committee on the Future of Primary Care in 1994:

> *Primary care is the provision of integrated, accessible health care services by clinicians who are accountable for addressing a large majority of personal health care needs, developing a sustained partnership with patients, and practicing in the context of family and community.*[2]

In explicating this definition, the IOM avoided specifying the type of provider or location of service required to provide primary care. Instead, the statement emphasized characteristics of clinicians and systems, such as the ability to provide care that addresses health and social needs as well as illness management, cultural competence, and ability to work in the context of an individual's social network. Other structural aspects of care were also emphasized such as the provision or coordination of care for most of an individual's needs, acting as a point of entry to the healthcare system, and the persistence of relationships over time.[2]

The importance of identifying oneself, or one's profession, as able to offer primary care services can easily be seen in the economic consequences of direct patient access as opposed to requirements for referral or restrictions on authority to treat. For clinicians such as midwives and other women's health practitioners, the recognized ability to treat an expanded range of conditions affects state and institutional scope of practice, prescriptive authority, third-party reimbursement, and a host of other pragmatic business survival factors. A small study published in 2002 indicated that midwives identified lack of reimbursement, institutional policies, state laws, and public perception of scope of care as barriers to their providing primary care.[3] And as Phillippi and Barger pointed out in 2015, state limitations on scope of practice, uneven and incomplete recognition as primary care providers by the federal government, and insurance reimbursement continue to be barriers.[4]

A growing body of literature has examined quality and cost issues when midwives or nurse practitioners provide primary care. Although each of the studies has flaws, they have consistently demonstrated overall equivalence in quality and possible cost savings.[5-8] The factors that attract many women to midwifery care, such as longer visits or more time for discussion, may offset financial savings. However, to the extent that interventions in primary care decrease the impact of chronic disease, that money may be well spent.

Midwifery Scope of Practice

Regardless of the credentialing or financial benefits that might accrue from midwives' identification as primary care clinicians, the traditional scope of midwifery (maternity cycle care) did not meet the definition. Whether midwives could reasonably act in this role was addressed by the American College of Nurse-Midwives (ACNM) in its 1992 position statement, "Certified Nurse Midwives and Certified Midwives as Primary Care Providers/Case Managers."[9] Appropriate populations for midwifery primary care were identified as healthy women and newborns, and the focus on health maintenance was emphasized. In 2012, following enactment of the Patient Protection and Affordable Care Act (ACA), the ACNM reaffirmed the role midwives can play in the position statement, "Midwives Are Primary Care Providers and Leaders of Maternity Care Homes."[10]

The "Core Competencies for Basic Midwifery Practice"—a document defining the scope of basic midwifery education—include the knowledge and skills required to assess, diagnose, and treat conditions beyond the maternity cycle and well women's gynecologic concerns.[11] The expected scope of practice includes health promotion and disease prevention, immunizations, diagnosis

and treatment of common self-limited health problems, and management of mild to moderate chronic conditions such as asthma or obesity.[11]

Women's Health as Primary Care Practice

Clinicians whose focus is on women's health care are often de facto primary care providers. Many healthy women choose to see their gynecologic provider for primary care on a regular basis, where prenatal care and ongoing reproductive health care have established a trust relationship. Even as recommendations around management of cancer screening have changed, consultation regarding contraceptive and procreative plans, the effects of hormonal changes during menopause, and sexual health remain integral parts of providing care for women. Midwives already provide health screening, preventive health recommendations, and counseling about lifestyle changes to women. In addition, during pregnancy, many clinicians defer to the obstetric provider for the management of many health concerns, probably because the "extra patient" complicates choices of therapy or medication.

A key component of primary care is health maintenance. This is accomplished in several ways: through counseling and education to decrease lifestyle risks and promote health, disease prevention, and regular general healthcare examinations. But beyond health maintenance, how are midwives active in primary care?

The task analysis undertaken periodically by the American Midwifery Certification Board evaluates congruence between education and practice to support the certification examination's validity. Apart from these periodic assessments, there is little literature that directly evaluates the participation of midwives in primary care. Data collected from midwives attending the ACNM

Annual Meeting in 1993 identified obesity, anemia, and upper respiratory and gastrointestinal infections as primary care diagnoses managed by more than 80% of midwives.[12] Murphy has reported that for gynecologic patients seen by midwives, blood pressure evaluation and assessment of medication use were common; cholesterol assessment and determination of rubella immunity were provided by more than half of the clinicians.[13] Those services provided to the fewest women included other immunizations. About half of the midwives asked women about other sources of primary care. Midwives identified lifestyle and psychosocial issues as counseling issues commonly addressed in their practice. The counseling services least often reported as provided included injury prevention, seatbelt use, and work-related risks.[13]

Midwives surveyed by Stuart and Oshio most commonly reported that their formal education included material related to acute respiratory, gastrointestinal, and genitourinary problems and hematologic and metabolic conditions.[3] Knowledge of behavioral, psychosocial, and sexual conditions was also reported by a large majority of the respondents. In each case, a somewhat smaller percentage managed these conditions independently.

A 2011 report on community health centers included a small number of midwives and nurse practitioners.[14] While the midwifery care provided was predominately for reproductive needs, 42% reported serving as a primary care provider for their patients, of whom approximately 18% had one or more chronic conditions.

The 2012 Task Analysis by the American Midwifery Certification Board found that almost half of recently certified midwives were providing primary care and managing most conditions that were diagnosed either independently or collaboratively.[15] More than 50% of respondents indicated they provided independent management

for concerns ranging from anemia and asthma to skin infections, respiratory infections, and common gastrointestinal complaints.[15]

The Clinical Scope of Primary Care

Reviewing the commonly identified problems, screening tests, and counseling during primary care visits helps to establish a basis for deciding when and to whom midwives can offer primary care services. Adult women on average have more than four office visits per year.[16] Women are seen more frequently than men, whites more often than blacks, and elderly women more often than young women (excluding pregnancy).[17] In contrast, African Americans have more visits to hospital outpatient departments than do whites, and those between 45 and 64 years of age are more likely to be seen there than those over 65 (who presumably have a source of care through Medicare).[18] Approximately 40% of visits by women are for acute care, 30% for management of a chronic condition, and 23% for preventive care.[19]

The federal government regularly reports on common diagnoses seen in ambulatory care. The National Ambulatory Medical Care Survey (NAMCS) reports comprehensive access and diagnosis data every 5 years in addition to yearly summaries.[17] These reports help identify the "substantial majority" of health problems a primary care clinician should be able to identify and manage or refer appropriately. However, data for nurse practitioner and midwife visits include only 1.2% of reported primary care visits.

Common symptoms described as reasons for office visits include cough; pain, whether specified or general; fatigue; and malaise. **Table 1-1** lists some of the most commonly identified diagnoses for women during an office visit, outside of reproductive care.[17,20,21] Obesity is rarely

Table 1-1 Common Diagnoses During Office Visits for Women

Acute upper respiratory infection (URI), sinusitis, pharyngitis

Asthma

Lower respiratory infection, bronchitis, pneumonia

Essential hypertension

Headache, migraine

Diabetes mellitus

Depression, anxiety, other mental health

Joint pain

Back pain

Urinary tract infection

Lipid abnormality

Hypothyroidism

Viral infections

Skin lesions or rashes

Data from National Center for Health Statistics. National Ambulatory Medical Care Survey: 2012 State and National Summary Tables. Available from: http://www.cdc.gov/nchs/data/ahcd/namcs_summary/2012_namcs_web_tables.pdf. Accessed February 11, 2016; St Sauver J, Warner DO, Yawn BP, Jacobson DJ, McGree MF, Pankratz JJ, et al. Why patients visit their doctors: assessing the most prevalent conditions in a defined American population. *Mayo Clin Proc.* 2013;88:56-67; Wändell P, Carlsson AC, Wettermark B, Lord G, Cars T, Ljunggren G. Most common diseases diagnosed in primary care in Stockholm, Sweden, in 2011. *Fam Pract.* 2013;30(5):506-513.

included on a list of reasons for visits, although in 2010 the majority of American women were either overweight or obese; this includes 27.9% who were classified as overweight (body mass index [BMI] of 25.0-29.9) and 35.5% who were classified as obese (BMI of 30.0 or more).[22]

Among the screening or general evaluation services provided during office visits, weight measurement and blood pressure evaluation are by far the most common. The NAMCS reports on selected examinations during primary care visits. For women, the most commonly reported were skin (16.4%), pelvic (10.7%), and breast (7.8%); of note, depression screening was performed less than 2% of the time.[17] Selected educational topics included nutritional counseling (7.1%), exercise (4.9%), tobacco cessation, and injury prevention.[17] When one considers the obesity rate among US women, the fact that nutritional information was provided only 7% of the time, and exercise recommendations of all types made < 5%, the need for increased counseling appears evident. The ACA has additionally mandated a series of preventive services specific to women's health.[23] These are shown in **Table 1-2**.

More than 50% of women take one or more medications. The most common prescriptions among nonpregnant women of childbearing age include oral contraceptives, levothyroxine, albuterol, acetaminophen, hydrocodone, and selective serotonin reuptake inhibitors (SSRIs). Pregnant women are less likely to take prescription medications other than prenatal vitamins, but 1 in 4 reported taking medications that included treatment for asthma, allergies, and diabetes; antibiotics; and levothyroxine.[24] In one study in Minnesota that worked from pharmacy records, women age 19-29 years were prescribed antibiotics, contraceptives, antidepressants, opioid analgesics, and antiasthmatics most commonly; women age 30-49 received antidepressants and antibiotics most frequently, followed by opioids, antiasthmatics, and medications for gastrointestinal disorders.[25]

While the preceding data identify a number of conditions that preclude the midwife or other women's health clinicians from acting as the primary source of medical care (e.g., insulin-dependent diabetics may require endocrinologist supervision), these women can be identified on history and physical examination, and then referred as necessary. Far more women need health

Table 1-2 Preventive Services Specific to Women Mandated by the ACA

Type of Preventive Service	HHS Guideline for Health Insurance Coverage	Frequency
Well-woman visits	Well-woman preventive care visit for adult women to obtain the recommended preventive services that are age and developmentally appropriate, including preconception care and many services necessary for prenatal care	Annual, although several visits may be needed to obtain all necessary recommended preventive services, depending on a woman's health status, health needs, and other risk factors.
Screening for gestational diabetes		In pregnant women between 24 and 28 weeks' gestation and at the first prenatal visit for pregnant women identified to be at high risk for diabetes.
HPV testing	High-risk human papillomavirus DNA testing in women with normal cytology results	Screening should begin at 30 years of age and should occur no more frequently than every 3 years.
Counseling for STIs	All sexually active women	Annual.
Counseling and screening for HIV	All sexually active women	Annual.
Contraceptive methods and counseling	All FDA-approved contraceptive methods, sterilization procedures, and patient education and counseling for all women with reproductive capacity	As prescribed.
Breastfeeding support, supplies, and counseling	Comprehensive lactation support and counseling by a trained provider during pregnancy and/or in the postpartum period, and costs for renting breastfeeding equipment	In conjunction with each birth.
Screening and counseling for interpersonal and domestic violence		Not specified.

FDA = Food and Drug Administration; HHS = US Department of Health and Human Services; HIV = human immunodeficiency virus; HPV = human papillomavirus; STI = sexually transmitted infection

Modified from Health Resources and Services Administration. Women's preventative service guidelines. Rockville, MD: US Department of Health and Human Services; 2011. Retrieved from: http://www.hrsa.gov/womensguidelines/

education, preventive services and screening, and general examinations that fall well within the midwife's scope of practice. The use of tools such as the *Choosing Wisely* campaign by the American Board of Internal Medicine and the US Preventive Services Task Force Guidelines can assist midwives and other health practitioners in effective decision making and counseling.

Chronic Diseases and Cause of Death

Prevention of chronic disease is a key component of primary care. Chronic diseases are linked to 7 of the "Top Ten" causes of mortality in the United States; about 50% of American adults have at least 1 chronic disease.[26] Women generally report an increased number of days of feeling physically or mentally unhealthy compared to men, and rates are higher among minority, low socioeconomic status, and poorly educated groups.[27] Increasingly, attention is paid to the role of modifiable risk factors—poor nutritional habits and physical inactivity (linked to overweight and obesity), tobacco and alcohol use, uncontrolled hypertension, and hyperlipidemia—in affecting the burden of chronic illness. It is unlikely that the overall disease burden can be reduced without improvements in these factors.[28]

Monitoring for causes of death from chronic diseases uses Centers for Disease Control and Prevention (CDC) indicators linked to key topics such as cancer, cardiovascular disease (CVD), diabetes, asthma, chronic obstructive pulmonary disease, renal disease, arthritis, and mental health. Lifestyle factors including nutrition; exercise; tobacco and alcohol use; oral health; and the "overarching" factors of poverty, education, and insurance status are also followed for their contribution to the development of diseases.[29]

Causes of death can be viewed in two ways, and most people are used to the report of disease states,

grouped into typical categories, such as "cancer" and "unintentional injuries" (**Table 1-3**).[30,31] These groupings allow for the comparison of relative contributions from broad categories; at the same time, they do not provide specifics. For example, if "malignant neoplasm of the trachea, bronchus, and lung" were a stand-alone category, rather than part of the broader category cancer, it would be the number 3 cause of death for some population groups.[30] Another way to consider the burden of disease is to show the contribution of factors that promote disease. Mokdad and colleagues reported on underlying factors that contributed to the official diagnostic cause of death, the "actual" cause, in 2000.[32] They found that lifestyle factors such as tobacco, alcohol, and drug use; poor diet and lack of exercise; and toxic agents including pollutants were direct contributors to more than 40% of all-cause mortality. Krueger and colleagues documented lack of a high school education as a contributor to mortality equal to current tobacco use, with a particular link to cardiovascular death.[33]

Disparities in Health Care

Having looked at common components of primary care visits and areas where health education and preventive measures can improve long-term health, midwives must also consider how disparities in health and access to health care can affect practice. One difficulty in studying the disparities found between racial and cultural groups is that US studies have historically used race as a marker for class or socioeconomic status.[34] Disparities in services sought and provided can be found across ethnic groups, age groups, rural versus urban locations, and economic strata. The World Health Organization states, "the social determinants of health are mostly responsible for health inequities—the unfair and avoidable differences in health status seen within and between countries."[35] The first National Healthcare

Table 1-3 Leading Causes of Death for Women, 2013*

Rank	15-19	20-24	25-34	35-44	45-54	55-64	65+	65-74	75-84	85+	All Ages
1	Unintentional injuries 40.4%	Unintentional injuries 40.3%	Unintentional injuries 29.9%	Cancer 24.6%	Cancer 33.3%	Cancer 38.3%	Heart disease 24.6%	Cancer 35.6%	Cancer 23.2%	Heart disease 28.7%	Heart disease 22.4%
2	Suicide 14.6%	Suicide 11.8%	Cancer 13.0%	Unintentional injuries 18.1%	Heart disease 14.8%	Heart disease 16.6%	Cancer 18.9%	Heart disease 18.2%	Heart disease 21.8%	Cancer 10.1%	Cancer 21.5%
3	Cancer 9.6%	Homicide 8.1%	Suicide 9.2%	Heart disease 12.0%	Unintentional injuries 9.7%	Chronic lower respiratory diseases 5.8%	Chronic lower respiratory diseases 6.6%	Chronic lower respiratory diseases 9.0%	Chronic lower respiratory diseases 8.2%	Alzheimer's disease 8.0%	Chronic lower respiratory diseases 6.1%
4	Homicide 6.2%	Cancer 7.7%	Heart disease 7.5%	Suicide 5.8%	Chronic liver disease 4.2%	Unintentional injuries 4.1%	Stroke 6.5%	Stroke 4.4%	Stroke 6.5%	Stroke 7.3%	Stroke 5.8%
5	Heart disease 3.9%	Heart disease 4.2%	Homicide 4.9%	Chronic liver disease 3.3%	Chronic lower respiratory diseases 3.6%	Diabetes 3.9%	Alzheimer's disease 5.7%	Diabetes 3.8%	Alzheimer's disease 4.6%	Chronic lower respiratory diseases 4.8%	Alzheimer's disease 4.6%
6	Birth defects 2.6%	Pregnancy complications 2.8%	Pregnancy complications 3.1%	Stroke 2.8%	Stroke 3.4%	Stroke 3.6%	Diabetes 2.7%	Kidney disease 2.1%	Diabetes 3.1%	Influenza & pneumonia 3.1%	Unintentional injuries 3.8%
7	Pregnancy complications 1.5%	Birth defects 1.4%	Diabetes 2.0%	Diabetes 2.8%	Diabetes 3.2%	Chronic liver disease 2.6%	Influenza & pneumonia 2.6%	Unintentional injuries 2.0%	Influenza & pneumonia 2.2%	Unintentional injuries 2.4%	Diabetes 2.8%
8	Influenza & pneumonia 1.2%	Diabetes 1.2%	Chronic liver disease 1.7%	Homicide 2.1%	Suicide 3.2%	Septicemia 1.9%	Unintentional injuries 2.2%	Septicemia 1.9%	Unintentional injuries 2.1%	Diabetes 2.0%	Influenza & pneumonia 2.3%
9	Stroke 1.0%	Influenza & pneumonia 1.0%	Stroke 1.6%	Septicemia 1.6%	Septicemia 1.6%	Kidney disease 1.6%	Kidney disease 2.0%	Influenza & pneumonia 1.7%	Kidney disease 2.1%	Hypertension 1.9%	Kidney disease 1.8%
10	Chronic lower respiratory diseases 0.8%	Septicemia 1.0%	Influenza & pneumonia 1.4%	Influenza & pneumonia 1.6%	Influenza & pneumonia 1.4%	Influenza & pneumonia 1.5%	Hypertension 1.6%	Alzheimer's disease 1.3%	Septicemia 1.8%	Kidney disease 1.9%	Septicemia 1.6%

*Percentages represent total deaths in the age group due to the cause indicated. Some terms have been shortened from those used in the National Vital Statistics Report. To learn more, visit Mortality Tables at http://www.cdc.gov/nchs/nvss/mortality_tables.htm or http://www.cdc.gov/nchs/deaths.htm (HHS, CDC, NCHS).

Modified from Centers for Disease Control and Prevention. Leading causes of death in females 2013. Retrieved from: http://www.cdc.gov/Women/lcod/2013/WomenAll_2013.pdf. Accessed February 11, 2016.

Disparities Report noted, "there are complicated interrelationships between race, ethnicity, and socioeconomic status that may result in healthcare disparities."[36(p8)] Those disparities remain more than a decade later, as evidenced in a 2014 report on health disparities and quality, which found that many measures of access and quality were unimproved or worsening.[37] Within racially and ethnically defined groups, those with less education, lower incomes, and working class jobs fare more poorly.

An illustration of the intertwining of risk factors and worsened outcomes can be seen in the case of CVD, the most important overall cause of death for women. Rates of CVD are higher among African American women than whites or Hispanics.[31] Multiple studies have documented that the factors associated with increased risk of cardiovascular death—obesity, uncontrolled hypertension, and diabetes mellitus—are increased among African Americans.[38-40]

Barriers to accessing care fall into categories that include structural/logistical, financial, and knowledge of available resources.[41] Among structural obstacles, including issues such as transportation and office locations and hours open, poverty and race both have been shown to negatively affect access. The issue is worse for women than for men. Financially, as many as 28% of uninsured women delayed seeking care as a direct result of cost in 2011, although that number drops precipitously to 8.8% among publicly insured women and 3.9% among those with private insurance.[22]

Having a usual source of care (defined as an office or health center) is also associated with improved access to services. Almost 90% of all women report having such a source of care. The percentage rises with age, influenced by Medicare access in the elderly, and is lower for Hispanic women.[22] The group most directly affected includes those ineligible for insurance under the

ACA, of whom only 54% reported having a usual source of care.[42] The ACA extended health coverage to approximately 14 million previously uninsured women through a combination of tax credits and Medicaid expansion. However, 20 states have not accepted federal money to expand Medicaid as of 2015, with the result that about 3 million women living in those states fall into a gap where they are neither covered by Medicaid nor are eligible for financial subsidies to purchase insurance.[42] They also do not have guaranteed access to the women's health services provided under the ACA.

Disparities in education about health needs and in treatment exist. Little change has occurred over time in the knowledge among members of an ethnic group about relative risks of specific health problems within their own group,[43] suggesting lack of health information provided by clinicians. Patients in racial/ethnic minorities have been shown to receive less information about their diagnoses and possible treatments compared to whites.[44]

The costs of health disparities are not just to the individual or their families. One study estimated the economic burden of health disparities to be greater than 1 trillion dollars between 2006 and 2009 in the United States. This included direct medical costs, indirect societal costs from chronic illness, disability and missed workdays, and premature death.[45]

Health equity has been defined as

attainment of the highest level of health for all people. Achieving health equity requires valuing everyone equally with focused and ongoing societal efforts to address avoidable inequalities, historical and contemporary injustices, and the elimination of health and health care disparities.[46]

Anyone who is interested in improving healthcare equity should consider these goals in evaluating their own clinical practice and ask questions such as: Have I asked all of my patients about immunizations? About violence? About substance abuse? How can I make my practice more accessible to women in the community? Am I treating my patients with as much respect as I would want to be treated? Am I listening to the women I serve? And, am I helping them work toward better health?

Cultural Competence in Practice

Simply knowing about disparities in health access and health care is not enough to make one an effective provider. Awareness of and respect for the diversity among women can help remove a common barrier to care. Culture has been defined as "a socially transmitted design for living which includes traditional values, beliefs, rituals, and behaviors."[22] Within groups there is diversity and change over time; cultures are not monolithic. Dunn describes the characteristics of any culture as dynamic, shared, learned, and integrated.[47] Other authors have suggested that healthcare providers form a culture based on a common set of knowledge and behaviors, including a use of language that is not common in the community,[48] and that medicine sees itself as culture-free, while identifying anyone with a different perspective as being "cultural."[49]

Several terms are used to describe the effort to function effectively as a caregiver for a woman of differing race or ethnicity. Whether it is called cultural awareness, cultural sensitivity, cultural humility, or some other term, cultural competence is the skill of learning, accepting, and appreciating cultural differences and similarities between groups, and being able to act on that understanding. Nunez suggested that the term *cross-cultural efficacy* is more appropriate than cultural competence, because it represents an understanding of equalities between cultures.[50] Whether one

uses efficacy or competence as a goal, the first barrier for many healthcare providers is recognizing that persons from different communities have different practices and belief systems, and that their reality, their truth, is based in those practices and beliefs. Lack of understanding on the part of the clinician is a barrier to care, both because it decreases the chance that data are collected, and because the patients can identify this as bias against their cultural or racial identity.

Race, education, source of care (defined as having a regular provider), and other variables all play a role in the patient's perception of bias from his or her providers, and that racial identity is a more powerful factor when asking about system bias. Regardless of education or financial status, non-white groups tended to perceive system bias based on cultural identity and use of English.[51] Among the specific factors suggesting a lack of cultural sensitivity to patients were a failure to provide ethnically sensitive office materials, such as illustrations or reading materials, and office staff behavior.[52] In this study, the language barrier was more important to Latinos, while environmental factors that suggested respect for African American culture were more important to African Americans. Other factors are also sources of potential bias in provider-patient encounters. Religious group, financial or educational status, obesity, substance use, or even sexual preference can lead to withdrawal and distancing by providers.

Other factors that primary care patients have identified as indicators of culturally sensitive care include people skills and effective communications, individualized treatment plans, and technical skill. Positive characteristics used to describe physician behavior in one study included listening, demonstrating concern, and good communication skills.[52] Beck and colleagues' review of the literature on patient-provider relations identified more than 20 nonverbal and verbal behaviors that had positive associations.[53] Among these were friendliness, courtesy, and empathy, which are behaviors that suggest acceptance of the person.

In medicine, providers also need to be respectful of the traditions and "folk illnesses" of their patients.[48] These issues may cause women to delay coming for care, utilize parallel care (medical plus traditional healers), or cause behaviors that the provider interprets as noncompliance when in fact the patient is following his or her own script for healing. Some illnesses do not fit a Western biomedical model, but are deeply rooted in cultural beliefs. Awareness and responsiveness to different cultural expectations can help to identify instances of parallel treatment, practices, and therapies that may be harmful, and to improve communication.

Having said all this, is cultural competence enough? There is limited evidence that cultural competence can erase the barriers to health quality caused by poverty, race, and lack of education.[54-56] Recall the definitions of primary care with which this chapter began and think about how to create a patient-centered care setting. It is often difficult for providers to actually listen and hear what the underlying barriers to adherence to treatment, or even attendance at a clinic, really are. True primary care requires not only awareness of one's culture, but of the family and community influences that impact the individual. Care has to begin where the woman is.

It has been recommended that an anti-racist approach needs to be taken, rather than one of cultural competence, and that white providers need to acknowledge and address issues of privilege and bias that affect perceptions of patients who are not similar in either ethnic or socioeconomic background.[57-59] Recent studies have found that particularly when white providers are working with black patients, implicit bias among providers is a factor in quality of communication and patient satisfaction.[59,60]

Conclusion

Primary care is a complex construct. It requires that care be available and that a clinician take the responsibility for paying attention to the whole person, not only one organ system or disease. It is best provided when the clinician can see across the divides of race, education, culture, and financial status, working to understand the individual and community network to provide care that works for the woman. Outreach and intervention strategies need to be tailored to each community, just as healthcare interventions are targeted at the individual to be most effective.

Many women rely on their midwife or other gynecologic caregiver to recognize and address all of their healthcare needs. Although the public perception of midwives is closely tied to birth and to care of healthy women, since the earliest days of Frontier Nursing Service American midwives have cared for women at risk from poor nutrition, poverty, and other socioeconomic problems. Midwives have continued to care for a population that is disproportionately adolescent, of color, immigrant, and poor.[61] When considering the focus on education, empowerment for shared decision making, psychosocial interventions, and lifestyle changes to improve health that are components of primary care, it is not surprising that midwives can be considered primary care providers. Because midwives are skilled at being "with women," they can evaluate the needs of women under their care, provide high-quality services, and refer women requiring more in-depth care to the appropriate consultants. Fulfilling that expectation—and triaging those who are not appropriate for midwifery primary care to a different clinician—requires knowledge. The basics of that knowledge are in the following chapters.

References

1. World Health Organization, UNICEF. Primary Health Care: Report of the International Conference on Primary Health Care, Alma-Ata, USSR, 6-12 September 1978/Jointly Sponsored by the World Health Organization and the United Nations Children's Fund; 1978.

2. Donaldson MS, Yordy KD, Lohr KN, Vanselow NA, eds. *Primary Care: America's Health in a New Era.* Washington, DC: National Academy Press; 1996.

3. Stuart D, Oshio S. Primary care in midwifery practice: a national survey. *J Midwifery Womens Health.* 2002;47(2):104-109.

4. Phillippi JC, Barger MK. Midwives as primary care providers for women. *J Midwifery Womens Health.* 2015;60:250-257.

5. Brown SA, Grimes DE. Meta analysis of nurse practitioners and nurse midwives in primary care. *Nurs Res.* 1995;44(5):332-339.

6. Kuo YF, Chen NW, Baillargeon J, Raji MA, Goodwin JS. Potentially preventable hospitalizations in Medicare patients with diabetes: a comparison of primary care provided by nurse practitioners versus physicians. *Med Care.* 2015;53(9):776-783.

7. Swan M, Ferguson S, Chang A, Larson E, Smaldone A. Quality of primary care by advanced practice nurses: a systematic review. *Int J Qual Health Care.* 2015;27(5):396-404.

8. Martin-Misener R, Harbman P, Donald F, Reid K, Kilpatrick K, Carter N, et al. Cost-effectiveness of nurse practitioners in primary and specialised ambulatory care: systematic review. *BMJ Open.* 2015;5(6):e007167.

9. American College of Nurse-Midwives. *Certified Nurse Midwives and Certified Midwives as Primary Care Providers/Case Managers.* Washington, DC: ACNM; 1992, revised 1997.

10. American College of Nurse-Midwives. *Midwives Are Primary Care Providers and Leaders of Maternity Care Homes.* Silver Spring, MD; 2012.

11. American College of Nurse-Midwives. *Core Competencies for Basic Midwifery Practice.* Silver Spring, MD; 2012.

12. Scupholme A, Carr KC. CNMs and primary care: practice models and types of services. *Quickening.* 1993;24(6):14.

13. Murphy PA. Primary care for women: health assessment, health promotion, and disease prevention services. *J Nurse-Midwifery.* 1996;41(2):83-91.

14. Hing E, Hooker RS. Community health centers: providers, patients, and content of care. *NCHS Data Brief.* 2011(65):1-8.

15. Hastings-Tolsma M, Emeis C, McFarlin B, Schmiege S. *Task Analysis: A Report of Midwifery Practice.* Linthicum, MD: American Midwifery Certification Board; 2012.

16. National Center for Health Statistics. *Health Care in America: Trends in Utilization 2004.* Hyattsville, MD: National Center for Health Statistics; 2004.

17. National Center for Health Statistics. National Ambulatory Medical Care Survey: 2012 State and National Summary Tables. Available from: http://www.cdc.gov/nchs/data/ahcd/namcs_summary/2012_namcs_web_tables.pdf. Accessed February 12, 2016.

18. Centers for Disease Control and Prevention. National Ambulatory Medical Care Survey Factsheet: Outpatient Department Visits. Available from: http://www.cdc.gov/nchs/data/ahcd/NHAMCS_2011_opd_factsheet.pdf. Accessed February 12, 2016.

19. Smedley BD, Stith AY, Nelson AR, eds. *Unequal Treatment: Confronting Racial and Ethnic Disparities in Health Care.* Washington, DC: National Academy Press; 2003.

20. Wändell P, Carlsson AC, Wettermark B, Lord G, Cars T, Ljunggren G. Most common diseases diagnosed in primary care in Stockholm, Sweden, in 2011. *Fam Pract.* 2013;30(5):506-513.

21. St Sauver J, Warner DO, Yawn BP, Jacobson DJ, McGree MF, Pankratz JJ, et al. Why patients visit their doctors: assessing the most prevalent conditions in a defined American population. *Mayo Clin Proc.* 2013;88:56-67.

22. US Department of Health and Human Services, Health Resources and Services Administration, Maternal and Child Health Bureau. *Womens Health USA 2013.* Rockville, MD: US Department of Health and Human Services, 2013.

23. US Department of Health and Human Services, Health Resources and Services Administration. Women's Preventive Services Guidelines. Available from: http://www.hrsa.gov/womensguidelines/. Accessed February 12, 2016.

24. Tinker SC, Broussard CS, Frey MT, Gilboa SM. Prevalence of prescription medication use among non-pregnant women of childbearing age and pregnant women in the United States—NHANES, 1999-2006. *Matern Child Health J.* 2015;19(5):1097-1106.

25. Zhong W, Maradit-Kremers H, St Sauver JL, Yawn BP, Ebbert JO, Roger VL, et al. Age and sex patterns of drug prescribing in a defined American population. *Mayo Clin Proc.* 2013;88:697-707.

26. Ward BW, Schiller JS, Goodman RA. Multiple chronic conditions among US adults: a 2012 update. *Prev Chronic Dis.* 2014;11:130389.

27. Centers for Disease Control and Prevention. CDC Health Disparities & Inequalities Report 2013. Available from: http://www.cdc.gov/minorityhealth/CHDIReport.html#Factsheet. Accessed February 12, 2016.

28. Bauer UE, Briss PA, Goodman RA, Bowman BA. Prevention of chronic disease in the 21st century: elimination of the leading preventable causes of premature death and disability in the USA. *Lancet.* 2014;384(9937):45-52.

29. Holt JB, Huston SL, Heidari K, Schwartz R, Gollmar CW, Tran A, et al. Indicators for chronic disease surveillance—United States, 2013. *MMWR Recomm Rep.* 2015;64(RR-01):1-246.

30. Heron M. Deaths: Leading causes for 2011. *Natl Vital Stat Rep.* 2015;64(7). Hyattsville, MD: National Center for Health Statistics. Available from: http://www.cdc.gov/nchs/data/nvsr/nvsr64/nvsr64_07.pdf. Accessed February 12, 2016.

31. Centers for Disease Control and Prevention. Leading causes of death in females 2013. Available from: http://www.cdc.gov/Women/lcod/2013/WomenAll_2013.pdf. Accessed February 12, 2016.

32. Mokdad AH, Marks JS, Stroup DF, Gerberding JL. Actual causes of death in the United States, 2000. *JAMA.* 2004;291(10):1238-1246.

33. Krueger PM, Tran MK, Hummer RA, Chang VW. Mortality attributable to low levels of education in the United States. *PLoS One.* 2015;10(7):e0131809.

34. Navarro V. Race or class versus race and class: mortality differentials in the United States. In: Lee PR, Carroll LE, eds. *The Nation's Health.* 5th ed. Sudbury, MA: Jones and Bartlett Publishers; 1997:32-36.

35. World Health Organization. Social determinants of health. Available from: http://www.who.int/social_determinants/sdh_definition/en/index.html. Accessed February 12, 2016.

36. Agency for Healthcare Quality and Research. *The National Healthcare Disparities Report.* Rockville, MD: US Department of Health and Human Services; 2003.

37. Agency for Healthcare Research and Quality. 2014 National Healthcare Quality & Disparities Report. Rockville, MD: Agency for Healthcare Research and Quality; 2015. Available from: http://www.ahrq.gov/research/findings/nhqrdr/nhqdr14/index.html. Accessed February 13, 2016.

38. Gebreab SY, Diez Roux AV, Brenner AB, Hickson DA, Sims M, Subramanyam M, et al. The impact of lifecourse socioeconomic position on cardiovascular disease events in African Americans: the Jackson Heart Study. *J Am Heart Assoc.* 2015;4(6):e001553.

39. Sharma S, Malarcher AM, Giles WH, Myers G. Racial, ethnic and socioeconomic disparities in the clustering of cardiovascular disease risk factors. *Ethn Dis.* 2004;14(1):43-48.

40. Mensah GA, Mokdad AH, Ford ES, Greenlund KJ, Croft JB. State of disparities in cardiovascular health in the United States. *Circulation.* 2005;111(10):1233-1241.

41. Carrillo JE, Carrillo VA, Perez HR, Salas-Lopez D, Natale-Pereira A, Byron AT. Defining and targeting health care access barriers. *J Health Care Poor Underserved.* 2011;22(2):562-575.

42. National Women's Law Center. States Must Close the Gap: Low-Income Women Need Health Insurance. Washington, DC: National Women's Law Center; 2014. Available from: http://www.nwlc.org/sites/default/files/pdfs/new_nwlc_mindthegap_updateoct2014.pdf. Accessed February 13, 2016.

43. Benz JK, Espinosa O, Welsh V, Fontes A. Awareness of racial and ethnic health disparities has improved only modestly over a decade. *Health Aff.* 2011;30:101860-7.

44. Lin MY, Kressin NR. Race/ethnicity and Americans' experiences with treatment decision making. *Patient Educ Couns.* 2015;S0738-3991(15)30025-2.

45. LaVeist TA, Gaskin DJ, Richard P. *The Economic Burden of Health Inequalities in the United States.* Washington, DC: Joint Center for Political and Economic Studies; 2009.

46. National Partnership for Action. Health Equity & Disparities. US Department of Health and Human Services. Available from: http://minorityhealth.hhs.gov/npa/templates/browse.aspx?lvl=1&lvlid=34. Accessed February 13, 2016.

47. Dunn AM. Cultural competence and the primary care provider. *J Pediatr Health Care.* 2002;16:105-11.

48. Pachter LM. Culture and clinical care: folk illness beliefs and their implications for health care delivery. *JAMA.* 1994;271:690-694.

49. Taylor JS. Confronting "culture" in medicine's "culture of no culture." *Acad Med.* 2003;78:555-559.

50. Nunez AE. Transforming cultural competence into cross cultural efficacy in women's health education. *Acad Med.* 2000;75:1071-1080.

51. Johnson RL, Saha S, Arbelaez JJ, Beach MC, Cooper LA. Racial and ethnic differences in patient perceptions of bias and cultural competence in health care. *J Gen Intern Med.* 2004;19:101-110.

52. Tucker CM, Herman KC, Pedersen TR, Higley B, Montrichard M, Ivery P. Cultural sensitivity in physician-patient relationships. *Med Care.* 2003;41: 859-870.

53. Beck RS, Daughtridge R, Sloane PD. Physician-patient communication in the primary care office: a systematic review. *J Am Board Fam Pract.* 2002; 15:25-38.

54. Lie DA, Lee-Rey E, Gomez A, Bereknyei S, Braddock CH. Does cultural competency training of health professionals improve patient outcomes? A systematic review and proposed algorithm for future research. *J Gen Intern Med.* 2011;14(3):317-325.

55. Truong M, Paradies Y, Priest N. Interventions to improve cultural competency in healthcare: a systematic review of reviews. *BMC Health Serv Res.* 2014;14:99.

56. Drevdahl DJ, Canales MK, Dorcy KS. Of goldfish tanks and moonlight tricks: can cultural competency ameliorate health disparities? *Adv Nurs Sci.* 2008;31(1):13-27.

57. Malat J. The appeal and problems of a cultural competence approach to reducing racial disparities. *J Gen Intern Med.* 2013;28(5):605-607.

58. Blair IV, Steiner JF, Fairclough DL, Hanratty R, Price DW, Hirsh HK, et al. Clinicians' implicit ethnic/racial bias and perceptions of care among Black and Latino patients. *Ann Fam Med.* 2013;11(1):43-52.

59. Saha S, Korthuis PT, Cohn JA, Sharp VL, Moore RD, Beach MC. Primary care provider cultural competence and racial disparities in HIV care and outcomes. *J Gen Intern Med.* 2013;28(5):622-629.

60. Schaa KL, Roter DL, Biesecker BB, Cooper LA, Erby LH. Genetic counselors' implicit racial attitudes and their relationship to communication. *Health Psychol.* 2015;34(2):111-119.

61. Declerq ER, Williams DR, Koontz AM, Paine LL, Streit EL, McKloskey L. Serving women in need: nurse-midwifery practice in the United States. *J Midwifery Womens Health.* 2001;46(1):11-16.

CHAPTER 2

GENERAL HEALTH EXAMINATION

Barbara K. Hackley

The annual physical exam was promoted as a valuable service for the general population beginning in the early 20th century and became an entrenched healthcare practice by the 1960s.[1] It has historically consisted of: 1) a health history; 2) a physical examination; 3) laboratory evaluation; 4) assessment of lifestyle, behavioral, and physical factors that increase the risk of chronic disease or death; and 5) the provision of immunizations. Because the history, physical examination, and testing are addressed within each chapter focusing on an organ or system, this chapter places most emphasis on the screening and vaccination recommendations for adult women.

Annual Health Exam

The utility of the annual examination has been debated for a number of years. Opponents of this practice are concerned about the expense of annual assessments, the low yield and intrusiveness of the physical examination, and the waste of valuable resources (time of highly skilled clinicians) that could be better used to increase access

to care for acutely and chronically ill individuals rather than for asymptomatic well individuals.[2-4] In contrast, proponents of the annual exam cite the importance of developing an ongoing trusting relationship between patient and clinician, the value of reassurance to the patient from a comprehensive assessment, the safety of the physical examination relative to more invasive testing, and the need to remain well versed in recognizing normal variants in physical examination finding.[5-7]

Little evidence is available about the effectiveness of the annual physical examination. The bulk of the evidence has evaluated the utility of particular screening practices, such as blood pressure, obesity, or sexually transmitted infection (STI) risk, in specific high-risk populations. Little research has been directed at evaluating the annual physical examination as a comprehensive entity for the general population. In a systematic review of the literature, Boulware and colleagues identified more than 7000 articles published between 1973 and 2006 on the potential benefits and risks of the periodic health assessment including improvements in patient attitudes (knowledge, satisfaction, trust, respect, and alleviation of worry), behavioral outcomes (health habits, motivation to change, adherence, and continuity), clinical (proximal and distal) outcomes, resource use and costs, and public health (family and community health, prevention of communicable disease). The authors concluded, based on an evaluation of the best available evidence consisting of 21 higher quality studies, that the periodic health examination was associated with higher receipt of preventive health services and reduced patient worry, but had mixed effect on other clinical outcomes and costs.[8] However, their results were undermined by the heterogeneity of outcomes measured. A more recent study found that repeated periodic healthcare examinations over 10 years were associated with significantly lower risk of all-cause mortality in both men and women.[9] The evidence is mixed and insufficient in quantity and quality to determine the most effective approach to providing clinical care to well adults.

With the demise of the annual Pap smear, the utility of the annual well-woman examination is also being questioned as to its purpose and effectiveness.[10,11] The evidence on the benefit of the pelvic exam in asymptomatic women is limited, with the exception of cervical cancer screening.[12] Noninvasive tests using urine samples can now reliably detect most sexually transmitted diseases. As a result, various authorities are proposing different approaches to care. The American College of Physicians found that the evidence does not support the use of periodic pelvic examinations in asymptomatic average-risk women except for cervical cancer screening.[12] However, because the evidence does not refute the benefit of an annual pelvic examination, the American College of Obstetricians and Gynecologists (ACOG) reaffirmed its recommendation to include an external and internal pelvic examination as part of the routine annual well-woman examination for women older than 21 years of age in 2014.[13]

All authorities agree on the importance of regular screening for risk factors that can undermine the health and wellbeing of women, adherence to the recommended immunization schedule, and timely care of symptomatic women. The following sections of this chapter discuss screenings and immunizations recommended for women across the lifespan.

Screening Tests

Effective screening tests can save lives by identifying preclinical stages of disease, which offers the opportunity to intervene early enough in the course of the disease to avert death and disability. Screening is expensive and has limited effectiveness unless certain criteria are met. Screening programs generally target those who are most at risk. Disagreements exist on which groups to target, which tests to use, and how frequently to screen. Professional groups, such as the American Cancer Society (ACS) and ACOG, and national authorities, such as the US Preventive Services Task Force (USPSTF), issue recommendations depending on their risk-benefit analyses of the efficacy and cost of screening, as well as the prevalence, morbidity, and mortality associated with the disease in question. Each authority also issues periodic updates as new information becomes available. This chapter is not meant to provide clinicians with the most current recommendations issued by various authorities; rather, it presents the background needed to be able to evaluate screening recommendations and to gain an understanding of the diversity of opinion held by various authorities. Table 2-1 lists Internet resources that can help providers stay updated on changes in recommendations issued by leading authorities.

Criteria for Successful Screening Programs

For a screening program to significantly reduce the negative health consequences of a specific disease, the condition being considered must

Table 2-1 Internet Resources

Agency	Resource	Website
ACOG	Well-Woman Recommendations (by age)	http://www.acog.org/About-ACOG/ACOG-Departments/Annual-Womens-Health-Care/Well-Woman-Recommendations
AHRQ ePSS Widget	Downloadable app that allows the provider to enter patient specific data (e.g., age, gender, risk factors) to identify recommendations for a particular woman	http://epss.ahrq.gov/PDA/widget.jsp
National Guideline Clearinghouse	Searchable collection of guidelines issued by different authorities	http://www.guideline.gov
USPSTF	Searchable recommendations released by the USPSTF	http://www.uspreventiveservicestaskforce.org/BrowseRec/Index

ACOG = American College of Obstetricians and Gynecologists, AHRQ = Agency for Healthcare Research and Quality, USPSTF = United States Preventive Services Task Force

meet several criteria (**Table 2-2**). First, the disease in question must cause substantial morbidity or mortality in a significant percentage of the population. Second, prevention or treatment options that can effectively reduce the likelihood of disease progression must be available. Third, a screening test must be available that is inexpensive, reliable, effective, and acceptable to patients. Use of the screening test must identify illness when the disease is asymptomatic. Early intervention must result in improved outcomes compared to care begun when the disease is clinically obvious.

Screening programs that do not meet these criteria will be less effective and, in some cases, worthless. Screening can also be potentially harmful if

Table 2-2 Criteria for an Effective Screening Test

Condition	Screening Test
• Common • Associated with significant morbidity and/or mortality • Intervention in preclinical stage of illness can prevent disease progression and sequelae • Early intervention leads to improved outcomes compared to those achieved with treatment started later in the course of the disease	• Available • Inexpensive • Accurate • Reliable • Acceptable to patients • Able to pick up disease earlier than routine clinical care

further evaluation of abnormal results requires the use of invasive tests. For example, ovarian cancer is the leading cause of reproductive-related cancer mortality in women.[14] It is usually asymptomatic and commonly clinically detected late in the course of the disease. Survival rates are higher if cancer is detected early. Unfortunately, while ovarian cancer meets some of the criteria necessary for effective screening programs, it does not meet all of them—it lacks an effective screening test. Screening tests used in the detection of ovarian cancer (serum CA-125 and transvaginal sonograms) have a high false-positive rate (10%) and a positive predictive value of less than 1%. Further, as many as one-third of women with false-positive results undergo unneeded follow-up surgery.[15] Therefore, no authorities currently recommend screening for ovarian cancer in asymptomatic individuals unless genetic risk factors are present.

Other conditions, such as colorectal cancer, do meet all of the necessary criteria, but may be detected using screening tests (fecal occult blood testing, sigmoidoscopy, and colonoscopy) that are less acceptable to patients. Adherence to screening is low, but rising, and varies by demographic factors. In 2000, only one-third of the adult population over age 50 were screening appropriately for colon cancer.[16] In 2013, just over 50% of individuals between 50 and 75 years of age had been screened.[17] However, screening rates are lower in younger compared to older individuals (59% in individuals 50 to 64 years vs. 76% in individuals between 65 and 75 years), in those with less education (39% in individuals with less than a high school education vs. 72% in college-educated individuals), those with lower incomes (47% of those with income < $ 15,000 vs. 73% in individuals with incomes of > $75,000), and among Hispanics (51%) compared to non-Hispanic individuals (65%).[18] Failure to convince enough at-risk individuals to obtain screening tests will lower the effectiveness of a screening program.

Accuracy of Screening Tests

The accuracy of screening tests is determined by their sensitivity, specificity, positive predictive value, and negative predictive value. Sensitivity answers the question, "If the disease is present, will the test be positive?", whereas specificity answers the question, "If the disease is absent, will the test be negative?" Sensitivity refers to the likelihood that the screening test will be positive if an individual has the disease. Specificity is the opposite; it describes the likelihood that the test will be negative if the individual is healthy. However, sensitivity and specificity are of less clinical value to providers than positive or negative predictive values. From a provider's perspective, the more important questions are, "If the test is positive, does the patient have the disease?" (positive predictive value) and "If the test is negative, is the patient disease-free?" (negative predictive value). **Table 2-3** describes the combination of possible answers to these questions in a 2 × 2 table. This 2 × 2 table can then be used to define the criteria used to describe the accuracy of a screening test: sensitivity, specificity, positive predictive value, and negative predictive value (**Table 2-4**).

In addition to having high sensitivity and specificity, a good screening test must be reliable. Values should be consistent across time so that differences are assumed to be because of the presence or absence of disease, and are not related to factors such as normal diurnal fluctuations, changes in diet or activity level, variations in laboratory techniques or personnel, or other external factors.

Table 2-3 Screening Test Results: A 2 × 2 Table

Test	Disease Present	Disease Absent
Positive	A = True Positive	B = False Positive
Negative	C = False Negative	D = True Negative

Table 2-4 Definitions: Values Used to Describe the Accuracy of Screening Tests

Value	Definition	Formula
Sensitivity	If the disease is present, will the test be positive?	A/ A & C or True Positive/Disease Present
Specificity	If the disease is absent, will the test be negative?	D/ B & D or True Negative/ Disease Absent
Positive Predictive Value	If the test is positive, will the disease be present?	A/ A & B or True Positive/ All Positive Tests
Negative Predictive Value	If the test is negative, will the disease be absent?	D/ C & D or True Negative/ All Negative Tests

Impact of Disease Prevalence

Disease prevalence has a direct and powerful impact on the success of screening programs. Prevalence is more important than the quality of the screening test, the seriousness of the disease, or the effectiveness of treatment. Disease conditions that are more prevalent can be more readily identified by screening tests and will have higher positive and negative predictive values, even if the screening test used has relatively poor sensitivity and specificity. For example, the positive predictive value of a screening test is 95% for a condition that occurs in 50% of the population and if the screening test used has a sensitivity and specificity of 95%. However, if prevalence is lower and affects only 5% of the population, this same excellent screening test can detect only 50% of individuals with the disease (**Table 2-5**).[19]

Prevalence also affects whether any interventions implemented as a result of screening are likely to improve health outcomes. Less effective interventions targeting more prevalent diseases

Table 2-5 Impact of Prevalence on Positive Predictive Value

Prevalence (%)	Sensitivity 90% Specificity 90%	Sensitivity 95% Specificity 95%	Sensitivity 99% Specificity 99%
0.1	0.9	1.9	9.0
1	8.3	16.1	50
2	15.5	27.9	66.9
5	32.1	50	83.9
50	90	95	99

Data from Selection and interpretation of diagnostic tests. In: Goroll A, May L, Mulley A, (eds.). Primary Care Medicine. 4th ed. Philadelphia: Lippincott Williams & Wilkins; 2000; Akobeng AK. Understanding diagnostic tests 1: sensitivity, specificity and predictive values. Acta Paediatr. 2007; 96:338-341. DOI:10.1111/j.1651-2227.2006.00180.x; Johns Hopkins Bloomberg School of Public Health.

Table 2-6 Deaths Prevented as a Function of Disease Prevalence and Treatment Effectiveness

Reduction in Mortality with Intervention	Deaths per Year from Target Population	Total Deaths Prevented with Intervention
50%	10	5
1%	100,000	1000

Reproduced from USPSTF. Guide to clinical preventive services: report of the US Preventive Services Task Force (2nd ed). Baltimore, MD: Williams & Wilkins; 1996.

improve health at the population level better than more effective interventions for less common diseases.[20] Few deaths will be prevented if a disease is rare, even if highly effective interventions exist. Therefore, authorities such as the USPSTF whose recommendations are based on population rather than individual health considerations do not recommend screening for rare diseases even if highly effective treatment is available. See **Table 2-6** for examples illustrating how the numbers of deaths prevented vary as a function of disease prevalence and intervention effectiveness.

Prevalence has such strong influence on the effectiveness of screening programs that many authorities recommend directing screening efforts to subpopulations at higher risk of a particular health problem rather than to the general population. Guidelines commonly recommend that particular screening strategies be directed to subgroups based on their age, lifestyle, or risk profile.

Biases in Screening Tests

Screening tests are subject to biases, such as lead-time and length-time biases, which make screening tests appear to be effective in improving health outcomes when, in fact, they are not. Lead-time bias occurs when a screening test identifies a disease earlier than usual clinical care, but

treatment begun earlier does not improve outcomes. Screening tests for cancer, for example, may falsely appear to improve survival rates by allowing earlier detection, thereby increasing the length of time from detection to death, but they do not truly increase survival (**Figure 2-1**).

Length-time bias is also problematic. This bias is present if screening identifies only slowly progressing or more benign forms of a condition, which are more likely to have better outcomes, and miss more aggressive forms. Treatment for indolent forms of the disease may appear to, but will not actually improve outcomes, if most of the deaths occur with more aggressive disease. For example, controversy over the effectiveness of prostate cancer screening is due to differences in interpretations of the effect of length-time bias on the success of prostate cancer screening (**Figure 2-2**).

Recommendations of Various Organizations

Many professional and national organizations issue screening guidelines. These guidelines differ in many ways, including what conditions should be screened, what tests should be used, which groups should be targeted, when screening tests should be initiated, and how often (if at all) they should be repeated. These differences reflect an organization's cost-effectiveness analysis as well as its underlying interest. Determining the incidence and health impact of disease, the accuracy of a particular screening test, or the effectiveness of early treatment in preventing death and disability is not an exact science. Using more conservative or more liberal estimates of these numbers can dramatically change the cost-benefit equation. In addition, only limited resources are available for health care in general and screening in particular. It may be that healthcare dollars and provider and patient time devoted to marginally effective screening programs are better used in other ways.

Differences exist in the way organizations evaluate these competing demands. For example,

Figure 2-1 Algorithm showing lead-time bias.

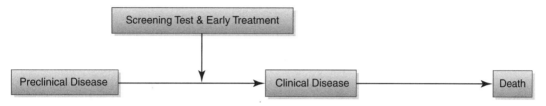

A. Effective Screening Test

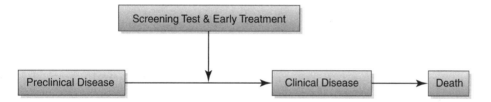

B. Lead-Time Bias

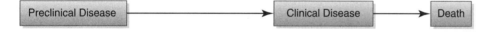

C. Natural Course of Disease with Care Starting at Symptomatic Stage

Figure 2-2 Algorithm showing length-time bias.

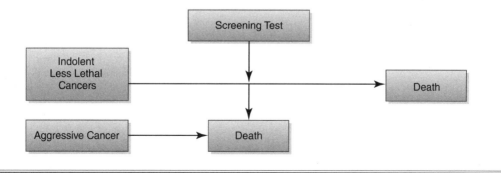

the USPSTF makes recommendations based on population benefit, whereas others, such as the ACS and the National Osteoporosis Foundation, are concerned about the impact of one condition. In general, therefore, the USPSTF tends to issue more conservative screening recommendations, while condition-specific organizations tend to be more aggressive in their recommendations. **Table 2-7** compares the recommendations issued by different authorities for adolescent women against those recommended by ACOG; **Table 2-8** compares recommendations for adult women.[21-24]

Table 2-7 Adolescent Healthcare Visit: Comparison of ACOG Recommendations to Other Authorities

Categories	Components	Organizations		
		ACOG	AAFP	USPSTF
Timing	Onset	13-15 years		
	Frequency	Yearly		
History	Health status, family history	R		
Physical	BMI	R	B	B
	Blood pressure	R	I	I
	Tanner staging	R		
	Abdominal exam	R		
	Additional physical and/or pelvic as clinically indicated	R		
Counseling/ Assessment	Alcohol	R		B ≥ 18 years I < 18 years
	Illicit drug use	R	I	I
	Smoking	R	B	B
	Diet and physical activity	R		
	Emotional, physical, sexual abuse	R		
	Gender identity, sexual orientation, and sexual practices	R		
	STI and pregnancy prevention	R		B
	Acquaintance rape prevention	R		
	Personal goal development	R		
	School and peer relationships	R		
	Depressive symptoms	R	B*	B*
	Suicide	R		I
	Injury prevention	R		
	Skin cancer prevention	R	B if fair skinned	B if fair skinned

Categories	Components	Organizations		
		ACOG	AAFP	USPSTF
Laboratory	Piercings and tattooing	R		
	Anemia (CBC)			
	Cholesterol screening			I
	Diabetes			
	Gonorrhea/chlamydia	R		B
	HIV	R	A if ≥ 18 years	A if ≥ 15 years

AAFP = American Academy of Family Physicians; ACOG = American College of Obstetricians and Gynecologists; BMI = body mass index; CBC = complete blood count; HIV = human immunodeficiency virus; STI = sexually transmitted infection; USPSTF = US Preventive Services Task Force.

A = recommends without reservation, net benefit substantial; B = offer service, benefits are likely to be moderate; B* = offer services if support services are in place; I = insufficient evidence to know if intervention if effective, even if behavior is desirable; R = recommends, no grade attached.

Data from American College of Obstetricians and Gynecologists. Well-Woman Recommendations. Available at: http://www .acog.org/About-ACOG/ACOG-Departments/Annual-Womens-Health-Care/Well-Woman-Recommendations. Accessed November 12, 2015; American Academy of Family Physicians. Recommendations by topic: Infants, children, and adolescents. Available at: http://www.aafp.org/patient-care/clinical-recommendations/children.html. Accessed February 16, 2016; US Preventive Services Task Force. USPSTF A and B Recommendations. 2015. Available at: http://www.uspreventiveservicestaskforce .org/Page/Name/uspstf-a-and-b-recommendations/. Accessed November 12, 2015.

Table 2-8 Healthcare Visit, Adult Women

Categories	Components	Organizations		
		ACOG[a,b]	AAFP[c]	USPSTF[d]
Timing	Frequency	Yearly	Not specified	Not specified
History	Health status, family history	R		
Physical	BMI	R	A	
	Blood pressure	R	A	A, annually if > 40 years or high risk factors
	Neck/thyroid	R		
	Breast	R	I	I
	Abdominal exam	R		
	Pelvic	R[1], periodic		
	Additional physical as clinically indicated	R		

(continues)

Table 2-8 Healthcare Visit, Adult Women (*continued*)

Categories	Components	ACOG[a,b]	AAFP[c]	USPSTF[d]
			Organizations	
Counseling/ Assessment	Alcohol	R	B	B
	Illicit drug use	R	I	I
	Smoking	R	A	A
	Diet and physical activity	R	B, if risk factors	B, if risk factors
	Emotional, physical, sexual abuse	R	B, women of reproductive age I, elderly	B, women of reproductive age I, elderly
	Acquaintance rape prevention	R		
	Sexual function	R		
	Preconception counseling	R		
	Folic acid supple- mentation, cal- cium intake	R		
	STI and pregnancy prevention	R		B, adolescents and at-risk women
	Depressive symptoms	R	Only if supportive services are in place	B, if supportive services are in place C, if no services are available
	Suicide	R		I
	Injury prevention	R		
	Family function	R		
	Skin cancer prevention	R	B, up to age 24 years	B, $<$ 24 years and fair-skinned
	High-risk behaviors	R		
	Work satisfaction, lifestyle, stress	R		
	Sleep disorders	R		
	Breast self-examination	R^2, if risk factors	D, low-risk women	D

Categories	Components	Organizations		
		ACOG[a,b]	AAFP[c]	USPSTF[d]
	Urinary or fecal incontinence	R		
	Pelvic prolapse	R, if > 40 years		
	Menopausal symptoms	R, if > 40 years		
Laboratory	Anemia (CBC)	R[3], if risk factors		
	Breast cancer screening	R, age $\geq$ 50 years, yearly mammogram; earlier if risk factors[2]	B, between 50 and 74 years, every 2 years	B, between 50 and 74 years, every 2 years C, before age 50 I $\geq$ 75 years
	Cervical cancer screening	R[4], age $\geq$ 21 years, periodic	A, same as ACOG	A, same as ACOG
	Colon cancer screening	R[5], age $\geq$ 45 if African American and $\geq$ 50 years in general population, periodic; earlier if risk factors present	A, 50 to 75 years, periodic; no specific recommendation for African Americans	A, 50 to 75 years; periodic
	Diabetes	R[6], age $\geq$ 45 years, every 3 years; earlier if risk factors	B, only if has sustained BP > 130/80	B, ages 40 to 70 years if BMI $\geq$ 25 kg/m^2; every 3 years
	Dyslipidemia screening	R[7], age $\geq$ 45 years, every 5 years; earlier if risk factors	A, age $\geq$ 45 years, with risk factors B, 20 to 45 years, with risk factors	A, age $\geq$ 45 years, with risk factors B, 20 to 45 years, with risk factors
	Gonorrhea/ chlamydia	R[8], if < 25 years or risk factors	B, < 25 years or high-risk behavior	B, < 25 years or high-risk behavior
	Hepatitis C	R[9], once, if born in 1945-1965 or if risk factors	B, 1 time or if risk factors	B, once, if born in 1945-1965 or if risk factors
	HIV	R[10], if risk factors	A, if between 18 and 65 years	A, between 15 and 65 years of age

(continues)

Table 2-8 Healthcare Visit, Adult Women (*continued*)

Categories	Components	Organizations		
		ACOG[a,b]	AAFP[c]	USPSTF[d]
	Osteoporosis (bone mineral density testing)	R[11], age ≥ 65 years; earlier if risk factors present	B ≥ 65 years; earlier if risk factors	B ≥ 65 years; earlier if risk factors
	Thyroid function	R[12], ≥ 65 years; earlier if risk factors present	I	I

AAFP = American Academy of Family Physicians; ACOG= American College of Obstetricians and Gynecologists; BMI = body mass index; BP = blood pressure; CBC = complete blood count; HIV = human immunodeficiency virus; STI = sexually transmitted infection; USPSTF = US Preventive Services Task Force.

A = recommends without reservation, net benefit substantial; B = offer service, benefits are likely to be moderate; B* = offer services if support services are in place; I = insufficient evidence to know if intervention if effective, even if behavior is desirable; R= recommends, no grade attached.

R[1] Pelvic examinations may be discontinued at over age 65 years if a woman's age or health condition is such that she would not seek treatment for any identified conditions.

R[2] ACOG breast cancer risk factors: Recommend breast self-exam if lifetime breast cancer risk of ≥ 20%, women with BRCA1 or BRCA2 mutations, women with first-degree relatives with BRAC mutations who are untested, personal high-risk biopsy including atypical hyperplasia and lobular carcinoma in situ, personal receipt of thoracic irradiation.[b] Recommend mammogram if first-degree relative or multiple relatives with premenopausal breast cancer or breast and ovarian cancers, women with positive BRCA tests, personal history of high-risk biopsy results, or irradiation between 10 and 30 years of age.[b]

R[3] ACOG anemia risk factors: Ancestry (Caribbean, Latin American, Asian, Mediterranean, or African), heavy menstrual flow.[b]

R[4] ACOG cervical cancer screening: Recommendations vary by age: onset age 21 years; ages 21 to 29 years every 3 years with cytology alone; age 30 to 65 every 5 years with cytology and human papillomavirus (HPV) co-testing (preferred); stop at > 65 years if adequate screening and no history of ≥ CIN 2.[e]

R[5] ACOG recommendations: Colonoscopy preferred, every 10 years. Colon cancer risk factors: colorectal cancer or adenomatous polyps in first degree relative younger than 60 years or in 2 or more first-degree relatives of any age; family history of familial adenomatous polyposis or hereditary nonpolyposis colon cancer; personal history of colorectal cancer, adenomatous polyps, inflammatory bowel disease, chronic ulcerative colitis, or Crohn's disease.[b]

R[6] ACOG diabetes risk factors: Overweight or obese, first-degree relative with diabetes, physical inactivity, high-risk race/ethnicity (African American, Hispanic, Latina, Native American, Asian American), history of gestational diabetes or birth of a baby > 9 lbs, high-density lipoprotein (HDL) < 35 mg/dL, triglycerides > 250 mg/dL, polycystic ovarian syndrome (PCOS), history of having preeclampsia and delivering prematurely or recurrent preeclampsia in several pregnancies.[b]

R[7] ACOG cardiovascular risk factors: Family history of premature cardiovascular disease; personal history of cardiovascular disease, obesity, or diabetes; presence of multiple risk factors; history of having preeclampsia and delivering prematurely or recurrent preeclampsia in several pregnancies.[b]

R[8] ACOG gonorrhea/chlamydia risk factors: < 25 years of age, history of multiple partners or partner with multiple partners, sexual contact with culture-proven STI, repeated STIs in past, drug use, commercial sex work, inconsistent condom use.[b]

R[9] ACOG risk factors for hepatitis C: HIV infection; history of injecting illegal drugs; recipient of clotting factor concentrate before 1987; long-term hemodialysis; persistently abnormal alanine aminotransferase levels; recipient of blood, blood products, or organ transplant before 1992; occupational, percutaneous, or mucosal exposure to hepatitis C-positive blood.[b]

R[10] ACOG HIV risk factors: More than 1 sexual partner since last test or a sexual partner with more than 1 partner, diagnosed with another STI in the last year, intravenous drug use, exchange sex for drugs or money, residence in area with high prevalence of HIV, blood transfusion between 1978 and 1985, invasive cervical cancer, adolescent entering detention center.[b]

R[11] ACOG risk factors for earlier screening for osteoporosis: Medical history of bone fragility or causes of bone loss (medications or disease), weight less than 125 lbs, current smoker, alcoholism, or rheumatoid arthritis.[b]

R[12] ACOG risk factors for thyroid disease: Strong family history, dyslipidemia.[b]

[a] Data from American College of Obstetricians and Gynecologists. Well-Woman Recommendations. Available at: http://www.acog.org/About-ACOG/ACOG-Departments/Annual-Womens-Health-Care/Well-Woman-Recommendations. Accessed November 12, 2015.

[b] American College of Obstetricians and Gynecologists. High-Risk Factors. Available at: http://www.acog.org/About-ACOG/ACOG-Departments/Annual-Womens-Health-Care/Well-Woman-Recommendations/High-Risk-Factors. Accessed February 16, 2016.

[c] American Academy of Family Physicians. Recommendations by topic: Infants, children, and adolescents. Available at: http://www.aafp.org/patient-care/clinical-recommendations/children.html. Accessed February 16, 2016.

[d] US Preventive Services Task Force. USPSTF A and B Recommendations. 2015. Available at: http://www.uspreventiveservicestaskforce.org/Page/Name/uspstf-a-and-b-recommendations/. Accessed November 12, 2015.

[e] American College of Obstetricians and Gynecologists. ACOG practice bulletin no. 131: screening for cervical cancer. *Obstet Gynecol.* 2012;120(5):1222-38.

Over time, recommendations of different authorities are increasingly becoming aligned with each other, but differences do exist. ACOG recommends an annual health assessment, which includes a comprehensive psychosocial evaluation—issues not addressed by other authorities. ACOG also staunchly defends an annual mammogram and periodic pelvic examinations. Other experts recommend a comprehensive health assessment every 3 years or the use of multidisciplinary teams to help address a wider array of issues and to assist with the mundane tasks of completing a healthcare visit (documentation, medication refills, and referrals) that will free healthcare providers to be able to concentrate on the provision of medical care.[3,5]

Like ACOG, other authorities disagree with the recommendations set by the American Academy of Family Physicians and the USPSTF and recommend more aggressive and comprehensive screening. The American Thyroid Association recommends screening for thyroid dysfunction with a thyroid-stimulation hormone (TSH) test beginning at age 35 and every 5 years thereafter. The American Association of Clinical Endocrinologists suggests a low index of suspicion for thyroid dysfunction, particularly in women, and recommends screening in older women, age unspecified.[25] Similarly, the ACS makes the following suggestions: 1) offer mammograms to asymptomatic low-risk women between the ages of 40 and 44, 2) yearly mammograms between 45 and 54 years, and 3) reduce frequency of mammography to every 2 years beginning at age 55 years, but allow women to have the option of yearly mammograms if they prefer.[26] These disparate recommendations are confusing to patients and providers alike. To create a unified approach to care, ACOG convened a panel of experts representing more than 14 healthcare disciplines involved in the care of women and created a set of recommendations as outlined in Tables 2-7 and 2-8 on components of the well-woman visit, including screening, laboratory assessment, counseling, and immunizations. As these recommendations become incorporated into care, it is hoped that a more standardized approach to care will emerge.[27]

All clinicians must exercise clinical judgment when offering screening tests to their clients.

Screening can save lives. However, women who are considered at low risk may incur additional expense, discomfort, and worry during the evaluation of false-positive tests that can result from overzealous screening. In midwifery and women's health, striking the correct balance depends on understanding the prevalence and sequelae of the common health problems found in the communities in which a provider practices, an ability to evaluate the risk status of individual clients, and a willingness to devote time during a healthcare visit to these issues. Providers who do this will successfully improve the health of women while minimizing the risks and expense associated with screening.

Immunizations

Immunizations are widely acknowledged to be one of the most effective health interventions yet implemented. Declines of 99% or more in deaths related to vaccine-preventable illnesses have occurred for diphtheria, mumps, pertussis, and tetanus after vaccines against these diseases were widely adopted.[28] Further, endemic transmission in the United States has been eliminated for rubella infection and smallpox has been eradicated worldwide. These achievements have resulted from widespread public acceptance due to concentrated efforts on the part of manufacturers, public health infrastructure, and providers who recommend and administer vaccines to their patients. Thus, it is critical that women's health providers remain updated on new developments in the field and offer vaccines to the women in their care.

Immune Response

The immune system has two components, innate and adaptive, which work in concert to prevent infection. The innate system starts with the protection afforded by intact skin and mucous membranes and is augmented by the protection provided by chemical barriers (e.g., gastric acid in the stomach, anti-infective properties found in tears and saliva, commensal flora of the gastrointestinal [GI] and vaginal ecosystems that outcompete pathogens for nutrients) and processes that expel pathogens from the body (e.g., coughing, urination, and defecation).

If a pathogen breaches these defenses, the innate immune system, composed of the general defensive mechanisms of the immune system, is immediately and rapidly activated. This immune response is nonspecific. Defenses include circulating phagocytes (neutrophils, monocytes), nonspecific antibodies, complement proteins, interferon, and natural killer cells. The neutrophils are the first to respond; they are attracted to the area of injury from chemical signals released by damaged cells. Neutrophils release chemicals that trigger other components of the immune system, but their primary function is to ingest and kill pathogens. The monocytes circulate in the blood but also can enter into the tissue and become macrophages. They produce cytokines (which can signal a broader immune response), "present" bacterial antigens (which can trigger the adaptive immune system), and phagocytize pathogens. Phagocytosis triggers local inflammation, which increases local blood supply and fluid in the tissue and can induce fever. Thus, inflammation can lead to local and systemic responses that ultimately increase the numbers of phagocytes and clotting factors in the area, which can help confine the infection and promote healing. The complement system helps to mark the invading pathogens as foreign substances, attracting phagocytes to the pathogen. They also weaken the cell wall and induce bacterial cell lysis. Natural killer cells attach to the pathogen, weakening and rupturing its cell membranes. Interferon is also released as part of the innate response; its function is to help protect noninfected cells from becoming infected, thereby limiting the infection. It inhibits viral replication, enhances the function of macrophages and natural killer cells, and stimulates the production of antibodies. Working together, the processes of the innate immune response may be enough to eradicate pathogens and prevent infection. If not, the adaptive system will be triggered and amplify the immune response.

Unlike the innate immune system, the adaptive system is slower to respond but more specific and enduring. Exposure to a pathogen triggers the two components of the adaptive system, humoral and cellular immunity, and creates immunologic memory. Humoral immunity is responsible for long-term protection; its primary mechanism is to trigger the development of antibodies produced by B cells, but B cells also augment the innate immune system and increase its effectiveness. Cellular immunity is a result of the activity of T cells, which are produced in the bone marrow and mature in the thymus. The two major types of T cells, killer T cells (also known as cytotoxic T lymphocytes) and helper T cells, each play a different role. Killer T cells directly attack the infected cells and are particularly aggressive in eliminating cells infected with viruses and malignant cells. Helper T cells are essential in coordinating the overall immune response and stimulate other cells, such as B cells, needed for the body to mount an effective immune response. Antibodies produced by B cells recognize and combat viruses and bacteria upon entry into the body and so prevent infection. Antibodies prevent infection from developing and modify the course of infection once it is established by using several different mechanisms. Antibodies directed to surface antigens can cause viruses to aggregate, making them easier to clear out of the body by the immune system. Other kinds of antibodies change the structure of antigens, rendering them noninfectious. Others neutralize antigens, not by changing their structure, but by not allowing viruses to attach to human cells. Antibodies work synergistically and by doing so effectively attack viruses and bacteria. Both systems—cellular and

humoral—work together to inactivate pathogens and eliminate infected cells. Once infection is eradicated, levels of antibodies wane. Following re-exposure to an antigen, memory B cells (which circulate in the blood and are present in bone marrow) recognize the antigen and rapidly reproduce antibodies to levels high enough to prevent infection. This immunologic memory can last for years, sometimes for a lifetime, and provides long-term protection from infection.

Active vaccines work by exposing the immune system to a substance that triggers an immune response similar to that which occurs upon exposure to wild infection. Vaccines use a modified live antigen such as a virus or bacterium or a manufactured one with a structure very similar to the wild form. The essential qualities of a wild virus or bacterium are mimicked so that the immune system will create antibodies to these antigens without allowing an active infection to develop. Exposure to a vaccine triggers both humoral and cellular immunity and creates immunologic memory.

Vaccines provide either active or passive immunity. Active immunity is long-lasting because it triggers the immune system to develop antibodies. The protection afforded by passive immunization wanes as the antibodies provided by the vaccine die off; the immune system is not stimulated to produce antibodies with passive immunization. Examples of vaccines providing active immunity include measles, mumps, and rubella (MMR) vaccines; those providing passive immunity include vaccines containing immunoglobulin. Passive transmission of antibodies can also occur transplacentally from mother to fetus and by receipt of some blood products.

Types of Vaccinations

There are two basic types of immunizations: live attenuated and inactivated vaccines.[29] Live attenuated vaccines use weakened viruses and bacteria to induce low-level replication in the individual receiving the vaccine. The immune response from exposure to the low levels of viruses and bacteria after immunization with live attenuated vaccines is almost identical to that produced by wild infection. Occasionally, receipt of live attenuated vaccines results in clinical infection, but often these infections are much milder than wild infections and cause few problems. Because they are so effective, live attenuated vaccines can usually achieve an effective immune response with only one dose.

Inactivated vaccines are developed in several steps. First, live viruses and bacteria are modified so that they cannot reproduce, and then various portions (whole or fractional) of these inactivated viruses or bacteria are used to stimulate an immune response. Whole-cell inactivated vaccines (e.g., polio and hepatitis A) use the entire bacteria or virus. Fractional vaccines use subunits (e.g., hepatitis B, influenza, acellular pertussis, and human papillomavirus [HPV]), pure or conjugated polysaccharide components of bacterial cell walls (pneumococcal), or toxins produced by a bacterium (diphtheria, tetanus) to stimulate the immune system. Some fractional vaccines are also called recombinant vaccines, because they are genetically engineered by inserting a segment of the viral gene into the gene of a yeast cell, which then produces viral proteins. These proteins are extracted, purified, and used to create recombinant vaccines. Because no viral replication occurs with any inactivated vaccines, they are less effective than live attenuated vaccines and require multiple doses to induce an effective initial immune response and boosters to maintain adequate antibody levels thereafter.[29]

Of the inactivated vaccines, the pure polysaccharide vaccines have the least staying power—their protection is generally short lived. The immune response to pure polysaccharide vaccines is T cell independent, meaning that they stimulate B cells without the aid of T helper cells. Thus, the immune response is weaker (and often nonexistent in children younger than 2 years of age) and cannot be strengthened with booster shots. However, combining the polysaccharide with a protein molecule through a process called conjugation changes the immune response from T cell independent to T cell dependent and markedly improves the performance of the vaccine. Subsequently, the vaccine schedule for children, and in some cases for adults, has been adapted to preferentially use conjugated over pure polysaccharide vaccines.[29]

Vaccine Safety

As with all medications, the use of vaccines may result in unwanted effects. Up to 40% of all vaccinations may be associated with mild local reactions. Systemic symptoms such as fever and malaise are less common. More serious reactions can occur but are rare, and are commonly referred to as vaccine adverse events (VAE). VAEs can result from a reaction to any of the additives or immunologic components of the vaccine; from medication errors, such as reconstituting a vaccine with the wrong diluent or using poor technique during administration; or from errors made during the manufacturing process. VAEs also may be coincidental and unrelated to vaccine receipt.

Gaining, and maintaining, public trust in the safety of vaccines is dependent on having a robust system in place to monitor vaccine safety. The evaluation of vaccine safety is based on pre-licensure research and post-licensure surveillance. In order to receive Food and Drug Administration (FDA) approval for use, a vaccine must be evaluated by a series of pre-licensure research studies consisting of Phase 1, Phase 2, and Phase 3 clinical trials.[30] Phase 1 trials have few participants and are designed to determine whether an intervention passes minimal safety standards. Phase 2 trials are larger and designed to evaluate effectiveness, determine dosage, and identify the more frequent minor and major side effects. Phase 3 trials are the largest, often comprising more than 1000 participants, and help to further refine the dosage needed to maximize benefits and minimize risks, and to provide better data on the safety profiles of vaccines.[30] However, because serious reactions are rare, vaccine trials may need to include substantially more subjects than typical Phase 3 trials, making them very costly. For example, the second-generation rotavirus trials consisted of 60,000 subjects, which was necessary to confirm that intussusception (which occurred in 1 out of 10,000 children vaccinated with the original rotavirus vaccine) was not associated with the revised rotavirus vaccine.[30] Because VAEs are likely not to be picked up in pre-licensure trials, post-licensure surveillance is essential.

Post-licensure surveillance is conducted through several avenues. To be approved for licensure, the FDA sometimes also requires the manufacturer to conduct a Phase 4 trial, which is a continuation of the Phase 3 trial using a much larger cohort. While a large sample size helps identify other previously unrecognized reactions or subpopulations at increased risk of developing VAEs, it may still not be sufficiently large enough to pick up rare events.[31] For example, the relationship between the original rotavirus vaccine and bowel obstruction was not suspected to be a problem in pre-licensure trials of more than 17,000 individuals.[32,33] This relationship became evident only after 1.5 million doses were distributed and led to a recall of the vaccine.[34]

Trying to determine whether a reaction is truly a result of vaccine exposure or coincidental can be difficult. More severe and more immediate effects are most likely to be identified as possible vaccine-related reactions. Subtle or later developing reactions are more easily missed. Concern has been expressed in a few communities that receipt of some vaccines is related to the development of multiple sclerosis, autism, and other autoimmune disorders.[35] Others have suggested that receipt of

pertussis vaccine is associated with the development of severe neurologic damage in children.[36]

Vaccine-related safety concerns prompted the Institute of Medicine (IOM) to convene an expert panel to examine the safety of vaccines, initially in 1991,[37] and then again in response to more recent concerns in 2001-2004.[35] This expert panel, also known as the Immunization Safety Review Committee, has published a series of reports on the safety of individual vaccines, evaluating possible relationships between the receipt of specific vaccines and particular adverse events. The Immunization Safety Review Committee used the same methodology in all of its reports: first evaluating whether the relationships between various vaccines and VAEs were biologically plausible and then determining if there was enough available evidence of sufficient quality and quantity to assess if a causal relationship existed. The Immunization Safety Review Committee concluded that the evidence demonstrated 1) a causal relationship between the receipt of the 1976 Swine Flu vaccine and Guillain-Barré syndrome, 2) no relationship (favors rejection) of a relationship between influenza vaccination and multiple sclerosis, 3) no relationship between MMR vaccination or thimerosal-containing vaccines and autism, and 4) no relationship between childhood vaccines and sudden infant death syndrome (SIDS) for some vaccines. However, the data were insufficient in many other cases to draw firm conclusions.[35] Consequently, the Immunization Safety Review Committee made numerous recommendations directed toward policymakers, vaccine program implementers, healthcare professionals, and the lay public on suggested future activities on ways to improve surveillance, research, communication, and policy on vaccine safety.[35]

The IOM more recently summarized the state of the science on vaccine safety in a report issued in 2012. Its findings are incorporated into the tables on various vaccines found in this chapter.[38]

One program designed to improve vaccine safety monitoring is the Vaccine Adverse Event Reporting System (VAERS), a national passive reporting system, which was established in 1990; it is jointly administered by the Centers for Disease Control and Prevention (CDC) and the FDA.[39] Healthcare providers are mandated to report all suspected vaccine-related adverse events, but reports submitted by the general public are also accepted. These case reports are reviewed to determine if a suspected link exists between a vaccine and a specific adverse event, if problems are occurring in certain manufacturer lots, if rates of adverse events are increasing, or if a cluster of adverse events is noted. If potential problems are identified, further research is needed. Because the VAERS is a collection of case reports, it cannot prove causality; rather, VAERS data are used to generate hypotheses to be evaluated by other research modalities. Two systems that can evaluate hypotheses generated by VAERS data are large linked data sets (LLDS), such as the Vaccine Safety Datalink, and the Clinical Immunization Safety Assessment (CISA) network.[30] These systems complement each other and can be used to answer different kinds of research questions.

The Vaccine Safety Datalink is a collaboration between the CDC's Immunization Safety Office and nine healthcare organizations. The Vaccine Safety Datalink pulls together electronic health data from each participating site on vaccines received and the health status of individuals receiving vaccination.[40] Consequently, it can better answer questions on the incidence of specific vaccine-related adverse events, the normal background incidence of these reactions in patients who have not recently received a vaccine, and subgroups at higher risks of vaccine-related complications. It can also help monitor the safety of newly introduced vaccines or changes in the recommended vaccine schedule.[30] For example, the Vaccine Safety Datalink helped to identify that febrile seizures occurred at a higher rate after administration of the newly combined measles-mumps-rubella-varicella (MMRV) vaccine compared to the simultaneous injection of two separate vaccines, MMR and the varicella vaccine in children.[41]

However, while the Vaccine Safety Datalink is a substantial improvement in the vaccine safety net, it does have problems that undermine the quality of the data it can provide. Data may not be completely accurate as information is being collected, not for research purposes, but as part of routine health care. Errors may occur in coding.[42] Reactions too minor to warrant medical attention will be lost to analysis. Nor are these data sets likely to include a sufficient number of unvaccinated individuals who can serve as controls.[42] Because nearly 95% of the US population has received recommended childhood vaccinations,[43] relatively few unvaccinated controls are available. In addition, these individuals may be significantly different in their genetic makeup, lifestyle, or environmental exposures from the general public. Therefore, the Vaccine Safety Datalink is best at identifying problems with new vaccines or with changes in recommendations on the initiation or use of older ones. Because of the lack of a vaccine-naïve control group, large linked data sets, such as the Vaccine Safety Datalink, cannot easily answer lingering questions regarding the safety of older vaccines already in widespread use. Over time it may be able to shed light on the risks of cumulative vaccine exposure or about the relationship between vaccine receipt and the future development of autoimmune disorders. Large long-term longitudinal studies are needed to answer these latter questions, which can be expensive and difficult to conduct. However, despite these limitations, large linked data sets are a significant improvement that allows a more sophisticated analysis of vaccine safety than was previously available.

The CISA Project, established in 2001, is a network of designated referral centers and is designed to serve several purposes.[30,44] First, it helps develop research protocols for clinical evaluation, diagnosis, and management of vaccine-associated adverse events. Second, it assists in developing evidence-based protocols for vaccination of individuals at higher risk of experiencing an adverse event. Third, it acts as a resource for clinical vaccine safety inquiries and during public health emergencies such as pandemics. Finally, because of the standardized scrutiny each case reported to the CISA network receives, the CISA network may be able to identify differences in the genetic makeup, environmental exposures, or physiology of individuals that may predispose them to the development of vaccine-related reactions.[30,44] Identifying idiosyncratic differences that predispose individuals to VAEs may be particularly useful in the future development of safer vaccines.

For post-surveillance to be most effective, all providers who order or administer vaccines need to report potential adverse reactions of any degree to VAERS and seek further advice from the CISA network if needed. Because the background incidence of many reactions attributed to vaccines, such as Guillain-Barré syndrome, autism, or multiple sclerosis, is unknown, it is very difficult or impossible to quantify the relationship between vaccine receipt and these events. Consequently, VAERS data are often quoted as a surrogate measure of prevalence. For example, the rate of serious VAEs associated with hepatitis A vaccine has been reported to be 1.4 VAEs per 100,000 distributed doses.[45] This statistic does not describe a causal relationship, only an association. However, it is useful in counseling patients to have some understanding of how rare VAEs are thought to be. The use of VAERs data in this fashion can only be accurate if all suspected reactions are reported. **Table 2-9** lists the websites where VAERS reporting forms and other vaccine safety-related information can be obtained.

Table 2-9 Vaccine Safety Internet Resources

Resource	Description	Website
Advisory Committee on Immunization Practices Vaccine Statements	Detailed description of individual vaccines: recommended schedule, side effects, safety profile, and more	http://www.immunize.org/acip/
Immunization Action Coalition	Patient information, vaccine information statements available in different languages	http://www.immunize.org/new/
Travelers' Health: Destinations	Updated list of vaccinations recommended by the CDC, which can vary by age of traveler and destination	http://wwwnc.cdc.gov/travel/destinations/list
National Vaccine Injury Compensation Program	Details on program and how to file a claim for a vaccine-related injury	http://www.hrsa.gov/vaccinecompensation/index.html
VAERS Data Reporting Central	Data reporting forms, consultation available	https://vaers.hhs.gov/professionals/index

CDC = Centers for Disease Control and Prevention, VAERS = Vaccine Adverse Event Reporting System

Communicating Vaccine Risk

Unlike medications used to treat already-established disease, vaccines are given to healthy individuals to protect against future infection. Future exposure to a vaccine-preventable illness may or may not occur, and, even if exposure occurs, infection may not develop. Because vaccines may not be necessary to protect an individual's health, particularly if the prevalence of disease or its virulence is low, vaccines must adhere to the highest level of safety. Even rare reactions may make some individuals reluctant to accept vaccination.[46-48] If enough individuals refuse to participate in community inoculation, the ability of vaccines to protect the general public will decline.

Vaccines provide individual protection, but they also induce herd immunity when enough individuals are protected. Herd immunity protects unvaccinated individuals by disrupting transmission. If a vaccine-preventable illness enters a community with high levels of immunity, only a few isolated cases may develop. Transmission does not occur, and the infection dies out. However, if infection enters a community with uneven or no vaccination coverage, infection can be transmitted to unvaccinated individuals and lead to widespread illness. The level of community acceptance needed to induce herd immunity varies depending on the inherent effectiveness of the vaccine, the prevalence and virulence of infection, and the mode of transmission.[49,50] For example, it is thought that approximately 70% of the population needs to be vaccinated against diphtheria,[51] 80% against rubella and mumps,[49] and 95% against pertussis and measles[49] to induce herd immunity against these viral infections. Therefore, while the decision to be vaccinated is made by the individual, the individual's decision to accept or reject vaccination affects the health of the entire community. In areas where vaccination levels waned, such as in Japan and parts of the former Soviet Union,

vaccine-preventable illnesses rose, in some cases to epidemic levels.[46,52,53]

The perception of the risks and benefits related to vaccination differs depending on whether they are viewed from the individual or societal perspective.[54] From the individual perspective, vaccines provide protection but also are associated with minor side effects and some very rare but serious risks. From the societal perspective, vaccines carry no risk. They promote the general health of the community because large-scale acceptance leads to herd immunity, which protects those individuals who cannot afford or do not have access to immunizations, those whose immunity has unknowingly waned, and those who cannot be immunized because other medical problems place them at higher risk of vaccine-related complications. However, because the risks of vaccination are borne by the individual, some may decide against immunization and rely on chance or on the protection afforded by herd immunity.[55] Others may decide to be vaccinated for their own individual protection, as well as for the public good. Still others do not actively evaluate their choices and simply follow the example of the majority of individuals around them. Individuals accept or reject vaccinations because of differences in their underlying beliefs about the importance of individual rights versus the public good, their understanding and preference for various types and degrees of risk, and their interpretation of the statistics used to describe the risks and benefits of vaccination.[55]

Understanding the underlying values affecting decision making and the ways that individuals evaluate risk is essential in order to provide the counseling needed to help women decide whether they want to receive, or have their family members receive, vaccinations.[56] In general, individuals contemplating a choice among "risky" options will be more likely to choose an intervention where the associated risks are familiar, voluntary, and natural.[55,57] Risks that are human-made—that is, they result from an imposed choice or are unknown and unquantified—are less acceptable. Individuals are also more likely to accept vaccination if it provides protection against catastrophic events, such as death or severe disability, even if these events are rare.

Other values affect vaccine decision making. Individuals will have different preferences for risks associated with omission or commission.[54,55] Does a woman prefer to expose her child to the potential risk of a serious reaction associated with receipt of a vaccine, or does she prefer the risks associated with contracting a vaccine-preventable illness? To a certain extent, the preference for risks associated with omission or commission is based on a woman's understanding of the frequency of the risk that her child could contract a vaccine-preventable illness.[57] Individuals differ in their perception of the meaning of statistics used to describe these events.[57] In addition, health providers have their own set of values and ways of interpreting the data used to describe the benefits and risks of vaccines, which can color their discussion of these issues with their clients.[57] Often healthcare providers couch their explanations in evidence-based reasoning, whereas the public may process information through a different philosophical lens.[58]

After weighing all the pros and cons, some women will decide against immunization either for themselves or their families. These women often experience pressure from other health professionals and from institutions such as schools, workplaces, and childcare centers to accept vaccination. Women need to be counseled in an accepting manner about the risks associated with various infections, the likelihood that infection with a vaccine-preventable infection will occur, and the types and frequency of vaccine-related side effects. Tables 2-13 to 2-20 (presented later in this chapter) describe commonly used vaccines in adults and the presentation and risks associated with vaccine-preventable diseases. These tables can be used to help women understand the risks associated with vaccine-preventable diseases and weigh them against the effectiveness and safety of commonly used vaccinations.

Women who choose not to vaccinate their children can request a school waiver so that their children do not have to comply with state immunization requirements in order to attend school. Each state has established specific regulations governing eligibility, what vaccines are covered, and the exact steps an individual must follow in order to be deemed exempt from vaccine requirements. All states grant medical exemptions; 48 states also grant exemptions for religious or personal beliefs. Fewer states (19) offer exemptions for personal beliefs.[49] Only a small percentage of families request personal exemptions, but these requests rose nationally from 0.99 in 1991 to 2.45% in 2004, respectively,[49] before declining slightly to 1.9% in 2012.[59] In consequence, states such as California are repealing these exemptions and developing policies that will extend mandatory vaccination policies for daycares and preschool programs.[60]

Women who decide to forgo immunizations should be informed that herd immunity provides limited protection from vaccine-preventable illnesses. Several studies have shown that unimmunized children are more likely to contract pertussis and measles than immunized children, and they can spread infection to already immunized children whose immunity has lapsed due to primary vaccine failure or waning antibody levels. In studies of school-aged children, children who had been exempted from vaccination were 22[61] to 35 times[62] more likely to develop measles and 6 times more likely to develop pertussis.[61] In addition, Feikin and colleagues found that 11% of vaccinated children who developed measles acquired their infection through exposure to an unimmunized child.[61] However, the overall incidence of infection remained low. The annual incidence of measles in unvaccinated children was 32 cases per 100,000 compared to 1.4 cases per 100,000 for vaccinated children; the incidence of pertussis was 80 cases per 100,000 for unvaccinated children and 13 cases per 100,000 for vaccinated children.[61] More recently, a multi-state outbreak of measles in 2014 was sparked by children who acquired measles while visiting Disneyland and then transmitted it to others in 24 states and the District of Columbia.[63]

Principles of Vaccination

Proper administration of vaccines is critical. Using improper technique, spacing vaccine boosters incorrectly, or administering vaccines simultaneously with antibody-containing products can all undermine the effectiveness of vaccines. Following a few essential principles can ensure that vaccines will provide long-lived immunity.

GIVE VACCINES SIMULTANEOUSLY WHEN POSSIBLE

Simultaneous administration is often recommended because it is more practical. The simultaneous administration of vaccines (e.g., giving MMR, varicella, and tetanus all at the same visit) will not impair the immune response to any of the vaccines commonly used in adult practice. Nor does the safety profile of vaccines seem to change with simultaneous administration. The immune response to vaccines administered simultaneously is robust and confers long-lasting protection. Compared to having the patient return for repeated vaccinations of single products, simultaneous administration is more likely to result in the timely completion of any needed immunization series.

When immunizations are not given simultaneously, correct timing becomes important. Incorrect timing of vaccine administration may interfere with the immune response, leaving the patient vulnerable to vaccine-preventable diseases. Inactivated vaccines are not affected by nonsimultaneous administration, but live viral vaccines are. If two live parenteral viral vaccines, such as the MMR and varicella vaccines, or the live nasal influenza vaccine are not given simultaneously, they should be administered a minimum of 4 weeks apart. Giving live viral vaccines too close together will inhibit the immune response of the second vaccine. In this case, either the second vaccine should be repeated or the woman should have serologic confirmation that immunity developed.[29]

SPACE BOOSTERS CORRECTLY

The immune response also can be inhibited by starting a vaccine series too early or by too close spacing of boosters. Both live and inactivated vaccines can be affected by these errors. Recommendations for what age to start a vaccine series, the number of doses needed in the primary series, and the need for subsequent boosters are based on such considerations as when exposure is expected to occur, the physiology of the immune response, and the maturity of the immune system. Childhood vaccine series start as early as birth and as late as 15 months. Beginning at an earlier age than recommended for the specific vaccine will result in inadequate antibody levels because the immune system is too immature to mount a permanent response. If multiple doses are required, adherence to the recommended time intervals between doses is also important. Immunologic memory is induced only by repeated separate exposures to an antigen. Boosters given at longer intervals than recommended will still induce an adequate immune response.[29] Giving vaccines too close together will not "boost" the immune system because too early administration of a second dose will not be recognized as a separate event.

Because the types of vaccines and the number of vaccines needed to complete a primary series is different for adults than for children, the management of adults whose records indicate that vaccines were given incorrectly also differs. For example, a primary series of tetanus vaccine for children consists of a total of five doses, whereas the adult primary series consists of only three. Therefore, adults who did not receive a primary series of tetanus vaccine in childhood do not need to "make up" missed doses and need to receive only three doses to complete their primary series.

Recommendations regarding the management of spacing errors are the same for children and adults. Vaccines requiring multiple doses should not be given at shorter time intervals than recommended. If this occurs, the dose given too early should not be counted as part of the series and should be repeated at the correct time. Boosters given at longer intervals than recommended still induce an appropriate response and may be counted as part of the series. In this case, the vaccine series does not need to be restarted no matter how much time has elapsed between doses.[29]

Table 2-10 shows an adult immunization schedule and describes the types and timing of vaccines recommended for general use in adults. Adults who will be traveling to areas of the world where vaccine-preventable illnesses not commonly seen in the United States occur should consult resources provided by their local health department or the CDC website on Travelers' Health for current travel recommendations as these recommendations are constantly updated.

USE PROPER TECHNIQUE

Correct administration of vaccine products requires that proper technique be used. Some vaccines should be administered intramuscularly and others subcutaneously to work effectively. Some vaccines, such as measles, require that their distribution and administration follow "cold chain" principles for temperature regulation. Other vaccines require that they be stored only at room temperature. Failure to keep vaccines at the proper temperature during each step of the distribution process, from the manufacturer to the patient, can result in loss of vaccine potency. Consequently, practices that provide immunizations to their clients need to follow all manufacturers' instructions on the correct handling and storage for each specific vaccine.[64]

Vaccines should not be coadministered with products that can inhibit the immune response. Passive acquisition of antibodies through receipt of immunoglobulins, whole blood, or other blood products can reduce the effectiveness of some vaccines when both products are administered simultaneously. Inactivated vaccines are not affected; however, the immune response of live antigen vaccines can be compromised if they are given too close to the receipt of antibody-containing products. If the vaccine is given first, then 2 or more weeks should elapse before an antibody-containing product is given. If an antibody-containing product is given first, then 3 or more months should elapse before receipt of a live antigen vaccine. Allowing a minimum interval between receipt of an antibody-containing product and a live antigen vaccine will permit levels of passively acquired antibodies to decline to low enough levels so that the development of a permanent immune response will not be affected. The recommended window of time needed to elapse before immunizing with a live antigen vaccine differs according to which type of antibody-containing product was given (**Table 2-11**).[64]

In obstetrical practice, one time that a woman might need both a live viral vaccine and an antibody-containing product would be the Rh-negative woman who needs both rubella vaccine and an Rh immune globulin (RhoGAM) injection postpartum. However, the levels of antibodies found in RhoGAM are so low that they are not thought to interfere with the development of an effective immune response to the rubella vaccine in most cases. Even in cases where a postpartum blood transfusion is needed, the CDC recommends vaccinating rubella-susceptible women.[65] Postpartum immunization with the rubella vaccine is a critical strategy used to reduce the incidence of infection and congenital rubella syndrome. Serologic confirmation of immunity is suggested by the Advisory Committee on Immunization Practices (ACIP) when a woman receives RhoGAM or other antibody-containing products after her delivery.[65] The timing of serologic confirmation varies according to which antibody-containing product a woman received. If RhoGAM was given, serology should be obtained at 3 or more months postpartum (Table 2-11).[64]

Table 2-10 Adult Vaccine Schedule 2015

Recommended Adult Immunization Schedule—United States - 2015

Note: See on-line adult immunization at CDC for notes on when and how to immunize.

Recommended adult immunization schedule, by vaccine and age group[1]

Vaccine / Age Group ▶	19-21 years	22-26 years	27-49 years	50-59 years	60-64 years	≥ 65 years
Influenza*[2]	1 dose annually					
Tetanus, diphtheria, pertussis (Td/Tdap)*[3]	Substitute 1-time dose of Tdap for Td booster; then boost with Td every 10 yrs					
Varicella*[4]	2 doses					
Human papillomavirus (HPV) Female*[5]	3 doses	3 doses				
Human papillomavirus (HPV) Male*[5]	3 doses	3 doses				
Zoster[6]					1 dose	1 dose
Measles, mumps, rubella (MMR)*[7]	1 or 2 doses					
Pneumococcal 13-valent conjugate (PCV13)*[8]						1 dose
Pneumococcal 23-valent polysaccharide (PPSV23)[8]			1 or 2 doses			1 dose
Meningococcal*[9]	1 or more doses					
Hepatitis A*[10]	2 doses					
Hepatitis B*[11]	3 doses					
Haemophilus influenzae type b (Hib)*[12]	1 or 3 doses					

*Covered by the Vaccine Injury Compensation Program

- For all persons in this category who meet the age requirements and who lack documentation of vaccination or have no evidence of previous infection; zoster vaccine recommended regardless of prior episode of zoster
- Recommended if some other risk factor is present (e.g., on the basis of medical, occupational, lifestyle, or other indication)
- No recommendation

Report all clinically significant postvaccination reactions to the Vaccine Adverse Event Reporting System (VAERS). Reporting forms and instructions on filing a VAERS report are available at www.vaers.hhs.gov or by telephone, 800-822-7967.

Information on how to file a Vaccine Injury Compensation Program claim is available at www.hrsa.gov/vaccinecompensation or by telephone, 800-338-2382. To file a claim for vaccine injury, contact the U.S. Court of Federal Claims, 717 Madison Place, N.W., Washington, D.C. 20005; telephone, 202-357-6400.

Additional information about the vaccines in this schedule, extent of available data, and contraindications for vaccination is also available at www.cdc.gov/vaccines or from the CDC-INFO Contact Center at 800-CDC-INFO (800-232-4636) in English and Spanish, 8:00 a.m. - 8:00 p.m. Eastern Time, Monday - Friday, excluding holidays.

Use of trade names and commercial sources is for identification only and does not imply endorsement by the U.S. Department of Health and Human Services.

The recommendations in this schedule were approved by the Centers for Disease Control and Prevention's (CDC) Advisory Committee on Immunization Practices (ACIP), the American Academy of Family Physicians (AAFP), the America College of Physicians (ACP), American College of Obstetricians and Gynecologists (ACOG) and American College of Nurse-Midwives (ACNM).

Table 2-11 Spacing of Live Antigen Vaccines After Receipt of Antibody-Containing Products

Antibody-Containing Products	Months Needed to Elapse Before Vaccinating with Live Vaccine
Varicella immunoglobulin	5
Hepatitis B immunoglobulin	3
Packed red blood cells	6
Whole blood	6
Plasma/platelet products	7

Data from Kroger AT, Sumaya CV, Pickering LK, Atkinson WL. General recommendations on immunization: recommendations by the Advisory Committee on Immunization Practices (ACIP). *MMWR.* 2011;60(RR02):1-60.

SCREEN FOR CONTRAINDICATIONS TO RECEIVING VACCINES

Very few true contraindications exist for vaccine receipt. Vaccines have been inappropriately withheld for many reasons. These missed opportunities are among the most common reasons why individuals may not be adequately immunized. According to the CDC, the only absolute contraindication to any vaccine is an anaphylactic reaction to a vaccine or a vaccine component, such as egg proteins, neomycin, and gelatin. Because influenza and yellow fever vaccines contain egg proteins, individuals with severe allergic reactions (generalized hives, itching of the mouth or throat, shortness of breath, hypotension, or shock) to eggs should not receive these vaccines. Historically, egg allergy has been thought to be responsible for allergic reactions after the receipt of the MMR vaccine. However, more recently, ACIP concluded that eggs are unlikely to be a cause of allergic reactions to MMR, because the MMR vaccine utilizes chick embryos, rather than eggs, in its manufacturing process. Gelatin,

another component of MMR and other vaccines (influenza, varicella, and zoster),[66] is thought to be a more likely cause of allergic reactions after receipt of MMR.[29] A reasonable way to discern those who can safely receive vaccination is to inquire about a woman's reaction to eating eggs; those who have no reaction can safely receive the yellow fever and influenza vaccines.[64]

Other components of concern include neomycin and latex. Most individuals with allergies to these substances develop contact dermatitis, not anaphylaxis, after exposure. Neomycin is contained in some vaccines, including hepatitis A, influenza, MMR, varicella, and zoster vaccines.[66] Latex and latex derivatives (natural rubber latex and dry natural rubber) are used in the manufacture of medical gloves, intravenous (IV) tubing, vaccine vials, and syringes. Those who experience only contact dermatitis may receive vaccines containing neomycin or packaged in vials containing latex without concern; however, those who have had an anaphylactic reaction should not receive vaccines that contain the offending substance(s).[64] Those who experience anaphylactic reactions from exposure to latex should not receive vaccines supplied in vials or syringes that contain natural rubber of any type.[64] Clinicians should carefully read the package inserts that come with vaccine products for details before administering vaccinations to individuals with allergies to vaccine components.

Conditions such as immunosuppression or pregnancy can also affect which vaccines are recommended. See the sections that follow for more details.

Other situations may occur that are labeled precautionary. Vaccines may be given in these cases if the chance of acquiring a vaccine-preventable illness is high, but withholding the vaccine until the precautionary condition or situation resolves is preferable. Precautions listed by the CDC include the following:[67]

- A condition that increases the likelihood that a VAE may occur or could increase the severity of a VAE
- A condition or situation that may inhibit the immune response to a vaccine

Table 2-12 Appropriate and Inappropriate Reasons to Withhold Some Vaccines

Appropriate Reasons	Inappropriate Reasons
• Pregnancy for some vaccines* • Moderate or severe illness • Anaphylactic reaction to vaccine or vaccine components (eggs, neomycin, and gelatin among others) • Personal history of severe immunosuppression may be a contraindication for some vaccines*	• Pregnancy in the household • Breastfeeding • Mild illness • Need for multiple vaccines • Nonspecific allergies

* See section on pregnancy and immunosuppression for further details.

Data from Kroger AT, Sumaya CV, Pickering LK, Atkinson WL. General recommendations on immunization: recommendations by the Advisory Committee on Immunization Practices (ACIP). *MMWR.* 2011;60(RR02):1-60.

• A moderate-to-severe illness is present at the time of the visit. Vaccination should be deferred until the illness has resolved. These individuals do not seem to be at higher risk of impaired immunity or vaccine reactions; rather, the underlying illness may make the recognition of a VAE, particularly fever, more difficult to ascertain.

Before administering vaccines, the clinician should ask a few screening questions regarding conditions that would make vaccine receipt problematic. Patients should be queried about allergies, particularly food allergies; whether they and/or anyone living in their household have problems with their immune system; if they ever had any reaction to the receipt of any other vaccines; their current state of health; and the likelihood they could be pregnant. **Table 2-12** summarizes the conditions that impact the decision to administer vaccines.[62]

When a Vaccine History Is Unknown

Three approaches are acceptable for women whose immunization status is unknown.[62] The provider can determine immunity by obtaining serologic titers and administer vaccine(s) if low titers indicate a vaccine is needed. Testing for titers is expensive but will avoid unnecessary vaccine administration.

However, giving a vaccine without documenting immunity is acceptable if no contraindications are present. This approach may be less expensive and easier to implement than obtaining titers. The third approach is to obtain immunization records from school and medical records, analyze these records to determine what vaccinations are needed, and immunize accordingly. This approach will avoid unneeded vaccination, but will be more difficult and time-consuming to implement. Clinicians should discuss these options with their clients and suggest the one that best meets the needs of the client and the system in which care is provided.

Commonly Used Adult Vaccines

The specific vaccines recommended for general use in adults vary according to age, exposure potential, vaccine history, and the presence of underlying medical conditions. The discussion in the following subsections of this chapter briefly covers the presentation and complications associated with vaccine-preventable diseases and focuses on issues specific to vaccinations commonly given to adults in the United States. Readers should also refer to the tables on specific vaccine-preventable diseases and their corresponding vaccines for details on the risks associated with vaccine-preventable disease and the indications, schedule, and risks associated with vaccination.

Hepatitis A and B Vaccines

Hepatitis infections, regardless of type, present similarly. Infected individuals first report general malaise, anorexia, nausea and vomiting, fever, headache, myalgias, and right upper quadrant pain. Jaundice typically develops 3 to 10 days after symptom onset and may be preceded by dark urine. Recovery may be prolonged with malaise and fatigue persisting for several weeks or months.[29] Despite these similarities, the sequelae of infections are markedly different between hepatitis A and B infections, with corresponding different recommendations regarding vaccination.

Hepatitis A is caused by a picornavirus and is commonly transmitted through the fecal-oral route. The virus replicates in the liver and is excreted in the feces, beginning 2 weeks before symptom onset and continuing up to 3 weeks after the infection becomes clinically recognizable. High-risk groups include international travelers to areas with poor sanitation, users of illicit drugs, and men who have sex with men (MSM). Certain individuals can play a substantial role in transmission. Infected food handlers can unwittingly transmit infection to a large number of individuals if proper sanitation and food preparation standards are not followed. Infected children, who are often asymptomatic, can also pass on infection to other family members and caregivers.[29]

Hepatitis A vaccines, introduced in 1996, were initially recommended for use in high-risk groups as previously described and in children living in communities in the Western United States with high prevalence rates. Over the intervening years, ACIP gradually expanded its recommendations and ultimately recommended hepatitis A vaccination to all children beginning in 2006.[29] Adults who are at risk of infection should also be vaccinated.[68,69] (See **Table 2-13**.) Because infection confers lifelong immunity and vaccination induces long-term durable protection, serology tests can be performed to determine the need for vaccination in high-risk patients. Alternatively, vaccination can be given immediately without serologic testing because reactions to hepatitis A vaccines are very rare.

Hepatitis B vaccines have been available since 1981. The vaccine in current use is a recombinant vaccine, which is formed by inserting the hepatitis B antigen into Baker yeast cells. These yeast cells produce hepatitis B antigen (HBAg), which is then harvested, purified, and used as a basis for the vaccine. The final product contains no infectious components and is incapable of causing active infection. For adults, hepatitis B vaccine is available in two formulations: a single agent containing only hepatitis B or a combined product containing both hepatitis A and hepatitis B vaccines. The single agent product is approved for use in both adolescents and adults, whereas the combined product (Twinrix) is approved for use in individuals older than 18 years. Both formulations are recommended for use in previously unvaccinated individuals at high risk of acquiring infection or who are at higher risk of severe disease or complications if infected (Table 2-13).[29,70]

Since 1991, the CDC has recommended a multifaceted approach to eliminating hepatitis B infection in the United States, including universal screening of pregnant women, immunoprophylaxis of exposed newborns, routine vaccination of all infants, and catch-up vaccination of high-risk adolescents and adults. These efforts have resulted in significant declines in the number of cases reported to the CDC. More than 25,000 new cases of hepatitis B were reported each year to the CDC in the mid-1980s, dropping to just over 3000 new cases in 2013.[71]

Infection is still endemic in many parts of the world (particularly Sub-Saharan Africa, East Asia, Oceania, and Andean Latin America) despite dramatic increases in the global uptake of hepatitis B vaccination.[72] High-prevalence areas are defined

Table 2-13 Hepatitis Infections and Vaccines

	Infection			Vaccine			
Pathogen	Incubation/ Presentation	Complications	Vaccine Agent/ Schedule	Vaccine Efficacy	Vaccine Contraindications/ Precautions	Vaccine-Associated Side Effects
Hepatitis A[a,b,c,d]	**Incubation** 28 days **Presentation** Abrupt onset of malaise, headache, fever, discomfort, nausea, anorexia, dark urine, and jaundice Recovery almost always complete Lifetime immunity after infection	Severe complications are rare	**Type Hepatitis A** Inactivated whole-cell vaccine **Indications** All children Adults at risk of infection: international travelers to high-risk areas, MSM, illicit drug users, occupational risk (work with primates), chronic conditions (clotting factor disorder, chronic liver disease), close contact with international adoptees **Schedule** 2-dose schedule, 0 and 6 months	Nearly 100% after 2 doses Immunity likely to persist for at least 15 to 25 years Has strong anamnestic anti-hepatitis B response	**Contraindications** Allergy to vaccine or vaccine component **Precautions** Moderate to severe illness	**Local reactions** 20-50% **Severe** Rarely reported, not quantifiable

| Hepatitis B[a,e,f] | Incubation 45 to 160 days
Presentation Nonspecific symptoms of malaise, fever, headache, and myalgia but up to 50% of infections are asymptomatic | Most resolve completely
Fulminant hepatitis occurs in 1-2% of cases and has a case fatality of 63-93%
Chronic infection develops in 5% of adults
Chronic infection associated with cirrhosis and cancer | **Type Hepatitis B** Inactivated recombinant vaccine
Indications All children
Unvaccinated high-risk adults (household contacts and sexual partners of hepatitis B-positive individuals, multiple sexual partners defined as more than 1 partner in the last 6 months, MSM, recent intravenous drug use, healthcare workers, diabetics, HIV infection, renal disease, residents and staff of facilities for developmentally disabled adults, international traveler to parts of the world with high prevalence rates | 95% effective
Duration of immunity ≥ 20 years | **Contraindications** Allergy to vaccine or vaccine component (including yeast)
Precautions Moderate to severe illness | Case reports suggest that alopecia may be associated with hepatitis B vaccination, although an unpublished case-control study found no association
Anaphylaxis |

(continues)

Table 2-13 Hepatitis Infections and Vaccines *(continued)*

Infection			Vaccine			
Pathogen	Incubation/ Presentation	Complications	Vaccine Agent/ Schedule	Vaccine Efficacy	Vaccine Contraindications/ Precautions	Vaccine-Associated Side Effects
			Schedule 3 doses: 0, 1, 6 months			
			Accelerated schedule: 0, 1, 2 months			
			Type Hepatitis A and B Combines both vaccines			
			Indications Same as for parent vaccines			
			Schedule 3 doses: 0, 1, 6 months			

[a] Data from Centers for Disease Control and Prevention. *Epidemiology and Prevention of Vaccine-Preventable Diseases*. 13th ed. Washington, DC: Public Health Foundation; 2015.

[b] Fiore AE, Wasley A, Bell BP. Prevention of hepatitis A through active or passive immunization: recommendations of the Advisory Committee on Immunization Practices. *MMWR*. 2006;RR 07(55):1-23.

[c] Centers for Disease Control and Prevention. Updated recommendations from the Advisory Committee on Immunization Practices (ACIP) for use of hepatitis A vaccine in close contacts of newly arriving international adoptees. *MMWR*. 2009;58(36):1006-7.

[d] Murphy TV, Feinstone SM, Bell BP. Hepatitis A vaccines. In: Plotkin SA, Orenstein WA, Offit PA, eds. *Vaccines*. 6th ed. Elsevier; 2013.

[e] Institute of Medicine. *Adverse Effects of Vaccines: Evidence and Causality*. Washington, DC: National Academies Press; 2012.

[f] Centers for Disease Control and Prevention. 2014 final pertussis surveillance report. 2015. Available at: http://www.cdc.gov/pertussis/downloads/pertuss-surv-report-2014.pdf. Accessed December 6, 2015.

as locations where more than 8% of the population is hepatitis B surface antigen positive, moderate prevalence is between 2% and 7%, and low prevalence is below 2%. In areas of the world with high prevalence, more than 60% of the population become acutely infected,[29] often in infancy or during childhood, and 8% develop chronic infection. In areas of low prevalence, less than 20% become acutely infected, most often in adulthood, and chronic infection is present in fewer than 1% of individuals.[29]

Women from endemic areas of the world may not have received hepatitis B vaccination in their native country and need to be screened for evidence of active or past infection and immunized as appropriate. Serologic markers that can help indicate whether a woman needs to be immunized are hepatitis B core antibody (HBcAb), hepatitis B surface antibody (HBsAb), and HBAg. Individuals who are immune will test positive for one or both of the antibodies (HBcAb, HBsAb) and negative for the antigen (HBAg). Those who acquired immunity via vaccination usually test positive for HBsAb, whereas those who acquired immunity from resolved infection usually test positive for HBcAb. Individuals who are chronically infected test negative for antibodies (HBcAb, HBsAb) and positive for antigen (HBAg).

A number of potential VAEs related to hepatitis B vaccines have been investigated since the mid-1990s. Concerns were raised in France in the mid-1990s about a potential relationship between the receipt of hepatitis B vaccines and multiple sclerosis and resulted in routine hepatitis B vaccination being dropped from school health clinics in France despite assertions from the World Health Organization (WHO) that the vaccine was safe.[73,74] After an intensive review of the available research, the Immunization Safety Review Committee released a report in 2002 agreeing with this assessment.[74] A number of follow-up studies have also reported no

relationship between hepatitis B vaccines and demyelinating disease in the general population[75] or with relapse in those already diagnosed with multiple sclerosis.[76]

Another safety issue of concern in the late 1990s was whether incorporating hepatitis B vaccines into the infant immunization schedule would raise infants' exposure to mercury to unsafe levels. Many vaccines, including the hepatitis B vaccine, have historically used thimerosal, which contains mercury, as a preservative. It was added to multidose vials of many vaccines to prevent bacterial contamination.[74] Until 1991, the only vaccine given to infants that contained thimerosal was the diphtheria, tetanus, pertussis (DTP) vaccine, but in 1991, hepatitis B and *Haemophilus influenzae* type b (HIB) vaccines, both of which contained thimerosal, were recommended for routine use in infants younger than 1 year of age.[74] This expanded immunization schedule was estimated by the FDA to increase the exposure of infants younger than 6 months to mercury levels that exceeded Environmental Protection Agency (EPA) body-weight recommendations.[74] The FDA recommended that vaccine manufacturers remove mercury from vaccines or justify why its continued use was necessary. In 1999, the American Academy of Pediatrics and the Public Health Service released a statement recommending that thimerosal-free vaccines be used wherever possible, but stated that the risks of disease outweighed the risks of vaccination and concluded that thimerosal-containing vaccines were acceptable if thimerosal-free alternatives were not available.[77]

To what degree, if any, thimerosal is related to neurodevelopmental damage is still being debated. A recent case-control study based on VAERS data found increasing odds of neurodevelopmental disorders (pervasive developmental disorders, developmental delay, tic disorders, and hyperkinetic syndrome) with increasing number of thimerosal-containing vaccines given in the first 6 months of life.[78] Another study of VAERS data reported no discernible patterns between cumulative exposure to thimerosal-containing vaccines on 42 neuropsychologic outcomes in children between 7 and 10 years of age (N = 1047).[79]

Since mid-2001, vaccines administered to children are either thimerosal-free or contain only trace amounts.[64,80] Thimerosal is present in some adult vaccines (some formulations of Td, meningococcal, and multidose influenza).[80] One of the reasons put forward by some scientists about these differing results is the difficulty in accounting for vaccine exposures, particularly if international samples are used, because vaccine schedules can differ from one country to another; the difficulty in accounting for confounding variables; the need to amass large sample sizes when evaluating rare events; and the biases that researchers may harbor that inadvertently influence the outcomes.[81] Certainly, the bulk of the evidence to date supports the safety of hepatitis B vaccination, although vigilance must be maintained to ensure vaccine safety.

HPV Vaccines

Human papilloma viral infections are common and usually resolve without sequelae. Unfortunately, persistent infection is associated with almost all cervical cancers, 90% of anal cancers, and more than 70% of cancers of the vulva, vagina, penis, and oropharynx.[29] Three HPV vaccines are currently available in the United States: HPV 2 (Cervarix) targeting HPV 16 and 18 licensed in 2009;[82] HPV 4 (Gardasil) targeting HPV types 16, 18, 6, and 11 licensed in 2006;[83] and HPV 9 (Gardasil 9) targeting HPV types 16, 18, 6, 11, 31, 33, 45, 52, and 58 licensed in 2015.[84]

While 15 or more viral types are thought to cause cervical disease, HPV vaccines target those most commonly associated with symptomatic disease and/or those thought to be most virulent for cervical cancer. Types 6 and 11 (included in

HPV 4 and HPV 9 vaccines) are responsible for causing 90% of genital warts.[29] HPV types 16 and 18, which are targeted by all HPV vaccines, are estimated to cause 64% of all invasive HPV-associated cancers. The newest vaccine adds on protection against 5 other HPV types (31, 33, 45, 52, and 58), which account for another 10% of invasive cancers in the United States.[84] The viral types included in the HPV 9 vaccine, if used globally, would also substantially reduce cervical cancer worldwide since these strains are prevalent in areas of the world (China, South America, and Africa) where the burden of cervical cancer is particularly high.[85] However, no current vaccines protect against other carcinogenic strains (35, 39, 51, 56, and 59), which are associated with approximately 5-6% of cervical cancers globally.[85] Use of the HPV 9 vaccine is likely to be more beneficial for women in parts of the world where they are more likely to be infected with oncogenic HPV strains other than 16 and 18.[86,87]

While increasing use of HPV vaccines is anticipated to significantly reduce the burden of HPV-related disease, the exact impact of HPV vaccines will depend on a number of factors. Widespread uptake of vaccination is needed to reduce the incidence of disease, which currently is estimated to infect 33% of adolescents, 54% of women between 20 and 24 years of age, and 39% of women age 50 to 59.[88] Second, it will depend on whether the reductions in subclinical infections and cancer precursors seen in pre- and post-licensure trials will translate in the future to fewer cervical cancers. This can occur only if vaccination results in long-term protection. Studies have documented sustained antibody titers for 6 to 8 years.[89,90] Third, the projections are based on the assumption that other oncogenic types not targeted by vaccination will remain low. Consequently, it will be many years before the extent of the benefits related to HPV vaccination can be accurately quantified.[91] See **Table 2-14** for a description of HPV infections and vaccines.

Table 2-14 HPV Vaccines

	Infection			Vaccine			
Pathogen	Incubation/ Presentation	Complications	Vaccine Agent/ Schedule	Vaccine Efficacy	Vaccine Contraindications/ Precautions	Vaccine- Associated Side Effects
HPV[a,b,c,d,e,f]	**Incubation** 28 days **Presentation** Usually asymptomatic and self-limited	Anogenital warts Respiratory papillomas Cervical cancer precursors Cancer of the vagina, cervix, anus, and oropharynx	**Type** Inactivated vaccine using recombinant technology to produce virus-like particles Three formulations 1) HPV 2: types 16, 18 Schedule: 0, 1-2, 6 months All girls, age 11-12, up to 25 years if missed or incomplete series 2) HPV 4: types 16, 18, 6, 11 Schedule: 0, 1-2, 6 months All girls and all boys age 11-12, up to 26 years in women and age 21 in men if missed or	93-99% in women 75-89% in men	**Contraindications** Allergy to vaccine or components (contains yeast) Pregnancy **Precautions** Severe to moderate illness	**Local reactions** Local reactions, 20-90% Fever 10-13% **Severe** anaphylaxis

(continues)

Table 2-14 HPV Vaccines *(continued)*

Infection			Vaccine			
Pathogen	Incubation/ Presentation	Complications	Vaccine Agent/ Schedule	Vaccine Efficacy	Vaccine Contraindications/ Precautions	Vaccine- Associated Side Effects
			incomplete series. May extend vaccination in men up to age 26 if immunocompromised or if engage in sex with men 3) HPV 9: types 16, 18, 6, 11, 31, 33, 45, 52, 58 Schedule: 0, 1-2, 6 months Same as HPV 4 vaccines			

[a] Data from Centers for Disease Control and Prevention. *Epidemiology and Prevention of Vaccine-Preventable Diseases.* 13th ed. Washington, DC: Public Health Foundation; 2015.

[b] Institute of Medicine. *Adverse Effects of Vaccines: Evidence and Causality.* Washington, DC: National Academies Press; 2012.

[c] Centers for Disease Control and Prevention. FDA licensure of bivalent human papillomavirus vaccine (HPV2, Cervarix) for use in females and updated HPV vaccination; Recommendations from the Advisory Committee on Immunization Practices. *MMWR.* 2010;59(20):626-8.

[d] Markowitz LE, Dunne EF, Saraiya M, Lawson HW, Chesson H, Unger ER. Quadrivalent human papillomavirus vaccine: recommendations of the Advisory Committee on Immunization Practices. *MMWR.* 2007;56:1-24.

[e] Petrosky E, Bocchini JA, Hariri S, Chesson H, Curtis CR, Saraiya M, et al. Use of 9-valent human papillomavirus (HPV) vaccine: updated HPV vaccination: recommendations of the Advisory Committee on Immunization Practices. *MMWR.* 2015;64(11):300-4.

[f] Centers for Disease Control and Prevention. FDA licensure of quadrivalent human papillomavirus vaccine (HPV4, Gardasil) for use in males and guidance from the Advisory Committee on Immunization Practices. *MMWR.* 2010;59(20):630-2.

As a relatively new set of vaccines, HPV vaccines are undergoing ongoing scrutiny. Reports of syncope post-vaccination in adolescents increased between 2005 and 2007 compared to the prior 2 years in the VAERS system. These events were particularly common in young adolescent females and coincided with the increase in adolescent vaccination with tetanus-diphtheria-acellular pertussis (Tdap), meningococcal, and HPV vaccines. Some of these episodes of syncope were associated with injury.[92] In a follow-up study, 6% of the 3174 cases reported to VAERS in the 3 years after licensure were deemed serious; the most common conditions reported were Guillain-Barré syndrome and seizures.[93] A follow-up study based on VAERS data did not find any relationship between HPV vaccines and Guillain-Barré syndrome.[94]

Influenza Vaccines

The influenza virus has three subtypes: A, B, and C.[29] Influenza A infects humans and animals and causes moderate to severe illness. Subtypes of influenza A are described in terms of the hemagglutinin (H) and neuraminidase (N) proteins on the viral surface, of which there are a total of 144 possible combinations. Influenza B also infects humans but generally causes milder disease. Influenza C rarely infects humans; when infection occurs, it tends to be subclinical.

Influenza viruses constantly evolve. Minor changes in subtypes are called antigenic drift; major changes are called antigenic shifts. Both changes can lead to epidemics, but antigenic shifts, which generally result from genetic recombination between influenza A viruses that infect humans and birds, can lead to pandemics. Pandemics (disease that infects a region, country, or that is global) spread along travel routes and have high attack rates in all age groups. While disease severity tends to remain unchanged, because so many more individuals are infected during pandemics, mortality can be high.[29]

Each year, the influenza vaccine is reformulated to match the subtypes expected to be circulating during the flu season. The ideal time to vaccinate is in October and November, before the start of the flu season that typically runs from November to March. If a good match exists between the current vaccine and circulating subtypes, vaccine efficacy is high (90%) in healthy young adults.[95] Influenza vaccine is less effective, even with a good match, in the frail elderly, but can mitigate the severity of infection. Use of the influenza vaccine in the elderly is estimated to prevent infection in only 30-40% of recipients, but is 50-60% effective in preventing hospitalization and 80% effective in preventing death.[95] (See **Table 2-15**.)

The influenza vaccine comes in two basic formulations: inactivated influenza vaccine (TIV) and live attenuated influenza vaccine (LAIV).[96] Several versions of TIVs are available:

- TIV, trivalent, standard dose (Afluria, Fluvirin, Fluzone)
- TIV, trivalent, high dose (Fluzone High-Dose)
- TIV, quadrivalent, standard dose (Fluarix, FluLaval, Fluzone)
- TIV, cell-culture-based, standard dose (Flucelvax)
- Recombinant influenza vaccine, trivalent (Flublok)

These products differ by included subtypes, dose, processes used to create the vaccine, and recommendations for use. In 2015-2016, Trivalent vaccines contain type A (H1N1), type A (H3N2), and type B; the quadrivalent vaccines include an additional type B subunit.[29] High-dose trivalent influenza vaccines are licensed for use in individuals 65 years or older and contain 4 times as much hemagglutinin as the regular formulation of Fluzone for adults.[29] Some are administered by nasal spray, injection (intramuscular or intradermal), single injection, or by injector jet. The

Table 2-15 Influenza Vaccines

	Infection		Vaccine		
Pathogen	Incubation/ Presentation	Complications	Vaccine Agent/ Schedule	Vaccine Efficacy	Vaccine Contraindications/ Precautions	Vaccine- Associated Side Effects
Influenza[a,b]	**Incubation** 2 days, range 1 to 4 days **Presentation** Only 50% experience a classic presenta- tion: abrupt onset of fe- ver, malaise, myalgia, cough, and sore throat.	Secondary bacterial infections Myocarditis Worsening of asthma or chronic bronchitis Deaths 0.5-1 per 1000 cases, primarily in the elderly	**Type Influenza "shot"** Inactivated virus, various formula- tions. See text. **Indications** Can be used in any- one older than 6 months. **Schedule** Every year	With a good match between the vaccine and the strains of influenza in circula- tion, the influenza vaccine will prevent illness in 90% of adults and 30-40% of the frail elderly. Vaccine use among the elderly reduces the risk of hos- pitalization by 50-60% and of death by 80%. Immunity lasts less than 1 year.	**Contraindications** Anaphylactic al- lergy to eggs or other vaccine component (can use recombi- nant formula- tions, see text) **Precautions** Severe to moderate illness History of Guil- lain-Barré syn- drome within 6 weeks of receipt of influenza vaccine	Fever, malaise, myalgias, and chills have been reported in < 1% Anaphylaxis

Type		Contraindications	
Type Influenza Nasal Spray Live attenuated influenza vaccine (LAIV) administered via nasal spray **Indications** Only given to healthy individuals between ages of 5 and 49 years **Schedule** Every year	Same	**Contraindications** Anaphylactic allergy to eggs or other vaccine component Age > 50 years Pregnancy **Precautions** Severe to moderate illness History of Guillain-Barré syndrome within 6 weeks of receipt of influenza vaccine	Cough, runny nose, nasal congestion, sore throat, chills in 10-40%

[a] Data from Centers for Disease Control and Prevention. *Epidemiology and Prevention of Vaccine-Preventable Diseases.* 13th ed. Washington, DC: Public Health Foundation; 2015.

[b] Institute of Medicine. *Adverse Effects of Vaccines: Evidence and Causality.* Washington, DC: National Academies Press; 2012.

CDC does not recommend any one product over another, as long as the proper product is given based on age and risk considerations.[96]

The trivalent LAIV, approved for use in 2003, is administered as a nasal spray. While the efficacy is similar for both LAIV and TIVs, recommendations on who should receive them differ significantly. Viral shedding has occurred for 2 to 3 days after receipt of LAIV vaccine but not after receipt of the TIV vaccine.[97,98] Consequently, LAIV has the potential to cause clinical illness in the recipient and to be spread to close contacts, but studies to date indicate that this rarely occurs. In a study of transmissibility of the LAIV in a childcare setting, the probability of acquiring vaccine virus after close contact with a vaccinated child was only 0.58-2.4%.[97,98] Because there is a remote possibility that clinical illness and/or transmission may occur with LAIV, the ACIP recommends that the use of LAIV be limited to healthy individuals between ages 5 and 49 years. In contrast, TIV is approved for use in individuals age 6 months or older and in those with underlying medical conditions, HIV-infected individuals, and pregnant women. Both vaccines may be given to family members and close personal contacts of individuals with mild-to-moderate immunosuppression; those in contact with individuals with severe immunosuppression requiring protective care in a hospital should receive the TIV vaccine.[96]

All influenza vaccines, except recombinant and cell-culture vaccines, are grown in chicken eggs and contain trace amounts of egg protein. Caution should be used in vaccinating individuals if they have developed hives, swelling of the lips or tongue, acute respiratory distress, or collapse after ingesting eggs. According to 2015 CDC recommendations, these individuals are best immunized with recombinant vaccines.[96] Those with milder symptoms such as hives can receive an inactivated vaccine.[99] Because serious reactions have been reported to VAERS in individuals who are allergic to eggs after receiving influenza vaccines, it is prudent to closely read the vaccine product insert and consult with a vaccine expert as needed, prior to vaccination, to confirm which products can safely be used.

Measles, Mumps, Rubella (MMR) Vaccines

Despite a nearly 80% decline in the global numbers of measles cases since 2000 due to increasing use of immunizations, measles infection remains one of the leading causes of death and disability in children younger than 5 years of age worldwide.[100] Measles is highly infectious; the highest rates of complications occur in individuals younger than 5 years of age or older than 20 years. Infection can lead to diarrhea, otitis media, and pneumonia. Other less common complications include encephalitis, seizures, and subacute sclerosing panencephalitis (SSP). SSP, while rare, can be devastating. It is a degenerative disease of the central nervous system (CNS) that slowly progresses from intellectual and behavioral impairment to ataxia, myoclonic seizures, and ultimately death.[101]

A number of organizations—the American Red Cross, CDC, United Nations Children's Emergency Fund (UNICEF), United Nations Foundation, and WHO—have set an ambitious plan to eradicate measles and rubella by 2020.[102] Measles has many of the attributes that make it amenable to eradication: 1) the only reservoir is humans; 2) a highly effective and affordable vaccine has been developed; 3) subclinical infections are rare, making diagnosis easier; and 4) serologic tests are available that can confirm infection and/or immunity, making it possible to monitor success and pinpoint geographical areas or at-risk populations that may require further vaccine coverage. Significant progress toward worldwide eradication has been made, particularly in the Americas, which eliminated measles in 2002. However, importation of measles from other parts of the world remains a constant threat.[103] In fact, 96% of the cases reported to the CDC in 2015 were import related, from countries such as Azerbaijan, China, Germany, India, Indonesia, Kyrgyzstan, Pakistan, Qatar, Singapore, and United Arab Emirates.[104]

While vaccine coverage is high in the United States, rubella vaccine use is uneven in other parts of the world. According to a surveillance report issued by WHO in 2015, the Americas were declared free of endemic rubella, but cases were reported in the European and Western Pacific regions and increasing in the Southeast Asia and African regions. Despite expanding vaccine coverage globally, importation into the United States is possible, particularly into immigrant communities with lower immunity levels.[105] In the 1990s, prior to widespread adoption of rubella vaccine in the Americas, most cases in the United States occurred in Hispanic adults who had immigrated from parts of the world where rubella vaccine was not commonly given.[106]

Rubella is rare in the United States but remains of major concern because of the devastating consequences for the fetus from maternal infection during pregnancy. Maternal infection in pregnancy is associated with major congenital defects such as deafness, cardiac anomalies, microcephaly, mental retardation, cataracts, glaucoma, and other problems. The probability that infection will lead to congenital defects varies by stage of pregnancy. Up to 85% or more of fetuses will be affected if infection occurs during the first trimester and 20% in the second trimester.[107,108]

The mumps vaccine is commonly given as a combined product containing the measles and rubella and/or varicella vaccines. Mumps is caused by a paramyxovirus. Its initial presentation is nonspecific and similar to that seen in upper respiratory infections. Forty percent or more

of infected individuals will develop parotitis. More serious complications are rare but can include orchitis, oophoritis, pancreatitis, and hearing loss. Serious side effects associated with use of the mumps vaccine are rare. One study based on VAERS data from 1990 to 2003 estimated that 1 case of hearing loss was reported per 6 to 8 million distributed doses.[109]

Vaccines against measles, mumps, and rubella are available as combined products. Because these vaccines are live attenuated viral vaccines, they are highly effective and in general need only one dose to achieve long-lasting immunity, although additional doses may be needed for consistent protection. As live vaccines, they are contraindicated for use in pregnancy and in some circumstances for immunosuppressed individuals. Side effects and adverse reactions are uncommon but can result from exposure to vaccine components or from viral replication, which rarely leads to clinical disease (**Table 2-16**).

Meningococcal Vaccine

Neisseria meningitidis is the most common cause of bacterial meningitis in the United States. It primarily affects young children younger than 5 years, adolescents, and individuals older than 65 years.[110] Strains of *Neisseria meningitidis* can be classified by the structure of the surrounding polysaccharide capsule. Thirteen distinct capsules have been described, but five serogroups (A, B, C, Y, and W) cause almost all invasive disease.[29] In the United States, B, C, and Y serogroups account for 90% of all infections.[110]

Two types of vaccines are available: polysaccharide and conjugate. Until February 2005, the only vaccine recommended for use in adults was a polysaccharide vaccine. It was recommended for use in high-risk groups (college freshmen, travelers to areas of the world where *Neisseria meningitidis* is endemic, in individuals at higher risk of exposure

Table 2-16 Measles-Mumps-Rubella Vaccines (MMR)

	Infection		Vaccine			
Pathogen	Incubation/Presentation	Complications	Vaccine Agent/Schedule	Vaccine Efficacy	Vaccine Contraindications/Precautions	Vaccine-Associated Side Effects
Measles[a,b,c,d]	**Incubation** 10 to 12 days to prodrome, 14 days to rash **Presentation** Prodrome of fever, cough, runny nose. Next develops Koplik spots, which are pathognomonic of measles. They are bluish-white spots surrounded by erythema found on the buccal membranes. As they fade, a rash begins behind the ears, neck, and hairline	Otitis media 7% Pneumonia 6% Encephalitis 0.1% Seizures 0.6% Thrombocytopenia 1 out of 3000 cases Subacute sclerosing panencephalitis rare Case fatality rate 1-2 deaths per 1000 reported cases	**Type** Live virus vaccine available as measles-mumps-rubella (MMR) or combined also with varicella (MMRV) **Indications** All children **Schedule** *Children* 2 doses 1, 4-6 years *Adults* All adults born in 1957 or later require at least 1 dose. If unimmunized or a member of high-risk group (i.e., healthcare workers, travelers to foreign countries, college	95% efficacy after 1 dose 99% after 2 doses Duration usually lifelong	**Contraindications** Severe allergic reaction to vaccine or its components (neomycin, gelatin) Pregnancy Severe immunosuppression or on high-dose immunosuppressive therapy **Precautions** Moderate or severe acute illness Egg allergy is no longer considered a contraindication	**Local reactions** Fever in 5-15% and rash in 5% of recipients, usually seen 7 to 10 days after vaccination **Severe** Thrombocytopenia 1: 30,000 doses Measles inclusion-body encephalitis (case reports, occurred only in immunocompromised individuals. In 1 case, measles vaccine strain was identified.)[e-g]

Disease	Presentation	Complications	Vaccine	Efficacy/Duration	Contraindications	Adverse Reactions/Notes
	and spreads downward from the face and outward to feet. Rash is maculopapular and initially blanches under pressure, but by 3 to 4 days does not blanch when pressed. Rash fades in same order in which it appears.		students) then complete a 2-dose series 0, 1 month		Prior history of thrombocytopenic purpura or thrombocytopenia (applies to measles component) Personal or family history (parents, siblings) of seizure (applies only to MMRV) Recent receipt of Immunoglobulin or blood product	Death from vaccine-induced infection (5 deaths in > 200 million doses of administered vaccine) has occurred only in severely immunocompromised individuals[h] Anaphylaxis See rubella and mumps sections in text if giving MMR.
Mumps[a,d,i]	**Incubation** 12 to 25 days **Presentation** Prodrome is nonspecific and includes low-grade fever, malaise, anorexia, and headache.	Orchitis in 12-66% of postpubertal males, sterility is rare Oophoritis occurs in 5% of postpubertal females, sterility unaffected Deafness in 1 per 20,000 cases	**Type** See notes under measles. Given as MMR or MMRV **Indications** All children and unimmunized adults **Schedule** Unimmunized adults need 2 doses.	88% efficacy after 2 doses Duration probably lifelong	See measles.	Usually given as MMR. Most reactions to MMR are attributed to either measles or rubella component.

(continues)

Table 2-16 Measles-Mumps-Rubella Vaccines (MMR) (continued)

| Pathogen | Infection | | Vaccine | | | |
	Incubation/ Presentation	Complications	Vaccine Agent/ Schedule	Vaccine Efficacy	Vaccine Contraindications/ Precautions	Vaccine-Associated Side Effects
	Parotitis occurs in 31-65% of cases and can be unilateral or bilateral. Between 15-27% of cases are asymptomatic.	Encephalitis 1 out of 300 to 6000 cases Death is rare, 2 out of 10,000 cases				Case reports of hearing loss after receipt of mumps vaccines, very rare.[j] Allergic reactions
Rubella[a,d]	**Incubation** Average 14 days, range 12 to 23 days **Presentation** Symptoms can be mild. Up to 50% of cases are subclinical. Nonspecific prodrome of low-grade fever, malaise, and URI symptoms, progresses	Arthritis/ arthralgia in 70% of women, rare in children and men Encephalitis occurs in 1 out of 6000 cases, more common in women Thrombocyto-penia in 1 out of 3000 cases, more common in children	**Type** See notes under measles. Vaccine in current use in United States is RA 27/3 Available as MMR or MMRV **Indications** All children and unimmunized adults **Schedule** Unimmunized adults need 1 dose.	95% Duration usually lifelong	See measles.	Commonly given as MMR. Most reactions thought to be due to measles component. Rubella component thought to cause fever, lymph-adenopathy, and arthral-gia; 25% of susceptible

women develop arthralgia, 10% develop acute arthritis.

Transient peripheral neuritic complaints

Collagen disease

to rash beginning on day 2 to 6 after onset of symptoms. Rash is fainter than in measles, but has similar head-to-toe progression. Rash lasts about 3 days. Lymphadenopathy common

[a] Data from Centers for Disease Control and Prevention. *Epidemiology and Prevention of Vaccine-Preventable Diseases*. 13th ed. Washington, DC: Public Health Foundation; 2015.

[b] Institute of Medicine. *Adverse Effects of Vaccines: Evidence and Causality*. Washington, DC: National Academies Press; 2012.

[c] Moss W. Measles (Rubeola) In: Longo D, Fauci A, Kasper D, Hauser S, Jameson J, Loscalzo J, eds. *Harrison's Principles of Internal Medicine*. 18th ed. New York, NY: McGraw-Hill; 2012.

[d] McLean HQ, Parker Fiebelkorn A, Temte JL, Wallace GS. Prevention of measles, rubella, congenital rubella syndrome, and mumps, 2013: summary recommendations of the Advisory Committee on Immunization Practices. *MMWR.* 2013;62(RR 04):1-34.

[e] Poon T, Tchertkoff V, Win H. Subacute measles encephalitis with AIDS diagnosed by fine needle aspiration biopsy. A case report. *Acta Cytol.* 1998;42:729-33.

[f] Bitnun A, Shannon P, Durward A, et al. Measles inclusion-body encephalitis caused by the vaccine strain of measles virus. *Clin Infect Dis.* 1999;29:855-61.

[g] Baram T, Gonzalez-Gomez I, Xie Z, et al. Subacute sclerosing panencephalitis in an infant: diagnostic role of viral genome analysis. *Ann Neurol.* 1994;36:103-8.

[h] Centers for Disease Control and Prevention. Update: vaccine side effects, adverse reactions, contraindications, and precautions: recommendations of the Advisory Committee on Immunization Practices. *MMWR.* 1996;45(RR 12):1-35.

[i] Rubin S, Carbone K. Mumps. In: Longo D, Fauci A, Kasper D, Hauser S, Jameson J, Loscalzo J, eds. *Harrison's Principles of Internal Medicine*. 18th ed. New York, NY: McGraw-Hill; 2012.

[j] Asatryan A, Pool V, Chen R, Kohl K, Davis R, Iskander J, et al. Live attenuated measles and mumps viral strain-containing vaccines and hearing loss: Vaccine Adverse Event Reporting System (VAERS), United States, 1990-2003. *Vaccine.* 2008;26(9):1166-72.

or complications) and in the control of outbreaks. While one dose confers protection in more than 90% of recipients, antibody levels wane 2 to 3 years after receipt. Repeat doses do not increase antibody levels and may induce a hyporesponsive reaction resulting in reduced protection.[110]

The newest vaccines, the quadrivalent conjugate vaccines such as Menactra, were designed to create a more durable level of protection. The conjugate vaccines vary by the serotype they target (quadrivalent-ACYW vs. bivalent-CY) and the substance used for conjugation (diphtheria toxoid vs. CRM_{197}, a naturally occurring, nontoxic form of diphtheria toxin). Conjugation changes the immunologic pathway induced by vaccination from a T cell-independent to a T cell-dependent one, resulting in a more robust initial response and stronger anamnestic response upon re-exposure. However, in practice the protection afforded by conjugate vaccines also wanes, but not as quickly. Therefore, booster doses are recommended 5 years after the first dose for individuals whose risk status remains high.[110]

Historically, available vaccines have targeted A, C, Y, and W, but not B, serogroups. However, two new vaccines directed against B serotypes were recently approved for use in individuals ages 10 to 25: MenB-FHbp (Trumenba, three-dose series) and MenB-4C (Bexsero, two-dose series). ACIP has stated that adolescents ages 16 to 23 years (ages 16 to 18 are preferred) may be immunized with either of the recently approved meningococcal vaccines if desired to provide short-term protection and that MenB can be administered to those > 10 years of age at increased risk.[111,112] These newer vaccines may also be used to control outbreaks with serogroup B.[113] (See **Table 2-17.**)

Pneumococcal Vaccines

Infection with *Streptococcus pneumoniae* causes 36% of all cases of community-acquired pneumonia and 50% of all cases of bacterial meningitis in adults.[29] More than 90 serotypes have been identified, which are classified into 23 serogroups based on the characteristics of their surrounding polysaccharide capsules.[114] The polysaccharide capsules provide protection from phagocytosis by the host (unless there are pneumococcal type-specific antibodies present). Vaccine effectiveness varies by geographical location and age, depending on how prevalent the vaccine-related serotypes are in a particular community and age group. Not only are there regional differences in the prevalence of certain serotypes, but also the distribution of serotypes differs by age. It is estimated that the pneumococcal polysaccharide vaccine (PPSV) directed against 23 serotypes protects against infection in 84% of cases in young children younger than 5 years of age, 76% of individuals 18 to 64 years, and 65% of those 65 years of age or older.[110]

Pneumococcal vaccines are changing the epidemiology of pneumococcal infections. Infections due to serotypes covered by vaccines have dropped dramatically—by 90%. Non-vaccine serotypes have increased, but overall not enough to offset the reductions in vaccine-targeted serotypes in most studies. Pneumococcal vaccines also seem to have beneficial indirect effects, reducing nasal carriage in immunized infants, who are often an asymptomatic reservoir of disease. This protects adults from infection. Further, many of the serotypes targeted by vaccines have high rates of antibiotic resistance; use of pneumococcal vaccines has reduced rates of antibiotic-resistant infection.[115]

Invasive pneumococcal disease is most common in children under 2 years of age and in adults 65 years or older. ACIP recommends routinely vaccinating individuals in these age groups as well as all individuals regardless of age who have underlying chronic illness or immunosuppression. Recently, ACIP expanded its recommendations to include more common conditions such as asthma and smoking.[29]

Table 2-17 Meningococcal Vaccine

	Infection			Vaccine			
Pathogen	Incubation/ Presentation	Complications	Vaccine Agent/ Schedule	Vaccine Efficacy	Vaccine Contraindications/ Precautions	Vaccine- Associated Side Effects
Meningitis[a,b]	**Incubation** 3 to 4 days, range 2 to 10 days **Presentation** Sudden onset of headache, fever, and stiff neck Other symptoms such as photophobia, nausea, vomiting, and altered mental status are common.	Sepsis in 5–20% of invasive infections Pneumonia in 5–15% Arthritis in 2% Case fatality rates 9–12% Up to 20% of survivors have permanent disability	**Type** Inactivated Three available vaccines 1) Meningococcal quadrivalent conjugate (Menactra, Menveo) 2) Meningococcal polysaccharide vaccine (Menomune) 3) Serogroup B meningococcal vaccines (Bexsero, Trumenba) **Indications** For adolescents/ Young adults: Quadrivalent conjugate vaccines are included in childhood	Clinical effectiveness > 85% for serogroups A and C. Efficacy assumed but not documented for Y and W-135 subgroups. Clinical protection lasts a minimum of 3 years.	**Contraindications** Allergy to vaccine or its components (Note that some meningococcal vaccines contain diphtheria toxoid.) **Precautions** Moderate to severe illness History of Guillain-Barré (controversial if true precaution)	Local reactions Fever Anaphylaxis

(continues)

Table 2-17 Meningococcal Vaccine *(continued)*

	Infection		Vaccine		
Pathogen	Incubation/ Presentation	Complications	Vaccine Agent/ Schedule	Vaccine Efficacy	Vaccine Contraindications/ Precautions	Vaccine- Associated Side Effects
			schedule, 2 doses: age 11 and booster at age 16

Adolescents and young adults age 16 to 23 years may also be vaccinated with a sero-group B vaccine (Bexsero, Tru-menba), higher risk teens/young adults should be vaccinated.

For adults: Meningococcal quadrivalent conjugate (Menactra, Menveo) | | | |

2 doses (0, 2 months) for adults with persistent complement component deficiencies

1 dose to high-risk individuals (military recruits, outbreak control, travel to countries where infection is endemic)

Booster in 5 years if risk continues

Meningococcal polysaccharide vaccine (Menomune)

Adults ≥ 56 years never vaccinated who require a single dose

a Data from Centers for Disease Control and Prevention. *Epidemiology and Prevention of Vaccine-Preventable Diseases*. 13th ed. Washington, DC: Public Health Foundation; 2015.

b Institute of Medicine. *Adverse Effects of Vaccines: Evidence and Causality*. Washington, DC: National Academies Press; 2012.

Two types of vaccines are available: conjugate and polysaccharide. Conjugate vaccines are recommended for children and polysaccharide vaccines for adults. The antibody response to polysaccharide vaccine is poor in children under 2 years of age, but robust after receipt of the conjugate vaccine. However, while the newer conjugate vaccines have increased the number of serotypes they contain from 7 to 13, they still cover a more limited number of serotypes compared to the 29 covered by polysaccharide vaccines. Polysaccharide vaccines are preferred for use in adults, who are able to mount a more effective response, because they increase protection against disease. Some adults may have less than an optimal antibody response, particularly the elderly and adults with underlying medical conditions, particularly immunosuppression. ACIP recommends that pneumococcal vaccine be administered even to those unlikely to mount a full and sustained antibody response, because most recipients are afforded some level of protection from infection.[29,116]

Antibody levels decline over 5 to 10 years and can decline faster in those individuals whose initial response was poor. Revaccination is recommended for those at the highest risk of complications from infection. High-risk individuals who are candidates for revaccination are those with asplenia, transplants, chronic renal failure, nephritic syndrome, or immunosuppression. These individuals should receive a 1-time booster 5 or more years after receipt of their original pneumococcal vaccine.[116] (**Table 2-18**)

Tetanus, Diphtheria, Acellular Pertussis (Tdap) Vaccine

Toxins released by *Clostridium tetani* cause tetanus. The infection can lead to paralysis, laryngospasm, hypertension, and fractures.[29] Infection occurs when the organism, commonly found in soil, enters the body usually through minor (scratches,

minor cuts) or major (puncture) injuries or chronic wounds (diabetic ulcers). Adults are the most at risk.[29] While immune levels remain high for up to 20 years after vaccination,[117] many adults do not receive booster shots and their immune levels wane over time. Between 2001 and 2008, individuals 65 years or older were almost 3 times more likely to be infected with tetanus and 9 times more likely to die of infection than individuals younger than 65 years.[118] Others at higher risk of contracting infection include diabetics (15.4% of cases) and IV drug users (15.3% of cases).[118]

Many pregnant women are not protected from tetanus. In a survey of more than 200 pregnant women in 2000, Kalaça and colleagues found that 35% of subjects had no serologic evidence of immunity to tetanus.[119] In 2013, only 62.9% of adults between 19 and 49 years of age had received a tetanus-containing vaccine in the last 10 years.[120] Despite low levels of vaccine coverage, neonatal infection is rare in the United States; only two cases of neonatal tetanus have been reported in the United States since 1989. One occurred in a child born to a Mexican woman who had resided in the United States for several years, received prenatal care, and delivered in a US hospital, yet never received the tetanus vaccine.[121]

Providers need to be aware of the immunization practices of the countries of origin of the women in their care. Many countries primarily target pregnant women, whereas in the United States adults have generally received a complete series in childhood. There has been more than a 90% reduction in deaths due to neonatal tetanus worldwide from 1999 to 2015 thanks to a worldwide campaign championed by UNICEF and WHO.[122] However, as of 2012, neonatal tetanus was still occurring primarily in parts of Sub-Saharan Africa (e.g., Cameroon, Central African Republic, Chad, Democratic Republic of the Congo, Equatorial Guinea, Ethiopia, Nigeria, Somalia, and South Sudan), Southeast Asia (e.g., Afghanistan, Cambodia, parts of India and

Table 2-18 Pneumococcal Vaccines

	Infection		Vaccine			
Pathogen	Incubation/ Presentation	Complications	Vaccine Agent/ Schedule	Vaccine Efficacy	Vaccine Contraindications/ Precautions	Vaccine-Associated Side Effects
Pneumococcal infections[a]	**Incubation** 1 to 3 days **Presentation** Varies in severity from mild to severe disease. Classified as noninvasive (otitis media, sinusitis, nonbacteremic pneumonia) or invasive, meaning that the pneumococcus invades a normally sterile space, (i.e., bacteremic pneumonia or meningitis)	Bacteremia in 25-30% Bacterial meningitis (Severe, generalized, gradual-onset headache, fever, and nausea, stiff neck, confusion) Pneumococcal pneumonia (Abrupt onset of fever, chills, and rigor. Also can present with pleuritic chest pain, productive cough, dyspnea, tachypnea, hypoxia, tachycardia, malaise, and weakness)	**Type** Inactivated **Adults ≥ 65 years** Pneumococcal vaccine naive 0: Conjugate vaccine, PCV-13 6 month: Polysaccharide, PPSV-23 If PSSV-23 given first, wait 1 year before vaccinating with PCV-13 **Adults 19-64 years** Adults with certain chronic conditions or immunosuppression should be vaccinated with a combination of PCV-13 and PPSV-23. See ACIP guidelines.	PPSV 60-70% PPSV 90% against invasive disease in children, 75% in adults	**Contraindications** Allergy **Precautions** Pregnancy Safety is unknown. Women at high risk for pneumococcal infection can be vaccinated in pregnancy. Allergy to vaccine or its components Moderate to severe illness	**PPSV** Local reactions occur in 30-50% of recipients. Fever, myalgias, and other moderate systemic reactions occur in < 1% of recipients. Serious adverse events are rare. **PCV** 5-49% local reactions 24-35% fever Rare febrile seizures, both

ACIP = Advisory Committee on Immunization Practices; PCV = polysaccharide conjugate vaccine; PPSV = pneumococcal polysaccharide vaccine

[a] Data from Centers for Disease Control and Prevention. *Epidemiology and Prevention of Vaccine-Preventable Disease.* 13th ed. Washington, DC: Public Health Foundation; 2015.

Indonesia, and Pakistan), and Haiti.[123] Women's health providers should be cognizant of global patterns of vaccine-preventable diseases, query women about their vaccine history, and update vaccinations as needed.

The other case of neonatal tetanus occurred in an infant born to an American woman who had never received the vaccine due to personal beliefs.[124] Exposure was thought to occur via inappropriate cord care, which led to subsequent infection. Both of these cases point out the importance of ensuring that pregnant women are protected from tetanus and, if vaccination is not acceptable to a client, that mothers receive instruction on appropriate ways to clean and wrap the umbilical cord for infants after birth.

Wound Management

Wound management to prevent tetanus after an injury will depend on the individual's vaccine history and seriousness of the wound. Minor wounds do not require any tetanus vaccination or prophylaxis in an individual who is fully immunized with a three-dose series and has received all needed follow-up boosters. However, if the individual's vaccine series is incomplete, then the individual with a minor wound should receive a tetanus vaccine, preferably Tdap, if the individual has not received a dose of Tdap in the past. More serious wounds require more aggressive care. At-risk wounds are considered to be those that are contaminated with dirt, feces, soil, and saliva; puncture wounds; avulsions; and wounds resulting from crushing, missiles, burns, and frostbite.[29,125] If the tetanus vaccine history is unknown or if the individual has received fewer than three doses, then more severe wounds require both tetanus vaccination and tetanus immunoglobulin. If the primary series is complete, then the individual should be vaccinated (preferably with Tdap if she has not received a dose previously) if more than 5 years have elapsed since her last dose.[29]

The tetanus vaccine is usually combined with diphtheria (Td) and in some formulations pertussis (Tdap) vaccines and given to adults and adolescents as Td or Tdap.[29] Other formulations, such as the DT, DPT, and DTaP vaccines, are available but are given only to young children. Currently, the recommended adult primary series consists of three doses of Td with boosters every 10 years and a one-time Tdap catch-up dose. Patients do not require more frequent doses except in special circumstances such as an injury or pregnancy.[29] However, expanded use of Tdap is under consideration by ACIP. The recommended adult schedule is likely to change in the upcoming years. Clinicians should monitor for changing recommendations.

Diphtheria

Diphtheria is much more common than tetanus and is easily spread via person-to-person contact from infected respiratory secretions. It can infect any mucous membrane and is classified as anterior nasal diphtheria (which can mimic the common cold, at least initially, before a white membrane forms over the nasal septum), pharyngeal and tonsillar (which are the most common form of diphtheria and associated with significant disease), laryngeal (which affects only this site or can be an extension of pharyngeal/tonsillar infection), skin (uncommon in the United States, but can occur most commonly in homeless persons), and genital (rare).[29]

Diphtheria vaccines are only offered as combination products (e.g., Td or Tdap). While diphtheria is extremely rare in the United States, it still occurs in other parts of the world. The immunization coverage rate with at least three doses of childhood vaccine (DTP3) is now estimated to be approximately 85% worldwide and has been associated with dramatic drops in infections. Parts of the Caribbean, Sub-Saharan Africa, and the Middle East are estimated to have less than 50% coverage of the infant series. Even fewer adults are up to date with vaccination.[126] Continuing to immunize here in the United States with a diphtheria-containing vaccine is as an effective approach to keeping diphtheria under control. Epidemics have occurred in countries with low vaccine coverage rates such as in Eastern Europe in the 1990s when immunization levels fell in the aftermath of the dissolution of the Soviet Union.[52]

Boosters are recommended every 10 years. The longevity of protection after vaccination is unknown. One study estimated the half-life of diphtheria antibodies to be 19 years.[127] Another seroprevalence study reported that one-third of patients presenting to the emergency department had no protection against diphtheria.[128] Further, the peak incidence of pertussis in the epidemic in the 1990s in Moscow occurred in children age 5 to 10 years and in adults age 30 to 50 years.[52] Taken together, these studies highlight the importance of ongoing boosters for adults. Although little evidence is available to determine the ideal spacing of boosters, decennial boosters provide good disease control.

Pertussis-Containing Vaccines

Pertussis-containing vaccines were first licensed for use in adolescents and adults in 2005, although they have been included in the childhood schedule since the 1950s.[29] Despite widespread vaccine coverage in children, pertussis infection is the only vaccine-preventable illness that has been increasing in recent years.[129] Since Tdap was approved, ACIP has released 8 different recommendations on vaccinating adolescents, adults, healthcare workers, and pregnant women in an attempt to gain control over pertussis infection in the United States.[125,130-131]

Unfortunately, the effectiveness of the pertussis acellular vaccine appears to be short-lived. In a cross-sectional study conducted during the 2012 Washington State pertussis epidemic, protective levels of antibody declined rapidly after vaccination; adolescents vaccinated solely with acellular vaccines had protective levels of antibodies of 73% at < 12 months, 55% at 12 to 23 months, and 34% at 24 to 47 months after vaccination with acellular vaccines.[132] Currently, ACIP is considering the use of Tdap as the preferred 10-year booster, rather than Td, in an attempt to better control the infection.[133]

Of greatest concern is the control of infection in young children. Almost all deaths related to pertussis infection occur in infants, particularly in those younger than 3 months of age. Pertussis-related encephalopathy is highly predictive of a poor outcome: One-third of children with encephalopathy die, one-third will have permanent neurologic sequelae, and only one-third recover completely.[134] See the section, *Pregnancy,* under *Immunizations in Special Populations,* later in this chapter for further details.

Because Td has long been included in the adult immunization schedule, it is possible to study whether acellular pertussis-containing vaccines (Tdap) differ in their safety from Td vaccines. A prospective cohort study from the VAERS network compared VAEs reported in adolescents and adults who received Tdap (N = 276,284) between 2005 and 2008 to a historical control group (N = 890,000) who received Td vaccination between 2000 and 2004.[135] No differences were seen in encephalopathy, paralytic syndromes, seizures, cranial nerve disorders, and Guillain-Barré syndrome between the two products. However, this study only had the power to detect a relative risk of 4-5 for Guillain-Barré syndrome and 1.5-2 for other outcomes.[135] Another cohort study compared adolescents (age 10 to 18 years) vaccinated with Tdap (N = 13,427) to a historical cohort control (N = 12,509) in the Kaiser Permanente System. No differences were noted between the two vaccines in reported rates of chronic diseases such as diabetes, thyroiditis, vasculitis, and lupus.[136] These studies provide reassurance about the safety of Tdap relative to Td vaccines. (See **Table 2-19.**)

Table 2-19 Tetanus-Diphtheria-Pertussis Infections and Vaccines

	Infection		Vaccine			
Pathogen	Incubation/Presentation	Complications	Vaccine Agent/Schedule	Vaccine Efficacy	Vaccine Contraindications/Precautions	Vaccine-Associated Side Effects
Tetanus[a]	**Incubation** 3 to 21 days **Presentation** 80% of cases are generalized tetanus, which presents with lockjaw, stiff neck, difficulty swallowing, laryngospasm, muscle spasms, and fever. Recovery usually complete; may take months. Infection does not confer immunity.	Fractures from severe muscle spasms Aspiration pneumonia 10% case fatality rate, highest in elderly	**Type** Toxoid **Indications** All adults **Schedule** Td: tetanus-diphtheria Primary adult series if not completed in childhood: 3 doses: 0, 4-8 weeks apart, 3rd dose 6-12 months after the 2nd dose Booster 10 years with Td or Tdap (see below)	Tetanus toxoid has a clinical efficacy approaching 100%. Immunity lasts minimum of 10 years, likely longer for many individuals.	**Contraindications** Severe allergic reaction to prior dose **Precautions** Moderate to severe illness History of Guillain-Barré syndrome within 6 weeks after a prior dose of tetanus toxoid-containing vaccine Progressive neurologic disorder until the condition has stabilized	**Local reactions** Erythema, induration, pain common Fever less common **Arthus-like reactions** (Extensive painful swelling 2 to 8 hours after injection). Most common in those with very high antitoxin levels from frequent immunization. People with arthus-like reactions should not receive boosters more often than every 10 years.

Severe

Very rarely, brachial neuritis (0.5 to 1 case per 100,000 recipients of tetanus toxoid)[a]

Possible

Guillain-Barré syndrome in susceptible individuals based on one case report.[b,c,d]

Likely no to low risk of cranial neuropathies or Guillain-Barré syndrome in the general public after receipt of vaccine. One study reported a higher number of cases than expected for these conditions, making ongoing surveillance critical in detecting any relationships between Guillain-Barré and cranial neuropathies and vaccine use.[135]

(continues)

Table 2-19 Tetanus-Diphtheria-Pertussis Infections and Vaccines *(continued)*

Pathogen	Infection		Vaccine			
	Incubation/Presentation	Complications	Vaccine Agent/Schedule	Vaccine Efficacy	Vaccine Contraindications/Precautions	Vaccine-Associated Side Effects
Diphtheria[a,g]	**Incubation** 2 to 5 days **Presentation** Commonly infects tonsils and pharynx. Begins with malaise, sore throat, low-grade fever, progressing to development of blue-white membrane covering tonsils and soft palate. Covering turns to	Myocarditis and abnormal cardiac rhythms Neuritis Paralysis of muscles of soft palate, eyes, limbs, and diaphragm Pneumonia Case fatality rate is 5–10%.	**Type** Toxoid **Indications** All adults **Schedule** Given as a combination product. For adults the primary series consists of 3 doses, followed by boosters every 10 years.	Nearly 95%, longevity unknown, likely to be approximately 10 years	See precautions under tetanus.	Crude reporting rate of 10.2 VAEs per 100,000 doses, temporal but not causal relationship[e] Anaphylaxis[f] Because always given as a combined product, unable to distinguish reactions due to the diphtheria component from the tetanus component

grey-green to black in color. If larynx involved, membrane can cause airway obstruction.

Pertussis[a]	Incubation 7 to 10 days **Presentation** Initially similar to the common cold with runny nose, low-grade fever, and mild cough then progresses to paroxysms of coughing, worse at night. Paroxysmal stage lasts between 1 and 6 weeks with gradual recovery thereafter. Secondary pneumonia Neurologic complications more common in infants than adults Case fatality rate low in adults, high in infants < 1 year of age	80-85%	**Type** Acellular **Indications** All adults Pregnancy **Schedule** Tdap 1-time catch-up dose for adolescents ages 11 to 18 years and adults 19 years or older Tdap in pregnancy Booster, to be determined. Under discussion by ACIP to consider more frequent use of Tdap in adults	**Contraindications** Severe allergy Encephalopathy not due to another identifiable cause occurring within 7 days after vaccination with a pertussis-containing vaccine **Precautions** History of Guillain-Barré syndrome within 6 weeks after a prior dose of tetanus toxoid-containing vaccine Progressive neurologic disorder until the condition has stabilized	**Local Reactions** Pain, redness, swelling common Fever less common **Severe** Adverse reactions occur at approximately the same rate as with Td alone (without acellular pertussis vaccine)[h,i] Crude reporting rate of 10.2 VAEs per 100,000 doses of Tdap, temporal but not causal relationship[e]

(continues)

Table 2-19 Tetanus-Diphtheria-Pertussis Infections and Vaccines *(continued)*

Infection			Vaccine			
Pathogen	Incubation/ Presentation	Complications	Vaccine Agent/ Schedule	Vaccine Efficacy	Vaccine Contraindications/ Precautions	Vaccine-Associated Side Effects
					History of a severe local reaction (Arthus reaction) following a prior dose of a tetanus- and/or diphtheria toxoid-containing vaccine	
					Moderate or severe acute illness	

[a] Data from Centers for Disease Control and Prevention. *Epidemiology and Prevention of Vaccine-Preventable Diseases.* 13th ed. Washington, DC: Public Health Foundation; 2015.

[b] Kretsinger K, Broder KR, Cortese MM, Joyce MP, Ortega-Sanchez I, Lee GM, et al. Preventing tetanus, diphtheria, and pertussis among adults: use of tetanus toxoid, reduced diphtheria toxoid and acellular pertussis vaccine recommendations of the Advisory Committee on Immunization Practices (ACIP) and recommendation of ACIP, supported by the Healthcare Infection Control Practices Advisory Committee (HICPAC), for use of Tdap among health-care personnel. *MMWR Recomm Rep.* 2006;55(RR-17):1-37.

[c] Pollard J, Selby G. Relapsing neuropathy due to tetanus toxoid: report of a case. *J Neurol Sci.* 1978;37:113-25.

[d] Stratton K, Howe C, Johnston R. Adverse events associated with childhood vaccines other than pertussis and rubella: summary of a report from the Institute of Medicine. *JAMA* 1994;271:1602-5.

[e] Chang S, O'Connor PM, Slade BA, Woo EJ. US Postlicensure safety surveillance for adolescent and adult tetanus, diphtheria and acellular pertussis vaccines: 2005-2007. *Vaccine.* 2013;31(10):1447-52.

[f] Institute of Medicine. *Adverse Effects of Vaccines: Evidence and Causality.* Washington, DC: National Academies Press; 2012.

[g] Amanna IJ, Carlson NE, Slifka MK. Duration of humoral immunity to common viral and vaccine antigens. *N Engl J Med.* 2007;357(19):1903-1915.

[h] Yih WK, Nordin JD, Kulldorff M, Lewis E, Lieu TA, Shi P, et al. An assessment of the safety of adolescent and adult tetanus-diphtheria-acellular pertussis (Tdap) vaccine, using active surveillance for adverse events in the Vaccine Safety Datalink. *Vaccine.* 2009;27(32):4257-62.

[i] Klein NP, Hansen J, Lewis E, Lyon L, Nguyen B, Black S, et al. Post-marketing safety evaluation of a tetanus toxoid, reduced diphtheria toxoid and 3-component acellular pertussis vaccine administered to a cohort of adolescents in a United States health maintenance organization. *Pediatr Infect Dis J.* 2010;29(7):613-7.

Varicella and Zoster Vaccines

Historically, varicella has been endemic in the United States. It was a childhood infection estimated to cause 4 million cases a year.[137] The disease is generally mild and self-limited, particularly in children. Adults are more likely to experience severe disease, and are 25 times more likely to die of varicella-related complications than children.[137] The varicella vaccine is highly effective, reducing reported cases by 90% since 1995, although older adults who were never immunized may still be vulnerable.[137] Consequently, all adults should be screened and offered varicella vaccine as appropriate.

The decision on whether immunization is needed is based on patient history. Unlike other vaccine-preventable illnesses, varicella causes few subclinical infections and has a distinctive rash, making it easy to recognize and diagnose. In the pre-vaccine era, serologic studies confirmed that relying on patient history was a reasonable approach. In one study, more than 97% of those who gave a history of having had varicella had seropositive titers indicating immunity. Even those with a negative history were likely to be immune: 71-93% of these individuals were seropositive.[138] Therefore, if a woman was born before 1980 and gives a history of varicella, neither serological confirmation of immunity or vaccination is needed.[139] Those born later are unlikely to have been exposed to wild infection and may need to complete a two-dose series if the series was not completed in childhood.

In addition to causing chickenpox, the varicella zoster virus also can cause herpes zoster. Varicella virus lies dormant in the dorsal root ganglia after the primary infection resolves. If the virus becomes reactivated, it travels down the nerves to the skin resulting in a painful vesicular rash. This rash typically presents in a classic pattern, following the distribution of the affected dermatome.[140] Not all individuals infected with varicella develop zoster. The likelihood seems to be increased in those who were infected at a young age (in utero or younger than 18 months of age) and in immuno-compromised individuals.[138] Herpes zoster is rare in childhood if infection occurs after 18 months and increases with age.[138] The incidence has been reported to be 2.5 per 1000 in people 20 to 50 years of age, rising to 7.8 cases per 1000 in individuals older than 60 years.[141] Post-herpetic neuralgia or pain that resolves slowly (sometimes as long as 1 year) after resolution of the rash is an uncommon but debilitating complication. It occurs more often in older adults, increasing from 3-4% in individuals age 30 to 49 years to 21% in those between 60 and 70 years of age to 34% in those older than 80 years.[141]

To date, preliminary evidence seems to indicate that use of the varicella vaccine may be protective against the development of herpes zoster. The incidence of herpes zoster in vaccinated children from VAERS reports is 2.6 cases per 100,000 distributed doses compared to 68 cases in healthy children younger than 20 years of age per 100,000 person-years after natural infection.[142] More recent evidence supports this finding—that herpes zoster is less common in children after vaccination than after infection with wild virus.[143] However, it is unclear what impact varicella vaccination has had on the incidence of herpes zoster in the elderly. The rates of herpes zoster are increasing, beginning before the introduction of the vaccine, perhaps due to age-related risk from increased longevity.[144] Beginning in 2008, ACIP recommended the use of the herpes zoster vaccine (Zostavax) in adults 60 years of age or older to prevent herpes zoster.[145] The herpes zoster vaccine is a live, attenuated strain of the same type used in the varicella vaccine, but has at least 14 times the potency of single-antigen varicella vaccines.[140] See **Table 2-20** for a description of varicella-related infections and vaccines.

Table 2-20 Varicella and Zoster Vaccines

	Infection			Vaccine		
Pathogen	Incubation/ Presentation	Complications	Vaccine Agent/ Schedule	Vaccine Efficacy	Vaccine Contraindications/ Precautions	Vaccine-Associated Side Effects
Varicella[a,b,c]	**Incubation** 14 to 16 days **Presentation** Prodrome of malaise and fever for 1 to 2 days before rash. Rash usually starts on head, progresses to trunk, and then to extremities with lesions concentrated on trunk. Rash evolves from macules to papules to vesicles to crusting. All stages of lesions can be present at the same time. Lesions	Generally mild and self-limited Complications much more common in adults than in children Secondary bacterial skin infection Pneumonia Acute cerebellar ataxia in 1 out of 4000 cases Encephalitis without ataxia in 1 out of 33,000 cases Herpes zoster	**Type** Attenuated live virus vaccine **Indications** Persons who did not complete a 2-dose series **Schedule** 0, 4-8 weeks	94-99% after 2 doses	**Contraindications** Pregnancy **Severe** immunosuppression or high-dose systemic corticosteroid therapy (consult as recommendations vary by condition and degree of immunosuppression) Family history of congenital or hereditary immunodeficiency in first-degree relatives unless immunocompetence of recipient has been confirmed Cancers affecting lymphatic system or bone marrow	Fever Varicelliform rash after dose 1 was 3%, compared with 1% after dose 2. Breakthrough infection in which vaccinated individuals develop varicella > 42 days after receipt of vaccine. Rarely, varicella vaccine virus is associated with pneumonia, hepatitis, severe disseminated varicella infection, encephalitis.

	Clinical features	Type / Indications / Schedule	Efficacy	Contraindications / Precautions	Adverse effects
	also present on mouth, vagina, and mucous membranes.			**Precautions** Moderate or severe illness Thrombocytopenia Recent administration of blood, blood products, or immunoglobulins	Rarely, transmission of vaccine virus to other healthy or immuno-compromised individuals Rarely, herpes zoster from varicella vaccine virus
Zoster[d,e]	Reactivation of latent varicella virus from the sensory nerve ganglia Unilateral rash over 1 or 2 dermatomes Postherpetic neuralgia Herpes zoster ophthalmicus Transmission to other susceptible contacts	**Type** Attenuated live virus vaccine **Indications** All individuals ≥ 60 years **Schedule** 1-time dose	39-51% for herpes zoster 60-66% for postherpetic neuralgia	**Contraindications** Allergy to vaccine, vaccine component (gelatin, neomycin) Primary or acquired immunodeficiency Pregnancy **Precautions** Moderate to severe infection	Rare, varicella virus vaccine rash Rare, arthritis Rare, alopecia

[a] Data from Centers for Disease Control and Prevention. *Epidemiology and Prevention of Vaccine-Preventable Diseases*. 13th ed. Washington, DC: Public Health Foundation; 2015.

[b] Institute of Medicine. *Adverse Effects of Vaccines: Evidence and Causality*. Washington, DC: National Academies Press; 2012.

[c] Marin M, Güris D, Chaves SS, Schmid S, Seward JF. Prevention of varicella: recommendations of the Advisory Committee on Immunization Practices (ACIP). *MMWR*. 2007;56(RR-04):1-40.

[d] Centers for Disease Control and Prevention. Update on recommendations for use of herpes zoster vaccine. *MMWR*. 2014;63(33):729-31.

[e] Lai Y, Yew Y. Severe autoimmune adverse events post herpes zoster vaccine: a case-control study of adverse events in a national database. *J Drugs Dermatol*. 2015;14(7):681-4.

Immunization in Special Populations

Pregnancy

All inactivated vaccines are considered safe in pregnancy. Live viral vaccines should be avoided. Live viral vaccines induce low-level replication similar to that seen in wild infection and could theoretically cause infection in the fetus.[146] Rubella vaccine is of most concern because wild infection in the mother can lead to fetal infection and the development of congenital rubella syndrome in a significant percentage of infected fetuses. In the pre-vaccine era, congenital rubella infection occurred in 80% of children born to mothers infected in the first trimester and 25% of those whose mothers were infected in the second trimester.[147] Between 1971 and 1989, the CDC followed 324 women who received the rubella vaccine between 3 months before conception and the third month of pregnancy.[148] None of the infants born to these women had congenital rubella syndrome, and only five had serologic evidence of subclinical infection.[148] Therefore, women who inadvertently receive the vaccine during pregnancy should be informed of these theoretical risks but should not be advised to terminate their pregnancy.[65] Pre-vaccination pregnancy tests are not recommended; however, women should be advised to avoid pregnancy for 1 month after receiving the vaccine.[64]

No cases of adverse fetal effects have been documented after receipt of mumps, measles, or varicella vaccines.[65] Exposure to these live viral vaccines during pregnancy is of less concern because adverse fetal effects are rarely seen after wild infection, making it unlikely that exposure to these vaccines will increase the risk of poor outcomes. Measles and mump infections in pregnancy are not thought to lead to significant increases in birth defects, although they may increase the risk of preterm delivery, spontaneous abortion, and intrauterine growth restriction.[65] Maternal infection with varicella during pregnancy can lead to congenital varicella syndrome in exposed fetuses, which can present with skin lesions, limb hypoplasia, cataracts, microphthalmia, and other malformations.[149] However, the incidence of congenital varicella syndrome is low and has been estimated to occur in 0.4% of infants born to mothers infected in the first trimester and 2% of infants exposed before 20 weeks of pregnancy.[149,150] Infants exposed to maternal infection between 5 days before and up to 2 days after birth are at high risk of developing a fulminant varicella infection, which occurs in 17-30% of exposed infants.[139,150] Because the virulence of the attenuated strain used in the varicella vaccine is much less than that of wild virus, fetuses exposed to the vaccine are unlikely to be affected. Women should be advised to avoid pregnancy for 1 month after receipt of the vaccine, but those who inadvertently received the varicella vaccine 1 month before conception or in pregnancy do not need to be advised to terminate their pregnancy.[139]

Beginning in 1995 until the varicella registry was closed in 2013, 96 pregnant women inadvertently vaccinated with varicella- or zoster-containing vaccines in the first half of pregnancy were reported to the Varivax Pregnancy Registry.[151] None had any evidence of congenital varicella. However, while these results are reassuring, the number of women reported to the registry was too small to accurately quantify the risk, if any, of exposure to varicella and zoster vaccines in pregnancy. The CDC estimates that another 271 women exposed to varicella and zoster vaccines are needed to be able to quantify the risk, because the risk of congenital varicella infection, if it were to occur, is likely to be substantially less frequent after vaccine exposure than exposure to wild infection.[151] Women who are exposed to the varicella or zoster vaccines in the month before pregnancy and/or early pregnancy should be reported to VAERS (see Table 2-9 for the contact information).

Unlike the live viral vaccines, which are avoided in pregnancy, two vaccines—the influenza and Tdap vaccines—are actively promoted for use in pregnancy by ACIP. Influenza infection is associated with higher rates of hospitalization in pregnant women compared to nonpregnant women of similar ages, particularly in the latter stages of pregnancy and in those with underlying comorbidities such as asthma.[152-155] It may also be associated with poorer fetal and neonatal outcomes. One meta-analysis of 22 observational studies on the relationship between maternal flu or flu-like illness in the first trimester and fetal outcomes found that exposed fetuses were more likely to have congenital anomalies of any type (OR 2, 95% CI 1.62-2.48) compared to unexposed fetuses. Risks were highest for neural tube defects (OR 3.33, 95% CI 2.05-5.40), cleft lip (OR 3.12, 95% CI 2.20-4.42), and hydrocephaly (OR 5.74, 95% CI 1.10-30.0).[156] Infants born to severely ill women hospitalized for influenza during the 2009 pandemic were more likely to deliver prematurely or to be small for gestational age (SGA) at birth.[157] It is unknown if these associations are due to high fever, which accompanies influenza infection, or the influenza virus itself. Infants younger than 6 months of age with influenza are twice as likely to require hospitalization and are more likely to die of influenza-related complications than older infants and children.[158] ACIP and ACOG both recommend immunization against influenza in pregnancy.

ACIP recommends vaccinating women with the TIV, but not the live attenuated nasal vaccine, as early as possible during the flu season without reference to gestational age. Cohort studies have shown that vaccination is unlikely to be associated with adverse outcomes such as spontaneous abortion, preterm delivery, SGA, or stillbirth.[159,160] However, not all studies concur; some report that vaccination is associated with lower risk of preterm birth (AOR 0.75, 95% CI 0.60-0.94)[161] or SGA,[160] while other studies report increased risk of preterm birth, particularly if vaccination occurs during the first or second trimester of pregnancy (HR 3.28, 95% CI 1.25-8.63).[162] Because the complications associated with infection do not increase substantially until the second or third trimester of pregnancy, vaccination can safely be deferred for low-risk women in the first trimester of pregnancy until the beginning of the second trimester.

An advantage of waiting until later to vaccinate with TIV is that maternal immunization in the later stages of pregnancy appears to protect the newborn from infection. A significantly higher percentage of infants born to mothers who were immunized in pregnancy have serologic evidence of antibodies against influenza compared to those infants born to unimmunized mothers, 75%[163] to 86%[164] versus 18%[163] to 33%,[164] respectively. Further, another large randomized controlled trial (N = 2116) found that vaccination in the second or third trimester of pregnancy was associated with reduced rates of influenza infection in the first 6 months after birth in infants of influenza-vaccinated mothers (1.9%) compared to infants of placebo-vaccinated mothers (3.6%, $p = .01$).[165]

The other vaccine recommended to be given during pregnancy—primarily to protect the newborn rather than the mother—is the adult pertussis-containing vaccine, Tdap. After falling dramatically with the introduction of the childhood pertussis vaccine in the late 1940s, the numbers of individuals infected with pertussis have risen sharply in recent years.[166,167] Improvements in the availability and accuracy of diagnostic testing certainly explain a significant part of the increase in cases,[168] but other factors have contributed to the rise in infection and have increased the vulnerability of newborns. First, the newest version of the pertussis vaccine (the acellular pertussis vaccine) provides less than optimal protection. It was adopted because it causes significantly fewer reactions than the original whole-cell vaccine; however, its immunogenicity is weaker and wanes more rapidly. Immunity appears to last as long as 6 years for acellular pertussis vaccines and 10 to 14 years for whole-cell vaccines compared to 20 years or more after wild infection.[169] However, for some individuals, immunity can wane as early as 4 to 5 years after vaccine receipt.

Second, the current recommended vaccination schedule leaves many individuals vulnerable to infection. The childhood schedule begins at 2 months of age and ends at 4 to 6 years. A follow-up booster is recommended at 11 to 12 years and every 10 years thereafter. It is estimated that only 17% of adults older than 19 years have received a Tdap vaccine.[120] A large reservoir of infection is likely to be present among older adolescents and adults, who can potentially expose young infants.[170] In a comprehensive review of the literature, Wiley and colleagues reported that across 7 studies the most common source of infant infection was a parent (range 39-57%) or sibling (range 16-43%).[170] It is not surprising that in 2013 and 2014, 12.8% of reported cases occurred in infants younger than 1 year of age and 33.8% in children between 11 and 19 years of age. Nine out of the 13 deaths from pertussis in this time period occurred in infants less than a year old, mostly in the first 3 months of life.[171]

Several strategies are being proposed to better protect infants against pertussis infection. These strategies include catch-up doses of Tdap for adolescents and adults; cocooning, ensuring vaccination of individuals living with or caring for young infants; and vaccination of pregnant women. The CDC first recommended a one-time catch-up dose of Tdap for adolescents and adults 19 to 24 years of age in 2006.[125,131] ACIP also recommends that women be vaccinated before or immediately after pregnancy, and advised that adults younger than 65 years who anticipate or have close contacts with infants younger than 1 year of age should also be vaccinated.[125]

In 2010, ACIP expanded its recommendation to include a one-time catch-up dose for adults older than 65 years who have contact with young infants and an optional dose for older adults without contact with young infants.[172] In 2012, ACIP expanded its recommendations to include a one-time catch-up dose for all older adults, whether or not they had contact with children.[133]

ACIP began recommending immunization with pertussis vaccines in pregnant women in 2011. Vaccination was recommended after 20 weeks of pregnancy for women who previously had never received Tdap. Then in 2012, ACIP recommended vaccinating all pregnant women in the third trimester of every pregnancy.[173] The rationale set forth by ACIP supporting this recommendation included difficulties in getting sufficient numbers of individuals in the infant's social network immunized,[174] limited protection afforded by maternal postpartum vaccination,[175] and lower pertussis antibody levels in infants whose mothers were immunized within 2 years before the start of their pregnancy compared to women who were immunized in their most recent pregnancy.[176] These assumptions are based on limited evidence at this time.

Several outstanding issues need to be addressed before the most optimal strategy for protecting infants can be determined. Tetanus and diphtheria vaccines have long been used in the developed world to protect infants from neonatal tetanus, but were never studied in pre- or post-licensure trials. Only a handful of cases of women receiving Tdap in pregnancy have been reported to the VAERS data set.[177] The limited data available suggest that Tdap is safe,[178] but it is possible that more frequent administration of Tdap could increase VAEs, because tetanus-containing vaccines are much more reactive than other vaccines. There could be a mismatch with pertussis vaccines needing to be boosted more frequently than tetanus vaccines because pertussis immunity usually wanes within 4–5 years; tetanus vaccines induce long-term immunity against tetanus for 10 to 20 years or more[117] and are required every 10 years. Immunizing more frequently with Tdap could help control pertussis but could at the same time increase the risk of over-immunizing against tetanus and precipitate reactions to the tetanus component of the vaccine. Further, it is unclear how vaccination in pregnancy will affect the immune response of infants once they start their own vaccine series at 2 months of age. Some studies suggest that maternal immunization may blunt the infant's response to future pertussis (as well as other) vaccines, but more research is needed to determine if this is a valid concern.[179] In addition, it is unknown what level of maternal antibodies is needed in the newborn to prevent pertussis infection. Nor is it known how long maternal antibodies will last and if the protection they provide will last until the infant's vaccine series starts at 2 months. Perhaps earlier infant vaccination before 2 months of age would better protect the infant. Lastly, it is unclear which strategy, or combination of strategies, would be most cost effective. Models have come to opposing conclusions with some predicting that adolescent immunization alone is the best option, while others predict that cocooning or maternal immunization strategies are more cost effective.[179,180] Very few, if any, studies have yet been conducted on any of these proposed interventions.[181] Because research in this area is rapidly emerging, clinicians will need to stay abreast of new developments on pertussis vaccination.

LACTATION

All vaccines can safely be given during lactation. While live viral vaccines replicate in the mother's body, there is little evidence that any vaccine virus other than rubella is excreted in human milk. There are only a few reports in the literature linking the presence of virus in human milk to infection in the infant, and the resulting infections

have been well tolerated. Therefore, ACIP recommends that breastfeeding mothers and their infants follow the routine adult and childhood immunization schedule.[64]

Pregnancy and early postpartum provide an ideal opportunity to catch up on needed vaccines. It is a time when many women, including those who would otherwise not seek health care, are seen repeatedly over a relatively short time span in the same institution or practice. Many vaccines needed by adults require boosters, and most are safe to administer in pregnancy or in the early postpartum period. The vaccines of particular concern for women during this time period are tetanus, hepatitis B, rubella, and varicella.

IMMUNOSUPPRESSIVE CONDITIONS

Severe immunosuppression can be caused by cancer, chemotherapy, human immunodeficiency virus (HIV) infection, or high-dose corticosteroid use, and less commonly can be found in some congenital disorders. Inactivated, recombinant, subunit, polysaccharide, conjugate, and toxoid vaccines commonly used in the United States can safely be given to all immunocompromised individuals, although response to vaccination may be suboptimal.[64]

Live viral vaccines can be problematic for immunosuppressed individuals depending on the cause and severity of immunosuppression. They may be contraindicated in those with severe immunosuppression because uncontrolled replication of vaccine virus can occur with some vaccines and cause vaccine-virus infections. For example, deaths from vaccine-related infections have occurred in severely immunocompromised HIV-positive individuals after receipt of live-viral oral polio and live-viral measles vaccination. Most individuals with milder immunosuppression can receive most live vaccines. Although the immune response may not be as robust at that seen in healthy, immunocompetent vaccine recipients, individuals with immunosuppression benefit from whatever protection vaccines can induce. Recommendations vary by vaccine, by level of immunosuppression, and by underlying cause. Clinicians should consult an expert in immunizations in situations where it is unclear what immunizations are needed or whether immunizations are safe.

The two most common situations that women's health providers may encounter are managing immunizations for HIV-positive women and those on high-dose corticosteroids. ACIP states that corticosteroid therapy is not a contraindication when they are used short term (i.e., < 14 days); at a low to moderate dose (< 20 mg of prednisone or equivalent per day); administered long term, but on an alternate-day schedule with short-acting preparations; or topically (skin or eyes), inhaled, or by intraarticular, bursal, or tendon injection. Immunization should be delayed for a minimum of a month if high-dose corticosteroids are used for more than 14 days.[64]

Ensuring that asymptomatic HIV-positive individuals and others receive vaccines at a time when the immune system is healthy enough to mount an effective response may protect these individuals from serious infection later when their immune system begins to fail. Immunosuppressed individuals are at higher risk of complications secondary to pneumococcal, influenza, and meningococcal infections and should be vaccinated against these diseases.[64] Current guidelines recommend vaccination with the pneumococcal conjugate vaccine (Prevnar-13) at the time of HIV diagnosis followed by polysaccharide pneumococcal vaccine, PPV-23. PPV-23 is then repeated 5 years post-HIV diagnosis and then again at 65 years of age or older. Other vaccines of concern for individuals with HIV include hepatitis B (which should be given if the individual has no serologic evidence of immunity), hepatitis A (given to all with risk factors for disease and can be considered in all others), and herpes simplex virus (if not given earlier and age requirements are met). Live viral vaccines (MMR, varicella, and zoster) can be considered in individuals whose CD_4 count is $\geq$ 200 cells/mm. However, the live viral influenza vaccine should not be used; the TIV is just as immunologic and safer in individuals with immunosuppression.[182]

In addition, household contacts of immunocompromised individuals should follow the standard adult immunization schedule and receive vaccines as needed for their own health. The only exceptions are that they should not be vaccinated with smallpox vaccine and should take precautions in the rare event they develop a rash after receipt of the varicella vaccine; a rash is a sign they have developed a more pronounced infection than usual and may be at risk for transferring varicella-vaccine virus to others.[182] In addition, household members caring for infants after receipt of rotavirus vaccination should employ good handwashing techniques to avoid transmitting rotavirus-vaccine virus to others.[182] These situations are rare. Adherence to the vaccine schedule for household members may partially protect family members with immunosuppression by reducing exposures to vaccine-preventable illness.

References

1. Han P. Historical changes in the objectives of the periodic health examination. *Ann Intern Med.* 1997;127(10):910-917.
2. Hawkes CH. I've stopped examining patients! *Pract Neurol.* 2009;9(4):192-194.
3. Mehrotra A, Prochazka A. Improving value in health care—Against the annual physical. *N Engl J Med.* 2015;373(16):1485-1487.
4. Patel K. Is clinical examination dead? *BMJ.* 2013;346.

5. Goroll AH. Toward trusting therapeutic relationships—In favor of the annual physical. *N Engl J Med*. 2015;373(16):1487-1489.
6. Richardson B. Clinical examination is essential to reduce overdiagnosis and overtreatment. *BMJ*. 2014;348.
7. Warlow C. Why I have not stopped examining patients. *Pract Neurol*. 2010;10(3):126-128.
8. Boulware LE, Marinopoulos S, Phillips KA, Hwang CW, Maynor K, Merenstein D, et al. Systematic review: the value of the periodic health evaluation. *Ann Intern Med*. 2007;146(4):289-300.
9. Henny J, Paulus A, Helfenstein M, Godefroy T, Guéguen R. Relationship between the achievement of successive periodic health examinations and the risk of dying. Appraisal of a prevention scheme. *J Epidemiol Community Health*. 2012;66(12):1092-1096.
10. Westhoff CL, Jones HE, Guiahi M. Do new guidelines and technology make the routine pelvic examination obsolete? *J Womens Health*. 2011;20(1):5-10.
11. MacLaughlin KL, Faubion SS, Long ME, Pruthi S, Casey PM. Should the annual pelvic examination go the way of annual cervical cytology? *Womens Health*. 2014;10(4):373-384.
12. Bloomfield HE, Olson A, Greer N, Cantor A, MacDonald R, Rutks I, et al. Screening pelvic examinations in asymptomatic, average-risk adult women: an evidence report for a clinical practice guideline from the American College of Physicians. *Ann Intern Med*. 2014;16(1):46-53.
13. American College of Obstetricians and Gynecologists. Committee Opinion Number 534 Well Woman Visit. 2012. Available at: http://www.acog.org/Resources-And-Publications/Committee-Opinions/Committee-on-Gynecologic-Practice/Well-Woman-Visit. Accessed November 21, 2015.
14. Centers for Disease Control and Prevention. Ovarian cancer statistics. 2015. Available at: http://www.cdc.gov/cancer/ovarian/statistics/index.htm. Accessed November 12, 2015.
15. Moyer V. US Preventive Services Task Force. Screening for ovarian cancer: U.S. Preventive Services Task Force reaffirmation recommendation statement. *Ann Intern Med*. 2012;157:900-904.
16. Swan J, Breen N, Coates RJ, Rimer BK, Lee NC. Progress in cancer screening practices in the United States: results from the 2000 National Health Interview Survey. *Cancer*. 2003;97(6):1528-1541.
17. Healthy People. Clinical Preventive Services: Latest Data: Colorectal Cancer Screening (C-16). Available at: http://www.healthypeople.gov/2020/leading-health-indicators/2020-lhi-topics/

18. Steele CB, Rim SH, Joseph DA, King JB, Seeff LC. Colorectal cancer incidence and screening—United States, 2008 and 2010. *MMWR*. 2013;62(3):53-60.
19. Selection and interpretation of diagnostic tests. In: Goroll A, May L, Mulley A, eds. *Primary Care Medicine*. 4th ed. Philadelphia, PA: Lippincott Williams & Wilkins; 2000.
20. US Preventive Services Task Force. Introduction: Methodology Table 4. *Guide to Clinical Preventive Services*. Baltimore, MD: Williams & Wilkins; 1998.
21. American Academy of Family Physicians. Recommendations by topic: Infants, children, and adolescents. Available at: http://www.aafp.org/patient-care/clinical-recommendations/children.html. Accessed February 16, 2016.
22. American College of Obstetricians and Gynecologists. Well-Woman Recommendations. Available at: http://www.acog.org/About-ACOG/ACOG-Departments/Annual-Womens-Health-Care/Well-Woman-Recommendations. Accessed November 12, 2015.
23. US Preventive Services Task Force. USPSTF A and B Recommendations. 2015. Available at: http://www.uspreventiveservicestaskforce.org/Page/Name/uspstf-a-and-b-recommendations/. Accessed November 12, 2015.
24. American College of Obstetricians and Gynecologists. ACOG practice bulletin no. 131: screening for cervical cancer. *Obstet Gynecol*. 2012;120(5):1222-1238.
25. Garber J, Garber R, Cobin H, Gharib J, Hennessey I, Klein J, et al. Clinical practice guidelines for hypothyroidism in adults: cosponsored by the American Association of Clinical Endocrinologists and the American Thyroid Association. *Thyroid*. 2012;22(12):1200-1235.
26. American Cancer Society. Recommendations for early breast cancer detection in women without breast symptoms. 2015. Available at: http://www.cancer.org/cancer/breastcancer/moreinformation/breastcancerearlydetection/breast-cancer-early-detection-acs-recs. Accessed February 16, 2016.
27. Conry J, Brown H. Well-woman task force: components of the well-woman visit. *Obstet Gynecol*. 2015;126(4):697-701.
28. Roush S, Murphy T, Vaccine-Preventable Disease Table Working Group. Historical comparisons of morbidity and mortality for vaccine-preventable diseases in the United States. *JAMA*. 2007;18:2155-2163.
29. Centers for Disease Control and Prevention. *Epidemiology and Prevention of Vaccine-Preventable*

Diseases. 13th ed. Washington, DC: Public Health Foundation; 2015.

30. Offit PA, DeStefano F. Vaccine safety. In: Plotkin SA, Orenstein WA, Offit PA, eds. *Vaccines*. 6th ed. Elsevier; 2013.

31. Jacobson R, Adeqbenro A, Pankratz S, Poland G. Adverse events and vaccination—the lack of power and predictability of infrequent events in pre-licensure study. *Vaccine*. 2001;19(17-19):2428-2433.

32. Advisory Committee on Immunization Practices. Rotavirus vaccine for the prevention of rotavirus gastroenteritis among children, recommendations of the Advisory Committee on Immunization Practices (ACIP). *MMWR Recomm Rep*. 1999;48(RR-2):1-23.

33. Centers for Disease Control and Prevention. Intussusception among recipients of rotavirus vaccine—United States, 1998-1999. *MMWR*. 1999;48(27):577-581.

34. Centers for Disease Control and Prevention. Withdrawal of rotavirus vaccine. *MMWR*. 1999;48(43):1007.

35. Institute of Medicine (IOM). Immunization Safety Review. Available at: http://iom.nationalacademies.org/Activities/PublicHealth/ImmunizationSafety.aspx. Accessed November 12, 2015.

36. Rock A. The lethal dangers of the billion-dollar vaccine business. *Money*. 1996:148-164.

37. Institute of Medicine. *Adverse Effects of Pertussis and Rubella Vaccines*. Washington, DC: National Academy Press; 1991.

38. Institute of Medicine. *Adverse Effects of Vaccines: Evidence and Causality*. Washington, DC: National Academies Press; 2012.

39. Vaccine Adverse Event Reporting System (VAERS). About the VAERS program. Available at: https://vaers.hhs.gov/index/about/index. Accessed February 16, 2016.

40. Centers for Disease Control and Prevention. Vaccine Safety Datalink (VSD). 2015. Available at: http://www.cdc.gov/vaccinesafety/ensuringsafety/monitoring/vsd/index.html. Accessed November 20, 2015.

41. Klein N, Fireman B, Yih W, Lewis E, Kulldorff M, Ray P, et al. Measles-mumps-rubella-varicella combination vaccine and the risk of febrile seizures. *Pediatrics*. 2010;128(1):e1-8.

42. McNeil MM, Gee J, Weintraub ES, Belongia EA, Lee GM, Glanz JM, et al. The Vaccine Safety Datalink: successes and challenges monitoring vaccine safety. *Vaccine*. 2014;32(42):5390-5398.

43. Seither R, Calhoun K, Knighton CL, Mellerson J, Meador S, Tippins A, et al. Vaccination coverage among children in kindergarten—United States,

2014-15 school year. *MMWR*. 2015;64(33):897-904.

44. Centers for Disease Control and Prevention. Clinical Immunization Safety Assessment (CISA) Project. Available at: http://www.cdc.gov/vaccinesafety/ensuringsafety/monitoring/cisa/index.html. Accessed February 16, 2016.

45. Advisory Committee on Immunization Practices. Prevention of hepatitis A through active or passive immunization. *MMWR*. 1999;48(RR 12):1-37.

46. Gangarosa E, Galazka A, Wolfe C, Phillips L, Gangarosa R, Miller E, et al. Impact of anti-vaccine movements on pertussis control: the untold story. *Lancet*. 1998;351(9099):356-361.

47. Reagan L. Show us the science: an exclusive mothering report on the Second International Public Conference of the National Vaccine Information Center. *Mothering*. 2001;March/April:38-55.

48. National Vaccine Information Center. The Health Liberty Revolution to Save Our Children. Available at: http://www.nvic.org/NVIC-Vaccine-News/October-2015/health-liberty-revolution-to-save-our-children.aspx. Accessed November 22, 2015.

49. Diekema DS. Personal belief exemptions from school vaccination requirements. *Annu Rev Public Health*. 2014;35(1):275-292.

50. De Jong M, Bouma A. Herd immunity after vaccination: how to quantify it and how to use it to halt disease. *Vaccine*. 2001;19(17-19):2722-2728.

51. Dadswell J. Susceptibility to diphtheria. *Lancet*. 1978;1(8061):428-430.

52. Galazka AM, Robertson SE, Oblapenko G. Resurgence of diphtheria. *Eur J Epidemiol*. 1995;11(1):95-105.

53. Galazka A, Robertson S. Diphtheria: changing patterns in the developing world and the industrialized world. *Eur J Epidemiol*. 1995;11(1):107-117.

54. Fine P, Clarkson J. Individual versus public priorities in the determination of optimal vaccination policies. *Am J Epidemiol*. 1986;124:1012-1020.

55. Risk communication and vaccination: summary of a workshop. In: Evans G, Bostrom A, Johnston R, Fisher B, Stoto M, eds. *Risk Communication and Vaccination*. Washington, DC: National Academy Press; 1997.

56. Chen R, Hibbs B. Vaccine safety: current and future challenges. *Pediatr Ann*. 1998;27(7):445-455.

57. Ball L, Evans G, Bostrom A. Risky business: challenges in vaccine risk communication. *Pediatrics*. 1998;101(3):453-458.

58. Browne M, Thomson P, Justus Rockloff M, Pennycook G. Going against the herd: psychological and cultural factors underlying the 'vaccination confidence gap.' *PLoS One*. 2015;10(9):e0132562.

59. Centers for Disease Control and Prevention. Vaccination coverage among children in kindergarten—United States, 2012-13 school year. *MMWR.* 2013;62(30):607-612.

60. Wang E, Clymer J, Davis-Hayes C, Buttenheim A. Nonmedical exemptions from school immunization requirements: a systematic review. *Am J Public Health.* 2014;104:e62-e84.

61. Feikin D, Lezotte D, Hamman R, Salmon D, Chen R, Hoffman R. Individual and community risks of measles and pertussis associated with personal exemptions to immunization. *JAMA.* 2000;284(24):3145-3150.

62. Salmon D, Haber M, Gangarosa E, Phillips L, Smith N, Chen R. Health consequences of religious and philosophical exemptions from immunization laws: individual and societal risk of measles. *JAMA.* 1999;282(1):47-53.

63. Centers for Disease Control and Prevention. Measles outbreaks and cases. 2015. Available at: http://www.cdc.gov/measles/cases-outbreaks.html. Accessed February 16, 2016.

64. Kroger AT, Sumaya CV, Pickering LK, Atkinson WL. General recommendations on immunizations: recommendations by the Advisory Committee on Immunization Practices. *MMWR.* 2011;60(RR02):1-60.

65. McLean HQ, Fiebelkorn AP, Temte JL, Wallace GS. Prevention of measles, rubella, congenital rubella syndrome, and mumps, 2013: summary recommendations of the Advisory Committee on Immunization Practices (ACIP). *MMWR.* 2013;62(RR-04):1-34.

66. Centers for Disease Control and Prevention. Appendix B vaccine excipient & media summary. In: Hamborsky J, Kroger A, Wolfe S, eds. *Epidemiology and Prevention of Vaccine-Preventable Diseases.* 13th ed. Washington, DC: Public Health Foundation; 2015.

67. Centers for Disease Control and Prevention. Contraindications and precautions to commonly used vaccines in adults. 2015. Available at: http://www.cdc.gov/vaccines/schedules/hcp/imz/adult-contraindications.html. Accessed February 16, 2016.

68. Fiore AE, Wasley A, Bell BP. Prevention of hepatitis A through active or passive immunization: recommendations of the Advisory Committee on Immunization Practices. *MMWR.* 2006;55(RR-07):1-23.

69. Centers for Disease Control and Prevention. Updated recommendations from the Advisory Committee on Immunization Practices (ACIP) for use of hepatitis A vaccine in close contacts of newly arriving international adoptees. *MMWR.* 2009;58(36):1006-1007.

70. Mast EE, Fiore AE, Weinbaum CM, Alter MJ, Bell BP, et al. A comprehensive immunization strategy to eliminate transmission of hepatitis B virus infection in the United States: recommendations of the Advisory Committee on Immunization Practices. *MMWR.* 2006;55(RR 16):2-26.

71. Centers for Disease Control and Prevention. Viral Hepatitis Statistics and Surveillance. 2015. Available at: http://www.cdc.gov/hepatitis/statistics/index.htm. Accessed December 9, 2015.

72. Ott JJ, Stevens GA, Groeger J, Wiersma ST. Global epidemiology of hepatitis B virus infection: new estimates of age-specific HBsAg seroprevalence and endemicity. *Vaccine.* 2012;30(12):2212-2219.

73. World Health Organization. The Global Advisory Committee on Vaccine Safety rejects association between hepatitis B vaccination and multiple sclerosis (MS). 2002. Available at: http://www.who.int/vaccine_safety/committee/topics/hepatitisb/ms/en/. Accessed December 6, 2015.

74. Institute of Medicine, Immunization Safety Review Committee, Stratton K, Almario D, McCormick MC, eds. *Immunization Safety Review: Hepatitis B Vaccine and Demyelinating Neurological Disorders.* Washington, DC: National Academies Press; 2002.

75. Martínez-Sernández V, Figueiras A. Central nervous system demyelinating diseases and recombinant hepatitis B vaccination: a critical systematic review of scientific production. *J Neurol.* 2013;260(8):1951-1959.

76. Confavreux C, Suissa S, Saddier P, Bourdès V, Vukusic S. Vaccinations and the risk of relapse in multiple sclerosis. Vaccines in Multiple Sclerosis Study Group. *N Engl J Med.* 2001;344(5):319-326.

77. Centers for Disease Control and Prevention. Thimerosal in vaccines: a joint statement of the American Academy of Pediatrics and the Public Health Service. *MMWR.* 1999;48(26):563-565.

78. Geier D, Hooker B, Kern J, King P, Sykes L, Geier M. A dose-response relationship between organic mercury exposure from thimerosal-containing vaccines and neurodevelopmental disorders. *Int J Environ Res Public Health.* 2014;11(9):9156-9170.

79. Thompson WW, Price C, Goodson B, Shay DK, Benson P, Hinrichsen VL, et al. Early thimerosal exposure and neuropsychological outcomes at 7 to 10 Years. *N Engl J Med.* 2007;357(13):1281-1292.

80. Food and Drug Administration. Thimerosal in Vaccines. 2015. Available at: http://www.fda.gov/BiologicsBloodVaccines/SafetyAvailability/VaccineSafety/UCM096228. Accessed December 11, 2015.

81. Hooker B, Kern J, Geier D, Haley B, Sykes L, King P, et al. Methodological issues and evidence of malfeasance in research purporting to show thimerosal in vaccines is safe. *Biomed Res Int.* 2014:247218.

82. Centers for Disease Control and Prevention. FDA licensure of bivalent human papillomavirus vaccine (HPV2, Cervarix) for use in females and updated HPV vaccination; Recommendations from the Advisory Committee on Immunization Practices. *MMWR.* 2010;59(20):626-628.

83. Markowitz LE, Dunne EF, Saraiya M, Lawson HW, Chesson H, Unger ER. Quadrivalent human papillomavirus vaccine: recommendations of the Advisory Committee on Immunization Practices. *MMWR.* 2007;56:1-24.

84. Petrosky E, Bocchini JA, Hariri S, Chesson H, Curtis CR, Saraiya M, et al. Use of 9-valent human papillomavirus (HPV) vaccine: updated HPV vaccination: recommendations of the Advisory Committee on Immunization Practices. *MMWR.* 2015;64(11):300-304.

85. Li N, Franceschi S, Howell-Jones R, Snijders PJ, Clifford GM. Human papillomavirus type distribution in 30,848 invasive cervical cancers worldwide: variation by geographical region, histological type and year of publication. *Int J Cancer.* 2011;128:927-935.

86. Saraiya M, Unger ER, Thompson TD, Lynch CF, Hernandez BY, Lyu CW, et al. US assessment of HPV types in cancers: implications for current and 9-valent HPV vaccines. *J Natl Cancer Inst.* 2015;107(6):djv086.

87. Serrano B, Alemany L, Ruiz PA, Tous S, Lima MA, Bruni L, et al. Potential impact of a 9-valent HPV vaccine in HPV-related cervical disease in 4 emerging countries (Brazil, Mexico, India and China). *Cancer Epidemiol.* 2014;38(6):748-756.

88. Satterwhite CL, Torrone E, Meites E, Dunne EF, Mahajan R, Ocfemia M, et al. Sexually transmitted infections among US women and men: prevalence and incidence estimates, 2008. *Sex Transm Dis.* 2013;40(3):187-193.

89. Ferris D, Samakoses R, Block SL, Lazcano-Ponce E, Alberto Restrepo J, Reisinger KS, et al. Long-term study of a quadrivalent human papillomavirus vaccine. *Pediatrics.* 2014;134(3):e657-e665.

90. Luna J, Plata M, Gonzalez M, Correa A, Maldonado I, Nossa C, et al. Long-term follow-up observation of the safety, immunogenicity, and effectiveness of Gardasil™ in adult women. *PLoS One.* 2013;8(12):e83431.

91. Julius JM, Ramondeta L, Tipton KA, Lal LS, Schneider K, Smith JA. Clinical perspectives on the role of the human papillomavirus vaccine in the prevention of cancer. *Pharmacotherapy.* 2011;31(3):280-297.

92. Centers for Disease Control and Prevention. Syncope after vaccination—United States, January 2005-July 2007. *MMWR.* 2008;57(17):457-460.

93. Borja-Hart NL, Benavides S, Christensen C. Human papillomavirus vaccine safety in pediatric patients: an evaluation of the Vaccine Adverse Event Reporting System. *Ann Pharmacother.* 2009; 43:356-359.

94. Ojha R, Jackson B, Tota J, Offutt-Powell T, Singh K, Bae S. Guillain-Barre syndrome following quadrivalent human papillomavirus vaccination among vaccine-eligible individuals in the United States. *Hum Vaccin Immunother.* 2014;10(1):232-237.

95. Centers for Disease Control and Prevention. Influenza. In: Atkinson W, Hamborski J, Wolfe C, eds. *Epidemiology and Prevention of Vaccine-Preventable Diseases.* 8th ed. Waldorf, MD: Public Health Foundation; 2004.

96. Centers for Disease Control and Prevention. Prevention and control of influenza with vaccines: recommendations of the Advisory Committee on Immunization Practices, United States, 2015-16 Influenza Season. *MMWR.* 2015;64(30):818-825.

97. Vesikari T. eaR, double-blind, placebo-controlled trial of the safety, transmissibility and phenotypic stability of a live, attenuated, cold-adapted influenza virus vaccine (CAIV-T) in children attending day care [Abstract G-450]. Presented at the 41st Annual Interscience Conference on Antimicrobial Agents and Chemotherapy (ICAAC), Chicago, IL, 2001.

98. Harper SA, Fukuda K, Uyeki TM, Cox NJ, Bridges CB. Prevention and control of influenza: recommendations of the Advisory Committee on Immunization Practices. *MMWR.* 2004;53(RR06): 1-40.

99. Des Roches A, Paradis L, Gagnon R, Lemire C, Begin P, Carr S, et al. Egg-allergic patients can be safely vaccinated against influenza. *J Allergy Clin Immunol.* 2012;130:1213-1216.e1.

100. World Health Organization. Measles. 2015. Available at: http://www.who.int/mediacentre/factsheets/fs286/en/. Accessed December 11, 2015.

101. Moss W. Measles (Rubeola) In: Longo D, Fauci A, Kasper D, Hauser S, Jameson J, Loscalzo J, eds. *Harrison's Principles of Internal Medicine.* 18th ed. New York, NY: McGraw-Hill; 2012.

102. Global Measles and Rubella Strategic Plan: 2012-2010. Available at: http://www.measlesrubellainitiative.org/wp-content/uploads/2013/06/Measles-Rubella-Strategic-Plan.pdf. Accessed December 11, 2015.

103. Centers for Disease Control and Prevention. Global control and regional elimination of measles, 2000-2011. *MMWR.* 2013;62(2):27-31.

104. Centers for Disease Control and Prevention. Measles—United States, January 4-April 2, 2015. *MMWR.* 2015;64(14):373-376.

105. Grant GB, Reef SE, Dabbagh A, Gacic-Dobo M, Strebel PM. Rubella and congenital rubella syndrome control and elimination—global progress, 2000-2014. *Wkly Epidemiol Rec.* 2015; 39(90):510-516.

106. Centers for Disease Control and Prevention. Rubella among Hispanic adults—Kansas, 1998, and Nebraska, 1999. *MMWR.* 2000;49(11):225-228.

107. Zimmerman LA, Reef SE. Rubella (German Measles). In: Longo D, Fauci A, Kasper D, Hauser S, Jameson J, Loscalzo J, eds. *Harrison's Principles of Internal Medicine.* 18th ed. New York, NY: McGraw-Hill; 2012.

108. McLean HQ, Parker Fiebelkorn A, Temte JL, Wallace GS. Prevention of measles, rubella, congenital rubella syndrome, and mumps, 2013: summary recommendations of the Advisory Committee on Immunization Practices. *MMWR.* 2013;62 (RR 04):1-34.

109. Asatryan A, Pool V, Chen R, Kohl K, Davis R, Iskander J, et al. Live attenuated measles and mumps viral strain-containing vaccines and hearing loss: Vaccine Adverse Event Reporting System (VAERS), United States, 1990-2003. *Vaccine.* 2008;26(9): 1166-1172.

110. Cohn AC, MacNeil JR, Clark TA, Ortega-Sanchez IR, Briere EZ, Meissner HC, et al. Prevention and control of meningococcal disease: recommendations of the Advisory Committee on Immunization Practices. *MMWR.* 2013;62(RR 02):1-22.

111. Folaranmi T, Rubin L, Martin SW, Patel M, MacNeil JR. Use of serogroup B meningococcal vaccines in persons aged ≥10 years at increased risk for serogroup B meningococcal disease: recommendations of the Advisory Committee on Immunization Practices, 2015. *MMWR.* 2015;64: 608-612.

112. MacNeil JR, Rubin L, Folaranmi T, Ortega-Sanchez IR, Patel M, Martin SW. Use of serogroup B meningococcal vaccines in adolescents and young adults: recommendations of the Advisory Committee on Immunization Practices, 2015. *MMWR.* 2015;64:1171-1176.

113. Centers for Disease Control and Prevention. Use of serogroup B meningococcal vaccines in adolescents and young adults: recommendations of the Advisory Committee on Immunization Practices, 2015. *MMWR.* 2015;64(41):1171-1176.

114. Goldblatt D, O'Brien KL. Pneumococcal infections. In: Longo D, Fauci A, Kasper D, Hauser S, Jameson J, Loscalzo J, eds. *Harrison's Internal Medicine.* 8th ed. New York, NY: McGraw-Hill; 2012.

115. Pilishvili T, Bennett NM. Pneumococcal disease prevention among adults: strategies for the use of pneumococcal vaccines. *Vaccine.* 2015;33(Suppl 4): D60-5.

116. Centers for Disease Control and Prevention. Use of 13-valent pneumococcal conjugate vaccine and 23-valent pneumococcal polysaccharide vaccine for adults with immunocompromising conditions: recommendations of the Advisory Committee on Immunization Practices. *MMWR.* 2012; 61(40):816-819.

117. Simonsen O, Badsberg J, Kjeldsen K, Møller-Madsen B, Heron I. The fall-off in serum concentration of tetanus antitoxin after primary and booster vaccination. *Acta Pathol Microbiol Scand C.* 1986;94:77-82.

118. Centers for Disease Control and Prevention. Tetanus surveillance—United States, 2001-2008. *MMWR.* 2011;60(12):365-369.

119. Kalaça S, Yalçin M, Simşek YS. Missed opportunities for tetanus vaccination in pregnant women, and factors associated with seropositivity. *Public Health.* 2004;18(5):377-382.

120. Williams WW, Lu P-J, O'Halloran A, Bridges CB, Kim DK, Pilishvili T, et al. Vaccination coverage among adults, excluding influenza vaccination—United States, 2013. *MMWR.* 2015;64(04):95-102.

121. Craig A, Reed G, Mohon R, Quick M, Swarner O, Moore W, et al. Neonatal tetanus in the United States: a sentinel event in the foreign born. *Pediatr Infect Dis J.* 1997;16(10):955-959.

122. UNICEF. Elimination of maternal and neonatal tetanus. 2015. Available at: http://www.unicef.org/health/index_43509.html. Accessed December 6, 2015.

123. World Health Organization Western Pacific Region. Tetanus. 2012. Available at: http://www.wpro.who.int/mediacentre/factsheets/fs_20120307_tetanus/en/. Accessed December 6, 2015.

124. Centers for Disease Control and Prevention. Neonatal tetanus—Montana. *MMWR.* 1998;47(43): 928-930.

125. Kretsinger K, Broder KR, Cortese MM, Joyce MP, Ortega-Sanchez I, Lee GM, et al. Preventing tetanus, diphtheria, and pertussis among adults: use of tetanus toxoid, reduced diphtheria toxoid and acellular pertussis vaccine recommendations of the Advisory Committee on Immunization Practices (ACIP) and recommendation of ACIP, supported

by the Healthcare Infection Control Practices Advisory Committee (HICPAC), for use of Tdap among health-care personnel. *MMWR Recomm Rep.* 2006;55(RR-17):1-37.

126. World Health Organization. Immunization, Vaccines and Biologicals: Diphtheria 2014. 2014. Available at: http://www.who.int/immunization/monitoring_surveillance/burden/diphtheria/en/. Accessed December 6, 2015.

127. Amanna IJ, Carlson NE, Slifka MK. Duration of humoral immunity to common viral and vaccine antigens. *N Engl J Med.* 2007;357(19): 1903-1915.

128. Alagappan K, Rennie W, Kwiatkowski T, Narang V. Antibody protection to diphtheria in geriatric patients: need for ED compliance with immunization guidelines. *Ann Emerg Med.* 1997;30(4):455-458.

129. Centers for Disease Control and Prevention. Pertussis (Whooping Cough): Surveillance and Reporting. 2015. Available at: http://www.cdc.gov/pertussis/surv-reporting.html. Accessed February 16, 2016.

130. Centers for Disease Control and Prevention. Updated recommendations for use of tetanus toxoid, reduced diphtheria toxoid and acellular pertussis vaccine (Tdap) in pregnant women and persons who have or anticipate having close contact with an infant aged <12 months—Advisory Committee on Immunization Practices. *MMWR.* 2011;60(41):1424-1426.

131. Broder KR, Cortese MM, Iskander JK, Kretsinger K, Slade BA, Brown KH, et al. Preventing tetanus, diphtheria, and pertussis among adolescents: use of tetanus toxoid, reduced diphtheria toxoid and acellular pertussis vaccines: recommendations of the Advisory Committee on Immunization Practices. *MMWR Recomm Rep.* 2006;55(RR 03):1-34.

132. Acosta AM, DeBolt C, Tasslimi A, Lewis M, Stewart LK, Misegades LK, et al. Tdap vaccine effectiveness in adolescents during the 2012 Washington state pertussis epidemic. *Pediatrics.* 2015;135(6):981-989.

133. Centers for Disease Control and Prevention. Updated recommendations for use of tetanus toxoid, reduced diphtheria toxoid, and acellular pertussis (Tdap) vaccine in adults aged 65 years and older—Advisory Committee on Immunization Practices. *MMWR.* 2012;61(25):468-470.

134. Edwards K, Decker M. Pertussis. In: Plotkin SA, Orenstein WA, Offit PA, eds. *Vaccines.* 6th ed. Elsevier; 2013.

135. Yih WK, Nordin JD, Kulldorff M, Lewis E, Lieu TA, Shi P, et al. An assessment of the safety of adolescent and adult tetanus-diphtheria-acellular pertussis (Tdap) vaccine, using active surveillance for adverse events in the Vaccine Safety Datalink. *Vaccine.* 2009;27(32):4257-4262.

136. Klein NP, Hansen J, Lewis E, Lyon L, Nguyen B, Black S, et al. Post-marketing safety evaluation of a tetanus toxoid, reduced diphtheria toxoid and 3-component acellular pertussis vaccine administered to a cohort of adolescents in a United States health maintenance organization. *Pediatr Infect Dis J.* 2010;29(7):613-617.

137. Marin M, Güris D, Chaves SS, Schmid S, Seward JF. Prevention of varicella. *MMWR.* 2007;56 (RR 4):1-40.

138. Centers for Disease Control and Prevention. Prevention of varicella: recommendations of the Advisory Committee on Immunization Practices. *MMWR.* 1996;45(RR 11):1-25.

139. Marin M, Güris D, Chaves SS, Schmid S, Seward JF. Prevention of varicella: recommendations of the Advisory Committee on Immunization Practices (ACIP). *MMWR.* 2007;56(RR-04):1-40.

140. Centers for Disease Control and Prevention. Prevention of herpes zoster: recommendations of the Advisory Committee on Immunization Practices. *MMWR.* 2008;57(5):1-30.

141. Arvin A. Varicella-zoster virus. In: Knipe D, Howley P, Griffin D, Lamb R, Martin M, Roizman B, et al., eds. *Fields Virology.* 4 ed. Baltimore, MD: Lippincott Williams & Wilkins; 2001.

142. Centers for Disease Control and Prevention. Prevention of varicella: updated recommendations of the Advisory Committee on Immunization Practices. *MMWR.* 1999;48(RR 06):1-5.

143. Wen S-Y, Liu W-L. Epidemiology of pediatric herpes zoster after varicella infection: a population-based study. *Pediatrics.* 2015;135(3):e566-e571.

144. Leung J, Harpaz R, Molinari N, Jumaan A, Zhou F. Herpes zoster incidence among insured persons in the United States, 1993-2006: evaluation of impact of varicella vaccination. *Clin Infect Dis.* 2011;52(3):332-340.

145. Centers for Disease Control and Prevention. Update on recommendations for use of herpes zoster vaccine. *MMWR.* 2014;63(33):729-731.

146. Centers for Disease Control and Prevention. Rubella vaccination during pregnancy—United States, 1971-1988. *MMWR.* 1989;38:289-293.

147. Miller E, Cradock-Watson J, Pollock T. Consequences of confirmed maternal rubella at successive stages of pregnancy. *Lancet.* 1982;2(8302):781-784.

148. Advisory Committee on Immunization Practices. Measles, mumps, and rubella-vaccine use and strategies for elimination of measles, rubella,

and congenital rubella syndrome and control of mumps: recommendations of the Advisory Committee on Immunization Practices. *MMWR*. 1998;47(RR-8):1-57.

149. Sauerbrei A, Wutzler P. The congenital varicella syndrome. *J Perinatol*. 2000;20(8 Pt 1):548-554.

150. Shrim A, Koren G, Yudin MH, Farine D. Management of varicella infection (chickenpox) in pregnancy. *J Obstet Gynaecol Can*. 2012;34(3):287-292.

151. Marin M, Willis ED, Marko A, Rasmussen SA, Bialek SR, Dana A. Closure of varicella-zoster virus-containing vaccines pregnancy registry—United States, 2013. *MMWR*. 2014;63(33):732-733.

152. Hartert TV, Neuzil KM, Shintani AK, Mitchel Jr EF, Snowden MS, Wood LB, et al. Maternal morbidity and perinatal outcomes among pregnant women with respiratory hospitalizations during influenza season. *Am J Obstet Gynecol*. 2003;189(6):1705-1712.

153. Jamieson, DJ, Honein M, Rasmussen S, Williams J. H1N1 2009 influenza virus infection during pregnancy in the USA. *Lancet*. 2009;374:451-458.

154. Van Kerkhove MD, Vandemaele KA, Shinde V, Jaramillo-Gutierrez G, Koukounari A, Donnelly CA, et al. Risk factors for severe outcomes following 2009 influenza A (H1N1) infection: a global pooled analysis. *PLoS Med*. 2011;8(7):e1001053.

155. Dodds L, McNeil S, Fell D, Allen VA, Coombs A, Scott J, et al. Impact of influenza exposure on rates of hospital admissions and physician visits because of respiratory illness among pregnant women. *CMAJ*. 2007;178:463-468.

156. Luteijn JM, Brown MJ, Dolk H. Influenza and congenital anomalies: a systematic review and meta-analysis. *Hum Reprod*. 2014;29(4):809-823.

157. Centers for Disease Control and Prevention. Maternal and infant outcomes among severely ill pregnant and postpartum women with 2009 pandemic influenza A (H1N1)—United States, April 2009-August 2010. *MMWR*. 2011;60(35):1193-1196.

158. Rasmussen SA, Jamieson DJ, Uyeki TM. Effects of influenza on pregnant women and infants. *Am J Obstet Gynecol*. 2012;207(Suppl 3):S3-8.

159. Kharbanda EO, Vazquez-Benitez G, Lipkind H, Naleway A, Lee G, Nordin JD, et al. Inactivated influenza vaccine during pregnancy and risks for adverse obstetric events. *Obstet Gynecol*. 2013;122(3):659-667.

160. Beau AB, Hurault-Delarue C, Vidal S, Guitard C, Vayssière C, Petiot D, et al. Pandemic A/H1N1 influenza vaccination during pregnancy: a comparative study using the EFEMERIS database. *Vaccine*. 2014;32(11):1254-1258.

161. Legge A, Dodds L, MacDonald NE, Scott J, McNeil S. Rates and determinants of seasonal influenza vaccination in pregnancy and association with neonatal outcomes. *CMAJ*. 2014;186(4):E157-E164.

162. Chambers CD, Johnson D, Xu R, Luo Y, Louik C, Mitchell AA, et al. Risks and safety of pandemic H1N1 influenza vaccine in pregnancy: birth defects, spontaneous abortion, preterm delivery, and small for gestational age infants. *Vaccine*. 2013;31(44):5026-5032.

163. Puleston R, Bugg G, Hoschler K, Konje J, Thornton J, Stephenson I, et al. Observational study to investigate vertically acquired passive immunity in babies of mothers vaccinated against H1N1during pregnancy. *Health Technol Assess*. 2010;14(55):1-82.

164. Blanchard-Rohner G, Meier S, Bel M, Combescure C, Othenin-Girard V, Swali R, et al. Influenza vaccination given at least 2 weeks before delivery to pregnant women facilitates transmission of seroprotective influenza-specific antibodies to the newborn. *Pediatr Infect Dis J*. 2013;32(12):1374-1380.

165. Madhi SA, Cutland CL, Kuwanda L, Weinberg A, Hugo A, Jones S, et al. Influenza vaccination of pregnant women and protection of their infants. *N Engl J Med*. 2014;371(10):918-931.

166. Centers for Disease Control and Prevention. Pertussis—United States. *MMWR*. 2002;51(4):997-2000.

167. Spector TB, Maziarz EK. Pertussis. *Med Clin North Am*. 2013;97(4):537-552.

168. Cherry JD. Epidemic pertussis in 2012—The resurgence of a vaccine-preventable disease. *N Engl J Med*. 2012;367(9):785-787.

169. Wendelboe AM, Van Rie A, Salmaso S, Englund JA. Duration of immunity against pertussis after natural infection or vaccination. *Pediatr Infect Dis J*. 2005;24(5):S58-S61.

170. Wiley KE, Zuo Y, Macartney KK, McIntyre PB. Sources of pertussis infection in young infants: a review of key evidence informing targeting of the cocoon strategy. *Vaccine*. 2013;31(4):618-625.

171. Centers for Disease Control and Prevention. 2014 final pertussis surveillance report. 2015. Available at: http://www.cdc.gov/pertussis/downloads/pertuss-surv-report-2014.pdf. Accessed December 6, 2015.

172. Centers for Disease Control and Prevention. Updated recommendations for use of tetanus toxoid, reduced diphtheria toxoid and acellular pertussis (Tdap) vaccine from the Advisory Committee on Immunization Practices, 2010. *MMWR*. 2011;60(1):13-15.

173. Centers for Disease Control and Prevention. Updated recommendations for use of tetanus toxoid, reduced diphtheria toxoid, and acellular pertussis vaccine (Tdap) in pregnant women—Advisory Committee on Immunization Practices (ACIP), 2012. *MMWR*. 2013;62(07):131-135.

174. Urwyler P, Heininger U. Protecting newborns from pertussis - the challenge of complete cocooning. *BMC Infect Dis*. 2014;14:397.

175. Castagnini LA, Healy CM, Rench MA, Wootton SH, Munoz FM, Baker CJ. Impact of maternal postpartum tetanus and diphtheria toxoids and acellular pertussis immunization on infant pertussis infection. *Clin Infect Dis*. 2012;54(1):78-84.

176. Healy CM, Rench MA, Baker CJ. Importance of timing of maternal combined tetanus, diphtheria, and acellular pertussis (Tdap) immunization and protection of young infants. *Clin Infect Dis*. 2013;56(4):539-544.

177. Kharbanda E, Vazquez-Benitez G, Lipkind H, et al. Receipt of pertussis vaccine during pregnancy across 7 Vaccine Safety Datalink sites. *Prev Med*. 2014;67:316-9.

178. Donegan K, King B, Bryan P. Safety of pertussis vaccination in pregnant women in UK: observational study. *BMJ*. 2014;349.

179. Chiappini E, Stival A, Galli L, de Martino M. Pertussis re-emergence in the post-vaccination era. *BMC Infect Dis*. 2013;13(151).

180. Terranella A, Beeler Asay GR, Messonnier ML, Clark TA, Liang JL. Pregnancy dose Tdap and postpartum cocooning to prevent infant pertussis: a decision analysis. *Pediatrics*. 2013;131(6):e1748-e1756.

181. Rivero-Santana A, Cuéllar-Pompa L, Sánchez-Gómez LM, Perestelo-Pérez L, Serrano-Aguilar P. Effectiveness and cost-effectiveness of different immunization strategies against whooping cough to reduce child morbidity and mortality. *Health Policy*. 2014;115(1):82-91.

182. Crum-Cianflone N, Wallace M. Vaccination in HIV-infected adults. *AIDS Patient Care STDS*. 2014;28(8):397-410.

CHAPTER 3

ENVIRONMENTAL HEALTH

Katie Huffling

A significant increase in the incidence of acute and chronic health conditions such as asthma, obesity, infertility, autism, and certain types of cancers has been seen since the 1970's.[1] The environment has been shown to play a crucial role in the complex process of disease formation. Assessing for environmental exposures and providing anticipatory guidance are key components in providing quality care and preventing disease. Women's healthcare providers are central to the primary care of women, and need to keep abreast of environmental health risks and their impacts on human health. The purposes of this chapter are to introduce environmental health into the clinician's consciousness and offer a guide to appropriate resources to improve care.

Why Women's Healthcare Professionals?

The term *environment* includes industrial and agricultural chemicals, food and nutrients, pharmaceuticals, physical agents such as heat and radiation, social and economic factors, lifestyle choices and substance abuse, and byproducts of industrial processes (e.g., dioxin). Environmental exposures can occur anywhere—at home, in the workplace, in schools, in healthcare settings—and are often influenced by social, economic, and cultural factors (e.g., income, housing, and food sources and preparation). Exposures to environmental hazards can be chronic, such as poor indoor air quality, or acute, such as an industrial accident. The ubiquitous nature of this exposure is highlighted in an analysis of data from the 2003–2004 National Health and Nutrition Examination Survey (NHANES): 99% of pregnant women in the United States are exposed to at least 43 different chemicals during their pregnancy.[2] The Environmental Working Group has identified 232 toxic chemicals in the cord blood of infants, indicating in utero exposures.[3] As the public and the healthcare community are increasingly aware of the hazards of environmental toxin exposure, emphasis is placed on identifying risk factors, developing prevention strategies, and translating knowledge into practice to prevent human illness.

Historically, women have been assessed for environmental exposures during the first prenatal

visit, when questions about substance and tobacco use, occupation, and medication usage are
asked. However, assessing for exposures only after
a woman is pregnant increases the likelihood that
the fetus has already experienced environmental
assaults. By assessing for environmental exposures preconception and periodically across the
lifespan, healthcare providers can have a significant
impact on reducing exposures and negative health
impacts. Healthcare providers are responsible for
their knowledge of environmental health and how
to use this knowledge in practices. Because healthcare providers generally have strong credibility
with the public, they have both the opportunity
and the responsibility to aid in the prevention of
problems related to exposure to environmental
toxins. Additionally, because women's healthcare
providers have multiple visits with women during
pregnancy and provide continuity of care before,
between, and after pregnancies, they are in a prime
position to have a positive effect on the health of
women and children. Careful history taking and
physical evaluation, laboratory screening, and anticipatory guidance are all tools to identify and
treat problems. In 2013, the American College of
Obstetricians and Gynecologists issued a Committee Opinion recognizing reduction of environmental exposures as a "critical area of intervention"
for reproductive healthcare professionals.[4] The
American College of Nurse-Midwives has also af-
firmed that midwives and reproductive healthcare
professionals have an ethical and professional responsibility to address environmental exposures
in their clients due to the increasing evidence of
health impacts from these exposures.[5]

In addition to answering questions, clinicians
need to assess risks within the home, at work, and
in the community. Women's healthcare providers
need to respond to the expanding research showing adverse effects of environmental exposures
and to address women's concerns regarding pertinent and sensitive issues such as breast cancer and
the safety of breastfeeding.

Scope of the Issue

As scientific evidence has mounted that environmental exposures negatively impact human
health, new areas of inquiry have emerged. These
include endocrine-disrupting chemicals (EDCs),
the timing of exposures, and epigenetics. EDCs
are chemicals that "interfere with the production, transport, metabolism, binding, action, or
elimination of natural hormones in the body that
are responsible for the maintenance of homeostasis and the regulation of the developmental
processes."[6] Just as naturally occurring hormones
are biologically active at very small doses, EDCs
can disrupt hormone signaling at very small
doses and cause negative health impacts such as
decreased fertility, abnormal reproductive organ
development, and poor pregnancy outcomes.[6]
Examples of EDCs discussed in this chapter include bisphenol A (BPA), phthalates, and some
types of pesticides.

The timing of exposures is also significant.
During fetal development, there are critical
windows of susceptibility in which exposure to
chemicals can have lasting, profound impacts on
health. These windows occur at times of rapid
cell growth and differentiation, when chemicals
can interrupt the carefully orchestrated sequence
of events. Some of these impacts are readily apparent, such as seen with congenital abnormalities, while others may be subtler and the affects
not apparent for years after the exposure, such as
with increased susceptibility to certain types of
cancers, obesity, neurodevelopmental disabilities,
and fertility issues.

One of the most famous examples of fetal origins of adult disease is seen with prenatal exposure
to the EDC diethylstilbestrol (DES), a synthetic
estrogen that was prescribed to pregnant women
from 1938–1971. DES was falsely believed to
prevent spontaneous abortion, preterm labor,
and other pregnancy complications. DES interferes with fetal reproductive tract differentiation,

and females exposed in utero have an increased risk of clear-cell adenocarcinoma of the vagina and cervix, reproductive tract abnormalities, poor pregnancy outcomes, infertility, and may have an increased risk of breast cancer, although this finding is less clear.[6,7] Males exposed to DES in utero may have genital tract abnormalities such as undescended testicles; there is also a possible link to prostate and testicular cancer.[7] Some evidence exists that these reproductive tract effects may be passed on to the subsequent generation, DES granddaughters and grandsons, with a greater risk of menstrual irregularities, infertility, and cancer.[6]

It is not only during fetal growth that there is risk from EDCs and other environmental exposures. Other important developmental periods include the early postnatal period, childhood, and adolescence. For example, girls who are exposed to EDCs that mimic estrogen prior to puberty, when the breast tissue is very sensitive to low levels of estrogen, have an increased risk of developing breast cancer later in life.[8] The Endocrine Disruption Exchange (TEDX) has developed resources to use when investigating EDCs and timing of exposures. The TEDX Critical Windows of Development Web application is an interactive timeline that links the timing of normal human development to research on low-dose and/or endocrine-disrupting chemicals.[9]

Epigenetics refers to changes in the structure of deoxyribonucleic acid (DNA). These changes do not alter the DNA sequence but change how cells interact with that gene, as shown in **Figure 3-1**. These changes are also heritable and can be passed from one generation to the next. Stress, diet, and exposures to environmental contaminants can all cause epigenetic changes. In utero exposures can also cause epigenetic changes that lead to increased susceptibility to cancers, obesity, and heart disease.[10,11]

Since the 1950s, both the number and total amount of chemicals being produced have increased exponentially, with more than 84,000 chemicals now registered for use in the United States.[12] These chemicals are regulated by the US Environmental Protection Agency (EPA) under the Toxic Substances Control Act (TSCA) of 1976. When TSCA was passed, it grandfathered in more than 60,000 chemicals already on the market and approved them as safe for use.

Unlike pharmaceuticals, chemicals regulated by TSCA do not have to be tested for safety before being placed on the market. The EPA has required comprehensive safety testing to be performed on only 200 of the chemicals regulated under TSCA and has restricted the use of only five of these chemicals. The EPA must prove that a chemical is harmful, as opposed to a company proving a chemical is safe, before going into the marketplace, and this burden of proof has been set so high that the EPA was unsuccessful in restricting asbestos, a known human carcinogen. TSCA also allows manufacturers to keep chemical ingredients secret. Approximately 20% of chemicals are classified as trade secrets. This lack of transparency hinders providers' ability to document health impacts of exposures.

In contrast to the United States, the European Union passed the Registration, Evaluation, Authorisation and Restriction of Chemicals (REACH) regulation in 2005.[13] This regulation is touted as the strictest chemical regulation law in the world and requires manufacturers to prove their chemicals are safe. It also addresses substances of very high concern (SVHC), which are categorized due to their potential to harm human health or the environment. The use of these chemicals is strictly regulated, and replaced in most cases with a safer alternative. REACH encourages innovation and the production of safer products. This type of regulatory action will significantly decrease exposures to harmful chemicals and prevent harm to human health and the environment.

Besides assessing for and addressing environmental exposures, healthcare providers also

Figure 3-1 Epigenetic mechanisms and health endpoints.

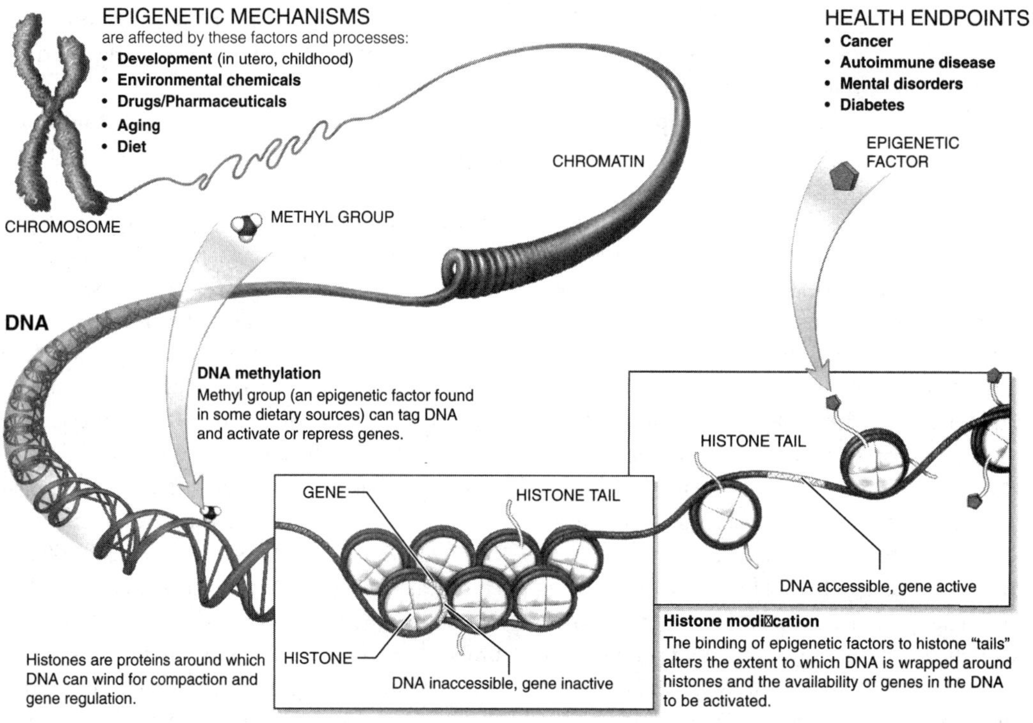

EPIGENETIC MECHANISMS
are affected by these factors and processes:
• **Development** (in utero, childhood)
• **Environmental chemicals**
• **Drugs/Pharmaceuticals**
• **Aging**
• **Diet**

CHROMOSOME

METHYL GROUP

CHROMATIN

DNA

DNA methylation
Methyl group (an epigenetic factor found in some dietary sources) can tag DNA and activate or repress genes.

HEALTH ENDPOINTS
• **Cancer**
• **Autoimmune disease**
• **Mental disorders**
• **Diabetes**

EPIGENETIC FACTOR

HISTONE TAIL

DNA accessible, gene active

GENE

HISTONE TAIL

Histones are proteins around which DNA can wind for compaction and gene regulation.

HISTONE

DNA inaccessible, gene inactive

Histone modification
The binding of epigenetic factors to histone "tails" alters the extent to which DNA is wrapped around histones and the availability of genes in the DNA to be activated.

Reproduced from National Center for Biotechnology Information. Epigenomics help. Bethesda, MD: Author; Published January 20, 2011. Retrieved from: http://www.ncbi.nlm.nih.gov/books/NBK45788/.

need to be involved in policy change. There is only so much that individuals can do to reduce their exposure without regulatory action. These policy changes may include reforming TSCA to be more protective of health like REACH, enforcing and strengthening clean air and water regulations, and addressing climate change. The American Nurses Association has been a leader in incorporating environmental health into the standards for advanced practice nurses and has passed a number of resolutions addressing environmental health principles, chemical exposures, healthy foods, and clean energy choices.[14]

Clinical Care

Prevention is essential to healthcare sustainability and is a key component to addressing many chronic diseases. Most chronic diseases arise from a complex array of factors including intrinsic genetic susceptibility, environmental exposures, behavior, age, and stage of development. Examples of diseases whose development may be attributed to environmental factors include:

• Reproductive impacts (infertility, reproductive tract abnormalities, poor pregnancy outcomes)

- Cancer (breast, prostate, kidney, thyroid, childhood cancers)
- Congenital anomalies (cleft palate, cardiac defects, hypospadias)
- Learning and developmental disabilities (autism, attention deficit hyperactivity disorder [ADHD])
- Lung disease (asthma, asbestosis)
- Cardiovascular disease
- Obesity
- Endocrine disorders (type 2 diabetes)

The women's healthcare provider's responsibility, relative to environmental health, is to understand and apply the knowledge and risks related to environmental exposures. Anticipatory guidance, counseling, and referral are ways that environmental health practice is implemented. With the majority of practices now utilizing electronic health records, an opportunity exists to streamline the assessment of environmental exposures and provide anticipatory guidance. For example, a decision tree can be created that will direct the provider in follow-up questions if an exposure is identified, provide recommendations for referrals, and automatically print out teaching sheets for the patient. The use of this technology can help increase provider confidence and encourage the incorporation of environmental health into standard practice.

Assessment of Risk

Assessment of risk, which includes a health history of the patient, should be made at initial healthcare visits and updated at subsequent visits as indicated (see **Table 3-1**). Questions about a woman's environment are basic to the health history. This is particularly true for women who might become pregnant or who have unexplained symptoms. Preconception visits always should include environmental screening, because the effects of exposure to environmental toxins vary depending on the developmental stage of the fetus.[9]

Environmental exposures can trigger illnesses or cause exacerbations of underlying medical conditions. For example, in respiratory illnesses such

Table 3-1 Contents of Healthcare Visits Relative to Environmental Health

Visit Type	Environmental History	Focused Environmental History	Anticipatory Guidance	Focused Physical Exam*	Appropriate Laboratory/ Procedures	Appropriate Consultation or Referral
Preconception	X		X	X	X	X
Initial Prenatal	X		X	X	X	X
Prenatal		X	X	X	X	X
Interconceptional	X		X	X	X	X
Post-Childbearing	X		X	X	X	X
Illness	X		X	X	X	X

An "X" indicates that these visits should include the particular action.

* Includes appropriate screenings for cancer depending on age, history, family history, and other factors, such as breast examination and mammogram.

Box 3-1 Evaluation for Environmental Exposure

- Are the symptoms present or worse in certain locations (e.g., the workplace)?
- What is the timing of the symptoms (e.g., every day, only during the week, only on weekends)?
- When did the symptoms begin?
- Is there something else associated with the symptoms (e.g., a particular activity)?
- Does anyone else that you know have the same symptom(s)?
  - If yes, who are they or how are they associated with you?

---

as asthma and other airway diseases, environmental tobacco smoke (ETS) is the most commonly associated environmental toxin. Lead poisoning may present with recurrent abdominal pain, seizures, irritability, constipation, developmental delays, or unexplained coma.[15] Most often, because there are not symptoms that immediately suggest an environmental cause, it is important to actively consider environment when presented with a case that has atypical symptoms or that is unresponsive to treatment. In contrast, many environmental exposures may not present with acute symptoms. Effects such as increased cancer risk occur most often with chronic low-level exposures.

Some questions to ask are similar to those used to evaluate pain and are shown in **Box 3-1**.

History and Physical Examination

An environmental health history that was developed for use with women of childbearing age is shown in **Table 3-2**.[16] This easy-to-use tool assesses for common exposures that impact reproductive health and provides actions that women can implement. The form can be given to the woman as she is filling out other health history paperwork. It provides her with basic information and recommends ways to reduce exposures.

By providing basic information during the assessment process, environmental teaching is streamlined. The tool can be modified based on

regional concerns and can be expanded to include other environmental health questions, such as occupational exposures. Any warning signs need further investigation and may require consultation or referral. It should be used as any health history tool is used, allowing the provider to focus the remainder of the patient encounter on the most likely risks.

The Agency for Toxic Substances and Disease Registry (ATSDR) has developed a mnemonic, I PREPARE, to use when developing customized questions and to prompt guidance and educational materials (see **Box 3-2**).[17]

This tool is especially useful in eliciting information about possible workplace exposures. Workplace exposure questions from I PREPARE include those shown in **Box 3-3**.

The physical examination includes careful evaluation of any potential risks identified in the history. For many providers, this will mean increased awareness of common symptoms related to environmental health risks, some of which are addressed specifically in this chapter. Areas of concern may require laboratory testing, consultation, or referral for evaluation by an expert in environmental health.

Laboratory

Laboratory testing is of limited value in environmental health, particularly in the primary healthcare setting. Specific laboratory tests that identify exposures are not available for many suspected

Table 3-2 Environmental Exposure Assessment

The growing fetus can be particularly sensitive to many of the chemicals a woman is exposed to in her daily life. However, there are many ways that a woman who is pregnant, or thinking of becoming pregnant, can reduce her risk of exposures to these chemicals. This assessment will help you identify some of these risks and give you suggestions on how you can minimize your exposure. If you have specific questions or would like more information put a check at the "?" box and discuss this assessment with your healthcare provider.

Name: _____

Date: _____

Question	Yes	No	?	Why Do We Ask This Question?	Steps to Reduce Risks
Was your house/apartment built before 1978? Has your home been tested for lead?				Buildings built before 1978 may contain lead paint. Lead can cause damage to the brain and neurologic system. Babies and children are especially sensitive to these effects.	• If your home was built before 1978, it should be tested for lead. • Maintain your home to prevent paint from chipping or peeling. Chipping paint may release lead into the air.
Does your home have a smoke detector? Does your home have a carbon monoxide detector?				Carbon monoxide is an odorless, colorless gas that is harmful to human health. Having working smoke and carbon monoxide detectors in your home can help save lives.	• Smoke detectors should be on all floors and in bedrooms. • There should be a carbon monoxide detector on all levels in a home with a combustion-heating source (uses a flame to produce heat) or a garage.
Has your home been tested for radon?				Radon is a cancer-causing gas and is the second leading cause of lung cancer.	• All homes should be tested for radon. Testing is easy and inexpensive.

© davidhurjak/Shutterstock

© Dennis Cox/Shutterstock

(continues)

Table 3-2 Environmental Exposure Assessment *(continued)*

Question	Yes	No	?	Why Do We Ask This Question?	Steps to Reduce Risks
Does your home water come from a well? Do you live in an older home or building?				Well water should be tested routinely for contaminants. Pipes in some older homes may contain lead.	• Have your well water tested. • Run the tap for at least 60 seconds to flush out sitting water and always start with cold water for cooking. • Use a home water filter that removes lead.
Do you use pesticides (chemicals used to kill insects, rodents, weeds): In your home? In your yard? On your pets? This includes flea collars, dips, once-a-month products. At your workplace? If yes, what:				Many chemicals in pesticides are suspected of being harmful to the fetus. They may also cause health problems in infants, children, and even adults. There are alternatives to using pesticides, such as Integrated Pest Management (IPM), which is being used in many workplaces and homes. This method of pest control works through a variety of methods so that fewer pesticides need to be used.	• Eliminate items that attract pests. Keep surfaces clean of food residues, keep food in containers or in the fridge, and keep trash contained. • Use less toxic methods of pest control such as sticky traps and boric acid. • Take off your shoes when you enter the house to avoid tracking in pesticides, lead, and other toxins through the house.

© GraphicsRF/Shutterstock

© DeiMosz/Shutterstock

Do you smoke (cigarettes, cigars, pot, other substances)?

Smoke contains chemicals that can be harmful to the growing fetus. Some of these can make the baby grow too slowly, develop asthma, or have learning problems after birth. Infants and children are also very sensitive to these chemicals.

- Make your home and car smoke free.
- Do not allow family, visitors, or childcare providers to smoke in your home or car.
- If you smell smoke, it means you're breathing in smoke.

Is smoking allowed in your home, car, or workplace?

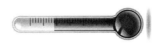

© PiXXart/Shutterstock

Is there a mercury thermometer in your home?

Do you use traditional or cultural remedies that contain mercury or mercurio as an ingredient?

Do you use compact fluorescent light (CFL) bulbs? These are energy-efficient bulbs used in place of standard light bulbs.

Mercury exposure during pregnancy can cause problems with how the fetus's brain and nervous system develop.

- Use only non-mercury thermometers.
- Do not use mercury-containing remedies.
- CFLs contain a small amount of mercury. Do not throw mercury-containing products in the trash. Contact your local trash collector for instructions on safe disposal.

© meaculpa_1/Shutterstock

(continues)

Table 3-2 Environmental Exposure Assessment *(continued)*

Question	Yes	No	?	Why Do We Ask This Question?	Steps to Reduce Risks
Do you come in contact with chemicals at home or where you work, such as cleaning supplies, medications, or other chemicals? If yes, what: Do you use air fresheners, plug-ins, or incense? Do you use strong-smelling/fragrant personal care products, such as perfume, deodorant, nail polishes?				Some chemicals require special handling or may not be safe to use while pregnant. Products that have strong scents or fragrance as an ingredient may contain chemicals that have been linked with negative health effects, such as cancer and infertility.	• Practice safe handling techniques if using chemicals in the workplace and discuss with your healthcare provider if they need to be avoided during pregnancy. • Use natural or green cleaners if possible and wear gloves when cleaning to avoid getting cleaners on your skin. • Minimize use of air fresheners and incense. • Decrease the number of personal care products you use. Avoid strong-smelling personal care products and purchase fragrance-free if possible.
Do you eat fish? If yes, how often: What kind(s):				Fish is a great food to eat while pregnant. However, some fish contain higher levels of mercury and need to be avoided by pregnant women, toddlers, and children. Do not eat shark, swordfish, king mackerel, or tilefish as they have high levels of mercury.	• Most fish contain some mercury. Usually, the larger the fish, the more mercury they contain. Fish with low levels of mercury include shrimp, pollock, tilapia, and salmon. • Avoid albacore tuna while pregnant and eat only 1–2 cans of chunk light tuna per week.

© AWesleyFloyd/Shutterstock

© Viktorija Reuta/Shutterstock

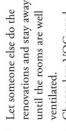	Do you eat fresh fruits and vegetables? If yes, how often: Do you eat locally grown or organic produce? If yes, how often:	Fresh fruits and vegetables are an important part of a healthy diet. Produce grown organically is grown without the use of pesticides. Locally grown produce may be grown with fewer pesticides even if it is not labeled organic.	Try to buy organic apples, bell peppers, celery, spinach, peaches, nectarines, kale, grapes, potatoes, cherries, blueberries, and strawberries.

© Alkestida/Shutterstock

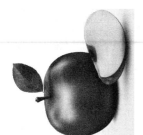	Do you use water bottles or baby bottles made out of polycarbonate plastic (a hard and clear plastic or labeled #7)? Do you eat canned foods, soups, or baby formula? Do you microwave your food in plastic?	Polycarbonate plastic and many food can liners contain bisphenol A (BPA), a chemical that may interfere with how hormones work in the body. Avoid using these plastics and, if needed, purchase plastics labeled BPA-free. Microwaving in plastic containers may cause chemicals in the plastic to go into the food.	• Avoid using polycarbonate plastic and look for plastics labeled BPA-free. • Choose fresh or frozen products instead of canned, and use powdered baby formula instead of liquid. • Microwave in glass or ceramic if possible.

© Yershov Oleksandr/Shutterstock

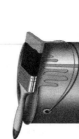	Are you planning on doing any renovations, including painting, in your home while you are pregnant?	The dust from paint, sheet rock, and other building materials can contain lead and other toxins that can be breathed in. Some home improvement products contain chemicals called volatile organic compounds (VOCs), which can cause breathing problems.	• Let someone else do the renovations and stay away until the rooms are well ventilated. • Choose low-VOC products if possible.

© Nasared/Shutterstock

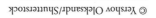

Box 3-2 I PREPARE

I—Investigate potential exposures

P—Present work

R—Residence

E—Environmental concerns

P—Past work

A—Activities

R—Referrals and resources

E—Educate

Data from Agency for Toxic Substances and Disease Registry. Environmental exposure history. Atlanta, GA: US Department of Health and Human Services; n.d. Retrieved from: http://www.atsdr.cdc.gov/asbestos/site-kit/docs/IPrepareCard.pdf; Paranzino GK, Butterfield P, Nastoff T, Ranger C. I PREPARE: Development and clinical utility of an environmental exposure history mnemonic. *AAOHN J.* 2005;53:37-42.

Box 3-3 Evaluation Related to Work Exposures

At present workplace:

- Are you exposed to solvents, dust, fumes, radiation, loud noise, pesticides, or other chemicals?
- Are work clothes worn at home?
- Do you wear personal protective gear?
- Do your coworkers have similar health problems?

Past workplace:

- What are your past work experiences?
- Have you ever been in the military, worked on a farm, or done seasonal work?

---

toxins, nor would they be particularly useful in guiding practice. Many of these tests are extremely expensive and are unlikely to be covered by insurance. Exceptions include tests for lead and mercury levels, although normal blood levels do not exclude mercury poisoning. Even if such tests were readily available, few, if any, treatments exist that can effectively eliminate toxins from the body or mitigate their short- or long-term effects.

Diagnosis, Treatment, and Referral

Depending on the type of exposure, the Pediatric Environmental Health Specialty Units (PEHSUs) are an excellent resource on the health impacts, diagnosis, and management of exposures. There are PEHSUs located throughout the United States, and while they are focused on children's health, many of these centers are staffed with reproductive healthcare professionals as well as toxicologists.[18] The local or state health department is another resource for information on particular environmental hazards and individual exposures (thus aiding in diagnosis). Health department staff can also assist with locating appropriate consultants. As with any diagnosis when environmental risks are present, a plan should be developed that includes further testing, consultation, referral, and other interventions, as appropriate.

Anticipatory Guidance

Many of the toxins to which women are exposed have no treatment other than prevention of further exposure. Therefore, anticipatory guidance is the key intervention in clinical practice. The guidance given depends on the reason for the healthcare visit and individual characteristics such as the patient's childbearing status. For example, a preconception visit would focus on past and present environmental risks such as chemical exposures and ways to avoid exposures at home and the workplace. The woman could be counseled on risks to the fetus associated with chemical exposures and given tools and resources to decrease these exposures. To address the realities of a busy practice as well as the enormity of discussion or intervention for possible environmental exposures, an assessment tool that incorporates both assessment and guidance, such as the one provided in Table 3-2, could be used. Practices may also develop a packet of information that could be given to patients on environmental exposures. There are many scientifically accurate resources already developed that could be added to such a packet and Web resources such as those provided in **Tables 3-3** and **3-4**.

The Environment and Patient Care—Issues and Foundation

The concept of environmental justice has emerged, because environmental pollutants in the United States disproportionately affect lower socioeconomic groups. Environmental justice is achieved when everyone enjoys the same degree of protection from environmental health hazards and has equal access to a healthy environment in which to live, learn, and work.[19]

Women's healthcare providers have an opportunity to move this environmental justice and environmental health agenda forward by continuing to provide services to and advocate for vulnerable populations. Approximately 70% of the women and newborns seen by midwives are considered vulnerable by virtue of age, socioeconomic status, education, ethnicity, or place of residence. Many of the women served by midwives in the United States receive public sources of insurance coverage indicating near or at poverty level. Such populations often have the least access to information that can help them to make informed decisions about their health care. These same populations also share many of the same characteristics as the communities served by environmental justice grants made by the federal government.[20]

Two issues are particularly relevant to women's healthcare providers and their clients: breastfeeding and breast cancer.

Breastfeeding

The benefits of breastfeeding are substantial for both the infant and the mother. The American Academy of Pediatrics highlights that breastfed infants are less likely to develop illnesses such as pneumonia, diarrhea, ear infections, bacterial meningitis, bacteremia, urinary infections, type 1 and type 2 diabetes, and childhood obesity.[20] Other clearly demonstrated benefits include maternal health improvements such as reduction in postpartum bleeding, earlier return to prepregnancy weight, reduced risk of premenopausal breast cancer, and reduced risk of osteoporosis. However, human milk is not invulnerable to environmental toxins:

The goodness of breast milk—and indeed a mother's very ability to produce it—is compromised by the presence of toxic chemicals in the human food chain. The question is not whether we should feed our babies chemically contaminated, yet clearly superior, breast milk or chemically uncontaminated, yet clearly inferior, formula. The question is, what do we need to do to get chemical contaminants out of breast milk?[21]

Biomonitoring studies offer evidence that some of the most persistent pollutants in the

Table 3-3 Environmental Health Resources

Resource	Explanation	Website
Alliance of Nurses for Healthy Environments	Leading nursing organization focusing on environmental health. Website has a number of resources: assessment tools, eTextbook, information on environmental contaminants and health impacts, and can be used to connect with other nurses interested in environmental health.	http://www.enviRN.org
Health Care Without Harm (HCWH)	HCWH has a wide array of publications, information, and programs on many of the health hazards encountered in health care. Additionally, this organization provides many opportunities for healthcare providers to become involved in making health care safer for patients, families, and communities.	http://www.noharm.org
U.S. Environmental Protection Agency	Excellent website and publications relevant to almost all aspects discussed in this chapter, including environmental justice, pregnancy and children's health, reproductive health, and endocrine disruptor screening program.	http://www.epa.gov/ Environmental Justice: http://www.epa.gov/environmentaljustice/ Endocrine Disruptor Screening Program: http://www.epa.gov/endocrine-disruption/endocrine-disruptor-screening-program-edsp-overview Office of Children's Health Protection: http://www.epa.gov/children/
National Institute of Environmental Health Sciences (NIEHS)	NIEHS funds research on environmental health and provides resources for scientists, healthcare providers, and the public. Informational materials for children and adults are also provided.	http://www.niehs.nih.gov/
Breast Cancer Fund	Dedicated to preventing breast cancer by exposing and eliminating environmental causes of breast cancer. Website has the latest science and recommendations to prevent exposures.	http://breastcancerfund.org/
Environmental Work Group (EWG)	Advocacy organization that produces excellent resources for consumers. EWG has a number of tools to help consumers choose safe products.	http://www.ewg.org

Pediatric Environmental Health, 3rd Edition[15]	Geared toward the pediatrician, although also very relevant to women's healthcare providers. Lists of toxins. Very good discussion of communication of risk to clients as well as how to advocate for environmental policy.	See extensive resource list at the end of the book: http://ebooks.aappublications.org/content/pediatric-environmental-health-3rd-edition
National Library of Medicine	Excellent environmental resources. LactMed database has extensive information on drugs and chemicals and their impacts on breastfeeding	TOXNET Database (toxicology, hazardous chemicals, environmental health, and toxic releases): http://toxnet.nlm.nih.gov/ Environmental Health and Toxicology: http://sis.nlm.nih.gov/enviro.html Drugs and Lactation Database (LactMed): http://toxnet.nlm.nih.gov/newtoxnet/lactmed.htm
Agency for Toxic Substances and Disease Registry (ATSDR)	Website has a number of great resources for healthcare providers. These include case studies that are self-instructional continuing education primers and excellent information on the toxicity of specific chemicals.	http://www.atsdr.cdc.gov/ Case Studies in Environmental Medicine http://www.atsdr.cdc.gov/csem/csem.html I PREPARE pocket card: http://www.atsdr.cdc.gov/asbestos/site-kit/docs/IPrepareCard.pdf
Collaborative on Health and the Environment	International collaborative whose mission is to maintain a dialogue and foster collaboration on environmental factors affecting human health.	http://www.healthandenvironment.org The Ecology of Breast Cancer http://www.healthandenvironment.org/uploads/docs/EcologyOfBC_Intro.pdf
Organization of Teratology Information Specialists (OTIS)	Nonprofit organization of physicians, genetics counselors, and others dedicated to dissemination of information about environmental risks during pregnancy.	http://mothertobaby.org/
Migrant Clinicians Network	Tools for assessment and management of acute exposure, patient materials.	http://www.migrantclinician.org
Beyond Pesticides	Low and nontoxic pesticide resources.	http://www.beyondpesticides.org
The Endocrine Disruption Exchange (TEDX)	Nonprofit dedicated to collecting and sharing information on endocrine-disrupting chemicals.	http://www.endocrinedisruption.org

Table 3-4 Resources from Environmental Organizations

- Program on Reproductive Health and the Environment—a great patient handout, "Toxic Matters":
  http://prhe.ucsf.edu/prhe/toxicmatters.html
- MotherToBaby, "Mold and Pregnancy":
  https://mothertobaby.org/fact-sheets/mold-pregnancy/pdf/
- Centers for Disease Control and Prevention, "Mold: Basic Facts":
  http://www.cdc.gov/mold/faqs.htm
- Natural Resources Defense Council, "Guide to Protecting Your Family's Health—Mercury in Fish":
  http://www.nrdc.org/health/effects/mercury/walletcard.pdf
- Environmental Working Group, "Skin Deep Cosmetics Database":
  http://www.ewg.org/skindeep/
- Environmental Working Group, "Shoppers Guide to Pesticides in Produce":
  http://www.ewg.org/foodnews/
- Environmental Working Group, "Guide to Healthy Cleaning":
  http://www.ewg.org/guides/cleaners
- American Academy of Pediatrics, *Pediatric Environmental Health*, 3rd ed:
  http://ebooks.aappublications.org/content/pediatric-environmental-health-3rd-edition
- Women's Voices for the Earth, ingredients in cleaning products:
  http://www.womensvoices.org
- Women's Voices for the Earth, less toxic cleaning product recipes:
  http://www.womensvoices.org/protect-your-health/cleaning-products/green-cleaning-recipes/
- Beyond Pesticides, how to get rid of specific pests:
  http://www.beyondpesticides.org/resources/managesafe/choose-a-pest
- Beyond Pesticides, less toxic pesticides:
  http://www.beyondpesticides.org/
- National Institute of Environmental Health Sciences, children's online materials on environmental health:
  http://kids.niehs.nih.gov/
- Breast Cancer Fund, canned foods to avoid wallet card:
  http://www.breastcancerfund.org/assets/pdfs/tips-fact-sheets/tip-card-ten-canned-foods-to.pdf

environment are expressed in human breast milk.[2,22] However, the evidence is limited by the lack of consistency in protocol development, techniques used for collection, and analyses.[23,24] What are the implications of this evidence for the prospective mother? What are the risks and benefits of breastfeeding in light of this evidence? Are the same contaminants present in cow's milk, soy products, and/or infant formula? It is imperative that midwives and other women's healthcare providers understand the possible health implications of the contaminants as they relate to the many benefits that breastfeeding affords both the baby and the mother.

The contaminants being measured include, but are not limited to, heavy metals such as lead and mercury, chlorinated pesticides (including DDT), flame retardants, BPA, phthalates, synthetic fragrances such as musks, various industrial chemicals, fungicides, furans, and other pesticides. Many of these chemicals are persistent in the environment and bioaccumulate as they move up the food chain. Breastfed infants are at the pinnacle of the food chain as they derive all of their sustenance from another human, who is already at the top of the food chain, and are the final destination of these contaminants.[25] Many of these same chemicals are lipophilic, meaning they are easily stored in body fat and with contin-ued exposure and due to their lengthy half-lives bioaccumulate in adipose tissue. When a woman breastfeeds, these chemicals are released from fat cells into her breast milk and then into the infant. Contaminants have been found in breast milk of women from countries from around the world as diverse as Vietnam, the United States, the Netherlands, and Kazakhstan.

Studies have examined trends in the composition and concentrations of these chemicals in human milk. Other studies have looked at the daily intakes and body burdens of various chemicals in infants and the adverse effects that these chemicals may pose to the infant in utero and postnatally. Overwhelmingly, studies comparing breast- and bottle-fed infants who were also exposed in utero to environmental contaminants, have found that breastfeeding provides a protective effect and counteracts negative developmental outcomes from in utero exposures. Boersma and Lanting studied cognitive development in children exposed prenatally to polychlorinated biphenyls (PCBs) and dioxins.[26] The authors found that breastfeeding had a beneficial effect on cognitive development, fluency of movement, and quality of movement when measured at 18 and 42 months and 6 years of age when compared to formula feeding. The authors show "evidence that breastfeeding counteracts the adverse developmental effects of PCBs and dioxins." In a 2006 study by Eskenazi and colleagues, the researchers also found protective effects of breastfeeding when women had high prenatal exposures to the pesticides DDT and DDE.[27] Neurodevelopmental studies can have significant confounders as children age, such as home environment and maternal IQ, and as stated by Nickerson, "both human and animal studies have demonstrated the persistent organic pollutants and other pollutants rarely occur individually, and the effects of these chemicals are quite complex, as are the neurodevelopmental processes of humans."[28]

Human milk substitutes may not be safe from environmental contaminants either. Cow's milk–based infant formulas may contain chemical and hormone residues, antibiotics, and bovine growth hormone. Recent analyses of the most widely used formulas in the United Kingdom contained aluminum contamination at levels at least twice the level recommended by the European Union for drinking water.[29] Milk- and soy-based formulas are also subject to industrial poisoning accidents, such as the melamine-contaminated formula that resulted in 3 deaths and more than 13,000 hospitalizations in China, as well as preparation errors.[30] In addition to the occasions when these formulas are watered down in an attempt to save on cost, another concern is that the product may be reconstituted with water contaminated with diarrhea-causing bacteria, pesticides, or heavy metals. These issues are particularly relevant for the developing world.

In predominantly agricultural Midwestern states, many bottle-fed infants may be exposed to the pesticide atrazine when formula is reconstituted with contaminated tap water. Infant hair manganese levels are also high in formula-fed infants because of the high content of this element in infant formulas, especially soy-based formulas. Elevated levels of manganese may be associated with various attention problems in children. Infant soy products have high levels of phytoestrogens, which could have endocrine-disrupting effects.[31] They may also be made from genetically altered soy, the effects of which are unknown.

Researchers as well as national and international public health organizations currently agree that the benefits of breastfeeding far outweigh the possible risks that may or may not be associated with contaminants in human breast milk. In 2007, the World Health Organization (WHO), as part of their breast milk biomonitoring protocols stated, "Evidence for the health advantages of breastfeeding and scientific evidence to support breastfeeding has continued to increase. . . . On a population basis, exclusive breastfeeding for six months is the recommended feeding mode for the vast majority of infants."[32]

Breast milk contamination tends to be a frequent topic in the popular press. Clinicians need to be prepared to counsel patients on the importance of breastfeeding and the positive health benefits for both mother and child. The majority of exposures to the chemicals of concern and breastfeeding occur through the diet, so preconception diet counseling, such as reducing intake of animal fats and avoiding contaminated fish, is an important component to preconception visits.

Breast Cancer

Once primarily a disease of women beyond childbearing age, breast cancer is increasingly being seen in women in their 20s and 30s. In the 1940s, a woman's lifetime risk of breast cancer was 1 in 22. Today, it is 1 in 8.[33] Worldwide, breast cancer is the most commonly diagnosed form of cancer and is the leading cause of cancer-related deaths among women.[34] Environmental/lifestyle risk factors for breast cancer include:

- Recent oral contraceptive use (risk disappears within 4 years after discontinuation of use)
- Combination hormone therapy
- Alcohol consumption
- Exposure to environmental tobacco smoke (ETS)
- Exposure to radiation, especially to the chest

Genetics and family history make up only 5–10% of breast cancer diagnoses, so researchers are now investigating environmental factors as an important component in the etiology of the disease.[34] The Interagency Breast Cancer and Environmental Research Coordinating Committee highlights that "prevention is the key to reducing the burden of breast cancer" and addressing environmental exposures is an essential component of prevention.[35] A number of exposure sources to chemicals linked to breast cancer are from EDCs in cleaning products, pesticides, prescription drugs, and fuels. Seemingly innocuous sources include some cosmetics, plastic wrap on food (a source of phthalates), personal care items such as deodorant, and some fragrances. Lifestyle factors that can reduce the risk of breast cancer include weight loss, nutritional focus on plant-based diet, and moderate exercise 30–60 minutes, 5–7 days a week.[36,37]

Common Environmental Risks

This section reviews common toxins that are particularly hazardous to women, fetuses, and children. Some of the information about specific toxins focuses on effects on children because they are disproportionately affected by these toxins due to their developmental stages and behaviors (e.g., hand-to-mouth activity and rapidly developing body systems).

Molds

Among the common molds that affect human health are *Cladosporium*, *Penicillium*, *Aspergillus*, *Alternaria*, and *Stachybotrys chartarum* (black mold).

SOURCES OF EXPOSURE

Molds can enter the home via doorways, windows, ventilation systems, water pipes, and heating or air conditioning units. Mold thrives in damp areas such as unventilated bathrooms, flooded basements, and greenhouses and other areas where indoor plants are grown. Different types of mold can grow in paint, paper or cardboard, carpet, and on other household surfaces.

ROUTES OF CONTAMINATION

Exposure to molds can occur via inhalation and direct physical contact.

LEVELS OF EXPOSURE FOR CONCERN

Most of the effects of exposure to mold are in the mucous membranes of the respiratory system, eyes, nose, and throat. The clinical effects can be allergic (e.g., sneezing, eye irritation, rhinitis, coughing, and wheezing) or toxic. Immunocompromised individuals and those with chronic respiratory illness may be at risk of worsening respiratory status with chronic mold exposure.[38] Toxic effects are secondary to inhalation of mycotoxins, which are lipid-soluble and readily absorbed by the airways. Childhood asthma has been linked to infant exposure to high household mold levels.[39] In several cases, pulmonary hemorrhage in young infants was found to be associated with molds, particularly with exposure to *Stachybotrys chartarum*.[40,41] Neurologic impacts, such as fatigue, headaches, and difficulty concentrating, may also be seen.[15]

WAYS TO MINIMIZE EXPOSURE

On a day-to-day basis, household cleaning should address common areas of mold growth, such as wet bathroom walls and sink drains. Use of household dehumidifiers may also decrease mold burden in humid areas. Water and all water-damaged items should be removed within 24 hours of a flood or leak as a preventive intervention. If some mold is already present, the affected area needs to be washed with soap and water, and then with a solution of 1 part bleach to 10 parts water. Protective gloves and eyewear should be worn for any cleanup activities. Doors and windows should be opened to provide fresh air.

IMPACT ON PREGNANCY, LACTATION, AND THE FETUS

There have been no human studies evaluating the impacts of mold exposures on pregnancy or lactation. The Organization of Teratology Information Specialists (OTIS) reports there is no established risk to pregnancy and lactation from mold exposure.[42]

Mercury

SOURCES OF EXPOSURE

Mercury is a neurotoxic heavy metal. It occurs in three forms: the metallic element, inorganic salts, and organic compounds of which the most dangerous is methylmercury. In the metallic form, mercury has industrial uses that include thermometers, batteries, and fluorescent lighting. Exposure to elemental mercury is primarily by fume inhalation after an accidental spill. Inorganic mercury salts are found in some over-the-counter drugs and herbal remedies.

The primary source of environmental mercury in the United States is combustion of coal for energy production. Steel production and waste incinerators also contribute.[43] Mercury is released into the air and then deposited onto land and water surfaces, where it remains indefinitely. Methylmercury, the most toxic organic form, is produced by environmental interaction with carbon; the most common exposure of humans to methylmercury is eating contaminated fish.[44]

A reference dose (RfD) is an amount determined to be safe on the basis of available toxicity information and used to provide a basis for establishing safety standards and guidelines. The mercury RfD is based on mercury levels in the cord blood of children in the Faroe Islands (the population of these islands has a relatively high level of fish consumption); levels at or below this RfD are recommended to prevent neurodevelopmental effects from fetal and childhood exposures.

DIAGNOSIS

Diagnosis of mercury poisoning is made by history and physical examination. Some signs and symptoms are tremors, impaired vision and hearing, paralysis, insomnia, emotional instability, developmental deficits during fetal development, and attention deficit and developmental delays during childhood. Laboratory testing may demonstrate elevated blood mercury, although normal blood levels do not exclude mercury poisoning.[15] Women with elevated mercury levels may not exhibit any symptoms, and in these women it is only through a diet or environmental health history that exposures will be discovered.

TREATMENT

The treatment for exposure to mercury is to eliminate the source. Although chelating agents have been used for treatment of elemental and inorganic mercury poisoning, it is not clear whether this treatment helps. There is no chelating agent approved by the US Food and Drug Administration (FDA) that is effective for organic (methylmercury) poisoning.[45]

Preventing mercury intake is the only way to prevent its effects. As there are potential neurotoxic risks to the fetus and child, fish consumption advisories for pregnant women, for women of childbearing age, and for children are in place in the United States. Fish intake during pregnancy is encouraged, due to the positive impacts of omega-3 fatty acids on fetal neurodevelopment, but women need to be advised on making smart seafood choices so they reduce mercury exposure. The FDA and the EPA advise women of childbearing age, pregnant and nursing women, and young children to avoid some types of fish and shellfish. Their recommendations are:[46]

- Do not eat shark, swordfish, king mackerel, or tilefish.
- Eat up to 12 ounces (two average meals) a week of a variety of fish and shellfish that are lower in mercury. Examples of these are shrimp, canned light tuna, salmon, pollock, and catfish. Because albacore ("white") tuna has more mercury than canned light tuna, only up to 6 ounces of this tuna should be eaten per week.

- Check local advisories about the safety of fish caught in local lakes, rivers, and coastal areas. If no advice is available, eat up to 6 ounces per week of fish caught from local waters, but do not consume any other fish during that week.

Recent data show that albacore tuna may contain much higher levels of mercury, so providers may find it prudent to recommend completely avoiding albacore.[47]

IMPACT ON HEALTH, INCLUDING PREGNANCY, LACTATION, AND THE FETUS

Mercury attacks the central nervous system, kidneys, and lungs. Ingested methylmercury (via fish consumption) crosses the placenta easily, causing decreased IQ levels and adverse neurobehavioral effects.[15] Organic mercury, a powerful teratogen, causes disruption of the normal patterns of neuronal migration and nerve cell histology in the developing brain. Among the gradually developing symptoms are psychomotor retardation, blindness, deafness, and seizures. In 2013, the EPA estimated that 1.4 million women had blood mercury concentrations high enough to place their unborn children at risk of learning disabilities.[43] Based on the US birth rate, 75,000 newborns are at risk each year due to in utero methylmercury exposure.

Polyvinyl Chloride Plastic, Phthalates

Polyvinyl chloride (PVC) is a chlorinated plastic. The use of PVC plastic leads to environmental contamination by dioxin and di-2-ethylhexyl phthalate (DEHP), each of which has different toxic effects. Phthalates are anti-androgenic EDCs. They can impact hormone levels, lower the age of puberty in girls, and increase risk of pregnancy loss.[48] Male infants exposed to phthalates in utero appear to be especially sensitive to the endocrine-disrupting effects with increased risk of nipple retention, decreased ano-genital distance (a measure of feminization of external genitalia), and cryptorchidism.[49] Animal studies have shown that prenatal exposure in rodents substantially increased their risk of breast cancer later in life.[50] Children with high phthalate exposure show evidence of higher asthma and allergy rates as well as adverse effects on fetal growth, cognitive development, and obesity.[51-53] Among adults, higher rates of type 2 diabetes and cardiovascular disease have been shown.[54-56]

SOURCES OF EXPOSURE FOR DIOXIN AND DEHP (PHTHALATES)

Dioxin is created when PVC is manufactured and when materials that contain chlorine are burned. For example, when PVC is burned in a medical or municipal waste incinerator, dioxin is emitted into the air. Dioxin first came to the attention of the US public via Agent Orange, which was used as a defoliant during the Vietnam War. US soldiers and Vietnamese exposed to dioxin now exhibit a number of different illnesses including chronic lymphocytic leukemia, soft-tissue sarcoma, Hodgkin's disease, and chloracne. Long-term exposure to dioxin is linked to impaired immune functioning, endocrine disruption, reproductive effects, and neurologic impacts.[56] The WHO International Agency for Research on Cancer (IARC) has classified dioxin as a known human carcinogen.[57]

PVC plastic is made soft and flexible for most applications by the addition of DEHP. It is widely used by the food and construction industries, as well as in health care. PVC medical products are between 20% and 80% DEHP by weight. Some common sources of dioxin and/or DEHP are:

- Building products (wall and floor coverings, carpet backing, piping, vinyl shower curtains)
- Personal care products—phthalates are added as a fragrance stabilizer (lotions, cosmetics, hair products, nail polish, perfume)
- Children's toys (teething rings, children's meal toy products)
- Food preparation and packaging (plastic wraps, plastic containers, vinyl gloves for food workers)
- Medical products such as intravenous bags and tubing, and other tubing used in dialysis, cardiopulmonary bypass, and enteral and total parenteral nutrition (TPN; the packaging for the product should state if the product contains DEHP.)

ROUTES OF CONTAMINATION

Humans ingest dioxin in food after particles are distributed via incineration into the atmosphere by wind and rain. These particles become lodged in soil, lakes, and rivers, and settle on plants. When humans consume contaminated fish, meat, and dairy products, the bio-accumulative dioxin dose that an animal incurred over its lifespan and stored in its fatty tissue is also ingested. Additionally, the fats in human milk can store dioxin. Inhalation of airborne dioxin particles can also lead to exposure.

DEHP plasticizer is not chemically bound to PVC. During medical procedures with DEHP-containing products, the chemical can be absorbed into the human body when in contact with fluids such as blood, plasma, and drug solutions, or it can be released and migrate when the device is heated. The rate of migration depends on the storage conditions (temperature of the fluid contacting the device, the amount of fluid, the contact time, the extent of shaking or flow rate of the fluid) and the lipophilicity of the fluid.[58]

LEVELS OF EXPOSURE FOR CONCERN

Dioxin is a potent carcinogen at very low levels of exposure, and even daily exposures of dioxin measured in picograms or nanograms can cause toxic effects, including endocrine disruption. In 2012, the EPA released an RfD of dioxin of

0.7 picogram/kg/day. Based on this RfD, adults and children under the age of 5 years currently exceed this exposure level.[59] The general population, through ordinary dietary exposures, carries a current body burden of dioxin that is near or above the levels that cause adverse effects in animal tests.[59] Dioxin levels are falling due to regulatory improvements; however, they still are not at safe levels.[60]

Daily human exposure to DEHP in the United States is significant, but occupational and clinical exposures from DEHP-plasticized medical devices (e.g., blood bags, hemodialysis tubing, nasogastric feeding tubes) further increase body burden levels.

Ways to Minimize Exposure to Dioxin and DEHP

The 2008 Consumer Product Safety Improvement Act prohibited the use of DEHP and certain other phthalates in children's toys and products.[61] To avoid exposure to PVC, dioxin, and phthalates, women are counseled to:

- Choose products not made with vinyl for children's toys, food containers, car seats, crib bumpers, wallpaper, wall coverings, and flooring. If a vinyl product must be used, choose one that is phthalate free.
- Avoid burning PVC (#3) plastic.
- Avoid cooking/microwaving food in plastic containers or with plastic cling wrap.
- Avoid putting plastic in the dishwasher.
- Eat fewer fatty foods (e.g., cheese, red meats, whole milk).
- Avoid personal care products made with phthalates. Avoid all personal care products with "fragrance" on the ingredient list. And limit the total number of products used.

Additionally, healthcare workers can work to prevent the spread of DEHP by advocating that their healthcare facility use alternatives to those products manufactured with DEHP.

Impact on Pregnancy, Lactation, and the Fetus

There is no known way to lower body burdens of toxins generated by PVCs other than to avoid exposure. Thus far, the infant morbidity attributable to exposure to these compounds is believed to come from prenatal exposure to maternal body burden rather than from exposure through breast milk.[3] These effects include lower developmental and intelligence scores, including lower psychomotor scores from newborns. Some nursing infants may be exposed to dioxin levels at high concentrations. However, the long-term impact of exposure to dioxin from breast milk seems to be minimal. While shorter-term studies have shown an association between breast milk intake and adverse cognitive function from dioxin exposure, longer-term studies do not. Long-term studies following breast-fed and formula-fed infants have found an association between pregnancy maternal body burden and poorer cognitive function, but no association between type of feeding and dioxin-related damage.[25,48,57] Therefore, there is *no* recommendation to avoid breastfeeding infants due to dioxin exposure in the mother. Rather, the emphasis should be on reducing the body burden by minimizing exposure to these chemicals.

Based on its earlier safety assessment of DEHP, the FDA issued a public health notification in 2002 that has been updated as recently as 2015, recommending that alternatives to DEHP-containing products be used when procedures that have a high risk of leaching DEHP into the body are performed on male newborns, pregnant women carrying male fetuses, and peripubertal males.[62] These include neonatal TPN with lipids, multiple procedures on sick infants, hemodialysis in prepubescent males, and enteral nutrition for pregnant or lactating females and peripubertal males.

Lead

Lead is a naturally occurring element. Blood levels are low in the absence of industrial activities or other sources indicated as follows.

SOURCES OF EXPOSURE

In the United States, the chief sources of lead exposure for children have been airborne (mainly from leaded gasoline combustion) and inhalation or ingestion of leaded chips or dust from lead-based paints. Lead levels in human milk are low; lead has also been found in canned formula and evaporated milk.[15]

ROUTES OF CONTAMINATION

The most common way that lead poisoning occurs, particularly in children, is through the unintentional ingestion of lead-containing particles, such as lead dust from paint or soil, in water (including public drinking water) or foreign bodies. Lead can also be inhaled as fumes and absorbed via the pulmonary tract.

LEVELS OF EXPOSURE FOR CONCERN

In 2012 the Centers for Disease Control and Prevention (CDC) Advisory Committee on Childhood Lead Poisoning issues new prevention recommendations, based on the premise that no lead level is safe for children and the neurologic effects of lead exposure are permanent; 5 mcg/dL be used as the reference level.[63] Previously, parents may or may not have been told the testing results if a child's blood lead levels were below 10 mcg/dL. This left a large number of children being chronically exposed to lead in the 5–10 mcg/dL range. By identifying children with measurable amounts of lead in their blood parents, healthcare providers, and public health officials can take earlier action to reduce lead exposures. In 2010, the CDC issued "Guidelines for the Identification and Management of Lead Exposure in Pregnant and Lactating Women."[64] While there has been a significant decrease in US blood lead levels, 1% of pregnant women still have blood lead levels 5 mcg/dL or more. See **Figure 3-2** for management recommendations for women of childbearing age and during pregnancy and lactation. All women should be screened for exposures and blood lead levels should be checked if a risk is identified.[64,65] Routine testing for most populations is not recommended.

WAYS TO MINIMIZE EXPOSURE

The public should know the lead level in local tap water sources. This is especially important for infants who are being fed formula reconstituted with tap water. Additionally, prevention of ingestion or inhalation (lead-based paint chips and fuels) is important. Other risk factors for lead exposure are listed in **Box 3-4**. Women can be encouraged to consume adequate amounts of calcium, iron, and zinc and vitamins C, D, and E in order minimize lead absorption from the environment and release of lead from bony body stores. Women should also be screened for pica behavior, because cases of lead poisoning have been reported in women consuming lead-contaminated pottery and soil.[64] Ensuring adequate intake of vitamin C, iron, and calcium may be of even greater importance in these women, because it may minimize further lead exposure from endogenous and exogenous sources.

IMPACT ON PREGNANCY, LACTATION, THE FETUS, AND CHILDREN

Lead levels in human milk are low. Laws enacted in the 1970s that banned lead in gasoline and paint have led to substantial decreases in blood lead levels. Fatal lead encephalopathy has virtually disappeared. However, while lead poisoning is less common, it still occurs, particularly in infants and children living in older substandard housing, in those who emigrated

Figure 3-2 Summary of public health actions in women of childbearing age and pregnant and lactating women based on blood lead levels.

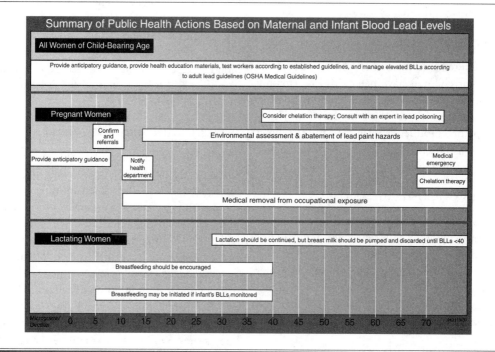

Modified from Centers for Disease Control and Prevention. Guidelines for the identification and management of lead exposure in pregnant and lactating women. Atlanta, GA: US Department of Health and Human Services; 2010. Retrieved from: http://www.cdc.gov/nceh/lead/publications/leadandpregnancy2010.pdf. Accessed February 17, 2016.

from parts of the world where lead exposures are high, and in pregnant women who engage in pica behavior (i.e., eating abnormal things like ash and chalk).

In the human body, the main repository for lead is bone, where the turnover rate is approximately 25 to 30 years. Chronic lead exposure results in significant accumulation of lead in the skeleton. During pregnancy, lactation, and the perimenopausal transition, calcium turnover is greatly increased, which may trigger a release of lead stores from bone. The main effect on children is damage to the central nervous system. Elevated lead levels during pregnancy increase the risk of low birth weight, spontaneous abortion, and gestational hypertension.[64] Health effects of chronic low-level exposure in women include hypertension and other cardiac impacts, poor reproductive outcomes, cognitive decline, and decreased renal function.[64]

Flame Retardants

Halogenated flame retardants (HFRs) are chemicals added to products to make them more resistant to heat and flames, such as polybrominated diphenyl ethers (PBDEs), chlorinated tris, hexabromocyclododecane (HBCD), and

---

Box 3-4 Risk Factors for Lead Exposure in Pregnant and Lactating Women

- Recent immigration from or residency in areas where ambient lead contamination is high (leaded gasoline, industrial exposure)
- Living near a point source of lead, such as lead mines, smelters, or battery-recycling plants (even if the establishment is closed)
- Working with lead or living with someone who does
- Using lead-glazed ceramic pottery to cook, store, or serve food; usually made by traditional methods and imported outside the normal commercial channels
- Eating nonfood substances (pica)
- Using alternative or complementary medicines, herbs, or therapies
- Using imported cosmetics (such as kohl or surma) or certain food products and spices that might be contaminated
- Engaging in certain high-risk hobbies or recreational activities
- Renovating or remodeling older homes by removing lead-based paint or dust without lead hazard controls in place
- Consuming drinking water from lead-lined or lead-contaminated pipes
- Having a history of previous lead exposure or evidence of elevated body burden of lead, particularly those who are deficient in certain key nutrients (calcium, iron)
- Living with someone identified with an elevated lead level

Modified from Centers for Disease Control and Prevention. Guidelines for the identification and management of lead exposure in pregnant and lactating women. Atlanta, GA: US Department of Health and Human Services; 2010. Available at: http://www.cdc.gov/nceh/lead/publications/leadandpregnancy2010.pdf. Accessed February 17, 2016.

---

tetrabromobisphenol A (TBBPA). HFRs are added to a wide range of products, including electronics, furniture, appliances, building materials, and child care products. The levels of HFRs in the US population are up to 20 times higher than in other countries, and biomonitoring studies have found flame retardants in almost all of the US population.[67] One of the reasons that there is such widespread exposure is the flammability standards created in the 1970s to reduce fire deaths from cigarette-related fires. Instead of creating safer cigarettes, these standards focused on the highly flammable polyurethane foam found in furniture and require large amounts of flame retardants to be added to foam furniture in order to meet the standard. These flame retardants have not reduced fire severity and have instead caused widespread exposure to harmful chemicals. Besides the toxicity inherent in these chemicals, they also produce dioxins and furans across their entire lifecycle.

HFRs tend to be lipophilic and bioaccumulative, building up in the body over time. HFRs have been shown to have a number of harmful human health effects. These include:[67]

- Neurodevelopmental effects: Children exposed in utero are at increased risk for autism, ADHD, decreased IQ, and poor motor development.
- Endocrine-disrupting effects: People in homes with higher HFR levels were found to have lower thyroid hormone levels and lower prolactin levels. Males may have lower testosterone levels and children whose mothers have high PBDE levels during pregnancy had lower thyroid hormone levels. There is also an increased risk of diabetes and obesity.
- Reproductive issues: HFRs may decrease sperm counts, increase time to conception, and increase risk of cryptorchidism. There is

also an increased risk of poor pregnancy outcomes including low birth weight, preterm
delivery, and stillbirth.
• Cancer.

Sources of Exposure

Due to the widespread use of HFRs, they are
ubiquitous in the environment and are found in
air, dust, soil, and food. House dust and food are
significant sources of exposure. When HFRs are
burned, such as in a house fire, they produce dioxins. The elevated cancer rates among firefight-
ers are thought to be related to dioxin exposure.[67]

Routes of Contamination

The most common route of ingestion is through
food and accidental ingestion of house dust. Exposure through house dust is of particular concern
for children who are more likely to be crawling
and playing on the floor and because of their
hand-to-mouth activities. Many of the HFRs are
lipophilic and are excreted during breastfeeding.
A 2005 study found US human milk PBDE levels to be 35 to 500 times higher than in other
countries.[68] The two main types of PBDEs were
removed from the market in 2005 due to health
concerns, and if the experiences of other countries that removed PBDE from use are an indication, breast milk levels will decline significantly
over time. HFRs are also found in higher levels in
low-income and minority populations. HFR exposure is also an environmental justice issue. This
is exemplified by a study of women in California
that found low-income and African American
and Latina women had the highest levels of HFRs
worldwide.[69]

Levels of Exposure for Concern

US residents are exposed to significant amounts
of HFRs every day. While there are ways to

minimize these exposures, regulatory action must
be taken that does not require the use of toxic
chemicals in order to pass flammability standards. The main regulation impacting the use
of flame retardants in foam furniture, California
TB 117, was recently updated and went into effect on January 1, 2014.[70] TB 117-2013 will allow
companies to pass these flammability standards
without using flame retardants in soft furnishings, such as couches. However, it is not required
and manufacturers may choose to continue adding these chemicals to their products. Public engagement is needed to pressure manufacturers to
discontinue the use of these toxic chemicals.

Ways to Minimize Exposure

There are a number of ways to reduce exposures:

• Vacuum frequently and use a high-efficiency
  particulate arresting (HEPA) filter.
• Wet mop floors and damp dust furniture
  regularly.
• Wash hands frequently and always before
  eating.
• Avoid polyurethane foam products. Look for
  TB 117-2013 label on foam products and buy
  those marked "contains no added flame retar-
  dant chemicals". If the label is not marked,
  contact the manufacturer and inquire. Do
  not buy products with flame retardants added
  to the foam. This is especially true for infant
  and child products, such as nursing pillows,
  changing pads, and strollers.
• Replace furniture with crumbling foam cushions and make sure foam is covered by fabric.

Bisphenol A

BPA is a chemical that was first developed
as a synthetic estrogen. It is one of the most
widely studied EDCs and is frequently used as
an example of how low doses of chemicals can

impact the endocrine system and produce negative health impacts.

Sources of Exposure

The use of BPA worldwide has doubled since the early 2000s. It is used in polycarbonate plastic, epoxy linings in food and drink cans, PVC, dental sealants, food packaging, and thermal receipts. BPA is an unstable compound that readily leeches out of these products. BPA has been banned from baby bottles and infant formula packaging in the United States. BPA was found in almost all of the urine samples in the latest NHANES data, indicating close to universal exposure.[66] In an unfortunate example of how TSCA has failed to protect human health, as BPA has been removed from products due to the health concerns and public pressure, other chemicals, such as bisphenol S, have been added to products without prior health and safety testing. There is increasing evidence that many products labeled as BPA free still leak estrogen-affecting chemicals.[71,72]

Routes of Contamination

BPA is found in ambient air, house dust, and drinking water and a significant source of exposure is through food sources. BPA readily leeches out of food can linings, especially into acidic and fatty food. Studies have shown rapid increases in BPA blood and urine levels with ingestion of foods and beverages packaged in BPA-containing materials.[73] BPA can also enter the body through skin exposure, such as when handling thermal paper receipts.

Levels of Exposure for Concern

Health impacts of BPA exposure can occur at extremely low doses, especially with fetal exposures. Health impacts seen at low doses include increased risk of breast and prostate cancer, cardiovascular disease, spontaneous abortion, low birth weight, infertility, sexual dysfunction, altered metabolism and obesity, diabetes, immune dysfunction, and neurodevelopmental impacts.[66,73,74]

Ways to Minimize Exposure

There are many ways to minimize exposure to BPA and other estrogen disruptors. Providers can counsel their patients to:

- Limit the use of canned foods. Use fresh fruits and vegetables when possible and frozen when not.
- Avoid plastic food storage containers. Switch to glass or metal.
- Switch to dry beans instead of canned.
- Avoid handling thermal receipts. Do not recycle thermal receipts, because the BPA gets into the recycled paper products.

Pesticides

A pesticide is any substance used to kill an animal or organism. These include insecticides, herbicides, fungicides, and fumigants. The majority of these pesticides work by disrupting reproductive or neurologic function. It is not surprising then that many of the health impacts of pesticide exposures in humans show negative reproductive and neurologic effects. Pesticide use has grown considerably since the 1940s, with less than 200 million pounds used per year in 1945, to more than 1.1 billion pounds being used every year in the United States in 2006–2007.[75]

Sources of Exposure

Exposures can occur through residues on food; pesticide application in the home, workplace, or community; agricultural uses (worker exposure and air and water drift); breastfeeding; and water contamination. Children and the growing fetus are especially vulnerable to these exposures.

Children eat more fruits and vegetables, pound for pound, than adults, and due to their greater time spent on the ground playing and hand-to-mouth activities, they may ingest pesticides tracked into the home or used in the home for pest reduction. Many pesticides readily cross the placenta.

ROUTES OF CONTAMINATION

Exposure can occur through three routes: inhalation, ingestion, and dermal exposures. Agricultural workers and pesticide applicators need to be especially careful when using pesticides and wear appropriate protective equipment. By law, Material Safety Data Sheets, which provide information on proper handling, use, and protective equipment needed, need to be available for employees for each chemical being used.

LEVELS OF EXPOSURE FOR CONCERN

Evidence is increasingly pointing to prenatal exposures to pesticides being particularly damaging to neurologic development. In a study in California's Central Valley, researchers found that when women were exposed to organochlorine pesticides early in pregnancy, the risk of autism among their children increased sharply.[76] In another study of fetal exposures to the pesticide chlorpyrifos, researchers found significant structural changes to the brain in areas related to language, attention, emotions, and control.[77] Other health impacts of fetal and childhood exposures include increased risk of some types of cancers, birth defects (related to seasonal, agricultural, and other work exposures), early puberty, obesity, diabetes, and asthma. Pesticide exposures have also been linked to breast cancer, lymphoma, decreased sperm counts, endocrine disruption, and difficulty conceiving.[6,15,78] Symptoms of acute exposures include headaches, dizziness, nausea and vomiting, and skin irritation. Serious acute exposures can result in difficulty breathing, seizures, and even death.

WAYS TO MINIMIZE EXPOSURE

Providers should recommend the following to minimize exposure to pesticides:

- Pesticides applicators should be instructed not to wear their work shoes into the home, and their clothes should be washed and stored separately from others in the household. The Migrant Clinicians Network has a number of resources for clinicians, including assessment and management tools for acute pesticide exposures and patient education materials especially geared toward agricultural workers and their families
- Encourage use of Integrated Pest Management (IPM) in the home and workplace. IPM can even be used in the healthcare setting. It is common-sense approach that focuses on keeping food and water away from pests, keeping pests out, and using the least toxic pesticides if needed. For non- and low-toxic pest management techniques, see Beyond Pesticides in Tables 3-3 and 3-4.
- If the client has to use pesticides in the home (such as individuals living in apartments that spray periodically), they should make sure all food, food-preparation items, and toys are stored (not on counters). Especially during pregnancy, they should try to stay out of the home for at least 24 hours. They should wash all counters when they return.
- Some fruits and vegetables contain higher levels or greater numbers of pesticides than others. Washing fruits and vegetables is usually not enough to remove the pesticides. If possible, clients should be encouraged to buy organic fruits and vegetables that have the highest levels while buying conventionally grown produce that has the lowest pesticide levels (**Table 3-5**).

Table 3-5 Shopping Guide to Avoid Pesticides

Highest levels/greatest number/most toxic pesticides—try to buy organic	Low levels of pesticides—okay to buy conventionally grown
• Apples	• Asparagus
• Celery	• Avocados
• Cherry tomatoes	• Cabbage
• Cucumbers	• Cantaloupe
• Grapes	• Sweet corn
• Hot peppers	• Eggplant
• Imported nectarines	• Grapefruit
• Kale/collard greens	• Kiwi
• Peaches	• Mangoes
• Potatoes	• Mushrooms
• Spinach	• Onions
• Strawberries	• Papayas
• Summer squash	• Pineapples
• Sweet bell peppers	• Sweet peas (frozen)
	• Sweet potatoes

Data from Environmental Working Group. Shopper's guide to pesticides in produce. Washington, DC: Author. 2013. Retrieved from: https://www.ewg.org/foodnews/.

Climate Change

Due to human activities, the climate is changing. We are now seeing more frequent extreme weather events such as flooding and drought, heat waves, more intense hurricanes and storms, and wildfires. Disease vectors are changing, and in many areas air pollution is on the rise. Women, children, the elderly, and the poor are groups that are disproportionately affected by the health impacts of climate change.[79] In the 2015 Lancet Commission on Health and Climate Change report, the study authors note "Given the potential of climate change to reverse the health gains from economic development, and the health co-benefits that accrue from actions for a sustainable economy, tackling climate change could be the greatest global health opportunity of this century."[80] See **Table 3-6** for a review of how climate change impacts weather events and human health, as described by the CDC.[81]

Women's healthcare providers need to be able to provide anticipatory guidance to clients around impacts of climate change, such as being aware of the potential for mold following floods or counseling patients to limit outdoor activities on hot days when ozone levels could negatively impact respiratory function. Healthcare providers also need to participate in climate change discussions and policies and make sure that health is at the forefront of policy decisions.

Conclusion

Environmental health is an often unrecognized public health concern, and primary care providers can play a vital role in educating women about the problem and its effect on both adults and children. This education extends beyond the assessment and referral of patients for the possible ill effects of environmental hazards. Ideally, it includes anticipatory counseling, which can minimize exposure and guide healthy choices.

Table 3-6 Centers for Disease Control: Weather Events, Health Effects, and Populations Most Affected

Weather Event	Health Effects	Populations Most Affected
Heat waves	Heat stress	Extremes of age, athletes, people with respiratory disease
Extreme weather events, (rain, hurricane, tornado, flooding)	Injuries, drowning	Coastal, low-lying land dwellers, low socioeconomic status (SES)
Droughts, floods, increased mean temperature	Vector-, food- and water-borne diseases	Multiple populations at risk
Sea-level rise	Injuries, drowning, water and soil salinization, ecosystem and economic disruption	Coastal, low SES
Drought, ecosystem migration	Food and water shortages, malnutrition	Low SES, elderly, children
Extreme weather events, drought	Mass population movement, international conflict	General population
Increases in ground-level ozone, airborne allergens and other pollutants	Respiratory disease exacerbations (chronic obstructive pulmonary disease, asthma, allergic rhinitis, bronchitis)	Elderly, children, those with respiratory disease
Climate change generally; extreme events	Mental health	Young, displaced, agricultural sector, low SES

Reproduced from Centers for Disease Control and Prevention. CDC policy on climate change and public health. Atlanta, GA: US Department of Health and Human Services; n.d. Retrieved from: http://www.cdc.gov/climateandhealth/pubs /Climate_Change_Policy.pdf. Accessed February 17, 2016.

References

1. Safer Chemicals, Healthy Families. Chemicals and our health: Why recent science is a call to action. 2012. Available at: http://saferchemicals.org/health-report/. Accessed February 21, 2016.
2. Woodruff TJ, Zota AR, Schwartz JM. Environmental chemicals in pregnant women in the United States: NHANES 2003–2004. *Environ Health Perspect.* 2011;119:878-885.
3. Environmental Working Group. Toxic chemicals found in minority cord blood. 2009. Available at: http://www.ewg.org/news/news-releases/2009/12/02/toxic-chemicals-found-minority-cord-blood. Accessed February 17, 2016.
4. American College of Obstetricians and Gynecologists. Committee Opinion No. 575. Exposure to toxic environmental agents. *Obstet Gynecol.* 2013;122:931-5.
5. American College of Nurse-Midwives. The Effect of Environmental Toxins on Reproductive and Developmental Health. http://www.midwife.org/ACNM/files/ACNMLibraryData/UPLOADFILENAME/000000000292/Environmental-Toxins-June-2015.pdf. Approved June 2015. Accessed November 29, 2015.
6. Woodruff TJ, Carlson A, Schwartz JM, Giudice LC. Proceedings of the summit on environmental

challenges to reproductive health and fertility: executive summary. *Fertil Steril.* 2008;89:281-300.

7. National Cancer Institute. Diethylstilbestrol (DES) and Cancer. Available at: http://www.cancer.gov/cancertopics/factsheet/Risk/DES. Accessed February 17, 2016.

8. Aksglaede L, Juul A, Leffers H, Skakkebaek N, Andersson A. The sensitivity of the child to sex steroids: possible impact of exogenous estrogens. *Hum Reprod Update.* 2006;12:341-349.

9. The Endocrine Disruption Exchange. Prenatal origins of endocrine disruption: Critical windows of development. 2013. Available at: http://endocrinedisruption.org/prenatal-origins-of-endocrine-disruption/critical-windows-of-development/timeline-test/. Accessed February 17, 2016.

10. National Center for Biotechnology Information. Epigenomics help. 2011. Available at: http://www.ncbi.nlm.nih.gov/books/NBK45788/. Accessed February 17, 2016.

11. Barouki R1, Gluckman PD, Grandjean P, Hanson M, Heindel JJ. Developmental origins of non-communicable disease: implications for research and public health. *Environ Health.* 2012;11:42.

12. US Environmental Protection Agency. TSCA Chemical Substance Inventory. Available at: http://www.epa.gov/oppt/existingchemicals/pubs/tscainventory/basic.html. Accessed February 17, 2016.

13. European Chemicals Agency. REACH. Available at: echa.europa.eu/regulations/reach. Accessed February 21, 2016.

14. American Nurses Association House of Delegates. Resolution Index. Available at: http://ananet.nursingworld.org/Main-Menu/Governance/HOD-Delegates/Reference-Process-2012/Resolution-Index_1.aspx. Accessed February 17, 2016.

15. Etzel RA, ed. *Pediatric Environmental Health.* 3rd ed. Elk Grove Village, IL: American Academy of Pediatrics; 2012.

16. Huffling, K. Preconception-Prenatal Assessment. 2011. Available at: http://envirn.org/pg/file/read/26122/preconceptionprenatal-assessment. Accessed February 17, 2016.

17. Paranzino GK, Butterfield P, Nastoff T, Ranger C. I PREPARE: Development and clinical utility of an environmental exposure history mnemonic. *AAOHN J.* 2005;53:37-42.

18. Pediatric Environmental Health Specialty Units. Published 2015. Available at: http://www.pehsu.net/. Accessed February 21, 2016.

19. US Environmental Protection Agency. Environmental justice. Available at: http://www3.epa.gov/environmentaljustice/. Accessed February 17, 2016.

20. American Academy of Pediatrics. AAP policy on breastfeeding and use of human milk. Available at: http://www2.aap.org/breastfeeding/policyOnBreastfeedingAndUseOfHumanMilk.html. Accessed February 17, 2016.

21. Steingraber S. *Having Faith: An Ecologist's Journey to Motherhood.* Cambridge, MA: Perseus Publishing; 2001.

22. Solomon GM, Weiss PM. Chemical contaminants in breast milk: time trends and regional variability. *Environ Health Perspect.* 2002;110(6):A339-347.

23. Renfrew MJ, Hay AM, Shelton N, Law G, Wallis S, Madden S, et al. Assessing levels of contaminants in breast milk: methodological issues and a framework for future research. *Paediatr Perinat Epidemiol.* 2008;22(1):72-86.

24. Landrigan PJ, Sonawane B, Mattison D, McCally M, Garg A. Chemical contaminants in breast milk and their impacts on children's health: an overview. *Environ Health Perspect.* 2002;110(6):A313-A315.

25. Mead MN. Contaminants in human milk: weighing the risks against the benefits of breastfeeding. *Environ Health Persp.* 2008;116:A427-434.

26. Boersma ER, Lanting CI. Environmental exposure to polychlorinated biphenyls (PCBs) and dioxins. Consequences for longterm neurological and cognitive development of the child lactation. *Adv Exp Med Biol.* 2000;478:271-287.

27. Eskenazi B, Marks AR, Bradman A, Fenster L, Johnson C, Barr DB, et al. In utero exposure to dichlorodiphenyltrichloroethane (DDT) and dichlorodiphenyldichloroethylene (DDE) and neurodevelopment among young Mexican American children. *Pediatrics.* 2006;118:233-241.

28. Nickerson K. Environmental contaminants in breast milk. *J Midwifery Womens Health.* 2006;51:26-34.

29. Chuchu N, Patel B, Sebastian B, Exley C. The aluminium content of infant formulas remains too high. *BMC Pediatr.* 2013;13:162.

30. World Health Organization. Outbreak news. Melamine contamination, China. *Wkly Epidemiol Rec.* 2008;83:358.

31. Barrett JR. Children's health: Sour news for soy formula? *Environ Health Perspect.* 2005;113:A302.

32. World Health Organization. Fourth WHO-Coordinated survey of human milk for persistent organic pollutants in cooperation with UNEP Guidelines for developing a national protocol. 2007. Available at: http://www.who.int/foodsafety/chem/POPprotocol.pdf. Accessed February 17, 2016.

33. Schettler T. Ecology of breast cancer: The promise of prevention and the hope for healing. 2013. Available at: http://www.healthandenvironment.org/uploads/docs/EcologyOfBC_Intro.pdf. Accessed February 17, 2016.

34. Jemal A, Bray F, Center MM, Ferlay J, Ward E, Forman D. Global cancer statistics. *CA Cancer J Clin.* 2011;61:69-90.

35. Interagency Breast Cancer and Environmental Research Coordinating Committee. Breast cancer and the environment: Prioritizing prevention. 2003. Available at: http://www.niehs.nih.gov/about/assets/docs/ibcercc_full_508.pdf. Accessed February 17, 2016.

36. Brody JG, Rudel RA, Michels KB, Moysich KB, Bernstein L, Attfield KR, et al. Environmental pollutants, diet, physical activity, body size, and breast cancer: where do we stand in research to identify opportunities for prevention? *Cancer.* 2007;109 (12 Suppl):2627-2634.

37. Ledesma N. Women's Health Matters: Nutrition & Breast Cancer. Available at: http://cancer.ucsf.edu/_docs/crc/nutrition_breast.pdf. Accessed February 17, 2016.

38. National Institute of Environmental Health Science. Mold. Available at: http://www.niehs.nih.gov/health/topics/agents/mold/index.cfm. Accessed February 17, 2016.

39. Reponen T, Vesper S, Levin L, Johansson E, Ryan P, Burkle J, et al. High environmental relative moldiness index during infancy as a predictor of asthma at 7 years of age. *Ann Allergy Asthma Immunol.* 107(2):120-126.

40. Centers for Disease Control and Prevention. Update: pulmonary hemorrhage/hemosiderosis among infants. *MMWR.* 2000;49:180-184.

41. Weiss A, Chidekel AS. Acute pulmonary hemorrhage in a Delaware infant after exposure to *Stachybotrys atra. Del Med J.* 2002;74:363-368.

42. Organization of Teratology Information Specialists (OTIS). Mold and Pregnancy. Available at: http://www.mothertobaby.org/files/Mold.pdf. Accessed February 17, 2016.

43. US Environmental Protection Agency. How people are exposed to mercury. Available at: http://www.epa.gov/mercury/how-people-are-exposed-mercury. Accessed February 17, 2016.

44. Natural Resources Defense Council. Mercury contamination in fish: A guide to staying healthy and fighting back. Available at: http://www.nrdc.org/health/effects/mercury/sources.asp. Accessed February 17, 2016.

45. Risher JF, Amler SN. Mercury exposure: evaluation and intervention the inappropriate use of chelating agents in the diagnosis and treatment of putative mercury poisoning. *Neurotoxicology.* 2005;26(4):691-699.

46. US Food and Drug Association, US Environmental Protection Agency. What you need to know about mercury in fish and shellfish. 2004. Available at: http://www.fda.gov/food/resourcesforyou/consumers/ucm110591.htm. Accessed February 17, 2016.

47. Consumer Reports. Mercury in canned tuna still a concern. New tests reinforce a need for some people to limit consumption. 2011. Available at: http://www.consumerreports.org/cro/magazine-archive/2011/january/food/mercury-in-tuna/overview/index.htm. Accessed February 17, 2016.

48. Health Care Without Harm. Aggregate exposures to phthalates in humans. 2002. Available at: http://noharm.org/lib/downloads/pvc/Agg_Exposures_to_Phthalates.pdf. Accessed February 17, 2016.

49. Barrett JR. Phthalates and baby boys: potential disruption of human genital development. *Environ Health Perspect.* 2005;113(8):A542.

50. Breast Cancer Fund. Phthalates. State of the evidence on phthalates. 2013. Available at: http://www.breastcancerfund.org/clear-science/radiation-chemicals-and-breast-cancer/phthalates.html. Accessed February 17, 2016.

51. Braun JM, Sathyanarayana S, Hauser R. Phthalate exposure and children's health. *Curr Opin Pediatr.* 2013;25(2):247-254.

52. Patandin S, Lanting CI, Mulder PG, Boersma ER, Sauer PJ, Weisglas-Kuperus N. Effects of environmental exposure to polychlorinated biphenyls and dioxins on cognitive abilities in Dutch children at 42 months of age. *J Pediatr.* 1999;134:33-41.

53. DiVall SA. The influence of endocrine disruptors on growth and development of children. *Curr Opin Endocrinol Diabetes Obes.* 2013;20(1):50-5.

54. Lind PM, Zethelius B, Lind L. Circulating levels of phthalate metabolites are associated with prevalent diabetes in the elderly. *Diabetes Care.* 2012;35(7):1519-1524.

55. Boas M, Feldt-Rasmussen U, Main KM. Thyroid effects of endocrine disrupting chemicals. *Mol Cell Endocrinol.* 2012;355(2):240-248.

56. Lind PM, Lind L. Circulating levels of bisphenol A and phthalates are related to carotid atherosclerosis in the elderly. *Atherosclerosis.* 2011;218(1):207-213.

57. World Health Organization. Dioxins and their effects on human health. Available at: http://www.who.int/mediacentre/factsheets/fs225/en/. Accessed February 17, 2016.

58. Koopman-Esseboom C, Weisglas-Kuperus N, de Ridder MA, Van der Paauw CG, Tuinstra LG, Sauer PJ. Effects of polychlorinated biphenyl/dioxin exposure and feeding type on infants'

mental and psychomotor development. *J Pediatr.* 1996;97(5):700-706.

59. Center for Health, Environment and Justice. Dioxin Levels in Food—Where's the Beef? Available at: http://chej.org/2013/06/dioxin-levels-in-food-wheres-the-beef/. Accessed February 17, 2016.

60. Vogt R, Bennett D, Cassady D, Frost J, Ritz B, Hertz-Picciotto I. Cancer and non-cancer health effects from food contaminant exposures for children and adults in California: a risk assessment. *Environ Health.* 2012;11:83.

61. Consumer Product Safety Improvement Act of 2008. PUBLIC LAW 110–314. Available at: http://www.cpsc.gov//PageFiles/113865/cpsia.pdf. Accessed February 21, 2016.

62. Food and Drug Administration. FDA Public Health Notification: PVC Devices Containing the Plasticizer DEHP. Available at: http://www.fda.gov/MedicalDevices/Safety/AlertsandNotices/PublicHealthNotifications/ucm062182.htm. Accessed February 28, 2015.

63. Advisory Committee for Childhood Lead Poisoning Prevention of the Centers for Disease Control and Prevention. Low level lead exposure harms children: A renewed call for primary prevention. 2012. Available at: http://www.cdc.gov/nceh/lead/ACCLPP/Final_Document_030712.pdf. Accessed February 17, 2016.

64. Centers for Disease Control and Prevention. Guidelines for the identification and management of lead exposure in pregnant and lactating women. 2010. Available at: http://www.cdc.gov/nceh/lead/publications/leadandpregnancy2010.pdf. Accessed February 17, 2016.

65. American College of Obstetricians and Gynecologists. Committee Opinion Number 533. Lead screening during pregnancy and lactation. Atlanta, GA: US Department of Health and Human Services; 2012. Available at: https://www.acog.org/-/media/Committee%20Opinions/Committee%20on%20Obstetric%20Practice/co533.pdf?dmc=1&ts=20131215T1736260137. Accessed February 17, 2016.

66. Centers for Disease Control and Prevention. Fourth Report on Human Exposure to Environmental Chemicals, 2009. Atlanta, GA: US Department of Health and Human Services, Centers for Disease Control and Prevention. Available at: http://www.cdc.gov/exposurereport/. Accessed February 17, 2016.

67. Shaw SD, Blum A, Weber R, Kannan K, Rich D, Lucas D, et al. Halogenated flame retardants: do the fire safety benefits justify the risks? *Rev Environ Health.* 2010;25:261-305.

68. Kotz A, Malisch R, Kypke K, Oehme M. PBDE, PBDD/F and mixed chlorinated-brominated PXDD/F in pooled human milk samples from different countries. *Organohalogen Compounds.* 2005;67:1540-1544.

69. Zota AR, Park JS, Wang Y, Petreas M, Zoeller RT, Woodruff TJ. Polybrominated diphenyl ethers, hydroxylated polybrominated diphenyl ethers, and measures of thyroid function in second trimester pregnant women in California. *Environ Sci Technol.* 2011;45:7896-7905.

70. California Department of Consumer Affairs. Department of Home Furnishings and Thermal Insulation. Technical Bulletin 117. Requirements, Test Procedure and Apparatus for Testing the Flame Retardance of Resilient Filling Materials Used in Upholstered Furniture. 2000. Available at: http://www.bhfti.ca.gov/industry/117.pdf. Accessed February 17, 2016.

71. Yang CZ, Yaniger SI, Jordan VC, Klein DJ, Bittner GD. Most plastic products release estrogenic chemicals: a potential health problem that can be solved. *Environ Health Perspect.* 2011;119(7):989-996.

72. Bittner GD, Yang CZ, Stoner MA. Estrogenic chemicals often leach from BPA-free plastic products that are replacements for BPA-containing polycarbonate products. *Environ Health.* 2014;13(1):41.

73. Thayer KA, Heindel JJ, Bucher JR, Gallo MA. Role of environmental chemicals in diabetes and obesity: a National Toxicology Program workshop review. *Environ Health Perspect.* 2012;120(6):779-789.

74. Breast Cancer Fund. Bisphenol A. State of the evidence on bisphenol A. Available at: http://www.breastcancerfund.org/clear-science/radiation-chemicals-and-breast-cancer/bisphenol-a.html. Accessed February 17, 2016.

75. Environmental Protection Agency. 2006–2007 Pesticide Market Estimates: Usage. Available at: http://www.epa.gov/pesticides/pesticides-industry-sales-and-usage-2006-and-2007-market-estimates. Accessed February 21, 2016.

76. Roberts EM, English PB, Grether JK, Indham GC, Somberg, L, Wolff, C. Maternal residence near agricultural pesticide applications and autism spectrum disorders among children in the California Central Valley. *Environ Health Perspect.* 2007;115:1482-1489.

77. Rauh VA, Perera FP, Horton MK, Whyatt RM, Bansal R, Hao X, et al. Brain anomalies in children exposed prenatally to a common organophosphate pesticide. *Proc Natl Acad Sci U S A.* 2012;109:7871-7876.

78. Pesticide Action Network. A generation in jeopardy. How pesticides are undermining our children's health and intelligence. 2013. Available at: http://www.panna.org/sites/default/files/KidsHealthReportOct2012.pdf. Accessed February 17, 2016.

79. Centers for Disease Control and Prevention. CDC Policy on Climate Change and Public Health. Available at: http://www.cdc.gov/climateandhealth/pubs/Climate_Change_Policy.pdf. Accessed February 17, 2016.

80. Watts N, Adger WN, Agnolucci P, Blackstock J, Byass P, Cai W, et al. Health and climate change: policy responses to protect public health. *Lancet.* 2015;386(10006):1861-1914.

81. Centers for Disease Control and Prevention. Climate Effects on Health. http://www.cdc.gov/climateandhealth/effects/. Published October 2, 2015. Accessed February 21, 2016.

CHAPTER 4

SLEEP DISORDERS

Janet Beardsley | Jennifer G. Hensley | Julia Lange Kessler

The third edition of the *International Classification of Sleep Disorders* (ICSD-3) identifies 6–8 categories of sleep disorders that include more than 37 specific conditions, not including their subtypes.[1] This chapter provides in-depth coverage of the most common sleep disorders: insomnia, sleep disorder breathing such as obstructive sleep apnea (OSA), and restless legs syndrome (RLS).

Introduction

Adequate sleep is critical to survival, although the functions of sleep are not completely known.[2,3] What we do know is that it is a time of restoration and that sleep, or sleep-like behavior, is seen not only in mammals and birds but also in reptiles, amphibians, fish, and invertebrates.[4] Such a highly conserved function, from an evolutionary standpoint, is obviously extremely important, and yet this is an area of health that is often overlooked by both the individual and the clinician.[5]

According to the American Academy of Sleep Medicine (AASM) and the Sleep Research Society, healthy sleep means the absence of sleep disorders, adequate hours in duration, good

sleep quality, sleep regularity, and appropriate timing.[6] However, about 50% of women who completed the 2014 Sleep Health Index survey by the National Sleep Foundation reported either insomnia or difficulty remaining asleep.[7] Inadequate sleep is associated with significant adverse health consequences, including depression, diabetes, obesity and cardiovascular diseases of hypertension, stroke, and heart disease, as well as daytime cognitive impairment with potential adverse outcomes.[6] Loss of sleep can occur from external disruption and decreased hours, or it can be the result of treatable sleep disorders. It is important for the clinician to 1) recognize the signs and symptoms of sleep disorders, inadequate sleep, or poor sleep quality, and 2) to be able to identify, treat, or refer as needed.

Current recommendations from the AASM and the Sleep Research Society include 7 or more hours of sleep per night on a regular basis for adults 18 to 60 years old to maintain optimal health.[6] Significant individual variation in sleep habits and duration of sleep is common, and sleep patterns change throughout the lifespan due to illness, pregnancy, breastfeeding, childcare and caretaking, illness, stress, and emotions.[8] Some conditions that disrupt sleep may be treatable, allowing the individual to attain or regain healthy, restful sleep. Identification of sleep disturbance and implementation of interventions to improve sleep quality can have a dramatic positive effect on the individual's health and are an essential part of providing primary care. This chapter outlines common sleep disruptions and disorders and provides guidelines for recognition, evaluation, management, and referral.

Since the early 20th century, there have been increasing efforts to understand the physiology of sleep, the effects of sleep on overall health, and causes of sleep disruption and its consequences. The research in this area has increased dramatically since the 1960s, and the field of sleep medicine emerged in the late 20th century with the founding of what would become the AASM.[3] The first version of ICSD, was published in 1990, and the latest edition, the ICSD-3, was released in 2014.[1]

Sleep Loss, Health, and Safety

Sleep disorders and sleep deprivation are associated with an increase in adverse health outcomes. Inadequate or poor quality sleep has been associated with an increased risk of hypertension and diabetes, weakened immune system, depression, anxiety, alcohol use, cardiac disease, and cancers.[9-11] Inadequate sleep also leads to a delay in psychomotor vigilance and has been implicated in accidents associated with major human and environmental disasters, including meltdowns of the nuclear reactors at Three Mile Island and Chernobyl, the Exxon Valdez Oil spill, and the Union Carbide chemical spill in Bhopal, India.[5] Adequate and restful sleep is essential to wellbeing and daytime functioning without impairment. Adequate sleep is defined in **Table 4-1**.

Increased incidence of motor vehicle crashes has been related to both short-term and chronic sleep deprivation. The AAA Foundation data analysis from the National Highway Safety Administration annual estimates includes approximately 328,000 crashes with 6400 deaths and 109,000 injuries related to drowsy drivers.[12] Drowsy driving, including after an "extended-hour call shift" (greater than or equal to 24 hours), has been identified as a significant risk factor for healthcare providers. A national survey conducted between 2002 and 2003 reported that medical interns, subsequent to an extended-hour call shift, were in 2.3% more motor vehicle crashes than nondrowsy drivers, including near-miss accidents. For each extended-hour call shift per month, the risk of a motor vehicle accident increased 9.1%, near-miss

Table 4-1 Normal Sleep

Normal Sleep Activity	Normal Time
Total sleep time (TST)	8–8.5 hours
Sleep onset after head hits pillow or sleep onset latency (SOL)	Less than 30 minutes
Number of awakenings from sleep or wake after sleep onset (WASO)	Fewer than 7, falling back to sleep in less than 30 minutes each time
Awakening in the morning	Within 30 minutes before desired time

Data from Kryger MH, Roth T, Dement WC. *Principles and Practice of Sleep Medicine.* 5th ed. St. Louis, MO: Elsevier-Saunders; 2011:1766.

accidents were five times more likely, and the odds of a documented crash were more than doubled. Interns who worked five or more extended-hour call shifts reported a significant increase in their risk of falling asleep while driving and while stopped in traffic.[13]

Work and career demands are a common cause of acute and chronic sleep deprivation. Reviewing data from the National Health Interview survey, Luckhaupt and colleagues found that 30% of American workers reported short sleep duration of less than 6 hours per night.[14] The expanding prevalence of cell phones, beepers, electronic devices, and online access to job-related resources has expanded the possibilities for work to impinge on home life and sleep time. In addition, the spectrum of light from electronic screens can cause a disruption in the circadian rhythm, compounding the opportunity for inadequate sleep already compromised in the 21st century.

Loss of sleep, whether from external factors, inadequate sleep hours, or a sleep disorder, has enormous consequences for both the individual and society. It is important for the clinician to recognize a sleep disorder, manage and treat it, or provide a referral.

Physiology of Sleep

Sleep-Wake Cycles

Borbély proposed a Two-Process Model of Sleep Regulation.[15] Process S is the homeostatic drive for sleep—the longer awake, the sleepier the body becomes. Process C is the circadian rhythm that resets approximately every 24 hours. (See **Figure 4-1**.) The circadian rhythm, or internal sleep-wake timing system, is largely determined by daylight and darkness, as well as genetics, but is influenced by external forces such as work schedule, latitude, and being sighted or nonsighted. Circadian rhythm disorders occur when the internal timing system is out of sync with external forces.

Figure 4-1 Borbély's Two-Process Model.

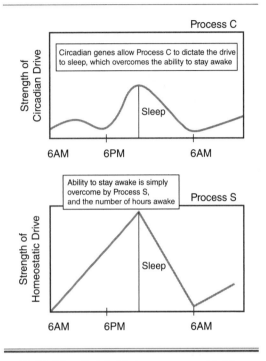

Modified from Borbély AA. A two process model of sleep regulation. *Hum Neurobiol.* 1982;1(3):195-204.

Circadian rhythms, hormone levels, neurochemicals, and the daylight–darkness cycles are significant factors that help promote healthy sleep. An individual circadian rhythm is the *internal clock* that resets every 24 hours to entrain (or synchronize) and regulate sleep-wake (restoration-activity). Circadian rhythms that do not comply with sleep onset around 10 p.m. and wake onset around 6 a.m. include advanced and delayed sleep-wake disorders.[8,15] (See **Figure 4-2**.)

Although sleep is a time of restoration for most body systems and critical to health and mental wellbeing, the brain remains in an active state. The "sleep-wake cycle" is managed by internal and external forces, but the most obvious method

Figure 4-2 Circadian rhythm examples.

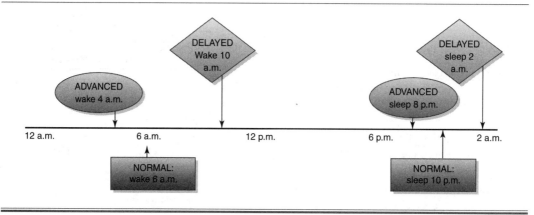

Data from Kryger MH, Roth T, Dement WC. *Principles and Practice of Sleep Medicine.* 5th ed. St. Louis, MO: Elsevier-Saunders; 2011.

of control is the *circadian rhythm*, which is synchronized by light, especially natural daylight.[16,17] Aging results in the loss of neurons in the suprachiasmatic nucleus and an eventual change in the circadian rhythm. Individuals over 50 years of age are often affected by advance sleep phasing, or falling asleep earlier and getting up earlier.[11] At any age, a disrupted circadian rhythm can cause acute and chronic adverse effects such as nonrestful sleep, metabolism dysfunction, cognitive impairment, cardiovascular abnormalities, and gastrointestinal and genitourinary dysfunctions.[17]

Natural daylight is the "zeitgeber," or synchronizer, for the circadian rhythm. As light is directed to the retina during the daylight hours, the suprachiasmatic nucleus signals the pineal gland, through the superior cervical ganglion, to inhibit the production of the hormone, *melatonin*, which is one of the most important hormones of sleep regulation.[18] In darkness this inhibition is turned off and melatonin is released, which initiates the drive for sleep.[19] With the advent of electric lights, the timing and release of melatonin have significantly changed sleep patterns.[16] Adjusting

exposure to the light stimulus can be an important part of sleep regulation and aid in improving sleep quality. This is discussed more later in this chapter.

A second hormone directly involved in controlling wakefulness and sleep is *cortisol*. Levels of cortisol, which promotes wakefulness, are highest in the morning. Cortisol levels steadily decrease during the day, which then helps allow other factors initiate the drive for sleep. Numerous neurochemicals and genes are involved in the regulation of sleep, many of which the science of sleep has only begun to understand. Here the major two players, *melatonin* and *cortisol*, have been introduced.[18] (See **Table 4-2** and **Figure 4-3** for more detail about the influences on sleep.)

Sleep Stages

Sleep is divided into two categories: non-rapid eye movement (NREM) and rapid eye movement (REM), which cycle every 60 to 90 minutes, or 4 to 6 times throughout the night[18] (**Table 4-3**). Research has led to recategorization of NREM sleep from stages 1 to 4 into 1 to 3. In an adult,

Table 4-2 Chemical/Environmental Stimuli Related to Sleep

Sleep Inhibiting	Sleep Promoting
Acetylcholine (AcCH)	Adenosine
Cortisol	Daylight
Dopamine (DA)	Decreased core body temperature (CBT)
Epinephrine (E)	CBT lowest 2 hours before awakening
Caffeine	Gamma aminobutyric acid (GABA)
Histamine (HA)	Galanin
Hypocretin/orexin (ORX)	Melatonin
Norepinephrine (NE)	
Serotonin (5-HT)	

Data from Kryger MH, Roth T, Dement WC. *Principles and Practice of Sleep Medicine.* 5th ed. Philadelphia, PA: Elsevier/Saunders; 2011.

Figure 4-3 Physiologic interactions affecting sleep.

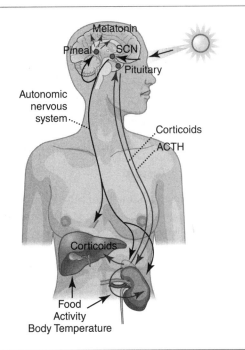

sleep will typically begin with NREM stages 1 and 2 and last approximately 30 minutes. Stage 1 (beginning to sleep) is considered light sleep or "between being awake and asleep" and lasts from 1 to 10 minutes. It is easy to wake from stage 1, and the individual may not even be aware of having fallen asleep. Stage 1 can be seen as a transitional sleep stage throughout the night. However, a high proportion of stage 1 sleep indicates significantly disrupted sleep. As the individual becomes more disengaged from his or her surroundings, the body slips into stage 2 NREM sleep, breathing and heart rate become steady, and the body temperature begins to drop. Stage 3 NREM sleep is slow-wave (as seen on electroencephalogram [EEG]) or restorative sleep when blood flow to the muscles is increased, growth and tissue repair occurs, and energy is restored.[20]

REM sleep is the active dream state and critical for memory consolidation and processing what has been taken in during wakefulness. As the body enters REM and dreaming, the eyes begin to dart back and forth, but the body enters a state of atonia to keep the individual from acting

Table 4-3 Sleep Stages

Stage of Sleep	Purpose
N1: Drowsy–awake • "Alpha" waves"	• Beginning of relaxation, in between awake and sleep • Hypnagogic jerks = sense of falling
N2: Deepening sleep	• Brain waves slow, onset of sleep, RR & HR regular, temp ↓ • No eye movements
N3: Deep sleep • "Slow wave" or delta waves • Previously N3 and N4 • Hard to arouse	• No eye movements • No muscle activity but ↑ blood supply to muscles, ↓ BP and RR • Growth and repair of tissues, energy is restored • Restorative sleep (↓ sympathetic tone, ↓ NE, ↓E)
REM tonic	• No eye movements • Suppression of muscle tone with active brain, body relaxed (atonic)
REM phasic	• Activated brain in a paralyzed body so as not to act out dreams • SNS bursts (↑ HR, BP [up to 40 mmHg], RR) • Conjugate eye movements • More vivid and active dreams

BP = blood pressure, E = epinephrine, HR = heart rate, NE = norpinephrine, REM = rapid eye movement, RR = resting rate, SNS = sympathetic nervous system

Data from Kryger MH, Roth T, Dement WC. *Principles and Practice of Sleep Medicine*. 5th ed. St. Louis, MO: Elsevier-Saunders; 2011.

out dreams.[18] When an individual who is otherwise asleep acts out a dream, there is the real risk of harm to self or others. Episodes of dream enactment can occur as a result of sleep deprivation; untreated sleep apnea; narcolepsy; and under the influence of alcohol, medications (especially selective serotonin reuptake inhibitors [SSRIs]), and other substance use or abuse.[1] In such cases, further investigation is warranted because of risk of injury to the individual or bed partner and to learn more about sleep disruption and disturbance indicated by the dream enactment.

In its most dramatic presentation, this is known as REM behavior disorder (RBD) and may be associated with Parkinson disease. RBD is different from somnambulism, or sleepwalking, which occurs during stage 3 NREM.[1,18] It is typically seen in men over the age of 50 and should not be confused with dream enactment

alone. These parasomnias and sleep-related motor disorders are beyond the scope of this chapter, and the interested reader is referred to a sleep text.

Metabolic Changes During Sleep

Thermoregulation

Human thermoregulation is comprised of a homeothermal core and a poikilothermic shell (ability to change with environmental temperature). During the day and early evening (or wake cycle), the thermoregulatory system of the body keeps the temperature at a steady state. Between 6 p.m. and 8 p.m., it peaks and then begins to decrease, which is thought to help bring on the drive for sleep.[18] During sleep the body systems slow down, less

Table 4-4 The 10 Commandments of Sleep Hygiene

1. Set a consistent bedtime and an awakening time.
2. If you are in the habit of taking naps, try not to exceed 45 minutes of daytime sleep.
3. Avoid excessive alcohol ingestion 4 hours before bedtime, and do not smoke.
4. Avoid caffeine 6 hours before bedtime. This includes coffee, tea, sodas, and chocolate.
5. Avoid heavy, spicy, or sugary foods 4 hours before bedtime. A light snack before bed is acceptable.
6. Exercise regularly, but not right before bed.
7. Use comfortable bedding.
8. Find a comfortable temperature setting for sleeping, and keep the room well ventilated.
9. Block out all distracting noise, and eliminate as much light as possible.
10. Reserve the bed for sleep. Don't use the bedroom as an office, workroom, or recreation room.

Modified from American Sleep Apnea Association. 10 commandments of healthy sleep. Washington, DC: Author; 2015. Retrieved from: http://www.sleepapnea.org/learn/healthy-sleep/ten-commandments.html.

heat is generated, and during REM sleep the skeletal muscles become atonic. This leads to a drop in temperature of 1° to 2°F. This is especially notable in the 2 hours prior to waking, when an individual is most likely to require additional bedding to keep warm. Because core temperature is so strongly connected to an individual's ability to fall asleep and stay asleep—that is, the easier it is for the body temperature to drop—the easier it is for the individual to fall asleep. The "10 Commandments of Sleep Hygiene" (**Table 4-4**) recommend a "cool" sleep environment, preferably 62°F.

Respiratory and Cardiovascular

NREM sleep, compared with the wake cycle of the day, allows for rest of the pulmonary and cardiovascular systems. There is a decrease in breathing rate, heart rate, and blood pressure, plus a sustained regularity of respiration. During normal sleep, an individual's blood pressure decreases by approximately 15% (both diastolic and systolic), which is known as "nocturnal dipping." When the blood pressure does not "dip" during sleep, the risk for

developing heart disease is increased. Sleep disruptions and OSA can both contribute to a lack of nocturnal dipping in blood pressure.[18,21] During REM sleep and dreaming, breathing and heart rate increase again and become variable, which may account for early morning sudden cardiac death.[22]

Endocrine

Many hormones are released and affected by the sleep-wake cycle beyond those related directly to sleep; these include those related to appetite (leptin and ghrelin) and to growth (human growth hormone [HGH]). HGH is characterized as being stable throughout the day with abrupt secretory episodes. The most consistently occurring episode happens within the first hour after the onset of sleep. In adults, HGH released during sleep contributes to necessary restoration and repair of tissue. Aging leads to a significant drop in HGH levels, which matches the decreased time spent in NREM and REM sleep cycles in older age.[18]

Sleep deprivation can contribute directly to weight gain and diabetes.[23,24] The hormones leptin and ghrelin play a role in an individual's feelings of hunger (ghrelin) and fullness (leptin). Studies done to test the effect of sleep deprivation on appetite and physical activity found that subjects with sleep deprivation of just 2 to 3 hours had elevated levels of leptin and ghrelin, which led to increases in appetite and decreases in exercise.[25] Insulin resistance is also increased in a sleep-deprived state, even from a single night of only 4 hours of sleep duration, which in turn increases the risk of diabetes and metabolic syndrome.[24]

Common Symptoms of Sleep Disorders

A good night's sleep should lead to awakening in the morning with a feeling of being refreshed (restorative sleep) and ready to "take on the day." There should be no lapses into sleep during the waking hours. Common symptoms of sleep disruption include difficulty with sleep initiation and/or maintenance, excessive daytime sleepiness, nonrestorative sleep, snoring, memory and concentration issues, mood swings and irritability, depression and anxiety, and nocturia. External factors such as stress, lifestyle, overactive mind, menopause, both acute and chronic illness, and side effects from medications can have significant adverse impacts on sleep and initiation of sleep. Excessive daytime sleepiness, or hypersomnia, can lead to daytime impairment, one example of which includes safety issues with driving. Nonrestorative sleep can manifest as vague tiredness, inability to stay awake, and/or rapid onset of sleep (less than 5 minutes after sitting or lying quietly). Sleep disruption may be intermittent or may represent a more significant condition such as OSA.

Recognition of the symptoms of disrupted sleep is the most important step for the clinician. Many women believe that fatigue, insomnia, nocturia, multiple awakenings during the night, and excessive daytime somnolence are symptoms of their overly busy days that are to be tolerated, rather than indications of a possible, treatable sleep disorder. To begin a sleep assessment, the clinician should assess symptoms and sleep patterns. There are many validated tools for the identification of sleep disorders, but clinicians can start with a few simple questions to evaluate for sleep disorders (see **Figure 4-4**).

Specific Sleep Conditions

The ICSD-3 lists 5 basic categories for sleep disorders: 1) insomnia, 2) sleep-related breathing disorders, 3) central disorders of hypersomnolence, 4) circadian rhythm sleep-wake disorders, 5) parasomnias, and 6) sleep-related movement disorders.[1] While many sleep disorders present as vague complaints such as difficulty sleeping, daytime sleepiness, fatigue, and irritability, this chapter should help the clinician to recognize sleep disorders, use specific tools to help diagnose, consider treatments available, and when to refer to a sleep specialist.

Insomnia

DEFINITION, TYPES, AND EPIDEMIOLOGY (*INTERNATIONAL CLASSIFICATION OF DISEASES, TENTH REVISION, CLINICAL MODIFICATION*)

"Insomnia is the inability to fall asleep or stay asleep despite adequate opportunity to do so."[26(p683)] Insomnia is defined by the AASM as "persistent difficulty with 1) sleep initiation, 2) duration, 3) consolidation, or quality that occurs despite adequate opportunity and circumstances for sleep, and results in some form of daytime impairment"[1(p19)] Daytime impairment includes, but is not limited to, fatigue, irritability, cognitive impairment, and excessive daytime sleepiness, all of which may cause the patient to seek treatment. Misdiagnosis and mismanagement of the disorder can worsen the symptoms.

Figure 4-4 Questions to rule out a sleep disorder in 20 seconds.

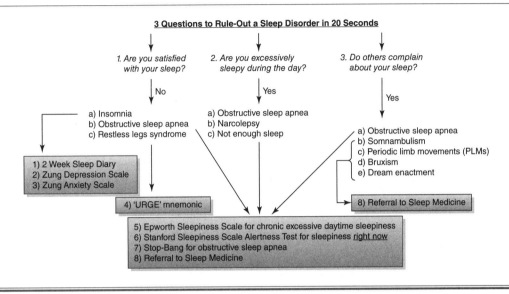

Data from Reite M, Weissberg M, Ruddy J. *Clinical Manual for Evaluation and Treatment of Sleep Disorders.* Arlington, VA: American Psychiatric Publishing; 2009; Kryger MH, Roth T, and Dement WC. *Principles and Practice of Sleep Medicine.* 5th ed. St. Louis, MO: Elsevier-Saunders; 2011.

The ICSD-3 recognizes three types of insomnia: chronic, short-term or transient, and other.[1] There is considerable overlap in symptoms of the chronic insomnia subtypes; it is helpful for the clinician to understand the differences between these. Diagnostic criteria for each type of insomnia and subtypes of chronic insomnia are found in **Tables 4-5** and **4-6**.

Chronic insomnia affects 10% of the general population, and difficulty sleeping must be present at least 3 times per week for 3 consecutive months.[1,27] Short-term insomnia affects an additional 30–35% of the population. Other insomnia does not meet criteria for either, but symptoms are severe enough to warrant clinical intervention. All types of insomnia occur more frequently in individuals with psychiatric or medical comorbidities, women, the aged, those of lower socioeconomic status, and shift workers. Short-term insomnia

can progress to chronic insomnia if not addressed and treated.

Difficulty with sleep initiation, duration, and consolidation is important to understand in terms of 1) difficulty falling asleep, 2) staying asleep, 3) the number of nighttime awakenings and why, 4) how long it takes to fall back to sleep, 5) early morning awakenings, and 6) the overall number of minutes actually asleep. (See Table 4-1 for normal sleep characteristics.) The timing during the night that difficulty with sleep occurs may provide important information for differential diagnoses. Difficulty falling asleep could point to a circadian rhythm disorder while nighttime awakenings could point to gastroesophageal reflux or sleep-disordered breathing. A 2-week sleep diary will provide the clinician with a visual representation of the patient's sleep patterns over a 14-day period. See **Figure 4-5**.

Table 4-5 Classification of Insomnia

Chronic Insomnia Disorder

ICD-9-CM code: 307.42 ICD-10-CM code: F51.01

Alternate Names

Chronic insomnia, primary insomnia, secondary insomnia, comorbid insomnia, disorder of initiating and maintaining sleep, behavioral insomnia of childhood, sleep-onset association disorder, limit-setting sleep disorder.

Diagnostic Criteria

Criteria A-F must be met

A. The patient reports, or the patient's parent or caregiver observes, one or more of the following:
   1. Difficulty initiating sleep.
   2. Difficulty maintaining sleep.
   3. Waking up earlier than desired.
   4. Resistance to going to bed on appropriate schedule.
   5. Difficulty sleeping without parent or caregiver intervention.

B. The patient reports, or the patient's parent or caregiver observes, one or more of the following related to the nighttime sleep difficulty:
   1. Fatigue/malaise.
   2. Attention, concentration, or memory impairment.
   3. Impaired social, family, occupational, or academic performance
   4. Mood disturbance/irritability.
   5. Daytime sleepiness.
   6. Behavioral problems (e.g., hyperactivity, impulsivity, aggression).
   7. Reduced motivation/energy/initiative.
   8. Proneness for errors/accidents.
   9. Concerns about or dissatisfaction with sleep.

C. The reported sleep/wake complaints cannot be explained purely by inadequate opportunity (i.e., enough time is allotted for sleep) or inadequate circumstances (i.e., the environment is safe, dark, quiet, and comfortable) for sleep.

D. The sleep disturbance and associated daytime symptoms occur at least three times per week.

E. The sleep disturbance and associated daytime symptoms have been present for at least three months.

F. The sleep/wake difficulty is not better explained by another sleep disorder.

Notes

1. Reports of difficulties initiating sleep, difficulties maintaining sleep, or waking up too early can be seen in all age groups. Resistance going to bed on an appropriate schedule and difficulty sleeping without parent or caregiver intervention is seen most commonly in children and older adults who require the supervision of a caretaker due to a significant level of functional impairment (e.g., those with dementia).

2. Some patients with chronic insomnia may show recurrent episodes of sleep/wake difficulties lasting several weeks at a time over several years, yet not meet the three-month duration criterion for any single such episode. Nonetheless, these patients should be assigned a diagnosis of chronic insomnia disorder, given the persistence of their intermittent sleep difficulties over time.

Table 4-5 Classification of Insomnia (*Continued*)

3. Some patients who use hypnotic medications regularly may sleep well and not meet the criteria for an insomnia disorder when they take such medications. However, in the absence of such medications these same patients may meet the above criteria. This diagnosis would apply to those patients particularly if they present clinically and voice concerns about their inability to sleep without their sleep medications.
4. Many comorbid conditions such as chronic pain disorders or gastroesophageal reflux disease (GERD) may cause the sleep/wake complaints delineated here. When such conditions are the sole cause of the sleep difficulty, a separate insomnia diagnosis may not apply. However, in many patients such conditions are chronic and are not the sole cause of sleep difficulty. Key determining factors in the decision to invoke a separate insomnia diagnosis include: "How much of the time does the sleep difficulty arise as a result of factors directly attributable to the comorbid condition (e.g., pain or GERD)?" or "Are there times that the sleep/wake complaints occur in the absence of these factors?" "Have perpetuating cognitive or behavioral factors (e.g., negative expectations, conditioned arousal, sleep-disruptive habits) arisen, suggesting an autonomous aspect to the ongoing insomnia?" If there is evidence that the patient's sleep/ wake complaints are not solely caused by the medical condition, and those sleep/wake complaints seem to merit separate treatment attention, then a diagnosis of chronic insomnia disorder should be made.

Modified from American Academy of Sleep Medicine. *The International Classification of Sleep Disorders.* 3rd ed. Darien, IL: American Academy of Sleep Medicine; 2014; Schutte-Rodin S, Broch L, Buysse D, Dorsey C, Sateia M. Clinical guideline for the evaluation and management of chronic insomnia in adults. *J Clin Sleep Med.* 2008;4(5):487-504.

Table 4-6 Chronic Insomnia Subtypes

Chronic Insomnia Subtype	Possible Predisposing Factor(s)
Psychophysiologic	1. Learned bad sleep behavior 2. Hyperarousal (worry, genetics)
Idiopathic (lifelong)	1. Learned bad sleep behavior 2. Genetics
Paradoxical	Objectively patient sleeps more than subjectively reported
Inadequate sleep	Not sleeping enough although there is adequate time to sleep
Insomnia due to psychiatric disorder	1. Anxiety 2. Depression 3. Other psychiatric disorder
Insomnia due to a medical condition	Medical conditions: arthritis, chronic pain syndromes, etc.
Insomnia due to medications or substances	Medications/substances that adversely impact sleep

Data from Kryger MH, Roth T, Dement WC. *Principles and Practice of Sleep Medicine.* 5th ed. St. Louis, MO: Elsevier-Saunders; 2011:1766; American Academy of Sleep Medicine. *The International Classification of Sleep Disorders.* 3rd ed. Darien, IL: American Academy of Sleep Medicine; 2014.

Figure 4-5 Two-week sleep diary.

TWO WEEK SLEEP DIARY

INSTRUCTIONS:
1. Write the date, day of the week, and type of day: Work, School, Day Off, or Vacation.
2. Put the letter "C" in the box when you have coffee, cola or tea. Put "M" when you take any medicine. Put "A" when you drink alcohol. Put "E" when you exercise.
3. Put a line (I) to show when you go to bed. Shade in the box that shows when you think you fell asleep.
4. Shade in all the boxes that show when you are asleep at night or when you take a nap during the day.
5. Leave boxes unshaded to show when you wake up at night and when you are awake during the day.

SAMPLE ENTRY BELOW: On a Monday when I worked, I logged on my lunch break at 1 PM, had a glass of wine with dinner at 6 PM, fell asleep watching TV from 7 to 8 PM, went to bed at 10:30 PM, fell asleep around Midnight, woke up and couldn't got back to sleep at about 4 AM, went back to sleep from 5 to 7 AM, and had coffee and medicine at 7:00 in the morning.

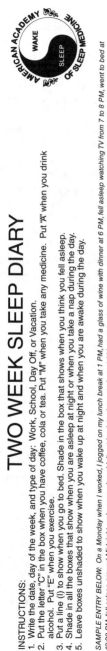

Etiology

Insomnia has long been considered a state of hyperarousal with possible contributions from the hypothalamic-pituitary-adrenal axis (increased cortisol is a known alerting hormone), a reduction in hippocampal volume (an area of the brain responsible for inhibition, such as inhibition of wakefulness), a decrease in gamma-aminobutyric acid (a depressant), and genetics.[18] While much of insomnia is not well understood, Spielman's "3 Ps" model presents a foundation for not only understanding its pathophysiology but also its treatment.[18,28] The 3 Ps model describes insomnia in terms of predisposing factors, precipitating factors, and perpetuating factors—the 3 Ps.

Predisposing factors may or may not be modifiable and include genetics, learned bad sleep behaviors and associations (e.g., eating in bed, TV on in bedroom), circadian rhythm predisposition (e.g., "owl" or "lark"), inadequate coping mechanisms for stress, advancing age, female gender, and work schedule. Precipitating factors are situational (stressful job), environmental (noisy neighborhood), medical (new cancer diagnosis), psychiatric (anxiety or depression), or medications side effects. Perpetuating factors, such as continued poor sleep habits and misconceptions about sleep, may be modifiable and have been successfully treated with cognitive behavioral therapy for insomnia (CBT-i).[29]

Essential History

The past medical/surgical history should be comprehensive and include psychiatric disorders, particularly anxiety and depression. The clinician should focus on the predisposing, precipitating, and perpetuating factors associated with insomnia. **Table** 4-7 lists questions specific to a history of insomnia that complement the review of systems. Social history includes questions regarding occupation, hours worked, smoking, and alcohol consumption. The medication history should include all medications in the past year plus over-the-counter products and herbal remedies, because an alerting medication/substance started within the year may have precipitated difficulty initiating sleep and led to insomnia symptoms.

If the clinician is worried about comorbid anxiety and depression, there are several easy-to-administer-in-the-clinical-setting tools, such as the Two-Question Screen for Depression (PHQ-2), the Edinburgh Postnatal Depression Scale, and the Generalized Anxiety Disorder Screening Tool (GAD-7).

Table 4-7 History for Insomnia

Questions for Patient	Rationale
Baseline information for sleep habits	
What type of work do you do?	These questions speak to the patient's
What shift do you work?	ability to have adequate time for
How many hours per week do you work?	sleep. Children and pets in the
Do you sleep alone or with a partner?	bed can cause multiple awaken-
Do you have children?	ings from sleep.
How many children do you have, and what are their ages?	
Do you have pets?	
How many pets do you have, and where do they sleep?	
Describe your sleeping space to me: What furniture is in the room? What is the temperature? Is it light or dark in the room? Is there a TV?	Speaks to lack of sleep hygiene

(Continues)

Table 4-7 History for Insomnia (*Continued*)

Questions for Patient	Rationale
Ask each question twice regarding: 1) sleep during the workweek and 2) sleep when off work	
What time do you go to bed?	Comparing sleep routines during the
What time do you wake up and get out of bed?	workweek and when off work can
How many hours do you spend in bed total?	help the clinician determine:
How many hours do you think you actually sleep?	1. Circadian rhythm preference
Do you have trouble falling asleep?	(owl/lark) and synchronicity with
Do you have difficulty staying asleep?	work schedule
How many times do you wake up during the night?	2. If the patient is making up for
Why do you wake up during the night?	lost sleep during the workweek or
How many minutes or hours until you fall back to sleep?	when off work
Do you ever wake up before you want to, or before the alarm clock?	3. The possibility of another sleep
When you wake up, do you feel refreshed and ready for the day?	disorder
Do you take naps?	
Other questions to help understand your insomnia:	
Have you traveled recently?	Jet lag and altitude will resolve after a
Have you been at high altitude recently?	few days.
Have you ever fallen asleep driving? If so, how many times in the last week?	Examines daytime sleepiness
Do you use tobacco? If so, what types, and what times of the day?	Alerting agents will adversely impact sleep; the sedative effects of alco-
Do you do "recreational" drugs? If so, what types, and what times of the day?	hol wear off in the early morning hours, leaving the patient with
Do you drink alcohol? If so, how much alcohol do you drink, and at what time is your last drink?	"early morning awakenings."
Do you drink caffeine (any form)? If so, how much, and at what times of the day?	
How many minutes or hours does it take to fall asleep?	

Data from Kryger MH, Roth T, Dement WC. *Principles and Practice of Sleep Medicine*. 5th ed. St. Louis, MO: Elsevier-Saunders; 2011:1766.

Other tools that can be used in assessing the degree of impairment for insomnia include the Insomnia Severity Index (**Table 4-8**), the Epworth Sleepiness Scale, and the Two-Week Sleep Diary (Figure 4-5) mentioned earlier. The Epworth Sleepiness Scale asks about whether the individual is more likely to fall into a doze, as opposed to feeling tired under eight common conditions that range from sitting quietly reading or watching television, to brief pauses while driving, to sitting in a car or at a movie for an extended period of time. Each item is scored from 0–3, with a higher score reflecting increased likelihood of dozing off.

Scores above 10 are considered to indicate increased risk of excessive sleepiness. The Epworth Sleepiness Scale, although validated for OSA, may help determine the extent of daytime impairment due to the insomnia complaints. The sleep diary, completed after an initial visit, is essential for evaluation of time to bed, time asleep, wake time, and total time asleep.

Physical

There is no specific physical examination that assists with the diagnosis of insomnia. Insomnia is

Table 4-8 The Insomnia Severity Index

Insomnia Severity Index					
0–7 = No clinically significant insomnia	0	1	2	3	4
8–14 = Subthreshold insomnia					
15–21 = Clinically moderate insomnia					
22–28 = Clinical severely insomnia					
1. Rate current severity of insomnia					
a. Difficulty falling asleep	None	Mild	Moderate	Severe	Very severe
b. Difficulty staying asleep	None	Mild	Moderate	Severe	Very severe
c. Problem waking up too early	None	Mild	Moderate	Severe	Very severe
2. How satisfied/dissatisfied are you with your current sleep pattern?	Not at all	Barely	Somewhat	Much	Very much
3. To what extent do you consider your sleep problem to interfere with your daily functioning?	Not at all	Barely	Somewhat	Much	Very much
4. How noticeable to others do you think your sleeping problem is in terms of impairing the quality of your life?	Not at all	Barely	Somewhat	Much	Very much
5. How worried/distressed are you about your current problem?	Not at all	Barely	Somewhat	Much	Very much

Reprinted from Bastien CH, Vallières A, Morin CM. Validation of the Insomnia Severity Index as an outcome measure for insomnia research. *Sleep Med.* 2001;2(4):297-307. Copyright 2001, with permission from Elsevier.

often a comorbidity with OSA, and the clinician may choose to measure the patient's neck circumference, examine the oropharynx for a crowded airway, and administer the STOP-BANG questionnaire,[30] which requires physical examination data (see **Table 4-9**).

LABORATORY/IMAGING

There is no laboratory or imaging workup that will assist the clinician with the diagnosis of insomnia. Polysomnography (sleep study) is not beneficial. Use of actigraphy (gross motion sensor tracking) for a 1-week period will provide objective data for the patient's subjective complaints and may be ordered by a specialist as part of a comprehensive evaluation.

TREATMENTS FOR INSOMNIA

Most of us will have nights of sleeplessness (family, health, work, and/or school situations). How many nights of sleeplessness and how we deal with the situation are crucial to the difference between "other" or short-term insomnia and chronic insomnia. While other and short-term insomnia treatment may only require reassurance that sleep routines should be restored once the situation has resolved, intermittent use of short-acting sleep aids may be useful. Chronic insomnia is best treated without sleep aids, and CBT-i is recommended.[27] CBT-i can be delivered by trained sleep specialists, other healthcare professionals (registered nurses, physician assistants, nurse practitioners), or the patient herself via the Internet (e.g., at http://shuti.me/).

Table 4-9 STOP-BANG Questionnaire

1. Snoring: Do you snore loudly (loud enough to be heard through closed doors)?
   Yes   No

2. Tired: Do you often feel tired, fatigued, or sleepy during daytime?
   Yes   No

3. Observed: Has anyone observed you stop breathing during your sleep?
   Yes   No

4. Blood pressure: Do you have or are you being treated for high blood pressure?
   Yes   No

5. Body Mass Index (BMI): BMI more than 35 kg/m^2?
   Yes   No

6. Age: Age over 50 years old?
   Yes   No

7. Neck circumference: Neck circumference greater than 40 cm?
   Yes   No

8. Gender: Male?
   Yes   No

High risk of obstructive sleep apnea: Yes to 3 or more questions

Low risk of obstructive sleep apnea: Yes to fewer than 3 questions

Reproduced from Chung F, Subramanyam R, Liao P, Sasaki E, Shapiro C, Sun Y. High STOP-Bang score indicates a high probability of obstructive sleep apnoea. *Br J Anaesth*. 2012;108(5):768-775. By permission of Oxford University Press.

Using the 3 Ps model, and assuming perpetuating factors play a large role in chronic insomnia, CBT-i challenges misconceptions about sleep and misperceptions about insomnia. CBT-i includes four aspects: stimulus control, sleep restriction, relaxation, and sleep hygiene. Stimulus control is the single most effective aspect of CBT-i and includes: 1) going to bed only when sleepy, 2) getting out of bed after 20 minutes if not asleep and repeating as necessary, 3) use of the bed and bedroom only for sleep and sex (no TV, no food, no studying), 4) getting up at the same time every morning, and 5) no napping.

Sleep restriction is imposed so that time in bed is limited to sleeping only and not "trying to fall asleep." For example, if the woman goes to bed at 9 p.m. so she can get 8 hours of sleep before needing to rise for work at 5 a.m., but falls asleep at 11 p.m., she is prescribed consistent time to bed at 11 p.m. and rise time at 5 a.m. until she begins to fall asleep within 30 minutes. This creates an uncomfortable mild sleep deprivation in the short term. Once falling asleep and staying asleep are consistent throughout the prescribed times, bedtime is moved backward to extend sleep time. *Relaxation* is prescribed when in bed and can be taught as progressive muscle relaxation or mindfulness. Sleep hygiene includes use of the 10 Commandments of Sleep Hygiene (Table 4-4), individualized to the lifestyle of the patient. **Figure** 4-6, The 3 Ps and CBT-i, summarizes the diagnosis and management of insomnia. CBT-i is useful for adolescents, women during pregnancy and menopause, and the elderly.

Figure 4-6 The 3 Ps and CBT-i.

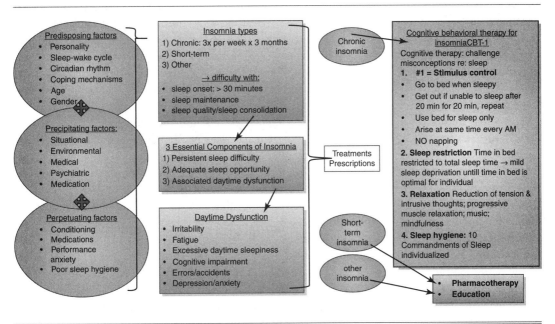

Data from Schutte-Rodin S, Broch L, Buysse D, Dorsey C, Sateia M. Clinical guideline for the evaluation and management of chronic insomnia in adults. *J Clin Sleep Med*. 2008;4(5):487-504; Spielman AJ, Caruso LS, Glovinsky PB. A behavioral perspective on insomnia treatment. *Psychiatr Clin North Am*. 1987;10(4):541-53; American Academy of Sleep Medicine. *The International Classification of Sleep Disorders*. 3rd ed. Darien, IL: American Academy of Sleep Medicine; 2014.

ADOLESCENTS

Adequate and restorative sleep (about 9 hours per night) during adolescence can be threatened by a normal shift in sleep patterns due to hormonal changes that force the sleep-wake cycles forward, and by early start times for school.[18,31] Traditional sleep patterns (e.g., sleep at 10 p.m. and rise at 7 a.m.) become difficult. Inadequate sleep may adversely impact school performance and manifest as behavior problems such as inattention, irritability, hyperactivity, lack of impulse control, or depression. When compounded by caffeine ingested during the day to maintain wakefulness and nighttime use of electronic devices, both of which are stimulating and counteract the body's normal rise in melatonin to help the adolescent fall asleep, maintaining healthy sleep during adolescence is challenging.[31]

Four to 9.5% of adolescents suffer from insomnia, and if unhealthy sleep habits are not addressed during adolescence, these can become the predisposing factors for chronic sleep problems.[32] Naps may become necessary to make up for lost sleep. CBT-i has been shown to help improve sleep habits in teens.

PREGNANCY AND LACTATION

Insomnia symptoms affect up to 61% of women during pregnancy and are far more common in the third trimester as the common discomforts of pregnancy increase (backache, nocturia, fetal movements).[33] Women prone to hyperarousability and worry might experience the most sleep disruption. Inadequate sleep impairs daytime functioning and quality of life, but severe sleep deprivation (less than 5 to 6 hours of sleep per night) has been associated with longer labors, an increased rate of operative delivery, and abnormal glucose metabolism/gestational diabetes.[34-37] CBT-i is useful during pregnancy, as are naps. The incidence of sleep-disordered breathing also increases in late pregnancy and should be considered with new-onset sleep difficulty in the second and third trimesters, especially if accompanied by snoring.

A newborn in the home who breastfeeds every 2 to 3 hours can be challenging for a woman and her family used to 8 hours of uninterrupted sleep. A breastfeeding woman can be encouraged that, at 3 months, she will likely sleep 1 hour more and experience more slow-wave or restorative sleep than her formula-feeding counterpart. The postpartum period is a time for coinciding maternal and newborn sleep schedules—that is, mother should nap when the newborn is asleep.

MENOPAUSE

Half of menopausal women will experience sleep disturbances and daytime fatigue.[38] The exact cause of menopausal sleep disturbance is unknown, but hot flashes and night sweats are known to interrupt nighttime sleep; however, difficulty initiating sleep is the most common complaint. Sleep hygiene, CBT-I, and/or sleep aids may help the menopausal woman, but only after she has treatment for vasomotor symptoms.[38,39] Sleep apnea also increases in frequency after menopause and may be a factor in sleep disturbance.[38]

MANAGEMENT

The woman should be presented with the 10 Commandments of Sleep Hygiene (Table 4-4) and have the recommendations individualized to her lifestyle. As sleep hygiene is essential for healthy sleep, but in and of itself is not an adequate treatment for insomnia, CBT-i should be offered if the condition warrants it. Once the patient has made a commitment to CBI-i, she must not deviate for even one night. Sleep restriction

can be particularly difficult, as it will cause a mild sleep deprivation in the beginning, and should be started during a time of decreased stress, such as during a vacation. All medications may have a next-day sedating effect, and the patient who uses sleep aids should be warned of the side effects and risks, especially drowsy driving.

Pharmacologic therapies for insomnia should always be used in conjunction with behavioral changes, because the former addresses the immediate lack of sleep and the latter addresses the chronic lack of sleep. Sleep aids should be used at the lowest dose and for the shortest period appropriate. They do not replace therapeutic approaches that deal with underlying causes of sleep loss.

Pharmacologic treatments fall into the following categories: 1) supplements; 2) benzodiazepine gamma aminobutyric acid receptor agonists, including a) benzodiazepines b) non-benzodiazepines; 3) melatonin receptor agonists; 4) orexin receptor antagonists; 5) histamine receptor antagonists; and 6) sedating antidepressants. See **Table 4-10** for pharmacologic treatments for insomnia.

During pregnancy and lactation, nonpharmacologic treatments such as CBT-i and naps should be encouraged.[33]

Sleep-Disordered Breathing

DEFINITION, TYPES, AND EPIDEMIOLOGY

In some forms of sleep-disordered breathing, respirations are abnormal when the individual is awake as well as during sleep, but these disorders are typically characterized by abnormal respirations during sleep. ICSD-3 groups sleep-disordered breathing under four categories: OSA disorders, central sleep apnea disorders, sleep-related hypoventilation disorders, and sleep-related hypoxemia disorder.[1]

The common forms of sleep-disordered breathing fall under the obstructive disorders, which include snoring, upper airway resistance syndrome

Table 4-10 Pharmacologic Agents for Sleep

Drug	Name	Dosing	Mechanism of Action	Side Effects
Melatonin	Melatonin	0.3 mg to "phase shift" 1–10 mg as hypnotic	Supplement	Headache, hangover
Melatonin receptor agonist	Ramelteon (Rozerem)	8 mg at sleep onset Long-term use	Binds to and stimulates melatonin receptors 1 and 2	Headache, ↑ prolactin, ↓ testosterone
Benzodiazepines	Flurazepam (Dalmane)	15–30 mg Long acting (> 24 hours)	Stimulation of the GABA system	Rebound insomnia; somnolence; dependence; tolerance; complex sleep-related behaviors, such as sleep eating
	Temazepam (Restoril)	15–30 mg Intermediate acting		
	Triazolam (Halcion)	0.125–0.25 mg Short acting		
Benzodiazepines receptor agonists	Zolpidem/Zolpidem CR* (Ambien)	5 mg/6.25 mg* Short acting		
	Zaleplon (Sonata)	5–10 mg Ultra short acting		
	Eszopiclone (Lunesta)	1–3 mg Intermediate acting		
Sedating antidepressants	Trazodone	50–150 mg	Blocks alerting serotonin and norepinephrine	Dry mouth, blurred vision, constipation, drowsiness, orthostatic hypotension, weight gain, cardiotoxicity
	Amitriptyline	25–50 mg		
	Mirtazapine (Remeron)	15–30 mg		
Histamine-receptor antagonists	Diphenhydramine (Benadryl)	50–100 mg	Blocks alerting effects of histamine	Next-day drowsiness; paradoxical reaction
	Doxylamine	6.25–25 mg		
	Doxepin (Sinequan or Silenor)	25–250 mg For chronic insomnia		
Orexin-receptor antagonist	Suvorexant (Belsomra)	5–20 mg	Blocks orexin, the central promoter of wakefulness	Next-day drowsiness; abnormal thoughts and behaviors

Data from Schutte-Rodin S, Broch L, Buysse D, Dorsey C, Sateia M. Clinical guideline for the evaluation and management of chronic insomnia in adults. *J Clin Sleep Med.* 2008;4(5):487–504.

(UARS), OSA, and mixed sleep apnea.[9] Snoring, UARS, and OSA are all characterized by an obstruction or partial obstruction of the upper airway. In OSA and UARS, diminished or absent airflow results in a decrease in oxygen saturation. This desaturation triggers an arousal from sleep to a state of wakefulness or to a lighter stage of sleep. The resulting disruption in sleep continuity contributes to symptoms of daytime somnolence and fatigue, which are frequently seen in the presence of sleep-disordered breathing disorders.

Central and mixed sleep apneas are characterized by a reduction or cessation of breathing efforts, which may or may not be accompanied by an obstructive event. Central sleep apnea can be seen as the result of cardiac disease, neurologic disorders, and high altitude.[1]

Sleep-related hypoventilation is commonly seen as a medication effect but may also be associated with congenital disorders, medical disorders, and morbid obesity, which can also cause hypoventilation while awake. Approximately 80–90% of patients with obesity hypoventilation syndrome have comorbid OSA,[1] which likely contributes to the myth that only the morbidly obese suffer from OSA.

Sleep-related hypoxemia disorder occurs when a patient has low oxygen saturation levels at night of less than 88% for greater than or equal to 5 minutes total during the night. Other forms of sleep-disordered breathing, which can contribute to oxygen desaturation, must first be ruled out before a diagnosis of sleep-related hypoxemia can be made. In sleep-related hypoxemia disorder, sleep apnea or hypoventilation may be present, but these conditions are not the primary cause of the hypoxemia seen during sleep.

All sleep apnea can result in sleep fragmentation and can lead to sleep-related hypoxia. Awareness of sleep apnea has been increasing since the 1980s when it was first realized that OSA was not limited to individuals with morbid obesity.[40] The landmark paper on the prevalence of OSA in the general population was the Wisconsin Cohort Study, written by Young and colleagues and published in 1993.[40] In this study of Wisconsin state employees ages 30–60 years old, the researchers found a 9% prevalence of sleep-disordered breathing in women and 24% prevalence in men. The estimate of prevalence in women was much higher than suspected at that time, when the ratio of male-to-female referral rates was 10:1 in sleep medicine clinics. Recent reports suggest an increasing incidence of sleep-disordered breathing and sleep apnea since the Wisconsin data were originally published, corresponding with the obesity epidemic in the United States.[41] Moderate to severe sleep apnea can have significant long-term health consequences, including heart disease, hypertension, diabetes, depression, and increased rates of motor vehicle accidents. It is important for the primary care provider to identify the signs of sleep-disordered breathing, particularly because these issues are frequently underrecognized in women.[40-43]

Sleep apnea is measured both by apneic events, with full cessation of airflow, and also by desaturation events, which may be caused by shallow and/or restricted breathing episodes. The severity of sleep apnea is categorized by the frequency of apneas, defined as 10 seconds with no airflow, and hypoxias, defined as a greater than 3–4% oxygen desaturation. Milder forms of OSA, such as UARS, still have restriction or obstruction of airflow accompanied by oxygen desaturations but do not meet the criteria for sleep apnea. These respiratory effort–related arousals (RERAs) cause subtle but disruptive arousals from sleep. Individuals with UARS can have significant symptoms of sleep deprivation and daytime somnolence. In obstructive and central sleep apnea, the number of apneic events and the number of desaturation/hypopneic events per hour determine the severity of the diagnosis.

This section focuses on the OSAs, as these disorders are the most common and may be initially evaluated and managed by the primary care practitioner. Other forms of sleep-disordered breathing, if suspected, should be referred to a sleep specialist for further evaluation.

SNORING

Snoring as an isolated symptom is not considered a sleep disorder, but it is frequently associated with OSA and warrants further investigation. Snoring is caused by a restriction of airflow, which causes concussion of the tissues in the nose and/or throat. Snoring, by itself, is a mild form of sleep-disordered breathing. It can also be a sign of more serious issues, such as OSA and UARS. According to the Wisconsin Cohort Study, 24% of adult women between the ages of 30 and 60 reported habitual snoring.[40] The incidence increases with aging, obesity, nasal obstruction, and substances that cause muscle relaxation including alcohol, narcotics, and muscle relaxers.[1] Pregnancy also increases the risk of snoring and sleep apnea.[44] In transient or intermittent snoring, the nasal passages may be constricted by allergic reactions or sinus infections. Chronic obstruction can be caused polyps or physical defects. The soft palate or uvula may extend into the airway. Snoring tends to increase in frequency and volume during stage N3 and REM sleep. Obesity and swollen tonsils and adenoids can affect the volume of tissue in the throat, leading to an increase in snoring. Sleep position may further narrow the airway, with the greatest restriction typically seen in the supine position. It is important to rule out OSA and UARS, which are chronic conditions with significant health risks and may require continuous positive airway pressure (CPAP) for effective treatment. Any individual who reports habitual snoring along with symptoms of daytime sleepiness/fatigue or possible observed pauses in their breathing during sleep needs a referral for a sleep study to evaluate for OSA or UARS. Patients who report snoring who also have cardiovascular disease, especially hypertension, coronary artery disease, and atrial fibrillation, are at an increased risk of OSA even if they do not complain of daytime somnolence. They also need to be referred for a sleep study to rule out OSA. Patients who snore are at risk for developing OSA as they age or gain weight.[1]

UPPER AIRWAY RESISTANCE SYNDROME (UARS)

This condition is considered a mild form of OSA in the ICSD-3 classification system, but is often described as a distinct diagnosis from OSA.[1] The pathophysiologies of UARS and OSA are the same, differing in degree of severity. UARS is found when there is restriction in the upper airway, causing a decrease in oxygen saturation and paused or diminished airflow, which causes an arousal from sleep. This can be a full awakening or a shift from deep sleep to a lighter sleep. These episodes are called RERAs and can cause significant sleep disruption and fragmentation. UARS can be seen by itself or in conjunction with OSA, sometimes explaining the significant daytime symptoms for individuals with an otherwise mild sleep apnea diagnosis.[45-47] According to the AASM, scoring of RERAs is optional on diagnostic sleep studies, which can lead to underestimation of the severity of sleep-disordered breathing and failure to diagnose UARS.[48] Some insurance companies, including Medicare, do not cover the use of positive airway pressure (PAP) for the treatment of UARS, although this treatment can be very effective for symptomatic individuals. Untreated UARS is associated with daytime fatigue and sleepiness, insomnia, and depression.[45,49] Evaluation for this form of sleep-disordered breathing should be considered in any woman complaining of significant sleep disruption and may be seen more commonly in the premenopausal woman with a normal body mass index (BMI) and complaints of sleep disturbance than full-blown sleep apnea.[42,50]

Obstructive Sleep Apnea (OSA)

OSA is a more significant form of sleep-disordered breathing, and it also occurs when there is restriction or cessation of airflow during sleep. Untreated sleep apnea has been associated with hypertension, coronary artery disease, stroke, congestive heart failure, diabetes, depression, arrhythmia such as atrial fibrillation, and increased rates of motor vehicle accidents, cancer, and all-cause mortality even when controlling for comorbid factors.[1,51-55] On a polysomnogram (PGM) or home sleep study, breathing efforts are seen in chest expansion, but airflow is restricted or absent. Sleep apnea is defined by the number of apneic and hypopneic events per hour of sleep. Apnea is a full 10 seconds of no airflow from the nose or mouth. Hypopnea occurs when there is a diminished or absent airflow of briefer duration, accompanied by a drop in oxygen saturation, typically 3–4%. These events can occur in all four stages of sleep, but are less frequently seen during stage N3. Apneas and hypopneas typically worsen during REM sleep and when the individual is in the supine position. Oxygen saturations usually improve after normal breathing resumes following arousal, unless there is underlying respiratory disease. Most individuals will wake feeling their sleep was not refreshing, regardless of length. Snoring and observed pauses may or may not be reported. These apneic episodes increase in frequency following sedating substances such as alcohol, drugs, and medication. Increasing weight also increases the incidence of sleep apnea, although 30–40% of individuals with OSA are not overweight.[1] The diagnostic criterion, an Apnea-Hypopnea Index (AHI) of less than five events per hour, is considered a negative/normal. An AHI between 5 and 15 events per hour is mild sleep apnea, 15–30 events per hour are moderate sleep apnea, and greater than 30 events per hour indicate severe sleep apnea. There may also be a significant number of RERAs, causing additional sleep disruption. Adding all apnea, hypopnea, and RERA events is typically reported as the respiratory disturbance index, or RDI. Unfortunately, the RDI is sometimes also reported as an AHI equivalent, and these terms may be used interchangeably on sleep studies.[48]

OSA is more common in women than previously recognized, with rates increasing with age and BMI. Menopause also increases the frequency of OSA. Current estimates of OSA frequency in women are as follows: 3% between the ages of 30 and 49 years old, increasing to 9% for women 50–70 years old. However, this rate changes dramatically with increasing BMI. In 30- to 49-year-old women, a BMI between 25 and 29.9 increases the rates of mild to moderate OSA to 4.5%. A BMI of 30–39.9 causes the rate to rise to 13.5% for women 30–49 years old. For women with a BMI greater than 40, the estimated rate of mild to severe OSA is 43% in women ages 30–49. Women over the age of 50 with a BMI less than 25 still have an estimated 9.3% risk of mild to severe OSA. This increases to 20% with a BMI between 30 and 39.9, and OSA occurs in 68% of women over the age of 50 with a BMI greater than or equal to 40.[41,56]

Sleep apnea is often underrecognized in women, particularly younger women, who often present with different, less "classic" symptoms than men. Women are less likely to complain of excessive sleepiness and more likely to report insomnia, poor sleep quality, and fatigue.[42,57] Younger, non-obese women are less likely to be recognized as being at risk for OSA and may be inappropriately treated for years for their symptoms alone before receiving a full sleep evaluation.[58] Of the women in the Wisconsin Cohort who were found to have moderate to severe sleep apnea, 93% had not previously been diagnosed.[43,59] Normal weight (BMI less than 25) premenopausal women with sleep-disordered breathing may present with concerns of depression, insomnia, or parasomnia.[42] Women under the age of 30 with sleep-disordered breathing are less likely to report snoring, observed pauses in breathing, or gasping. They are also more likely to have structural factors that cause airway constriction, such as retrognathia, a crowded oropharynx, and nasal obstruction.[58]

In pregnancy, changes in the upper airway increase the risks of sleep-disordered breathing and OSA. The frequency of snoring rises in the third trimester as the size of the upper airway decreases. There is also a decrease in the respiratory functional residual capacity, and 30% of pregnant women develop gestational rhinitis.[60,61] These physiologic changes all increase the risks of developing some form of sleep-disordered breathing, either snoring, OSA, or UARS. Rates of sleep-disordered breathing in pregnancy are estimated to be between 15% and 35%, but true prevalence has not been adequately documented.[62,63] A recent meta-analysis of research on OSA in pregnancy found an association with complications such as preeclampsia and gestational diabetes.[63] OSA has also been associated with significant adverse pregnancy outcomes, including increased neonatal intensive care unit admissions, severe maternal morbidity, cardiovascular morbidity, and even maternal death.[62]

Despite the increasing evidence, screening for sleep-disordered breathing is not part of routine prenatal evaluation. Bourjeily and colleagues reported on a survey conducted to evaluate the frequency of sleep-disordered breathing evaluation in prenatal care.[64] The researchers found that nurse-midwives and nurse practitioners were more likely to ask prenatal patients about sleep quality than physician providers. However, providers and patients reported only a 3–5% rate of questions related to snoring during prenatal visits, although patients reported snoring incidence of 32%. In this study population, 44% were overweight and 21.7% were obese, known factors for increased sleep-disordered breathing.

OSA often presents with complaints of insomnia, and the clinical symptoms of sleep apnea and insomnia frequently overlap. In a review of studies examining comorbid insomnia and OSA, Luyster and colleagues found that 39–58% of patients with OSA also report insomnia, and 29–67% of patients with insomnia have an AHI greater than 5, indicating at least mild OSA.[65]

Women who present with insomnia, particularly mid-cycle insomnia (difficulty with insomnia after waking during the night) should also be assessed for the possibility of sleep apnea. Effective treatment of sleep-disordered breathing can be a critical part of treating insomnia symptoms—if the patient is presenting with comorbid sleep-disordered breathing.[65-67]

Essential History, Physical, and Testing

History Numerous medical conditions have been associated with OSA, indicate an increased risk, and should trigger further investigation.[1,51,68] These are shown in **Table 4-11**. In addition, a positive family history of these conditions and/or diagnosis of sleep-disordered breathing and being of Japanese or Chinese ancestry, which increases risk even in the absence of obesity—likely due to facial and airway structure—are risk factors.[1]

Common Symptoms Associated with Sleep-Disordered Breathing Patient history of apneic events during sleep may be difficult to identify. Despite the severe degree of sleep disruption caused, apneic events may not be recognized by the person experiencing them or their bed partners. Traditional symptoms of loud snoring and gasping awake may not be present, with nighttime OSA symptoms manifesting only as frequent awakenings, nocturnal gastroesophageal reflux disease (GERD), night sweats, or frequent nocturia. The symptoms listed in **Table 4-12** have all been associated with sleep-disordered breathing and may be seen alone or in the presence of

Table 4-11 Conditions Associated with OSA

Obesity
Polycystic ovarian syndrome
Hypertension
Hyperlipidemia
Hypothyroidism
Stroke
Coronary artery disease/myocardial infarction
Atrial fibrillation
Type 2 diabetes
Gastroesophageal reflux disease (GERD)
Depression and anxiety
Gestational diabetes or gestational hypertension
    during a prior pregnancy
Current pregnancy

Data from American Academy of Sleep Medicine. *The International Classification of Sleep Disorders.* 3rd ed. Darien, IL: American Academy of Sleep Medicine; 2014; Epstein LJ, Kristo D, Strollo PJ, Jr, Friedman N, Malhotra A, Patil SP, et al. Clinical guideline for the evaluation, management and long-term care of obstructive sleep apnea in adults. *J Clin Sleep Med.* 2009;5(3):263-76; Facco F, L. Sleep-disordered breathing and pregnancy. *Semin Perinatol.* 2011;35(6):335-9. doi:10.1053/j.semperi.2011.05.018.

Table 4-12 Symptoms Associated with OSA

Snoring (may or may not be present!)
Fatigue
Excessive daytime sleepiness/somnolence
Waking feeling unrefreshed or as if one has not
    slept at all
Observed pauses in breathing during sleep
Waking feeling short of breath or gasping
Night sweats
Frequent nocturia
Difficulty with memory and concentration
Irritability
Morning headaches
Nocturnal heartburn/gastroesophageal reflux
    disease
Frequent awakenings during the night/sleep
    fragmentation/maintenance insomnia/"being a
    light sleeper"
Decreased libido
Restless sleep
Motor parasomnias induced by breathing episodes,
    including sleepwalking, sleep terrors, sleep
    eating, confusional arousals, arousals from rapid
    eye movement (REM) sleep mimicking REM
    sleep behavior disorder

Data from American Academy of Sleep Medicine. *The International Classification of Sleep Disorders.* 3rd ed. Darien, IL: American Academy of Sleep Medicine; 2014; Epstein LJ, Kristo D, Strollo PJ, Jr, Friedman N, Malhotra A, Patil SP, et al. Clinical guideline for the evaluation, management and long-term care of obstructive sleep apnea in adults. *J Clin Sleep Med.* 2009;5(3):263-76.

others symptoms. Consideration for OSA screening should be given to any woman presenting with the symptoms shown in Table 4-12.[1,51,68]

It is important to differentiate OSA from insomnia, as management differs; however, the symptoms overlap, as shown in **Figure 4-7**.

CLINICAL AND PHYSICAL FINDINGS   Unlike most sleep disorders, OSA is associated with several findings on physical exam. These include a BMI equal to or over 35, a neck circumference > 16 inches in women (> 17 inches in men), retrognathia/recessed jawline, hypertension, crowded oropharynx/Mallampati score greater than III or IV, and current pregnancy, particularly second or third trimester.[51,68]

SCREENING TOOLS   The STOP-BANG Tool[30] is a simple questionnaire that can be used in clinical offices to screen for OSA. Like the Epworth Sleepiness Scale and Berlin Questionnaire, it has been validated as a predictor of OSA in the adult population. Three positive answers have a high sensitivity for severe OSA (87%), but poor specificity. When two of the first four (STOP) questions are positive, and the patient has a BMI

Figure 4-7 Differentiation Between OSA and Insomnia

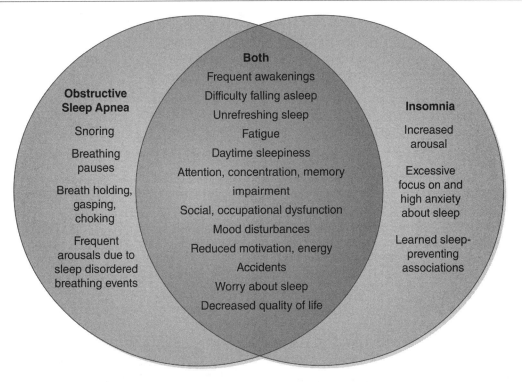

Both
Frequent awakenings
Difficulty falling asleep
Unrefreshing sleep
Fatigue
Daytime sleepiness
Attention, concentration, memory impairment
Social, occupational dysfunction
Mood disturbances
Reduced motivation, energy
Accidents
Worry about sleep
Decreased quality of life

Obstructive Sleep Apnea
Snoring
Breathing pauses
Breath holding, gasping, choking
Frequent arousals due to sleep disordered breathing events

Insomnia
Increased arousal
Excessive focus on and high anxiety about sleep
Learned sleep-preventing associations

Reproduced with permission of American Academy of Sleep Medicine, from Luyster FS, Buysse DJ, Strollo PJ,Jr. Comorbid insomnia and obstructive sleep apnea: challenges for clinical practice and research. *J Clin Sleep Med*. 2010;6(2):196-204. Permission conveyed through Copyright Clearance Center, Inc.

> 35, neck circumference > 40 cm, or is male, specificity is improved (85%, 79%, and 77% respectively).[69]

Common sleep apnea screening tools have been shown not to be valid in the pregnant population when tested against polysomnography.[61,70,71] In the pregnant population, the following components of these questionnaires were correlated with subsequent diagnosis of sleep apnea with PSG testing: frequent snoring, pre-pregnant BMI greater than 30, preexisting chronic hypertension, and age older than 35 years.[70] Pre-pregnancy obesity and onset of snoring in the second trimester and/or significant weight gain during pregnancy are also predictive of sleep apnea in the second and third trimesters of pregnancy.[61]

DIAGNOSIS

Diagnosis of sleep-disordered breathing is made through a formal sleep study, which may be initiated by referral to a sleep specialist but can also be ordered by the primary care provider in some situations. Sleep studies can occur either in the form of an in-lab PSG or an out-of-center sleep test (OCST) or home sleep apnea test (HSAT, also referred to as portable monitors, or PMs).

Table 4-13 Criteria for OSA from ICSD-3

According to the ICSD-3, in order to meet the diagnostic criteria for obstructive sleep apnea, the patient must meet both A and B *or* meet C:

A. The presence of one or more of the following:
1. The patient complains of sleepiness, nonrestorative sleep, fatigue, or insomnia symptoms.
2. The patient wakes with breath holding, gasping, or choking.
3. The bed partner or other observer reports habitual snoring, breathing interruptions, or both during the patient's sleep.
4. The patient has been diagnosed with hypertension, a mood disorder, cognitive dysfunction, coronary artery disease, stroke, congestive heart failure, atrial fibrillation, or type 2 diabetes mellitus.

B. Polysomnography (PSG) or home sleep apnea testing/out-of-center sleep testing (HSAT or OCST) demonstrates:
1. Five or more predominantly obstructive respiratory events (obstructive and mixed apneas, hypopneas, or respiratory effort–related arousals [RERAs]) per hour of sleep during a PSG or per hour of monitoring (OCST).

OR

C. PSG or OCST demonstrates:
1. Fifteen or more predominantly obstructive respiratory events (apneas, hypopneas, or RERAs) per hour of sleep during a PSG or per hour of monitoring (OCST).

Reproduced from American Academy of Sleep Medicine. *The International Classification of Sleep Disorders.* 3rd ed. Darien, IL: American Academy of Sleep Medicine; 2014:297.

In-lab PSG studies can be used to evaluate for other forms of sleep disorders, while home testing assesses only for sleep apnea.[51] Home sleep studies tend to underestimate the severity of sleep-disordered breathing, because RERAs cannot be identified on a home sleep study. Any woman with a negative home study who has significant symptoms or a high clinical suspicion for sleep apnea should be considered for referral to a sleep specialist for further evaluation and in-lab PSG testing.[9,72] Criteria for diagnosis of OSA are shown in **Table 4-13**.

The differential diagnosis of OSA involves both milder conditions and more severe forms of apnea, including the following:

- Isolated snoring without obstructive apneas, hypoxias, or RERAs on sleep testing, without other symptoms suggestive of breathing-related sleep disturbance

- Sleep-related hypoxia or hypoventilation disorders that show desaturations in the absence of apneic events
- Obesity hypoventilation syndrome, as described earlier, which displays daytime symptoms including hypercapnia
- Central sleep apnea either as a separate entity or in conjunction with OSA
- Other sleep disorders that can cause excessive daytime sleepiness, including narcolepsy, idiopathic hypersomnia, and insufficient sleep time
- Medical conditions causing nocturnal dyspnea including congestive heart failure, angina, nocturnal panic attacks, GERD, and asthma

MANAGEMENT WITH POSITIVE AIRWAY PRESSURE

PAP, such as CPAP or bilevel positive airway pressure (BPAP or BiPAP), is the treatment of choice for mild, moderate, and severe sleep apnea.[51] This option should be offered to all patients when a diagnosis has been made, especially to those complaining of daytime symptoms. PAP can be initiated through a therapeutic PSG study to assess optimal PAP settings; recently, auto-titrating PAP devices at home have been used to initiate therapy. Out-of-center auto-titrating treatment initiation at home is not appropriate for individuals with congestive heart failure, chronic obstructive pulmonary disease, central sleep apnea types, or hypoventilation syndromes.[51] The efficacy of PAP therapy is assessed by ongoing evaluation of symptom improvement, stability, or recrudescence. Improvement in breathing episodes and the AHI can be monitored through the data collected by the PAP devices on a nightly basis. Adjustments in pressure settings may be needed with weight gain or loss or if the AHI remains at or returns to a level above five events per hour. Regular replacement of supplies such as masks, tubing, and filters is important to minimize leak and maximize efficacy of therapy. Proper mask fit and pressures are essential elements to improve tolerance and compliance, and a well-trained sleep technologist or durable medical equipment (DME) service provider can be an invaluable resource in assisting with mask fit. Use of the humidifier and addressing any issues with nasal congestion can also be crucial for tolerance and adherence.[51] Early and ongoing assessment of PAP therapy for efficacy assessment, utilization patterns, and patient education is an important part of successful treatment and positive outcomes.

OTHER THERAPEUTIC OPTIONS

Lifestyle and behavioral changes can sometimes help with UARS and mild OSA. These interventions include weight loss, exercise, avoiding the supine position for sleep, elevating the head of the bed, and avoiding sedating substances such as alcohol and medication before sleep. However, although weight loss is recommended for any individual with sleep apnea and an elevated BMI, this intervention should be combined with more immediate and effective treatments. After significant weight loss of 10% or more, a repeat PSG study is recommended if the patient wishes to discontinue PAP to ensure resolution of sleep apnea with weight loss alone. If lifestyle and behavioral changes are chosen as a primary intervention, ongoing assessment of symptoms is recommended to assess efficacy.[51]

Oral mandibular advancement devices can be worn to improve snoring, upper airway resistance, and sleep apnea. Unfitted devices are commercially available and may be helpful for individuals complaining of primary snoring, after sleep apnea has been ruled out. A custom-fit, titratable oral device managed by a qualified sleep medicine–trained dentist may be recommended for patients with mild to moderate sleep apnea who are intolerant of CPAP therapy. Follow-up sleep study is recommended after the oral appliance has been adjusted to confirm treatment efficacy. Ongoing follow up with a qualified sleep-trained dentist is advised to monitor for changes in dental structure side effects over time.[73] For overall reduction of OSA events, CPAP is a more effective intervention than an oral appliance.[73]

Surgical interventions were the first methods available to treat OSA, with the placement of a tracheotomy in the most severe circumstances. Current surgical interventions can address constriction or obstruction in the following areas: nasal passages, oral/oropharynx/nasopharynx, hypopharynx, larynx, or globally with maximal mandibular advancement or bariatric surgery in children (tonsillar hypertrophy may be a significant factor for sleep apnea, but this is not generally true in adults). Surgical procedures to the airway are generally considered a secondary treatment when the patient has been intolerant of PAP. Bariatric surgery, for appropriate individuals, can be quite effective for improving or resolving OSA through weight loss. Ongoing assessment due to high remission rates is recommended,[51] and patients who have significant weight loss should be counseled that age and menopause can increase rates of sleep apnea and they may be at risk for the return of symptoms over time.

MEDICATION

There is no effective pharmacologic intervention for sleep apnea, unless treating a medical cause such as hypothyroidism or acromegaly. The use of nasal corticosteroid sprays may be beneficial for women with chronic rhinitis and UARS, or those with OSA who are having difficulty tolerating CPAP therapy. Saline nasal washes and rinses are also beneficial for the reduction of chronic rhinitis symptoms. Supplemental oxygen is not effective as a primary treatment for sleep apnea, and when used by itself may worsen nocturnal hypercapnia.[51]

EVALUATION AND MANAGEMENT DURING PREGNANCY AND LACTATION

Because of the increasing evidence that untreated sleep apnea can have significant complications during pregnancy, evaluation of risk for sleep-disordered breathing should be a high priority. Women with a pre-pregnant BMI greater than 35 and neck circumference greater than 16 inches or a history of essential hypertension should be considered at risk for sleep-disordered breathing. An early sleep study may be warranted. The frequency of sleep-disordered breathing increases in the second and third trimesters, and the onset of snoring, frequent sleep disruptions, inability to sleep, or sleeping in the recliner should also be indications for further evaluation.

Women who enter pregnancy with known sleep apnea are at risk for developing pregnancy-related hypertension and gestational diabetes, particularly if the sleep apnea is untreated or undertreated. Early testing for gestational diabetes and a glucose tolerance test between 24 and 28 weeks are recommended. If a woman with known sleep apnea is untreated, she should be referred to a specialist to initiate treatment as early in pregnancy as possible.[74]

All pregnant women with mild, moderate, or severe sleep apnea should be treated with PAP therapy to minimize adverse outcomes for mother and fetus.[74,75]

REFERRAL/CONSULTATION

When available, referral to a sleep medicine provider is recommended as soon as a suspicion that a woman has risk factors and symptoms for sleep-disordered breathing is identified. Because pregnancy evaluations can be needed in a very time-limited fashion, early establishment of relationships with your local sleep medicine providers can be invaluable for timely referral, evaluation, and treatment during pregnancy. In the absence of local sleep specialists, out-of-center sleep studies can also be ordered through local DME providers or online services. PAP equipment and supplies are typically provided through local DME services and are also available through online services.

Central Disorders of Hypersomnolence—Narcolepsy

Narcolepsy is a chronic neurologic disorder that causes sleep-wake dysregulation as aspects of sleep intrude into wakefulness. Research links the cause of narcolepsy to lack of or a deficiency in the neurotransmitter hypocretin/orexin in the hypothalamus, which is thought to play a major role in the regulation of wakefulness.[76] It is equally diagnosed in men and women.

Narcolepsy remains underdiagnosed. When not treated, narcolepsy can cause significant daytime impairment. A patient who experiences narcolepsy does not sleep more than usual, but requires sleep at different times during the day. An irresistible sleep attack can occur at any time of the day and may last a few seconds to several minutes. It can also result in poor sleep quality from frequent awakenings during nighttime sleep. Narcolepsy can occur with or without cataplexy.[1]

Cataplexy is a sudden weakness of the muscles of the body, particularly the legs but also the face and neck, which can be triggered by strong emotions, especially laughing.[77] Approximately 64–70% of those with narcolepsy experience cataplexy.[1,78]

Narcolepsy may cause a strange, "dreamlike experience" before falling asleep or waking up, causing the patient to believe it was a hallucination. During this time, there is usually temporary paralysis (atonia) of the body. The "hallucination(s)" and atonia are similar to what is found during REM sleep and dreaming. A tetrad of symptoms assists the clinician with the possible diagnosis of narcolepsy.[78] See **Figure 4-8**.

Narcolepsy is the third most frequently diagnosed sleep disorder, after OAS and RLS, in sleep specialty centers. The prevalence of narcolepsy is estimated at 0.05–0.18% of the worldwide population, most frequently appearing in adolescence. It sometimes follows a streptococcal or H1N1 infection, which may indicate an autoimmune component to the pathophysiology of narcolepsy.[1,78] If there is a suspicion of narcolepsy, the woman should be referred to a sleep specialist; the disorder and its treatment are complex and beyond the scope of this chapter.

Circadian Rhythm Sleep-Wake Disorder

Chronobiology is the study of biologic rhythms; human biologic functions are dictated by circadian rhythms, which are reset approximately every 24 hours. A "normal" circadian rhythm that demands sleep at 10 p.m. and awakening at 6 a.m. will demonstrate biologic functions as shown in **Figure 4-9**. An advanced sleep-wake phase circadian rhythm, seen in aging due to loss of neurons in the suprachiasmatic nuclei, will demonstrate a chronobiologic morningness preference and pull all biologic functions earlier on the 24-hour clock. A delayed sleep-wake phase circadian rhythm, often seen in adolescents, will demonstrate a chronobiologic eveningness preference and push all

Figure 4-8 Narcolepsy symptoms.

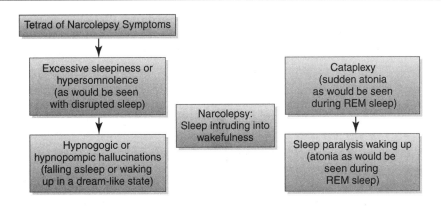

Data from Kryger MH, Roth T, Dement WC. *Principles and Practice of Sleep Medicine.* 5th ed. St. Louis, MO: Elsevier-Saunders; 2011; American Academy of Sleep Medicine. *The International Classification of Sleep Disorders.* 3rd ed. Darien, IL: American Academy of Sleep Medicine; 2014.

Figure 4-9 Example of a chronobiologic clock.

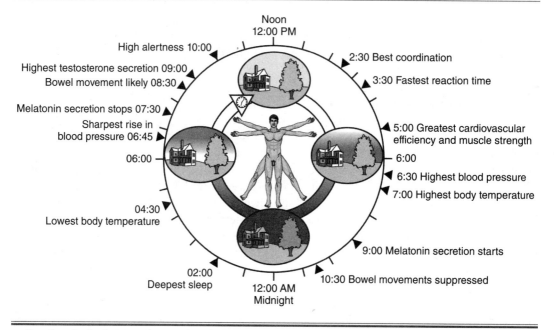

Data from Smolensky M, Lamberg L. *The Body Clock Guide to Better Health*. New York, NY: Henry Holt and Company; 2000.

biologic functions later on the 24-hour clock. Chronobiologic preference can be inferred from such validated tools as the Horne and Ostberg Morningness-Eveningness Questionnaire.[79] This tool can be accessed online for individuals to use. Understanding morningness-eveningness preferences can assist the clinician to diagnose an advanced or delayed sleep-wake phase disorder.

In addition to chronobiologic preferences, circadian rhythms are impacted by 24-hour lighting, shift work, and global travel. These disruptions can negatively impact the internal clock leading to sleep disruption with adverse mental, emotional, and physical changes. These circadian rhythm disorders (CRD) mimic insomnia disorders discussed in the section on insomnia earlier in this chapter. All of them are characterized by a chronic or recurrent pattern of sleep-wake

cycle disruption that is due to alteration of the endogenous circadian timing or misalignment between an individual's endogenous circadian rhythm and the sleep-wake cycle required by their travel, work, or personal schedule. That disruption produces symptoms of insomnia or excessive sleepiness and leads to distress or impairment of mental, physical, social, or other areas of daily function. The most common CRD the clinician is likely to diagnose include delayed sleep-wake phase disorder, advanced sleep-wake phase disorder, shift work sleep disorder, and jet lag. Delayed Sleep-Wake Phase Disorder typically has onset in adolescence and affects 7–16% of the general population. It can be characterized as an "eveningness" chronotype. Daytime sleepiness is noted, along with improved sleep when the individual is not on a work or school schedule and can sleep on a delayed cycle. Complaints include difficulty falling asleep and waking at a desired or required clock time. Three months symptom duration is required.[1] Advanced Sleep-Wake Phase Disorder, in contrast, is a "morningness" chronotype. It affects 1–7% of the population, with prevalence increasing with age. Individuals present with difficulty staying awake in the evening and with sleeping until the expected time to awake over a period of at least three months. Improved sleep occurs when the person is allowed to sleep on their advanced cycle.[1]

Shift Work Sleep Disorder affects those whose work schedules are set in shifts that overlap their normal sleep hours. About 1 in 5 workers in developed countries are on such shifts and estimates of prevalence for Shift Work Sleep Disorder range from a low of 2–5% to as high as 10–38%. Complaints include insomnia or excessive sleepiness and a reduction in total sleep hours associated with a recurring work schedule that overlaps normal sleep hours. Symptoms must last for three months and be associated with the shift work schedule during that time.[1] Jet Lag Disorder is more time limited that the three previous conditions. It is a complaint of insomnia or excessive daytime sleepiness accompanied by a reduction in total sleep associated with transmeridian jet travel across at least two time zones. Additional symptoms within 1 to 2 days of travel can include functional impairment, malaise, and somatic symptoms such as GI disturbance.[1]

The criteria for these and other circadian rhythm disorders are detailed in the International Classification of Sleep Disorders published by the American Academy of Sleep Medicine.[1]

Parasomnias

According to the ICSD-3, parasomnias are undesirable physical events or experiences occurring as one falls asleep, during sleep, or as one arouses.[1] These are not the same as sleep movement disorders, such as RLS or bruxism (grinding teeth during sleep). Parasomnias occur both during REM sleep and non-REM sleep and can be very alarming to both the individuals having the experience and to their household members. Commonly recognized phenomena include sleepwalking, sleep talking, and dream enactment. Less common and sometimes frightening episodes such as sleep paralysis, exploding head syndrome (abrupt awakening with the sense of a sudden loud noise or explosion in the head, which is not associated with significant complaints of pain), sleep-related hallucinations, and night terrors also occur. Isolated, rare episodes of some parasomnias can be normal, while recurrent episodes are associated with other forms of sleep disorders such as acute or chronic sleep deprivation, sleep apnea, or narcolepsy. Some medications and medical conditions can also trigger parasomnias, and alcohol and substance use or abuse should also be considered as potential triggers.[1]

Evaluation of a woman who presents with complaints of parasomnia is best referred to a sleep medicine specialist. However, discussion of safety issues, particularly with sleepwalking or dream enactment that has provoked injury in the past, is an important part of the initial evaluation. Parasomnias are sometimes associated with other forms of sleep disorders, such as narcolepsy or OSA, and may improve with the treatment of the primary sleep disruption or disorder.

Sleep-Related Movement Disorders—Restless Legs Syndrome/ Willis-Ekbom Disease

DEFINITION, TYPES, AND EPIDEMIOLOGY

RLS is also known as Willis-Ekbom disease (WED) in the United States. RLS is a neurologic *sensorimotor* disorder characterized by unpleasant sensations, typically of the lower legs, that create an overwhelming urge to move the affected limbs. It becomes clinically significant when the symptoms cause distress or impairment in day-time functioning for the patient.

The natural course of RLS may be remitting or may progress, with spreading of the paresthesias to the torso, arms, and face. RLS symptoms follow a circadian pattern, beginning in the early evening, peaking during the night, and becoming quiescent in the morning hours. Symptoms mirror the circadian nadir levels of serum dopamine and iron.[80,81] RLS adversely impacts quality of sleep and can lead to impairment in mental, physical, social, occupational, educational, behavioral, sexual, or other important areas of functioning.[1,81] Although the exact pathophysiology for RLS is not understood, the current theory of central nervous system dopamine dysfunction and low levels of iron in the brain seem to be validated by research.

RLS affects all ethnicities and children, but is more prevalent in the Caucasian population, in women, during pregnancy, in the elderly, and in persons with chronic renal disease.[1] Prevalence rates vary from 5–15% in the general population to 15–25% in the pregnant population. Genetics may play a strong role in the development of RLS, and six potential risk factor genes have been identified.[82] RLS can be seen in patients as a primary disease or related to a medical condition. Clinically significant RLS can range from intermittent symptoms that occur less than twice per week to chronic, persistent symptoms that occur at least twice per week to refractory symptoms that are unresponsive to monotherapy with first-line agents such as the dopaminergics and require "add-on" treatment.[80,82] If the disease progresses, symptoms may be experienced throughout the day and the night. Eighty to 90% of patients with RLS also suffer motor symptoms known periodic limb movements (PLMs), which occur both day and night and which include, but are not limited to, involuntary jerking of the knee. PLMs at night lead to arousals from sleep, further adversely impacting a good night's sleep.[1]

According the International Restless Legs Syndrome Study Group (IRLSSG), the diagnosis of RLS is made clinically based on five criteria: 1) the patient must have an urge to move the legs due to uncomfortable and unpleasant sensations, 2) the symptoms must begin or worsen during periods of rest or inactivity, 3) the symptoms must be partially or totally relieved by getting up and moving, 4) the symptoms must begin predominantly in the evening or night rather than during the day, and 5) the symptoms cannot be explained by other pathologies. Three additional criteria may help to make the diagnosis: the patient experiences PLMs, there is a family history, and the patient has responded to dopaminergic therapy in the past with symptom alleviation.[80]

ESSENTIAL HISTORY

A current or past medical history should focus on chronic diseases, such as kidney failure, or diabetes, which may require treatment along with the diagnosis and treatment of RLS. The medication history should focus on those medications known to antagonize dopamine synthesis in the central nervous system, including antiemetics, decongestants, antihistamines, cough suppressants, calcium channel blockers, and antidepressants.[81] These are listed in **Table 4-14**.

As part of the review of systems, the five diagnostic criteria can be asked using the "URGES" mnemonic in **Table 4-15**.

PHYSICAL

A neuromuscular examination of the lower extremities for sensation, motor coordination, and strength will reveal no deficits. Differential diagnoses, known as "RLS mimics," should be considered and treated appropriately: sore leg muscles, ligament sprain/tendon strain, positional ischemia (numbness) or discomfort, dermatitis, bruises, leg cramps, positional neuropathy, myalgias, venous

Table 4-14 Medications That Aggravate Symptoms of RLS

Classification of Drug	Specific Drug	Consider Change to/Comments
Antihistamines	Diphenhydramine (Benadryl)	Loratadine (Claritin)
Antiemetics	Metoclopramide (Reglan)	Ondansetron (Zofran)
	Promethazine (Phenergan)	
	Prochlorperazine (Compazine)	
	Chlorpromazine (Thorazine)	
Antipsychotics	Haloperidol (Haldol)	Consult with psych-mental
	Phenothiazines	health
Calcium channel blockers	Nifedipine (Procardia)	Other antihypertensive
	Verapamil (Calan)	
Cough suppressants	Dextromethorphan	Tessalon Perles
		Codeine without Phenergan
Decongestants	Pseudoephedrine (Sudafed)	Neti pot or nasal rinse
Noradrenergic and specific serotonergic antidepressants (NaSSA)	Mirtazapine (Remeron)	Bupropion (Wellbutrin)
	Venlafaxine (Effexor)	
Selective serotonin reuptake inhibitors (SSRIs)	Paroxetine (Paxil)	Bupropion (Wellbutrin)
	Sertraline (Zoloft),	
	Fluoxetine (Prozac), etc.	
Tricyclic antidepressants (TCAs)	Imipramine (Tofranil)	Bupropion (Wellbutrin)
	Amitriptyline (Elavil), etc.	
Foods and habits	Coffee	
	Chocolate	
	Red wine	
	Tobacco	

Data from Picchietti DL, Hensley JG, Bainbridge JL, et al. Consensus clinical practice guidelines for the diagnosis and treatment of restless legs syndrome/Willis-Ekbom disease during pregnancy and lactation. *Sleep Med Rev.* 2015; 22: 64-77. doi:S1087-0792(14)00119-1 [pii]

stasis, post-thrombotic syndrome, leg edema, arthritis, and habitual foot tapping.[1]

LABORATORY/IMAGING

RLS is a clinical diagnosis; there is no imaging or blood test that will confirm the diagnosis. A PSG is not necessary for the diagnosis of RLS. Patients diagnosed with RLS should have a serum ferritin level drawn and be started on iron repletion therapy if the value is < 75 mcg/L.[82] Ferrous sulfate 325 mg with vitamin C 500 mg

three times daily is the most cost-effective combination. Many patients experience constipation as a side effect of iron therapy and should receive anticipatory guidance regarding bowel hygiene.

MANAGEMENT

Treatment of RLS must be individualized. Offering nonpharmacologic treatments as first-line treatment is prudent, because the pharmacologic treatments, although the most efficacious, are not

Table 4-15 URGES

1. Do you have sensations in your legs that give you an urge to get up and move? _____Yes _____No

2. Do these sensations become stronger at rest, such as sitting still or lying down? _____Yes _____No

3. When you get up and move (walk), do the sensations in your legs go away completely? _____Yes _____No

4. Do these leg sensations start in the early evening and continue into the night? _____Yes _____No

5. Do you have any medical conditions that could cause your restless legs syndrome (RLS) symptoms, or are you on any medications that could unmask or worsen your RLS? (question with clinician guidance) _____Yes _____No

If you answered yes to the questions above:

6. Do your legs jerk on their own? (What does your bed partner say at night?) _____Yes _____No

7. Do these leg sensations disturb your overall sleep? _____Yes _____No

8. If so, how many hours of total sleep per night do you get? _____

9. Is there anyone in your family who also has these leg sensations? _____Yes _____No

10. Did you experience these leg sensations during a pregnancy? _____Yes _____No _____N/A

Data from Aurora RN, Kristo DA, Bista SR, Rowley JA, Zak RS, Casey KR . . . American Academy of Sleep Medicine. The treatment of restless legs syndrome and periodic limb movement disorder in adults—an update for 2012: Practice parameters with an evidence-based systematic review and meta-analyses: An American Academy of Sleep Medicine clinical practice guideline. *Sleep.* 2012;35(8):1039-1062. doi:10.5665/sleep.1988

without side effects. When developing a plan of management with the patient, the clinician should never underestimate the power of placebo effect or therapeutic presence. Many patients simply want to know that they are not "crazy" and that the symptoms are not "just in their heads." The clinician who confirms that RLS is a real disease and listens to the patient may be providing more of a therapeutic treatment than medication.

LIFESTYLE

Avoidance of RLS "triggers" such as alcohol, caffeine, chocolate, and tobacco, all of which antagonize dopamine and decrease absorption of iron from the stomach, may help manage mild to moderate symptoms. If low iron stores have been documented by a serum ferritin level, high-iron foods or iron supplementation may help. Relief measures include setting a time to go to bed and a time to rise each morning, moderate exercise during the day but not before bed, massaging the legs, warm or hot baths, or use of a heating pad or ice packs to the lower legs at time of sleep. Other nonpharmacologic treatments include yoga, cognitive behavior training and stimulus control, hypnosis, near-infrared therapy, sequential compression devices, intercourse, and acupuncture.[80] None of these will eliminate the disease or recurring symptoms, but they may help the patient who prefers no medication. For more restless nights, the use of mind-stimulating devices, such as online gaming, may help attenuate the symptoms.

MEDICATIONS

A change from more to less dopamine antagonizing medications may be indicated. It is wise to provide a list of RLS triggers, as many patients may be unaware of what they consume that antagonizes dopamine.

The Medical Advisory Board of the Restless Legs Syndrome Foundation advises the following when considering pharmacologic treatment: 1) intermittent RLS ($\leq$ two times per week), medication only as needed; 2) chronic-persistent RLS ($\geq$ two times per week), daily treatment beginning with a low-dose dopaminergic; and 3) refractory RLS (incomplete response to dopaminergic monotherapy), medication adjustment and/or adjunct medications.[81]

Medication management of RLS can be summed up in 3 steps: 1) avoidance of aggravating medications and triggers, 2) iron repletion, and 3) pharmacotherapy known to attenuate symptoms. Pharmacotherapy is generally effective for the treatment of RLS and PLMs and falls into the following categories: 1) dopaminergics, 2) alpha-2 delta ligand anticonvulsants, 3) sedative-hypnotics and benzodiazepines/benzodiazepine receptor agonists, 4) one alpha adrenergic, and 5) opioids. Not all are US Food and Drug Administration (FDA)–approved for the treatment of RLS; some are used "off-label." Dopaminergics are rated as having the highest evidence for efficacy by the AASM.[82,83] See **Table 4-16** for details.

Patient Instructions

The patient should follow instructions and take medications as indicated. Patients started on dopaminergics should be cautioned about dizziness (due to a decrease in blood pressure) and the potential for unmasking compulsive behaviors such as gambling, shopping, and eating. Although dopaminergics are the most effective, they can cause augmentation or worsening of RLS symptoms earlier in the evening, which should be reported to the clinician.

Referral/Consultation

Referral to a sleep specialist should be considered if the patient's symptoms worsen despite iron repletion, if symptoms do not respond to nonpharmacologic therapies, if symptoms persist despite a change from more to less dopamine antagonizing, or if medical therapy has failed.

Management During Pregnancy and Lactation

The pregnant patient may find comfort in knowing RLS symptoms generally resolve within 1 month postpartum. RLS during pregnancy, however, is a risk factor for development of the disease during a subsequent pregnancy or later in life.[84]

A 2-year project was sanctioned by the IRLSSG to determine safe and efficacious treatments for RLS during pregnancy and lactation. Many medications pose a real or potential risk to the fetus and newborn. For pregnant women whose symptoms are not controlled with iron repletion and nonpharmacologic therapies, carbidopa-levodopa, clonazepam, or oxycodone can be used sparingly after the first trimester. During lactation, women can be offered gabapentin or clonazepam.[80] Use of pharmacotherapeutics should be at the lowest dose for the shortest period of time.

Summary

This chapter has given an overview of sleep and sleep disorders in women's health for primary care providers. Sleep is an important and often overlooked part of health. The goal of this chapter was to guide initial evaluation and management, and identification of those women who should be referred to a sleep medicine provider. There are many excellent resources available in print and online for providers and patients who are searching for additional information.

Table 4-16 Treatment of RLS

Non-pregnant	Medication	Dosing/24 hours	Comments
Dopaminergics	Pramipexole (Mirapex)	0.125 mg up to 0.5 mg up to max 1.0 mg	• Risk of augmentation • Slow titration to avoid orthostatic hypotension
	Ropinirole (Requip)	0.25 mg up to max 4 mg	• Take 1 hour before symptom onset
	Carbidopa-levodopa ER (Sinemet)	Initial 12.5/50 mg up to 25/100 mg to max 50/200 mg	• Nausea
	Rotigotine patch (Neupro)	1 mg patch/24 hours max 3 mg/24 hours	• Compulsivity
Anticonvulsants	Gabapentin (Neurontin)	300 mg Max 3600 mg	
	Gabapentin enacarbil (Horizant)	600 mg Max 1200 mg	
	Pregabalin (Lyrica)	100 mg Max 450 mg	
Non-benzodiazepine sedative hypnotics	Eszopiclone (Lunesta)	1 mg Max 3 mg	• Warn about sleep-related, drug-induced behaviors such as eating
	Zaleplon (Sonata)	5 mg Max 10 mg	
	Zolpidem (Ambien)	5 mg Max 10 mg	
Benzodiazepines	Clonazepam (Klonopin)	0.25 mg Max 4 mg	
	Temazepam (Restoril)	7.5 mg Max 30 mg	
Alpha adrenergic	Clonidine	0.1 mg Max 4 mg	• Risk of orthostatic hypotension
Opioids	Codeine	15 mg Max 120 mg	• Consider addictive potential
	Oxycodone	5 mg Max 20 mg	• Have patient sign Chronic Opioid Use Consent Form
	Oxycodone XR	10 mg Max 30 mg	
	Hydrocodone	5 mg Max 30 mg	
	Methadone	5 mg Max 40 mg	
	Tramadol	50 mg Max 400 mg	

Pregnant	Medication	Dosing	Comments after first trimester
	Carbidopa-levodopa ER (Sinemet)	12.5/50–200 mg	
	Clonazepam (low dose)	0.25–1 mg	Neonatal abstinence syndrome a potential in high doses
	Oxycodone (low dose)	2.5–5 mg	

Lactation	Medication	Dosing	Comments
Anticonvulsant	Gabapentin (Neurontin)	300–900 mg	
Benzodiazepine	Clonazepam (low dose)	0.25–1 mg	Maternal drowsiness and inability to care for newborn in high doses

Data from Picchietti DL, Hensley JG, Bainbridge JL, et al. Consensus clinical practice guidelines for the diagnosis and treatment of restless legs syndrome/Willis-Ekbom disease during pregnancy and lactation. *Sleep Med Rev.* 2015; 22: 64–77.doi:S1087-0792(14)00119-1.

Online Resources

1. American Academy of Sleep Medicine—provides access to the most up-to-date clinical practice guidelines for sleep disorders: http://www.AASMnet.org
2. Horne and Ostberg Morningness-Eveningness Questionnaire: http://www.cet-hosting.com/limesurvey/?sid=61524
3. National Sleep Foundation provides general information for providers and patients on sleep and sleep disorders: https://sleepfoundation.org/
4. Online program for cognitive behavioral therapy for insomnia: http://shuti.me/
5. Restless Legs Syndrome Foundation provides information for providers and patients on restless leg syndrome/WED: http://www.RLS.org

References

1. American Academy of Sleep Medicine. *The International Classification of Sleep Disorders*. 3rd ed. Darien, IL: American Academy of Sleep Medicine; 2014:297.
2. Bonnet MH. Acute sleep deprivation. In: Kryger MH, Roth T, Dement WC, eds. *Principles and Practice of Sleep Medicine*. 4th ed. Philadelphia, PA: Elsevier Saunders; 2005:51-66.
3. Shepard JW, Jr, Buysse DJ, Chesson AL, Jr, Dement WC, Goldberg R, Guilleminault C, et al. History of the development of sleep medicine in the United States. *J Clin Sleep Med*. 2005;1(1):61-82.
4. Tobler I. Phylogeny of sleep regulation. In: Kryger MH, Roth T, Dement WC, eds. *Principles and Practice of Sleep Medicine*. 4th ed. Philadelphia, PA: Elsevier/Saunders; 2005:77-90.
5. Colten HR, Altevogt BM, eds.; Institute of Medicine (US) Committee on Sleep Medicine and Research, ed. *Sleep Disorders and Sleep Deprivation: An Unmet Public Health Problem*. Washington, DC: National Academies Press; 2006. Available at: http://www.ncbi.nlm.nih.gov/books/NBK19960/. Accessed February 29, 2016.
6. Consensus Conference Panel, Watson NF, Badr MS, Belenky G, Bilwise DL, Buxton OM, et al. Joint consensus statement of the American Academy of Sleep Medicine and Sleep Research Society on the recommended amount of sleep for a healthy adult: methodology and discussion. *J Clin Sleep Med*. 2015;11(8):931-952. doi: 10.5664/jcsm.4950.
7. National Sleep Foundation. 2014 Sleep Health Index. Available at: https://sleepfoundation.org/sites/default/files/2014%20Sleep%20Health%20Index-FINAL_0.PDF. Accessed February 29, 2016.
8. Jenni OG, Carskadon MA. Life cycles: Infants to adolescents. In: Amlaner CJ, Fuller PM, eds. *SRS Basics of Sleep Guide*. 2nd ed. Westchester, IL: Sleep Research Society; 2009:33-41.
9. Darukhanavala A, Booth JN, 3rd, Bromley L, Whitmore H, Imperial J, Penev PD. Changes in insulin secretion and action in adults with familial risk for type 2 diabetes who curtail their sleep. *Diabetes Care*. 2011;34(10):2259-2264. doi: 10.2337/dc11-0777.
10. Rod NH, Kumari M, Lange T, Kivimaki M, Shipley M, Ferrie J. The joint effect of sleep duration and disturbed sleep on cause-specific mortality: results from the Whitehall II cohort study. *PLoS One*. 2014;9(4):e91965. doi: 10.1371/journal.pone.0091965.
11. von Ruesten A, Weikert C, Fietze I, Boeing H. Association of sleep duration with chronic diseases in the European prospective investigation into cancer and nutrition (EPIC)-Potsdam study. *PLoS One*. 2012;7(1):e30972. doi: 10.1371/journal.pone.0030972.
12. Teft BC. Prevalence of motor vehicle crashes involving drowsy drivers, United States, 2009-2013. AAA Foundation for Traffic Safety website. 2014. Available at: https://www.aaafoundation.org/sites/default/files/AAAFoundation-DrowsyDriving-Nov2014.pdf. Accessed February 29, 2016.
13. Barger LK, Cade BE, Ayas NT, Cronin JW, Rosner B, Speizer FE, et al. Extended work shifts and the risk of motor vehicle crashes among interns. *N Engl J Med*. 2005;352(2):125-134. doi: 352/2/125 [pii].
14. Luckhaupt SE, Tak S, Calvert GM. The prevalence of short sleep duration by industry and occupation in the national health interview survey. *Sleep*. 2010;33(2):149-159.
15. Borbély AA. A two process model of sleep regulation. *Hum Neurobiol*. 1982;1(3):195-204.
16. Stevens RG, Zhu Y. Electric light, particularly at night, disrupts human circadian rhythmicity: is that a problem? *Philos Trans R Soc Lond B Biol Sci*. 2015;370(1667):10.1098/rstb.2014.0120. doi: 10.1098/rstb.2014.0120.
17. Zhu L, Zee PC. Circadian rhythm sleep disorders. *Neurol Clin*. 2012;30(4):1167-91. doi: 10.1016/j.ncl.2012.08.011.

18. Kryger MH, Roth T, Dement WC. *Principles and Practice of Sleep Medicine.* 5th ed. Philadelphia, PA: Elsevier/Saunders; 2011:1766.
19. Scheer FA, Cajochen C, Turek FW, Czeisler CA. Melatonin in the regulation of sleep and circadian rhythms. In: Kryger MH, Roth T, Dement WC, eds. *Principles and Practice of Sleep Medicine.* 4th ed. Philadelphia, PA: Elsevier/Saunders; 2005.
20. Carskadon MA, Dement WC. Normal human sleep: An overview. In: Kryger MH, Roth T, Dement WC, eds. *Principles and Practice of Sleep Medicine.* 4th ed. Philadelphia, PA: Elsevier/Saunders; 2005:13-23.
21. Cappuccio F, Miller MA, Lockley SW. *Sleep, Health, and Society: From Aetiology to Public Health.* New York, NY: Oxford University Press; 2010:471.
22. Cappuccio F, Miller MA. The epidemiology of sleep and cardiovascular risk and disease. In: Cappuccio F, Miller MA, Lockley SW, eds. *Sleep, Health, and Society: From Aetiology to Public Health.* New York, NY: Oxford University Press; 2010:83-110.
23. Depner CM, Stothard ER, Wright KP, Jr. Metabolic consequences of sleep and circadian disorders. *Curr Diab Rep.* 2014;14(7):507. doi: 10.1007/s11892-014-0507-z.
24. Nedeltcheva AV, Scheer FA. Metabolic effects of sleep disruption, links to obesity and diabetes. *Curr Opin Endocrinol Diabetes Obes.* 2014;21(4):293-8. doi: 10.1097/MED.0000000000000082.
25. Broussard J, Knutson KL. Sleep and metabolic disease. In: Cappuccio F, Miller MA, Lockley SW, eds. *Sleep, Health, and Society: From Aetiology to Public Health.* New York, NY: Oxford University Press; 2010:111-140.
26. Khoury J, Doghramji K. Primary sleep disorders. *Psychiatr Clin North Am.* 2015;38(4):683-704.
27. Schutte-Rodin S, Broch L, Buysse D, Dorsey C, Sateia M. Clinical guideline for the evaluation and management of chronic insomnia in adults. *J Clin Sleep Med.* 2008;4(5):487-504.
28. Spielman AJ, Caruso LS, Glovinsky PB. A behavioral perspective on insomnia treatment. *Psychiatr Clin North Am.* 1987;10(4):541-553.
29. Morin CM, Bootzin RR, Buysse DJ, Edinger JD, Espie CA, Lichstein KL. Psychological and behavioral treatment of insomnia: update of the recent evidence (1998–2004). *Sleep.* 2006;29(11):1398-1414.
30. Chung F, Yegneswaran B, Liao P, Vairavanathan S, Islam S, Khajehdehi A, et al. STOP questionnaire: a tool to screen patients for obstructive sleep apnea. *Anesthesiology.* 2008;108(5):812-821.
31. National Sleep Foundation. *2006 Sleep in America Poll: Adolescents and Sleep: Summary of Findings.* Washington, DC: National Sleep Foundation; 2006. Available at: https://sleepfoundation.org/sites/default/files/2006_summary_of_findings.pdf. Accessed March 1, 2016.
32. Schlarb AA, Liddle CC, Hautzinger M. JuSt—a multimodal program for treatment of insomnia in adolescents: a pilot study. *Nat Sci Sleep.* 2010;3:13-20. doi: 10.2147/NSS.S14493.
33. Abbott SM, Attarian H, Zee PC. Sleep disorders in perinatal women. *Best Pract Res Clin Obstet Gynaecol.* 2014;28(1):159-168. doi: 10.1016/j.bpobgyn.2013.09.003.
34. Lee KA, Gay CL. Sleep in late pregnancy predicts length of labor and type of delivery. *Am J Obstet Gynecol.* 2004;191(6):2041-2046. doi: S0002937804005745 [pii].
35. Chang JJ, Pien GW, Duntley SP, Macones GA. Sleep deprivation during pregnancy and maternal and fetal outcomes: is there a relationship? *Sleep Med Rev.* 2010;14(2):107-114. doi: 10.1016/j.smrv.2009.05.001.
36. Izci-Balserak B, Pien GW. Sleep-disordered breathing and pregnancy: potential mechanisms and evidence for maternal and fetal morbidity. *Curr Opin Pulm Med.* 2010;16(6):574-582. doi: 10.1097/MCP.0b013e32833f0d55.
37. Izci-Balserak B, Pien GW. The relationship and potential mechanistic pathways between sleep disturbances and maternal hyperglycemia. *Curr Diab Rep.* 2014;14(2):459. doi: 10.1007/s11892-013-0459-8.
38. Hall MH, Kline CE, Nowakowski S. Insomnia and sleep apnea in midlife women: prevalence and consequences to health and functioning. *F1000Prime Rep.* 2015;7:63. eCollection 2015. doi: 10.12703/P7-63.
39. Nowakowski S, Meliska CJ, Martinez LF, Parry BL. Sleep and menopause. *Curr Neurol Neurosci Rep.* 2009;9(2):165-172.
40. Young T, Palta M, Dempsey J, Skatrud J, Weber S, Badr S. The occurrence of sleep-disordered breathing among middle-aged adults. *N Engl J Med.* 1993;328(17):1230-1235. doi: 10.1056/NEJM199304293281704.
41. Peppard PE, Young T, Barnet JH, Palta M, Hagen EW, Hla KM. Increased prevalence of sleep-disordered breathing in adults. *Am J Epidemiol.* 2013;177(9):1006-1014. doi: 10.1093/aje/kws342.
42. Tantrakul V, Guilleminault C. Chronic sleep complaints in premenopausal women and their association with sleep-disordered breathing. *Lung.* 2009;187(2):82-92. doi: 10.1007/s00408-009-9137-7.
43. Tantrakul V, Park CS, Guilleminault C. Sleep-disordered breathing in premenopausal women: differences between younger (less than 30 years old) and older women. *Sleep Med.* 2012;13(6):656-662. doi: 10.1016/j.sleep.2012.02.008.
44. O'Brien LM, Bullough AS, Owusu JT, Tremblay KA, Brincat CA, Chames MC, et al. Pregnancy-onset habitual snoring, gestational hypertension, and preeclampsia: prospective cohort study. *Am J Obstet Gynecol.* 2012;207(6):487.e1-9. doi: 10.1016/j.ajog.2012.08.034.

45. Gold AR, Gold MS, Harris KW, Espeleta VJ, Amin MM, Broderick JE. Hypersomnolence, insomnia and the pathophysiology of upper airway resistance syndrome. *Sleep Med.* 2008;9(6):675-683. doi: S1389-9457(07)00315-2 [pii].

46. Stoohs RA, Philip P, Andries D, Finlayson EV, Guilleminault C. Reaction time performance in upper airway resistance syndrome versus obstructive sleep apnea syndrome. *Sleep Med.* 2009;10(9):1000-1004. doi: 10.1016/j.sleep.2008.11.005.

47. Stoohs RA, Knaack L, Blum HC, Janicki J, Hohenhorst W. Differences in clinical features of upper airway resistance syndrome, primary snoring, and obstructive sleep apnea/hypopnea syndrome. *Sleep Med.* 2008;9(2):121-8. doi: S1389-9457(07)00084-6 [pii].

48. Krakow B, Krakow J, Ulibarri VA, McIver ND. Frequency and accuracy of "RERA" and "RDI" terms in the *Journal of Clinical Sleep Medicine* from 2006 through 2012. *J Clin Sleep Med.* 2014;10(2):121-4.

49. Guilleminault C, Kirisoglu C, Poyares D, Palombini L, Leger D, Farid-Moayer M, et al. Upper airway resistance syndrome: a long-term outcome study. *J Psychiatr Res.* 2006;40(3):273-9. doi: S0022-3956(05)00045-2 [pii].

50. Kristo DA, Lettieri CJ, Andrada T, Taylor Y, Eliasson AH. Silent upper airway resistance syndrome: prevalence in a mixed military population. *Chest.* 2005;127(5):1654-7. doi: 127/5/1654 [pii].

51. Epstein LJ, Kristo D, Strollo PJ, Jr, Friedman N, Malhotra A, Patil SP, et al. Clinical guideline for the evaluation, management and long-term care of obstructive sleep apnea in adults. *J Clin Sleep Med.* 2009;5(3):263-276.

52. American Academy of Sleep Medicine Board of Directors, Watson NF, Morgenthaler T, Chervin R, Carden K, Kirsch D, et al. Confronting drowsy driving: the American Academy of Sleep Medicine Perspective. *J Clin Sleep Med.* 2015;11(11):1335-6. doi: 10.5664/jcsm.5200.

53. Nieto FJ, Peppard PE, Young T, Finn L, Hla KM, Farre R. Sleep-disordered breathing and cancer mortality: results from the Wisconsin Sleep Cohort study. *Am J Respir Crit Care Med.* 2012;186(2):190-194. doi: 10.1164/rccm.201201-0130OC.

54. Young T, Finn L, Peppard PE, Szklo-Coxe M, Austin D, Nieto FJ, et al. Sleep disordered breathing and mortality: eighteen-year follow-up of the Wisconsin Sleep Cohort. *Sleep.* 2008;31(8):1071-1078.

55. Young T, Palta M, Dempsey J, Peppard PE, Nieto FJ, Hla KM. Burden of sleep apnea: rationale, design, and major findings of the Wisconsin Sleep Cohort study. *WMJ.* 2009;108(5):246-249.

56. Young T, Finn L, Austin D, Peterson A. Menopausal status and sleep-disordered breathing in the Wisconsin Sleep Cohort study. *Am J Respir Crit Care Med.* 2003;167(9):1181-1185. doi: 10.1164/rccm.200209-1055OC.

57. Young T. Rationale, design and findings from the Wisconsin Sleep Cohort study: toward understanding the total societal burden of sleep disordered breathing. *Sleep Med Clin.* 2009;4(1):37-46. doi: 10.1016/j.jsmc.2008.11.003.

58. Facco F, L. Sleep-disordered breathing and pregnancy. *Semin Perinatol.* 2011;35(6):335-339. doi: 10.1053/j.semperi.2011.05.018.

59. Young T, Evans L, Finn L, Palta M. Estimation of the clinically diagnosed proportion of sleep apnea syndrome in middle-aged men and women. *Sleep.* 1997;20(9):705-706.

60. Wilson DL, Walker SP, Fung AM, O'Donoghue F, Barnes M, Howard M. Can we predict sleep-disordered breathing in pregnancy? The clinical utility of symptoms. *J Sleep Res.* 2013;22(6):670-678. doi: 10.1111/jsr.12063.

61. Tantrakul V, Sirijanchune P, Panburana P, et al. Screening of obstructive sleep apnea during pregnancy: differences in predictive values of questionnaires across trimesters. *J Clin Sleep Med.* 2015;11(2):157-163. doi: 10.5664/jcsm.4464.

62. Louis J, Auckley D, Miladinovic B, Shepherd A, Mencin P, Kumar D, et al. Perinatal outcomes associated with obstructive sleep apnea in obese pregnant women. *Obstet Gynecol.* 2012;120(5):1085-1092. doi: http://10.1097/AOG.0b013e31826eb9d8.

63. Pamidi S, Pinto LM, Marc I, Benedetti A, Schwartzman K, Kimoff RJ. Maternal sleep-disordered breathing and adverse pregnancy outcomes: A systematic review and metaanalysis. *Obstet Gynecol.* 2014;210(1):52.e1-14. doi: http://dx.doi.org.ezproxy.lib.umb.edu/10.1016/j.ajog.2013.07.033.

64. Bourjeily G, Raker C, Paglia MJ, Ankner G, O'Connor K. Patient and provider perceptions of sleep disordered breathing assessment during prenatal care: a survey-based observational study. *Ther Adv Respir Dis.* 2012;6(4):211-9. doi: 10.1177/1753465812444958.

65. Luyster FS, Buysse DJ, Strollo PJ, Jr. Comorbid insomnia and obstructive sleep apnea: challenges for clinical practice and research. *J Clin Sleep Med.* 2010;6(2):196-204.

66. Pigeon WR, Sateia MJ. Is insomnia a breathing disorder? *Sleep.* 2012;35(12):1589-1590. doi: 10.5665/sleep.2222.

67. Björnsdóttir E, Janson C, Sigurdsson JF, Gehrman P, Perlis M, Juliusson S, et al. Symptoms of insomnia among patients with obstructive sleep apnea before and after two years of positive airway pressure treatment. *Sleep.* 2013;36(12):1901-1909. doi: 10.5665/sleep.3226.

68. Stansbury RC, Strollo PJ. Clinical manifestations of sleep apnea. *J Thorac Dis*. 2015;7(9):E298-310. doi: 10.3978/j.issn.2072-1439.2015.09.13.
69. Chung F, Yang Y, Brown R, Liao P. Alternative scoring models of STOP-Bang questionnaire improve specificity to detect undiagnosed obstructive sleep apnea. *J Clin Sleep Med*. 2014;10(9):951-958.
70. Facco FL, Ouyang DW, Zee PC, Grobman WA. Development of a pregnancy-specific screening tool for sleep apnea. *J Clin Sleep Med*. 2012;8(4):389-394. doi: 10.5664/jcsm.2030.
71. Wilson DL, Walker SP, Fung AM, O'Donoghue F, Barnes M, Howard M. Can we predict sleep-disordered breathing in pregnancy? The clinical utility of symptoms. *J Sleep Res*. 2013;22(6):670-678. doi: 10.1111/jsr.12063.
72. Kapoor M, Greenough G. Home sleep tests for obstructive sleep apnea (OSA). *J Am Board Fam Med*. 2015;28:504-9. doi:10.3122/jabfm.2015.04.140266.
73. Ramar K, Dort LC, Katz SG, Lettieri CJ, Harrod CG, Thomas SM, et al. Clinical practice guideline for the treatment of obstructive sleep apnea and snoring with oral appliance therapy: an update for 2015. *J Clin Sleep Med*. 2015;11(7):773-827. doi: jc-00186-15 [pii].
74. Louis J, Auckley D, Bolden N. Management of obstructive sleep apnea in pregnant women. *Obstet Gynecol*. 2012;119(4):864-868. doi: 10.1097/AOG.0b013e31824c0c2f.
75. Facco FL. Sleep-disordered breathing and pregnancy. *Semin Perinatol*. 2011;35(6):335-339. doi: http://dx.doi.org.ezproxy.lib.umb.edu/10.1053/j.semperi.2011.05.018.
76. Siegel JM. REM sleep. In: Dement MHKRC, ed. *Principles and Practice of Sleep Medicine*. 4th ed. Philadelphia, PA: Saunders/Elsevier; 2005:120-135. http://dx.doi.org.ezproxy.lib.umb.edu/10.1016/B0-72-160797-7/50017-3
77. Fraigne JJ, Torontali ZA, Snow MB, Peever JH. REM sleep at its core—circuits, neurotransmitters, and pathophysiology. *Front Neurol*. 2015;6:123. doi: 10.3389/fneur.2015.00123.
78. Thorpy MJ, Dauvilliers Y. Clinical and practical considerations in the pharmacologic management of narcolepsy. *Sleep Med*. 2015;16(1):9-18. doi: 10.1016/j.sleep.2014.10.002.
79. Horne JA, Ostberg O. A self-assessment questionnaire to determine morningness-eveningness in human circadian rhythms. *Int J Chronobiol*. 1976;4(2):97-110.
80. Allen RP, Picchietti DL, Garcia-Borreguero D, Ondo WG, Walters AS, Winkelman JW, et al. Restless legs syndrome/Willis-Ekbom disease diagnostic criteria: updated international restless legs syndrome study group (IRLSSG) consensus criteria—history, rationale, description, and significance. *Sleep Med*.2014;15(8):860-873.doi:10.1016/j.sleep.2014.03.025.
81. Becker PM, Novak M. Diagnosis, comorbidities, and management of restless legs syndrome. *Curr Med Res Opin*. 2014;30(8):1441-1460. doi: 10.1185/03007995.2014.918029.
82. Willis-Ekbom Disease Foundation. WED/RLS medical bulletin: A publication for healthcare providers. Available at: http://www.rls.org/about-rls/publications. Accessed March 1, 2016.
83. Aurora RN, Kristo DA, Bista SR, Rowley JA, Zak RS, Casey KR, et al. The treatment of restless legs syndrome and periodic limb movement disorder in adults—an update for 2012: practice parameters with an evidence-based systematic review and meta-analyses: an American Academy of Sleep Medicine clinical practice guideline. *Sleep*. 2012;35(8):1039-1062. doi: 10.5665/sleep.1988.
84. Hensley JG. Leg cramps and restless legs syndrome during pregnancy. *J Midwifery Womens Health*. 2009;54(3):211-218.

CHAPTER 5

MENTAL ILLNESS IN PRIMARY WOMEN'S HEALTH CARE

Barbara W. Graves

Mental illness profoundly affects women and their families. Anxiety and mood disorders are the most prevalent psychiatric diagnoses, and these disorders are diagnosed more frequently in women than in men. In women, depression alone has a lifetime prevalence of about 21% and is believed to be the leading cause of disease-related disability for women worldwide.[1] The lifetime prevalence of common mental health disorders as determined by a survey of more than 9000 English-speaking Americans is presented in **Figure 5-1**.

Patients with mental illness often suffer from other medical conditions and tend to be frequent utilizers of outpatient care.[2,3] Mental illness can complicate the treatment of other conditions by clouding the patient's thought processes, impairing her ability to make good decisions and to act in her own best interest.

Mental disorders are multifactorial in origin, with genetic,[4] epigenetic, and environmental factors all playing a role in the development of mental illness. Both prenatal and early-life stress influence mental health in later life.[5] The relative importance of biology versus environment seems to vary among the different illnesses. Bipolar disorder generally requires a genetic predisposition to the illness, while personality disorders are regarded as developing from learned behaviors. Psychiatric disorders tend to run in families, partly because of genetic vulnerability but also because of the environmental contribution of affected family members.

Gender and Mental Health

Women who have a biologic susceptibility to mental illness are likely to become symptomatic when they encounter the stressful events of a typical life. They appear to be more vulnerable than men to environmental stress, and not only when faced with life-threatening trauma. The hormonal shifts of puberty, menstruation, and childbearing or the stress of parenthood and intimate relationships can have significant effects on the neurologic and immune systems of women.

Figure 5-1 Lifetime prevalence of selected DSM-IV disorders from the World Mental Health Survey version of the Composite International Diagnostic Interview.

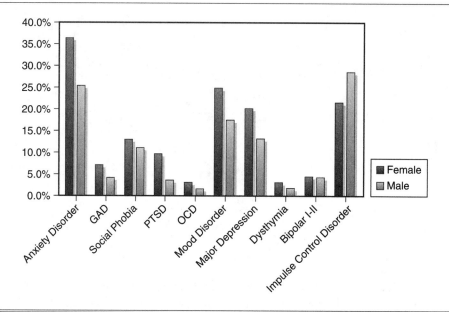

Data from Kessler RC, Berglund P, Demler O, Jin R, Merikangas KR, Walters EE. Lifetime prevalence and age-of-onset distributions of DSM-IV disorders in the National Comorbidity Survey Replication. *Arch Gen Psychiatry.* 2005;62:593-602.

Women are also more likely than men to experience somatic symptoms when they are anxious or depressed.[6] Patients often report appetite changes, sleep disturbances, fatigue, and pain rather than emotional distress.[7] Mental illness significantly impairs a woman's relationships with others and can threaten her interactions with her children. Maternal mental illness adversely affects even very young infants.

Depressed mothers do not engage with their infants as fully as healthy mothers. With limited maternal feedback, their babies are less likely to seek interaction with others.[8] According to recent meta-analyses, children of depressed mothers show developmental and cognitive delays, and more conduct and behavior disorders later in childhood than children whose mothers were not depressed. These problems persisted in children studied up to age 18 and were in direct proportion to the severity of the mother's illness.[9,10]

Each episode of mental illness makes the patient more vulnerable to the next. The individual's threshold for illness becomes progressively lower with each succeeding exposure to stress or trauma. The first episode of illness may be triggered by a sexual assault, the death of a loved one, or the hormonal shifts of pregnancy. The patient recovers with time, but a lesser degree of trauma may produce more distress than the first. Over a woman's lifetime, episodes can become more frequent, more severe, and more resistant to treatment. Untreated—or inadequately treated—mental illness will lead to increasing disability over the patient's lifetime.[11] Clinicians must identify signs of illness and engage their patients in effective treatment in order to minimize the cascading severity of their disease.

Presentations of Mental Illness Through the Life Cycle

Women's reproductive landmarks—pregnancy, childbirth, menarche, menopause—are often the very events that can trigger or worsen mental illness. Women's health providers need to be aware of how mental illness may present throughout a woman's life in order to appropriately identify, treat, and refer their patients. Mental disorders discussed in this chapter include those most often seen in primary women's health care. A number of well-known diagnoses (e.g., schizophrenia and dissociative disorders) are less common, and the reader is referred to the psychiatric literature for more information.

MENSTRUATION

Premenstrual symptoms are most commonly reported by women in their 20s and 30s, but may appear at any time. Emotional distress that varies through the menstrual cycle includes the familiar gynecologic diagnosis of premenstrual syndrome (PMS) as well as the psychiatric condition known as premenstrual dysphoric disorder (PMDD). Considering the relative incidences of mood disorders and PMDDs, women who experience cyclic emotional distress are more likely to have an exacerbation of an underlying mental illness than a "pure" premenstrual disorder.

A woman with a known psychiatric illness may request help from her primary or gynecologic provider in managing menstrual symptoms. In such a case, consultation with a mental health provider will validate the patient's experience and provide her with coordinated care.

SEXUAL BEHAVIOR AND CONTRACEPTION

Mental illness can affect a woman's ability to engage in safe sexual and contraceptive practices. Any of the mental illnesses can impair cognition and increase confusion about making choices, and an affected patient may require lengthy visits and repeated explanations. She may still make decisions that lead to a pregnancy or sexually transmitted infection that are—to the patient—unexpected. When a patient reports that she is participating in risky sexual behavior, it is important to consider that an underlying mental illness may be impairing her judgment. In addition to the cognitive slowing that is a hallmark of depression, bipolar disorder or personality disorders may lead to impulsive behaviors, while eating disorders and posttraumatic stress disorder (PTSD) often feature self-injurious behavior.

THE CHILDBEARING YEARS: PREGNANCY AND POSTPARTUM

Women are especially at risk to develop mood disorders and anxiety disorders during their childbearing years. The first year postpartum is the time when a woman is most likely to be hospitalized for psychiatric illness. With an estimated incidence between 5% and 25% of all mothers who have recently delivered, postpartum depression is the most common medical problem following childbirth.[12] Postpartum psychosis occurs once or twice per 1000 births and carries a significant risk of infanticide or suicide.[13]

The most significant risk factor for mental illness in pregnancy and postpartum is a history of previous mental illness in the patient or her family. Bipolar disorder in the patient or a family member is the single strongest predictor of psychosis in the postpartum period. The initial patient history is the most powerful tool for identifying risks. Because illness during pregnancy predicts postpartum illness, clinicians need to continue screening for symptoms as pregnancy progresses and throughout postpartum care.

MENOPAUSE

The decade before menopause is another time of vulnerability for development of mood disorders, particularly depression. As women mature, the accumulated stresses of life begin to wear down neurologic defenses. A woman who gives a history of premenstrual distress, dysphoric mood with hormonal contraceptives, postpartum illness, or any prior episode of mental illness is particularly at risk to develop psychiatric illness in middle age. Women can also experience a new onset of mental illness (including bipolar disorder and schizophrenia) as they enter middle age.

Essential History, Physical, and Laboratory Evaluation

Given the devastating impact that maternal depression and other mental health conditions can have on the health and wellbeing of mothers and children, women's health providers need to screen, treat, and refer affected women as appropriate. While often the diagnosis is clear after a careful history, on occasion physical and laboratory findings may help pinpoint an underlying medical condition masquerading as a mental health condition or can help pinpoint a specific mental health condition.

History

A careful clinical interview is the most powerful diagnostic tool for identifying current mental illness and risk factors that predict vulnerability to future illness. The thorough medical, surgical, family, obstetric, social, and psychiatric histories are each critical to identifying potential psychiatric disorders. Along with the physical examination and laboratory investigations, the

interview can be integrated into a routine office visit. **Table 5-1** offers suggestions for information about the patient's mental health at each phase of an office visit.

Women often avoid talking about their emotional health for fear that clinicians will be judgmental or unsympathetic. A clinician who is comfortable asking questions about mental illness and encourages the patient to tell her story will obtain the most useful information and be most helpful to the patient. The knowledge base and perspective that a midwife or an obstetrics and gynecology (OB/GYN) provider offer may be uniquely useful, because many mental health providers are not experts in women's health issues.

PSYCHIATRIC HISTORY

The single strongest predictor of future mental illness is past mental illness. Although medical history forms typically include a standard query about whether the patient has a history of mental illness, these items produce many false-negative responses. Rather than rely on such standard histories, clinicians should include direct and specific questions in every patient interview. Following the principle of beginning with less intrusive questions, the patient's history of physical illness and treatment should come first. As the patient and clinician become more comfortable with each other, the following six questions should be asked. These questions are in increasing order of intrusiveness and specificity for serious mental illness. A positive response to one question should be followed by the next:

1. Have you ever had trouble with feeling anxious or depressed?
   Depression and anxiety are common problems and are relatively easy to talk about. Start here and continue inquiring about other problems. Ask about past diagnoses and whether they seemed reasonable to the patient.

Table 5-1 Elements of Mental Health Assessment in a Primary Care Visit

Area of Assessment	Data	Rationale
Chief Complaint: Current Health Status	Emotional distress Stressful events Medications and prescribers; diagnosis and duration of use Habits	Patients may report their own illness. Stress can trigger mental illness. Medications can trigger mental symptoms. Use of or withdrawal from substances can trigger mental symptoms.
Review of Systems	Headaches, gastrointestinal disturbances, fatigue, disordered sleep, changes in cognition or memory, appetite derangements, chronic pain	Can be somatic or neurochemical manifestations of psychiatric illness.
Patient History	1. Have you ever had trouble with feeling anxious or depressed? 2. Have you ever been in therapy? 3. Have you ever taken medication for emotional troubles? 4. Have you ever been hospitalized or gone to the emergency room for emotional troubles? 5. Have you ever thought of hurting yourself? 6. Have you had any thoughts like that recently?	When taking the patient's history, ask about physical health first to build rapport, and then begin asking about mental health. The questions are in order of increasing intrusiveness and specificity for serious mental illness. Ask them in the order given; a positive response to one should be followed by the next.
Family History	1. Have any of the women in your family had emotional troubles after childbirth? 2. Has anyone in your family had trouble with mental illness? 3. Do you think that anyone in your family may have been bipolar or manic depressive? 4. Has anyone in your family attempted suicide? 5. Does anyone in your family have a substance problem?	Mental illness can be familial and the history should include grandparents, aunts, uncles, cousins, nieces, and nephews. Proceed as for the patient history above.
Physical Exam	Physical appearance: grooming, gait, tics, speech Mental Status: appearing sad or anxious; impaired cognition, insight, memory Body mass index, especially changes since last visit Head, ears, eyes, nose, and throat: thyroid, dental condition Skin: signs of self-injury Pain or "difficult exam"	Changes or inconsistencies can suggest emotional distress or neurologic disturbance. These are key indicators of mental functioning. Body mass index can be a marker for eating disorders, depression, drug use, and other problems. Thyroid disease can trigger psychiatric symptoms; women with sex abuse histories often avoid dental exams. Scars, burns, cuts, or extensive piercings may indicate parasuicidal behaviors. May be a sign of previous abuse; may be somatization of emotional distress.
Laboratory Studies	Complete blood count Thyroid function tests Glucose tolerance screening Drug screening; metabolic screening for liver, adrenocortical, and renal function Blood levels of psychotropic meds, as indicated by the prescriber If an eating disorder is suspected: serum electrolytes, liver function tests, bone density assessment, and electrocardiogram	Rule out anemia. Thyroid disease can cause psychiatric symptoms. Diabetes has a high comorbidity with depression. If history indicates, order these tests to check on toxicity or malfunction that could cause symptoms. Check with the prescriber and follow serum levels where indicated. Blood tests can reveal metabolic malfunction if eating disorder is suspected; work in consultation with the patient's primary providers if the diagnosis is known.

2. Have you ever been in therapy?

   Ask whether the therapy was helpful and why (or if) it was stopped. Ask for dates, duration, type of therapy, and provider(s) seen.

3. Have you ever taken medication for emotional troubles?

   Ask whether the medicine was helpful and whether there were any problems with it. List all medications, dosages, duration, and reasons why (or if) discontinued. It is also helpful to know the prescriber's credentials.

4. Have you ever been hospitalized or gone to the emergency room to treat emotional troubles? Hospitalization indicates a serious episode. Ask about diagnosis, treatment, institution, duration, and outcome.

5. Have you ever thought of hurting yourself? Did she have a plan? What method(s) did she try? What stopped her?

6. Have you had any thoughts like that recently? This provides an opening to talk about how likely she is to hurt herself or someone else. A woman who admits to having "bad thoughts" must contract for safety. **Box 5-1** offers suggestions on how to approach this topic.

Even in the absence of a formal diagnosis, the clinician should also take note of behavior and events that suggest mental illness. This includes risky sexual behavior, poor decision making, interpersonal conflicts, and inappropriate relationships.

FAMILY HISTORY

As with the patient history, the family history should begin with inquiries about physical health. Many mental illnesses have a strong genetic component, and a family history of mental illness should be as wide-ranging as any other genetic history. Before asking about mental health issues, the clinician should clarify to the patient that these questions include grandparents, aunts, uncles, cousins, nieces, and nephews. Be specific and include these questions in the following order:

1. Have any of the women in your family had emotional troubles during or after childbirth? This is the least intrusive inquiry about mental illness, especially in the context of an obstetric or preconception visit. Family members may have used such terms as "nervous breakdown," "nerve trouble," or "that postpartum" in

---

Box 5-1 A Contract for Safety

If a patient reports that she is having thoughts of hurting herself or others, you must ask her to contract for safety. In this context, "safety" means that she will not act upon an urge to hurt herself or another person. A woman who has been in therapy or been hospitalized for psychiatric illness understands what is meant by "contracting for safety," but you may have to explain what you mean very specifically to a patient who has not been in treatment before.

   Ask these questions in the order given:

1. *Are you safe now?*
2. *If you have any thoughts of hurting yourself or others, you must call me. If you can't wait for me to call back, you must call 9-1-1 and go to the hospital.*
   Can you promise me you will do that?
3. *Can you promise that you will not act on any urge to hurt yourself or someone else?*

A negative answer to any of these questions requires your immediate action to ensure the patient's safety. Psychiatric emergency protocols for your practice should be spelled out and adhered to just as they would be for any other medical emergency.

describing their difficulties. The patient should be encouraged to describe such episodes in her own way.

2. Has anyone in your family had trouble with emotional problems? Been hospitalized for mental illness?

   As with the previous question, the patient should be encouraged to describe diagnoses and treatment however she can. When a serious illness is described, it is important to sympathize with the devastating effect it has had on the family.

3. Do you think anyone in your family might have been bipolar or manic-depressive?

   In previous generations, bipolar illness was often not diagnosed or treated as such. If an older relative had times of high energy, sleeplessness, and grand ideas that alternated with periods of feeling low and miserable, bipolar illness can be presumed.

4. Has anyone in your family attempted suicide? Succeeded?

   This question is a very sensitive indicator of a history of severe illness, especially undiagnosed or untreated bipolar disorder. A family history of suicide is troubling to family members, and patients are generally grateful when a clinician opens the topic for discussion.

5. Does anyone in your family have a substance problem? How about alcohol?

   Substance use can be either a cause or an effect of mental illness. Direct questioning elicits the best information on the social history. Specific, yet open-ended questions such as "How many cigarettes per day?", "When was your last drink?", and "How many people have you have sex with during the last 6 months?" can be useful.

REVIEW OF SYSTEMS

Problems such as chronic headaches, gastrointestinal (GI) disturbances, fatigue, disordered sleep, changes in cognition or memory, appetite derangements, or chronic pain may be signs of psychiatric illness. If workups have not shown physical causes for the patient's distress, particularly if she's been told that, "it's all in my head," she may be experiencing psychomotor, cognitive, or somatic manifestations of an underlying mental disorder.

Life events, including recent surgery or current medical illness, often trigger or exacerbate psychiatric symptoms. **Table 5-2** includes factors that can be either comorbid with or causes of psychiatric illness. Medication reconciliation should include herbs, hormones, supplements, vitamin preparations, and over-the-counter (OTC) medications. Even OTC medications and antibiotics have been known to trigger symptoms. A patient's report of emotional disturbance while taking a particular medication should be considered to be just as serious as a report of drug allergy.

Physical Examination

Specific findings from the routine physical can contribute to the suspicion of a mental illness. Many women with mental illness may be appropriately dressed and appear to have a normal affect. Some women who are depressed may look sad and withdrawn, or present with psychomotor slowing and confusion. Anxious women may be physically tense and fidgety, asking many questions and demanding constant reassurance. Women with longstanding mental illness often look worn down and older than their age. Their appearance may be unkempt and their grooming inconsistent with their resources. Such outward signs of distress are particularly significant if they are a change from the patient's previous appearance; such changes may indicate a new onset of psychiatric illness.

Changes in body mass index (BMI) can also raise suspicions of possible mental illness. Significant weight loss in an adult or a failure to gain in a growing teenager suggests anorexia nervosa, which ranks among the deadliest of psychiatric disorders. Obesity may indicate bulimia or another eating disorder. Weight gain can also accompany depression; hypomanic or manic episodes

Table 5-2 Conditions and Medications That May Be Associated with Mental Illness

Medical Conditions	Endocrine: thyroid disorder, adrenocortical disorder, diabetes mellitus
	Neurologic: migraine, multiple sclerosis, epilepsy
	Rheumatologic: fibromyalgia, chronic fatigue, lupus, rheumatoid arthritis
	Cancers
	Gastrointestinal: irritable bowel syndrome
	Cardiovascular disease
	Substance use
	Medications
	Hormonal preparations, including contraceptives and hormone replacement therapy
	Psychotropic medications, including benzodiazepines and neuroleptics
	Cardiac drugs, including beta blockers and antihypertensives
	Corticosteroids, either systemic or topical preparations
	Isoretinoin (Accutane)

Note: A patient history of emotional disturbance while taking a particular medication is just as serious as a drug allergy and should be documented in the medical record.

may be associated with weight loss. Anxiety can either suppress appetite or trigger overeating of "comfort" foods.

An enlarged thyroid gland should be noted and followed by a thyroid function test (TFT), as part of the laboratory workup. Thyroid disease can trigger psychiatric symptoms and should be suspected whenever a woman complains of emotional distress. Thyroid function can also change during pregnancy and especially postpartum; a woman with a history of psychiatric or thyroid disease in herself or her family should have thyroid testing during each trimester and postpartum.

Poor dental condition may be associated with eating disorders or substance abuse. Acidic vomitus wears away dental enamel and can inflame mucosal tissue. Methamphetamine users have severe dental caries, a result both of drug effects and lifestyle changes (poor hygiene, cravings for sugary foods, grinding teeth). Women who have experienced oral sexual abuse typically avoid dental examinations and treatment.

Physical signs of self-injury are varied. The forearms and anterior thighs are the most frequent sites for cuts, burns, and self-tattoos. Multiple short, straight scars are typical of razor cuts. Scars or tattoos on the wrists may be concealed by decorative cuffs or bracelets. Genital self-injury can include cutting and piercing, or the perianal injuries resulting from purging behaviors. It is reasonable to ask about such signs during the course of an examination: "How did this happen?" The patient may readily explain an accidental injury, or she may be embarrassed and hesitant to answer. She may honestly not know how the injuries happened if they occurred when she was not conscious of her actions. Although the woman may discount the seriousness of self-injuries, they are considered to be para-suicidal gestures associated with a guarded long-term prognosis.[14]

A woman who somaticizes her emotional distress may show signs of pain or guarding during a general physical exam, even if no cause for the pain is apparent. It is important to acknowledge the patient's discomfort and not to dismiss it with, "I can't find anything wrong."

If a woman cannot tolerate a routine pelvic exam, she may have suffered previous sexual trauma or injury. It is best not to pursue questioning after a "difficult" exam, especially if the patient has already given a negative response to routine queries about abuse. If the woman does in fact suffer from PTSD, talking about it can trigger her symptoms, including panic and dissociation. It is well to remember that many instances of vaginismus and vulvodynia, for example, are not at all related to abusive experiences.

Laboratory Studies

Unfortunately, there are no specific diagnostic studies for mental illness. Laboratory findings can be helpful, however, in detecting metabolic disorders and other conditions that can cause or masquerade as mental illness. Certain tests can be done as indicated:

- Complete blood count (CBC) can rule out anemia as a cause of fatigue.
- TFTs should be performed when any mental illness is suspected. TFTs should be followed through pregnancy and postpartum, especially in women with a history of psychiatric or thyroid illness.
- Glucose tolerance screening identifies uncontrolled diabetes as a cause of somatic symptoms.
- Drug screening and liver, adrenocortical, and renal function tests are needed when indicated by history.
- If the patient is on psychotropic medication, check with her prescriber to determine whether blood levels should be followed, especially during pregnancy.
- If an eating disorder is suspected, then perform a test for serum electrolytes, liver function tests (LFTs), and bone density assessment, in consultation with the primary providers.

Mental Disorders Commonly Seen in Primary Care

Psychiatric diagnoses are based primarily on observations of behavior. Unlike the disciplines of medicine and surgery, which can base diagnoses on measurable phenomena and laboratory or imaging studies, psychiatry describes the behavior and thought processes of its patients. To minimize the subjectivity and confusion that can result from such a diagnostic process, the American Psychiatric Association publishes standard diagnostic criteria and minutely detailed descriptive codes of recognized disorders. The *Diagnostic and Statistical Manual of Mental Disorders, Fifth Edition*[15] (DSM-5), published in 2013, is used by mental health professionals to describe and diagnose psychiatric disorders.

The DSM-5 diagnostic codes are different from those in the International Classification of Diseases (ICD-10), which are used by other health clinicians to codify diseases for research or billing. Primary care providers bill for services using the ICD classification and ICD-10 codes. The increased number of codes in ICD-10 now allows for more specificity in diagnoses than its previous editions. DSM-5 will continue to be used as the basis for diagnosis and contains the data to assign an ICD-10 code. DSM-5 is the diagnostic standard that guides the presentation of mental health disorders in this chapter. Each category of mental illness presented in this chapter has subcategories where the disorder is related to either substance use or a medical diagnosis. These subcategories reinforce the importance of evaluating mental health within the perspective of the entire individual. The discussions that follow address the diagnosis of disorders in the absence of substance abuse or a medical condition causing the disorder, such as cocaine or hypothyroidism leading to mania.

Mood Disorders

Prior to the release of DSM-5, unipolar and bipolar diagnoses were grouped together as one category of mental illness. The developers of DSM-5 opted to recognize the distinctions in terms of symptoms and genetic contribution, and currently present two distinct categories of mood disorders: depressive disorders and bipolar and related disorders.[15] Because women with either bipolar or unipolar mood disorders may present with depression, it is useful to have a strategy, such as the algorithm in **Figure 5-2**, to distinguish between the two. This algorithm builds on the nine questions of the Patient Health Questionnaire-2 (PHQ-2) (described later) by adding an additional question concerning prior manic episodes.

DEPRESSIVE DISORDERS

The list of depressive disorders has expanded beyond the traditional disorders of major depressive episode, dysthymia (now included in the diagnosis of persistent depressive disorder), and unspecified depressive disorder. For the first time, perimenstrual dysphoric syndrome has been recognized as a distinct diagnostic entity, which is discussed later in the section on menstrual mood disorders. **Table 5-3** lists the depressive disorders.

Figure 5-2 Differential diagnoses of mood disorders.

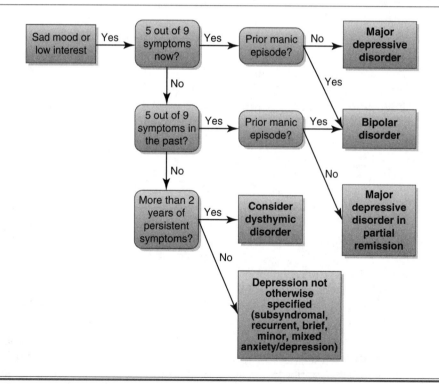

Reproduced from US Department of Health and Human Services. *Depression in Primary Care: Volume 1. Detection and diagnosis.* AHCPR Publication No. 93–0550. Rockville, MD: Agency for Health Care Policy and Research; 1993:20.

Table 5-3 Depressive Disorders

Previously included in DSM-IV
Major depressive disorder
Persistent mood disorder (dysthymia)
Unspecified depressive disorder

Added in DSM-5
Disruptive mood dysregulation disorder
Premenstrual dysphoric syndrome
Substance-/medication-induced depressive disorder
Depressive disorder due to another medical condition
Other specified depressive disorder

Data from American Psychiatric Association. *Diagnostic and Statistical Manual of Mental Disorders*. 5th ed. Arlington, VA: American Psychiatric Association; 2013; American Psychiatric Association. *Diagnostic and Statistical Manual of Mental Disorders*. 4th ed. Text Revision. Arlington, VA: American Psychiatric Association; 2000.

Major Depressive Disorder The phrase, "I'm depressed," is probably the most frequently heard psychiatric complaint. In addition to feeling sad or low, the patient suffering from depression may also report sleep disturbances, lack of energy, appetite changes, digestive difficulties, headaches, and unexplained bodily pains. Anxiety frequently accompanies depression, and patients may report feeling irritable, worried, or frustrated rather than blue.

Presentation While some women may present with a chief complaint of depression, many who are depressed do not report changes in mood, but instead seek help for memory loss, weight gain or loss, or decreased libido. They may become preoccupied with physical complaints, feelings of guilt or hopelessness, and—in extreme cases—suicidal thoughts or hallucinations. The clinician may notice a woman's slowed thinking, poor concentration and retention, confusion, and vague or contradictory decision making during the course of a routine visit. A sad or tearful appearance, slowed speech and delayed responses to questions,

or an anxious look with agitated gestures are signs that the patient is not well. She may also demand frequent, lengthy visits and multiple workups for problems that others would take in stride.

A history of depression in response to a previous trauma or change is a warning that recurrence is likely. Patients often dismiss their prior depressive episodes as "situational" or "stress related," and discount the likelihood that they will ever be troubled again. But any episode of depression indicates that the patient has a biologic vulnerability that may well cause a recurrence during subsequent periods of life stress. The clinician must keep in mind that depression is qualitatively the same no matter what triggered it, and any prior episode requires vigilance to anticipate a relapse. Postpartum depression is a major depressive episode occurring in the postpartum period and is addressed later in the chapter.

Screening The 2016 US Preventive Services Task Force (USPSTF) recommendation on screening for depression recommends routine screening for depression in adults and reinforces the importance of systems to ensure accurate diagnosis and adequate treatment and follow up.[16] The incorporation of routine screening for depression offers a unique opportunity for primary care clinicians to identify individuals with depressive disorders. This provider may also be in the unique position of providing targeted, time-limited counseling based on an ongoing therapeutic relationship. This relationship provides an opportunity to advise the woman on behaviors that improve depression, such as engaging in a realistic exercise program[17] and engaging in pleasurable activities. Bright-light therapy, which has been shown to be effective in treating depression, can also be recommended by the primary care clinician.[17,18]

While several screening tools are available, one of the simplest is the PHQ-2, with a sensitivity of 97% (95% CI, 83–99%) and a specificity of 67% (95% CI, 62–72%), displayed in **Table 5-4**.[19] This tool is available to the public free of charge. A score of 3 would suggest the need for further evaluation. Further evaluation using a focused interview is needed to determine whether referral to a mental health professional is warranted.

Diagnosis A careful clinical interview may be all that is needed for diagnosis. **Box 5-2** lists a mnemonic SIGECAPS—sleep, interest, guilt, energy, concentration, appetite, psychomotor, suicide—which includes the diagnostic criteria for major depression. A more structured assessment is the Patient Health Questionnaire (PHQ-9), provided

---

Table 5-4 Two-Question Screen for Depression (PHQ-2)

Over the last two weeks, how often have you been bothered by any of the following problems?	Not at all	Several days	More than half the days	Nearly every day
1. Little interest or pleasure in doing things	0	1	2	3
2. Feeling down, depressed, or hopeless	0	1	2	3

Reproduced from Pfizer. Patient Health Questionnaire-9 (PHQ-9). Retrieved from phqscreeners.com.

Box 5-2 Major Depression and Dysthymia

Major Depression: Symptoms (SIGECAPS)
Symptoms must include either depressed mood or anhedonia (lack of interest) *plus* any of the following symptoms (to total 5 symptoms), which occur nearly every day for at least 2 weeks, and are severe enough to impede function:
1. *S*leep disorder (insomnia or hypersomnia)
2. *I*nterest deficit or a lack of feeling pleasure
3. *G*uilt (worthlessness, hopelessness, regret)
4. *E*nergy deficit (fatigue or loss of energy nearly every day)
5. *C*oncentration deficit
6. *A*ppetite disorder (increased or decreased), unplanned weight loss or gain
7. *P*sychomotor retardation or agitation
8. *S*uicidality (recurrent thoughts of death)
There has never been a manic or hypomanic episode.
  Symptoms are not attributable to a medical condition or substance use.
  Must be qualified as single or recurrent, the severity, remission status, and the presence of psychotic symptoms.

Dysthymia: Symptoms
A. Depressed mood for most of the day, for more days than not, as indicated either by subjective account or observation by others, for at least 2 years.
B. Presence of ≥ 2 of the symptoms listed under major depression.
C. There has never been a manic or hypomanic episode.

Data from American Psychiatric Association. *Diagnostic and Statistical Manual of Mental Disorders.* 5th ed. Arlington, VA: American Psychiatric Association; 2013; Hackley B, Sharma C, Kedzior A, Sreenivarsan S. Managing mental health conditions in primary care settings. *J Midwifery Womens Health.* 2010;55:9-19.

in **Table 5-5**. The PHQ-9 has the advantage of providing a numeric score that can be followed to evaluate treatment success. Any person expressing thoughts of self-harm or harming another requires emergent psychiatric evaluation.

Treatment Major depression is an episodic disease that tends to recur throughout one's life. It can be treated, often to full remission of symptoms. Although combined psychotherapy and pharmacotherapy are the most effective at achieving remission and preventing relapses, one approach or the other may be favored by the patient.[20,21] Treatment with either psychotherapy or pharmacotherapy alone achieves similar rates of remission. Some women find that medication alone makes them feel as if they can handle life's problems and that they don't want to talk to anyone. Others prefer to "talk things through" with someone but consider medication to be a sign of weakness. Individuals who have not responded to a single modality of therapy should be referred for combination therapy.[22] The treatment goal for depression is to have a 50% reduction in symptoms within 10–12 weeks.[23]

Table 5-5 Patient Health Questionnaire (PHQ-9)

Over the last 2 weeks, how often have you been or had: (use "√" to indicate your answer)	Not at all	Several days	More than half the days	Nearly every day
1. Little interest or pleasure in doing things	0	1	2	3
2. Feeling down, depressed, or hopeless	0	1	2	3
3. Trouble falling or staying asleep, or sleeping too much	0	1	2	3
4. Feeling tired or having little energy	0	1	2	3
5. Poor appetite or overeating	0	1	2	3
6. Feeling bad about yourself or that you are a failure or have let yourself or your family down	0	1	2	3
7. Trouble concentrating on things, such as reading the newspaper or watching television	0	1	2	3
8. Moving or speaking so slowly that other people could have noticed; or the opposite—being so fidgety or restless that you have been moving around a lot more than usual	0	1	2	3
9. Thoughts that you would be better off dead, or of hurting yourself	0	1	2	3
	Add columns TOTAL			
10. If you checked off any problems, how difficult have these problems made it for you to do your work, take care of things at home, or get along with other people?	Not difficult at all Somewhat difficult Very difficult Extremely difficult			

(continues)

Table 5-5 Patient Health Questionnaire (PHQ-9) *(continued)*

Interpretation of Total Score

Total Score	Depression Severity
1–4	Minimal depression
5–9	Mild depression
10–14	Moderate depression
15–19	Moderately severe depression
20–27	Severe depression

Consider a depressive disorder if there are at least 4 √s in the shaded section (including Questions #1 and #2). Add score to determine severity.

Consider major depressive disorder if there are at least 5 √s in the shaded section (one of which corresponds to Question #1 or #2).

Consider other depressive disorder if there are 2–4 √s in the shaded section (one of which corresponds to Question #1 or #2).

Question # 10 Note: All responses should be verified by the clinician. Diagnoses of major depressive disorder or other depressive disorder also require impairment of social, occupational, or other important areas of functioning (Question #10) and ruling out normal bereavement, a history of a manic episode (bipolar disorder), and a physical disorder, medication, or other drug as the biological cause of the depressive symptoms.

Reproduced from Pfizer. Patient Health Questionnaire-9 (PHQ-9). Retrieved from phqscreeners.com.

Prior to initiating treatment for depression, especially pharmacotherapy, it is important to distinguish between unipolar depression and the depressive phase of a bipolar illness. A detailed description of bipolar is presented later in this chapter. **Box 5-3** describes the diagnostic criteria for mania and hypomania. Other important signs to screen for include a history of taking multiple antidepressants without improvement, previous suicide attempts, and a history of agitation or irritability while taking antidepresants in the past.[24] Antidepressant drugs typically trigger manic episodes in bipolar patients.[17] Any depressed woman with a history suspicious of previous manic states or family bipolar illness must have a medication evaluation by a mental health clinician who is skilled in the management of mood-stabilizing medication regimens.

Evidence-based guidelines are available to assist the the primary care provider in the management of depression. Three useful tools available on the Internet include the Depression Management Tool Kit,[25] the Institute for Clinical Systems Improvement guidelines for Major Depression in Adults and Primary Care,[17] and the IMPACT evidence-based depression care.[26] Each of these systems use the PHQ-9 both to diagnose depression and to track improvement with treatment. They also recommend collaboration with a mental health provider.

The IMPACT model, developed by the University of Washington Advancing Integrated Mental Health Solutions Center, is an example of a well-integrated team approach in the management of persons who are diagnosed with depression.[27] Implementation of collaborative care

---

Box 5-3 Bipolar Disorder

Diagnosis includes major depression *and* history of mania (bipolar I) or hypomania (bipolar II), leading to a marked impairment in occupational function, social activities or relationships; may lead to hospitalization or psychotic features. The manic phase must last a minimum of 7 days.

Symptoms of Mania
- Inflated self-esteem or grandiosity
- Decreased need for sleep
- More talkative than usual or pressure to continue talking
- Flight of ideas or feels thoughts are racing, agitation
- High energy, irritability, or pleasure seeking

Must have 3 symptoms (or 4 if only symptom is irritability) during the time of mood disturbance

Hypomania
- Lasts a minimum of 4 days
- Briefer duration and less severe symptoms
- Associated with unequivocal change in functioning that differs from normal function for that individual
- Is not severe enough to cause marked impairment in social or occupational functioning
- Not associated with psychosis

Data from American Psychiatric Association. *Diagnostic and Statistical Manual of Mental Disorders.* 5th ed. Arlington, VA: American Psychiatric Association; 2013; Hackley B, Sharma C, Kedzior A, Sreenivasan S. Managing mental health conditions in primary care settings. *J Midwifery Womens Health.* 2010;55(1):9-19.

using this model, involving a case manager (either a specially trained nurse or social worker) and a psychiatrist, has been found to improve outcomes when compared to usual care.[28] The case manager is responsible for educating the woman about depression, monitoring symptoms, and coaching her in behavioral activation and pleasant event scheduling and physical activity. Behavioral activation refers to helping the woman identify things/activities that give her pleasure and encouraging her to take part in an increasing number of them daily. The case manager may provide initial adjustments to medication dosages. The case manager is also useful in coordinating referrals and reinforcing follow through. The psychiatric consultant is available for any specific concerns, including reviewing cases that are not responding to treatment.

Whether or not the primary care providers practice within a collaborative care model, any clinician who opts to care for depressed individuals has the responsibility to continue to follow the response to complete remission, because adequate treatment decreases the risk of relapse. **Table 5-6** offers guidelines for initiating treatment based on initial PHQ-9 scores.

Inadequate treatment has been a continuing concern. Tamburrino, Nagel, and Lynch followed 94 participants with depressive disorders who were being managed by their primary care providers and found that about 75% of participants did not have their medications adjusted during the 12-week study period, despite having scores on the Beck Depression Inventory-II that indicated moderate depression.[29] Repeating the PHQ-9 (Table 5-3) or other tool that was used

Table 5-6 Translating PHQ-9 Depression Scores into Practice

PHQ-9 Symptoms and Impairment	PHQ-9 Severity	Provisional Diagnosis	Treatment Recommendations
1 to 4 symptoms, functional impairment	5–9	Mild or minimal depressive symptoms	• Education to call if deteriorates • Physical activity • Behavioral activation • If no improvement after 1 or more months, consider referral to behavioral health for evaluation
2 to 4 symptoms, question 1 or 2+, functional impairment	10–14	Mild major depression	• Pharmacotherapy or psychotherapy • Education • Physical activity • Behavioral activation • Initially consider weekly contacts to ensure adequate engagement, then at least monthly
≥ 5 symptoms, question 1 or 2+, functional impairment	15–19	Moderate major depression	• Pharmacotherapy and/or psychotherapy • Education • Physical activity • Behavioral activation • Initially consider weekly contacts to ensure adequate engagement, then minimum every 2–4 weeks
≥ 5 symptoms, question 1 or 2+, functional impairment	≥ 20	Severe major depression	• Pharmacotherapy necessary and psychotherapy when patient able to participate • Education • Physical activity • Behavioral activation • Weekly contacts until less severe

for the initial diagnosis will assess the individual's ongoing symptoms. Close follow up is essential, and increases or adjustments to medication are often necessary. If the individual does not improve despite changes in medication, then referral to a mental healthcare provider is indicated. Although most primary care providers are not in a position to provide ongoing psychotherapy for their patients, their responsibility for follow up continues. Even after referral to a mental health specialist, the provider is responsible for follow up and needs to

reinforce the treatment plan jointly developed by the mental healthcare provider and patient.

Many women are reluctant to enter into psychotherapy, dreading a long-term, unfocused process. In fact, most psychotherapeutic regimes for depression are short term. Cognitive behavioral therapy (CBT), problem-solving therapy, short-term psychodynamic therapy, and interpersonal therapy all have comparable outcomes.[17] Early studies of Internet-delivered psychotherapy with guidance from a therapist have been promising.

Self-guided Internet-delivered psychotherapy also has been shown to have some benefits.[30]

Pharmacotherapy Many depressed individuals will opt to initiate pharmacologic treatment rather than counseling. As discussed earlier, it is critical that the clinician has ruled out bipolar disorder prior to initiating pharmacotherapy, because treatment with an antidepressant may trigger mania,[17] suicidal ideation, or psychosis.[24]

Dopamine, serotonin, and norepinephrine are the three major neurotransmitters that modulate mood. **Figure 5-3** illustrates the effects and interactions of these neurotransmitters. The first-line pharmacotherapies for depression, including selective serotonin reuptake inhibitors (SSRIs), norepinephrine and dopamine reuptake inhibitors (NDRIs), and serotonin norepinephrine reuptake inhibitors (SNRIs), act to modify the levels of these three neurotransmitters.[31-33] Bupropion (Wellbutrin, Zyban), an NDRI, has fewer adverse effects on sexual function, but lowers the threshold for seizures and should not be used with other medications that also lower seizure threshold or by individuals with risk factors for seizures. Bupropion differs from the SSRIs in that it is of no benefit on anxiety and may even aggravate anxiety.[33]

Other classes of drugs that have been used in the past and that may be prescribed by psychiatric clinicians include monoamine oxidase inhibitors (MAOIs) and tricyclics. These medications have a narrow therapeutic range, potential for high toxicity, and serious interactions with many foods

Figure 5-3 Role of dopamine, norepinephrine, and serotonin.

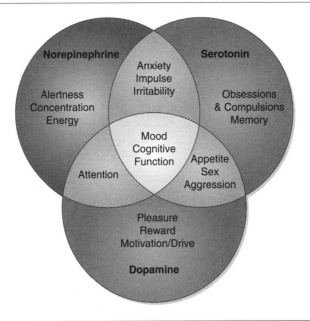

and other medications. Few primary care providers have the expertise to prescribe and manage these drugs.

SSRIs are metabolized through the CPY450 enzyme system and, as such, interact with other medications that are also metabolized by the same systems. Some of the specific medications that are known to interact with the second-generation antidepressants include older antidepressants such as tricyclic antidepressants, digoxin (Lanoxin), warfarin (Coumadin), anticonvulsants, and theophylline (Theo-Dur).[24] Prior to prescribing any psychotropic medication, the clinician is responsible for reviewing all medications the patient is taking to avoid potentially serious interactions.

Excess serotonin levels can lead to serotonin syndrome, a rare but potentially life-threatening reaction that results from excess serotonergic activity. In 2005 there were 8585 cases reported with moderate to major, but not life-threatening, effects and 118 deaths due to serotonin syndrome.[34] It can possibly occur in response to therapeutic dosing of an SSRI or SNRI, but more often is either a complication of drug–drug interactions or overdose. Combining treatment with more than one SSRI or SNRI, MAOIs, lithium, or concurrent use of St. John's wort may precititate serotonin syndrome. Other classes of drugs, such as the antiemetics metoclopromide and ondansetron, triptans, anticonvulsants, and some opioids, also have serotonergic activity.[35] High doses of tramadol have led to serotonin syndrome in individuals concurrently taking SSRIs or SNRIs.[36] Many recreational drugs, including amphetamines, cocaine, and ecstasy, can also trigger serotonin syndrome. A classic triad of symptoms, not all of which may be present in any given individual, includes autonomic instability, neuromuscular signs, and cognitive behavioral signs. Specific manifestations include fever, hyperreflexia, diarrhea, diaphoresis, myoclonus, tremor, agitation, confusion, or hypomania.[35,37] Persons who are suspected of experiencing serotonin syndrome should be directed to the emergency room.[32,33,35]

Various SSRIs, SNRIs, or NDRIs have not been shown to differ significantly in efficacy.[32,33] Individual medications in these classes do, however, have different side effect profiles as summarized in **Table 5-7**. The choice of medication to initiate therapy is made based on patient preference, past successful treatment with a given medication, and predominate symptoms that accompany the depression. For example, all the SSRIs may be associated with weight gain, but fluoxetine (Prozac) is more stimulating/activating than sertraline (Zoloft).[25,27] Fluoxetine might be a better choice for someone with hypersomnia and low energy. As a group, the SNRIs are less frequently associated with weight gain than the SSRIs.[31] Abrupt discontinuation of SSRIs or SNRIs usually leads to symptoms of serotonin withdrawal (or discontinuation) syndrome, which include dizziness, ataxia, agitation, headache, tremor, and confusion.[24,31] Fluoxetine has the longest half-life of the second-generation antidepressants and may be the most appropriate medication for those who may be less able to take their pills consistently.

Initiating Pharmacotherapy. Once the diagnosis of major depression has been made and bipolar disorder ruled out, the decision to begin psychotropic medication is made jointly with the woman. Initiating treatment with SSRIs or SNRIs often causes GI upset, jitteriness, and headache as the body adapts to the higher increased levels of neurotransmittors. These side effects usually resolve within approximately 2 weeks as the receptors are downregulated. For this reason, the starting dose for psychotropic drugs should be at a low dose for the first 2 weeks to minimize these symptoms. The lower starting dose, when accompanied by anticipatory guidance, will improve the likelihood of the patient continuing the medication.

Table 5-7 Antidepressant Medications for Use by Primary Care Providers

Generic Agent (Brand Name)	Starting Dose (mg)	Range (mg per day)	Side Effect Profile	Pharmacokinetic Half-life
SSRIs				
Citalopram (Celexa)	10–20	20–40	Minimal CYP 450 interactions. Caution QTc prolongation. Good choice for anxiety. May have fewer sexual side effects than other SSRIs; weight gain common, more likely after 6 months of use. Maintain initial dose for 4 weeks before increase.	35-hour half-life and few metabolites, therefore missing a dose can cause serotonin withdrawal symptoms
Escitalopram (Lexapro)	10	10–20	Minimal CYP 450 interactions. Good choice for anxiety. Increase to 20 mg if partial response after 4 weeks. More sexual side effects compared to citalopram in the short term, no long-term difference; weight gain common, more likely after 6 months of use.	Short half-life of 27–32 hours, therefore missing a dose can cause serotonin withdrawal symptoms
Fluoxetine (Prozac)	10–20	20–80	Maintain at 20 mg/day for 4–6 weeks, then 30 mg for 2–4 weeks before additional increases. Weight gain common, more likely after 6 months of use; sexual side effects, More activating than other SSRIs.	Longer half-life of 3–4 days and long elimination of active metabolites, making withdrawal symptoms the least likely of all SSRIs
Paroxetine (Paxil)	20	20–60	Maintain at 20 mg before dose increase, then may increase dose by 10 mg every week to max 50 mg/day. Weight gain more likely than with other SSRIs; sexual side effects may be more common in the short term, may be sedating.	Short half-life and no active metabolites, significant serotonin withdrawal symptoms
Sertraline (Zoloft)	50	50–200	Limited CYP 450 interactions. Mildly activating. Maintain 50 mg for 4 weeks, then may increase in 25-mg increments weekly. Weight gain common, more likely after 6 months of use; sexual side effects.	Half-life of 2–4 days and some minimally active metabolites, so withdrawal symptoms are less likely

(continues)

Table 5-7 Antidepressant Medications for Use by Primary Care Providers *(continued)*

Generic Agent (Brand Name)	Starting Dose (mg)	Range (mg per day)	Side Effect Profile	Pharmacokinetic Half-life
NDRIs				
Bupropion (Wellbutrin or Zyban)	200 (in 2 divided doses)	100–150 tid May increase to 100 mg tid after 7 days.	Contraindicated in history of seizure disorder or traumatic brain injury. May be stimulating. No sexual side effects; weight-neutral or minor weight loss.	Half-life is 29 hours for sustained release; withdrawal symptoms not reported
Bupropion SR 12 hr	100	150–200 bid Increase to 150 mg bid after 7 days.		
SNRIs				
Duloxetine (Cymbalta)	20–30	20–60 mg as 1 or 2 doses/day	Weight-neutral in the short term, uncertain if weight gain in the long term; fewer sexual side effects than some SSRIs in the short term, no long-term difference; monitor BP. Also used for neuropathic pain.	Half-life of 12 hours; withdrawal symptoms reported, but frequency unknown
Venlafaxine (Effexor)	37.5	75–300 in 2–3 divided doses	Weight-neutral; fewer sexual side effects than SSRIs; increases blood pressure in a dose-dependent fashion. More agitating, more GI symptoms than SSRIs.	Withdrawal symptoms reported, but frequency unknown

Data from Hackley B, Sharma C, Kedzior A, Sreenivasan S. Managing mental health conditions in primary care settings. *J Midwifery Womens Health*. 2010; 55:9–19; The MacArthur Initiative on Depression and Primary Care Depression Management Toolkit. 2009; AIMS Center. Commonly Prescribed Psychotropic Medications. Seattle, WA: University of Washington; 2013. Retrieved from: https://aims.uw.edu/resource-library/commonly-prescribed-psychotropic-medications

As the lethargy associated with major depression begins to lift, the risk of suicide and suicide attempts can increase during the first 1 to 2 months after beginning treatment with SSRIs, especially in adolescents and young adults. Close monitoring is indicated during this time.

Most individuals who begin these medications will require adjustments to the initial dose. The American College of Physicians recommends an encounter either in person or by telephone to monitor medication effects within 1 to 2 weeks after initiating therapy.[32] At this time, the clinician can explore whether the woman has filled the prescription, begun taking it, is continuing the medication, and, if not, what the barriers are to doing so. An assessment of side effects and evaluation for any suicidal thoughts also is included in this encounter.

Follow Up While some depressed women may experience an improvement in their depression by their 1- to 2-week encounter, many will not appreciate a response until 6 or more weeks after beginning medication. It is recommended to reassess depressive symptoms 4 to 8 weeks after initiating therapy. An assessment of compliance, barriers to compliance, and side effects is completed at this time. Use of the screening tool that was used during the initial diagnosis allows the provider and woman to see an objective, quantifiable response to the therapy. The goal of therapy is complete remission from depression, which would mean a score of < 5 on the PHQ-9. **Table 5-8** provides guidance for alterations in management based on the patient response to the PHQ-9.

Undertreatment of depression is common. If the woman has noticed partial response to treatment, the dosage of the initial medication may be increased. If the woman has less than a 25% decrease in symptoms, an increase in the dose is the most appropriate next step. Often an individual will require a "stepped" increase in dose to reach a dosage level that falls within the therapeutic range. Stepping up in incremental stages minimizes side effects. However, if relief is not achieved after reaching a therapeutic level, a referral for concurrent psychotherapy should be considered. Switching to another medication

Table 5-8 Using the PHQ-9 to Assess Clinical Response to Treatment

Change in Score	Response Level	If antidepressants chosen Review after 4 weeks	If therapy chosen Review after 6 weeks
Drop of 5 points from baseline	Adequate	Maintain dose, review in 4 weeks	Continue current schedule, review in 4 weeks
Drop of 2–4 points from baseline	Possibly inadequate	Consider increase in medication dose	Continue current schedule, share PHQ with psychiatrist as consult
Drop of 1 point or no change or increase	Inadequate	Consider increase or second medication, consider adding counseling or referral for consultation with psychiatrist	If satisfied in counseling setting, consider adding antidepressant If unsatisfied with counseling, review options for treatment and refer appropriately

Reproduced from The Macarthur Initiative on Depression & Primary Care. Depression management tool kit; 2009. Retrieved from: http://www.integration.samhsa.gov/clinical-practice/macarthur_depression_toolkit.pdf. Accessed 8 May 2016.

is another option. Monthly monitoring is continued until full remission is achieved; at this point, follow-up visits can be scheduled every 2 to 3 months. However, if complete remission is not achieved, a consultation with a psychiatric provider is indicated.

Between 20% and 85% of depressed individuals experience a second episode of depression within 2 years of the initial episode.[33] Continuing antidepressant therapy for at least 4 to 9 months after remission lowers the risk of a relapse. Some individuals are at high risk for relapses, such as those with dysthymia, repeated episodes of major depression, or a family history of mood disorders, and will benefit from long-term maintenance therapy. These patients should be encouraged to continue therapy for a minimum of 2 years, during which time provider–patient interactions may take place every 3–12 months as long as the mental health status is stable.[17,33] When a decision is made to discontinue psychotropic medications, the dose should be tapered over several weeks to months in order to avoid serotonin withdrawal syndrome.[17] Discussion regarding tapering the medication due to the risks associated with abrupt withdrawal, even if the patient is dicontinuing the therapy without consulting the provider, is an important component of ongoing medication management.

Dysthymia   While major depression is an acute illness that runs an episodic course, dysthymia is characterized by chronic low-grade symptoms. Dysthymia can include sleep and appetite disturbances, poor concentration, and fatigue, but the symptoms are not severe enough to meet the diagnostic criteria for major depression and the patient has no thoughts of self-injury. In some cases, the patient's mood may become normal temporarily in response to positive environmental circumstances, then return to the usual low mood and energy when events are less favorable. Many individuals with dysthymia also experience one or more episodes of major depression.[38]

Presentation   Dysthymic women typically do not report feeling depressed. Rather, they take their low energy, poor sleep, weight gain, chronic pains, and feelings of isolation and low self-esteem for granted. It is the chronic pattern over years—of never quite feeling up to life, even when offered support and opportunity—that reveals the underlying disorder.

Diagnosis   A diagnosis of dysthymia is more likely to be suggested by the observant clinician than by the woman herself. The patient thinks of her dysthymia as a normal state, because that is how she has always felt. She may seek treatment for an acute depressive or anxious episode, then discontinue treatment when she feels "better" and sink back into a familiar state of low mood and somatic discomforts. This familiarity can make the dysthymic woman resist diagnosis and treatment more adamantly than if she was acutely depressed.

Dysthymic women are particularly vulnerable to developing major depressive episodes and anxiety disorders (including PTSD) in response to life crises. Hormone changes can also trigger severe symptoms. Dysthymia, like major depression, is often seen in women who have thyroid disease, migraine, chronic fatigue syndrome, fibromyalgia, and chronic pelvic pain.

Treatment   Whereas psychotherapy and pharmacotherapy achieve comparable results for those with major depression, pharmacotherapy has been shown to be more effective in the treatment of dysthymia.[39,40] Pharmacotherapy for women with dysthymia differs from an acute mood episode in that medication may be a lifelong undertaking. Discontinuation may leave the patient vulnerable to acute relapses or recurring and varied somatic illness. Some women realize quickly that they feel better with treatment and eagerly ask how long they can stay on the medication. Others discontinue medication as soon as they feel a little better and then slide back into their usual state. They may go through several cycles of treatment, discontinuation, and relapse before accepting a diagnosis of dysthymia and making a commitment to effective treatment.

BIPOLAR AND RELATED DISORDERS

In addition to bipolar I and bipolar II disorders, this category includes cyclothymic disorder, which features symptoms similar to the bipolar disorders that do not meet diagnostic criteria for mania, hypomania, or major depression. Bipolar disorders are often misdiagnosed as depressive disorders by primary care providers. Clues to bipolar disorders include poor functioning in social and work arenas, risky behaviors, and legal issues. A family history of bipolar disorder and treatment failures with antidepressants also increase the chance of a bipolar diagnosis.[41] The diagnostic criteria for bipolar disorder are presented in Box 5-3.

The diagnosis and pharmacologic management of bipolar disorders is complex and resource intensive. A wide variety of medications are used, including mood stabilizers, anticonvulsants, and atypical antipsychotics. In many cases multidrug therapy is needed. These drugs are often accompanied with multiple drug interactions. Bipolar patients are at risk for both psychosis and suicide.[42] The majority of primary care providers find it prudent to refer their patients with bipolar disorders to psychiatric providers.

Bipolar Disorder I Formerly called manic depression, bipolar disorder I is characterized by episodes of both low (depressed) and high (manic) mood, usually alternating with periods of normal mood. It is less common than unipolar depression, affecting perhaps 1% of the population.[43] Bipolar disorder I occurs equally often in men and women, but several variants of the illness are more common in women. The majority of individuals with bipolar disorder have a family history

of similar diagnoses. Women tend to experience more depressive episodes and "mixed mania," in which depressive symptoms are present during a manic episode. Bipolar women are also more likely to develop "rapid cycling," with four or more mood episodes each year, and to experience seasonal destabilization of mood.[44]

In women who have a genetic predisposition to bipolar illness, symptoms can be triggered by hormonal shifts in pregnancy and postpartum. Postpartum psychosis is currently believed to be a manifestation of bipolar illness.[45-47] Among bipolar patients, the most common cause of premature death is suicide.[48] Drug overdose and accidental injury also contribute to morbidity and mortality.

Presentation Episodes of mania involve an elevated, expansive mood accompanied by impaired decision making and poor insight. The patient may forget to eat and get little sleep, perceiving herself to be productive and inspired. Women may engage in compulsive shopping, gambling, sexual activity, or substance use while they are manic. Irritability and self-centeredness may lead to interpersonal conflicts and impaired functioning at work, especially if the illness deepens to include paranoid or psychotic features. Acute mania usually comes to the attention of the healthcare system when the patient requires control of symptoms or treatment of injuries.

A woman in the midst of a manic episode is unlikely to appear in the office for a primary care appointment. She has too many other, more exciting things to do. She will instead come in during a period of normal mood, or when she needs to deal with the consequences of risky behavior. During a depressed episode, the woman may recall her manic times as productive and positive and seek help to regain her "high functioning." It may be helpful to think of the manic "high" as an addiction: The woman is almost certain to cling to her symptoms and behavior. Patients in the grip of mania believe that they are experiencing brilliant inspirations or profound revelations that exempt them from the rules of ordinary behavior.

Bipolar patients often consider themselves cured once an acute episode has passed. They may discontinue medication and psychotherapy, and describe their illness as something in their past. Clinicians must remember that bipolar disorder, if correctly diagnosed, is a lifelong and potentially deadly illness that never remits spontaneously. Untreated, the episodes become more severe and mood changes more frequent over time. The clinician must be prepared for the next episode even if the patient is not.

Diagnosis Bipolar illness frequently goes unrecognized for years. Mania with psychotic features may be confused with schizophrenia, while depressive episodes are often mistaken for unipolar depression. It is usually the alert clinician, rather than the patient, who will identify the illness in the primary care setting.

A history of substance use, including alcohol dependence, may indicate attempts to self-medicate mood or irritability; episodic substance use is associated with periods of mania. The patient may also describe a history of school difficulties, frequent employment conflicts, and inappropriate relationships. Reproductive health clinicians will notice a history of risky sexual behavior, poor contraceptive choices, and ill-timed pregnancies. Extreme irritability or irrational behavior around menses may also be reported. Bipolar patients often give a history of unsuccessful antidepressant medication. Antidepressants typically trigger mania, irritability, and sleeplessness in bipolar individuals. Because bipolar illness has a strong genetic component, any family history of suicidal behavior, substance abuse, or psychiatric hospitalization suggests a vulnerability to bipolar illness.

There are three screening tests that may be useful in identifying individuals with bipolar disorder. The M-3 Checklist is a 23-item checklist that not only screens for bipolar disorder, but also

unipolar depression, PTSD, and anxiety disorders. The checklist is completed online and usually takes less than 5 minutes to complete. It is available in both English and Spanish for patients to complete online at http://whatsmym3.com.[49] A second screening tool is the Mood Disorder Questionnaire (MDQ), also completed by the client. The tool includes 13 initial questions. If the client responds yes to 7 of the 13 questions and then goes on to state that two or more of the symptoms occurred simultaneously, there is a high suspicion of bipolar. In a third question clients rate their functional impairment. The MDQ is available online at http://www.integration.samhsa.gov/images/res/MDQ.pdf. The third commonly used screening tool is the World Health Organization's World Mental Health Composite International Diagnostic Interview, version 3.0 (CIDI). The CIDI is a provider-administered interview consisting of two "stem" questions, which if answered positively, lead to an additional nine questions aimed at identifying symptoms of mania. The interview takes about 5 minutes to complete. The STABLE (*Sta*ndards for *Bi*polar *E*xcellence) Resource Kit is a compilation of screening and assessment tools that describes the MDA and CIDI in greater detail and is available online.[50]

Bipolar illness often occurs with other psychiatric illness, including anxiety and eating and personality disorders. It can be difficult to differentiate from attention-deficit/hyperactivity disorder (ADHD) and is often present in disorders of impulse control and conduct. Medical conditions that can trigger mania include: multiple sclerosis, cerebrovascular accidents, thyroid disease, and postpartum status. The causal mechanisms for this are unclear.

Treatment Treatment of bipolar disorder is beyond the scope of primary care providers in the absence of postgraduate education in psychiatric disorders. If there is a suspicion of bipolar illness, prompt referral to a psychiatric provider is indicated. The cornerstone of treatment is mood-stabilizing medication. The illness is biologic, and treatment is a lifelong necessity. While a patient may be stable on a single medication most of the time, usually several medications are needed to control acute episodes.

Lithium revolutionized the treatment of bipolar illness in the middle of the 20th century, and it remains the classic mood stabilizer today. Several other medications, notably the anticonvulsants, are also used to stabilize mood and as adjunct therapy. Antidepressants may be used as adjunct therapy, but they must not be prescribed without a mood stabilizer because of the risk of triggering manic episodes. Many anticonvulsants can interfere with the effectiveness of oral contraceptives (OCs), so alternative or second forms of contraception are recommended for women taking these medications.

Patient adherence to treatment is a particular challenge with bipolar illness. During periods of normal mood, the patient typically wants to discontinue treatment and consider herself "cured." During a depressive episode, she may ask her primary provider for an antidepressant prescription. When the emergency room psychiatrist restarts a mood stabilizer (or neuroleptic), there will be a risk of treatment resistance. Further, when mood stabilizers are discontinued, there is a significant risk that they will be ineffective when resumed.[51]

Bipolar illness is the single strongest predictor of postpartum psychosis. If a pregnant woman's history includes bipolar illness, she must be followed by a psychiatric provider who is skilled in the treatment of bipolar illness in pregnancy and postpartum. Discontinuing medication during pregnancy or postpartum increases the risk of relapse with mania or psychosis.

Bipolar Disorder II Bipolar disorder II is of particular importance to clinicians who care for women, because women are more likely to suffer from bipolar disorder II than men are. The clinical course of this disorder is dominated by periods of depression that alternate with episodes of hypomania, which involves elevated mood or irritability that does not qualify as fully manic. Like bipolar disorder I, it is a heritable condition of lifelong duration with a significant risk of morbidity and mortality.

Presentation Hypomanic episodes tend not to attract the professional intervention that full-blown mania requires, particularly because it may be perceived as "normal and productive" by the affected individual. A woman may experience hypomania as a time when she feels energized and alert. Needing less sleep and "comfort food" than when she is depressed, she may finally be able to lose weight or finish her dissertation. She lives in dread of the next bout of depression and tries to accomplish as much as possible before it flattens her again.

The patient usually recognizes her depression when an episode arrives. She may seek help for the depression and may have tried a number of antidepressant medications without relief. A woman may experience only depressive episodes for years, until a strong environmental stressor such as childbirth triggers a hypomanic episode.

Diagnosis Bipolar disorder II can be a diagnosis of exclusion. It is frequently identified when a depressed patient responds to antidepressant medication by becoming irritable or acting irrationally. She may describe the effect of an antidepressant as, "it made me crazy," or, "I wanted to jump out of my skin all the time." Sometimes, patients refuse to discuss their reaction to an antidepressant, saying only, "I just wasn't myself," and quickly changing the subject. Findings in the patient history and family history will be similar to those of bipolar disorder I, and the same screening criteria may be used.

Bipolar disorder II presents the same differential diagnoses and comorbidities as bipolar disorder I. Bipolar disorder II most often masquerades as a unipolar depressive disorder. Women usually have somatic or medical problems that may, initially, present more prominently than do their shifting moods.

Treatment   Mood stabilization is key to successful treatment, as discussed in the section on bipolar disorder I. Antidepressants should not be prescribed for women with bipolar disorder II, even when depression is the presenting symptom, because they typically trigger hypomanic episodes.

Anxiety Disorders

Anxiety is a state of apprehension and arousal that warns of impending danger; it is a lifesaving response that tells a person in danger to prepare for fight or flight. Anxiety is a universally experienced human emotion, but it becomes pathologic when it is out of proportion to any actual threat and leads to impairment of social, family, or occupational functioning.[15] There is a biologic predisposition to anxiety. Anxiety disorders are the most common psychiatric diagnoses and occur approximately twice as often in women than in men. Anxiety associated with coexisting depression is common, especially in women.[52,53] Early childhood abuse tends to cause anxiety in children, although years may pass before symptoms are recognized and correctly diagnosed.

The anxious person is "on edge" under ordinary circumstances, and what begins with periodic episodes of intense panic or irritability can eventually become a constant state of worry that needs no provocation to trigger autonomic arousal and physical symptoms. Anxious people demand constant reassurance from those around them, especially family and caregivers. Anxiety typically presents in the primary care office as digestive disturbance, disordered sleep, headache, or chest pain. Anxious patients tend to be frequent utilizers of emergency services, incurring multiple workups that show no physical cause of symptoms. Suggestions for differentiating between different stress disorders are presented in **Figure 5-4**.

Like mood disorders, anxiety disorders can be triggered by medical conditions, substance use, and many medications. Whenever new symptoms appear, it is important to check for changes in the patient's health, habits, and medications. It is also possible to have more than one anxiety disorder. A patient with PTSD may develop phobias and obsessive-compulsive behavior. Anxiety also accompanies other psychiatric conditions, and may be the distressed patient's impetus for seeking treatment. Some of the anxiety disorders, such as the specific phobias, can be readily treated to full remission. Others, including obsessive-compulsive disorder (OCD) and generalized anxiety disorder, can cause lifelong impairment despite multiple treatment strategies.

Routine screening for anxiety disorders is less common than screening for depression. As discussed earlier, the M-3 checklist, which can be completed by the client prior to an office visit, screens for depression, bipolar disorders, anxiety disorders, and PTSD. The Generalized Anxiety Disorder Screening Tool (GAD-7), as shown in **Table 5-9**, was initially developed to screen specifically for GAD, but has since been validated to screen for social anxiety, panic disorders, and PTSD.[54]

PANIC ATTACKS AND PANIC DISORDER

The hallmark of panic disorder is the panic attack, as described in **Box 5-4**. A first panic attack can be triggered by a physical stimulus such as noise or vibrations, or by emotional stress as in stage fright. The sufferer's overwhelming fear coupled with the intense physical discomfort makes a panic attack unforgettable. Anyone who has experienced a panic attack dreads the possibility of ever having another one. In panic disorder, the initial panic attacks are usually triggered by specific circumstances, but over time the attacks begin to appear spontaneously. The patient becomes increasingly fearful that another attack will appear and begins to structure her life around anticipating the next attack.

Panic disorder is categorized as occurring either with or without agoraphobia. Agoraphobic fears can cause patients to lead increasingly restricted lives, as they hesitate to participate in

Figure 5-4 Suggested scheme for exploration of a suspected anxiety disorder.

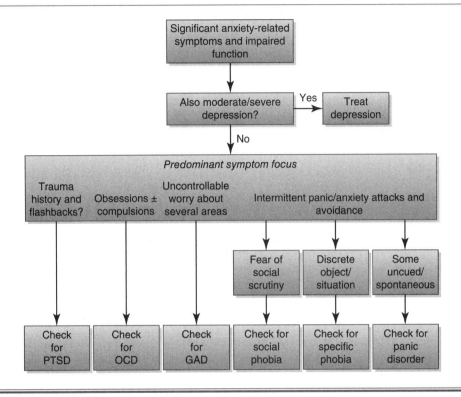

normal activities. In extreme cases, they are unable to leave the house at all.

PHOBIAS

A phobia is an excessive fear of a particular object or situation that persists for longer than 6 months.[15] Phobias may begin after a traumatic experience, such as a fear of dogs after having been bitten, and evolve into a pattern of avoidance that the patient recognizes as being excessive or unreasonable. Common specific phobias include: fears of heights, storms, or other environmental stimuli; invasive medical procedures or contamination; and certain situations such as being in an enclosed space. Phobias frequently occur with other anxiety disorders and can lead to a life with severely restricted activities and choices.

Social phobia, also known as social anxiety disorder, is a specific phobia where individuals avoid situations in which they fear that others may judge them to be inadequate. The physical signs of anxiety (trembling hands, shaky voice, muscle tension, and blushing) may be so embarrassing that they decline social invitations or even hesitate to engage in ordinary conversation with others. A vicious cycle may develop in which the anticipation of anxiety leads to symptoms that impair her social functioning, leading to further anxiety and avoidance.

Table 5-9 Generalized Anxiety Disorder Screening Tool (GAD-7)

Over the last 2 weeks, how often have you been bothered by the following problems?	Not at all	Several days	More than half the days	Nearly every day
1. Feeling nervous, anxious, or on edge	0	1	2	3
2. Not being able to stop or control worrying	0	1	2	3
3. Worrying too much about different things	0	1	2	3
4. Trouble relaxing	0	1	2	3
5. Being so restless that it is hard to sit still	0	1	2	3
6. Becoming easily annoyed or irritable	0	1	2	3
7. Feeling afraid as if something awful might happen	0	1	2	3
Total Score T_____ =		+	+	+

Scores of 5, 10, and 15 are cut-points for mild, moderate, and severe anxiety.
Further evaluation is recommended for a score of ≥ 10.
The GAD-2 uses the first 2 questions of the GAD-7, and a score of ≥ 3 suggests the presence of an anxiety disorder.

GENERALIZED ANXIETY DISORDER

Many women with GAD readily describe themselves as "worriers" and report that they have felt "nervous" for as long as they can remember. They experience excessive anxiety related to family, health, finances, work, or school. Most also suffer from depression or dysthymia, and sometimes agoraphobia or panic disorder. They may seek treatment for their physical symptoms for years without relief. GAD is associated with frequent somatic complaints, leading to frequent visits to the emergency room, primary care office, and absences from work.[55] When life crises and transitions occur, these women may develop more acute problems that require emergency mental health services; they then return to their usual level of functioning, with free-floating anxiety as a constant companion. Even a mild state of pervasive anxiety can disable the patient and impair her family life, becoming a lifelong pattern. GAD tends to run a chronic, persistent course that can be resistant to treatment over time. Even when appropriately treated, it has a lower likelihood of remission than other anxiety disorders.

OBSESSIVE-COMPULSIVE DISORDER

OCD is the presence of obsessions and/or compulsions that either consume more than an hour each day or cause significant distress or impairment in social, occupational, or other areas of functioning.[15] Obsessive thoughts are persistent, intrusive ideas or impulses that are inappropriate and cause distress. Most patients recognize that their obsessions are unreasonable and try to control such thoughts, often by repeating certain behaviors that aim to soothe their anxiety. Compulsive repetitions can include washing, checking, hoarding, and counting. Compulsive behaviors may evolve into elaborate rituals that lead to very rigid and limited lifestyles. Patients are often deeply ashamed of their thoughts and behaviors, and very secretive about their habits.[15]

OCD is usually recognized in late adolescence or early adulthood, but it may begin in childhood. The rate of OCD in those with first-degree relatives is twice that with unaffected families; in the case of childhood or adolescent onset, the rate is increased 10-fold.[15] It is among the most

---

Box 5-4 Panic Attacks and Panic Disorder

A. Recurrent unexpected panic attacks. A panic attack is an abrupt surge of intense fear or intense discomfort that reaches a peak within minutes, and during which time four (or more) of the following symptoms occur:
Note: The abrupt surge can occur from a calm state or an anxious state.
1. Palpitations, pounding heart, or accelerated heart rate.
2. Sweating.
3. Trembling or shaking.
4. Sensations of shortness of breath or smothering.
5. Feelings of choking.
6. Chest pain or discomfort.
7. Nausea or abdominal distress.
8. Feeling dizzy, unsteady, light-headed, or faint.
9. Chills or heat sensations.
10. Paresthesias (numbness or tingling sensations).
11. Derealization (feelings of unreality) or depersonalization (being detached from oneself).
12. Fear of losing control or "going crazy."
13. Fear of dying.
Note: Culture-specific symptoms (e.g. tinnitus, neck soreness, headache, uncontrollable screaming or crying) may be seen. Such symptoms should not count as one of the four symptoms.
B. At least one of the attacks has been followed by 1 month (or more) of one or both of the following:
1. Persistent concern or worry about additional panic attacks or their consequences (e.g., losing control, having a heart attack, "going crazy").
2. A significant maladaptive change in behavior related to the attacks (e.g., behaviors designed to avoid having panic attacks, such as avoidance of exercise or unfamiliar situations).
C. The disturbance is not attributable to the physiological effects of a substance (e.g., a drug of abuse, a medication) or another medical condition (e.g., hyperthyroidism, cardiopulmonary disorders).
D. The disturbance is not better explained by another mental disorder (e.g., the panic attacks do not occur only in response to feared social situations, as in social anxiety disorder; in response to circumscribed phobic objects or situations, as in specific phobia; in response to obsessions, as in obsessive-compulsive disorder; in response to reminders of traumatic events, as in posttraumatic stress disorder; or in response to separation from attachment figures, as in separation anxiety disorder).

Reproduced from American Psychiatric Association. *Diagnostic and Statistical Manual of Mental Disorders*. 5th ed. Arlington, VA: American Psychiatric Association; 2013.

---

disabling mental illnesses and can be difficult to treat. The longer it remains untreated, the poorer the prognosis.

TREATMENT OF ANXIETY DISORDERS

Both psychotherapy and pharmacotherapy can be useful in managing anxiety disorders. Unlike depressive disorders, individuals with anxiety disorders are more likely to opt for therapy rather than monotherapy with medication.[56] **Table 5-10** describes the recommendations for initial treatment of anxiety disorders from the British Association for Psychopharmacology.[53]

CBT is especially helpful in the treatment of anxiety disorders. It takes place in weekly sessions over 12 to 15 weeks, and has been found to be effective in reducing anxiety symptoms and improving quality of life.[57] Common areas that are addressed with CBT include behavioral activation, cognitive restructuring, psychoeducation, graded exposure, problem solving, assertiveness skills, and relapse prevention. Although not as effective as face-to-face therapy, many individuals

Table 5-10 Initial Treatment of Common Anxiety Disorders

Disorder	Psychotherapy	Pharmacotherapy	Comments
Generalized anxiety disorder	CBT Applied relaxation	SSRIs Some benzodiazepines: • Alprazolam • Diazepam • Lorazepam Pregabalin	Consider SSRI for first-line pharmacotherapy
Panic disorder	CBT	SSRIs Some benzodiazepines: • Alprazolam • Clonazepam • Diazepam • Lorazepam Avoid propranolol, buspirone, and bupropion	Consider SSRI for first-line pharmacotherapy
Specific phobia	Exposure techniques	SSRIs if have not responded to exposure techniques	
Social phobia (social anxiety disorder)	CBT more than exposure therapy	Most SSRIs Venlafaxine Some benzodiazepines: • Clonazepam	Consider SSRI for first-line pharmacotherapy Combined psycho/pharmacotherapy reduces risk of relapse
PTSD	Trauma-focused CBT EMDR	Paroxetine Sertraline Venlafaxine	Consider SSRI for first-line pharmacotherapy
OCD	Exposure therapy CBT Cognitive therapy		Consider SSRI for first-line pharmacotherapy Combined psycho/pharmacotherapy superior to monotherapy

CBT = cognitive behavioral therapy, EMDR = eye movement desensitization and reprocessing, OCD = obsessive-compulsive disorder, PTSD = posttraumatic stress disorder, SSRI = selective serotonin reuptake inhibitor

Data from Baldwin DS, Anderson IM, Nutt DJ, Allgulander C, Bandelow B, de Boer JA, et al. Evidence-based guidelines for the pharmacological treatment of anxiety disorders, post-traumatic stress disorder, and obsessive-compulsive disorder: a revision of the 2005 guidelines from the British Association for Psychopharmacology. *J Psychopharm*. 2014;28:403-439.

benefit from computer-based or Internet-based programs. A meta-analysis of 22 randomized controlled trials of computer therapy found that it was an acceptable alternative to face-to-face therapy, especially for those unable to access it otherwise.[58,59]

The recommended first-line pharmacotherapies for most anxiety disorders are the SSRIs and

SNRIs.[53,55,60] They have been well studied and are safe, efficacious, and well tolerated. As is true for depression, it may take up to 4 weeks for an individual to show a response. Lack of response by 6 weeks predicts a low chance of eventual reponse. Women need to be told that there may be a transient increased nervousness in the first few days of treatment, but that this usually passes within 2 weeks. The doses for the treatment of anxiety disorders are similar to those for depression. A low dose is prescribed for the first 2 weeks to minimize adverse symptoms, increasing the dose no more frequently than every 1 to 2 weeks. Drug counseling includes the importance of tapering the medication when it is discontinued. Treatment should continue for at least 12 months if the response to the medication has been adequate. If the response is inadequate, the provider may increase the same medication, switch to a different SSRI, recommend CBT, and/or refer to a prescribing mental health specialist who has experience with other pharmacotherapy, such as anticonvulsants including gabapentin (Neurontin) or pregabalin (Lyrica).[53,61]

Benzodiazepines, usually clonazepam (Klonopin), lorazepam (Ativan), or alprazolam (Xanax), may also be useful in the short term for individuals with significant impairment while waiting for the therapeutic effect of an SSRI. They may also be useful for the episodic treatment of panic disorder.[53] Although categorized as anticonvulsants, they are widely used to relieve anxiety, stop panic attacks, and induce sleep. Partly because of their strong potential for habituation and abuse, they are no longer favored as first-line maintenance therapy. A patient with a newly identified illness or crisis may be prescribed one of the longer-acting benzodiazepines, such as clonazepam (Klonopin) or lorazepam (Ativan), at the time she is started on an SSRI. She can then taper off the benzodiazepine as the SSRI starts to relieve her symptoms. A typical dose would be 0.50 mg clonazepam up to three times a day. The patient may take 1 to 2 mg at bedtime and break the scored tablets into 0.25 mg doses during the day, as needed to control her symptoms.

Benzodiazepines should be avoided in treating patients with a history of substance abuse. All patients should be warned of the risk of habituation and possible withdrawal symptoms. Common side effects can include, among other things, depression, confusion, drowsiness, dizziness, impaired coordination, amnesia, and nightmares. Clinicians should be wary of any situation in which the patient appears to be "shopping" for benzodiazepine refills. Pregabalin may be useful in assisting patients to discontinue benzodiazepines after long-term use.[62]

Early studies of benzodiazepine use in pregnancy identified risks of cleft palate when taken in the first trimester and a newborn withdrawal syndrome when taken at the end of pregnancy; prescribing during pregnancy is not recommended. Studies have found no serious adverse infant outcomes,[63,64] but liability can be an issue in prescribing these drugs. They are considered "probably safe" in lactation, making their short-term use for postpartum disorders a viable choice.

Stress Disorders

Acute stress disorder and posttraumatic stress syndrome are both reactions to a traumatic event; they differ in terms of the duration and degree of the stress reaction following the event. The diagnostic criteria are presented for both disorders in **Box 5-5**. Acute stress disorder is diagnosed during or immediately following a traumatic experience. Symptoms include emotional numbing, a reduced awareness of surroundings, a sense of unreality, and an inability to remember parts of the trauma. These disturbances in perception often prevent the patient from recognizing and seeking help for her problem. It is important for clinicians to take the initiative in observing a patient's response to a traumatic event and inquiring about

Box 5-5 Acute Stress Disorder and Posttraumatic Stress Syndrome in Adolescents and Adults

Features in Common

1. Exposure to actual or threatened death, serious injury, or sexual violence, either by direct experience, witnessing in person, learning of violent or accidental death or other traumatic event in a loved one, or repeated exposure to traumatic events.
2. Presence of intrusion symptoms, which may include distressing memories or dreams, flashbacks, and/or intense psychological or physiologic distress, in response to cues reminiscent of the traumatic event.
3. Avoidance of stimuli associated with the event.
4. Dissociative symptoms such as altered sense of reality or dissociative amnesia.
5. Alterations in arousal and reactivity, including sleep disturbances, irritability and outbursts, hypervigilance, difficulty concentrating, and exaggerated startle reflex.
6. Inability to experience positive emotions.
7. The disturbance causes clinically significant distress or impairment in social, occupational, or other areas of daily life.
8. The preceding symptoms are not attributable to use of substances, another medical condition or medication, or other psychiatric disorder (although may be associated with other comorbid mental disorders or substance use).

Distinguishing Features

1. Duration: Acute stress disorder lasts from 2 days to 1 month after the trauma; PTSD lasts more than 1 month. Many, but not all, who develop PTSD initially present with acute stress disorder.
2. Negative alterations in mood or cognition. Individuals with PTSD may experience persistent or negative beliefs about oneself, others, or the world; persistent sense of horror, fear, anger, guilt, or shame; an ongoing diminished interest in participation in significant activities; and feelings of detachment from others.

Data from American Psychiatric Association. *Diagnostic and Statistical Manual of Mental Disorders.* 5th ed. Arlington, VA: American Psychiatric Association; 2013.

symptoms. There is some evidence to support the prophylactic use of beta-blockers to prevent the development of full-blown PTSD. Intensive case management includes ensuring adequate nutrition and sound sleep for the patient, and initiating stress-reduction measures throughout the period of recovery.

Posttraumatic Stress Disorder

Most people who are exposed to life-threatening shock or stress will recover in due time, but vulnerable individuals can incur a lifetime of emotional and physical disability. PTSD begins with a triad of symptoms: 1) the constant emotional re-experiencing of the traumatic event, 2) avoidance of stimuli that are associated with the event, and 3) a persistent state of anxious vigilance after the stressful time has passed.

Each aspect of PTSD causes problems. Intrusive thoughts of the trauma cause disordered sleep and nightmares, and may compel the sufferer to talk obsessively about her experience, thereby reinforcing the trauma. To avoid stimuli that are related to the traumatic event, patients can develop phobic or compulsive patterns of behavior. *Avoidance* can include emotional numbing, which leads to impaired and distressing personal relationships. *Dissociation*, which is mentally detaching oneself from the present, is another means of escape. Dissociative disorders (including multiple personalities) may develop in response to traumatic stress.

Perhaps the most life-threatening aspect of PTSD is the constant state of autonomic arousal—the *hypervigilance* that is so familiar among war veterans and abuse survivors. Attempts to relieve the distress of constant anxiety can lead to substance use and other risk-seeking behavior. The constant alertness can precipitate the onset of hypertension, cardiovascular disease, and other chronic health problems.

The treatment of PTSD starts with symptom control. Initial medication regimens seek to prevent the deepening of neurologic trauma that happens with repetition of symptoms. Research had suggested that early treatment with beta-blockers such as propranolol (Inderal) might be able to prevent the PTSD triad from becoming established. A subsequent meta-analysis failed to find a benefit from propranolol, gabapentin, or antidepressants, but concluded there was a moderate benefit from the efficacy of hydrocortisone.[65] Medications used in other anxiety disorders (e.g., anxiolytics, antidepressants, and sleep aids) may be helpful in controlling symptoms to the point where the patient can learn effective behavioral interventions. Both eye movement desensitization and reprocessing (EMDR) and CBT have been helpful in the treatment of PTSD, with EMDR having slightly better results.[66] A recent adjunct to CBT has been introduced into the armamentarium of treatment options. D-cycloserine (DCS) is an antibiotic that was developed for the treatment of tuberculosis, but has been found to act as a "cognitive enhancer" for augmenting CBT. When used short term with CBT, DCS can augment extinction learning. This allows for a quicker response to the CBT, although the long-term benefits are comparable.[67] Patients must learn coping behaviors that help them manage their symptoms and avoid triggering stimuli.

Adjustment Disorders

When a life crisis causes more distress than expected, an adjustment disorder may be diagnosed. The DSM-5 specifies that symptoms begin within 3 months of a specific stressor and cause a significant impairment in daily functioning. Symptoms are expected to resolve within 6 months unless the stressor becomes chronic, as with a long-term medical illness. By definition, the symptoms of adjustment disorder do not represent bereavement (which is designated persistent complex bereavement disorder), nor are they severe enough to meet criteria for PTSD. Examples of triggering events may include breaking up with a partner, leaving home, financial crises, or serious illness. An adjustment disorder can include depressive or anxious symptoms or disturbed behavior, such as reckless driving or vandalism.[15] The diagnosis should be reconsidered, and other conditions suspected if symptoms change or do not resolve as expected.

Eating Disorders

The eating disorders involve a disturbance in eating behavior combined with a distorted perception of body shape and weight. Eating disorders are diagnosed far more frequently in women than in men, for reasons that seem to include social and cultural expectations as well as biologic vulnerability. Although relatively uncommon, with an estimated prevalence in females of 0.3% for anorexia nervosa (AN) and 1% for bulimia nervosa (BN), they contribute to significant societal costs due to treatment costs and loss of productivity.[68] Early sexual abuse increases the risk of developing an eating disorder.[69] Women with eating disorders share a deep preoccupation with self-image and self-esteem based on body shape and size, usually with extreme shame and secretiveness around their eating and purging habits. The two most common eating disorders are anorexia nervosa and bulimia nervosa.

Women with *anorexia nervosa* refuse to maintain a normal weight and obsessively fear becoming fat. They perceive themselves as being overweight even when their emaciated state is obvious to others. Patients restrict their food intake to lose even more weight. They may also induce vomiting or use diuretics, purgatives, or enemas. Medical complications caused by starvation and malnutrition can affect every body system, causing anorexia nervosa to have the highest mortality rate of any psychiatric disorder.[70] A recent meta-analysis concluded that anorexia is associated with a 5-fold risk of premature mortality and an 18-fold increased risk of death due to suicide compared to all 15- to 34-year-old females.[71] Lifelong disability or death can result from the medical complications of starvation.

Women with *bulimia* may be of normal weight or overweight; they do not experience the amenorrhea that accompanies anorexia. The alternation of binge eating and purging behaviors causes damage to a number of body systems, including the teeth and gums, esophagus, and the GI tract. The long-term outcome of bulimia is less well researched than that of anorexia, but studies suggest that it may have a very guarded prognosis because of its comorbidity with mood and personality disorders and the likelihood of recurrence throughout the patient's life.[72]

The diagnoses of *binge-eating disorder* and other specified feeding or eating disorder not otherwise specified are applied to a number of conditions that involve distorted body image and disturbed eating habits. Some patients have all the signs of anorexia except amenorrhea or engage in binge eating without the compensatory purging or restrictive behavior.[15]

Presentation

Individuals with anorexia nervosa are often brought to providers by relatives who are concerned with an excess weight loss. Individuals rarely self-refer because of their weight; when they do seek help, it is related to a somatic complaint related to their malnutrition.[15] Bulimia nervosa and binge eating, on the other hand, are often associated with other psychiatric illness such as mood and anxiety disorders, personality disorders, or substance abuse.[15] These are the most common presentations of eating disorders in primary care. Families may bring in the underweight teenager because of her amenorrhea; a depressed smoker may request an infertility workup; dental caries and damage may be noted on a routine exam; obesity may lead to a discussion that reveals alternating bingeing and restricting behaviors.

An increasingly frequent presentation of eating disorders is the *female athlete triad,* which includes disordered eating, amenorrhea, and osteoporosis. It is most common in disciplines that require a very slender appearance, such as gymnastics and ballet. Amenorrhea can be masked by OCs, which are frequently taken by young women to avoid bleeding during competition or performances.[73]

Diagnosis

Physical signs and symptoms and the laboratory workup for eating disorders are covered earlier in the section on essential evaluation. A thorough history is the most powerful screening tool. Two questions that can be integrated into routine interviews have been shown to be helpful in detecting bulimia:

1. Are you satisfied with your eating habits?
2. Do you ever eat in secret?

Anorexia should be suspected in underweight young women with delayed menarche, failure to menstruate other than with hormone withdrawal, or failure to gain weight as expected in adolescence or during pregnancy. The section on assessment describes laboratory testing, including electrocardiogram (EKG) and bone density. Consultation with the patient's primary care physician or pediatrician is essential.

TREATMENT

Treatment regimens for all of the eating disorders involve psychotherapy and medication by a qualified mental health team. The treatment of eating disorders is complicated by the patient's secrecy around her behavior and the frequent comorbidity with other psychiatric illness. Moderate to severe anorexia nervosa can constitute a medical emergency. Once an individual's medical condition has stabilized, intensive outpatient treatment has been shown to be as efficacious as prolonged inpatient therapy.[74,75] A comprehensive program involves a multidisciplinary team to provide both individual and family therapy. Because eating disorders tend to recur, clinicians caring for "recovered" patients must remain alert for signs of relapse during periods of life stress.

Anorexic women are generally infertile, but as they re-attain 90% of normal body weight, menses usually return. At that time ovulation and unexpected pregnancy may occur. Recent studies find that anorexic women experience more miscarriages, caesarean sections, premature births, and small-for-date babies than do controls.[76,77] Pregnant women with a history of eating disorder require comprehensive comanagement between obstetric and psychiatric personnel for optimal outcome. Women may be unwilling to be weighed, or to be questioned about eating habits, even when the pregnancy is progressing well in terms of fetal growth.

Bulimia may be treated on an outpatient basis. Psychotherapy involves individual or group cognitive-behavioral interventions designed to normalize patients' self-image and eating habits. Combined therapy with SSRI antidepressants has been shown to be more effective than either therapy alone.[78]

Personality Disorders

Personality disorders cause serious and complex impairments in the patient's ability to function in society, especially in interpersonal relationships. They typically develop before becoming an adult. Distorted perceptions of people and events, combined with impulsive behavior and labile moods, are disabling even though the patient may appear to be high functioning on a superficial level. Personality disorders have high comorbidity with other psychiatric diagnoses and can impair the patient's ability to recognize and participate in treatment of her other illnesses. They affect at least two of four areas: cognition, affectivity, interpersonal functioning, and impulse control.[15] They include many types and subtypes, several of which are more frequently diagnosed in women.

One of the more common conditions in this category is *borderline personality disorder*, with an estimated prevalence in primary care settings of about 6%, of which 75% are women.[15] Borderline personality disorder features unstable relationships such as idealizing a caregiver or potential partner at first, only to become angry at not being given enough attention; intensely labile moods; feelings of emptiness; and impulsive behavior. Borderline patients frequently have a history of ADHD and oppositional defiant disorder (ODD),[79] childhood abuse, and neglectful parenting.[80] The rate of suicide among patients with borderline personality is close to 10%; premature mortality from all causes is about 18%.[81]

"Borderline" can also be an informal term used by clinicians to describe patients who are demanding and manipulative, and who push the boundaries of professional relationships as they move from crisis to crisis and from provider to provider. When a psychiatric problem list includes the notation "with borderline features," it generally refers to behavior patterns that have tried the patience of caregivers, whether or not formal diagnostic criteria are met.

In the primary care setting, personality disorders can prevent the development of a trusting clinician–patient partnership. "Staff splitting" describes the patient's practice of being friendly and flattering to one staff member and argumentative or insulting to another. The patient may accept and cooperate with treatment one day while rejecting it the next. Such patients also tend to present "boundary" issues. They may ask that clinicians be available to them beyond regular work hours, seek reassurance that only certain people will be involved in their care, reject referrals to psychotherapy, and demand treatment or prescriptions that are outside the normal scope of primary care practice.

Treatment of personality disorders historically has been difficult and requires referral to a mental health provider. Medication has not been predictably helpful. Medication therapy of comorbid illness (typically including depression, PTSD, substance use, or bipolar disorders) can be compromised by the patient's impulsive behavior. Insight-oriented or supportive psychotherapy is not consistently useful. Various psychotherapy approaches have been developed specifically for the treatment of borderline personality disorder, including dialectical behavior therapy (DBT). DBT provides a structured program that can be used in individual or group therapy to help the patient learn new, more useful ways of perceiving herself and controlling her impulses, and was found to be more effective than client-centered therapy.[82]

Substance-Related Disorders

The DSM-5 disorders related to substances include deliberate drug abuse, side effects of medication use, toxin exposure, and substance withdrawal. Drug abuse can cause or be comorbid with psychiatric disturbances during intoxication or withdrawal.

Female Gender–Associated Mental Disorders

Menstrual Disorders

Women commonly report both physical and emotional changes around the time of their menses. When a patient's symptoms are severe enough to interfere with her daily life, the clinician must determine whether the situation represents the familiar gynecologic problem known as PMS, the psychiatric disorder referred to as PMDD, or the cyclic worsening of another mental illness around the time of menses. The differences among these three diagnoses are summarized in **Box 5-6**. The diagnoses of PMS and PMDD are grouped together in ICD-10 under the diagnosis of "N94.3 Premenstrual Tension Syndrome."

While women often blame their symptoms on abnormal "hormones," women with severe premenstrual mood swings tend to have normal hormone levels but an extreme neurologic sensitivity to fluctuations across their cycles. It is the neurochemical vulnerability, rather than any abnormality in gonadal functioning, that causes the troubling symptoms.[83]

PREMENSTRUAL SYNDROME

The concept of menstrual-related symptoms has been recognized for more than 80 years, and was first labeled premenstrual syndrome in the 1930s.[84] PMS includes a myriad of physical symptoms such as breast swelling and tenderness, acne, bloating and/or weight gain, headache or joint pain, and appetite alterations, and psychologic symptoms such as irritability, mood swings, crying spells, and depression.[85]

While the majority of women are believed to experience some premenstrual symptoms, most neither request nor need any specific treatment. A minority, however, do experience symptoms such

Box 5-6 Classification of Premenstrual Disorders

Core Premenstrual Disorders (Premenstrual Syndrome and Premenstrual Dysphoric Disorder)
Characteristics
Depend on the endocrine luteal phase events following ovulation. The primary characteristic is their timing; they occur in all or part of the 2-week premenstrual phase:
- Symptoms occur in ovulatory cycles.
- Symptoms are not specified—may be somatic and/or psychological.
- The number of symptoms is not specified.
- Symptoms recur in luteal phase.
- Symptoms must be prospectively rated over two cycles at minimum.
- Symptoms cause significant impairment.

Variant Premenstrual Disorders (Premenstrual Exacerbation, Non-Ovulatory Premenstrual Disorders, Progesterone-Induced Premenstrual Disorders, Premenstrual Disorders Without Menstruation)

Characteristics
- Symptoms of an underlying psychologic or somatic disorder significantly worsen in premenstrual phase.
- Women receiving exogenous progestogens may develop PMS symptoms as a form of progestin sensitivity.
- Symptoms arise from continued ovarian activity even though menstruation has been suppressed.
- Symptoms result (rarely) from ovarian activity other than those of ovulation.

Consensus on diagnostic criteria:
1. There is currently no imaging or biochemical test that is pathognomonic for PMDD.
2. Diagnosis is based on structured interview, self-report, and prospective recording of at least two menstrual cycles.
3. The individual must not receive treatment during the 2-month prospective rating of symptoms.

Modified from O'Brien PM, Backstrom T, Brown C, Dennerstein L, Endicott J, Epperson CN, et al. Towards a consensus on diagnostic criteria, measurement and trial design of the premenstrual disorders: the ISPMD Montreal consensus. *Arch Womens Mental Health.* 2011;14(1):13-21. With permission of Springer.

as migraine or emotional distress that impair their ability to carry on normal activities. It is also possible for other illnesses, such as seizure disorders or diabetes, to destabilize around the time of menses. Treatment of perimenstrual distress usually begins with trying to stabilize the woman's wellbeing; this includes interventions in nutrition, exercise, and general stress management. More aggressive treatment focuses on controlling the menstrual cycle, either by minimizing hormonal fluctuations or suppressing ovarian function altogether.

PREMENSTRUAL DYSPHORIC DISORDER

PMDD was recognized as a distinct condition for the first time in the DSM-5.[15] Current research indicates that its incidence in the general population is probably low, affecting perhaps 5% of women.[86] Because other mental illnesses are far more prevalent, a woman reporting premenstrual emotional distress is more likely to be experiencing an exacerbation of another mental illness around the time of menses.

As presented in **Box 5-7**, the DSM-5 criteria for diagnosing PMDD are more stringent than the criteria for PMS, requiring at least five

---

Box 5-7 Premenstrual Dysphoric Disorder Diagnostic Criteria

A. In the majority of menstrual cycles, at least five symptoms must be present in the final week before the onset of menses, start to *improve* within a few days after the onset of menses, and become *minimal* or absent in the week postmenses.
B. One (or more) of the following symptoms must be present:
   1. Marked affective lability (e.g., mood swings, feeling suddenly sad or tearful, or increase sensitivity to rejection).
   2. Marked irritability or anger or increased interpersonal conflicts.
   3. Marked depressed mood, feelings of hopelessness, or self-deprecating thoughts.
   4. Marked anxiety, tensions, and/or feelings of being keyed up or on edge.
C. One (ore more) of the following symptoms must additionally be present, to reach a total of *five* symptoms when combined with symptoms from Criterion B above.
   1. Decreased interest in usual activities (e.g., work, school, friends, hobbies).
   2. Subjective difficulty in concentration.
   3. Lethargy, easy fatigability, or marked lack of energy.
   4. Marked change in appetite; overeating; or specific food cravings.
   5. Hypersomnia or insomnia.
   6. A sense of being overwhelmed or out of control.
   7. Physical symptoms such as breast tenderness or swelling, joint or muscle pain, a sensation of "bloating," or weight gain.
      Note: The symptoms in Criteria A-C must have been met for most menstrual cycles that occurred in the preceding year.
D. The symptoms are associated with clinically significant distress or interference with work, school, usual social activities, or relationships with others (e.g., avoidance of social activities; decreased productivity and efficiency at work, school, or home).
E. The disturbance is not merely an exacerbation of the symptoms of another disorder, such as major depressive disorder, panic disorder, persistent depressive disorder (dysthymia), or a personality disorder (although it may co-occur with any of these disorders).
F. Criterion A should be confirmed by prospective daily ratings during at least two symptomatic cycles. (**Note:** The diagnosis may be made provisionally prior to this confirmation).
G. The symptoms are not attributable to the physiological effects of a substance (e.g., a drug of abuse, a medication, other treatment) or another medical condition (e.g., hyperthyroidism).

Reproduced from American Psychiatric Association. *Diagnostic and Statistical Manual of Mental Disorders*. 5th ed. Arlington, VA: American Psychiatric Association; 2013.

---

symptoms severe enough to disrupt normal functioning, only one of which may include physical complaints. Symptoms need not be present every month, but must be documented prospectively through at least two cycles and show complete remission during some portion of each cycle.

Psychiatrists studying PMDD currently describe several ways in which it appears to differ from mood disorders. The most common symptoms of PMDD are irritability and lability of mood, rather than feeling depressed or anxious.

Impaired social functioning may be the most common reason for seeking treatment, rather than subjective emotional distress. Antidepressant medication appears to relieve symptoms more quickly in PMDD than when treating other disorders, and may be effective when taken only in the second half of the menstrual cycle rather than daily.

Like other mental illnesses and PMS, PMDD seems to predict vulnerability to other psychiatric diagnoses. PMDD also appears to have a high comorbidity with mood and anxiety disorders.

Mental Illness with Perimenstrual Worsening of Symptoms

There are two common situations in which a woman with an underlying mental disorder presents with premenstrual distress. First, a woman who has a known mental illness may seek help for the management of perimenstrual exacerbation of her illness. She may not have told her psychiatric provider about her PMS, or her provider may have dismissed her complaints as being irrelevant to the management of her mental illness. More commonly, women seek treatment only for the period of exacerbation, blaming PMS or "my hormones" rather than acknowledging the possibility of a mental illness.

Three strategies are helpful in differentiating a "pure" premenstrual disorder from an underlying or comorbid mental illness:

1. Ask the patient to record her symptoms daily on a calendar, just as she would for any investigation of PMS. Emotional symptoms that are severe enough to impair functioning or cause distress and that do not abate for more than a few days at a time are not a premenstrual disorder.
2. Administer a standard depression screening tool during the early part of the patient's menstrual cycle, or weekly throughout the cycle. If the patient scores positive for depression at times not related to menses, a premenstrual disorder is not her primary diagnosis.
3. Suppress her ovulation, perhaps with several weeks of hormonal contraception. Symptoms that persist in the absence of an ovulatory cycle are not, by definition, premenstrual.

It is often clear to the clinician that the patient suffers from a mental illness, but the patient may only accept a diagnosis of PMS and be unwilling (or not yet ready) to acknowledge the full scope and implications of her problem. Happily, the evidence-based treatment of PMS, PMDD, and disorders of anxiety and depression is very similar.

Treatment

Pharmacologic treatment of premenstrual emotional distress has two aspects:

1. Control of cycles, thereby limiting hormonal fluctuations that trigger neurologic dysfunction
2. Enhancing neurologic resilience to hormonal changes via psychotropic medication

Control of Menstrual Cycles Hormonal contraceptives effectively eliminate ovulatory cycles. Hormonal fluctuations can be minimized by using a monophasic product in a continuous-therapy regimen. Extended or continuous use of combined OCs, the vaginal ring, or birth control patch provides a more steady state than does a monthly withdrawal. The only time endometrial growth occurs when using combined OCs is during the placebo week, so there is no increased risk of endometrial hyperplasia with extended or continuous use. Some women withdraw only twice a year. Some women may experience breakthrough bleeding with an extended regimen; this usually decreases the longer the woman is taking the pill.[87,88]

Mood changes on hormonal contraceptives are generally due to the progestin component of the pill. Medroxyprogesterone acetate, the first synthetic progestin and still widely available in oral and injectable forms, has been reported for years to trigger depressive symptoms.[89] Of the newer progestins, levonorgestrel and drospirenone tend to be the least likely to trigger adverse moods.[90] Drospirenone additionally can minimize fluid retention and other PMS symptoms and may be the first-choice OC formulation for women with mood disorders and for PMDD.[91]

Psychotropic Medication Extensive research supports the benefits of SSRI antidepressants for PMDD.[92] The US Food and Drug Administration (FDA) has recently approved fluoxetine (Prozac), sertraline (Zoloft), and paroxetine (Paxil) specifically for PMDD, although there is no evidence that the other SSRIs are not equally effective. SSRI use for premenstrual disorders differs from their use for depression in two significant ways:

1. They appear to be effective during the first month or two that they are taken, but when used as an antidepressant, they may take longer for a full effect.
2. They are often effective when taken cyclically, for the last week or two before expected menses, whereas they must be taken continuously for antidepressant effect. This regimen may also reduce the incidence of side effects such as sexual dysfunction. A woman may more readily accept the idea of taking medication for the week or two prior to menses (the weekly time-release form of fluoxetine [Prozac] requires only two pills, taken on days 14 and 21 of the cycle), than the prospect of daily medication for the foreseeable future. Episodic and continuous dosing have been found to be equally effective.[93]

Alternative Therapies for Premenstrual Disorders
There is some evidence that calcium supplementation and agnus castus (chasteberry) can improve premenstrual symptoms. CBT has shown some benefit, when compared to placebo, but is less effective than SSRIs.[94] Acupuncture and moxibustion were also found to decrease symptoms.[95]

Perinatal Mood Disorders

Pregnancy, childbirth, and adjusting to caring for a newborn can be fraught with situational stresses and emotional vulnerability. There are strong associations between the mental health of women and optimal outcomes of the pregnancy and birth, as well as to the cognitive and social development of the offspring. Women with mental illness struggle to negotiate the stresses of parenthood, and when they falter, their children—and other family members—may incur a lifetime of suffering as well.[96]

Many cultural traditions believe women are protected from dark thoughts and negative emotions during pregnancy. Often, women who did not feel the expected joy endured their distress quietly and in shame. Maternal anxiety also influences infant behaviors. In a 2003 study, infants of mothers with panic disorder showed more sleep disorders and higher levels of stress hormones than did infants of control mothers. It is as if the babies were anxious, too.[97] It is possible, however, to teach depressed mothers how to interact with their babies and coach them to elicit the responses that babies need.[98] The evidence supporting the long-term benefits of these interactions is less clear.[98]

Women are more likely to be diagnosed with a psychiatric disorder during their fertile years than at any other time in their lives. In addition, women are most vulnerable to psychiatric illness while they are pregnant or during the postpartum period.[99] Obstetric providers must be vigilant in identifying and ensuring treatment of psychiatric symptoms for pregnant women who have a history of mental illness or who are at significant risk of developing a mental illness.

Depression and/or Anxiety During Pregnancy

Approximately 10% to 20% of women will have major or minor depression during pregnancy, similar to the incidence in the general population. As when not pregnant, depressive and anxiety disorders are the most commonly diagnosed psychiatric conditions during pregnancy.[100] Untreated major depression and anxiety disorders can adversely affect the course and outcome of pregnancy.[101] The potential adverse outcomes are described in **Box 5-8**. Even mothers with a history of mental illness who feel well after childbirth tend to show more disengaged behavior toward their infants than do mothers without such a history. It is this disruption in the mother–infant bond that is believed to affect the infant's neurochemical and neuroendocrine development, with lasting effects.[102] Children of mothers who are depressed

---

Box 5-8 Risks of Untreated Depression and Anxiety During Pregnancy

1. Burden of disability directly due to the mental illness:
   Poor self-care, impaired judgment, self-medication with harmful drugs, insomnia, poor appetite and weight gain
2. Risks associated with treatment of mental illness:
   Anticonvulsant mood stabilizers are known teratogens; the potential effects of some other treatments are unknown.
3. Possible adverse effects of the illness on pregnancy:
   Increased risk for complications such as preeclampsia, fetal growth restriction, prematurity, miscarriage, and teratogenicity. The specific etiology and epidemiology of these risks have not yet been well characterized.
4. Antepartum mental illness predicts the worsening of illness postpartum:
   Increased risk for postpartum psychosis, postpartum obsessive-compulsive disorder, and suicide or infanticide.
5. Short- and long-term effects on offspring

Data from Meltzer-Brody S. New insights into perinatal depression: pathogenesis and treatment during pregnancy and postpartum. *Dialogues Clin Neurosci.* 2011;13:89-100. Yonkers KA, Gotman N, Smith MV, et al. Does antidepressant use attenuate the risk of a major depressive episode in pregnancy? *Epidemiology.* 2011;22:848-854; Hackley B. Antidepressant medication use in pregnancy. *J Midwifery Womens Health.* 2010;55:90-100.

---

during pregnancy exhibit short- and long-term adverse effects, such as increased cortisol levels, obesity, and internalizing and externalizing problems.[103] Most predictors for depression during the postpartum period can be identified during pregnancy, including depression or anxiety during pregnancy, stressful life effects and poor social support, or a history of depression at any other time in a woman's life.[104,105]

Anxiety per se is common during pregnancy and one must take care to differentiate the normal parental anxieties from genuinely disabling illness. Anxiety disorders can also develop de novo or be a result of relapse in a woman who had anxiety previously. A history of child abuse, poor social support, or previous episodes of anxiety increases the risk for GAD, which appears to have a prevalence of approximately 7% among pregnant women.[106] The effects of maternal stress and anxiety may begin before birth. Animal research shows that prenatal stress can affect learning, anxiety, and social behavior in the offspring.[107] Just as when not pregnant, women often experience comorbid psychiatric illness.

For example, recent studies of pregnant women who have screened positive for depression found that anxiety disorders were also present in about one-third of the women.[108] Obsessive-compulsive symptoms are not unusual during pregnancy and tend to become worse postpartum and be highly comorbid with depressive illness.[108]

SCREENING

Although a recent systemic review failed to find a benefit in routine screening for depression during pregnancy,[109] the American College of Obstetricians and Gynecologists (ACOG) has recommended universal screening for all pregnant women at least once during the pregnancy,[110] and the 2015 USPSTF draft recommendation on screening for depression also recommends routine pregnancy and postpartum screening.[16] Part of the debate about the value of routine screening centers on what happens after a woman has been identified as being depressed. If no action, such as behavioral counseling or pharmacotherapy, is taken, then little has been gained. Screening is only the first step in minimizing the impact of perinatal depression. Regardless of the choice to do routine or targeted screening, any woman who has risks for depression, or symptoms of depression, should be screened at least once and preferably two or three times during pregnancy. Some symptoms of prenatal depression include crying, weepiness, sleep problems, fatigue, and appetite disturbance, which also may be normal transient problems during pregnancy. Others, such as anhedonia, anxiety, and poor fetal attachment, are less common in the absence of depression. Formal screening to differentiate normal symptoms from major or minor depression is essential.

There are many screening tools for depression and other mood disorders. The M-3 Checklist screens for depression, anxiety, and bipolar disorder;[111] the PHQ-2 is a quick screen for depression;[112] and the GAD-2[54] can screen for anxiety. Several of these instruments have been validated for use during pregnancy and postpartum. These include the PHQ-2,[113,114] the Edinburgh Postnatal Depression Scale (EPDS),[115] the PHQ-9,[116, 117] and the Pregnancy Depression Scale.[115,118] Although the EPDS and the PHQ-9 have been shown to have comparable validity,[116] the EPDS is the most widely used and researched (see **Table 5-11**).[119] Additional screening for bipolar disorders is critical, because the treatment and prognosis for depression and bipolar disorders are quite different.

Elevations in thyroid-stimulating hormone (TSH), free T4, and thyroid autoantibodies have been associated with depression during pregnancy and postpartum.[111] A recent study by Sylven and colleagues found that an abnormal TSH at delivery was associated with a significant elevation in risk for postpartum depression at 6 months following birth (OR 11.30, 95% CI 1.93–66.11).[120] Thus, it is reasonable to include a TSH test in the evaluation of women for depression during and after pregnancy.

A complete history at the time of a first obstetric visit should inquire about previous episodes of mental illness in the pregnant woman or her family. If there is a history of prior mental illness, whenever possible the clinician should contact clinicians who have cared for the woman in the past to confirm her account, as it is the nature of mental illness to cloud the memory. Approximately 86% of women who discontinue antidepressant medication will relapse during pregnancy.[99] Similarly, approximately 85% of women with bipolar disorder who discontinue mood-stabilizing medication prior to pregnancy will have a relapse during pregnancy.[121] Several risk factors, such as onset of depression before age 18 years, individual or family history of suicide attempts, and multiple unsuccessful trials of antidepressant medications can often help to distinguish between unipolar and bipolar depression.[122]

TREATMENT OF DEPRESSION DURING PREGNANCY

Depression during pregnancy requires collaborative management between the woman, her provider, and mental health clinicians. The degree to which a provider will manage depression and anxiety varies depending on the severity of the presentation, the resources available to the clinician, and his or her level of expertise. Given that depression is common and often undertreated and that there is a shortage of mental health providers, some advocate that management of many mental health conditions by primary care providers is essential—and doable. Evidence has shown that counseling conducted by non-mental health providers is effective in reducing depressive symptoms.[123] However, others advocate that these issues are best managed by mental health providers and prefer to refer their patients for mental health care. Each provider will need to balance these approaches in his or her own practice.

Table 5-11 The Edinburgh Postnatal Depression Scale

1. I have been able to laugh and see the sunny side of things:	0	As much as I always could
	1	Not so much now
	2	Definitely not so much now
	3	Not at all
2. I have looked forward to things with enjoyment:	0	As much as I ever did
	1	Rather less than I used to
	2	Definitely less than I used to
	3	Hardly at all
3. I have blamed myself unnecessarily when things went wrong:	3	Yes, most of the time
	2	Yes, some of the time
	1	Not very often
	0	No, never
4. I have been anxious or worried for no good reason:	0	No, not at all
	1	Hardly ever
	2	Yes, sometimes
	3	Yes, very often
5. I have felt scared or panicky for no good reason:	0	No, not at all
	1	Hardly ever
	2	Yes, sometimes
	3	Yes, very often
6. Things have been getting on top of me:	3	Yes, most of the time I haven't been able to cope at all
	2	Yes, sometimes
	1	No, not very often
	0	No, not at all
7. I have been so unhappy that I have had difficulty sleeping:	3	Yes, most of the time
	2	Yes, quite often
	1	No, not very often
	0	No, not at all
8. I have felt sad or miserable:	3	Yes, most of the time
	2	Yes, quite often
	1	No, not very often
	0	No, not at all

(continues)

Table 5-11 The Edinburgh Postnatal Depression Scale *(continued)*

9. I have been so unhappy that I have been crying:	3	Yes, most of the time
	2	Yes, quite often
	1	Only occasionally
	0	No, never
10. The thought of harming myself has occurred to me:	3	Yes, quite often
	2	Sometimes
	1	Hardly ever
	0	Never

Patients complete the EPDS, and scores for each item are then totaled. Totals of 12 or more indicate clinical depression. Borderline scores of 9–11 warrant close follow up.

The choice of treatment is dictated by the severity of the illness, patient preference, and the likelihood of increased morbidity. Women with mild to moderate depression may find adequate relief from behavioral changes and psychotherapy alone.[124] Other women will do better with adjunctive treatment with antidepressant medication. Providers who are knowledgeable about depression and pharmacology of antidepressant medications may choose to prescribe these medications as primary care providers. However, to practice within a circle of safety, systems must be in place to ensure access to mental health resources and to provide continuity of care. Referral for counseling, if resources are available, is always helpful because combined therapy with psychotropic medication has been shown to have higher remission and lower relapse rates than treatment with either modality alone. Women who have multiple comorbidities such as bipolar disorder, eating disorders, and PTSD or who require complex medication regimens are best managed by a mental healthcare specialist. Prompt referral is needed for those with more serious presentations (e.g., suicidal ideation or a history of hospitalization). Urgent and immediate referral, potentially to the emergency room, is needed for those at high risk of suicide or homicide. Each provider should work within established institutional guidelines to ensure high-quality mental health care.

The choice to use medication during pregnancy is complicated by the potentially disparate needs of the mother and child. Treatment of the mother can prevent progression of disease. However, both treated and untreated disease pose risks for the exposed fetus and newborn. Balancing these benefits and risks is difficult and not always clear. Untreated depression is associated with adverse pregnancy and neonatal outcomes including preterm birth.[47] Women who are emotionally impaired are less likely to care for themselves during pregnancy and more likely to use substances such as nicotine and alcohol. Physiologically, recent research suggests that the disruption of the hypothalamic-pituitary-adrenal axis that occurs in depressive and anxiety disorders may directly affect fetal development in subtle ways, increase uterine irritability, and may increase the vulnerability of exposed fetuses to future depression and anxiety.[125,126]

On the other hand, antidepressant treatment of depression in pregnancy has been linked to potential teratogenic, fetal, and newborn complications, although the absolute risks are very small. Two large, population-based studies[127,128] came to conflicting conclusions about a possible link between first trimester SSRI use and structural cardiac defects.[129] In addition, several studies have investigated a potential link between SSRIs and persistent pulmonary hypertension of the newborn (PPHN), which was first identified in 2006.[130] A cohort study that included more than 100,000 women exposed to SSRIs calculated the adjusted odds ratio of 1.28 (95% CI 1.01–1.64) for PPHN. This is a more modest risk than that identified in previous studies; the absolute risk was 3.15/1000 women in comparison to 2.1/1000 women not exposed to SSRIs.[131] Between 10% and 30% of newborns exposed to SSRIs in utero will experience mild transient symptoms, including jitteriness, restlessness, and feeding difficulties.[132,133] Randomized controlled clinical trials are impossible to conduct on pregnant women, leaving clinicians to consider the conflicting findings of many observational, anecdotal, retrospective, and open trials. To date, no hard-and-fast rules have emerged despite a great deal of research.

Clinicians can help each woman to make an individual choice based on her illness, likely prognosis, and the results of a thorough informed consent. The components of informed consent prior to starting antidepressant medication should include discussing the risks of antidepressant use during pregnancy and lactation compared to the risks of no treatment or undertreatment. Resources are available to assist both the clinician and woman in decision making including reputable, evidence-based online resources about medication use during pregnancy and breastfeeding.

For example, the Massachusetts General Hospital (MGH) Center for Women's Mental Health offers online resources for both clinicians and patients that may help to allay concerns regarding the potential effects of using antidepressants while breastfeeding.[134] Another resource is the Organization of Teratology Information Specialists (OTIS), which is a network of teratology information services throughout the United States and Canada that provides information about exposure to medications during pregnancy and lacation. Motherisk, an affiliate of OTIS based out of the Hospital for Sick Children in Toronto is yet another online resource.[135] Both OTIS and Motherisk provide telephone consultations free of charge.

There is no evidence that any one individual SSRI works better during pregnancy than any other. Unless a woman's usual psychotropic regimen includes agents that are known to be harmful in pregnancy, the best medication for a pregnant woman to use is the one that keeps her well. When treating a relapse of depression during pregnancy, it is recommended that the clinician restart the medication that has worked well for the woman in the past. The choice of medication for new-onset illness is based on the same criteria as for nonpregnant women. Sertraline (Zoloft) and fluoxetine (Prozac) have been the most extensively studied, but with the exception of paroxetine (Paxil), none of the studies have demonstrated any risks or benefits of one SSRI over another.

Initial dosing regimens are similar to those for nonpregnant women, with several considerations. Hemodilution from blood volume expansion may necessitate progressively higher doses of medication as pregnancy progresses to achieve a stable clinical effect. Changes in gestational hormones can affect metabolism and excretion of medications during pregnancy, altering the effectiveness of a medication. These physiologic changes make it imperative that the provider monitor psychiatric symptoms frequently throughout pregnancy. In addition, some mental health clinicians are unaware of these physiologic changes, making it

even more important that there be close communication between the mental health provider and
the pregnancy care provider.

Bipolar Illness During Pregnancy

The majority of primary care providers would not
manage bipolar disorders during pregnancy but
should be informed of the psychiatric care their
patients are receiving. Mood stabilizers are crucial
for the management of bipolar illness in pregnancy
and prevention of postpartum mania and psychosis.
Lithium is the safest mood-stabilizing agent during
pregnancy, although it was formerly believed to have
a high incidence of fetal cardiac malformations. The
absolute risk of anomalies is now known to be low,
and patients can be reassured by fetal echocardiogram examinations.[136] Lithium has a narrow therapeutic window, and maternal serum levels should be
monitored during pregnancy. Hyperemesis in early
pregnancy and hemodilution in later pregnancy
can cause toxic high and subtherapeutic levels of
lithium, respectively. Serum levels should also be
followed during labor and postpartum; maternal
hydration status should be kept optimal.

Prevention of Postpartum Mental Illness

Primary and secondary prevention are always
preferable to dealing with acute or worsening illness. Identifying a vulnerability to postpartum
depression may allow an opportunity to intervene
early enough to prevent or minimize depression.
Most risk factors for postpartum mental illness
can be identified prior to the birth. Adolescents
are at almost twice the risk for postpartum depression compared to adult women. They are still
achieving their normal development tasks and
often have unrealistic expectations of motherhood and the demands of parenting. Adolescents
also tend to be more socially isolated from their
peers than adult mothers.[137] Immigrant women
may be a greater risk of postpartum depression,

depending on the circumstances of their immigration, their degree of social and language isolation, and whether they can engage in traditional
childbirth rituals.[137]

For women whose histories place them at elevated risk, there is evidence that starting prophylactic antidepressant medication in pregnancy or
immediately postpartum can dramatically reduce
the likelihood of postpartum illness.[138] Many
women try to get through pregnancy without
medication, even to the point of denying that they
are ill, but they may be receptive to the idea of
preventing postpartum illness. Considering medication in the third trimester can help the patient
feel prepared and in control, even if she ultimately
decides to "see how it goes" rather than take active
preventive measures.

Healthy behaviors can be fostered prior to
and during pregnancy. For example, counseling
regarding exercise, especially outdoors; healthy
eating; and good sleep habits can be reinforced
at each prenatal visit, not only for the physical
wellbeing of the pregnancy, but for the mother's
mental wellbeing. CenteringPregnancy* has been
shown to improve social support and is associated
with less risk of depression at 1 year postpartum
in women with high stress levels.[139,140] Other
support groups may also help women to develop
coping skills. Psychotherapy may help a woman
learn to identify and access sources of support
from family and friends, thus avoiding the development of postpartum depression. Women at
risk for postpartum depression who have a desire
to avoid medication may be especially receptive
to this advice.

Disordered sleep is common in late pregnancy,
but it is not benign and should be taken seriously.
A woman who is unable to fall asleep at bedtime,
has difficulty going back to sleep after getting up
to urinate, or wakes very early in the morning
and can't get back to sleep may be experiencing
somatic signs of anxiety or depression. There is
evidence that treatment for insomnia in the third

trimester decreases the risk of subsequent development of postpartum depression.[141] Simple sleep hygiene measures, along with an OTC antihistamine such as diphenhydramine (Benadryl), can prevent sleep deprivation from increasing the patient's vulnerability to postpartum stresses. Diphenhydramine should be avoided in individuals who have experienced a paradoxical reaction of stimulation rather than sedation.

Other products are available but the evidence on the safety of these products in pregnancy is limited. Hypnotic benzodiazepine receptor agonists are relatively new medications used for insomnia; they include zolpidem (Ambien), zopiclone (Zimovane), and zaleplon (Sonata). The limited research on these medications during pregnancy is reassuring that they are not teratogenic, although there may be an association with preterm birth.

Difficulty sleeping may also herald the presence of more serious psychopathology. If the woman reports poor sleep but does not feel tired during the day, hypomania or mania may be emerging.

Skin-to-skin contact is a simple, nonpharmacologic intervention that may reduce the risk for postpartum depression. Placing the newborn infant skin to skin with the mother is associated with many infant benefits, including more stable physiologic transition, less crying, and more restful sleep, that may in themselves decrease maternal stress. In a quasi-experimental study, Bigelow and colleagues evaluated the effects of continuing daily skin-to-skin contact throughout the first month.[142] Mothers giving birth in one of two hospitals were initially assigned to the skin-to-skin contact group; those giving birth at the second hospital were given routine care. Halfway through the study, the assignments of the hospitals were switched. Participants completed self-report depression scales at 1 week and at 1, 2, and 3 months postpartum. Mothers in the skin-to-skin contact group reported significantly lower scores on depression screening scales (i.e., the EPDS and Center for Epidemiologic Studies Depression Scale [CES-D]) at 1 week and 1 month. This benefit attenuated over time, and there were no clinically or statistically significant differences by 3 months postpartum.

Prevention of postpartum illness requires active measures for stress reduction following birth. Depending on the severity of the woman's illness or risk, certain measures should be considered, including minimizing visitors, phone calls, and other distractions and making plans that will allow for a mother's requirement for at least 5 consecutive hours of sleep in every 24-hour period, plus at least 3 additional hours. Arrangements for ensuring adequate sleep should be worked out during pregnancy. Some women will choose to bottle feed completely in order to safeguard their sleep time, and this decision should be supported. Some women may plan to breastfeed and pump milk for someone else to give the baby; if pumping is too stressful for the mother to cope with, formula feeds are preferable to maternal depression or mania.

Postpartum Mood Disorders

Birth is associated with massive biologic and psychosocial transitions. Estrogen levels decrease, and there is evidence of lower serotonergic activity following birth. Downregulation of the hypothalamic-pituitary-adrenal axis following birth may also contribute to a vulnerability to depression.[122] Most women tolerate these alterations with minimal effect on their mood. However, it is not surprising that childbirth can present a challenge to a new mother's mental health and wellbeing, especially if she has a personal or family history of depression or bipolar disorder, inadequate social support, and multiple stressors. Disturbances in sleep patterns and circadian rhythms occur in late pregnancy, but are even more common in the first few weeks after birth. Postpartum sleep disruption may both contribute to and be aggravated by depression.[143]

While the birth of an infant is generally a joyful event, most women experience postpartum mood swings. Postpartum mood disorders can range from the widespread "baby blues" to a full-blown psychosis. Postpartum suicide related to mood disorders accounts for 20% of all postpartum deaths.[144] Therefore, understanding how to distinquish between the various mental health presentations seen in the postpartum period is critical. A description of postpartum mood disorders is presented in **Table 5-12**.

Postpartum Blues

The most frequent alteration in mood in the postpartum period is postpartum blues, also known as baby or maternity blues, occurring in 50% to 75% of new mothers.[145] Early symptoms of crying, anxiety, emotional lability, irritability, and fatigue develop within the first 10 days after birth, with a peak onset of approximately 5 days.[145,146] Although postpartum blues are usually benign and self-limited, these mood changes can be frightening to a new mother. Anticipatory guidance can reassure mothers that they are not "going crazy" and that these mood swings are commonly experienced and usually resolve spontaneously within 10 to 14 days. Clinicians should advise women to seek further evaluation if these symptoms do not resolve within 2 weeks following birth, because up to 1 in 5 women with postpartum blues will develop a major depression. Women with a history of previous depression, PMDD, or interpersonal stressors have an increased risk for postpartum blues, as well as risk of the "blues" developing into a major depressive

Table 5-12 Common Clinical Features That Distinguish Among Postpartum Mood Disorders

Disorder	Onset	Duration	Common Symptoms	Degree of Disability
Postpartum blues	7–10 days after birth	< 2 weeks	Tears, sadness, labile mood, irritability, sense of being overwhelmed, frustration, fatigue	Mild to minimal, able to care for child, suicidal ideation unlikely
Postpartum depression	2 months to 1 year after birth	> 2 weeks	Anhedonia, sleep disturbance, feelings of loneliness and isolation or guilt, poor concentration, anxiety, somatic complaints	Severe, decreased bonding with infant, may need assistance to care for infant, may have suicidal ideation
Postpartum psychosis	2–4 weeks after birth	Mean ~40 days	Acute onset, delusional thoughts, hallucinations, paranoia, confusion, insomnia, delirium	High risk, also risk to child or children

Data from Graves BW, Johnson R. Mental health conditions. In: King TL, Brucker MC, Kriebs JM, Fahey JO, Gegor CL, Varney H, eds. *Varney's Midwifery*. 5th ed. Burlington, MA: Jones & Bartlett Learning; 2015; National Institute for Health Care Management. Identifying and Treating Maternal Depression: Strategies and Considerations for Health Plans. 2010. Available at: http://www.nihcm.org/pdf/FINAL_MaternalDepression6–7.pdf. Accessed February 28, 2016.

episode. If a new mother calls with concerns about her mood, it is good practice to ask the two questions of the PHQ-2 in the phone interview to explore whether she is also having pleasure and interest in things, or is feeling predominately down, depressed, or hopeless. If she reports anhedonia or depression more than rarely, an urgent visit is indicated to more thoroughly screen for postpartum depression.

POSTPARTUM DEPRESSION

Postpartum depression is a major depressive disorder that is distinguished from other major depression only by its timing. Symptoms can occur immediately after birth and up to a year after birth. Postpartum depression occurs in women of all cultures, ages, incomes, races, and ethnicities. The onset for postpartum depression peaks in the second month postpartum, and the risk continues up to 6 to 12 months.[12,145] The point prevalence of major and minor depression ranged from 6.5% to 12.9% through the first postpartum year, and as many as 19.2% of women will have a major depressive episode at some time during the first 3 months postpartum.[147] It is critical to rule out postpartum bipolar disorder, which can be severe and possibly lead to postpartum psychosis.

Effects of Postpartum Depression on the Family
Mothers are not alone in their risk for depression. Partners of depressed mothers are also at risk for depression, with up to 2.5 times the risk of developing depression when compared to those whose partners are not depressed.[148] Their offspring are also affected. Mothers who are depressed may be less responsive to their infants than mothers who are not depressed and less likely to engage in face-to-face interactions that contribute to infant communication skills. They also display less synchrony in their mother–baby interactions. Less time is spent reading, telling stories, touching and stroking, or singing to their infants.[149]

Untreated depression has been associated with impaired child development. Tactile contact with the infants influences the infants' sensitivity to pain, affect, and growth.[150] Studies find consistent evidence for the long-term effects of postpartum depression on subsequent childhood development and behavior. Children of mothers with postpartum depression have demonstrated poor cognitive funtioning, violent behaviors, and emotional maladjustment.[146]

Screening for Postpartum Depression Both the ACOG Committee on Obstetric Practice[110] and the USPSTF[16] recommend routine screening for postpartum depression. The efficacy of this screening depends on the ability to provide adequate treatment and follow up.[119]

Several tools are available to screen for postpartum depression. The EPDS, which was developed in the mid-1980s specifically for use in the postpartum period, consists of 10 items (Table 5-11). It is a self-report scale, is available for use free of charge, and has been validated for use both during pregnancy and postpartum. The Postpartum Depression Screening Scale (PDSS) is a second tool developed for use in the postpartum period. It is self-adminstered and is available as a long form of 35 items, or an abbreviated "short" form of 7 items. The PDSS also has been well validated and may be used to evaluate response to treatment in depressed women. The EPDS and PDSS both appear to be more accurate in identifying postpartum depression than generic screening tools for depression such as the CES-D or Beck Depression Inventory (BDI).[119] A major advantage of the EPDS over the PDSS is the ability to employ the tool free of charge; there is a charge for the PDSS manual and forms.

The PHQ-9 is another instrument that is gaining favor for screening for depression in the perinatal period. It has long been used in the general population and has more recently been validated for use during pregnancy and after birth.[114,116,117] It has the advantage of being able to compare how women are feeling in pregnancy and after birth to their scores at times unrelated to the perinatal period. Thus, the PHQ-9 can be used before, during, and after pregnancy to monitor fluctuations in symptoms over the long term. Its major disadvantage is that it does not include items that are specific to childbirth.

All OB/GYN practices should have a system in place to screen pregnant and postpartum women using a standardized screening instrument. The scale may be completed by the mother while waiting to be seen for a prenatal or postpartum appointment and reviewed with her by her provider.[115] A positive result on any screen should be followed up with a diagnostic evaluation in order to establish an accurate diagnosis. The tools described earlier do not differentiate between unipolar or bipolar depression, nor do they assess for anxiety. Therefore, women identified as being depressed should also be evaluated for a history or symptoms suggestive of mania or hypomania and anxiety. Suicidality and homicidality should also be assessed and, if present, require urgent referral and evaluation by a skilled mental health provider, potentially in the emergency room. While rare, a diagnosis of postpartum thyroiditis should be considered for depressed women, particularly for those with a history of autoimmune disorders.[151] Obtaining a TSH value can rule in or rule out this diagnosis.

Postpartum depression has bimodal peaks at 2 and 6 months postpartum, so the optimal time to screen for postpartum depression is between 2 weeks and 6 months postpartum.[146] Late onset of postpartum depression, after the 6-week checkup, can be more easily missed, unless it is recognized by the affected woman or her family or friends. For this reason, the American Academy of Pediatrics suggests that pediatricians have a low threshold of suspicion for parental depression and consider, at a minimum, asking parents the two questions in the PHQ-2.

Management of Postpartum Depression   Many states and professional organizations are either mandating or strongly encouraging providers to screen for postpartum depression, but identifying women with postpartum depression is only half the battle. Having in place systems of care for treatment and follow up is critical to improving the health of mothers and their families. Unfortunately, a minority of mothers who screen positive for depression are referred to mental health clinicians for treatment, and even fewer follow through with their care.[148] Thus, each woman's health provider will have to determine his or her own role in providing counseling services for women unwilling or unable to access mental health services. Some women's health providers will choose to provide ongoing counseling services using techniques such as CBT, problem-solving sessions, or supportive counseling. Others will prefer to refer to mental health specialists. However, ongoing contact with the affected woman is always beneficial, no matter what role the woman's health provider will assume, because the midwife or obstetrical provider is in the best position to maintain continuity with the mother—to reinforce ongoing treatment, even if the woman has been referred for management to a mental healthcare provider or primary care provider. Follow up by a known and trusted obstetric provider is likely to increase the chances of satisfactory treatment.

The decision to refer a woman to a mental health provider or to treat and follow the patient in the primary care setting is made after careful consideration of the provider's expertise, patient preference, and availability of outside resources. Women's health providers interested in honing their skills in mental health counseling can attend additional training. The Veterans Health Administration has instituted a pilot program training primary care providers to deliver brief CBT for their patients, with promising results.[152] Trained nurses and general family physicians have been shown to be as effective as mental health therapists in helping depressed individuals in the general population achieve remission.[123,153]

Other options exist including Internet-based interventions. While Internet-based CBT is not as effective as clinician-provided CBT, it may be an adjunct therapy for individuals who cannot or will not access mental health providers.[58] Women who access these resources can also receive ongoing support from their provider. The primary care provider can then act as a coach, supporting the patient in the journey through the process, rather than as a mental health clinician.

Accumulated data from many studies indicate that pyschotherapy is helpful for women with mild to moderate postpartum depression. The evidence most strongly supports the benefits of interpersonal psychotherapy, problem-solving therapy, and CBT.[154] Psychotherapy may be particularly attractive to lactating women who may prefer to avoid exposing their infants to antidepressant medication through breastmilk.[47]

Pharmacotherapy Antidepressant medications are another treatment option for postpartum depression once a diagnosis of bipolar disorder is excluded. The same considerations that make SSRIs the first-line antidepressants for major depression unrelated to childbirth make them the mainstay for pharmacologic treatment for postpartum depression. The choice of which SSRI to start is based on similar considerations as starting an SSRI at any other time, including patient preference and past response to any given medication. Any of the SSRIs listed in Table 5-7 can be considered for use postpartum.

Guidelines for postpartum antidepressant management are presented in **Figure 5-5**. A decision to begin an antidepressant is made jointly by the mother and her care provider after a thorough discussion of risks and benefits, including the potential effects of postpartum depression on her infant and any other children. Women who feel that a treatment decision has been imposed

on them are less likely to follow through with the treatment regimen.

Fortunately, research findings have been reassuring about the safety of using many of the antidepressants while breastfeeding. Serum levels have been found to be undetectable in breastfeeding infants whose mothers are taking sertraline (Zoloft), paroxetine (Paxil), and nortriptyline (a tricyclic antidepressant). Levels of fluoxetine and citalopram are detected in nursing infants, but these levels are extremely low.[155]

Reputable, evidence-based resources are available online that can help guide decision making about medication use during pregnancy and breastfeeding. As discussed earlier, the MGH Center for Women's Mental Health and Motherisk can be useful resources for both clinicians and mothers.

The approach to starting medication is to begin at a low dose for 4 to 7 days, then titrate doses upward until remission is achieved. Most women will need higher than the starting doses to achieve a therapeutic effect. Whichever tool was used to diagnose the depression, the same tool should be used to monitor response to treatment. Antidepressant therapy should be continued for 6 to 9 months after achieving remission. Once the decision is made to stop antidepressant medications, dosage should be tapered gradually downward. Abrupt cessation of medication can trigger unpleasant symptoms.

POSTPARTUM BIPOLAR DISORDER

Although the prevalence of bipolar disorder is low, there is a significant risk of relapse following birth in women who have the disorder. Women with a diagnosis of bipolar disorder are best cared for by a multidisciplinary team including a psychiatrist throughout the pregnancy and postpartum period in order to manage medications and decrease the chance of a relapse. Between 80% and 100% of women who discontinue their

Figure 5-5 Algorithm for pharmacologic therapy of postpartum major depression.

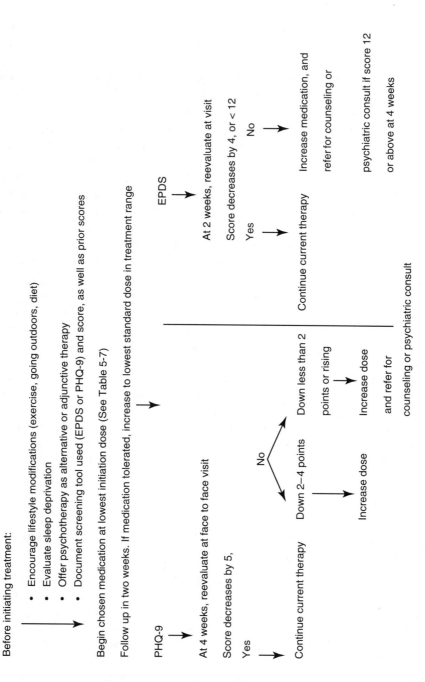

Before initiating treatment:

- Encourage lifestyle modifications (exercise, going outdoors, diet)
- Evaluate sleep deprivation
- Offer psychotherapy as alternative or adjunctive therapy
- Document screening tool used (EPDS or PHQ-9) and score, as well as prior scores

Begin chosen medication at lowest initiation dose (See Table 5-7)

Follow up in two weeks. If medication tolerated, increase to lowest standard dose in treatment range

PHQ-9

At 4 weeks, reevaluate at face to face visit

Score decreases by 5,

Yes

Continue current therapy

No

Down 2–4 points

Increase dose

Down less than 2 points or rising

Increase dose and refer for counseling or psychiatric consult

EPDS

At 2 weeks, reevaluate at visit

Score decreases by 4, or < 12

Yes

Continue current therapy

No

Increase medication, and refer for counseling or psychiatric consult if score 12 or above at 4 weeks

Reevaluate 2 to 4 weeks based on results and level of concern

Data from Hirst KP, Moutier, CY. Postpartum Major Depression. *Am Fam Physician*. 2010; 82(8): 926-933. Copyright© 2010 American Academy of Family Physicians. All rights reserved.

mood stabilizer medication during pregnancy experience a relapse. While the discontinuation of medication is the most important risk factor for relapse, the hormonal and circadian rhythm alterations that occur postpartum are also important factors. Women experiencing a relapse of their bipolar disorder postpartum often appear overly euphoric, talkative, and in need of less sleep. Conversely, they may present with the depressive symptoms. In extreme cases, it can devolve into postpartum psychosis. Any woman with a history of bipolar disorder or who exhibits signs of either mania or hypomania should be assessed by a psychiatric clinician.

Postpartum Psychosis

Postpartum psychosis is a rare and life-threatening emergency condition that requires immediate psychiatric evaluation; it is seen in 0.1% to 0.2% of patients. It may occur anytime in the first year postpartum. The incidence peaks during the first 2 weeks postpartum.[156] Women with bipolar disorder are at a much higher risk than other women. Active treatment of bipolar illness and protection of sleep are key elements in preventing mania and psychosis postpartum; such measures can reduce but not eliminate these risks. Autoimmune thyroid disease may also contribute to the development of postpartum psychosis. Bergink and colleagues recommend checking thyroperoxidase antibodies in women with bipolar disorder or a history of postpartum psychosis.[157] Women suffering from postpartum psychosis have a 4% to 5% risk of either suicide or infanticide.[148]

Postpartum Posttraumatic Stress Disorder

PTSD is a response to a traumatic event, followed by re-experiencing the event with nightmares, flashbacks, or other intrusive thoughts; avoidance of anything associated with the traumatic event and/or emotional numbing; and alterations in arousal such as sleep disturbance, difficulty concentrating, or aggressive behavior.[15] The reported incidence of postpartum PTSD varies from 1% to more than 7%, depending on the diagnostic tool that is used. Many more women suffer from "partial" PTSD, reporting re-experiencing and arousal and/or avoidance symptoms.[158] Some consider partial PTSD to be a normal response following a highly stressful experience, while others approach it as potentially impairing function that increases the risk for full-blown PTSD in the future.[159]

Women who have experienced childhood trauma, sexual abuse, depression, or PTSD preceding the pregnancy are at increased risk for postpartum PTSD.[158] Depression, anxiety, or a fear of childbirth during the pregnancy are also predictors of postpartum PTSD. The traumatic stressor for postpartum PTSD is birth trauma, "an event occurring during the labor and delivery process that involves actual or threatened serious injury or death to the mother or her infant."[160] It is the subjective perception of risk that predisposes women to PTSD rather than the absolute risk, and, in fact, women may perceive their births were traumatic despite the perception by the clinicians that everything was routine.[160] Negative emotions such as a negative experience of labor and birth and a loss of control are associated with PTSD just as much as emergency cesarean delivery and instrumental delivery. A perception of lack of support from either care providers or a partner also contributes to the risk for postpartum PTSD.[159]

Clinicians may identify women at high risk for postpartum PTSD by being alert to risk factors for signs of crisis, such as uncontrolled screaming, withdrawal, or dissociative behaviors. Early identification can provide the opportunity to offer more intensive support and communication during labor, and make an early referral if indicated. The limited studies that have been conducted suggest that many of the same therapies that are employed for PTSD in general have a benefit for postpartum PTSD. These include debriefing and counseling, CBT, and EMDR.[161]

Adjunctive Therapies for Mental Illness

In addition to psychotherapy and psychotropic medication, several other approaches to the treatment of mental illness have been evaluated:

1. *Essential fatty acids*: Initial research appeared supportive of the benefit of essential fatty acid supplements for decreasing psychiatric morbidity. Subsequent research has come to conflicting conclusions.[162,163] McNamara and colleagues propose that given the cost–benefit ratio, supplementation with long-chain omega-3 fatty acids 1 g/day in combination with docosahexaenoic acid (DHA) be considered as part of the management plan for individuals with depression or bipolar disorder.[163] The data supporting the benefit of essential fatty acids to prevent or treat depression during pregnancy or postpartum are conflicting.[164,165]

2. *Bright-light therapy*: Bright-light therapy, using a light box of 5000 to 10,000 lux for 30–60 minutes has been the treatment of choice for seasonal affective disorder. More recently, its efficacy for the treatment of nonseasonal depression and bipolar has been demonstrated. A subset of bipolar patients has developed mixed states. For those, individual midday therapy is recommended.[166,167] Particularly when combined with physical exercise, morning bright-light therapy appears to improve mood and can be used during pregnancy.

3. *Physical exercise*: Aerobic exercise and weight training have been used to improve mood and energy in various programs. Controlled trials demonstrate a small benefit.[168]

4. *Alternative biologics*: St. John's wort is probably the most extensively studied herbal preparation. Some studies have found St. John's wort to be more effective than placebo in mild-to-moderate depression, but more recent meta-analyses question the biases of these studies. Side effects of St. John's wort include headache, jitteriness, and worsening mood or mania. It also appears to reduce the bioavailability of several common prescription drugs, including cholesterol-lowering agents, cyclosporine, and OCs. It can dangerously potentiate the action of other psychotropic drugs. There are no current data on the safety of St. John's wort during pregnancy or lactation.[169]

Many patients are attracted to using natural remedies rather than prescription medication, but such products present problems with both efficacy and safety. The 1994 Dietary Supplement Health and Education Act exempts products sold as "herbals or supplements" from regulation by the FDA. Manufacturers are not required to prove safety or efficacy of these products, unlike the laws governing food, drug, and cosmetic products. The FDA can take action against a supplement only by proving that it is harmful, rather than requiring that the manufacturer prove it is safe, as is the case with prescription drugs.[170] Consequently, it is easy to recommend the use of unproven and unregulated products that are not covered by insurance.

Perhaps the greatest risk to the patient who tries natural substances is the risk of delaying effective treatment. A patient who chooses to treat her depression with, for example, St. John's wort can spend months using products of unproven usefulness. In the meantime, her symptoms can worsen, and she may eventually require more aggressive treatment than if she had used a standard regimen from the beginning. Natural remedies can be useful, however, as a first step toward self-care for patients who have difficulty accepting any treatment at all.

Referral and Consultation with Mental Health Clinicians

Several situations require that the patient be referred to one or more mental health clinicians (Table 5-13). If a patient presents with severe symptoms or if she is unable to contract for safety, the situation must be treated as a medical emergency and psychiatric treatment must be obtained to ensure her safety. Patients with severe mental illness who take multiple psychiatric medications should be in the care of a psychiatric clinician. Such a patient may describe herself as being "between providers" and ask for a medication refill or restart, or say that she is "more comfortable" getting her care from her primary women's health providers. This is not good practice. She should be referred to an appropriate mental health clinician.

A woman with a history of major mental illness should be referred for a psychiatric consultation before or during pregnancy. Her risk of a relapse during pregnancy or postpartum is significant, and establishing a therapeutic relationship will decrease her anxiety and lessen her stress during pregnancy and provide ready access to a skilled mental health clinician if the need arises postpartum. If she has been stable without treatment for years, referral is strongly encouraged but not mandatory.

Table 5-13 When to Refer

Referral Requirement	Examples	Reason
Psychiatric conditions	Severe depression Bipolar Disorder Eating Disorder, especially Anorexia Psychotic illness Substance abuse	Risk of self-harm is significant, also risk to others; impulsive acts; possible need for inpatient stabilization with team outpatient follow up.
Psychotropic medications	Mood stabilizers Antipsychotics Stimulants Non-benzodiazepine Anticonvulsants	These drugs have potential for severe and complex side effects and interactions, unsuitable for independent primary management.
History of major mental illness and pregnant or considering pregnancy	Asymptomatic and off medication	Risk of recurrence during pregnancy or postpartum is significant; consultation and evaluation are needed even without active treatment.

Medical emergency: Whenever a patient is unwilling to contract for safety, the situation must be considered a medical emergency and appropriate care ensured. These patients may need immediate evaluation in the psychiatric emergency room.

These situations require referral to appropriate mental health providers, even if the patient requests that her care be managed in the primary setting.

A patient's permission is necessary prior to referring a patient or consulting with her mental health clinicians. Some patients hesitate, fearing that intimate details of their psychotherapy will be shared. When it is explained that this would not happen, because clinicians are interested only in discussing the treatment plan and not the narrative content of visits, and the consent form specifies "to discuss treatment plan," receiving informed consent should not be a problem.

The professional culture of mental health clinicians encourages interdisciplinary cooperation. Once assured of the patient's consent to communicate, psychiatric providers welcome a team approach in planning for their patient's total care.

Conclusion

Millions of women are affected by mental illness. Many of them do not have access to a mental health community. Often, the primary or reproductive care provider is their only point of entry to the healthcare system. As a crucial component of primary care, providers must, at a minimum, screen for mental illness in their patients. Given the pervasive shortage of mental health providers, a large percentage of women, such as those with depression and anxiety, can be best served by their women's health provider or primary care physician who have developed the expertise to initiate and manage therapy, which can include pharmacotherapy and/or psychotherapy. If remission is not achieved, referral would then be indicated for more expert care. This approach is consistent with primary care management of other illnesses such as hypertension, asthma, and GI disorders. A smaller number of women will require management by mental health providers at the time that a mental health problem is identified, such as those with more complex or severe diagnoses. Providers must recognize the limits of their expertise and not exceed them. No provider works in a vacuum, and a collaborative team system offers the most accessible and cost-effective strategy to provide optimal care for women with mental illness.

Online Resources

1. My M3: http://whatsmym3.com
2. Mood Disorder Questionnaire: http://www.integration.samhsa.gov/images/res/MDQ.pdf
3. Depression Management Toolkit: http://otgateway.com/articles/13macarthurtoolkit.pdf
4. Dietary Supplements: www.fda.gov/food/dietarysupplements/usingdietarysupplements/ucm480069.htm

References

1. Kessler RC. Epidemiology of women and depression. *J Affect Disord.* 2003;74(1):5-13.
2. Bekhuis E, Boschloo L, Rosmalen JG, Schoevers RA. Differential associations of specific depressive and anxiety disorders with somatic symptoms. *J Psychosom Res.* 2015;78(2):116-122.
3. Greenberg PE, Fournier AA, Sisitsky T, Pike CT, Kessler RC. The economic burden of adults with major depressive disorder in the United States (2005 and 2010). *J Clin Psychiatry.* 2015;76(2):155-162.
4. Cross-Disorder Group of the Psychiatric Genomics C. Identification of risk loci with shared effects on five major psychiatric disorders: a genome-wide analysis. *Lancet.* 2013;381(9875):1371-1379.
5. Provencal N, Binder EB. The effects of early life stress on the epigenome: from the womb to adulthood and even before. *Exp Neurol.* 2015;268:10-20.
6. Mayor E. Gender roles and traits in stress and health. *Front Psychol.* 2015;6:779.
7. Gobinath AR, Mahmoud R, Galea LA. Influence of sex and stress exposure across the lifespan on endophenotypes of depression: focus on behavior, glucocorticoids, and hippocampus. *Front Neurosci.* 2014;8:420.
8. Weinberg MK, Tronick EZ. The impact of maternal psychiatric illness on infant development. *J Clin Psychiatry.* 1998;59(Suppl 2):53-61.
9. Bagner DM, Pettit JW, Lewinsohn PM, Seeley JR, Jaccard J. Disentangling the temporal relationship

between parental depressive symptoms and early child behavior problems: a transactional framework. *J Clin Child Adolesc Psychol.* 2013;42(1):78-90.

10. Beck CT. Maternal depression and child behaviour problems: a meta-analysis. *J Adv Nurs.* 1999;29(3): 623-629.

11. Post RM. Heading off depressive illness evolution and progression to treatment resistance. *Dialogues Clin Neurosci.* 2015;17(2):105-109.

12. Bobo WV, Yawn BP. Concise review for physicians and other clinicians: postpartum depression. *Mayo Clin Proc.* 2014;89(6):835-844.

13. Sit D, Rothschild AJ, Wisner KL. A review of postpartum psychosis. *J Womens Health.* 2006;15(4): 352-368.

14. Zahl DL, Hawton K. Repetition of deliberate self-harm and subsequent suicide risk: long-term follow-up study of 11,583 patients. *Br J Psychiatry.* 2004;185:70-75.

15. American Psychiatric Association. *Diagnostic and Statistical Manual of Mental Disorders.* 5th ed. Arlington, VA: American Psychiatric Association; 2013.

16. US Preventive Services Task Force. Depression in Adults: Screening; 2016. Available at: http://www.uspreventiveservicestaskforce.org/Page/Document/UpdateSummaryFinal/depression-in-adults-screening1?ds=1&s=depression. Accessed February 25, 2016.

17. Mitchell J, Trangle M, Degnan B, Gabert T, Haight B, Kessler D, et al; Institute for Clinical Systems Improvement. Health Care Guideline: Adult Depression in Primary Care Guideline. Available at: https://www.icsi.org/_asset/fnhdm3/Depr.pdf. Accessed February 25, 2016.

18. Freeman MP, Fava M, Lake J, Trivedi MH, Wisner KL, Mischoulon D. Complementary and alternative medicine in major depressive disorder: the American Psychiatric Association Task Force report. *J Clin Psychiatry.* 2010;71(6):669-681.

19. Arroll B, Khin N, Kerse N. Screening for depression in primary care with two verbally asked questions: cross sectional study. *BMJ.* 2003;327(7424):1144-1146.

20. Cuijpers P, Reynolds CF, 3rd, Donker T, Li J, Andersson G, Beekman A. Personalized treatment of adult depression: medication, psychotherapy, or both? A systematic review. *Depress Anxiety.* 2012;29(10): 855-864.

21. Cuijpers P, Sijbrandij M, Koole SL, Andersson G, Beekman AT, Reynolds CF, 3rd. Adding psychotherapy to antidepressant medication in depression and anxiety disorders: a meta-analysis. *World Psychiatry.* 2014;13(1):56-67.

22. National Collaborating Centre for Mental Health. *The NICE Guideline on the Management and Treatment of Depression in Adults* (updated edition). London, UK: National Institute for Health and Clinical Excellence; 2010.

23. Unutzer J, Park M. Strategies to improve the management of depression in primary care. *Primary Care.* 2012;39(2):415-431.

24. King T, Johnson R, Gamblian V. Mental health. In: King TL, Brucker MC, eds. *Pharmacology for Women's Health.* Sudbury, MA: Jones & Bartlett Learning; 2011.

25. The MacArthur Initiative on Depression and Primary Care. Depression Management Tool Kit. 2009. Available at: http://otgateway.com/articles/13macarthurtoolkit.pdf. Accessed February 25, 2016.

26. Unutzer J, Oisha S. *IMPACT Intervention Manual.* Los Angeles, CA: UCLA NPI, Health Services Research Center; 2004. Available at: http://impact-uw.org/files/IMPACT_Intervention_Manual.pdf. Accessed February 27, 2016.

27. AIMS Center. Advancing Integrated Mental Health Solutions. 2012. Available at: http://aims.uw.edu/. Accessed October 4, 2015.

28. Thota AB, Sipe TA, Byard GJ, Zometa CS, Hahn RA, McKnight-Eily LR, et al. Collaborative care to improve the management of depressive disorders: a community guide systematic review and meta-analysis. *Am J Prev Med.* 2012;42(5):525-538.

29. Tamburrino MB, Nagel RW, Lynch DJ. Managing antidepressants in primary care: physicians' treatment modifications. *Psychol Rep.* 2011;108(3):799-804.

30. Titov N. Internet-delivered psychotherapy for depression in adults. *Curr Opin Psychiatry.* 2011;24(1): 18-23.

31. Hackley B, Sharma C, Kedzior A, Sreenivasan S. Managing mental health conditions in primary care settings. *J Midwifery Womens Health.* 2010;55(1): 9-19.

32. Qaseem A, Snow V, Denberg TD, Forciea MA, Owens DK, Clinical Efficacy Assessment Subcommittee of American College of Physicians. Using second-generation antidepressants to treat depressive disorders: a clinical practice guideline from the American College of Physicians. *Ann Intern Med.* 2008;149(10):725-733.

33. American Psychiatric Association. Practice guideline for the treatment of patients with major depressive disorder. 3rd ed. 2010. Available at: http://psychiatryonline.org/pb/assets/raw/sitewide/practice_guidelines/guidelines/mdd.pdf. Accessed February 25, 2016.

34. Lai MW, Klein-Schwartz W, Rodgers GC, Abrams JY, Haber DA, Bronstein AC, et al. 2005 Annual Report of the American Association of Poison Control Centers' national poisoning and exposure database. *Clin Toxicol (Phila).* 2006;44(6-7):803-932.

35. Ables AZ, Nagubilli R. Prevention, recognition, and management of serotonin syndrome. *Am Fam Physician.* 2010;81(9):1139-1142.
36. Beakley BD, Kaye AM, Kaye AD. Tramadol, pharmacology, side effects, and serotonin syndrome: a review. *Pain Physician.* 2015;18(4):395-400.
37. Iqbal MM, Basil MJ, Kaplan J, Iqbal MT. Overview of serotonin syndrome. *Ann Clin Psychiatry.* 2012;24(4):310-318.
38. Rhebergen D, Beekman AT, de Graaf R, Nolen WA, Spijker J, Hoogendijk WJ, et al. Trajectories of recovery of social and physical functioning in major depression, dysthymic disorder and double depression: a 3-year follow-up. *J Affect Disord.* 2010;124(1-2):148-156.
39. Cuijpers P, van Straten A, Schuurmans J, van Oppen P, Hollon SD, Andersson G. Psychotherapy for chronic major depression and dysthymia: a meta-analysis. *Clin Psychol Rev.* 2010;30(1):51-62.
40. Hollon SD, Ponniah K. A review of empirically supported psychological therapies for mood disorders in adults. *Depress Anxiety.* 2010;27(10):891-932.
41. Culpepper L. Misdiagnosis of bipolar depression in primary care practices. *J Clin Psychiatry.* 2014;75(3):e05.
42. Culpepper L. The diagnosis and treatment of bipolar disorder: decision-making in primary care. *Prim Care Companion CNS Disord.* 2014;16(3).
43. Merikangas KR, Akiskal HS, Angst J, Greenberg PE, Hirschfeld RM, Petukhova M, et al. Lifetime and 12-month prevalence of bipolar spectrum disorder in the National Comorbidity Survey replication. *Arch Gen Psychiatry.* 2007;64(5):543-552.
44. Diflorio A, Jones I. Is sex important? Gender differences in bipolar disorder. *Int Rev Psychiatry.* 2010;22(5):437-452.
45. Chaudron LH, Pies RW. The relationship between postpartum psychosis and bipolar disorder: a review. *J Clin Psychiatry.* 2003;64(11):1284-1292.
46. Di Florio A, Forty L, Gordon-Smith K, Heron J, Jones L, Craddock N, et al. Perinatal episodes across the mood disorder spectrum. *JAMA Psychiatry.* 2013;70(2):168-175.
47. Meltzer-Brody S, Jones I. Optimizing the treatment of mood disorders in the perinatal period. *Dialogues Clin Neurosci.* 2015;17(2):207-218.
48. Latalova K, Kamaradova D, Prasko J. Suicide in bipolar disorder: a review. *Psychiatr Danub.* 2014;26(2):108-114.
49. Culpepper L. Pathways to the diagnosis of bipolar disorder. *J Fam Pract.* 2015;64(6 Suppl):S4-9.
50. STABLE. STABLE Resouce Toolkit. Available at: http://www.integration.samhsa.gov/images/res/STABLE_toolkit.pdf. Accessed February 25, 2016.
51. McIntyre RS. Evidence-based treatment of bipolar disorder, bipolar depression, and mixed features. *J Fam Pract.* 2015;64(6 Suppl):S16-23.
52. Kessler RC, Berglund P, Demler O, Jin R, Merikangas KR, Walters EE. Lifetime prevalence and age-of-onset distributions of DSM-IV disorders in the National Comorbidity Survey Replication. *Arch Gen Psychiatry.* 2005;62(6):593-602.
53. Baldwin DS, Anderson IM, Nutt DJ, Allgulander C, Bandelow B, den Boer JA, et al. Evidence-based pharmacological treatment of anxiety disorders, post-traumatic stress disorder and obsessive-compulsive disorder: a revision of the 2005 guidelines from the British Association for Psychopharmacology. *J Psychopharmacol.* 2014;28(5):403-439.
54. Kroenke K, Spitzer RL, Williams JB, Lowe B. The Patient Health Questionnaire Somatic, Anxiety, and Depressive Symptom Scales: a systematic review. *Gen Hosp Psychiatry.* 2010;32(4):345-359.
55. Karsnitz DB, Ward S. Spectrum of anxiety disorders: diagnosis and pharmacologic treatment. *J Midwifery Womens Health.* 2011;56(3):266-281.
56. Roy-Byrne P, Craske MG, Sullivan G, Rose RD, Edlund MJ, Lang AJ, et al. Delivery of evidence-based treatment for multiple anxiety disorders in primary care: a randomized controlled trial. *JAMA.* 2010;303(19):1921-1928.
57. Hofmann SG, Wu JQ, Boettcher H. Effect of cognitive-behavioral therapy for anxiety disorders on quality of life: a meta-analysis. *J Consult Clin Psychol.* 2014;82(3):375-391.
58. Hoifodt RS, Strom C, Kolstrup N, Eisemann M, Waterloo K. Effectiveness of cognitive behavioural therapy in primary health care: a review. *Fam Pract.* 2011;28(5):489-504.
59. Andrews G, Cuijpers P, Craske MG, McEvoy P, Titov N. Computer therapy for the anxiety and depressive disorders is effective, acceptable and practical health care: a meta-analysis. *PloS One.* 2010;5(10):e13196.
60. Bandelow B, Sher L, Bunevicius R, Hollander E, Kasper S, Zohar J, et al. Guidelines for the pharmacological treatment of anxiety disorders, obsessive-compulsive disorder and posttraumatic stress disorder in primary care. *Int J Psychiatry Clin Pract.* 2012;16(2):77-84.
61. Baldwin DS, den Boer JA, Lyndon G, Emir B, Schweizer E, Haswell H. Efficacy and safety of pregabalin in generalised anxiety disorder: a critical review of the literature. *J Psychopharmacol.* 2015;29(10):1047-1060.
62. Hadley SJ, Mandel FS, Schweizer E. Switching from long-term benzodiazepine therapy to pregabalin in patients with generalized anxiety disorder: a

double-blind, placebo-controlled trial. *J Psychopharmacol.* 2012;26(4):461-470.

63. Weinstock L, Cohen LS, Bailey JW, Blatman R, Rosenbaum JF. Obstetrical and neonatal outcome following clonazepam use during pregnancy: a case series. *Psychother Psychosom.* 2001;70(3):158-162.

64. Bellantuono C, Tofani S, Di Sciascio G, Santone G. Benzodiazepine exposure in pregnancy and risk of major malformations: a critical overview. *Gen Hosp Psychiatry.* 2013;35(1):3-8.

65. Amos T, Stein DJ, Ipser JC. Pharmacological interventions for preventing post-traumatic stress disorder (PTSD). *Cochrane Database Syst Rev.* 2014;7:CD006239.

66. Chen L, Zhang G, Hu M, Liang X. Eye movement desensitization and reprocessing versus cognitive-behavioral therapy for adult posttraumatic stress disorder: systematic review and meta-analysis. *J Nerv Ment Dis.* 2015;203(6):443-451.

67. Hofmann S, Wu JQ, Boettcher H. D-Cycloserine as an augmentation strategy for cognitive behavioral therapy of anxiety disorders. *Biol Mood Anxiety Disord.* 2013;3(1):11.

68. Mitchison D, Hay PJ. The epidemiology of eating disorders: genetic, environmental, and societal factors. *Clin Epidemiol.* 2014;6:89-97.

69. Madowitz J, Matheson BE, Liang J. The relationship between eating disorders and sexual trauma. *Eat Weight Disord.* 2015;20(3):281-293.

70. Brown C, Mehler PS. Medical complications of anorexia nervosa and their treatments: an update on some critical aspects. *Eat Weight Disord.* 2015; 20(4):419-425.

71. Keshaviah A, Edkins K, Hastings ER, Krishna M, Franko DL, Herzog DB, et al. Re-examining premature mortality in anorexia nervosa: a meta-analysis redux. *Compr Psychiatry.* 2014;55(8):1773-1784.

72. Keel PK, Mitchell JE, Miller KB, Davis TL, Crow SJ. Long-term outcome of bulimia nervosa. *Arch Gen Psychiatry.* 1999;56(1):63-69.

73. Javed A, Tebben PJ, Fischer PR, Lteif AN. Female athlete triad and its components: toward improved screening and management. *Mayo Clin Proc.* 2013;88(9):996-1009.

74. Gowers SG, Clark AF, Roberts C, Byford S, Barrett B, Griffiths A, et al. A randomised controlled multicentre trial of treatments for adolescent anorexia nervosa including assessment of cost-effectiveness and patient acceptability—the TOuCAN trial. *Health Technol Assess.* 2010;14(15):1-98.

75. Schmidt U, Oldershaw A, Jichi F, Sternheim L, Startup H, McIntosh V, et al. Out-patient psychological therapies for adults with anorexia nervosa: randomised controlled trial. *Br J Psychiatry.* 2012;201(5):392-399.

76. Koubaa S, Hallstrom T, Lindholm C, Hirschberg AL. Pregnancy and neonatal outcomes in women with eating disorders. *Obstet Gynecol.* 2005;105(2): 255-260.

77. Hoffman ER, Zerwas SC, Bulik CM. Reproductive issues in anorexia nervosa. *Expert Rev Obstet Gynecol.* 2011;6(4):403-414.

78. Flament MF, Bissada H, Spettigue W. Evidence-based pharmacotherapy of eating disorders. *Int J Neuropsychopharmacol.* 2012;15(2):189-207.

79. Stepp SD, Burke JD, Hipwell AE, Loeber R. Trajectories of attention deficit hyperactivity disorder and oppositional defiant disorder symptoms as precursors of borderline personality disorder symptoms in adolescent girls. *J Abnorm Child Psychol.* 2012;40(1):7-20.

80. Martin-Blanco A, Soler J, Villalta L, Feliu-Soler A, Elices M, Perez V, et al. Exploring the interaction between childhood maltreatment and temperamental traits on the severity of borderline personality disorder. *Compr Psychiatry.* 2014;55(2):311-318.

81. Paris J. Implications of long-term outcome research for the management of patients with borderline personality disorder. *Harv Rev Psychiatry.* 2002;10(6):315-323.

82. Stoffers JM, Vollm BA, Rucker G, Timmer A, Huband N, Lieb K. Psychological therapies for people with borderline personality disorder. *Cochrane Database Sys Rev.* 2012;8:CD005652.

83. Reid RL. Premenstrual Syndrome. In: De Groot LJ, Beck-Peccoz P, Chrousos G, Dungan K, Grossman A, Hershman JM, et al., eds. *Endotext.* South Dartmouth, MA: MDText.com, Inc; 2014.

84. O'Brien PM, Backstrom T, Brown C, Dennerstein L, Endicott J, Epperson CN, et al. Towards a consensus on diagnostic criteria, measurement and trial design of the premenstrual disorders: the ISPMD Montreal consensus. *Arch Womens Mental Health.* 2011;14(1):13-21.

85. US Department of Health and Human Services, Office on Women's Health. Premenstrual Syndrome. 2014. Available at: https://www.nlm.nih.gov/medlineplus/premenstrualsyndrome.html. Accessed February 28, 2016.

86. Epperson CN, Steiner M, Hartlage SA, Eriksson E, Schmidt PJ, Jones I, et al. Premenstrual dysphoric disorder: evidence for a new category for DSM-5. *Am J Psychiatry.* 2012;169(5):465-475.

87. Wright KP, Hammond C. Evaluation of extended and continuous use oral contraceptives. *Ther Clin Risk Manag.* 2008;4(5):905-911.

88. Edelman A, Micks E, Gallo MF, Jensen JT, Grimes DA. Continuous or extended cycle vs. cyclic use of combined hormonal contraceptives for contraception. *Cochrane Database Syst Rev.* 2014;7: CD004695.

89. Svendal G, Berk M, Pasco JA, Jacka FN, Lund A, Williams LJ. The use of hormonal contraceptive agents and mood disorders in women. *J Affect Disord.* 2012;140:92-96.

90. Freeman EW, Halbreich U, Grubb GS, Rapkin AJ, Skouby SO, Smith L, et al. An overview of four studies of a continuous oral contraceptive (levonorgestrel 90 mcg/ethinyl estradiol 20 mcg) on premenstrual dysphoric disorder and premenstrual syndrome. *Contraception.* 2012;85(5):437-445.

91. Rapkin AJ, Winer SA. The pharmacologic management of premenstrual dysphoric disorder. *Expert Opin Pharmacother.* 2008;9(3):429-445.

92. Nevatte T, O'Brien PM, Backstrom T, Brown C, Dennerstein L, Endicott J, et al. ISPMD consensus on the management of premenstrual disorders. *Arch Womens Mental Health.* 2013;16(4):279-291.

93. Brown J, PM OB, Marjoribanks J, Wyatt K. Selective serotonin reuptake inhibitors for premenstrual syndrome. *Cochrane Database Syst Rev.* 2009(2): CD001396.

94. Rapkin AJ, Lewis EI. Treatment of premenstrual dysphoric disorder. *Womens Health.* 2013;9(6): 537-556.

95. Jang SH, Kim DI, Choi MS. Effects and treatment methods of acupuncture and herbal medicine for premenstrual syndrome/premenstrual dysphoric disorder: systematic review. BMC *Complement Altern Med.* 2014;14:11.

96. Davalos DB, Yadon CA, Tregellas HC. Untreated prenatal maternal depression and the potential risks to offspring: a review. *Arch Womens Mental Health.* 2012;15(1):1-14.

97. Warren SL, Gunnar MR, Kagan J, Anders TF, Simmens SJ, Rones M, et al. Maternal panic disorder: infant temperament, neurophysiology, and parenting behaviors. *J Am Acad Child Adolesc Psychiatry.* 2003;42(7):814-825.

98. Tsivos ZL, Calam R, Sanders MR, Wittkowski A. Interventions for postnatal depression assessing the mother-infant relationship and child developmental outcomes: a systematic review. *Int J Womens Health.* 2015;7:429-447.

99. Cohen LS, Altshuler LL, Harlow BL, Nonacs R, Newport DJ, Viguera AC, et al. Relapse of major depression during pregnancy in women who maintain or discontinue antidepressant treatment. *JAMA.* 2006;295(5):499-507.

100. Kessler RC, Angermeyer M, Anthony JC, De Graf R, Demyttenaere K, Gasquet I, et al. Lifetime prevalence and age-of-onset distributions of mental disorders in the World Health Organization's World Mental Health Survey Initiative. *World Psychiatry.* 2007;6(3):168-176.

101. Meltzer-Brody S, Brandon A. It is time to focus on maternal mental health: optimising maternal and child health outcomes. *BJOG.* 2015;122(3):321.

102. Howell BR, Sanchez MM. Understanding behavioral effects of early life stress using the reactive scope and allostatic load models. *Dev Psychopathol.* 2011;23(4):1001-1016.

103. Gentile S. Untreated depression during pregnancy: short- and long-term effects in offspring. A systematic review. *Neuroscience.* 2015: S0306-4522(15)00811-8.

104. Robertson E, Grace S, Wallington T, Stewart DE. Antenatal risk factors for postpartum depression: a synthesis of recent literature. *Gen Hosp Psychiatry.* 2004;26(4):289-295.

105. Milgrom J, Gemmill AW, Bilszta JL, Hayes B, Barnett B, Brooks J, et al. Antenatal risk factors for postnatal depression: a large prospective study. *J Affect Disord.* 2008;108(1-2):147-157.

106. Buist A, Gotman N, Yonkers KA. Generalized anxiety disorder: course and risk factors in pregnancy. *J Affect Disord.* 2011;131(1-3):277-283.

107. Kofman O. The role of prenatal stress in the etiology of developmental behavioural disorders. *Neurosci Biobehav Rev.* 2002;26(4):457-470.

108. Chaudron LH, Nirodi N. The obsessive-compulsive spectrum in the perinatal period: a prospective pilot study. *Arch Womens Mental Health.* 2010;13(5):403-410.

109. Thombs BD, Arthurs E, Coronado-Montoya S, Roseman M, Delisle VC, Leavens A, et al. Depression screening and patient outcomes in pregnancy or postpartum: a systematic review. *J Psychosom Res.* 2014;76(6):433-446.

110. Committee on Obstetric Practice. The American College of Obstetricians and Gynecologists Committee Opinion no. 630. Screening for perinatal depression. *Obstet Gynecol.* 2015;125(5): 1268-1271.

111. Gaynes BN, DeVeaugh-Geiss J, Weir S, Gu H, MacPherson C, Schulberg HC, et al. Feasibility and diagnostic validity of the M-3 checklist: a brief, self-rated screen for depressive, bipolar, anxiety, and post-traumatic stress disorders in primary care. *Ann Fam Med.* 2010;8(2):160-169.

112. Arroll B, Goodyear-Smith F, Crengle S, Gunn J, Kerse N, Fishman T, et al. Validation of PHQ-2

and PHQ-9 to screen for major depression in the primary care population. *Ann Fam Med.* 2010;8(4): 348-353.

113. Bennett IM, Coco A, Coyne JC, Mitchell AJ, Nicholson J, Johnson E, et al. Efficiency of a two-item pre-screen to reduce the burden of depression screening in pregnancy and postpartum: an IMPLICIT network study. *J Am Board Fam Med.* 2008;21(4):317-325.

114. Smith MV, Gotman N, Lin H, Yonkers KA. Do the PHQ-8 and the PHQ-2 accurately screen for depressive disorders in a sample of pregnant women? *Gen Hosp Psychiatry.* 2010;32(5):544-548.

115. Cox JL, Holden JM, Sagovsky R. Detection of postnatal depression. Development of the 10-item Edinburgh Postnatal Depression Scale. *Br J Psychiatry.* 1987;150:782-786.

116. Flynn HA, Sexton M, Ratliff S, Porter K, Zivin K. Comparative performance of the Edinburgh Postnatal Depression Scale and the Patient Health Questionnaire-9 in pregnant and postpartum women seeking psychiatric services. *Psychiatry Res.* 2011;187(1-2):130-134.

117. Sidebottom AC, Harrison PA, Godecker A, Kim H. Validation of the Patient Health Questionnaire (PHQ)-9 for prenatal depression screening. *Arch Womens Mental Health.* 2012;15(5):367-374.

118. Altshuler LL, Cohen LS, Vitonis AF, Faraone SV, Harlow BL, Suri R, et al. The Pregnancy Depression Scale (PDS): a screening tool for depression in pregnancy. *Arch Womens Mental Health.* 2008;11(4):277-285.

119. Myers ER, Aubuchon-Endsley N, Bastian LA, Gierisch JM, Kemper AR, Swamy GK, et al. *Efficacy and Safety of Screening for Postpartum Depression [Internet] Executive Summary.* Rockville, MD: Agency for Healthcare Research and Quality; 2013.

120. Sylven SM, Elenis E, Michelakos T, Larsson A, Olovsson M, Poromaa IS, et al. Thyroid function tests at delivery and risk for postpartum depressive symptoms. *Psychoneuroendocrinology.* 2012; 38(7):1007-1013.

121. Viguera AC, Whitfield T, Baldessarini RJ, Newport DJ, Stowe Z, Reminick A, et al. Risk of recurrence in women with bipolar disorder during pregnancy: prospective study of mood stabilizer discontinuation. *Am J Psychiatry.* 2007;164(12):1817-1824; quiz 923.

122. Yonkers KA, Vigod S, Ross LE. Diagnosis, pathophysiology, and management of mood disorders in pregnant and postpartum women. *Obstet Gynecol.* 2011;117(4):961-977.

123. Ekers D, Murphy R, Archer J, Ebenezer C, Kemp D, Gilbody S. Nurse-delivered collaborative care for depression and long-term physical conditions: a systematic review and meta-analysis. *J Affect Disord.* 2013;149(1-3):14-22.

124. Yonkers KA, Blackwell KA, Glover J, Forray A. Antidepressant use in pregnant and postpartum women. *Annu Rev Clin Psychol.* 2014;10:369-392.

125. Sandman CA. Fetal exposure to placental corticotropin-releasing hormone (pCRH) programs developmental trajectories. *Peptides.* 2015;72:145-153.

126. Staneva A, Bogossian F, Pritchard M, Wittkowski A. The effects of maternal depression, anxiety, and perceived stress during pregnancy on preterm birth: a systematic review. *Women Birth.* 2015;28(3):179-193.

127. Huybrechts KF, Palmsten K, Avorn J, Cohen LS, Holmes LB, Franklin JM, et al. Antidepressant use in pregnancy and the risk of cardiac defects. *N Engl J Med.* 2014;370(25):2397-2407.

128. Wemakor A, Casson K, Garne E, Bakker M, Addor MC, Arriola L, et al. Selective serotonin reuptake inhibitor antidepressant use in first trimester pregnancy and risk of specific congenital anomalies: a European register-based study. *Eur J Epidemiol.* 2015;30(11):1187-1198.

129. Gentile S. Early pregnancy exposure to selective serotonin reuptake inhibitors, risks of major structural malformations, and hypothesized teratogenic mechanisms. *Expert Opin Drug Metab Toxicol.* 2015:11(10):1585-1597.

130. Chambers CD, Hernandez-Diaz S, Van Marter LJ, Werler MM, Louik C, Jones KL, et al. Selective serotonin-reuptake inhibitors and risk of persistent pulmonary hypertension of the newborn. *N Engl J Med.* 2006;354(6):579-587.

131. Huybrechts KF, Bateman BT, Palmsten K, Desai RJ, Patorno E, Gopalakrishnan C, et al. Antidepressant use late in pregnancy and risk of persistent pulmonary hypertension of the newborn. *JAMA.* 2015;313(21):2142-2151.

132. Jefferies AL, Canadian Paediatric Society F, Newborn C. Selective serotonin reuptake inhibitors in pregnancy and infant outcomes. *Paediatr Child Health.* 2011;16(9):562-563.

133. Leibovitch L, Rymer-Haskel N, Schushan-Eisen I, Kuint J, Strauss T, Maayan-Metzger A. Short-term neonatal outcome among term infants after in utero exposure to serotonin reuptake inhibitors. *Neonatology.* 2013;104(1):65-70.

134. Massachusetts General Hospital. MGH Center for Women's Mental Health. 2013. Available at: http://womensmentalhealth.org/. Accessed September 10, 2015.

135. The Hospital for Sick Children. MOTHERISK. 2015. Available at: http://motherisk.org/. Accessed September 10, 2015.

136. Gentile S. Lithium in pregnancy: the need to treat, the duty to ensure safety. *Expert Opin Drug Saf.* 2012;11(3):425-437.

137. Clare CA, Yeh J. Postpartum depression in special populations: a review. *Obstet Gynecol Surv.* 2012;67(5):313-323.

138. Wisner KL, Wheeler SB. Prevention of recurrent postpartum major depression. *Hosp Community Psychiatry.* 1994;45(12):1191-1196.

139. Ickovics JR, Reed E, Magriples U, Westdahl C, Schindler Rising S, Kershaw TS. Effects of group prenatal care on psychosocial risk in pregnancy: results from a randomised controlled trial. *Psychol Health.* 2011;26(2):235-250.

140. McNeil DA, Vekved M, Dolan SM, Siever J, Horn S, Tough SC. Getting more than they realized they needed: a qualitative study of women's experience of group prenatal care. *BMC Pregnancy Childbirth.* 2012;12:17.

141. Khazaie H, Ghadami MR, Knight DC, Emamian F, Tahmasian M. Insomnia treatment in the third trimester of pregnancy reduces postpartum depression symptoms: a randomized clinical trial. *Psychiatry Res.* 2013;210(3):901-905.

142. Bigelow A, Power M, MacLellan-Peters J, Alex M, McDonald C. Effect of mother/infant skin-to-skin contact on postpartum depressive symptoms and maternal physiological stress. *J Obstet Gynecol Neonatal Nurs.* 2012;41(3):369-382.

143. Lawson A, Murphy KE, Sloan E, Uleryk E, Dalfen A. The relationship between sleep and postpartum mental disorders: a systematic review. *J Affect Disord.* 2015;176:65-77.

144. Chesney E, Goodwin GM, Fazel S. Risks of all-cause and suicide mortality in mental disorders: a meta-review. *World Psychiatry.* 2014;13(2):153-160.

145. Beck CT. Postpartum depression: it isn't just the blues. *Am J Nurs.* 2006;106(5):40-50.

146. Pearlstein T, Howard M, Salisbury A, Zlotnick C. Postpartum depression. *Am J Obstet Gynecol.* 2009; 200(4):357-364.

147. Gavin NI, Gaynes BN, Lohr KN, Meltzer-Brody S, Gartlehner G, Swinson T. Perinatal depression: a systematic review of prevalence and incidence. *Obstet Gynecol.* 2005;106(5 Pt 1):1071-1083.

148. NIHCM Foundation. Identifying and Treating Maternal Depression: Strategies and Considerations for Health Plans. 2010. Available at: http://www.nihcm.org/pdf/FINAL_MaternalDepression6-7.pdf. Accessed February 28, 2016.

149. Field T. Postpartum depression effects on early interactions, parenting, and safety practices: a review. *Infant Behav Dev.* 2010;33(1):1-6.

150. Field T. Touch for socioemotional and physical well-being: a review. *Dev Rev.* 2010;30(4):367-383.

151. Stagnaro-Green A. Approach to the patient with postpartum thyroiditis. *J Clin Endocrinol Metab.* 2012;97(2):334-342.

152. Mignogna J, Hundt NE, Kauth MR, Kunik ME, Sorocco KH, Naik AD, et al. Implementing brief cognitive behavioral therapy in primary care: a pilot study. *Transl Behav Med.* 2014;4(2):175-183.

153. Hassink-Franke LJ, van Weel-Baumgarten EM, Wierda E, Engelen MW, Beek MM, Bor HH, et al. Effectiveness of problem-solving treatment by general practice registrars for patients with emotional symptoms. *Prim Health Care.* 2011;3(3): 181-189.

154. Barth J, Munder T, Gerger H, Nüesch E, Trelle S, Znoj H, et al. Comparative efficacy of seven psychotherapeutic interventions for patients with depression: a network meta-analysis. *PLoS Med.* 2013; 10(5):e1001454.

155. Hirst C, Calingaert B, Stanford R, Castellsague J. Use of long-acting beta-agonists and inhaled steroids in asthma: meta-analysis of observational studies. *J Asthma.* 2010;47(4):439-446.

156. Valdimarsdottir U, Hultman CM, Harlow B, Cnattingius S, Sparen P. Psychotic illness in first-time mothers with no previous psychiatric hospitalizations: a population-based study. *PLoS Med.* 2009;6(2):e13.

157. Bergink V, Bouvy PF, Vervoort JS, Koorengevel KM, Steegers EA, Kushner SA. Prevention of postpartum psychosis and mania in women at high risk. *Am J Psychiatry.* 2012;169(6):609-615.

158. Vossbeck-Elsebusch AN, Freisfeld C, Ehring T. Predictors of posttraumatic stress symptoms following childbirth. *BMC Psychiatry.* 2014;14:200.

159. Andersen LB, Melvaer LB, Videbech P, Lamont RF, Joergensen JS. Risk factors for developing post-traumatic stress disorder following childbirth: a systematic review. *Acta Obstet Gynecol Scand.* 2012;91(11):1261-1272.

160. Beck CT. Birth trauma: in the eye of the beholder. *Nurs Res.* 2004;53(1):28-35.

161. Lapp LK, Agbokou C, Peretti CS, Ferreri F. Management of post traumatic stress disorder after childbirth: a review. *J Psychosom Obstet Gynaecol* 2010;31(3):113-122.

162. Rakofsky JJ, Dunlop BW. Review of nutritional supplements for the treatment of bipolar depression. *Depress Anxiety.* 2014;31(5):379-390.

163. McNamara RK, Strawn JR. Role of long-chain omega-3 fatty acids in psychiatric practice. *PharmaNutrition.* 2013;1(2):41-49.

164. Dennis CL, Dowswell T. Interventions (other than pharmacological, psychosocial or psychological) for treating antenatal depression. *Cochrane Database Syst Rev.* 2013;7:CD006795.

165. Kaviani M, Saniee L, Azima S, Sharif F, Sayadi M. The effect of omega-3 fatty acid supplementation on maternal depression during pregnancy: a double blind randomized controlled clinical trial. *Int J Community Based Nurs Midwifery.* 2014;2(3):142-147.

166. Pail G, Huf W, Pjrek E, Winkler D, Willeit M, Praschak-Rieder N, et al. Bright-light therapy in the treatment of mood disorders. *Neuropsychobiology.* 2011;64(3):152-162.

167. Wirz-Justice A, Bader A, Frisch U, Stieglitz RD, Alder J, Bitzer J, et al. A randomized, double-blind, placebo-controlled study of light therapy for antepartum depression. *J Clin Psychiatry.* 2011;72(7):986-993.

168. Cooney GM, Dwan K, Greig CA, Lawlor DA, Rimer J, Waugh FR, et al. Exercise for depression. *Cochrane Database Syst Rev.* 2013;9:CD004366.

169. National Center for Complementary and Integrative Health. St John's Wort and Depression. Available at: https://nccih.nih.gov/health/stjohnswort/sjw-and-depression.htm. Accessed February 28, 2016.

170. US Food and Drug Administration. Questions and Answers on Dietary Supplements. Available at: www.fda.gov/food/dietarysupplements/usingdietarysupplements/ucm480069.htm. Accessed March 4, 2016.

CHAPTER 6

SUBSTANCE USE

Christine L. Savage | Deborah Finnell

Substance use has the potential to negatively impact the health of women at every stage of life. Healthcare providers play an essential role in preventing substance use–related adverse consequences across the continuum of use. Being able to effectively intervene includes knowledge of the prevalence of substance use in women from national, state, and local perspectives and the ability to distinguish between risky use and a substance use disorder (SUD). Armed with this information, the healthcare provider can choose appropriate evidenced-based interventions relevant to women aimed at the prevention of adverse health outcomes associated with substance use.

Substance use is the use of psychoactive substances including alcohol, tobacco, and drugs that have a pharmacologic effect on the brain and the central nervous system (CNS).[1] Effects include altered mood, perception, and change in level of consciousness. Substance use has the potential for harm above and beyond the development of an SUD. These harms include injury; alcohol-related organ pathologies; increased risk for cancer; transmission of communicable disease; and substance-related psychologic, social, and spiritual

consequences. The majority of the harm associated with alcohol, tobacco, and drug use is associated with at-risk use rather than with an SUD.[1-3] Because substance use can cause harm even without the existence of an SUD, the healthcare provider should view substance use as a continuum from low-risk use to the development of an SUD. The criteria for the diagnosis of an SUD in the recently released *Diagnostic and Statistical Manual of Mental Disorders, 5th Edition* (DSM-5) reflect this view through the framing of SUDs along a continuum from mild to severe.[4]

Substance Use Across the Continuum

Comprehending the impact of substance use on the health of women requires an understanding of the basic terms related to substance use. The use of substances occurs over a continuum from no use/low-risk use to at-risk/harmful use to use that meets the diagnostic criteria for an SUD (**Figure 6-1**). For some substances and/or populations, any use is considered at-risk use.

Figure 6-1 Continuum of use.

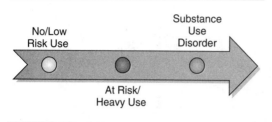

For example, any use of cocaine places the user at risk for adverse consequences, while alcohol use within the recommended limits in healthy adult women who are not pregnant is considered low risk. Thus, health risks associated with substance use in women vary across the lifespan, the amount of use, and the type of substance being used.

Level of Risk

Four aspects of substance use impact the level of risk. Frequency of substance use refers to how often the substance is used—daily, weekly, or monthly. Quantity of substance use refers to how much of the substance is consumed at a given time, and duration of substance use refers to how long the use has been taking place. Finally, pattern of substance use refers to use that is constant, that is, daily use, or use that is episodic, such as increased use on weekends with little or no use during the week. Understanding these four aspects can help the provider understand the level of risk and provide the underlying components related to the assessment of use.

Numerous terms are used to help differentiate the level of risk. For the purposes of this chapter, risk is divided into three main categories, no risk/low risk, at risk, and SUD. No-risk use is defined as no use of the substance or, in the case of alcohol, less than 3 drinks in the past 12 months. Low-risk use is defined as use that places the user at minimal risk for adverse consequences. At-risk use includes all use that places a person who does not meet the criteria for an SUD at risk for adverse consequences associated with the use of the substance. This category includes heavy use and heavy episodic use (also referred to as binge use) in persons without an SUD.

To help determine level of risk related to alcohol, the National Institute on Alcohol Abuse and Alcoholism (NIAAA) has published clinical guidelines that include recommended limits.[5] These limits are based on the definition of a standard drink as determined by the amount of alcohol contained in a beverage. Thus, a standard drink is equivalent to 12 fluid ounces (fl oz) of beer, 8–9 fl oz of malt liquor, 5 fl oz of table wine, and 1.5 fl oz of 80-proof spirits (hard liquor) (**Figure 6-2**).[6]

The recommended limits for women are no more than 3 drinks per occasion *and* no more than 7 drinks in 1 week compared to no more than 4 drinks per occasion *and* no more than 14 drinks per week for men. For adults 65 years and older, the recommended limit is 1 drink per day. NIAAA clarified that even within the limits, caution is needed (**Box 6-1**).[7] In the United States, 13% of women exceed the limits, drinking more than 7 drinks a week.[8] There is no safe level of use for tobacco or illicit drugs.

The final category of use, SUD, is defined by the diagnostic criteria set out by the American Psychiatric Association.[4] The new DSM-5 criteria use only one category, substance use disorder, in contrast to the previous two categories of abuse and dependence. Diagnosis occurs across a continuum that takes into account severity, evidence of physiologic dependence, and course of treatment to classify the disorder. The disorder can be established with or without physiologic dependence. Physiologic dependence is defined as evidence of tolerance or withdrawal.[4] The severity of the SUD is based on the number of the

Figure 6-2 Standard drink.

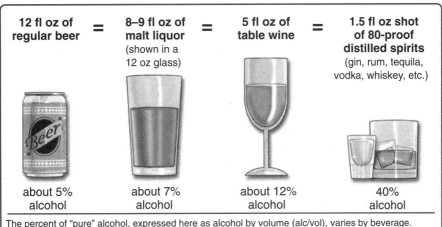

| 12 fl oz of regular beer | = | 8–9 fl oz of malt liquor (shown in a 12 oz glass) | = | 5 fl oz of table wine | = | 1.5 fl oz shot of 80-proof distilled spirits (gin, rum, tequila, vodka, whiskey, etc.) |

about 5% alcohol   about 7% alcohol   about 12% alcohol   40% alcohol

The percent of "pure" alcohol, expressed here as alcohol by volume (alc/vol), varies by beverage. Although the "standard" drink amounts are helpful for following health guidelines, they may not reflect customary serving sizes. In addition, while the alcohol concentrations listed are "typical," there is considerable variability in alcohol content within each type of beverage (e.g., beer, wine, distilled spirits).

Modified from National Institute on Alcohol Abuse and Alcoholism. What's a "standard" drink? Rethinking drinking: Alcohol & your health. http://rethinkingdrinking.niaaa.nih.gov/. n.d. Accessed April 14, 2016.

Box 6-1 NIAAA Recommendations Related to Low-Risk Drinking

For Women
No more than 3 drinks per occasion *and* no more than 7 drinks in 1 week.

To be determined to be low risk for alcohol use disorder, both the criteria for single-day and weekly limits must be met.

Even within these limits, health consequences can be seen if an individual drinks too quickly or has underlying medical conditions. To keep risk low, individual should be counseled to:

- Drink slowly
- Eat enough while drinking

Alcohol should be avoided completely if an individual:

- Plans to drive a vehicle or operate machinery
- Takes medications that interact with alcohol
- Has a medical condition that can be aggravated by alcohol
- Is pregnant or trying to become pregnant

Data from National Institute on Alcohol Abuse and Alcoholism. Drinking Levels Defined. http://www.niaaa.nih.gov/alcohol-health /overview-alcohol-consumption/moderate-binge-drinking. Accessed March 15, 2016.

Box 6-2 Diagnostic Criteria (DSM-5) for Substance Use Disorder

- Repeatedly unable to carry out major obligations at work, school, or home due to substance use
- Recurrent use of substances in physically hazardous situations
- Continued use despite persistent or recurring social or interpersonal problems caused or made worse by substance use
- Tolerance as defined by either a need for markedly increased amounts to achieve intoxication or desired effect or markedly diminished effect with continued use of the same amount
- Withdrawal manifesting as either characteristic syndrome *or* use of the substance to avoid withdrawal
- Using greater amounts or using over a longer time period than intended
- Persistent desire or unsuccessful efforts to cut down or control substance use
- Spending a lot of time obtaining, using, or recovering from using substances
- Stopping or reducing important social, occupational, or recreational activities due to substance use
- Consistent use of substances despite acknowledgment of persistent or recurrent physical or psychological difficulties from using substances
- Craving or a strong desire to use substances

Data from American Psychiatric Association. *Diagnostic and Statistical Manual of Mental Disorders.* 5th ed. Arlington, VA: American Psychiatric Association; 2013.

11 DSM-5 criteria (**Box 6-2**) endorsed. Two to three criteria indicate a mild disorder, four to five criteria indicate a moderate disorder, and six or more indicate a severe disorder.[4]

Types of Psychoactive Substances

All psychoactive substances that can lead to addiction increase dopamine levels in the brain through their interaction with different molecular targets by the various drug classes.[9] These actions will be discussed later in this chapter to convey how increases in dopamine levels translate into the pleasurable and reinforcing effects of various classes of drugs. Psychoactive substances can be classified in a variety of ways, including by chemical structure or by using the categories set by the US Drug Enforcement Administration schedules (i.e., Schedules I to V). Commonly accepted classifications include stimulants (e.g., cocaine, amphetamines, caffeine, nicotine), depressants or sedative hypnotics (e.g., alcohol, barbiturates, benzodiazepines), narcotics (e.g., heroin, morphine, hydrocodone, oxycodone), hallucinogens (e.g., lysergic acid diethylamide [LSD], phencyclidine

[PCP], ketamine, ecstasy), cannabis (e.g., marijuana, hashish), and inhalants (e.g., nitrous oxide, hydrocarbons). Numerous new psychoactive substances have appeared since the early 2000s, including beta-keto-amphetamines (cathinones), pyrrolidinophenones, tryptamines, and synthetic cannabinoids,[10] presenting ongoing challenges to providers for understanding the pharmacokinetic profiles of more recent psychoactive drugs.

Epidemiology of Substance Use in Women

The Centers for Disease Control and Prevention (CDC) website lists 11 national surveillance surveys that include data on substance use. The most often cited data come from the Behavioral Risk Factor Surveillance System (BRFSS), the National Survey on Drug Use and Health (NSDUH), the Pregnancy Risk Assessment Monitoring System, and the National Epidemiologic Survey on Alcohol and Related Conditions (NESARC). The NSDUH survey collects data on alcohol tobacco and illicit drug use. In this survey illicit drug use includes marijuana, cocaine, heroin, hallucinogens, and inhalants, as well as the nonmedical use of prescription-type pain relievers, tranquilizers, stimulants, and sedatives.

Some of the surveys collect data on any substance use; others collect data related to at-risk use such as heavy/episodic use, while others collect data to help determine the prevalence of SUDs. The data related to reported use can reflect any current use, use over the past 12 months, lifetime use, or heavy episodic (binge) use. Data are reported at the national, state, regional, and local levels. Surveillance data are also available from the World Health Organization (WHO). These data help healthcare providers understand the prevalence in the population to which they provide care and allow them to compare prevalence in their own region to other regions. The WHO also provides information on trends in use. For example, surveillance data helped to identify a rise in nonprescription use of opioids in women since the early 2000s.[1]

Women on the whole are less apt to use psychoactive substances than men. For example, twice as many men report binge drinking as women (30.9% vs. 15.7%). Despite this gap, the use of substances by women is concerning, with almost half of women age 12 or older reporting current alcohol use, 16.1% reporting tobacco use, and 7.3% reporting use of illicit drugs.[11] Understanding the prevalence of use and emerging trends can help healthcare providers develop and implement interventions aimed at the prevention of adverse health consequences associated with substance use and early identification of women at risk for these adverse consequences. Prevalence of use varies based on age, ethnicity, and geographic region.

Tobacco: Prevalence, Attributable Mortality

In the United States in 2014, 14.8% of women were current smokers; a steady decline has occurred since 2005.[12] A history of prior tobacco use increases the risk of certain adverse health outcomes even in women who are currently abstinent. According to data combined from 2010 and 2011, 17.6% of pregnant women reported smoking in the past month compared to 25.4% of women who were not pregnant (**Figure 6-3**).[12] Globally, 7% of all deaths in women are attributable to tobacco. Tobacco use accounts for 71% of all lung cancer deaths and 42% of all chronic obstructive pulmonary disease deaths.[13] In the United States the mortality rate is three times higher in men and women who smoked compared to those who never smoked.[14] Secondhand smoke also has a significant impact on mortality; it is associated with nearly 50,000 deaths in the United States each year and is one causative factor in sudden infant death syndrome.[15]

Alcohol: Prevalence, Attributable Mortality

In 2012, a little more than 50% of persons age 12 or older in the United States reported alcohol use in the past month. Women were slightly less apt to report current alcohol use than men (47.9% vs. 56.5%).[16] Globally, women are less apt to report alcohol use, but in some countries this gap between men and women is narrowing.[17] Of particular concern is the increase in at-risk drinking among women that includes both heavy episodic drinking and chronic drinking.[17] Among all US women age 12 or older, 15.7% reported heavy episodic drinking, but for women ages 18 to 25 the estimated rate of heavy episodic drinking was one-third (33.2%) (Figure 6-3).[16,18] Among adolescents ages 12 to 20, the rates of current use were almost the same, at a little under 25%. Females in this same age group were almost as likely to report heavy episodic drinking as males (14% vs. 16.5%) (**Figure 6-4**). Among pregnant women, 8.5% reported alcohol use during pregnancy, 2.7% reported heavy episodic drinking, and 0.3% reported heavy drinking.[16] Pregnant women ages 34–44 had the highest prevalence of alcohol use (14.3%).[19]

Figure 6-3 Women and alcohol use.

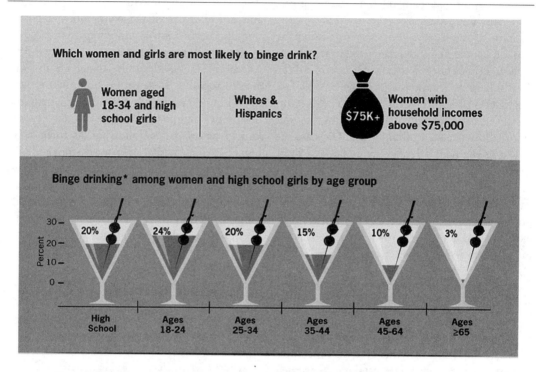

Binge drinking* by race/ethnicity among women and high school girls

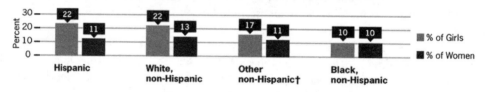

†Other non-Hispanic includes Asian, Native Hawaiian/other Pacific Islander, American Indian/Alaskan Native, and multiracial.

Binge drinking* among high school students reporting current alcohol use* by grade

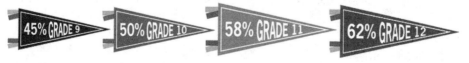

SOURCES: Behavioral Risk Factor Surveillance System (BRFSS) and Youth Risk Behavior Survey (YRBS), 2011.
*reported behavior in the past 30 days

Reproduced from Centers for Disease Control and Prevention. Vital signs: Binge drinking. CDC vital signs. http://www.cdc
.gov/vitalsigns/bingedrinkingfemale/index.html. January 8, 2013. Accessed April 14, 2016.

50% of the female alcohol-attributable cancer deaths being breast cancer deaths.[21]

Figure 6-4 Current, binge, and heavy alcohol use among those ages 12 to 20.

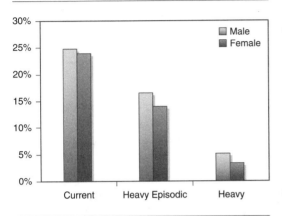

Data from Substance Abuse and Mental Health Services Administration. Results from the 2012 National Survey on Drug Use and Health: Summary of National Findings, NSDUH Series H-46, HHS Publication No. (SMA) 13-4795. Rockville, MD: Substance Abuse and Mental Health Services Administration; 2013.

Alcohol is associated with increased risk for morbidity and mortality and is in the top three risk factors for premature death globally.[20] Globally, alcohol accounts for approximately 5% of the disease burden and 5.9% of all deaths.[17] According to the WHO, alcohol results in 3.3 million deaths annually.[20] Alcohol accounts for more than 3% of all US cancer deaths with more than

Illicit Drugs: Prevalence, Attributable Mortality

Globally, between 3.4% and 6.6% of adults currently use illicit drugs. The most widely used are cannabis and amphetamine type stimulants.[22] In the United States, men are more apt to report illicit drug use (11.2%) than women (6.8%). Across different illicit drugs, the prevalence of current drug use is higher in males (**Table 6-1**).[16] According to pooled data from 2011 to 2012, 5.9% of pregnant women ages 15–44 reported that they had used illicit drugs. Men are more apt than women to report use of multiple drugs (9.6% vs. 5.0%).[16]

The most tangible evidence of mortality attributable to illicit drug use is overdose death, the leading cause of injury death in the United States.[23-24] Mortality associated with drug use is tied to three categories of risk: how drugs are administered (e.g., intravenous injection), the effect of the drug (e.g., the impact of cocaine on the cardiovascular system), and drug intoxication (e.g., accidental overdose).[24] Illicit drug use accounts for 0.8% of the global disability-adjusted life years.[25] Mortality attributable to illicit drug use in women includes increased risk for ectopic pregnancy[26] and prescription painkiller overdose.[27]

Table 6-1 Comparison of Use of Selected Illicit Drugs by Gender

Illicit Drug	Women: Lifetime	Men: Lifetime	Women: Past Year	Men: Past Year
Marijuana	38.1%	47.7%	9.2%	15.2%
Cocaine	11.1%	18.1%	1.0%	2.6%
Hallucinogens	17.6%	18.2%	1.1%	2.2%

Data from Substance Abuse and Mental Health Services Administration. Results from the 2012 National Survey on Drug Use and Health: Summary of National Findings, NSDUH Series H-46, HHS Publication No. (SMA) 13-4795. Rockville, MD: Substance Abuse and Mental Health Services Administration; 2013.

Figure 6-5 Comparison of substance use by ethnic groups.

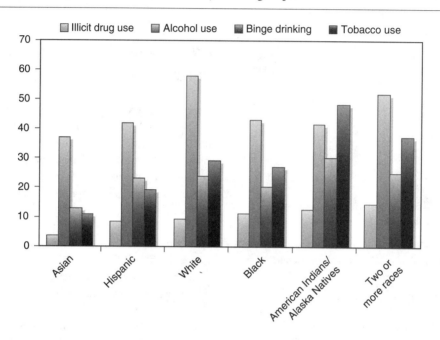

Substance Use in Women by Age and Ethnicity

The prevalence of substance use varies with age and ethnicity. The highest prevalence of tobacco, alcohol, and illicit drug use occurs in white persons (**Figure 6-5**).[16] The 18–25 age group is most apt to report substance use, with two-thirds reporting current alcohol use.[16] This age group is also most apt to report having been diagnosed with an SUD (18.9% vs. 7.0% of those age 26 and older).[16]

Emerging Issues

Since the early 2000s, there has been an increase in the nonprescription use of controlled substances resulting in the proliferation of pill mills. Another emerging issue is the rise in methamphetamine use. Methamphetamine use not only poses risk to the individual user, but also to the person's family and surrounding community due to environmental exposure to the toxic byproducts associated with the home manufacture of the drug. Finally, legalization of marijuana for medical use has occurred in a number of states across the United States. These new laws may have the unintended consequence of increasing the risk for developing an SUD.

Nonprescription Use of Controlled Substances

In the United States from 1990 to 2008, drug overdose tripled, with most of the deaths associated with prescription drugs (**Figure 6-6**).[27,28] There was

Figure 6-6 Trend in drug-related overdose deaths in women.

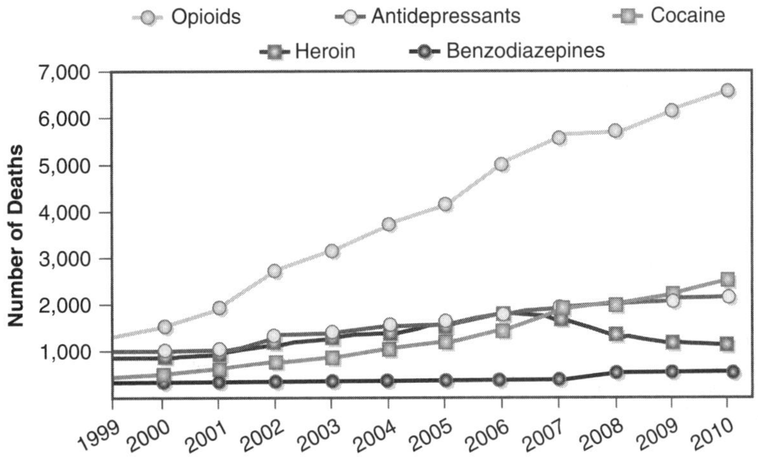

Reproduced from Centers for Disease Control and Prevention. Vital signs: prescription painkiller overdoses. CDC vital signs. http://www.cdc.gov/vitalsigns/PrescriptionPainkillerOverdoses/. July 2, 2013. Accessed April 14, 2016.

a 400% increase in these deaths in women compared to a 296% increase in men between 1999 and 2013.[27] Women are also being seen in the emergency department for prescription painkiller overdose (**Figure 6-7**).[28] Three out of four overdoses are due to nonmedical use of opioid painkillers. Nonmedical use of prescription drugs is defined as use of prescription drugs used for a purpose other than intended, often by someone other than the person for whom the medication was prescribed. Often the nonmedical use of opioids is combined with use of other substances, especially alcohol.[28] For every death associated with nonmedical use of prescription opioids, there are 825 nonmedical users. The majority of women (71.2%) obtain these drugs from a friend or a relative with or without permission. Another 17.3% obtain the opioids from a single doctor. Those at risk for nonmedical use of opioids include those who seek prescriptions from multiple providers ("doctor shopping"), those with a lower social economic status living in rural areas, and those with a history of at-risk substance use and/or a comorbid mental health disorder.[27-28]

Nonmedical use of prescription drugs also varies by area of the country. The two areas of the country with the highest prevalence are the Southwest and the Appalachian states. Healthcare providers can take action to prevent adverse consequences associated with nonprescription opioid use as described in **Box 6-3**.[28] In addition, providers should be aware of laws within their states in relation to prescription of opioids. Providers can advocate for implementation of laws within their states to prevent the operation of pain clinics that are actually "pill mills." Pill mills differ from legitimate pain management centers on a number of characteristics, including a cash-only/no insurance approach, no need for an appointment, no medical records, brief medical exams, sometimes armed guards, and the prescription of large doses of opioids outside of standard care practices. For example, in 2011 Florida passed an anti-pill mill law that helped to improve tracking of prescription of controlled substances and provide stricter regulations for the prescribing of these substances.

Figure 6-7 Prescription painkiller overdoses: A growing epidemic, especially among women.

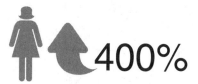

48,000

Nearly 48,000 women died of prescription painkiller* overdoses between 1999 and 2010.

400%

Deaths from prescription painkiller overdoses among women have increased more than 400% since 1999, compared to 265% among men.

30

For every woman who dies of a prescription painkiller overdose, 30 go to the emergency department for painkiller misuse or abuse.

*"Prescription painkillers" refers to opioid or narcotic pain relievers, including drugs such as Vicodin (hydrocodone), OxyContin (oxycodone), Opana (oxymorphone), and methadone.

Reproduced from Centers for Disease Control and Prevention. Vital signs: Prescriptions painkiller overdoses. CDC vital signs. http://www.cdc.gov/vitalsigns/PrescriptionPainkillerOverdoses/. July 2, 2013. Accessed April 14, 2016.

Box 6-3 CDC Recommendations to Healthcare Providers Related to Nonmedical Use of Opioids

- Recognize that women can be at risk of prescription drug overdose.
- Discuss pain treatment options, including ones that do not involve prescription drugs.
- Discuss the risks and benefits of taking prescription painkillers, especially during pregnancy. This includes when painkillers are taken for chronic conditions.
- Follow guidelines for responsible painkiller prescribing, including:
  - Screening and monitoring for substance abuse and mental health problems
  - Prescribing only the quantity needed based on appropriate pain diagnosis
  - Using patient–provider agreements combined with urine drug tests for people using prescription painkillers long term
  - Teaching patients how to safely use, store, and dispose of drugs
  - Avoiding combinations of prescription painkillers and benzodiazepines (e.g., Xanax and valium) unless there is a specific medical indication
- Talk with pregnant women who are dependent on prescription painkillers about treatment options, such as opioid agonist therapy.
- Use prescription drug monitoring programs (PDMPs)—electronic databases that track all controlled substance prescriptions in the state—to identify patients who may be improperly using prescription painkillers and other drugs.

Reproduced from Centers for Disease Control and Prevention. Vital signs: Prescription painkiller overdoses. CDC vital signs. http://www.cdc.gov/vitalsigns/PrescriptionPainkillerOverdoses/. July 2, 2013. Accessed May 24, 2014.

Methamphetamine

Another emerging trend in substance abuse since the early 2000s is methamphetamine use. There is considerable regional variability, with use occurring predominately in the west and the Midwest. There was a slight decrease in 2012, with 1.2 million (0.4%) of those age 12 or older reporting use within the past year.[29] The rate of use is close to the same for men and women.[30] Though the drug can be prescribed by healthcare providers, it has little therapeutic value. Both males and females report using methamphetamine because it increases their energy and enhances sexual performance. In addition, women stated they used it to help lose weight and to stay alert.[30,31]

For the most part, those who use methamphetamine obtain it through illegal labs. According to the National Institute on Drug Abuse, the use of methamphetamine over time directly impacts the functioning of the brain. Long-term use results in reduced motor skills and negatively impacts the ability to learn. There is also evidence that it affects the area of the brain that controls emotion and memory.[29]

Other adverse outcomes are the impacts that use has on the children who may accidentally ingest methamphetamine in the home. The manufacture of methamphetamine in a home lab also contaminates the home, creating an environmental and safety hazard. Children in the home are exposed to toxic environmental chemicals, as well as to the risk of fires and explosions.[32]

Legalization of Marijuana

As of fall 2013, 20 states had passed laws that legalized the use of marijuana for medical purposes. The majority (65%) passed those laws prior to 2009. Since 2008 there has been a significant rise in the reported use of daily or near-daily use of marijuana (**Figure 6-8**).[16] Men are more apt to report current marijuana use than women (9.6% vs 5.0%). This gender difference is vanishing with almost the same percent of females as males ages 12 to 17 reporting current marijuana use (**Figure 6-9**).[16] This increase may be due to the increased acceptance of use of this substance. To help determine if this may be the case, Cerda and colleagues conducted a secondary data analysis of the NESARC and found that the odds for marijuana use and having a marijuana SUD were almost twice as high in states that had legalized the use of marijuana compared to those that did not.[33] From a woman's health perspective, the use of marijuana increases the risk of multiple adverse health consequences including cancer and heart disease (**Box 6-4**).[34]

Figure 6-8 Trends in use of marijuana.

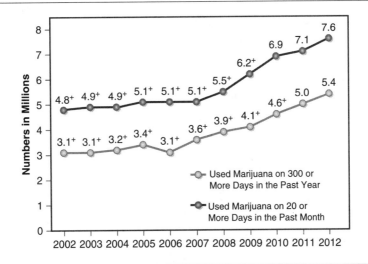

Data from Substance Abuse and Mental Health Services Administration. Results from the 2012 National Survey on Drug Use and Health: Summary of National Findings, NSDUH Series H-46, HHS Publication No. (SMA) 13-4795. Rockville, MD: Substance Abuse and Mental Health Services Administration; 2013.

Figure 6-9 Trends in marijuana use in females and males ages 12 to 17.

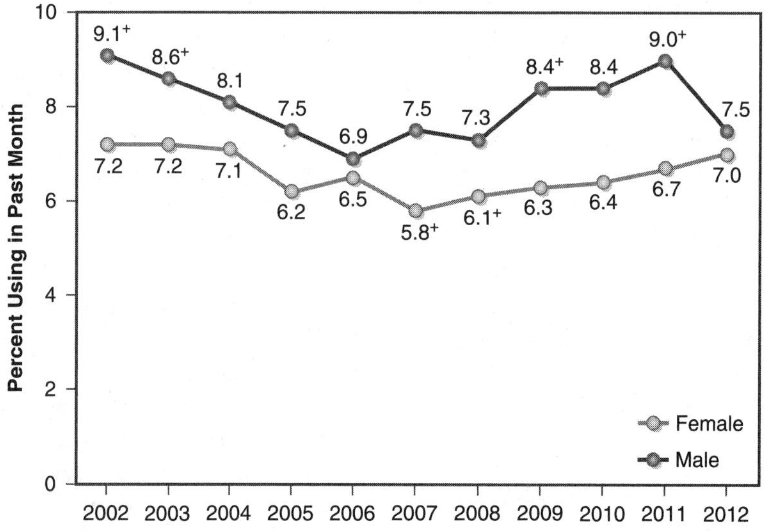

Data from Substance Abuse and Mental Health Services Administration. Results from the 2012 National Survey on Drug Use and Health: Summary of National Findings, NSDUH Series H-46, HHS Publication No. (SMA) 13-4795. Rockville, MD: Substance Abuse and Mental Health Services Administration; 2013.

Box 6-4 Health Risks Associated with Marijuana Use

- Withdrawal symptoms include irritability, trouble sleeping, decreased appetite, anxiety
- Problems with memory and learning
- Trouble with thinking and problem solving
- Loss of coordination, increased reaction time
- Anxiety and panic attacks
- Depression
- Hallucinations
- Possible effects on ability to learn and reason, when begun in adolescence
- Chronic cough, frequent URI, bronchitis
- Increased severity of mental illness such as schizophrenia
- In high doses paranoia and psychosis
- Possible associations include
  - Reduced ability of the immune system to fight disease
  - Lung and other upper aerodigestive cancers
  - Cardiovascular disease

Data from Volkow ND, Bale RD, Compotn WM, Weiss SRB. Adverse health effects of marijuana use. *N Engl J Med.* 2014;370(23), 2219-2227; National Institute on Drug Abuse. Commonly Abused Drug Charts. https://www.drugabuse.gov/drugs-abuse/commonly-abused-drugs-charts#marijuana. April 2016. Accessed May 5, 2016.

Neurobiologic Bases of Substance Use

Understanding the neurobiologic bases of substance use may help alter negative perceptions of and attitudes held by healthcare providers toward individuals affected by alcohol, nicotine, and other drugs.[35] However, this scientific evidence has not been widely disseminated, and SUDs remain highly stigmatized. This science-based information is important given the toxic effects of psychoactive substances on the developing and mature brain. At 7 weeks' gestation, the brainstem, cerebellum, and cerebrum of the human embryo are clearly visible.[36] While the basic structure of the child's brain is completed around 3 years of age, the prefrontal cortex is still developing into the teenage years and is fully developed at around 30 years of age.[36] Increases in myelination, initial arborization, and then pruning of gray matter are ongoing over 3 decades of life.[37] This process of neuronal maturation means that the developing brain is vulnerable to the neurotoxic effects of psychoactive substances.

This section discusses the neurobiologic bases of substance use to dependence. The common neural pathway for psychoactive substances underscores how initial voluntary use of psychoactive substances can eventually turn into automatic and compulsive use, characteristic of SUDs. A basic explanation is provided regarding the complex interplay between psychoactive substances and genetics. This discussion is aimed at helping providers understand why some people gravitate toward psychoactive substances in seeking pleasure or to relieve distress.

The Brain Reward System

A common feature of psychoactive substances is their ability to stimulate specific areas of the brain that activate pleasurable feelings of reward, motivation, and reinforcement. Collectively, this area of the brain is known as the brain reward system. Anatomically, it is known as the mesolimbic dopamine system. The mesolimbic dopamine system arises in the ventral tegmental area at the center of the brain. The ventral tegmental area is in close proximity to the amygdala, a component of the brain that has a significant role in processing negative and positive emotions.[38] The ventral tegmental area has neural connections to the forward part of the brain, through the nucleus accumbens.[39] Activation of the dopaminergic neurons located in the ventral tegmental area leads to increased release of dopamine in the nucleus accumbens. Importantly, these neurons are activated when an individual anticipates a reward such as any cue (e.g., seeing the actual substance) or consumption of the substance.[40] The medial prefrontal cortex functions as a final relay station in the mesolimbic system,[41] mediating the primary rewarding effects of reinforcing stimuli including drugs of abuse.[42] The mesolimbic dopamine system is where particular psychoactive substances have their primary impact (**Figure 6-10**).[43]

Dopamine is critical for the development of reward and motivation behaviors when individuals initiate substance use. Exposure to a substance releases dopamine and triggers a cascade of stimuli-response within the mesolimbic dopamine system. This initial flood of dopamine is associated with the subjective experience of pleasure; repeated exposure and subsequent flooding of dopamine leads to remodeling of the brain reward pathways. These morphologic changes are translated into the neurobiologic encoding of memories; these memories can be triggered by the substance itself or visual, auditory, or kinesthetic cues. The speed with which a psychoactive substance enters and leaves the brain is crucial for understanding its reinforcing effects. Pharmacokinetic studies show that peak levels in the human brain are reached within 10 minutes after intravenous administration, a fast uptake that is associated with intense euphoria.[9] The faster the uptake, the stronger the pleasure and the greater the reinforcing effects.[44]

Figure 6-10 Psychoactive substances and the mesolimbic dopamine system.

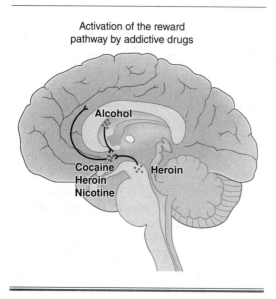

Activation of the reward
pathway by addictive drugs

Alcohol

Cocaine   Heroin
Heroin
Nicotine

Reproduced from National Institute for Drug Abuse. The neurobiology of drug addiction. Available at: http://www .drugabuse.gov/publications/teaching-packets/neurobiology -drug-addiction/section-iv-action-cocaine/7-summary -addictive-drugs-activate-reward. January 2007. Accessed March 15, 2016.

This response suggests a corresponding rapid increase in dopamine levels.

The transition from at-risk use to dependence is accompanied by physical characteristics such as craving, reduced ability to suppress drug seeking, and relapse. This transition occurs because there are cellular adaptations with repeated use of psychoactive substances, inducing reorganization in the circuitry of the brain. The pathophysiologic plasticity reduces the capacity of the prefrontal cortex to provide executive control for individuals when psychoactive substances are available.[45] These anatomic changes help explain the excessive motivational importance individuals place on seeking and using substances even in the face of serious adverse consequences. The temporal

progression of substance use leads to increased vulnerability to relapse. Changes in protein content or function often become greater with increasing periods of withdrawal from substances. For example, repeated alcohol exposures and withdrawals are capable of producing a persistent change in the CNS. In these vulnerable individuals, only a short period of drinking is necessary before tolerance develops and the effects of withdrawal become severe.[46]

While dopamine has a dominant role in the stimulus-response activation associated with substance use, other major neurotransmitter systems are impacted by substances. Inputs from the major inhibitory neurotransmitter gamma-aminobutyric acid (GABA) and the major excitatory neurotransmitter glutamate serve to balance excitation and inhibition in the CNS. In addition to the dopamine circuitry, these two neural circuits have a significant role in mediating the activation of goal-directed behavior related to psychoactive substance use.[45] These neurotransmitter receptors and transporters involved in the processes of drug reward and neuroplasticity have particular relevance for pharmacologic treatments, discussed later in this chapter.

Genetics and Epigenetics

There is a strong genetic component underlying the risk for developing SUDs. Heritability estimates for addiction from twin and adoption studies are approximately 30–60%.[47] It is likely that a vast number of genes operate through their influence either directly or indirectly on brain development, relevant neurotransmitter systems, drug metabolic pathways, neural circuitry, cellular physiology, behavioral patterns, the responses to the environmental stimuli, and an individual's personality traits.[48] An important discovery was that the expression of either high or low levels of particular dopamine receptors (D2) in the striatum predicted that controls (individuals with no psychoactive drug abuse) found the experience of a psychoactive drug aversive or pleasurable, respectively.[49] A paucity of dopamine receptors predisposed individuals to seek any substance that stimulates the dopaminergic system.[50] A test is under development to find the genetic antecedents of addiction. The genetic panel is based on science related to the discovery of alleles that impact the mesocorticolimbic system, including dopamine receptor genes, dopamine transporter genes, catechol-O-methyltransferase (COMT), serotonin transporter genes, mu opiate genes, monoamine oxidase-A, and GABA beta subunit genes.[50]

Chronic exposure to substances of abuse can alter gene expression in the ventral tegmental area, nucleus accumbens, and prefrontal cortex.[51] This dynamic process of epigenetics can induce stable and lasting changes in gene expression. The epigenetic regulation of genes related to addiction may underlie the lasting changes in neuronal and behavioral adaptations.[52] These changes and adaptations suggest that epigenetics is useful for understanding the processes that contribute to the chronic and relapsing nature of SUDs.

Application to Practice

Once introduced into the brain, substances have a powerful impact on the brain reward system. Repeated use of substances induces reorganization in the circuitry of the brain, resulting in behaviors that are characteristic of the brain being hijacked by the substance. By approaching patients with SUDs in the same objective manner as patients with biologically based chronic medical disorders, providers can provide objective and sensitive holistic care. Evidence-based patient education on the neurobiologic bases of substance use is a critical step toward treatment and recovery for this population.

Women-Specific Issues

There are gender-specific issues related to exposure to psychoactive substances. These include differences in physiology and adverse outcomes. In addition, there are special issues for women across the lifespan, particularly for women of childbearing age and women over the age of 65.

Women-Specific Physiology and Exposure to Psychoactive Substances

The basic neural systems discussed previously are similar in males and females. However, sex differences are present in how the neural systems are organized, activated, and connected with the rest of the brain.[53] Rodent models have been largely used to examine the effects of ovarian hormones on various parameters of psychoactive substance use. The neuroendocrine mechanisms across all phases of psychoactive substance use, from initiation to escalation of use, dependence, and relapse following abstinence are affected by ovarian hormone levels. These hormones impact dopamine neurotransmission in the nucleus accumbens. In turn, this results in an increase in dopamine production and a subsequent increase in the rewarding and psychomotor potency of psychoactive substances.[54] There is a dynamic fluctuation of estradiol and progesterone across an individual's cycle, day to day, month to month, year to year. These changing integrated fluctuations add further complexity in understanding the impact of psychoactive substance use beyond its pharmacokinetics and the amount, frequency, and duration of use.

Women have less total body water than men of comparable size. This biologic difference accounts for the higher blood-alcohol concentrations (BACs) for women after consuming equivalent amounts of alcohol as men.[55] Thus, "dose" adjustments for women are indicated. Another contributing factor for establishing standard alcohol limits for women relates to the metabolism of alcohol in the stomach and intestine, known as "first pass." Compared with men, women have lower levels or less activity of gastric alcohol dehydrogenase, so they metabolize less ethanol during this first pass.[55] There is conflicting evidence on rates of women's alcohol metabolism in the liver or elimination from the body.[55]

Addressing psychoactive substance use among women is critically important given their unique physiology, particularly related to sex hormones, proportionately less body water than men, and "first pass" metabolism rates. Additional evidence for concern is garnered from findings on gender differences in the general population and among treatment-seeking samples. The trajectory from initial substance use to dependence has been described as a downward spiral.[56] A "telescoping effect" has been described in which, compared with men, women have a more rapid progression to substance dependence. This course is characterized by an early onset of health and psychosocial consequences. This escalating effect of alcohol on women was described in the 1950s by Lisansky[57] and expanded more recently related to affirm this phenomenon for alcohol.[58] Similar patterns have been identified in women with opioid and cannabis dependence[59] and cocaine dependence.[58]

Adverse Health Consequences

Both men and women experience the emotional and physical consequences of alcohol and drugs on the human body. The negative health effects are wide ranging and include liver problems related to alcohol consumption, respiratory and lung cancer as a consequence of smoking, infections (e.g., HIV and hepatitis) acquired via injection of drugs or risky sexual practices, and memory/cognitive difficulties associated with marijuana use.[60] However, women have a greater susceptibility to health-related issues, because there is a shorter amount of time between the initial use and the development of physiologic problems

among women.[60] As such, clinicians need to be cognizant of this "telescoping effect" in women who are consuming alcohol and/or other drugs.

Additionally, women may present with associated gynecologic consequences. For example, substance use affects women's menstrual cycles, inducing increased cramping and heavier or lighter periods.[58] Women may use substances to alleviate discomforts associated with the ovarian cycle. Women may also experience amenorrhea, such as with opiate use or when taking methadone or other medications that induce the absence of menstrual cycles. Therefore, women of childbearing age may believe they are unable to conceive, and, if they become pregnant, they may be unaware that they are risking the health of the fetus. The information provided in **Table 6-2** can be used to educate women about the negative effects of various substances.

Women of Reproductive Age

Psychoactive substance use during pregnancy impacts the maternal-fetal dyad. Attending to substance use among women of reproductive age who are intending to become pregnant or are pregnant or those engaged in risky sexual activity is critically important given the negative immediate and long-term consequences for women and exposed children. Nearly all drugs that are consumed during pregnancy will enter, to some degree, the circulation of the fetus via passive diffusion across the placenta.[61] The direct effect of a psychoactive substance (and any drug) is dependent on the concentration of that drug in fetal circulation. At a time when women may be unaware of a pregnancy, use of substances in any amount can extend beyond risk to themselves to their unborn child. This timing is of concern because the major organs and the neurologic system of the human embryo develop in the first 2 months. **Table 6-3** lists some of the risks to the woman and to the fetus as a consequence of various psychoactive

Table 6-2 Physiologic Consequences Associated with Psychoactive Substance Use

Body System/Organ	Impact	Psychoactive Substance
Liver	Higher likelihood to develop alcoholic hepatitis and die from cirrhosis	Alcohol
	Increased risk of cancer of liver	Tobacco
Cardiovascular/Vascular	More likely to die prematurely from cardiac-related problems	Alcohol
	For ages 30 to 64 years, increased risk of hypertension with heavy consumption (15–21 units; 1 unit of alcohol is equivalent to half a pint of beer, 1 glass of wine, or 1 standard measure of spirits)	Alcohol
	Increased risk for ischemic stroke, subarachnoid hemorrhage, peripheral vascular atherosclerosis, abdominal aortic aneurysm rupture	Tobacco
	Heightened risk of chronic obstructive pulmonary disease and coronary heart disease	Tobacco
Respiratory	Heightened risk of pulmonary tuberculosis	Cocaine Heroin
	Heightened risk of recurrent pneumonia	Cocaine Heroin
	Increased risk of cancer of lung	Tobacco
	Premature decline in lung function	Tobacco
Gastrointestinal/ Urinary	Increased risk of peptic ulcers	Tobacco
	Increased risk of Crohn's disease	Tobacco
	Increased risk of cancer of esophagus, colon, bladder, kidney	Tobacco
Reproductive	Infertility	Alcohol (heavy drinking) Tobacco
	Painful and/or irregular menstruation	Alcohol Tobacco
	Risk for cancer of cervix	Alcohol Tobacco
	Risk for cancer of vagina	Alcohol
	Amenorrhea or irregular menstrual cycle	Heroin Tobacco Marijuana
	Increased risk of estrogen deficiency	Tobacco
	Younger onset of menopause	Tobacco

(continues)

Table 6-2 Physiologic Consequences Associated with Psychoactive Substance Use *(continued)*

Body System/Organ	Impact	Psychoactive Substance
Breast	Increased risk of breast cancer	Alcohol
Bone	Decreased bone density; increased risk for osteoporosis	Alcohol Tobacco
	Increased risk for hip fracture after menopause	Tobacco
Neurological/Brain	Declines in cognitive and motor function	Alcohol
	Deterioration in planning, visuospatial ability, working memory, psychomotor speed	Alcohol
	Significantly smaller volumes of gray and white matter, less hippocampal volume	Alcohol
	Peripheral neuropathy	Alcohol
	Appetite suppression	Methamphetamine
	Diminished sexual desire and performance	Heroin
Oral-facial	Jaw clenching (acute adverse effect)	Methamphetamine
	Dry mouth	Methamphetamine
	Increased risk of cancer of larynx	Tobacco

Note: Risks are in comparison to males with psychoactive substance use and/or healthy controls.

Reproduced from Hernandez-Avila CA, Rounsaville BJ, Kranzler HR. Opioid-, cannabis- and alcohol-dependent women show more rapid progression to substance abuse treatment. *Drug Alcohol Depend.* 2004;74(3):265-272. Copyright 2004 with permission from Elsevier.

substances, including tobacco, marijuana, alcohol, cocaine, and opioids.[62-64]

Older Women

Substance use in older women is associated with increased risk for adverse outcomes due to physiologic changes associated with aging. These risks are associated with changes in body mass water ratio, cognitive functioning, and increased physical frailty. Nutritional status also plays a role. In addition, sex differences exist among older adults, with women at increased vulnerability to the adverse effects of substances on the brain.[65]

ALCOHOL, AGE, AND NUTRITION

Acute and chronic alcohol ingestion may lead to a reduction of micronutrient absorption and manifest as deficiencies in thiamine, nicotinic acids, B vitamins, and folate.[66] Substance use of any type is associated with poorer quality dietary intake. For example, women who consume alcohol at higher levels may not only fail to eat thiamine-rich foods but may also be unable to adequately metabolize it due to alcohol's effect over time on the ability to absorb thiamine in the gastrointestinal tract and to metabolize thiamine at the cellular level. Thiamine deficiency facilitates excessive glutamate release, leading to neuronal damage resulting in

Table 6-3 Psychoactive Substance Use: Reproductive Risks to Childbearing Age/Pregnant Woman and Fetus

Psychoactive Substance	Adverse Risk to Woman	Adverse Risk to Fetus/Neonate
Tobacco	• Ectopic pregnancy • Premature rupture of membranes • Placental abruption • Placenta previa	• Stillbirth • Intrauterine growth restriction • Low birth weight • Birth defects (e.g., cleft lip or palate) • Sudden infant death syndrome • Developmental disorders (e.g., cerebral palsy, learning disabilities)
Marijuana	• Suppresses or increases serum luteinizing hormone levels in menstrual stage-specific manner	• Intrauterine restriction • Preterm birth • Developmental deficits into childhood • Predisposition to future substance use problems/disorders
Alcohol		• Intrauterine growth restriction • Brain damage • Skeletal malformations • Facial abnormalities • Preterm birth • Low birth weight • Vision problems • Hearing problems • Defects of the major organs • Failure to thrive
Cocaine	• Placental abruption • Premature rupture of membranes • Migraines • Seizures	• Preterm birth • Low birth weight • Intrauterine growth restriction • Small head circumference
Opioids	• Spontaneous abortion • Preeclampsia • Placental insufficiency • Abruptio placentae • Premature rupture of membranes • Chorioamnionitis • Postpartum hemorrhage • Septic thrombophlebitis	• Low birth weight • Small for gestational age • Intrauterine growth retardation • Congenital abnormalities (e.g., congenital heart disease) • Intrauterine passage of meconium • Intrauterine death • Low Apgar scores • Premature birth • Neonatal abstinence syndrome (with dysfunction in the nervous system, respiratory system, gastrointestinal system, and other regulatory systems)

Data from Kaltenbach K, Berghella V, Finnegan L. Opioid dependence during pregnancy: effects and management. *Obstet Gynecol Clin North Am*. 1998;25(1):139-151; Wang H, De SK, Maccarrone M. Jekyll and Hyde: two faces of cannabinoid signaling in male and female fertility. *Endocr Rev*. 2006;27(5):427-448; Wendell AD. Overview and epidemiology of substance abuse in pregnancy. *Clin Obstet Gynecol*. 2013;56(1):91–6.

conditions such as Wernicke-Korsakoff syndrome and Marchiafava-Bignami disease.[66,67]

The ability to metabolize substances is also affected by body composition. Compared with younger adults, older adults, especially older women, have less lean body mass and less body water. This mass-to-water ratio provides the rationale for alcohol consumption limits for healthy women and men over age 65 (i.e., no more than 3 standard drinks per occasion *and* no more than 7 standard drinks in 1 week).[6] Note that this recommendation specifies *healthy* older adults.

Substance Use and Comorbidity

Not only do the normal physiologic changes associated with aging make substance use riskier for older adults, but many older individuals are also more likely to have underlying medical conditions. Alcohol consumption among older adults increases the risk for cardiovascular disease; liver, pancreatic, and gastrointestinal diseases; cancer; pulmonary infections; decreased immune response; injury; and direct and indirect negative effects on the CNS.[66-68]

Older women with medical disorders who are on complex medication regimens are at even greater risk and thus should be consuming alcohol at lower levels or not at all. Older women are also more likely to experience a greater severity of pain and are more apt to have a psychiatric disorder. These factors put them at higher risk for being placed on medications that should not be used in conjunction with alcohol.[69] The interaction of age-related physiologic changes and poorer underlying health increases the chance that psychoactive substances, including some prescription medications, can trigger or exacerbate conditions such as hypertension, cardiac arrhythmia, myocardial infarction, cardiomyopathy, hemorrhagic stroke, malnutrition, or gastrointestinal bleeding; impair the immune system and reduce the capability to combat infection and cancer; lead to the development of cirrhosis and other liver diseases; and decrease bone density. Psychoactive substances can also worsen depression, anxiety, and other mental health problems.[68]

Social Implications— Gender Bias

Societal norms about substance use are changing as evidenced by the way that women are portrayed in advertisements for alcohol and tobacco. There also appears to be a cultural shift in that young women (12–20 years of age) are beginning to use substances at rates that are close to or in some cases higher than their male counterparts. These changes in societal norms pose significant challenges for women.

Advertising

In the 1970s, advertising of alcohol beverages shifted from depicting couples to a more masculine-focused approach that objectified women. With this shift came an increase in ads where women were depicted as "'admiring on-lookers' or as objects of sexual desire."[70(p393)] Thus, according to Towns, Parker, and Chase, advertisements that are aimed at male consumers of alcohol depict women's bodies as objects to be consumed; these ads are potentially dangerous due to the link between at-risk alcohol use and domestic violence.[70] One has only to search on the Internet for images of alcohol advertising and women to see multiple examples directed at men that depict women in provocative poses. There are also ads that target women presenting a before-and-after approach with the after picture presenting a sexually desirable woman, suggesting that women who drink will become more sexually desirable.[71] There is even an ad for "non-alcoholic" beer that depicts a woman exposing her pregnant belly with a glass of beer in her hand.

Researchers have examined the level of exposure to alcohol and cigarette advertising based on gender and age. In one study related to alcohol advertising in the Boston subway system, exposure to advertising promoting alcohol use was pervasive. On average, adults using the subway system were exposed to alcohol-related advertising slightly more than once a day. Every 5th to 12th grader using the subway system had even greater exposure, seeing on average 1.3 ads per day. Advertising was more extensive in higher-income areas; individuals, even adolescents, residing in these areas are more likely to have the means to pay for alcohol.[72] The tobacco industry reinforces the link between alcohol and tobacco use by depicting the concurrent use of alcohol and smoking in advertising.[73] In the 1970s the tobacco industry also purposefully targeted women through the creation of brands specifically for women such as Virginia Slims and tying the use of tobacco to women's liberation.

Adolescents are a frequent target of ads related to alcohol use;[71,74,75] magazines with higher adolescent readership tend to have more alcohol-related ads than those directed to adult readers.[76] Higher exposure to alcohol-related advertising is predictive of greater alcohol use in girls.[73] Minimizing adolescent exposure to alcohol and tobacco ads can be achieved through policy changes.[77] For example, the city of Philadelphia recently passed a law to ban alcohol advertisements on all city-owned property, including public bus shelters. Because most of the public school students are transported through the city bus system, this reduced student exposure.

Current advertising campaigns continue to depict women as objects of desire. Sex sells. Unfortunately, too few alternative views of women are available in the mass media. Counterbalancing how women are portrayed in alcohol and tobacco ads is challenging. One approach has been to use public service announcements (PSAs) including podcasts, videos, and posters. Posters with healthy alternative messaging are often located in the same areas that advertisements are placed such as buses, subways, and billboards. They are often also posted in doctors' offices, especially those that provide care to women.

Stigma

Traditionally, the use of substances by women has carried a certain stigma.[78] Where alcohol use by men might be acceptable as evidence of masculinity and even perceived as being humorous (e.g., *The Hangover* movies), women who consume alcohol the same way are considered loose and not feminine. In some states, women who use substances during pregnancy are subject to criminal prosecution. Fifteen states view substance abuse during pregnancy as child abuse, and three allow for involuntary commitment for behavioral health treatment.[79] Women who are diagnosed with SUDs are labeled "addicts" in contrast to women who have breast cancer for whom the only label used is "survivor." The SUD becomes the defining aspect of the person rather than remaining what it is—a treatable disorder.

Stigma directly impacts the ability of women to receive treatment; it results in women not seeking treatment and in healthcare providers being reluctant to provide it. Healthcare providers may have less empathy for those with SUDs than those with other chronic illnesses.[80,81] Stigma has also resulted in pharmaceutical companies engaging in less research and development on new therapies directed at the treatment of SUDs.[80,81] Because society "blames" the patient for the SUD, this can result in expressions of anger toward the substance user, withholding of help, avoidance, and implementation of coercive strategies, such as the mandatory SUD treatment required for pregnant women in three states.[78-80] Addressing stigma associated with at-risk use of psychoactive substances is critical to the building of effective interventions for women engaged in at-risk substance use.

Cultural Shift

The WHO report on alcohol demonstrates that a paradigm shift has occurred in the field of substance use. Substance use interventions now encompass prevention and early identification of at-risk alcohol and drug use rather than focusing solely on treatment of SUDs.[2,13] As the focus shifts to this broader view of substance use and its impact on health, healthcare providers will require knowledge and skills related to the full spectrum of the impact psychoactive substances have on health and how to prevent, identify, and intervene in a way that will reduce morbidity and mortality. Following this approach requires incorporating an upstream approach to intervention and includes skills related to screening, providing brief interventions (BIs), and referring to treatment when needed.

This shift is seen at a policy level in relation to tobacco use, with much of public health efforts aimed at prevention of tobacco use rather than treatment. Smoking in most public areas in the United States is no longer acceptable legally or socially. This is in stark contrast to the social acceptability of smoking in the 1950s and 1960s. There is also attention to reducing substance use in adolescents, especially the gateway substances of tobacco, marijuana, and alcohol. The parallel effort to legalize marijuana for treatment of pain may actually negatively impact the effort to reduce the use of marijuana for recreational purposes. However, the overall trend is to view substance use across the continuum of use and the lifespan and to reduce the harm associated with substance use.

Prevention Models

The emphasis today is prevention of harm associated with the use of substances as evidenced by the WHO 2014 report on alcohol.[13] Much of the harm associated with substance use occurs without the presence of an SUD. In women this is particularly important. For example, alcohol is associated with increased risk for injury and violence. Women who may have no individual risk may experience harm from others who are engaging in at-risk alcohol use that contributes to an increased risk of domestic violence or being involved in motor vehicle crashes.[82,83] Even moderate levels of alcohol consumption increase the risk of breast cancer.[84] Because risk occurs across the continuum, prevention efforts are not confined to identifying those with an SUD and providing treatment, but rather extend across the continuum of use.[84]

The Institute of Medicine Prevention Model

The Institute of Medicine recognized a need to develop a model of prevention for behavioral health that encompassed the entire continuum of use.[85] This model separated prevention from treatment and focused on target populations defined by risk for developing an SUD. There are three levels of prevention: 1) universal, 2) selective, and 3) indicated.

Universal Level of Prevention

The universal level targets the entire population regardless of risk. For example, the use of public service announcements aimed at informing women of the dangers of using alcohol during pregnancy targets all pregnant women regardless of whether they consume alcohol or not. These types of interventions focus on communicating to the general population the adverse health outcomes associated with the use of alcohol, tobacco, and other drugs. These interventions promote appropriate decision making and the development of social skills that help individuals, families, and communities to make healthy decisions regarding the use of substances.

SELECTIVE LEVEL OF PREVENTION

At the selective level of prevention, the goal is to provide interventions tailored to subgroups within a population that are at greater risk for harm based on biologic, psychologic, social, or environmental factors. A program at the local middle school to decrease early initiation of illicit drug use among adolescent girls, offered to girls with a history of truancy and poor grades, is an example of a selective prevention program. Participation in the program is not contingent on current use of alcohol, tobacco, or other drugs. Instead, members of the middle school population with risk factors associated with illicit drug use are asked to participate. The benefit of a selective prevention approach is that the intervention can be tailored to the specific characteristics of the identified at-risk group. For female populations, providing a selective prevention approach allows for taking into account issues such as age, gender, reproductive status, and the availability of drugs in their communities.

INDICATED LEVEL OF PREVENTION

At the indicated level of prevention, interventions target subgroups of the population who are at highest risk for development of SUDs, or who may be in the early stages of an SUD. Examples of indicated interventions include education programs such as driving under the influence education classes or the delivery of a BI (see information later in the chapter). The purpose of these interventions is to help the early user understand the possible consequences of their at-risk substance use, identify those with signs or symptoms of an SUD, and assist them in returning to no/low-risk use.

Harm Reduction Model

Globally, substance use prevention is presented within a harm reduction model. According to the San Francisco Department of Public Health,

Harm reduction is a public health philosophy, which promotes methods of reducing the physical, social, emotional, and economic harms associated with drug and alcohol use and other harmful behaviors on individuals and their community. Harm reduction methods and treatment goals are free of judgment or blame and directly involve the client in setting their own goals.[86]

This approach is congruent with the continuum of use and the fact that harm occurs even when a person does not have an SUD. It also aligns with the *Healthy People 2020* goals related to substance abuse.[87] From a public health perspective, harm reduction aims to reduce the harm for the community and the individual rather than focusing solely on achieving sobriety in individuals. This allows healthcare providers to assist those who may not be willing to stop engaging in at-risk substance use to begin to reduce the harm associated with the use. The underlying assumption of this model is that interventions associated with substance use are free of judgment or blame.[88]

Screening and Assessment

Screening for substance use is an essential component of assessment. Screening in this context is defined as using a tool to identify those who probably are engaged in at-risk substance use and those with a probable SUD. Early identification of problematic substance use is an essential first step in preventing harm associated with substance use. Identifying at-risk use provides the clinician with the means to intervene and prevent or reduce the harm related to substance use.

There are challenges when screening for at-risk substance use in women. Many screening tools were developed to help identify those who may have an SUD and consequently fail to identify those who are engaged in risky use but do not yet meet the criteria for an SUD. Many screening instruments do not routinely include items on consumption—specifically, quantity, frequency, duration, and/or pattern of substance use. This issue is especially important for women in their childbearing years, because substance use at any level has the potential to place a fetus at risk. Even screening tools specifically designed for pregnant women, such as the T-ACE, do not specifically ask about level and patterns of consumption.

Many screening tools have high validity and reliability in detecting SUDs (**Table 6-4**). When choosing a screening tool, it is important to select one that will detect the specific substance of concern. It is also important to determine how much time is available for the screening and what will be done with the results. If a patient screens positive for at-risk substance use, then further assessment is needed to determine if the woman may have an SUD. Those who screen positive should receive a BI appropriate to the level of risk (see Table 6-4) and if warranted a referral to treatment.

Screening for At-Risk Alcohol Use

Single screening questions are recommended for the evaluation of unhealthy alcohol use and other drug use. For example, a single-question tool for alcohol screening that is gender and age specific is, "How many times in the past year have you had 5 (men) or 4 (women and individuals over age 65) drinks or more in a day?" This question has a sensitivity of 82% and specificity of 79%.[89] In asking this question, it is essential to provide information about what is meant by "a drink" (see Figure 6-2). A response of one or more times triggers the need for further screening to ascertain frequency, quantity, and binge drinking over the past year.

The Alcohol Use Disorders Identification Test—Consumption (AUDIT-C)[0] is a psychometrically sound measure useful in identifying at-risk alcohol use.[90] Patients can fill out this three-question written instrument prior

to seeing the clinician, or the clinician can verbally administer it as part of the interview process. The first question addresses frequency (How often do you have a drink containing alcohol?), the second addresses quantity (How many drinks containing alcohol do you have on a typical day when you are drinking?), and the third question addresses binge drinking (How often do you have six or more drinks on one occasion?). There are five responses for each item with corresponding scores ranging from 0 to 4. A total score > 3 for women or men and women over age 65 years and > 4 for men reflects a positive screen. A score > 8 is suggestive of alcohol dependence.

A positive screen means that a more complete picture of the drinking pattern is needed. This entails asking, "On average, how many days a week do you have an alcoholic drink?" and, "On a typical day when you are drinking, how many [standard] drinks do you have?"[5] A total score is calculated by multiplying the two responses to determine the weekly average. The maximum limit for healthy women and healthy men over age 65 is no more than 3 drinks in a day *and* no more than 7 drinks in a week. For healthy men up to age 65, the maximum limit is no more than 4 drinks in a day *and* no more than 14 drinks in a week.[7] For example, a healthy woman who reports drinking 3 beers every day is within the daily limit but exceeding the weekly limit by having 21 beers per week. A healthy woman who reports drinking 3 beers on Friday night and 1 glass of wine on Saturday and Sunday has no more than 3 drinks in a day *and* no more than 5 drinks in a week. It is important to note that these maximum limits are for healthy men and women. Lower intake or abstinence is recommended for individuals who are taking medications that interact with alcohol or who have a health condition that is exacerbated by alcohol. Abstinence is recommended for women who are pregnant or considering becoming pregnant.

Table 6-4 Substance Use Screening Tools

Screening Tools	Gender Specific	ETOH and/or Drugs	Frequency	Pattern	Quantity	Psychosocial	Physical	# items
CAGE-C	No	ETOH	Yes	Yes	Yes	Yes	Yes	7
AUDIT	No	ETOH	Yes	Yes	Yes	Yes	Yes	10
AUDIT C	No	ETOH	Yes	Yes	Yes	No	No	3
CAGE	No	ETOH	No	No	No	Yes	Yes	4
NIAAA Single Question	No	ETOH	No	Yes	No	No	No	1
CRAFFT	No/adolescents	ETOH Drugs	No	No	No	Yes	Yes	7
TWEAK	Yes	ETOH	No	No	No	Yes	Yes	5
T-ACE	Yes/pregnant	ETOH	No	No	No	Yes	Yes	4
NIDA Quick Screen	No	ETOH Drugs Tobacco Nonmedical use	No	Yes	No	No	No	4
NIDA Modified ASSIST	No	ETOH Drugs Tobacco Nonmedical use	Yes	Yes	No	Yes	Yes	7
DAST	No	Drugs Nonmedical use	No	No	No	Yes	Yes	10

Data from National Institute on Drug Abuse. Chart of evidence-based screening tools for adults and adolescents. http://www.drugabuse.gov/nidamed-medical-health-professionals/tool-resources-your-practice/screening-assessment/screening-assessment-drug-testing-resources/additional-tools-screening-assessment-drug. September 2015. Accessed April 14, 2016; National Institute on Alcohol Abuse and Alcoholism. Screening tests. http://pubs.niaaa.nih.gov/publications/arh28-2/78–79.htm. n.d. Accessed April 14, 2016.

Screening for Drug Use Including Nonmedical Use of Prescription Medication

A single-question screen has also been established for drug use: "How many times in the past year have you used an illegal drug or used a prescription medication for nonmedical reasons?" This question has a sensitivity of 100% and specificity of 74%.[1] A response of 1 or more on this screening question triggers the need for further screening. The Drug Abuse Screening Test includes 10 items corresponding to problems related to drug misuse.[92] A total score is calculated based on yes (1 point) or no (0 points) responses. Scores of 1 to 2 indicate a low level, 3 to 5 a moderate level, and 6 to 8 a substantial level of problems.

Screening for Tobacco Use

The US Preventive Services Task Force (USPSTF) recommends that healthcare providers screen all patients for tobacco use, including current and past use.[93] Those who are currently using tobacco should be provided with information to assist with cessation. Asking about past use helps the clinician to identify those at increased risk for tobacco-related diseases.[93] To classify tobacco use, the woman should be asked if she currently uses tobacco products (cigarettes, cigars, or smokeless tobacco), and if so, the intensity of use (e.g., number of packs per day, number of cigars, number of dips). For those with previous use, the quit date should be determined.

Screening for Substance Use During Pregnancy

Screening for substance use during pregnancy involves two patients, the mother and child. Detection of any fetal exposure is important to help determine if the neonate will need to be screened

Figure 6-11 Screening for substance use during pregnancy.

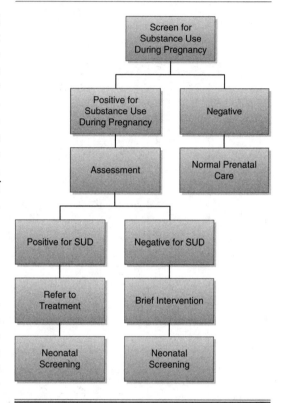

at birth. Any evidence of fetal exposure should trigger at minimum a BI (see section on BIs) and further assessment of the mother for a possible SUD and referral to treatment (**Figure 6-11**).

The Use of Biomarkers and Toxicology to Screen for Substance Use

Biomarkers are sometimes used to screen for substance use. If an alcohol use disorder is suspected or present, liver function tests may be helpful in detecting and monitoring the extent of the damage that alcohol use has had on the liver. Liver function tests, specifically the GGT (γ-glutamyl transpeptidase), aspartate aminotransferase (AST) and alanine aminotransferase (ALT) tests, are markers of tissue damage.[94] GGT is the most specific indicator of alcohol abuse. Other tests that should be considered when there is a concern about at-risk alcohol use are triglycerides and high-density lipoprotein (values are elevated with moderate levels of alcohol intake), complete blood count, renal function tests, and a complete lipid panel. However, these tests can be elevated in other diseases; therefore, abnormal results cannot be assumed to be due to substance use. Biomarkers have also been studied for their utility in detecting alcohol use during pregnancy. Though no single biologic marker for alcohol use has been found to have sufficient sensitivity and specificity, promising research is being conducted on both urine and blood biomarkers that could have utility to help detect alcohol use in the pregnant mother.[94,95]

Urine drug screens are the most common method for drug testing because of their ease for analysis. A typical drug panel screens for amphetamines, cocaine, opiates, PCP, and tetrahydrocannabinol (THC) and will detect drugs used within the last 24 to 48 hours depending on the half-life of the drug.[96] These five drugs have standardized cutoff values for positive and negative tests based on federal guidelines for employee testing programs. Other drugs may be added to this panel but are less likely to have standardized normative values, so the results must be interpreted with caution. Blood screens are also available and can test for a wider range of substances. Other tests can detect drug levels in saliva, sweat, or hair, but these tests are offered by only a few laboratories and are not commonly used. **Box 6-5** demonstrates persistence of positive results for various substances on toxicology screens.

Box 6-5 Persistence of Positive Results for Common Toxicology Screens

Alcohol: 3–10 hours

Amphetamines: 24–48 hours

Barbiturates: up to 6 weeks

Benzodiazepines: up to 6 weeks with high level of use

Cocaine: 2–4 days; up to 10–22 days with heavy use

Codeine: 1–2 days

Heroin: 1–2 days

Hydromorphone: 1–2 days

Methadone: 2–3 days

Morphine: 1–2 days

Phencyclidine (PCP): 1–8 days

Propoxyphene: 6–48 hours

Tetrahydrocannabinol (THC): 6–11 weeks with heavy use

Reproduced from U.S. National Library of Medicine. Toxicology screen. Medline Plus. http://www.nlm.nih.gov/medlineplus/ency/article/003578.htm. July 7, 2016. Accessed March 15, 2016.

Physical Assessment

Physiologic changes seen on the physical exam can vary depending on the substance or substances being used by an individual. The physical examination should include observations of the general appearance and behavior followed by a systematic head-to-toe assessment.

Minor impairment of judgment can occur with a BAC of 0.02–0.04% and lowering of inhibitions and impairment of reasoning and memory at 0.05–0.07%. Impairment in balance, speech, vision, reaction time, and hearing, as well as impairment of judgment and self-control correspond with a BAC of 0.08%–0.10%.

Heightened deep tendon reflexes and ankle clonus are indicative of profound CNS irritability that may be related to CNS depressant withdrawal. Other signs of CNS depressant withdrawal include significant increases or decreases in blood pressure and heart rate, increased body temperature, changes in mental status, presence of hallucinations, abdominal pain, and changes in responsiveness of pupils. The Clinical Institute Withdrawal Assessment, revised (CIWA-Ar) is a validated objective scale consisting of 10 items that measure withdrawal severity.[97] These 10 areas include agitation, anxiety, auditory disturbance, clouding of sensorium, headache, nausea/vomiting, paroxysmal sweating, tactile disturbances, tremor, and visual disturbances. The CIWA-Ar takes about 5 minutes to administer and is used to guide symptom-triggered pharmacologic management. The sum of all 10 areas provides a total score. Some nausea, anxiety, and headache reflect a score of 8 to 10 (mild), with higher scores reflecting moderate severity (10 to 15), and scores greater than 15 indicating marked autonomic activity, impending delirium tremens, and an urgency for pharmacologic treatment.

The intensity of opiate withdrawal is a function of the severity of physical dependence on opioids and the relative occupancy of the mu receptor.[98] The Clinical Opiate Withdrawal Scale (COWS) is an 11-item tool organized by symptoms including but not limited to pulse rate, sweating, tremors, and pupil size.[99] The COWS can be completed in about 2 minutes while talking with a patient and observing for opioid withdrawal signs. The sum of ratings for all 11 items provides a total score. Opiate withdrawal is not life threatening, but can be uncomfortable depending on the severity of symptoms. The COWS ratings range from 5 to 12 (mild), 13 to 24 (moderate), 25 to 36 (moderately severe), to greater than 36 (severe).

The severity and profile of stimulant withdrawal are related to dosage and duration of use. Typical withdrawal symptoms include disturbed sleep (hypersomnolence or insomnia), depressed mood, anxiety, agitation, reduced energy, and

vivid or unpleasant dreams. The hypothalamus-pituitary axis (HPA) activity is stimulated with use of these substances, adrenocorticotropin hormone (ACTH) and corticosteroid levels become elevated, and corticotropin-releasing factor (CRF) activity is increased; these physiologic changes explain the anxiogenic and stress-like symptoms accompanying withdrawal.[100] Thus, on physical assessment, elevations in systolic and diastolic blood pressure, heart rate, respiratory rate, and body temperature are expected. Individuals will exhibit increased motor activity, heightened alertness, and irritability, and they may report fatigue, depression, anxiety, poor concentration, paranoia, and hypersomnia or insomnia.[100] Physical examination findings that are suggestive of substance use or consequences are listed in **Table 6-5**.

Brief Interventions

A BI is a nonconfrontational, patient-centered approach that involves a conversation to raise awareness of alcohol-related consequences and motivate an individual toward behavior change.[101] A 5- to 15-minute BI can promote patients' understanding of the severity and extent of their substance use and motivate their behavior change.[102,103] The effectiveness of BI for alcohol consumption has informed the practice statement from the Committee on Health Care for Underserved Women of the American College of Obstetricians and Gynecologists.[104] A meta-analysis by Kaner and colleagues included 22 randomized controlled trials (RCTs) comparing BI treatment to control groups. This meta-analysis showed that participants receiving BI had lower alcohol consumption than the control group (mean difference: −38 grams/week, 95% confidence interval [CI]: −54 to −23) 1 year or more after the conclusion of the BI.[105] More recently, a systematic review of 24 systematic reviews, including 56 unique studies, focused on the impact of brief alcohol interventions in primary care.[106]

Table 6-5 Physical Examination Findings Suggestive of Substance Use or Consequences

System	Symptom
General	Odor: alcohol or tobacco on breath; marijuana or tobacco on clothing Poor nutritional status Poor personal hygiene
Mental Status Changes	Blackouts or periods of memory loss Nodding off, dozing, or falling asleep Agitation and/or delirium tremens Seizures Changes in levels of consciousness Visual or auditory hallucinations
Behavior	Intoxicated behavior during exam Slurred speech Staggering gait Scratching
Mood	Depressed, anxious, nervous, mood lability
Skin	Signs of physical injury Bruises Lacerations Scratches Burns Needle marks Skin abscesses Cellulitis Jaundice Palmar erythema Hair loss Diaphoresis Rash Puffy hands
Head, Eyes, Ears, Nose, Throat (HEENT)	Conjunctival irritation or injection Nystagmus—sedative/hypnotics, cannabis Mydriasis—stimulants, hallucinogens, or withdrawal from opiates Miosis—opioid use Inflamed nasal mucosa Perforated septum Rhinorrhea Dental caries, gingivitis
Cardiac	Murmurs Arrhythmias Chest pain Increased blood pressure
Abdominal	Diarrhea, constipation Hepatomegaly, splenomegaly, ascites

BIs were consistently effective in addressing hazardous and harmful alcohol use in primary care, particularly for middle-aged males, although the evidence for effectiveness in women was less clear.[106] The optimum length and intensity of BI are not well defined for women. In addition, the evidence on the effectiveness of BI for drug use has yet to be established.

Smoking cessation studies have compared physician brief advice or brief counseling with control or usual care. A meta-analysis by Stead and colleagues included 42 trials of more than 31,000 smokers, some of whom were at risk of specified diseases (chest disease, diabetes, ischemic heart disease), but most from unselected populations.[107] The most common setting for delivery of advice was primary care. Pooled data from 17 trials of brief advice versus no advice (or usual care) detected a significant increase in the rate of quitting (relative risk [RR] 1.66, 95% CI 1.42 to 1.94).[107] RCTs have been conducted to compare smoking cessation advice and/or counseling given by nurses with control or usual care. A meta-analysis pooling 35 RCTs reported that the intervention increased the likelihood of quitting (RR 1.29, 95% CI 1.20 to 1.39).[108]

A brief negotiated interview (BNI) provides a step-by-step guide for delivery of a BI. The BNI steps include raising the subject, providing feedback, enhancing motivation, and negotiating and advising.[109] **Table 6-6** provides information about the BNI steps and specific components. Examples are provided of scripts that can be used in the interview.

Referral to Treatment

Referral to treatment is indicated for individuals who are identified as having an SUD or are in need of specialty treatment. Healthcare providers need to be familiar with treatments that are accessible for their patients. The Substance Abuse and Mental Health Services Administration treatment locator, available on its website, can be used to find the closest services and treatment locations.[110] Most substance abuse treatment models have been developed for men and are based predominantly on male norms.[111] Merely changing a treatment program from mixed gender to women only does not necessarily affect treatment outcomes for women with SUDs.[112] Greenfield and colleagues reported that gender-specific treatment programming and interventions have been demonstrated to enhance treatment entry, retention, and outcomes among only certain subgroups of women.[112] However, additional research is needed to help design substance abuse treatment interventions that are effective for all women.

Supportive therapy is a beneficial approach for women with an SUD. Positive treatment outcomes for women are associated with variables related to the characteristics of the therapist, such as warmth, empathy, and the ability to stay connected during treatment crises.[60] Women also need a treatment environment that is supportive and safe with a therapeutic relationship that encompasses mutual respect, empathy, and compassion.[60]

Special programs have been developed for women who are at risk for alcohol-exposed pregnancies. One program, Project CHOICES (Changing High-Risk Alcohol Use and Increasing Contraception Effectiveness Study) was a model program promoted by the CDC.[113] Floyd and colleagues tested this model in an RCT of 830 nonpregnant women ages 18 to 44 at risk for alcohol-exposed pregnancy.[114] Participants were randomized to receive information plus a brief motivational intervention ($n = 416$) or to receive information only ($n = 414$). The brief motivational intervention consisted of four counseling sessions (employing motivational interviewing and cognitive behavioral strategies) and one contraception consultation and services visit. Across the follow-up period, the odds ratios (ORs) of

Table 6-6 Brief Negotiated Interview: Steps, Components, and Sample Script

Step	Components	Example
1. Raise the subject.	Establish rapport. Seek permission to introduce the subject. Present the subject in context of health risks.	*We address different health risks with our patients. Is it okay with you if we spend a few minutes talking about your use of [alcohol, tobacco, drugs]?*
2. Provide feedback.	Review results of screening. Summarize results. Compare/contrast with guidelines or recommendations. Make connections to risks and current health conditions.	*I'd like to review the results of the screening with you. Your responses to the questions show that you are at [no risk, low risk, moderate risk, high risk]. These are the recommendations for alcohol use (show graphic or communicate limits for drinking). No amount of drug use is safe. What connections do you see between your health condition/reason for health visit/ reason for admission and your drinking/drug use/nicotine use?*
3. Raise the subject.	Assess readiness to change behavior. Not Ready 1 2 3 4 5 6 7 8 9 10 Very Ready Develop discrepancy. Explore the good things [X] and the not-so-good things [Y] about the substance. Summarize.	*How ready are you on a scale of 1 to 10 to change your [alcohol, drug use, nicotine use] if 1 means not ready at all and 10 means very ready?* *So, you said a [repeat number]. Why that and not a [identify a number that is 2 or 3 lower than the number selected]?* *So, what would it take for you to get to a [identify a number that is 2 or 3 higher than the number selected]?* *Can you tell me some of the good things about [alcohol, drug use, nicotine use] for you? What are some of the not-so-good things?* *So, on the one hand you said [X] and on the other you said [Y]. So, where does that leave you?"*
4. Negotiate and advise.	Negotiate a goal: • Start with patient's ideas. • Help generate menu of options. • Encourage specificity. • Reiterate advice. Summarize. Arrange follow up. Thank patient.	*What do you see as the next step?* *What do you think will work for you?* *So, let me see if I can summarize the plan. [Provide summary.] Do I have that right?* *I'd like to schedule a follow-up appointment in [X time].*

being at reduced risk for alcohol-exposed pregnancy were twofold greater in the intervention group: 3 months, 2.31 (95% CI = 1.69–3.20); 6 months, 2.15 (CI = 1.52–3.06); 9 months, 2.11 (CI = 1.47–3.03).[114] Even if providers do not have access to this program, they can utilize the steps of the BNI, discussed earlier, and provide information about contraception.

The Early Start Program is another effective program. It was specifically developed to serve pregnant women in a managed care setting. Women who are identified to be at risk because of alcohol, tobacco, or other substance use are immediately referred to an Early Start specialist, located in the perinatal office setting.[115] The effect of Early Start on neonatal outcomes was evaluated among 6774 female Kaiser Permanente members who were screened by completing prenatal substance abuse screening questionnaires and urine toxicology screening tests. The study compared 4 groups: 1) 782 women with positive screens who were assessed and treated by Early Start; 2) 348 women with positive screens who were assessed by Early Start, but who had no follow-up treatment; 3) 262 women with positive screens and no further Early Start assessment or treatment; and 4) 5382 controls who screened negative. Infants of Group 1 women with positive screens assessed and treated by Early Start had assisted ventilation rates (1.5%) similar to infants of women who screened negative (1.4%), and lower than the Group 2 women who were screened and assessed (4.0%, $p = 0.01$) and Group 3 women who were only screened (3.1%, $p = 0.12$). Similar patterns were found for low birth weight and preterm delivery. Improved neonatal outcomes were found among babies whose mothers received substance abuse treatment integrated with prenatal care.[116] The results of these studies underscore the importance of screening and early identification of risk for women in general, and women who are

pregnant in particular. Additionally, this program highlights the need to refer women to specialty substance abuse treatment while ensuring ongoing prenatal care. Ideally, the substance abuse specialist will be an integral member of the healthcare team within the perinatal setting. Additional information about these two programs is presented in **Table 6-7.**

When referring women to treatment, it is important to proactively identify any barriers to treatment (e.g., cost, lack of transportation, child care) that could hinder effective linkage to, engagement in, and completion of specialty treatment. For example, based on data averaged across three annual National Surveys on Drug Use and Health, of those who needed treatment for alcohol disorders, the majority (87.4%) did not receive treatment and did not perceive a need for it.[117] Further, among those who did perceive a need for treatment, only 1 out of 7 accessed specialty SUD treatment in a 3-year period.[118] Women with SUDs are less likely, over the lifetime, to enter treatment compared to their male counterparts.[112]

Various strategies have been identified to close the gap in referral to treatment, and none are specific for women. One strategy is to disseminate the neuroscience behind SUDs. Integrating information about the neurobiologic base of alcohol disorders in conversations with at-risk individuals may reduce barriers to acceptance of referral to specialty treatment.[35] The manner in which a referral to further treatment is provided can have tremendous impact on whether the woman will actually receive services with the referral provider.

Pharmacology

Concurrent use of medications for SUDs with other treatment modalities is associated with better outcomes. Addressed here are medications used

Table 6-7 Model Programs for Promoting Maternal and Neonatal Outcomes

Program	CHOICES	Early Start
Description	Integrated behavioral intervention for prevention of prenatal alcohol exposure in women at high risk	Coordination of care between mental health and obstetric professionals in a service-delivery model for addressing substance abuse in pregnancy
Active ingredients	Motivational interviewing Cognitive-behavioral strategies	1) Placing a licensed substance abuse expert in the OB/GYN department whose appointments for assessment and treatment are linked to the patients' prenatal care appointments; 2) universally screening all women for drugs and alcohol by questionnaire and, with signed consent, by urine toxicology testing; 3) educating all providers and patients about the effects of drugs, alcohol, and cigarette use in pregnancy
Targets	Adoption of effective contraception Reduction of alcohol use	Neonatal and maternal outcomes
Format	Four manual-guided counseling sessions	Immediate referral of women identified as having some risk for alcohol, tobacco, or other drug use during pregnancy to the Early Start Specialist, who conducts an in-depth psychosocial assessment with the patient, concluding with diagnosis and care plan for follow up
Providers	Behavioral health counselors Family planning clinician (1 session)	Early Start specialist (licensed clinical social worker or marriage and family therapist), OB/GYN provider

Data from Velasquez MM, von Sternberg K, Parrish DE. CHOICES: an integrated behavioral intervention to prevent alcohol-exposed pregnancies among high-risk women in community settings. *Soc Work Public Health*. 2013;28(3–4):224-233. doi: 10.1080/19371918.2013.759011; Taillac C, Goler N, Armstrong MA, Haley K, Osejo V. Early start: an integrated model of substance abuse intervention for pregnant women. *Perm J*. 2007 Summer;11(3):5-11; Goler NC, Armstrong MA, Taillac CJ, Osejo VM. Substance abuse treatment linked with prenatal visits improves perinatal outcomes: a new standard. *J Perinatol*. 2008 September;28(9):597-603. doi: 10.1038/jp.2008.70. Epub 2008 Jun 26.

for three of the most commonly used substances: nicotine, alcohol, and opiates. These pharmacologic agents should not be viewed as stand-alone treatment, but rather provided in combination with BIs and longer-term counseling. **Table 6-8** lists the US Food and Drug Administration (FDA)–approved medications for nicotine, alcohol, and opiates; dosing range; actions; and special considerations for women, the fetus, and the neonate.

Table 6-8 Medications for Substance Abuse

Substance	Medication	Dose Range	Action	Special Considerations
Nicotine	Nicotine replacement therapy (NRT)	Over the counter: Gum/lozenge (2 and 4 mg strength) Transdermal patch (5–22 mg; 16 and 24 hour) Prescription: Nasal spray (prescribed for 3 months; should not exceed 6 months) Inhaler (4 to 20 cartridges/day)	Provides measured dose of nicotine through skin/mucosa	NRT may be safer than smoking in pregnancy.
Nicotine	Bupropion	150–300 mg PO daily	Weak inhibitor of dopamine and noradrenaline reuptake; has also been shown to antagonize nicotinic acetylcholine receptor function	Contraindicated in individuals with seizure disorder, monoamine oxidase (MAO) drug within 14 days, eating disorders, taking bupropion for depression
Nicotine	Varenicline	Begin 0.5 mg daily, increase to BID on day 3, increase slowly to 1 mg BID	Nicotine acetylcholine receptor partial agonist	Reduce dose for renal impairment. Serious neuropsychiatric events—changes in mood, suicidal ideation, irritability, hostility, completed suicide. Use cautiously in patients with psychiatric history; monitor closely.
Alcohol	Disulfiram	250 mg PO daily (range 125–500 mg)	Inhibits the enzyme acetaldehyde dehydrogenase (ALDH) from converting acetaldehyde to acetate. Acetaldehyde accumulation produces an aversive reaction.	When taking disulfiram, patient should carry card stating "On Disulfiram." Need to avoid exposure to alcohol in any form (e.g., aftershave, mouthwash, liquid medications, hand sanitizers) and read labels on foods and consumables. Contraindicated with drugs metabolized by cytochrome P450 enzymes (e.g., imipramine, warfarin, phenytoin, various benzodiazepines, omeprazole). Not recommended as first-line treatment. Not recommended for individuals with history of psychosis, cardiovascular disease, pulmonary disease, previous renal failure, diabetes, or those over the age of 60.

Alcohol	Naltrexone	Oral (ReVia): 50–100 mg daily IM (Vivitrol): 380 mg monthly	Competes with opiates for opioid receptors in the brain (i.e., opiate antagonist); reduces urge or desire to drink; if alcohol is consumed, decreases amount (due to antagonistic effect of the medication)	When taking naltrexone, patients should inform healthcare providers so possible interactions with other medications can be evaluated. Evaluate liver function prior to the onset of treatment and regularly during treatment. Ensure proper technique for IM; cellulitis has been reported.
Alcohol	Acamprosate	666 mg (2 tablets of 333 mg) PO 3 times per day	Mechanisms of action still lacking, but evidence suggests primary effect is to modulate glutamatergic transmission.	More effective if patient is abstinent when therapy starts. Considered when patient does not respond to naltrexone, or naltrexone is contraindicated. Excreted primarily by the kidneys (contraindicated in people with renal impairment). Does not appear to pharmacokinetically interact with alcohol or medications metabolized by the liver.
Opiates	Buprenorphine (Types: buprenorphine, mono product; and a tablet that combines buprenorphine with the opioid antagonist naloxone in a 1:4 ratio)	Induction typically then takes place over a 3-day period, beginning with either 2 mg or 4 mg, with a maximum dose of: • 8–12 mg on day 1 • 12–16 mg on day 2 • 16 mg up to 32 mg on day 3 Maintenance: 4–16 mg/day (max 24–32 mg)	Partial mu opioid receptor agonist and kappa-receptor antagonist	In pregnancy: Buprenorphine produces maternal outcomes similar to those associated with methadone. In neonates: Neonates exposed in utero to buprenorphine who are treated for neonatal abstinence syndrome (NAS) require, on average, a shorter duration of NAS treatment and less medication for the treatment of their NAS than neonates exposed in utero to methadone. Breastfeeding: The amount of buprenorphine or norbuprenorphine the infant receives via breast milk is only 1%.
Opiates	Methadone	Initial dose: determined by estimating the amount of opioid use and gauging the patient's response to administered methadone. 80–120 mg/day (higher for some individuals)	Full opioid agonist acting at the mu opioid receptor to displace opioids	QT prolongation may occur in higher doses.

BID = 2 times per day, IM = intramuscular, PO = per os/by mouth.

259

Smoking Cessation

The Agency for Healthcare Research and Quality (AHRQ) recommends "The 5 A's" behavioral counseling framework (ask, advise, assess, assist, and arrange) for engaging patients in smoking cessation.[119] Brief behavioral counseling sessions of less than 10 minutes and pharmacotherapy are effective in increasing the proportion of individuals who successfully quit and remain abstinent.[120] A systematic review of studies evaluating interventions for smoking cessation among hospitalized patients reported that adding pharmacotherapy, such as nicotine replacement therapy, bupropion, or varenicline, to a behavioral intervention increases quit rates more than placebo or no medication.[121] Combining pharmacotherapy with a behavioral intervention increases quit rates to a greater extent than counseling alone.[122,123] Women should be offered multiple modalities of care, because the chance of successfully quitting smoking increases dramatically with aggressive treatment.

Pharmacologic interventions appear to be most effective in helping highly addicted individuals stop smoking. Use of these products has been found to double or triple the quit rate in heavy smokers.[122] Whether lighter smokers should be offered pharmacologic support is unclear as evidence has not found that quit rates are improved with the use of smoking cessation products in individuals who smoke fewer than 10 cigarettes a day.[122] However, evidence does exist that can help direct treatment choices for heavier smokers.

Options for nicotine replacement include nicotine gum, transdermal nicotine (the patch), nasal sprays, and inhalers. Oral medications include bupropion and varenicline. Evidence suggests that treatment with varenicline alone is the most effective available monotherapy. Use of varenicline as a single agent is associated with quit rates of 33.2% (95% CI 28.9–37.8).[122] The use of several combination regimens has been shown to be associated with similar excellent quit rates: long-term patch use $\geq$ 14 weeks plus as-needed use of nicotine gum or spray (quit rate of 36.5%, 95% CI 28.6–45.3) and use of the patch plus bupropion (quit rate of 28.9%, 95% CI 23.5–35.1).[122]

Patients often benefit from using a variety of behavioral interventions in addition to medication. Common features of effective counseling interventions include: 1) provision by the women's care provider, 2) focus on identification and management of specific barriers to quitting, and 3) ongoing follow up and support.[122] Patients can be asked to keep a smoking diary that can be used to monitor the amount and the circumstances surrounding smoking. Some individuals prefer to wean slowly; others prefer to quit cold turkey. The following suggestions may be helpful in reducing a woman's daily number of cigarettes before quitting completely: 1) Smoke a different brand of cigarette of the same strength but different taste, or 2) remove the daily quota of cigarettes from the pack and place the remainder out of view, thereby reducing the temptation to smoke more. At the agreed-upon quit date, other techniques may be helpful such as throwing away ashtrays, matches, and lighters; changing or laundering curtains, bedspreads, or clothing, which can retain the smell of cigarette smoke; or identifying a smoking buddy who can lend support immediately as needed. Keeping the money usually spent on cigarettes in a money jar can be used to provide small rewards for success at quitting.

In pregnant women, the USPSTF recommends smoking cessation counseling augmented with messages and self-help materials tailored for women who are smoking during pregnancy.[95] Recommendations set by the AHRQ agree.[122] Use of nicotine replacement therapy and oral agents have not been shown to improve quit rates in pregnant women in most,[122,123] but not all[124] studies. A meta-analysis of five randomized clinical trials reported that use of nicotine replacement did not help women stop cigarette smoking (RR 1.63, 95% CI 0.85–3.14).[123] A more recent meta-analysis, which included a larger number of studies (*n* = 5 RCTs, 1 quasi-RCT, 1 prospective study), came to the opposite conclusion and found that nicotine replacement therapy improved quit rates by 80% (RR 1.80, 95% CI 1.32–2.44).[124] Nicotine replacement use was not associated with increased rates of low birth weight, preterm labor, perinatal mortality, fetal demise, spontaneous abortion, or admission to a neonatal intensive care unit.[123] In selected cases where counseling alone is insufficient to help women stop smoking in pregnancy, use of adjunctive nicotine replacement therapy can be considered.[122] No smoking cessation trials conducted with pregnant women have yet included bupropion or varenicline.[125]

Medications Used in the Treatment of Alcohol Abuse

The effectiveness of combining alcohol pharmacotherapy and counseling has also been established. The COMBINE (Combining Medications and Behavioral Interventions for Alcoholism) study demonstrated that using a medication such as naltrexone combined with a process called Medical Management is effective.[126] Medical Management employs several sessions that focus on education and strategies to promote abstinence as an option to treat moderate to severe alcoholism in various healthcare settings.[127] The majority of providers delivering Medical Management in the COMBINE study were nurses, followed by psychologists and residents.[128] An adapted version of the treatment manual for Medical Management is free and accessible online for clinicians interested in using this structured intervention.[129]

Medications Used in the Treatment of Opiate Addiction

Pharmacologic treatments for opiates, such as methadone and buprenorphine, are provided within the context of comprehensive care. Methadone maintenance treatment is provided through licensed methadone clinics. The Drug Addiction Treatment Act of 2000 provided the opportunity for the provision of office-based buprenorphine treatment.[130] Prescribing is restricted to qualified physicians who receive a DATA 2000 waiver. Additionally, prior to providing this office-based addiction treatment, physicians and other healthcare staff need to have appropriate training, experience, and comfort with opioid addiction treatment. Also, the medical practice must ensure continuity of treatment and the availability of comprehensive, community-based, psychosocial services.[131]

Mutual Self-Help Groups

Mutual support groups or self-help groups can be a primary source of behavior change or an adjunct to formal treatment. Twelve-Step programs such as Alcoholics Anonymous and Narcotics Anonymous have a long history of helping members who desire to stop using alcohol or drugs. However, the effectiveness of these programs is difficult to determine given that individuals who participate are a self-selected group. Member surveys conducted by Alcoholics Anonymous (*n* > 8000), Narcotics Anonymous (*n* = 11,723), and Cocaine Anonymous (*n* > 1000) report that about one-third of participants in each of the 3 programs have been abstinent between 1 and 5 years.[132] Donovan and colleagues highlight several key points from the literature that they recommend should be conveyed to patients: 1) beginning 12-step participation while in treatment is associated with better outcomes; 2) consistent, early, and frequent attendance and/or involvement is associated with better substance use outcomes; 3) engaging in other 12-step activities, such as getting a sponsor, doing service at meetings, and/or reading 12-step literature may be a better indicator of engagement and predictor of abstinence than mere attendance; and 4) continuing 12-step meeting involvement has been shown to lead to decreased utilization of mental health and substance abuse treatment and associated costs.[132] Clinicians should be aware that these 12-step mutual support groups are readily available, no-cost, community-based resources and make informed referrals to maximize the likelihood of engagement and positive outcomes.

Conclusion

Because substance use has the capacity to cause harm even without the existence of an SUD, healthcare providers should view substance use as a continuum from low-risk use to the development of an SUD. The early onset of health and psychosocial consequences associated with substance use among women commands special attention. Women's healthcare providers need to be particularly attentive to screening for substance use, and further assessment should be based on the identified risk level. BIs can be delivered during a single visit or across multiple contacts with women with a goal of reducing the associated harm. BIs to promote referral to treatment are also indicated to remove actual or potential barriers to treatment. Prescribing practitioners can offer medication within the scope of jurisdictional laws.

References

1. World Health Organization. Substance abuse. Available at: http://www.who.int/topics/substance_abuse/en/. Accessed March 15, 2016.
2. World Health Organization. Global strategy to reduce the harmful use of alcohol. 2010. Available at: http://www.who.int/substance_abuse/activities/gsrhua/en/index.html. Accessed March 15, 2016.
3. United Nations Office on Drugs and Crime. *World Drug Report 2012*. New York, NY: United Nations; 2012.
4. American Psychiatric Association. *Diagnostic and Statistical Manual of Mental Disorders*. 5th ed. Arlington, VA: American Psychiatric Association; 2013.
5. National Institute on Alcohol Abuse and Alcoholism. Helping patients who drink too much: a clinician's guide. Available at: http://pubs.niaaa.nih.gov/publications/Practitioner/CliniciansGuide2005/clinicians_guide.htm. Accessed March 15, 2016.
6. National Institute on Alcohol Abuse and Alcoholism. What is a standard drink? Available at: http://www.niaaa.nih.gov/alcohol-health/overview-alcohol-consumption/what-standard-drink. Accessed March 28, 2016.
7. National Institute on Alcohol Abuse and Alcoholism. Drinking levels defined. Available at: http://www.niaaa.nih.gov/alcohol-health/overview-alcohol-consumption/moderate-binge-drinking. Accessed March 15, 2016.
8. US Department of Health and Human Services, National Institute on Alcohol Abuse and Alcoholism. Alcohol: a women's health issue. 2008. Available at: http://pubs.niaaa.nih.gov/publications/brochurewomen/Woman_English.pdf. Accessed March 15, 2016.
9. Volkow ND, Fowler JS, Wang GJ, Baler R, Telang F. Imaging dopamine's role in drug abuse and addiction. *Neuropharmacology.* 2009;56:3-8.
10. Meyer MR, Peters FT. Analytical toxicology of emerging drugs of abuse—an update. *Ther Drug Monit.* 2012;34(6):615-621.
11. National Center for Health Statistics. Health, United States, 2014. Hyattsville, MD: National Center for Health Statistics; 2015. Available at: http://www.cdc.gov/nchs/hus.htm. Accessed March 29, 2015.
12. Centers for Disease Control and Prevention. Current Cigarette Smoking Among Adults—United States, 2005–2014. *MMWR.* 2015;64(44):1233-1240.

13. World Health Organization. WHO global report: mortality attributable to tobacco. Available at: http://www.who.int/tobacco/publications/surveillance/fact_sheet_mortality_report.pdf. Accessed March 15, 2016.

14. US Department of Health and Human Services. The Health Consequences of Smoking—50 Years of Progress. A Report of the Surgeon General. Atlanta, GA: US Department of Health and Human Services, Centers for Disease Control and Prevention, National Center for Chronic Disease Prevention and Health Promotion, Office on Smoking and Health; 2014.

15. Centers for Disease Control and Prevention. Smoking and tobacco use: health effects of secondhand smoke. Available at: http://www.cdc.gov/tobacco/data_statistics/fact_sheets/secondhand_smoke/health_effects/. Accessed March 15, 2016.

16. Substance Abuse and Mental Health Services Administration. Results from the 2012 National Survey on Drug Use and Health: Summary of National Findings, NSDUH Series H-46, HHS Publication No. (SMA) 13-4795. Rockville, MD: Substance Abuse and Mental Health Services Administration.

17. World Health Organization. Global status report on alcohol and health 2014. Available at: http://www.who.int/substance_abuse/publications/global_alcohol_report/en/. Accessed March 15, 2016.

18. Centers for Disease Control and Prevention. Alcohol use and binge drinking among women of childbearing age—United States 2006–2010. *MMWR.* 2012;61(28):534-538.

19. Dawson DA1, Grant BF, Stinson FS, Chou PS. Another look at heavy episodic drinking and alcohol use disorders among college and noncollege youth. *J Stud Alcohol.* 2004;65(4):477-488.

20. World Health Organization. Management of substance abuse: alcohol. Available at: http://www.who.int/substance_abuse/facts/alcohol/en/. Accessed March 15, 2016.

21. Nelson DE, Jarman DW, Rehm J, Greenfield TK, Rey G, Kerr WC, et al. Alcohol-attributable cancer deaths and years of potential life lost in the United States. *Am J Public Health.* 2013;103:641-648.

22. United Nations Office on Drugs and Crime. World Drug Report 2012. Available at: http://www.unodc.org/unodc/en/data-and-analysis/WDR-2012.html. Accessed March 15, 2016.

23. Straus MM, Ghitza UE, Tai B. Preventing deaths from rising opioid overdose in the US—the promise of naloxone antidote in community-based naloxone take-home programs. *Subst Abuse Rehabil.* 2013;4:1-13.

24. Centers for Disease Control and Prevention. Drug overdose in the United States: fact sheet. Available at: http://www.cdc.gov/homeandrecreationalsafety/overdose/facts.html. Accessed March 15, 2016.

25. Randall D, Roxburgh AD, Gibson AE, Degenhardt LJ. *Mortality among people who use illicit drugs* (NDARC Technical Report no. 301). Sydney, Australia: National Drug and Alcohol Research Centre; 2009.

26. Centers for Disease Control and Prevention. Ectopic pregnancy mortality—Florida 2009–2010. *MMWR.* 2012;61(06):106-109.

27. Centers for Disease Control and Prevention. Prescription painkiller overdoses. Available at: http://www.cdc.gov/vitalsigns/PrescriptionPainkiller Overdoses/. Accessed March 15, 2016.

28. Centers for Disease Control and Prevention. Policy impact: prescription painkiller overdoses. 2011. Available at: http://www.cdc.gov/drugoverdose/pdf/policyimpact-prescriptionpainkillerod-a.pdf/. Accessed March 28, 2016.

29. National Institute on Drug Abuse. Drug facts: methamphetamine. Available at: http://www.drugabuse.gov/publications/drugfacts/methamphetamine. Accessed March 15, 2016.

30. National Institute on Drug Abuse. What is the scope of methamphetamine abuse in the United States? Available at: http://www.drugabuse.gov/publications/research-reports/methamphetamine/what-scope-methamphetamine-abuse-in-united-states. Accessed March 15, 2016.

31. Venios K, Kelly JF. The rise, risks, and realities of methamphetamine use among women: implications for research, prevention and treatment. *J Addict Nurs.* 2010;21:14-21.

32. Substance Abuse and Mental Health Services Administration. Center for Behavioral Health Statistics and Quality. The TEDS Report: Gender Differences in Primary Substance of Abuse Across Age Groups. http://www.samhsa.gov/data/sites/default/files/sr077-gender-differences-2014.pdf. Accessed March 28, 2016.

33. Cerda M, Wall M, Keyes KM, Galea S, Hasin D. Medical marijuana laws in 50 states: investigating the relationship between state legalization of medical marijuana and marijuana use, abuse and dependence. *Drug Alcohol Depend.* 2012;120:22-27.

34. Volkow ND, Baler RD, Compton WM, Weiss SRB. Adverse health effects of marijuana use. *N Engl J Med.* 2014;370(23):2219-2227.

35. Finnell DS Nowzari S. Providing information about the neurobiology of alcohol use disorders to close the referral to treatment gap. *Nurs Clin North Am.* 2013;48(3):373-383.

36. Carter R. *The Human Brain Book.* New York, NY: DK Publishing; 2009.

37. Giedd JN. Structural magnetic resonance imaging of the adolescent brain. *Ann N Y Acad Sci.* 2004;1021(1):77-85.

38. Díaz-Mataix L, Tallot L, Doyère V. The amygdala: a potential player in timing CS-US intervals. *Behav Processes.* 2014;101:111-122.

39. Ikemoto S, Bonci A. Neurocircuitry of drug reward. *Neuropharmacology.* 2014;76(Pt B):329-341.

40. Müller UJ, Voges J, Steiner J, Galazky I, Heinze H-J, Möller M, et al. Deep brain stimulation of the nucleus accumbens for the treatment of addiction. *Ann N Y Acad Sci.* 2013;1282:119-128.

41. Pierce RC, Kumaresan V. The mesolimbic dopamine system: the final common pathway for the reinforcing effect of drugs of abuse? *Neurosci Biobehav Rev.* 2006;30(2):215-238.

42. Van den Oever MC, Spijke S, Smit AB, De Vries TJ. Prefrontal cortex plasticity mechanisms in drug seeking and relapse. *Neurosci Biobehav Rev.* 2010; 35(2):276-284.

43. National Institute for Drug Abuse. The neurobiology of drug addiction. Available at: http://www .drugabuse.gov/publications/teaching-packets/ neurobiology-drug-addiction/section-iv-action-cocaine/7-summary-addictive-drugs-activate-reward. Accessed March 15, 2016.

44. Balster RL, Schuster CR. Fixed-interval schedule of cocaine reinforcement: effect of dose and infusion duration. *J Exp Anal Behav.* 1973;20(1):119-129.

45. Kalivas PW, Volkow ND. The neural basis of addiction: a pathology of motivation and choice. *Am J Psychiatry.* 2005;162(8):1403-1413.

46. Littleton J. Neurochemical mechanisms underlying alcohol withdrawal. *Alcohol Health Res World.* 1998;22(1):13-24.

47. Bierut LJ. Genetic vulnerability and susceptibility to substance dependence. *Neuron.* 2011;69(4):618-627.

48. Volkow ND, Baler RD. Addiction science: uncovering neurobiological complexity. *Neuropharmacology.* 2014;76(Pt B):235-249.

49. Volkow ND, Wang G-J, Fowler JS, Thanos P, Logan J, Gatley SJ, et al. Brain DA D2 receptors predict reinforcing effects of stimulants in humans: replication study. *Synapse.* 2002;46(2):79-82.

50. Blum K, Oscar-Berman M, Barh D, Giordano J, Gold MS. Dopamine genetics and function in food and substance abuse. *J Genet Syndr Gene Ther.* 2013;4(121):1000121.

51. Renthal W, Nestler EJ. Epigenetic mechanisms in drug addiction. *Trends Mol Med.* 2008;14(8): 341-350.

52. Mahoub M, Monteggia LM. Epigenetics and psychiatry. *Neurotherapeutics.* 2013;10(4):734-741.

53. Becker JB, Perry AN, Westenbroek C. Sex differences in the neural mechanisms mediating addiction: a new synthesis and hypothesis. *Biol Sex Differ.* 2012;3(1):1-35.

54. Hedges VL, Staffend NA, Meisel RL. Neural mechanisms of reproduction in females as a predisposing factor for drug addiction. *Front Neuroendocrinol.* 2010;31(2):217-231.

55. Graham K, Wilsnack R, Dawson D, Vogeltanz N. Should alcohol consumption measures be adjusted for gender differences? *Addiction.* 1998;93(8): 1137-1147.

56. Koob GF, Le Moal M. Drug abuse: hedonic homeostatic dysregulation. *Science.* 1997;278(5335):52-8.

57. Lisansky ES. The woman alcoholic. *Ann Am Acad Polit Soc Sci.* 1958;315(1):73-81.

58. Haas AL, Peters RH. Development of substance abuse problems among drug-involved offenders: evidence for the telescoping effect. *J Subst Abuse.* 2000;12(3):241-253.

59. Hernandez-Avila CA, Rounsaville BJ, Kranzler HR. Opioid-, cannabis- and alcohol-dependent women show more rapid progression to substance abuse treatment. *Drug Alcohol Depend.* 2004;74(3): 265-272.

60. Substance Abuse and Mental Health Services Administration. *Substance Abuse Treatment: Addressing the Specific Needs of Women.* Treatment Improvement Protocol (TIP) Series, No. 51. HHS Publication No. (SMA) 13–4426. Rockville, MD: Substance Abuse and Mental Health Services Administration; 2009. Available at: http://store.samhsa.gov/product/TIP-51-Substance-Abuse-Treatment-Addressing-the-Specific-Needs-of-Women/SMA13–4426. Accessed March 15, 2016.

61. Syme MR, Paxton JW, Keelan JA. Drug transfer and metabolism by the human placenta. *Clin Pharmacokinet.* 2004;43(8):487-514.

62. Kaltenbach K, Berghella V, Finnegan L. Opioid dependence during pregnancy: effects and management. *Obstet Gynecol Clin North Am.* 1998;25(1): 139-151.

63. Wang H, De SK, Maccarrone M. Jekyll and Hyde: two faces of cannabinoid signaling in male and female fertility. *Endocr Rev.* 2006;27(5):427-448.

64. Wendell AD. Overview and epidemiology of substance abuse in pregnancy. *Clin Obstet Gynecol.* 2013;56(1):91-96.

65. Kapogiannis D, Kisser J, Davatzikos C, Ferrucci L, Metter J, Resnick SM. Alcohol consumption and premotor corpus callosum in older adults. *Eur Neuropsychopharmacol.* 2012;22(10):704-710.

66. Caputo F, Vignoli T, Leggio L, Addolorato G, Zol G, Bernardi M. Alcohol use disorders in the elderly: a brief overview from epidemiology to treatment options. *Exp Gerontol.* 2012;47(6):411-416.

67. Collella C, Savage CL, Whitmer K. Alcohol use in the elderly and risk for Wernicke-Korsakoff syndrome. *J Nurse Pract.* 2010;6(8):614-621.

68. Center for Substance Abuse Treatment. *Substance Abuse Among Older Adults.* Treatment Improvement Protocol (TIP) Series, No. 26. HHS Publication No. (SMA) 12–3918. Rockville, MD: Substance Abuse and Mental Health Services Administration; 1998.

69. Cicero TJ, Surratt HL, Kurtz S, Ellis MS, Inciardi JA. Patterns of prescription opioid abuse and comorbidity in an aging treatment population. *J Subst Abuse Treat.* 2012;42(1):87-94.

70. Towns AJ, Parker C, Chase P. Constructions of masculinity in alcohol advertising. *Addict Res Theory.* 2012;20(5):389-401.

71. Flegel K. Big alcohol catches up with adolescent girls. *CMAJ.* 2013;185(10):859.

72. Gentry E, Poirier K, Wilkinson T, Nhean S, Nybom J, Siegel M. Alcohol advertising at Boston subway stations: an assessment of exposure by race and socioeconomic status. *Am J Public Health.* 2011;101(10):1936-1941.

73. Jiang N, Ling PM. Reinforcement of smoking and drinking: tobacco marketing strategies with alcohol in the US. *Am J Public Health.* 2011;101(10):1942-1954.

74. Gerard JL, Dent CW, Stacy AW. Exposure to alcohol advertisements and teenage alcohol related problems. *Pediatrics.* 2013;131(2):e369-e3379.

75. Snyder LB, Milici FF, Slater M, Sun H, Strizhakova Y. Effects of alcohol advertising exposure on drinking among youth. *Arch Pediatr Adolesc Med.* 2006;160:18-24.

76. Garfield CF, Chung PJ, Rathouz PJ. Alcohol advertising in magazines and youth readership. *JAMA.* 2003;289(18):2424-2429.

77. Johns Hopkins Bloomberg School of Public Health Center on Alcohol Marketing and Youth. http://www.camy.org/resources/. Accessed March 29, 2016.

78. Carrigan PW, Watson, AC. The stigma of psychiatric disorders and the gender ethnicity and education of the perceiver. *Community Ment Health J.* 2007;43(5):439-458.

79. American College of Obstetricians and Gynecologists. ACOG Committee Opinion No. 473: substance abuse reporting and pregnancy: the role of the obstetrician-gynecologist. *Obstet Gynecol.* 2011;117: 200-201.

80. National Institute on Drug Abuse. Stigma of drug abuse. Available at: http://archives.drugabuse.gov/about/welcome/aboutdrugabuse/stigma/. Accessed March 15, 2016.

81. McKenna L, Boyle M, Brown T, Williams B, Mollory A, Lewis B, et al. Levels of empathy in undergraduate nursing students. *Int J Nurs Pract.* 2012;18:246-251.

82. Centers for Disease Control and Prevention. Intimate partner violence: risk and protective factors. Available at: http://www.cdc.gov/violenceprevention/intimatepartnerviolence/riskprotectivefactors.html. Accessed March 15, 2016.

83. Centers for Disease Control and Prevention. Injury Prevention and Control: Motor vehicle safety. Available at: http://www.cdc.gov/motorvehiclesafety/index.html. Accessed March 29, 2016.

84. Park S-Y, Kolonel LN, Lim U, White K, Henderson BE, Wilken LR. Alcohol consumption and breast cancer risk among women from five ethnic groups with light to moderate intakes: the Multiethnic Cohort Study. *Int J Cancer.* 2014;134:1504-1510.

85. Institute of Medicine Prevention Framework. Cited in: Springer F, Phillips Jl. The IOM Model: A Tool for Prevention Planning and Implementation. Available at: www.cars-rp.org/publications/Prevention%20Tactics/PT8.13.06.pdf Accessed March 29, 2016.

86. San Francisco Department of Public Health. Community Behavioral Health Services: Harm Reduction Policy. Available at: http://www.sfdph.org/dph/comupg/oservices/mentalHlth/SubstanceAbuse/Harm Reduction/default.asp. Accessed March 15, 2016.

87. US Department of Health and Human Services. Healthy People 2020 topics and objectives: substance abuse. Available at: http://www.healthypeople.gov/2020/topicsobjectives2020/overview.aspx?topicid=40. Accessed March 15, 2016.

88. Beirness DJ, Jesseman R, Notaradrea R, Perron M. Harm reduction: what's in a name? Canadian Centre on Substance Abuse; 2008. Available at: http://www.ccsa.ca/Resource%20Library/ccsa0115302008e.pdf. Accessed March 15, 2016.

89. Smith PC, Schmidt SM, Saitz R. Primary care validation of a single-question alcohol screening test. *J Gen Int Med* 2009;24(7):783-788.

90. Bradley KA, De Benedetti AF, Volk RJ, Williams EC, Frank D, Kivlahan DR. AUDIT-C as a brief screen for alcohol misuse in primary care. *Alcohol Clin Exp Res.* 2007;31(7):1208-1217.

91. Smith PC, Schmidt SM, Allensworth-Davies D, Saitz R. A single-question screening test for drug use in primary care. *Arch Intern Med.* 2010;170(13):1155-1160.

92. Yudko E, Lozhkina O, Fouts A. A comprehensive review of the psychometric properties of the Drug Abuse Screening Test. *J Subst Abuse Treat.* 2007;32(2):189-198.

93. US Preventive Services Task Force. Tobacco Smoking Cessation in Adults, Including Pregnant Women: Behavioral and Pharmacotherapy Interventions. Available at: http://www.uspreventiveservicestaskforce.org/Page/Document/UpdateSummaryFinal/tobacco-use-in-adults-and-pregnant-women-counseling-and-interventions1. Accessed March 29, 2016. http://www.uspreventiveservicestaskforce.org/uspstf09/tobacco/tobaccrs2.htm. Accessed March 15, 2016.

94. Bearer CF, Stoler JM, Cook JD, Carpenter SJ. Biomarkers of alcohol use in pregnancy. *Alcohol Res Health.* 2005;28(1):38-43.

95. Bakhireva LN, Savage DD. Focus on: biomarkers of fetal alcohol exposure and fetal alcohol effects. *Alcohol Res Health.* 2011;34(1):56-63.

96. Gitlow S. *Substance Use Disorders: A Practical Guide.* Philadelphia, PA: Lippincott Williams & Wilkins; 2001.

97. Sullivan JT, Sykora K, Schneiderman J, Naranjo CA, Sellers E. Assessment of alcohol withdrawal: the revised Clinical Institute Withdrawal Assessment for Alcohol scale (CIWA-Ar). *Br J Addict.* 1989; 84:1353-1357.

98. Scavone JL, Sterling RC, Van Bockstaele EJ. Cannabinoid and opioid interactions: implications for opiate dependence and withdrawal. *Neuroscience.* 2013;248:637-654.

99. Wesson DR, Ling W. The clinical opiate withdrawal scale (COWS). *J Psychoactive Drugs.* 2003;35(2): 253-259.

100. Kreek MJ, Levran O, Reed B, Schlussman SD, Zhou Y, Butelman ER. Opiate addiction and cocaine addiction: underlying molecular neurobiology and genetics. *J Clin Invest.* 2012;122(10):3387.

101. Sullivan E, Fleming M. *Tip 24: A Guide to Substance Abuse Services for Primary Care Clinicians.* Rockville, MD: US Department of Health and Human Services, Substance Abuse and Mental Health Services Administration, DHHS Publication No. (SMA); 1997.

102. Finnell DS. A clarion call for nurse-led SBIRT across the continuum of care. *Alcohol Clin Exp Res.* 2012;36:1134-1138.

103. Gebara CFP, Bhona FMC, Ronzani TM, Lourenço LM, Noto AR. Brief intervention and decrease of alcohol consumption among women: a systematic review. *Subst Abuse Treat Prev Policy.* 2013;8(1):31.

104. American College of Obstetricians and Gynecologists, Committee on Health Care for Underserved Women. At-risk drinking and alcohol dependence: obstetric and gynecologic implications. *Obstet Gynecol.* 2011;118(2):383-388.

105. Kaner EF, Dickinson HO, Beyer FR, Campbell F, Schlesinger C, Heather N, et al. Effectiveness of brief alcohol interventions in primary care populations. *Cochrane Database Syst Rev.* 2007(2): CD004148.

106. O'Donnell A, Anderson P, Newbury-Birch D, Schulte B, Schmidt C, Reimer J, et al. The impact of brief alcohol interventions in primary healthcare: a systematic review of reviews. *Alcohol Alcohol.* 2014;9(1):66-78.

107. Stead LF, Buitrago D, Preciado N, Sanchez G, Hartmann-Boyce J, Lancaster T. Physician advice for smoking cessation. *Cochrane Database Syst Rev.* 2013(5):CD000165.

108. Rice VH, Hartmann-Boyce J, Stead LF. Nursing interventions for smoking cessation. *Cochrane Database Syst Rev.* 2013(8):CD001188.

109. D'Onofrio G, Pantalon MV, Degutis LC, Fiellin DA, O'Connor PG. Development and implementation of an emergency practitioner–performed brief intervention for hazardous and harmful drinkers in the emergency department. *Acad Emerg Med.* 2005;12(3):249-256.

110. Substance Abuse and Mental Health Services Administration. Behavioral treatments and services. Available at: http://www.samhsa.gov/Treatment/. Accessed March 15, 2016.

111. Greenfield SF, Back SE, Lawson K, Brady KT. Substance abuse in women. *Psychiatr Clin North Am.* 2010;33(2):339-355.

112. Greenfield SF, Brooks AJ, Gordon SM, Green CA, Kropp F, McHugh RK, et al. Substance abuse treatment entry, retention, and outcome in women: a review of the literature. *Drug Alcohol Depend.* 2007;86(1):1-21.

113. Centers for Disease Control and Prevention. Preventing alcohol use during pregnancy: Project CHOICES. Available at: http://www.cdc.gov/ncbddd/fasd/documents/choices_onepager_-april2013.pdf. Accessed March 28, 2016.

114. Floyd RL, Sobell M, Velasquez MM, Ingersoll K, Nettleman M, Sobell L, et al. Preventing alcohol-exposed pregnancies: a randomized controlled trial. *Am J Prev Med.* 2007;32(1):1-10.

115. Armstrong MA, Lieberman L, Carpenter DM, Gonzales VM, Usatin MS, Newman L, et al. Early start: an obstetric clinic-based, perinatal substance

abuse intervention program. *Qual Manag Health Care*. 2001;9(2):6-15.

116. Armstrong MA, Osejo VG, Lieberman L, Carpenter DM, Pantoja PM, Escobar GJ. Perinatal substance abuse intervention in obstetric clinics decreases adverse neonatal outcomes. *J Perinatol*. 2003; 23(1):3-9.

117. Substance Abuse and Mental Health Services Administration, Office of Applied Studies. The NSDUH Report: Alcohol Treatment: Need, Utilization, and Barriers. 2009. Available at: http:// archive.samhsa.gov/data/2k9/AlcTX/AlcTX.htm. Accessed March 15, 2016.

118. Mojtabai R, Crum RM. Perceived unmet need for alcohol and drug use treatments and future use of services: results from a longitudinal study. *Drug Alcohol Depend*. 2013;127:59-64.

119. Agency for Healthcare Research and Quality. Five major steps to intervention (The "5 A's"). Available at: http://www.ahrq.gov/professionals/ clinicians-providers/guidelines-recommendations/ tobacco/5steps.html. Accessed March 15, 2016.

120. Agency for Healthcare Research and Quality. Helping Smokers Quit. May 2008. Rockville, MD: Agency for Healthcare Research and Quality; 2008. Available at: http://www.ahrq.gov/professionals/ clinicians-providers/guidelines-recommendations/ tobacco/clinicians/references/clinhlpsmkqt/index. html. Accessed March 15, 2016.

121. Rigotti NA, Clair C, Munafò MR, Stead LF. Interventions for smoking cessation in hospitalised patients. *Cochrane Database Syst Rev*. 2012(5):CD001837. doi: 10.1002/14651858.CD001837.pub3.

122. Agency for Healthcare Research and Quality. Treating Tobacco Use and Dependence. 2013. Available at: http://www.ahrq.gov/professionals/clinicians-providers/guidelines-recommendations/tobacco /clinicians/update/index.html. Accessed March 15, 2016.

123. Coleman T, Chamberlain C, Cooper S, Leonardi-Bee J. Efficacy and safety of nicotine replacement therapy for smoking cessation in pregnancy: systematic review and meta-analysis. *Addiction*. 2011;106(1):52-61.

124. Myung S, Ju W, Jung H, Park C, Oh S, Seo H, et al., for the Korean Meta-Analysis (KORMA) Study Group. Efficacy and safety of pharmacotherapy for smoking cessation among pregnant smokers: a meta-analysis. *BJOG*. 2012;119:1029-1039.

125. Coleman T, Chamberlain C, Davey MA, Cooper SE, Leonardi-Bee J. Pharmacological interventions for promoting smoking cessation during pregnancy. *Cochrane Database Syst Rev*. 2012(9):CD010078.

126. Anton RF, O'Malley SS, Ciraulo DA, et al; COMBINE Study Research Group. Combined pharmacotherapies and behavioral interventions for alcohol dependence: the COMBINE study: a randomized controlled trial. *JAMA*. 2006;295:2003-2017.

127. Pettinati HM, Matta ME. *Medical Management Treatment Manual: A Clinical Guide for Researchers and Clinicians Providing Pharmacotherapy for Alcohol Dependence* (Generic Version). Rockville, MD: US Department of Health and Human Services/ National Institutes of Health; 2010.

128. Savage C. Clinical Reviews: Pharmacotherapy for alcohol dependence, medical management and the role of nursing. *J Addict Nurs*. 2008;19(3):170-171.

129. Pettinati HM, Mattson ME. *Medical Management Treatment Manual: A Clinical Guide for Researchers and Clinicians Providing Pharmacotherapy for Alcohol Dependence*. 2010. Available at: http://pubs .niaaa.nih.gov/publications/MedicalManual/ MMManual.pdf. Accessed March 17, 2016.

130. Substance Abuse and Mental Health Administration. Drug Addiction Act of 2000. Available at: http://buprenorphine.samhsa.gov/data.html. Accessed March 15, 2016.

131. Substance Abuse and Mental Health Administration. *Tip 40: Clinical Guidelines for the Use of Buprenorphine in the Treatment of Opioid Addiction*. Rockville, MD: US Department of Health and Human Services; 2004.

132. Donovan DM, Ingalsbe MH, Benbow J, Daley DC. 12-step interventions and mutual support programs for substance use disorders: an overview. *Soc Work Public Health*. 2013;28(3-4):313-332.

CHAPTER 7

WOMEN AND VIOLENCE—ISSUES FOR PRIMARY CARE PROVIDERS

Jenna A. LoGiudice | Jan M. Kriebs

The Centers for Disease Control and Prevention (CDC) present a clear stance that "sexual violence against girls is a global human rights injustice of vast proportions with severe health and social consequences."[1] Sexual violence is defined as:

> any sexual act, attempt to obtain a sexual act, unwanted sexual comments or advances, or acts to traffic, or otherwise directed against a person's sexuality using coercion, by any person regardless of their relationship to the victim, in any setting. It includes rape, defined as the physically forced or otherwise coerced penetration of the vulva or anus with a penis, other body part or object.[2]

Violence against women is common and has far-reaching and long-lasting effects. A history of sexual violence puts women at risk for grave health consequences, such as anxiety and depression, substance abuse, sexually transmitted diseases (STDs), pregnancy complications such as preterm labor, and gynecologic issues.[3-5] Specifically, women with a history of sexual abuse often manifest systems of chronic pelvic and/or abdominal pain.[2] The Federal Bureau of Investigation in the late 1990s estimated that between one-third and one-half of all women in the United States would experience some form of physical violence during their lifetime.[6] More than one in three US women experience physical or sexual violence or stalking by an intimate partner.[3,7] New data reported by the United Nations found worldwide data that gave a figure of one in three women experiencing physical or sexual violence; when psychologic harm is included, nearly 50% of American women reported a lifetime history in this survey.[8] The number one in five is often quoted as the percentage of women who experience unwanted sexual activity, although this is a broad definition that includes touching as well as attempted assault. Data from the CDC support a high rate of violence against women, citing 18.3% lifetime incidence of forcibly attempted or completed sexual penetration or alcohol-/drug-related assault.[3] Nearly 1 in 4 (23.1%) college-aged women are affected by sexual violence.[9] Long-time family violence researcher Murray Straus stated that the American household is perhaps the most violent institution in the country, and that Americans generally face a greater risk of violence among people they know as opposed to strangers.[10] This is especially true for women. In addition, a woman who has experienced one type of abuse is more likely to experience at least one additional type of abuse, whether as a child or an adult, physical or emotional or sexual.[11]

Women who are in lesbian relationships, are bisexual, or are transgender also experience violence and rape. According to the 2010 National Intimate Partner and Sexual Violence Survey, lesbian women report higher rates of the spectrum of intimate partner violence (IPV) (4 in 10) than heterosexual women (1 in 3). Bisexual women experience a higher lifetime prevalence of rape and other intimate partner sexual violence (6 in 10) compared to heterosexual women and of any type of IPV, including stalking and physical violence, than women in lesbian or heterosexual relationships.[12] Transgender and bisexual individuals have higher rates of violence and discrimination than any other groups.[12,13]

Individuals who are moving through the profound life change of gender transformation so that their physical and hormonal self matches their internal gender identity are at high risk of violence in their lives, both from intimate partners and from strangers. The majority live with the aftermath of trauma and the fear of possible repeat victimization. At least 50% of transgender individuals are sexually abused or assaulted at some point in their lives; the prevalence of physical and sexual abuse may be as high as 66%.[14]

Individuals who have transitioned from male to female have increased mortality risk from substance abuse, human immunodeficiency virus (HIV), and suicide as well as homicide.[15] A significant majority of the murders of transgender individuals that are identified as hate crimes are of women of color.[16] According to the National Coalition of Anti-Violence Programs, (NCAVP) 2013 report on hate violence against lesbian, bisexual, transgender, queer, and HIV-affected communities, 72% of the victims of hate violence homicides in 2013 were transgender women, and 67% were transgender women of color.[17]

Men and women can be victimized as children or adults by family, friends, and strangers. In fact, nearly 2 million (1.7%) men in the United States have experienced sexual violence in the form of rape.[7] Women, however, experience more sexual assault and more violent IPV. Violence can be emotional, physical, sexual, or financial and often includes more than one type. No one is safe from abuse; it affects women of all ages, racial and ethnic groups, sexual orientations, and socioeconomic status. Survivors of violence, in all of its forms, are at risk for long-lasting physical and/or psychologic effects. From children who experience abuse to the elderly who may find themselves victimized by caregivers or strangers, violence and the threat of violence color the lives of many women.

Midwives and other women's health practitioners care for women across the lifespan and therefore will evaluate all types of violence, including abuse experienced as a child, adolescent, or adult; date or stranger rape; and ongoing IPV or family violence. Midwives must be aware of the healthcare needs of survivors. Research has demonstrated that survivors are likely to seek midwives for care, given the holistic approach of the midwifery model.[18-21] The midwifery model of care encourages women to be active participants in their own care and to make informed healthcare choices.[22] Midwives are often sought out for their family-centered, individualized, and patient-centered practices. A survivor of sexual abuse described, "I have felt safe in situations with the midwife that has provided care, just by some simple differences, like not having to completely undress. By them just being practical and flexible, giving me choices and options."[23(pp65,66)] The tenets of midwifery care are attractive to many women, especially survivors.

This chapter describes each of the types of violence that may occur in women's-lives and their potential clinical sequelae, including child abuse and neglect, sexual assault, and IPV. Theoretical explanations for why abuse occurs are presented with guidelines for assessing and managing abuse in practice.

Child Abuse and Neglect

Since 1973, US law has mandated reports of child abuse and neglect. The first recorded child abuse court case, brought against foster parents in New York City, was won based on the argument by the founder of the Society for the Prevention of Cruelty to Animals that children were part of the animal kingdom and deserved the same protection. From this beginning, states began to implement laws to offer children protection against abuse and neglect.[24] By the time the Child Abuse Prevention and Treatment Act (CAPTA) was passed in 1973, every state had some law regarding reporting of and response to child abuse and neglect. Federalizing the issue provided more funding for states and provided model laws for states to follow. All state laws have at least three similarities. They share the same general definitions of abuse and neglect, include mandated reporting requirements, and provide for anonymity and confidentiality. CAPTA defines abuse and neglect as:

> any recent act or failure to act on the part of a parent or caretaker which results in death, serious physical or emotional harm, sexual abuse or exploitation, or an act or failure to act which represents an imminent risk of serious harm.[25]

The definition further defines statutory rape as carnal knowledge occurring between persons having reached the age of majority with persons who have not yet reached the age of majority.

Though there are commonalities across state laws for definitions of abuse and neglect, these definitions remain problematic. Cultural differences regarding what constitutes punishment versus abuse are not easy to discern. Further, who is a mandated reporter and under what circumstance differs from state to state. In all 50 states, the District of Columbia, and Puerto Rico, healthcare professionals are mandated reporters of abuse, neglect, and/or sexual violence in anyone under the age of 18, and are required to report even suspicious (as opposed to proven) abuse.[26] In only two states, New Jersey and Wyoming, all persons are mandated reporters of abuse, neglect, and/or sexual violence in anyone under the age of 18.[26]

Prevalence

Estimates of child abuse and neglect rely primarily on reports to the US Department of Health and Human Services. In 2013, more than 3 million referrals for child abuse and neglect were accepted by social service agencies, representing 4.7% of all American children. Of those, 20% were confirmed to be abuse or neglect. More than a quarter of reported cases occurred in children between 0 and 3 years; nearly half of the children were 5 or younger. Slightly more cases involved girls than boys. African American children have the greatest risk, at 1.4%, while white and Hispanic children have victimization rates between 0.8% and 0.85%. Children often experience more than one type of abuse: 79.5% of victims were neglected, 18% were physically abused, and 9% were sexually abused. In addition, 10% of victims experienced such "other" types of maltreatment ranging from threats to parental substance use.[27] A meta-analysis that focused on the worldwide prevalence of sexual abuse revealed that in the United States and Canada, 20.1% of girls and 8.0% of boys experience childhood sexual abuse.[28]

Fatality statistics from both abuse and neglect of children show similar trends. The National Child Abuse and Neglect Data System reported slightly more than 1500 child fatalities in 2013, or just over 2 per 100,000 children.[27] Nearly three-quarters of all child fatalities occur in those younger than 3 years of age, with infants having the highest rate. Neglect and physical abuse are the most common factors in child mortality. Risk factors include violence in the home and financial instability. Most perpetrators are parents acting alone or with another individual.[27]

Due to underreporting, abuse and neglect reporting and fatalities data represent only the tip of the iceberg. Based on adults reporting about their own experiences as children, reasons for underreporting include the child's inability to recognize that what is happening is wrong or fear of what will happen if they "tell." Even when possible neglect or abuse is observed, personal and societal attitudes, relationship issues, or lack of knowledge about reporting may prevent an effective intervention.[29]

Etiology

It is difficult to distinguish co-occurring problems from causation in multifactorial issues such as child abuse. The Institute of Medicine research agenda for child abuse and neglect describes broad categories that may contribute to increased risk of abuse, although the evidence varies in strength.[29] Parental or individual factors include a family history of abuse and neglect, early childbearing, parental mental illness or substance abuse, and socioeconomic issues; childhood factors may include mental or physical disability. Familial factors include social isolation, IPV, poor parenting skills, and complex or unstable family arrangements (e.g., single parenting, multiple partners). Societal issues including poverty, unemployment, and distressed neighborhoods, as well as larger social issues such as attitudes toward personal violence and corporal punishment add to the complexity. The same study points out that little is known about protective factors—possibly including strong social networks—that might offset risk.[29]

Among theories that have been posited to explain childhood abuse and neglect are:

- Psychodynamic Theory stems from Freud's psychoanalytic approach. Current behaviors stem from unconscious cognitive and affective process; that is, much of mental disorders and adult behavior stems from childhood experiences. Therefore, abusers were most likely abused or witnessed abuse as children. Although Freud himself backed away from his conclusions that adult female "hysteria" was associated with actual childhood sexual experiences, he was the first to discuss concerns about childhood abuse openly. Modern psychoanalytic theory supports the relationship of unconscious stressors and current behavior.[30-32]

- Intergenerational Transmission Theory borrows from social learning theory and posits that children learn to be abusive by growing up with abuse. Sexual abuse and neglect have been linked to parental history by Widom and colleagues, while other studies see maternal physical abuse or repetitive abuse as predictive.[33-35] The same research suggests that current life events may be confounding factors.[34-36] Recently, research has suggested that there may be a bias favoring suspicion of prior victims of abuse when protective services reports occur.[33]

- Cognitive-Behavioral Theory identifies stages of interpretation and behavior rooted in unrealistic expectations that lead finally to abuse.[37]

- Transaction Theory poses that stress is what makes most families vulnerable to conflict, potentially increasing the risk of child abuse. This model generally follows three stages: Stage 1, in which the parent is stressed by life circumstances and is unable to fully cope with the child's behavior; Stage 2, when the parent has increasing difficulty managing and begins to blame the child; and Stage 3, when the parent begins to abuse the child. This is now presented as a combined Ecological/Transaction Model that relies on the four levels of individual, family, community, and culture/society to explain the dynamics that lead to abuse.[38]

Sequelae and Prevention

Further complicating the issue of child abuse is the difficulty in measuring rates of abuse, based on low reporting and multiple interpretations of events. While racial bias has been suspected in abuse reporting, higher levels of environmental risk factors are an alternative explanation for higher reported rates of child maltreatment.[39-41] Structured decision-making processes seem to improve analysis based on a holistic view of family environment, but different evaluators still may interpret events differently.[42] In order to decrease the disproportionately high rates among disadvantaged children, attention will need to be paid to social issues including individual and neighborhood poverty, support for young and single mothers, and access to community services.[39,41]

Sequelae may include psychosocial effects such as problems with socialization and interpersonal relationships, depressive and anxiety disorders, self-mutilation and suicide attempts, alcohol and drug abuse, eating disorders, posttraumatic stress disorder (PTSD), and risky behaviors. These may include teen delinquency and adult criminal behavior, and unsafe sexual behaviors that may result in unintended pregnancies, including teen pregnancy and/or STDs. Further, women growing up with abuse either as direct

victims or witnesses are more likely to abuse their own children and to be revictimized during their lifetimes.[43,44]

Violence Against Women

Rape and Sexual Assault

Rape was traditionally defined by the Bureau of Justice Statistics as "carnal knowledge (penile-vaginal penetration only) of a female forcibly and against her will."[45] Although men also experience sexual violence, this section addresses only the experiences of women. Since the mid-1990s, the federal code and most states have broadened this definition by:

- Including sexual penetration of any type, including vaginal, anal, and oral, and by penis, fingers, or objects
- Focusing on the offender's behaviors rather than the survivor's
- Restricting the use of a survivor's previous sexual history as evidence

Many states have also removed marital status as an exemption. Some states and the US Code have replaced the term *rape* with other terms such as *sexual abuse*, *sexual assault*, or *sexual battery*. Every midwife is responsible for knowing the legal definition of rape or sexual assault in her or his state. This information is essential in order to provide appropriate counseling and to comply with reporting requirements.

PREVALENCE

The most recent CDC estimate puts the lifetime prevalence of rape/sexual assault at an estimated 19.3% of women (> 23 million women). Completed forced penetration was experienced by about 11.5% of women. The annual incidence of rape in the most recent CDC report was 1.6%

of women (approximately 1.9 million women).[7] In that same survey, 5.5% of women reported an instance of any sexual victimization, and 4.2% reported being stalked within the previous year.[7] Multiracial and Native American women are at highest risk.[7] Most women who are raped or assaulted sexually know their perpetrator, and are often still in an intimate relationship with them; rape can also be a form of IPV.

Rates of sexual assault against women (including rape, attempted rape, or threat of rape) are highest among college-aged individuals, and higher among nonstudents than among current students.[46] Nearly 1 in 4 (23.1%) of college-aged women are affected by sexual violence.[9] Forty percent of women who have ever been raped were raped for the first time before they were 18.[7] Twelve percent were first raped when they were under 10 years of age.[3] A national study of high school students found that more than 10% of girls reported forced sexual activity.[47]

Most sexual assaults go unreported and therefore the perpetrator faces no punishment; in 2014 only 33.6% of rapes were reported to police.[48] Victims may be fearful of exposure of other parts of their lives. While rape shield laws have been imposed to prevent a woman's previous sexual activity from entering into a courtroom, this does not afford full protection. Victims often doubt themselves and question if they were partially at fault, perhaps thinking they were dressed provocatively, had too much to drink, or had placed themselves in a risky situation. Today, professionals recognize that rape is a crime of violence and not of passion; the victim's behavior never warrants the assault. However, societal messages are often mixed, and victims themselves may have conflicted emotions. A prominent trauma researcher, Judith Herman, additionally points out that society must come together and raise awareness of the crimes suffered by women and children in their own homes, and no longer turn a blind eye.[31] Awareness of the issue alone does not

promote justice for women. As a society, we must support survivors in their disclosures and provide care throughout their recovery process.

Etiology

Several theories attempt to explain why rape occurs:

- Sexual Assault and Male Dominance Theory states that rape is the result of social inequality between men and women. Men rape women to assert their male dominance and ensure female subordination. This theory claims that pornography and prostitution encourage rape, because they degrade women and portray them as subservient.
- Cultural Norm Theory posits that rape is learned behavior and is linked to a larger societal pattern of violence. According to this theory, rape is more prevalent in cultures where male physical prowess and honor are revered.
- The Biological Bases Theory of Sexual Assault suggests that reproductive drives, not violence, lead to rape. This theory states that rape is part of a biologic norm in that men are driven to have sex with as many women as possible to advance the species and their status. Women resist because they are biologically driven to mate with only a few chosen males. This latter theory is highly controversial because it relieves any responsibility for rape from the assailant.[49]

The first two theories view rape as an act of aggression and violence rather than an act of passion. This view underlies current rape laws and is generally more accepted. The CDC Rape Prevention and Education Program describes the factors precipitating sexual violence in an ecological model (**Figure 7-1**). When sexual assaults and rapes are considered in this way, the need for programs that address many aspects—from

Figure 7-1 The Ecological Model of Violence Prevention.

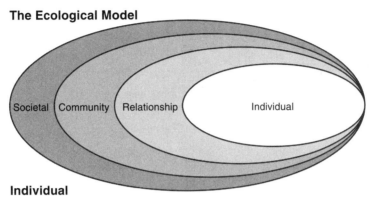

The Ecological Model

Individual
Identifies biological and personal history factors; such as age, education, income, substance use, or history of abuse, that increase the likelihood of becoming a victim or perpetrator of violence.

Relationship
Examines close relationships that may increase the risk of experiencing violence as a victim or perpetrator. A person's closest social circle—peers, partners and family members–influences their behavior and contributes to their range of experience.

Community
Explores the settings, such as schools, workplaces, and neighborhoods, in which social relationships occur and seeks to identify the characteristics of these settings that are associated with becoming victims or perpetrators of violence.

Societal
Looks at the broad societal factors, such as health, economic, educational and social policies, that help create a climate in which violence is encouraged or inhibited and help to maintain economic or social inequalities between groups in society.

Modified from Centers for Disease Control and Prevention. *Sexual violence prevention: beginning the dialogue.* Atlanta, GA: Centers for Disease Control and Prevention; Retrieved from: 2004. Available at: http://www.cdc.gov/violenceprevention/rpe/index.html. Accessed March 17, 2016.

community norms to personal responsibility to economic and social disparities—becomes clearer.

Sequelae

Regardless of the circumstances—where a woman was at the time of the rape, how she was dressed, or whether or not she was under the influence of any substances—no one has the right to force a woman into unwanted sexual activity.

In addition to the many physical, mental, and behavioral issues that may arise in the complex recovery from violence (see **Table 7-1**), specific sequelae to rape include PTSD, depressive and anxiety disorders, other phobias, lowered self-esteem, social adjustment problems, sexual dysfunction, and chronic pelvic pain.[50-67] This constellation of symptoms is sometimes referred to as rape trauma syndrome (RTS). PTSD is reported in 30–45% of women who have experienced a sexual assault.[68,69] Symptoms of PTSD include hyperarousal, re-experiencing the event, avoidance of triggers for remembering, and emotional numbing.

Table 7-1 Sequelae of Violence Against Girls and Women

Physical illness	Headache
	Asthma
	Hypertension
	Gastrointestinal disorders
	Obesity
	Diabetes
	Pelvic or abdominal pain
Reproductive health	Sexual dysfunction
	Unintended pregnancy
	Unsafe abortion
	Inadequate prenatal care
	Sexually transmitted infections including HIV
	Genital bruising or tears
	Traumatic fistulae
Mental health	Depression
	Mania
	Posttraumatic stress disorder
	Anxiety
	Sleep difficulties
	Somatic complaints
	Suicidal behavior
	Panic disorder
Behavioral issues	Unprotected sexual intercourse
	Early consensual sexual initiation
	Multiple partners
	Alcohol and drug abuse
	Tobacco use
	Violent antisocial behavior

Data from World Health Organization.[3,11,50-67]

RTS is variously described in 3–5 phases. As described by the Rape, Abuse and Incest National Network (RAINN), RTS includes the acute phase, outward adjustment phase, and resolution phase. The acute phase following a sexual attack or rape includes symptoms of overtly emotional expressions including agitation, crying, and anxiety; rigid self-control manifesting as decreased emotional expression; and disbelief or disorientation, with decreased memory and difficulty with daily tasks. The outward adjustment phase may include behaviors such as dramatization or minimization of the attack, refusal to discuss the issues, analysis, and/or flight, whether physically leaving the area where the rape occurred or altering other aspects of personal and work life. Women may experience flashbacks or labile emotional responses to daily life. In the third or resolution phase, women begin to adapt to their experience as part of their lives rather than as an overwhelming or central event.[70]

Studies have varied in determining who may seek rape care, but it is clear that a minority of women seek immediate care—21% in one recent study.[71] Resnick, in 2000, found that reporting the assault and "stereotypic" rape (i.e., stranger as perpetrator) and the threat of or actually experiencing injury were associated with seeking immediate care, as were minority status and fear of sexually transmitted infections (STIs) including HIV.[72] More recently, factors associated with seeking early medical care included black race, rape-related injury, concerns about STDs, pregnancy concerns, and reporting the incident to police.[71] In a survey by Amstadter, willingness to seek mental health care after a rape was associated with being white, unmarried, and having PTSD.[73] However, Darnell and colleagues reported that having a developmental or other disability, current mental illness, and being assaulted in public were associated with failure to follow up for psychiatric care, while a prior mental health condition, completing a forensic examination after the rape, and social support were associated with attending follow-up care.[74] A woman may be seen in a clinical setting at any time during her recovery, and may not initially acknowledge her assault; it is incumbent on women's health providers to actively assess for risk.

Responding appropriately to a history of rape, including an assessment of her recovery, can assist the woman in getting the care she needs at that moment. The survivor needs a safe and supportive environment to speak about the incident during each of these phases. Most female survivors indicate that they would like providers to ask about prior sexual violence.[32,75] The assessment and care for women both immediately following a sexual assault and during her recovery are discussed later in this chapter.

Intimate Partner Violence (IPV)

IPV includes physical violence, sexual violence, stalking, and psychologic aggression (including coercive tactics) by a current or former intimate partner (i.e., spouse, boyfriend/girlfriend, dating partner, or ongoing sexual partner).[76] Intimate partners include individuals who are currently in dating, cohabitating, or marital relationships, or those who have been in such relationships in the past. Heterosexual, gay, or lesbian couples all can experience IPV. IPV usually consists of multiple episodes over time and includes a range of tactics that may, or may not, be injurious and/or illegal. This combination of physical, sexual, psychologic, and financial controlling tactics results in fear as well as physical and psychologic harm to the victim and her children. IPV sets up a dynamic of power and control in the relationship. A power and control wheel illustrates the scope of behaviors and was developed, along with an Equality Wheel, by the Duluth Domestic Abuse Intervention Project, and can be purchased for use in clinical settings.[77]

PREVALENCE

More than 1 in 3 American women have experienced IPV during their lives.[3] One in 3 women has been violently attacked by an intimate partner and nearly 1 in 10 has experienced intimate partner rape. Approximately 5.9%, or almost 7.0 million women in the United States, reported experiencing these forms of violence by an intimate partner in the past 12 months.[3] While IPV cuts across all racial/ethnic, age, socioeconomic, and cultural lines, adolescent women and those living in poverty are at higher risk. Among ethnic or racial groups, black, Native American, and non-Hispanic mixed race women are at highest risk.[3] When psychologic aggression—expressive or coercive control—is assessed, nearly half of US women have experienced this at some point.[3] The evidence on whether IPV increases or decreases during pregnancy is conflicting; however, unplanned pregnancies, which account for half of all pregnancies, are a risk factor for IPV. Unintended pregnancy increases a woman's risk of IPV by 2.5 times when compared to an intended pregnancy.[78-80]

ETIOLOGY

IPV often follows a pattern that begins with social isolation and emotional degradation that leads to physical, sexual, and/or financial abuse and assault. In classic situations, the victim of the abuse has been manipulated and isolated to the point that she cannot recognize the abuse as such, so she minimizes the behavior or blames herself. The dual roles of unequal, gendered power relationships and the acceptance of violence as normative behavior have been posited as societal causes of IPV.[81] Other factors identified as personal-level risks include childhood abuse or trauma, substance use by the perpetrator, poverty, exposure to racism or sexism, absence of social support, and limited access to resources.[82] Use of alcohol or drugs by the woman may precede or result from abuse.[82]

The cycle of IPV was first described by psychologist Lenore Walker in her book *The Battered Woman*, currently in its third edition. She described, based on her interviews with women, a cycle that spirals through phases of tension building, violence, and loving contrition.[83] Since then, multiple theories have been proposed; perhaps the most useful because most inclusive is the socio-ecological model shown in Figure 7-1.

SEQUELAE

As with child abuse or sexual assault, women currently living with or having a history of abusive intimate relationships may experience common sequelae (Table 7-1). But unlike the woman who experiences a single sexual assault, women with IPV often experience persistent and prolonged abuse. This leads to a more complex clinical situation, with higher degrees of long-term adverse effects. In particular, rates of PTSD range as high as 84% in studies of women with IPV histories; depression and substance use may both contribute to the likelihood of experiencing IPV and increase as a result.[82] The pattern of sequelae is often referred to as battered woman syndrome, based on Walker's work.

For women living with violence, seeking help is complicated by the effects of IPV as a stigmatized condition. Overstreet and Quinn argue that stigma may be anticipatory, internalized, or cultural, and that each of these impacts the woman's efforts to seek help. Anticipatory stigma is the belief that one will be thought of as "less than" if an experience is revealed. Internalized stigma is the response belief by the woman that she should be ashamed, embarrassed, or that she may be responsible for her abuse. Cultural stigma is the response of others around her to her revelation that devalues her worth because she has been a victim.[84] This aspect is particularly important for clinicians to understand, because even inadvertent signals can make it more difficult for women to seek care.

Assessment and Care for Victims of Violence

Assessment

As many as 50% of women receiving reproductive health care may have experienced IPV.[85,86] The CDC reports that 35.6% of women in the United States have experienced IPV during their lifetime.[3] If screening is to be effective, it needs to be repeated and consistent, including all types of violence and asked of all women. Universal screening is the best way to eliminate bias—real or perceived. Many women do not reveal their histories until there is a level of trust with their provider, sometimes after several visits. The data on benefits of screening are mixed; harm from inquiring is not evident. The US Preventive Services Task Force (USPSTF) recommends screening women of reproductive age.[6] In contrast, the most recent Cochrane summary does not recommend universal screening, arguing that while identification is increased, re-victimization and other outcomes are not affected.[87] Klevens reported no benefit to health outcomes in a series of trials comparing simple provision of literature to screening plus resource provision.[88] The American College of Obstetricians and Gynecologists recommends repeated screening of women, at annual visits, when there is concern based on symptoms or requests for STI or pregnancy testing, during pregnancy "at the first prenatal visit, at least once per trimester, and at the postpartum checkup" as well as continually offering support and referral options.[89] The Institute of Medicine also promotes universally screening women for violence.[90] The American College of Nurse-Midwives states, "appropriate assessment, intervention and referral for violence against women should be an integral part of all health care services provided to women and techniques for this process should be included in all health professional education programs."[91] The significant percentage of women affected mandates screening, but dealing with the issues makes the demonstration of positive benefit challenging. It may be that the real good in screening is that recognition of IPV can be a force for societal change.

IPV screening should be done in a private setting, without partner or family members, including children, present. If translation is needed, it should never be provided by a family member or friend. Each practice should have a standard technique used by all providers, whether that is a self-assessment, staff or provider interview, or computer-based interview or questionnaire.[92-94] Women provided with a computer screen and

intervention in the emergency department reported that they still needed contact with a supportive, compassionate human, even though they found the computer screen acceptable.[94]

In a meta-synthesis on prenatal screening for IPV, LoGiudice reported that providers report barriers to universally screening women such as the patient's partner being present, variations of how and when to ask, feeling lost regarding the management/referral process when a patient does disclose, lack of time to address disclosures, and lack of education on the topic of IPV.[80] Every setting needs to develop techniques for screening and further assessment that meet the needs of privacy, empathy, and useful feedback.

There are validated research tools that screen for IPV; they are complex enough to have limited utility for general screening in busy clinical settings. The CDC reviewed available clinical screening tools and published the tools and existing evidence of their reliability in 2007.[95] None of the brief clinical tools included in Rabin's systematic review has proven to be ideal for both sensitivity and specificity. In addition, they differ in types of IPV screened and difficulty of use.[96]

It is best to use clear language and ask questions directly; however, carefully chosen wording is important. For example, asking a woman if she has been abused may yield a negative response because she does not identify a specific behavior as abusive. It is best to ask about behaviors and feelings. The seminal question for assessing IPV is to ask the client if she is ever afraid of her partner. Being fearful of one's partner is what separates the normal arguments that couples have from a dynamic involving coercion and fear.

Questions about abuse should be incorporated into the routine of history taking and preceded by the statement that all women in the practice are asked three questions as part of the normal history. The questions should be framed in a gender-neutral way, recognizing that whatever their sexual preference or gender identity, any woman may be at risk. Regardless of the answer, women need for their statements to be accepted without judgment. However, before asking for details, the woman needs to know that certain behaviors are illegal, and that if she has experienced these, the clinician must report them.

If one of the standardized tools is not chosen, what follows is a format that can be used for assessing violence of all types:

1. Generalize with an introduction, such as: "We ask everyone in our practice about risks to their health. That includes whether you have ever experienced certain kinds of harm. These questions can be sensitive, but they are important and I am asking them because they can affect your health."
2. Normalize with a statement, such as: "Many women I care for have experienced sexual violence or intimate partner violence. Have you ever experienced or are you experiencing these types of violence?"
3. Provide information about confidentiality and required reporting. Be specific about what the law requires (e.g., statutory rape). "Before you tell me any details, I need to let you know that I am required to report certain illegal activities, such as . . ."
4. Ask about specific types of abuse:
   - Do you ever feel threatened by or afraid of your partner?
   - Does he or she ever do anything to make you feel bad about yourself, like call you names or humiliate you in public?
   - Has anyone ever forced you to take part in any sexual activities that made you uncomfortable?
   - Has your partner refused to use a condom, taken away your birth control, or forced you to have an abortion?
   - Has anyone ever slapped, punched, kicked, bitten, or otherwise hurt you?

All staff members should have basic training in IPV prevention. Every practice member should have access to contacts for resources in the community as well as written material to offer the woman who discloses. These resources include counseling, housing, and support services. Many local, state, or nonprofit agencies can supply appropriate information, including cards small enough to tuck into a private place such as a shoe. The National Domestic Violence Hotline—800-799-SAFE (7233) and 800-787-3224 (TDD)—is available to women 24 hours a day. Futures Without Violence provides many materials, including *Addressing Intimate Partner Violence, Reproductive and Sexual Coercion: A Guide for Obstetric, Gynecologic and Reproductive Health Care Settings*, which can provide assistance with developing clinical practices.[97] Many cities and jurisdictions have police and judges trained in IPV issues, and court advocates may be available for the woman. The local battered woman's shelter, IPV coalitions, or police departments can provide this information about the ex parte system in the area. Ex parte refers to a safety or keep-away order prohibiting contact between the parties. See **Table 7-2** for a list of online resources.

Reporting Abuse

As stated earlier, it is the practitioner's responsibility to know the reporting requirements for his or her jurisdiction. The Futures Without Violence program has a *Compendium of State and U.S. Territory Statutes and Policies on Domestic Violence and Health Care* that can be accessed online.[98] Another important aspect of the law includes the time limits that may exist for prosecution. Many adults may begin to have memories of child abuse, particularly sexual abuse, later in life. The midwife should be prepared to advise the client as to her rights in this matter, or at least be able to access that information easily. This poses some

Table 7-2 Online Resources

Resource	URL	Description
Violence Against Women Network	http://www.vawnet.org/	A comprehensive and easily accessible online collection of full-text, searchable materials and resources on domestic violence, sexual violence, and related issues.
Centers for Disease Control and Prevention—Injury Prevention & Control: Division of Violence Prevention	http://www.cdc.gov/violenceprevention/index.html	Provides resources on multiple forms of violence, including the publication Preventing Multiple Forms of Violence: A Strategic Vision for Connecting the Dots available online at http://www.cdc.gov/violenceprevention/pdf/strategic_vision.pdf and information about ongoing initiatives
National Resource Center on Domestic Violence (NRCDV)	http://www.nrcdv.org	Provides a wide range of free, comprehensive and individualized technical assistance, training, and resource materials. Includes domestic violence intervention and prevention, community education and organizing, public policy and systems advocacy, and funding.
Family Violence Prevention & Services Resource Centers	http://www.acf.hhs.gov/programs/fysb/fv-centers	Parent site for NRCDV and other programs
National Sexual Violence Resource Center	http://www.nsvrc.org/	Collects and disseminates a wide range of resources on sexual violence including statistics, research, position statements, statutes, training curricula, prevention initiatives, and program information
National Network to End Domestic Violence	http://nnedv.org/	A membership and advocacy organization of state domestic violence coalitions, allied organizations, and supportive individuals
Futures Without Violence	http://www.futureswithoutviolence.org/	Advocacy organization providing training and policy work to end violence against women and children
Prevent Child Abuse America	http://www.preventchildabuse.org/	Membership organization; home of the National Center on Child Abuse Prevention
Child Welfare Information Gateway	https://www.childwelfare.gov/	Provides access to print and electronic publications, websites, databases, and online learning tools for improving child welfare practice, including resources that can be shared with families
Family Violence Prevention Fund	http://www.futureswithoutviolence.org	Compendium of State Statutes and U.S. Territories and Policies on Domestic Violence and Health Care: http://www.futureswithoutviolence.org/userfiles/file/HealthCare/Compendium%20Final.pdf
American College of Obstetricians and Gynecologists	Acog.org	Website has screening rubric and patient safety cards available for members, as well as a frequently asked questions page women can access. http://www.acog.org/Patients/FAQs/Domestic-Violence

difficulties, because fewer clients may disclose abuse if they do not want to face potential legal involvement. Each clinician will need to develop a personal approach to this type of assessment, balancing the risks and benefits of assessment with full disclosure.

Clinical Examination When Violence Is Suspected

During the physical examination, clues to ongoing abuse include the appearance of bruises and behavior of the client's partner. Any bruising should be questioned as to how it occurred. Important to note are:

- Bruises that appear to be defensive; for example, on the inside of the forearm or across the palms of the hands.
- Bruises that are incongruent with the client's history. Accidental bruising usually involves the hands, knees, shins, and top of the head. Bruises on the inside of the arms, on the back, or around the upper arms were probably intentionally inflicted.
- Bruises that carry characteristic marks such as those that look like a hand grabbing an upper arm, or carry an outline of a weapon such as an iron or cigarette.
- Bruises in various stages of healing. Just as with child abuse, a woman who is being repeatedly battered may have several bruises in various stages of healing on her body.
- Bruising on the thighs or genitals, or tissue tearing noted during the pelvic examination. Her response to being examined may also suggest current or prior abuse if she resists, dissociates during the exam, or flinches on being touched.

A more subtle indication of an abusive intimate relationship is a partner who appears overprotective. This type of partner wants to be present at every minute of every visit and may even speak for the woman. When such a partner is present, it is critical to find some time alone with the woman to assess the relationship. One way to do this is to escort the woman into the bathroom to "demonstrate how to collect a urine specimen" while politely excluding the partner.

Sexual Assault and Rape Evaluation

If the woman acknowledges rape or sexual assault, then exploring when the rape occurred, if she has previously disclosed this event, and whether she wants support at this time are all relevant issues. If the woman seeks supportive therapy or groups, it is best to refer her to a community resource. Many clinicians have neither the time nor the expertise to provide this service.

When a woman presents for care immediately following a sexual assault, she should be given information about the importance of having a sexual assault exam for evidence collection. She should be counseled that going through this type of exam does not mean that she must participate in legal activities but does have that option. Sexual assault nurse examiners (SANE) are generally available in communities, often within a hospital setting, with SANE-trained personnel and counselors.

Anticipatory guidance for a SANE exam includes counseling that evidence collection can be done for up to 72 hours after the incident using a Physical Evidence Recovery Kit. This involves collecting clothing worn at the time of the assault, combing through pubic and head hair to collect samples, taking swabs from all orifices that were involved in the assault, and perhaps performing a toxicology screen if the assailant used drugs. If the incident occurred more than 72 hours ago, the kit is no longer used. Evidence can still be collected, however, and important services rendered. Although the intent is always to conduct the examination in a way that will minimize further trauma, collecting evidence is a painstaking and invasive procedure. The client should know that she must give written consent to have this exam; she will need to surrender her clothing if it potentially contains biologic specimens that could be matched to an assailant.

If the woman refuses to have a SANE exam, then the midwife should assess and document injuries; perform baseline pregnancy, STD, and HIV screens; and offer emergency contraception. The woman's mental status should be evaluated and appropriate measures taken. Finally, the midwife should document all available details of the incident that might be used later should the client decide to pursue legal action. Photos and/ or use of a body map will be helpful with this type of documentation. Treatment at the time of evaluation includes empiric treatment for gonorrhea, chlamydia, and trichomoniasis; emergency contraception; hepatitis B vaccination and human papillomavirus (HPV) vaccination should be considered; and postexposure prophylaxis for HIV offered as indicated.[99]

Discussing the timing of screening for STIs is essential. The need for possible treatment of an infection already acquired, and/or prophylactic empiric treatment, should be balanced against the possibility that a woman will not return for follow-up care, when testing would be most appropriate. In most locations, evidence about prior sexual activity, including risk of infection, is limited during court proceedings. According to the CDC, if testing is done at the time of a post-assault examination, nucleic acid amplification testing (NAAT) for chlamydia, gonorrhea, and trichomoniasis and wet mount testing should be collected during the pelvic examination, and blood samples for hepatitis B, HIV, and syphilis should also be collected. Positive results will reflect infection prior to the attack.[99] Given that positive results reflect prior infection, it is advisable to treat survivors empirically and defer testing. A positive result indicating prior infection can be used against

the survivor if the case goes to trial. A pregnancy test should be performed and emergency contraception should be offered.

Victims often skip follow-up care. Homelessness, intimate partner assault, drug use, and psychiatric diagnoses increase the likelihood that someone will not return for care.[100] The CDC recommends 1- to 2-week follow up to review test results and test for gonorrhea, chlamydia, and trichomoniasis; 1–2 month evaluation for anogenital warts; repeat syphilis testing at 4–6 weeks and 3 months; and repeat HIV testing at 6 weeks, 3 months, and 6 months.[99]

Documentation

Documentation of abuse must contain the information needed to care for the woman, while recognizing that it may become part of a legal case. Medical records can be subpoenaed. Clear and thorough documentation offers more support for the client in the courtroom.

At the same time, preservation of confidentiality may require some alterations to procedures. Medical records may need to be separated so that notes documenting the abuse are kept separate. The record can be marked in a manner that tells other clinicians to look for the additional notes. These notes are then available for court support as necessary and help clinicians provide ongoing support and care for the survivor but pose less of a risk of breaching confidentiality.

Two other tools for documentation of physical abuse can be helpful: a body map and taking photographs. The body map can be used to record the location of bruises or other marks, and photographs can serve a similar purpose with even more detail and clarity. Keeping a digital camera in the clinic or office setting is useful. Certain guidelines, such as taking pictures from different angles, labeling each photo with the woman's name and date, and placing an object near the bruise or wound (e.g., a ruler or coin) before shooting the photograph will help with determining scale. It is important that a third party (or court) could be able to accurately view the immediate physical aftermath of the abuse long after the woman has healed.

Danger Assessment and Safety Planning

Safety planning is a critical aspect of caring for a woman in an abusive relationship. If the woman discloses a situation that sounds abusive, even if she is unwilling to label it as such, a safety assessment must be conducted to assist her in planning how to keep herself and her children safe should the situation escalate.

Safety planning can be lengthy and assess every aspect of the woman's life as well as her children's, or more succinct with an emphasis on recognizing increased danger and having a plan of response. Therefore, safety planning includes reviewing various situations where abuse may occur and identifying a plan to either avoid or respond to the situation in the safest way possible.

Safety planning may include disclosure about the abuse, and not every woman will be comfortable with providing that information. For example, safety assessment may mean letting neighbors know and asking them to call police if they hear sounds of loud fighting or physical altercation. Similarly, protecting children may involve disclosure to schools or daycare centers.

A plan to leave the situation safely should be developed. Each woman should have a bag prepared that includes a change of clothing for everyone in the family; identification for all members of the family; comfort items for children; keys to the house and car; other important items such as driver's license, insurance cards, birth certificates, and credit cards; and some cash. Each woman should identify someone she can go to if she and her children must leave quickly. She may keep her

bag with that person or outside the house somewhere that is both hidden and accessible. The process of safety planning is often helpful in that it allows the woman to acknowledge and address the abuse.

Abuse generally increases in frequency and severity over time, which increases the risk of lethality. Women must know that the act of leaving is potentially the most dangerous time in the relationship. If the abuser feels that he or she is losing control, then the need to control will escalate and this can translate into more severe forms of violence and even homicide. Therefore, leaving is something that must be taken very seriously. Women, of course, should leave immediately if they believe their life or their children's lives are threatened. Otherwise, having a plan for a safe place to go and having a "safety bag" prepacked will make leaving safely easier if it becomes necessary. **Table 7-3** suggests the types of assessments that should be part of danger assessment and safety planning.

Working with Survivors of Abuse

When assessing for abuse of any kind, the midwife must be prepared with a nonjudgmental and empathetic response that shows unequivocal support for the survivor. If the client has chosen to disclose abuse, the midwife must listen thoughtfully, show empathy, remind the client that it is not her fault, and offer appropriate resources and referrals.

If the client chooses not to disclose abuse and the midwife feels fairly certain that abuse is evident, it is acceptable to state that doubt to the client while not implying that she is lying. This type of response must be thought out. For example, if the woman describes a situation that is clearly abusive but doesn't acknowledge it as such, the midwife can say something like, "What you have described sounds like abuse to me. I would like to give you some resources that tell you more about

Table 7-3 Questions for Danger Assessment and Safety Planning

Assess the immediate safety of the victim.	Is there imminent danger? Where is the perpetrator now? Does the client want or need security at this time?
Assess the pattern and history of abuse.	What type of abuse has occurred? When does it happen?
Counsel regarding safety based on abuse patterns.	Make client aware that increased episodes and severity of abuse as well as certain types of abuse (specifically: sexual, use of weapons, and abuse of children) increases the risk of lethality.
Assess the client's plans at this time.	Is the client planning to stay in the relationship? Does she have adequate safety mechanisms in place? Is her "safety bag" packed? Does she have a plan for escape?
Assess the client's knowledge of resources.	Does she know about local support groups or shelters? Does she know about her legal rights and where to get an *ex parte* should she want one?
Assess the safety of the children.	Are the children being abused? Are they witnessing the abuse? Is she aware of resources for them? Has she noticed changes in their behavior? Does she have a safety plan that includes them?

abuse. Please know that I am here for you and we can talk more about this at a later date if you'd like." Even in the face of compelling evidence to the contrary, it is essential to meet the woman where she is in her process and not try to force her to see things that she is not yet ready to face.

Each client needs time to talk about her experience when she is ready to do so. It is important for the midwife to understand the limits in caring for abuse survivors who may need professional counseling. If memories of abuse are just re-emerging, as can happen when a woman is questioned during an outpatient visit or during the course of a pregnancy, she may need professional support while she acknowledges her history.

Another aspect of management, particularly with rape and sexual assault, is being sensitive to the client's potential unwillingness to disclose a perpetrator who is familiar to her. This may hinder her willingness to disclose the abuse or take legal action. Clients deserve full information about what it means to take legal action as well as the

time to consider all of the implications of disclosing a family member or friend as a sexual assaulter.

The Stages of Change Model, originally developed to assess the process of change in behaviors such as addictions, provides an effective way to form a response and offer appropriate stage-based counseling and resources for women living with abuse.[101] **Table 7-4** provides a framework for using this model to assess and respond to abuse, past or present, in a manner that may be most effective for assisting the survivor in moving to the next phase of change. Using this model meets survivors where they are emotionally, allows them to hear what is being offered, and assists them in moving to the next stage.

Women have identified both motivators and barriers to making change. In one focus group study, participants cited gaining knowledge, reaching an emotional or physical breaking point, and growing concern about children's safety as reasons to seek services.[102] Common barriers included pressure not to talk about IPV, failure

Table 7-4 Stages of Change Model: Abuse Assessment and Response

Stage	Evidence of Stage	Counseling Stage Appropriate	Stage Appropriate Resources
Pre-contemplation: Does not acknowledge that there is a problem.	Denies any abuse, past or present, even in the face of compelling evidence. For example, she may say that the bruises are a result of an accident.	"What you are describing to me would be considered abuse. If you ever want to discuss this with me further, I am always ready to listen."	Materials that define and describe abuse are helpful to give her a name for what is happening to her. The materials may contain links to more resources.
Contemplation: Beginning to acknowledge a problem exists but not ready to do anything about it.	May state something like, "I know there is a problem but what can I do? I can't leave because of the kids."	Respond with acceptance of the difficulties with leaving. Perform a safety assessment as part of counseling on how to remain safe within the relationship.	Phone numbers for a hotline and/or shelter or other community-based resources available if she needs to leave or wants more information.
Preparation: Is considering taking action and is gathering information to prepare for the action.	Client may say something like, "I am interested in seeking help with this situation. Do you have any contacts you can share?"	Warn the client that leaving can be the most dangerous time and counsel how to leave safely (if that is what she is considering).	Give names and numbers for community resources that address her issue (domestic violence shelters, therapists for child abuse, etc.).
Action: Client is taking action to change or address her situation.	She may report that she has left the situation and is staying with friends or at a shelter.	Support her decision and remind her what she needs to do to stay safe; repeat safety planning given her new situation.	Offer support groups; offer to see her more often if needed; referrals for any other assistance she may need for her and her family.
Maintenance	She may report that she has been back and forth but has been out of the situation for a month now and is feeling positive.	Offer support, remind her that relapse is a normal part of the process. Discuss what triggers relapse, offer comments accordingly.	Offer support groups and any resource materials that address the difficulties with staying away.

to recognize that violent behaviors were wrong, self-doubt, low self-esteem, financial constraints, difficulty with transportation, fear of loss, fear of perpetrator, and desire to protect the perpetrator.[102-104] Draucker and colleagues have described in a meta-synthesis four domains of healing: managing memories, relating to important others, seeking safety, and reevaluating self.[105] In order to be successful in moving forward, providers need to help women develop the resources to address each of these—whether it be developing social support that accepts and validates her lived experience, counseling, safety planning, identifying economic resources, or others. By working through each of these processes, women may be able to construct a healthier life view.

Trauma-Informed Care

Both as an organizational structure and as a treatment framework, trauma-informed care is a way to care for survivors of any type of trauma. Trauma-informed care was developed for use with men and women who have experienced violence and are now seeking help to recover.[106,107] Providing this care involves understanding, recognizing, and responding to the long-term effects of all types of trauma. Trauma-informed care also emphasizes safety, not only physical, but also psychologic and emotional, for both patients and providers. The framework aids survivors in rebuilding a sense of control and becoming empowered.[107]

This model of care is utilized in healthcare settings. Linden and Bell discussed their utilization of trauma-informed care when working with survivors of sexual abuse or of any other past trauma during pregnancy and childbirth.[108] Suggestions for the application of this model involve not only support, but shared decision making. The woman should be in control of the healthcare encounter. This control can be given by allowing the patient to remain in her own clothing and to provide input on the order in which the exam is conducted.

During a pelvic exam, a mirror should be offered to the woman to allow her to see what is happening to her body. Trauma-informed care strives to empower survivors and to improve their healthcare experience in order to aid in the recovery process.

Abuse During Pregnancy

Pregnancy and childbirth represent a distinctive part of a woman's lifecycle that are intrinsically linked to her overall physical and emotional health.[109] Childbearing has been identified as one of women's strongest learning experiences.[110] The experience may be negatively affected by a fear-mediated response due to past trauma, such as childhood or adult sexual abuse.[109,111]

Abuse within a relationship may presage an unintended pregnancy if reproductive coercion limits access to contraception.[112] Abuse during pregnancy poses its own special risks and dynamics. The exact incidence and risks associated with IPV in pregnancy are unclear. Incidence rates vary dramatically from study to study, reflecting differences in the definitions used to describe abuse, sample sizes, and characteristics as well as the method, timing, and frequency of screening. Worldwide, the prevalence of IPV during pregnancy ranges from 2% to 13.5%.[113]

Additional factors such as culture and pregnancy intendedness can affect the risk of abuse during pregnancy. For example, one study found that pregnancy protected women against abuse among some Latino cultures, whereas it seems to increase the risk of abuse among white women.[114] Why pregnancy would be protective in some circumstances and risky in others is unclear. Some theorists believe that because abuse is a situation of power and control, the abuser may feel as if he or she is losing some control over the pregnant woman. Abusers are thought to be immature and narcissistic. They may also be jealous of the attention a pregnant woman gives to her unborn baby. This jealousy may increase the risk of IPV. Why pregnancy may be a protector against abuse among some Latino cultures is not completely understood, but may reflect the role pregnancy plays in that culture.

It is well documented that unintended pregnancy is a risk factor for IPV. Unintended pregnancy increases a woman's risk of IPV by 2.5 times when compared to an intended pregnancy.[115] While it is difficult to ascertain which came first, more abuse is reported among women with unintended pregnancies, which represent half of all pregnancies.[115,116] This is particularly true for teens. In a seminal study of medical examiners' records of autopsies of women during their childbearing years, there was a statistically significant higher rate of murder in pregnant teenagers (15–19 years) than nonpregnant teenagers. Most of the teens were less than 21 weeks pregnant.[117] While the study design did not enable the authors to determine causality, the risk of homicide for pregnant teens seems apparent. Therefore, disclosing the results of a positive pregnancy test, to anyone, but particularly to teens should always be done in private.

Sequelae

For survivors, a sense of powerlessness reminiscent of past abuses can be caused by the lack of control experienced as the body physically changes during pregnancy. A history of sexual violence puts women at risk for serious health consequences during pregnancy, such as further violence, suicidal ideation, anxiety, depression, STDs, substance abuse, tobacco use, and pregnancy complications.[3,4] One of the most notable pregnancy complications affecting survivors of childhood sexual abuse is that they are more likely to have a preterm delivery, which is a severe complication of pregnancy with long-term implications for the child.[5] Survivors are also at significantly higher risk to currently be in an abusive relationship where they

or their child may be unsafe.[5] It is important also to screen survivors for suicidal ideation, given they are at increased risk.[5]

Indications of abuse during pregnancy may include low birth weight, prematurity, depression (including postpartum depression), excessive weight gain or loss, and a lack or sporadic use of prenatal care. These indications are also seen in women with a history of abuse who are currently safe. Women with a history of abuse are also more likely to have fear related to labor and birth.[111] Women with these pregnancy histories or who have difficulty with weight gain and general attendance to prenatal care during the pregnancy should be carefully screened and observed for abuse. As with nonpregnant survivors, smoking, drug, and alcohol use; repeated STDs; unintended pregnancies; pregnancy losses; "noncompliance" with treatment; and the other sequelae stated earlier all may be present. Although recognition of women at risk for current violence is important, providers should not screen based on symptoms alone or else they stand to leave out many women who are in danger. Universal screening of all women for violence, regardless of symptomology or presentation, is the recommendation.

Memories of childhood sexual abuse may begin to emerge during pregnancy, sometimes for the first time.[118] It is beneficial to assess for such an abuse history at least once each trimester, and more often if red flags begin to emerge. Signs of an abuse history may include poor attendance at prenatal visits, unrealistic fears, or, in extreme cases, total denial of the reality of labor and delivery. During the physical exam, the midwife should pay attention to signs of weight fluctuations, which can be either weight loss or gain; difficulty with pelvic exams, including disassociation; and scarring from potential self-mutilation or suicide attempts.

During the childbearing period, survivors have indicated they would like healthcare providers to screen them for abuse, to offer support, to allow them to be in control, and to inform them of what is occurring to their body.[32] During labor and birth, some survivors will experience flashbacks to the past abuses during vaginal exams, the epidural placement, or the delivery while others will compartmentalize the past from the current experience.[32] Providing trauma-informed care in the context of the childbearing period would help survivors to become empowered through their birth, in turn, helping them to heal.

Prevention of IPV

Prevention of abuse requires multiple layers of activity. These include empowering women to recognize and reject or leave abusive relationships, changing societal norms that permit violence as an acceptable behavior in relationships, and changing stressors such as poverty or disproportionate opportunities that disrupt relationships.[81] There is some evidence that advocacy work can produce benefits in terms of reduced violence and improved mental health among abused women.[119]

Elder Abuse

Elder abuse is the intentional maltreatment of an adult 60 years or older by either a caregiver or another person with whom there should be an expectation of trust. Just as with other age groups, this can be emotional/psychologic, physical, or sexual. Neglect, abandonment, and financial abuse of a dependent elder are also included in this definition.[120] The National Elder Mistreatment Study found that 10% of survey respondents reported possible abuse or neglect within the prior year. Correlates of mistreatment included low social support and exposure to previous traumatic events.[121] Correlates of increased risks include personal factors (cognitive impairment, behavioral problems, psychiatric or psychologic problems, functional dependency, poor physical health, low income, trauma or past abuse, ethnicity), caregiver burden or stress, psychiatric or psychologic problems of the perpetrator, relationship dysfunction, dependency of the perpetrator on the victim for support, social isolation, and shared housing.[122,123]

For women's health providers, the reason to be alert to elder abuse is the potential for its presentation in clinical practice. The USPSTF has not found sufficient evidence to support universal screening for abuse in the elderly[124] because the cognitive and physical decline associated with aging can make assessment difficult; comprehensive geriatric assessments should be performed by specialized clinicians.

However, history or physical examination findings may raise the possibility of abuse. Some of the items to consider when seeing an elder for care are shown in **Table 7-5**. Many of these items may also be explained by self-neglect, unintentional neglect by a nonresident caregiver, or by medical conditions affecting the health of the woman. For example, many older individuals bruise easily, have situational depression, or eat poorly leading to weight loss.[125,126] It is imperative that questions be asked in a nonthreatening manner, without the caregiver present.[126,127] For example, if malnutrition is suspected, a general question such as, "Who helps you with your meals?" could be followed with, "Does anyone refuse to give you food when you are hungry?" Or more generally, "Do you feel safe at home?" could be followed by, "Does anyone shout at you, hit you, touch you?"

When evaluating findings, the key points to assess are whether the explanation elicited makes sense, what community resources can be offered, and how they will be accepted. When elder abuse is suspected, referral to a geriatric physician or nurse practitioner is appropriate. If there is the appearance of immediate danger, hospital admission to allow more extensive evaluation and reporting to Adult Protective Services are warranted.[126,127] Requirements for reporting in each state can be accessed through the National Center on Elder

Table 7-5 Examples of Possible Findings in Elder Abuse

History	Depression, anxiety
	Insomnia
	Frequent bruising with varied stages of healing at one time
	Loss of appetite/weight loss
	Pelvic pain or discharge
	Burning or pain on urination
	Frequent falls
	Failure to maintain hygiene
	Lack of medication adherence
Physical examination	Extensive bruising
	Marks of physical injury such as welts, scratches, or restraint marks
	Facial injury
	Hair loss (traumatic)
	Physical withdrawal, discomfort, or reluctance to be examined
	Genital lesions, vaginal discharge, or bleeding
	Bruises on thighs, breasts, genitals
	Dehydration or malnutrition
Other	Wariness around caregiver
	Failure to seek care or missed appointments
	Lost or broken glasses, dentures not replaced
	Frequent emergency room visits
	Not able to manage activities of daily living
	Loss of financial control, bills not paid

Data from American College of Obstetricians and Gynecologists. Elder abuse and women's health. Committee Opinion No. 568. *Obstet Gynecol.* 2013;122:187-191; Collins KA. Elder maltreatment: a review. *Arch Pathol Lab Med.* 2006; 130(9):1294; Hoover RM, Polson M. Detecting elder abuse and neglect: assessment and intervention. *Am Fam Physician.* 2014;89(6):453-460.

Abuse (http://www.ncea.aoa.gov/stop_abuse/get_help/state/index.aspx). When abuse or neglect is not involved, the same national resource, or state and local agencies, can assist vulnerable older women to access needed resources.

Incarcerated Women

Although men far outnumber women both in the federal prison system and in local or state jails and prisons, women who are or have been incarcerated experience trauma that may have roots in prior abuse and increases the potential for future emotional and psychologic problems. In 2014, 113,000 women were in state or federal prisons; including women in local jails, more than 200,000 women were incarcerated.[128,129] More than 1 million women are involved in the correctional system when parole and probation are included. The number of women serving sentences greater than 1 year has increased; more than 100,000 were serving longer terms as of 2014. Individuals serving prison time are more likely to be poor, from a racial or ethnic minority, less educated, and in generally poor health.

Black women are now 2.8 times more likely than whites to be convicted, down from a 6:1 disparity in 2000.[130] Fifty-nine percent of women incarcerated in federal prison were serving terms for drug-related offenses, and 24% of those in state prisons.[129] Methamphetamine and prescription drug offenses have increased, as have rates of conviction for violent and property crimes.[130]

Men make up 93% of the prison population.[129] Historically, policies and programs have been developed based on male models. Beginning in 2003, the US National Institute of Corrections has been providing information and assessment tools to improve gender-responsiveness. Gender-responsiveness requires recognizing and developing systems that deal with women's issues and the realities of women offenders' lives.[131] In addition, the Prison Rape Elimination Act (PREA) has potential to improve the lives of female prisoners, who are disproportionately affected by sexual assault and harassment.[132]

Women in the prison system are likely to have minor children, and a majority of women were living with at least one child prior to their incarceration. Forty percent were single parents; the children are either placed with relatives or entered into foster care. Fifty-six percent of women in federal prison and 62% of those in state prisons have minor children.[133] Looked at from the child's perspective, 2.3% of all American children have an incarcerated parent.

Health Concerns

Women entering prison have high rates of victimization through prior sexual or physical abuse and of risky sex or sex work (defined as trading sex for drugs or money).[134-136] Kelly and colleagues reported child or adolescent rates of physical or sexual abuse to be nearly 65%, and current IPV to be 46%.[135] Raj and colleagues reported rates of childhood sexual abuse to be as high as 35%, with lower rates of adolescent or adult abuse.[136] McDaniels-Wilson and Belknap surveyed 391 women and found that 70% had experienced at least one event meeting a generally accepted definition of rape.[137] In the prison setting, more than 75% of staff on inmate sexual misconduct reports involve women victimized by male correctional officers.[128]

Childhood victimization is directly linked to adult mental illness, suicide attempts, and substance use among incarcerated women.[138] Mental health diagnoses in this population are also linked to higher rates of homelessness, foster care, and substance use.[139] Prior diagnoses commonly reported by women entering the jail or prison system include depression, schizophrenia, and bipolar disease. Additional symptoms identified in this population at high rates included anxiety, characteristics of borderline personality, somatization, and trauma-related symptoms.[135,140] The US Bureau of Justice estimates rates of prior mental illness among women at 61–75% depending on type of facility.[139]

Substance abuse, both current and prior, is also common in the prison population. Fazel and colleagues reviewed 13 studies and found reported rates of drug abuse or dependence from 30–60% and alcohol abuse or dependence of 10–24% among female prisoners.[141] Data from the Bureau of Justice Statistics in 2004 found 48–60% of women used drugs in the month prior to their offense.[142] Increases in the use of methamphetamines, most common among white women, have contributed to the rise in the incarceration rate for this group.[143]

Medical needs are increased among women prisoners, compared to the general population. Prior to incarceration, individuals are more likely to access emergency or hospital services than primary care, reflecting access, knowledge, and health needs.[143] Incarcerated women have high rates of hypertension, asthma, arthritis, cervical cancer, and hepatitis compared to the general population.[144] Infectious diseases, including STIs and HIV, are also present at high rates among incarcerated populations.[145-147]

Women's Health Care

The types and quality of health care available to individuals involved in the prison system vary. Improving prison health care is a complex issue, with as many facets as there are responsible jurisdictions. Data suggest that many prisoners receive limited or no medical care, or are off medications for part of their time.[148] However, the Federal Bureau of Prisons has detailed recommendations that include preventive services specific to women, including Pap testing, mammography, and STI screening[149] as do many state systems. Following release, women may lack access to health care and have continuing mental and physical health needs.[150] Soon after release, risk of death is increased, with drug overdose being a leading cause among women.[151]

Offering preventive care in the prison setting may be a valuable opportunity to reach underserved women. Beyond the psychologic, medical, and substance abuse care needed by incarcerated women, the following three areas offer opportunities to address health needs that are specific to women: contraception, STI and cancer screening, and pregnancy concerns.

CONTRACEPTION

Women entering the prison system have well documented risks for unintended pregnancy, and may have lacked the ability to negotiate safe sex and pregnancy prevention prior to incarceration. Many correctional facilities offer limited access prerelease or offer comprehensive counseling.[152] Lack of trust in the prison healthcare system, incorrect knowledge about contraceptive benefits and risks, difficulty with post-release access or discounting the possibility of release are factors that have been cited as discouraging women from choosing to use contraception.[153,154] Long-acting reversible contraceptives (LARC) should not be ruled out of prison programs; they are feasible and safe in this population.[155] Clarke and

colleagues found that the availability of a full range of options, coupled with nurse education on method use, increased prerelease use of effective contraceptives.[154]

STI AND CANCER SCREENING

High rates of STIs including HIV and HPV have been documented among women entering the prison system.[145-147] Limited use of barrier contraception contributes both to risk of infection and to risk of abnormal Pap smears. Studies place rates of reported cervical abnormalities as high as 40–50% among women entering a jail or prison,[156,157] while cervical cancer rates are 4–5 times that of the general population.[158] Women have cited a desire for preventive services while incarcerated. Educational sessions on HPV, vaccination, and STIs can be offered in small-group formats that promote discussion.[156,159]

PREGNANCY CONCERNS

Dignam and Adashi estimate the likelihood that a woman is pregnant during incarceration is 3–10%.[160] Being in the prison population for all or part of a pregnancy may actually benefit women, if there is access to qualified health care.[161,162] As might be expected, pregnant inmates have high degrees of prior stressors, as shown on Pregnancy Risk Assessment Monitory System (PRAMS) data, as well as high rates of tobacco use during pregnancy and substance or alcohol use prior to being incarcerated.[163] They are at increased risk for needing access to services such as the Special Supplemental Nutrition Program for Women, Infants, and Children (WIC) after release.[163]

Shackling is perhaps the most concerning aspect of pregnancy care in the jail or prison setting. The Federal Bureau of Prisons restricts shackling during labor, delivery, and postpartum to the minimum necessary if a woman is a flight risk or has violent behavior. As of 2014, 31 states and the District of Columbia do not have specific laws preventing shackling[160] in spite of the limitations imposed physically by late pregnancy, labor, and birth. The American College of Nurse-Midwives opposes shackling, absent specific risks, at any time during pregnancy, birth, or the immediate postpartum hospital stay.[161]

Programs Addressing These Challenges

Bloom and colleagues noted in their initial report on gender responsiveness that prison staffs often viewed women as difficult, or needy, and sought to clarify both the life experiences and risk factors that would underpin more effective programs for women prisoners.[131] Recommendations for gender-responsive care include addressing the lack of knowledge among prison staff about how men and women differ in communication and relationship styles. Dealing with trauma, substance abuse, and mental health needs requires gender-specific approaches to achieve best outcomes.[131,135] Implementation of PREA should help to reduce not only sexual assault but other forms of harassment and misconduct that disproportionately affect women. Midwives and other women's health practitioners already play a role in many prison settings, with examples that range from direct healthcare provision to educational programs to doula support in labor. Whether women prisoners are seen on site or at a private office, consideration of their vulnerabilities and risks will improve care.

A Final Note for Clinicians

Working with abuse survivors can be challenging in many ways. Addressing and creating solutions to any barriers that may exist to screening will identify more women either at risk or currently experiencing violence, and in turn aid in stopping the cycle of violence. Therefore, all clinicians must both receive education about screening during their training and continually educate themselves on services within their community for women experiencing violence. Adopting a universal screening policy and developing an open and accepting style will lead to identifying more abuse survivors. Clearly, this is desirable for the good that can come to the clients, but it may be challenging for the provider. It can be a heavy emotional burden to know this level of detail about clients' lives, leading to secondary traumatic stress.[164] Additionally, the midwife may feel some responsibility and concern for clients who are not yet ready to end an abusive situation or start legal action against a rapist or molester. It is important to maintain a client-centered focus, regardless of personal beliefs about what someone "should" do.

How one defines success in working with survivors is important. Success may not mean that the woman leaves the abusive relationship or seeks legal recourse for a rapist or perpetrator of previous incest. These may be long-term goals for some clients and not goals at all for others. It is the client's choice. The clinician's role is to actively listen and reflect, and add professional objective information that assists the client in her decision-making process.

Midwives and all healthcare providers are called to change the culture surrounding sexual abuse. For decades, the topic of sexual abuse has been "off limits," and the culture surrounding sexual abuse has been one of placing blame on the victim. Healthcare providers are called to challenge this culture of stigma and to break the silence on this issue. With an understanding of survivors' experiences, concrete changes can be made to the way in which health care is delivered in order to provide safe, therapeutic care to survivors, preventing potential re-victimization in the healthcare setting.

It is helpful to think of every possible action a woman takes as success. Consider the Stages of Change Model and what it takes for humans to move through painful situations. Having a long-term client finally admit to abuse is success. Getting someone to accept a brochure or phone number for a rape crisis center or IPV shelter is success. Maintaining an open, honest conversation with a client about her past or current abuse is success.

References

1. Centers for Disease Control and Prevention. Together for Girls: We Can End Sexual Violence. Available at: http://www.cdc.gov/ViolencePrevention/pdf/TogetherforGirlsBklt-a.pdf. Accessed March 17, 2016.

2. World Health Organization. Violence against women: Intimate partner and sexual violence against women. Fact sheet #239. Available at: http://www.who.int/mediacentre/factsheets/fs239/en/. Accessed March 17, 2016.

3. Black MC, Basile KC, Breiding MJ, Smith SG, Walters ML, Merrick MT, et al. *The National Intimate Partner and Sexual Violence Survey (NISVS): 2010 Summary Report.* Atlanta, GA: National Center for Injury Prevention and Control, Centers for Disease Control and Prevention; 2011.

4. Kendall-Tackett KA. Violence against women and the perinatal period: the impact of lifetime violence and abuse on pregnancy, postpartum, and breastfeeding. *Trauma Violence Abuse.* 2007;8(3):344-353. doi:10.1177/1524838007304406.

5. Leeners B, Rath W, Block E, Görres G, Tschudin S. Risk factors for unfavorable pregnancy outcome in women with adverse childhood experiences. *J Perinat Med.* 2014;42(2):171-178. doi:10.1515/jpm-2013-0003.

6. Tjaden P, Thoennes N. *Prevalence, Incidence, and Consequences of Violence Against Women: Findings from the National Violence against Women Survey.* Washington, DC: Department of Justice; 1998.

7. Breiding MJ, Smith SG, Basile KC, Walters ML, Chen J, Merrick MT. Prevalence and characteristics of sexual violence, stalking, and intimate partner violence victimization. National Intimate Partner and Sexual Violence Survey. United States 2011. *MMWR.* 2014;63(SS08):1-18. Available at: http://www.cdc.gov/mmwr/preview/mmwrhtml/ss6308a1.htm. Accessed March 17, 2016.

8. United Nations Statistics Division. The World's Women 2015: Trends and Statistics. Available at: http://unstats.un.org/unsd/gender/worldswomen.html. Accessed March 17, 2016.

9. Cantor D, Fisher B, Chibnall S, Townsend R. Report on the AUU campus climate survey on sexual assault and sexual misconduct. Available at: http://www.aau.edu/uploadedFiles/AAU_Publications/AAU_Reports/Sexual_Assault_Campus_Survey/Report on the AAU Campus Climate Survey on Sexual Assault and Sexual Misconduct.pdf. Accessed March 17, 2016.

10. Straus MA, Gelles RJ. *Behind Closed Doors. Violence in the American Family.* New York, NY: Anchor Press; 1981.

11. Chiu GR, Lutfey KE, Litman HJ, Link CL, Hall SA, McKinlay JB. Prevalence and overlap of childhood and adult physical, sexual, and emotional abuse: a descriptive analysis of results from the Boston Area Community Health (BACH) Survey. *Violence Vict.* 2013;28(3):381-402.

12. Walters ML, Chen J, Breiding MJ. *The National Intimate Partner and Sexual Violence Survey: 2010 Findings on Victimization by Sexual Orientation.* Atlanta, GA: National Center for Injury Prevention and Control, Centers for Disease Control and Prevention; 2013:18-20.

13. Jindasurat C, Waters E. *Lesbian, Gay, Bisexual, Transgender, Queer, and HIV-Affected Intimate Partner Violence in 2014.* New York, NY: National Coalition of Anti-Violence Programs; 2014.

14. Office for Victims of Crime. Responding to Transgender Victims of Sexual Assault. Available at: http://www.ovc.gov/pubs/forge/sexual_numbers.html. Accessed March 17, 2016.

15. Henk Asscheman H, Giltay EJ, Megens JAJ, de Ronde W, van Trotsenburg MAA, Gooren LJG. A long-term follow-up study of mortality in transsexuals receiving treatment with cross-sex hormones. *Eur J Endocrinol.* 2011;164:635-642. doi: 10.1530/EJE-10-1038.

16. Human Rights Campaign. Addressing Anti-Transgender Violence. Available at: http://www.hrc.org/resources/addressing-anti-transgender-violence-exploring-realities-challenges-and-sol. Accessed March 17, 2016.

17. Ahmed O, Jindasurat C. Lesbian, Gay, Bisexual, Transgender, Queer and HIV-affected Hate Violence 2013. National Coalition of Anti-Violence Programs. 2014. Available at: http://www.avp.org/storage/documents/2013_ncavp_hvreport_final.pdf. Accessed March 17, 2016.

18. Burian J. Helping survivors of sexual abuse through labor. *MCN Am J Matern Child Nurs.* 1995;20(5): 252-256.

19. Parratt J. The experience of childbirth for survivors of incest. *Midwifery.* 1994;10(1):26-39.

20. Rhodes N, Hutchinson S. Labor experiences of childhood sexual abuse survivors. *Birth.* 1994;21:213-220.

21. Seng JS, Sparbel KJH, Low LK, Killion C. Abuse-related posttraumatic stress and desired maternity care practices: women's perspectives. *J Midwifery Womens Health.* 2002;47(5):360-371.

22. King TL, Brucker MC, Kriebs JM, Fahey JO, Gegor CL, Varney H. *Varney's Midwifery.* 5th ed. Burlington, MA: Jones & Bartlett Learning; 2015.

23. Richmond KK. Being whole: Aligning personhoods to achieve successful childbirth with a history of childhood sexual abuse during perinatal services [dissertation]. University of San Diego; 2005.

24. New York Society for the Prevention of Cruelty to Children. History. Available at: http://www.nyspcc.org/about-the-new-york-society-for-the-prevention-of-cruelty-to-children/history/. Accessed March 28, 2016.

25. US Department of Health and Human Services. Administration for Children and Families. Child Abuse and Neglect. Available at: http://www.acf.hhs.gov/programs/cb/focus-areas/child-abuse-neglect. Accessed March 17, 2016.

26. Child Welfare Information Gateway. Mandatory reporters of child abuse and neglect. Washington, DC: US Department of Health and Human Services, Children's Bureau; 2014. Available at: https://www.childwelfare.gov/topics/systemwide/laws-policies/statutes/manda/. Accessed March 17, 2016.

27. Administration for Children and Families. *Child Maltreatment 2013.* Washington, DC: US Department of Health and Human Services; 2015.

28. Stoltenborgh M, van IJzendoorn MH, Euser EM, Bakermans-Kranenburg MJ. A global perspective on child sexual abuse: meta-analysis of prevalence around the world. *Child Maltreatment.* 2011;16(2):79-101.

29. Institute of Medicine, National Research Council. *New Directions in Child Abuse and Neglect Research.* Washington, DC: The National Academies Press; 2014. Available at: http://www.nap.edu/catalog/18331/new-directions-in-child-abuse-and-neglect-research. Accessed March 17, 2016.

30. Westen D. The scientific legacy of Sigmund Freud. Toward a psychodynamically informed psychological science. *Psychol Bull.* 1998;124:333-371.

31. Herman J. *Trauma and Recovery.* New York, NY: Basic Books; 1997.

32. LoGiudice JA, Beck CT. "It was the best of times, it was the worst of times": The lived experience of childbearing from survivors of sexual abuse. *J Midwifery Womens Health.* 2016; (in press).

33. Widom CS, Czaja SJ, DuMont KA. Intergenerational transmission of child abuse and neglect: real or detection bias? *Science.* 2015;347:1480-1485.

34. Berlin LJ, Appleyard K, Dodge KA. Intergenerational continuity in child maltreatment: mediating mechanisms and implications for prevention. *Child Dev.* 2011;82:162-176.

35. Pears KC, Capaldi DM. Intergenerational transmission of abuse: a two-generational prospective study of an at-risk sample. *Child Abuse Negl.* 2001;25: 1439-1461.

36. Thompson R. Exploring the link between maternal history of childhood victimization and child risk of maltreatment. *J Trauma Pract.* 2006;5:57-72.

37. Azar ST, Weinzierl KM. Child maltreatment and childhood injury research: a cognitive behavioral approach. *J Pediatr Psychol.* 2005;30(7):598-614.

38. Lynch M, Cicchetti D. An ecological-transactional analysis of children and contexts: the longitudinal interplay among child maltreatment, community violence, and children's symptomatology. *Dev Psychopathol.* 1998;10:235-257.

39. Drake B, Jolley JM, Lanier P, Fluke J, Barth RP, Jonson-Reid M. Racial bias in child protection? A comparison of competing explanations using national data. *Pediatrics.* 2011;127(3):471-478.

40. Putnam-Hornstein E, Needell B, King B, Johnson-Motoyama M. Racial and ethnic disparities: a population-based examination of risk factors for involvement with child protective services. *Child Abuse Negl.* 2013;37(1):33-46.

41. Lanier P, Maguire-Jack K, Walsh T, Drake B, Hubel G. Race and ethnic differences in early childhood maltreatment in the United States. *J Dev Behav Pediatr.* 2014;35(7):419-426.

42. Bartelink C, van Yperen TA, Ten Berge IJ. Deciding on child maltreatment: a literature review on methods that improve decision-making. *Child Abuse Negl.* 2015;S0145-2134(15):00231-00238.

43. Holz K. A practical approach to clients who are survivors of childhood sexual abuse. *J Nurs-Midwifery.* 1994;39(1):13-18.

44. Norman RE, Byambaa M, De R, Butchart A, Scott J, Vos T. The long-term health consequences of child

physical abuse, emotional abuse, and neglect: a systematic review and meta-analysis. Tomlinson M, ed. *PLoS Med.* 2012;9(11):e1001349. doi:10.1371/journal.pmed.1001349.

45. US Department of Justice. An updated definition of rape. Available at: https://www.justice.gov/opa/blog/updated-definition-rape. Accessed March 28, 2016.

46. Sinozich S, Langton L. Rape and Sexual Assault Victimization Among College-Age Females, 1995–2013. Washington, DC: US Department of Justice Bureau of Justice Statistics. Available at: http://www.bjs.gov/content/pub/pdf/rsavcaf9513.pdf. Accessed March 17, 2016.

47. Centers for Disease Control and Prevention. High School Youth Risk Behavior Survey 2013. Available at: https://nccd.cdc.gov/youthonline/App/Default.aspx?SID=HS. Accessed March 17, 2016.

48. Truman JL, Langton L. Criminal Victimization, 2014. Washington, DC: US Department of Justice Bureau of Justice Statistics; 2015. Available at: http://www.bjs.gov/index.cfm?ty=pbdetail&iid=5366. Accessed March 17, 2016.

49. Thornhill R, Palmer CT. Why men rape. *The Sciences.* 2000;Jan/Feb:30-36.

50. Centers for Disease Control and Prevention. *Sexual violence prevention: beginning the dialogue.* Atlanta, GA: Centers for Disease Control and Prevention; 2004. Available at: http://www.cdc.gov/violenceprevention/rpe/index.html. Accessed March 17, 2016.

51. World Health Organization. Understanding and Addressing Violence Against Women 2012. WHO/RHR/12.37. Available at: http://www.who.int/reproductivehealth/publications/violence/en/index.html. Accessed March 17, 2016.

52. Black MC. Intimate partner violence and adverse health consequences: Implications for clinicians. *Am J Lifestyle Med.* 2011;5:428-439.

53. Cloutier S, Martin S, Poole C. Sexual assault among North Carolina women: prevalence and health risk factors. *J Epidemiol Community Health.* 2002; 56:265-271.

54. Basile KC, Smith SG. Sexual violence victimization of women: prevalence, characteristics, and the role of public health and prevention. *Am J Lifestyle Med.* 2011;5:407-417.

55. Brown DW, Anda RF, Tiemeier H, Felitti VJ, Edwards VJ, Croft JB, et al. Adverse childhood experiences and the risk of premature mortality. *Am J Prev Med.* 2009;37(5):389-396.

56. Chartier MJ, Walker JR, Naimark B. Childhood abuse, adult health, and health care utilization: results from a representative community sample. *Am J Epidemiol.* 2007;165(9):1031-1038.

57. Hosser D, Raddatz S, Windzio M. Child maltreatment, revictimization, and violent behavior. *Violence Vict.* 2007;22(3):318-333.

58. Leserman J. Sexual abuse history: prevalence, health effects, mediators, and psychological treatment. *Psychosom Med.* 2005;67(6):906-915.

59. Link CL, Lutfey KE, Steers WD, McKinlay JB. Is abuse causally related to urologic symptoms? Results from the Boston Area Community Health (BACH) Survey. *Eur Urol.* 2007;52(2):397-406.

60. Lutfey KE, Link CL, Litman HJ, Rosen RC, McKinlay JB. An examination of the association of abuse (physical, sexual, or emotional) and female sexual dysfunction: results from the Boston Area Community Health Survey. *Fertil Steril.* 2008;90(4):957-964.

61. Molnar BE, Buka SL, Kessler RC. Child sexual abuse and subsequent psychopathology: results from the National Comorbidity Survey. *Am J Public Health.* 2001;91(5):753-760.

62. Paolucci EO, Genuis ML, Violato C. A meta-analysis of the published research on the effects of child sexual abuse. *J Psychol.* 2001;135(1):17-36.

63. Rich-Edwards JW, Spiegelman D, Lividoti Hibert EN, Jun HJ, Todd TJ, Kawachi I, et al. Abuse in childhood and adolescence as a predictor of type 2 diabetes in adult women. *Am J Prev Med.* 2010;39(6):529-536.

64. Sar V, Akyuz G, Dogan O. Prevalence of dissociative disorders among women in the general population. *Psychiatry Res.* 2007;149(1-3):169-176.

65. Seng JS, Sperlich M, Low LK. Mental health, demographic, and risk behavior profiles of pregnant survivors of childhood and adult abuse. *J Midwifery Womens Health.* 2008;53(6):511-521.

66. Smith SG, Breiding MJ. Chronic disease and health behaviours linked to experiences of non-consensual sex among women and men. *Public Health.* 2011; 125(9):653-659.

67. Talley NJ, Fett SL, Zinsmeister AR, Melton LJ. Gastrointestinal tract symptoms and self-reported abuse: a population-based study. *Gastroenterology.* 1994;107(4):1040-1049.

68. Resnick HS, Kilpatrick DG, Dansky BS, Saunders BE, Best CL. Prevalence of civilian trauma and post-traumatic stress disorder in a representative national sample of women. *J Consult Clin Psychol.* 1993; 61:984-991.

69. Kessler RC, Sonnega A, Bromet E, Hughes M, Nelson CB. Posttraumatic stress disorder in the National Comorbidity Survey. *Arch Gen Psychiatry.* 1995;52:1048-1060.

70. Rape Abuse and Incest National Network. Available at: https://rainn.org/. Accessed March 17, 2016.

71. Zinzow HM, Resnick HS, Barr SC, Danielson CK, Kilpatrick DG. Receipt of post-rape medical care in a national sample of female victims. *Am J Prev Med.* 2012;43(2):183-187.

72. Resnick HS, Holmes MM, Kilpatrick DG, Clum G, Acierno R, Best CL, et al. Predictors of post-rape medical care in a national sample of women. *Am J Prev Med.* 2000;19(4):214-219.

73. Amstadter AB, McCauley JL, Ruggiero KJ, Resnick HS, Kilpatrick DG. Service utilization and help seeking in a national sample of female rape victims. *Psychiatr Serv.* 2008;59(12):1450-1457.

74. Darnell D, Peterson R, Berliner L, Stewart T, Russo J, Whiteside L, et al. Factors associated with follow-up attendance among rape victims seen in acute medical care. *Psychiatry.* 2015;78(1): 89-101.

75. Robohm JS, Buttenheim M. The gynecological care experience of adult survivors of childhood sexual abuse: a preliminary investigation. *Womens Health.* 1996;24:59-75.

76. Breiding MJ, Basile KC, Smith SG, Black MC, Mahendra RR. *Intimate Partner Violence Surveillance: Uniform Definitions and Recommended Data Elements, Version 2.0.* Atlanta, GA: National Center for Injury Prevention and Control, Centers for Disease Control and Prevention; 2015.

77. Domestic Abuse Intervention Project. Power and Control Wheel. Available at: http://www.theduluthmodel.org/pdf/PowerandControl.pdf. Accessed March 17, 2016.

78. Goodwin MM, Gazmararian JA, Johnson CH, Gilbert BC, Saltzman LE. Pregnancy intendedness and physical abuse around the time of pregnancy: findings from the pregnancy risk assessment monitoring system, 1996-1997. PRAMS Working Group. Pregnancy Risk Assessment Monitoring System. *Matern Child Health J.* 2000;4(2):85-92.

79. Uscher-Pines L, Nelson DB. Neighborhood and individual-level violence and unintended pregnancy. *Urban Health.* 2010;87(4):677-687.

80. LoGiudice JA. Prenatal screening for intimate partner violence: a qualitative meta-synthesis. *Appl Nurs Res.* 2015;28(1):2-9.

81. Jewkes R. Intimate partner violence: causes and prevention. *Lancet.* 2002;359:1423-1429.

82. Hien D, Ruglass L. Interpersonal partner violence and women in the United States: an overview of prevalence rates, psychiatric correlates and consequences and barriers to help seeking. *Int J Law Psychiatry.* 2009;32(1):48-55.

83. Walker LEA. *The Battered Woman Syndrome.* 3rd ed. New York, NY: Springer Publishing Company; 2009.

84. Overstreet NM, Quinn DM. The Intimate Partner Violence Stigmatization Model and barriers to help-seeking. *Basic Appl Soc Psych.* 2013;35(1):109-122. doi:10.1080/01973533.2012.746599.

85. Miller E, Decker MR, Raj A, Reed E, Marable D, Silverman JG. Intimate partner violence and health care-seeking patterns among female users of urban adolescent clinics. *Matern Child Health J.* 2010;14(6):910-917.

86. Miller E, Decker MR, McCauley H, Tancredi DJ, Levenson RR, Silverman JG. Pregnancy coercion, intimate partner violence, and unintended pregnancy. *Contraception.* 2010;81(4):316-322.

87. O'Doherty L, Hegarty K, Ramsay J, Davidson LL, Feder G, Taft A. Screening women for intimate partner violence in healthcare settings. *Cochrane Database Syst Rev.* 2015;7:CD007007.

88. Klevens J, Kee R, Trick W, Garcia D, Angulo FR, Jones R, et al. Effect of screening for partner violence on women's quality of life: a randomized controlled trial. *JAMA.* 2012;308(7):681-689.

89. American College of Obstetricians and Gynecologists. Intimate partner violence. Committee Opinion No. 518. *Obstet Gynecol.* 2012;119:412-417.

90. Institute of Medicine. Clinical preventive services for women: closing the gaps. *Cochrane Database Syst Rev.* 2015;12:CD005043.

91. American College of Nurse-Midwives. *Violence against women.* Position Statement. September 2013.

92. Chen PH, Rovi S, Washington J, Jacobs A, Vega M, Pan KY, et al. Randomized comparison of 3 methods to screen for domestic violence in family practice. *Ann Fam Med.* 2007;5:430-435.

93. Ahmad F, Hogg-Johnson S, Stewart DE, Skinner HA, Glazier RH, Levinson W. Computer-assisted screening for intimate partner violence and control: a randomized trial. *Ann Intern Med.* 2009;151:93-102.

94. Choo E, Ranney M, Wetle T, Morrow K, Mello M, Squires D, et al. Attitudes toward computer interventions for partner abuse and drug use among women in the emergency department. *Addict Disord Their Treat.* 2015;14(2):95-104. doi:10.1097/ADT.0000000000000057.

95. Basile KC, Hertz MF, Back SE. *Intimate partner violence and sexual violence victimization assessment instruments for use in healthcare settings: Version 1.* Atlanta GA: Centers for Disease Control and Prevention, National Center for Injury Prevention and Control; 2007. Available at: http://www.cdc.gov/violenceprevention/pdf/ipv/ipvandsvscreening.pdf. Accessed March 17, 2016.

96. Rabin RF, Jennings JM, Campbell JC, Bair-Merritt MH. Intimate partner violence screening tools. *Am J Prev Med.* 2009;36(5):439-445.e4.

97. Chamberlain L, Levenson R. *Addressing Intimate Partner Violence, Reproductive and Sexual Coercion: A Guide for Obstetric, Gynecologic, and Reproductive Health Care Settings.* 3rd ed. 2013. Available at: https://secure3.convio.net/fvpf/site/Ecommerce/1928921300?VIEW_PRODUCT=true&product_id=1817&store_id=1241. Accessed March 17, 2016.

98. Futures without Violence. Compendium of State and U.S. Territory Statutes and Policies on Domestic Violence and Health Care, 2013. Available at: http://www.futureswithoutviolence.org/userfiles/file/HealthCare/Compendium%20Final%202013.pdf. Accessed March 17, 2016.

99. Centers for Disease Control and Prevention. Sexually transmitted diseases treatment guidelines, 2015. *MMWR Recomm Rep.* 2015;64(No. RR-3):1-137.

100. Ackerman DR, Sugar NF, Fine DN, Eckert LO. Sexual assault victims: factors associated with follow-up care. *Am J Obstet Gynecol.* 2006;194:1653-1659.

101. Prochaska JO, DiClemente CC, Norcross JC. In search of how people change. *Am Psychol.* 1992;47:1102-1104.

102. Petersen R, Moracco KE, Goldstein KM, Clark KA. Moving beyond disclosure: women's perspectives on barriers and motivators to seeking assistance for intimate partner violence. *Womens Health.* 2004;40(3):63-76.

103. Wilson KS, Silberberg MR, Brown AJ, Yaggy SD. Health needs and barriers to healthcare of women who have experienced intimate partner violence. *J Womens Health (Larchmt).* 2007;16(10):1485-1498.

104. Ford-Gilboe M, Varcoe C, Noh M, Wuest J, Hammerton J, Alhalal E, et al. Patterns and predictors of service use among women who have separated from an abusive partner. *J Fam Violence.* 2015;30(4):419-431. doi:10.1007/s10896-015-9688-8.

105. Draucker CB, Martsolf DS, Ross R, Cook CB, Stidham AW, Mweemba P. The essence of healing from sexual violence: a qualitative metasynthesis. *Res Nurs Health.* 2009;32(4):366-378. doi:10.1002/nur.20333.

106. Substance Abuse and Mental Health Services Administration (SAMHSA), National Center for Trauma-Informed Care. Trauma-informed approach and trauma-specific interventions. Available at: http://www.samhsa.gov/nctic/trauma-interventions. Accessed March 17, 2016.

107. The Trauma-Informed Care Project. Available at: http://www.traumainformedcareproject.org/index.php. Accessed March 17, 2016.

108. Linden J, Bell S. Sexual trauma: evaluation and management. A trauma informed care model. In Eckardt MJ,Sayegh R. 12th Annual Boston University School of Medicine Women's Health Conference: Women at Risk—A Special Program in Honor of International Women's Day 2012. Symposium conducted at the Boston University School of Medicine Continuing Education Program, Waltham, MA.

109. Schwerdtfeger KL, Wampler KS. Sexual trauma and pregnancy: a qualitative exploration of women's dual life experience. *Contemp Fam Ther.* 2009;31:100-122.

110. Belenky MF, Clinch BM, Goldberger NR, Tarule JM. *Women's Ways of Knowing.* New York, NY: Basic Books, Inc.; 1997.

111. Heimstad R, Dahloe R, Laache I, Skogvoll E, Schei B. Fear of childbirth and history of abuse: implications for pregnancy and delivery. *Acta Obset Gynecol Scand.* 2006;85:435-440.

112. Miller E, McCauley HL, Tancredi DJ, Decker MR, Anderson H, Silverman JG. Recent reproductive coercion and unintended pregnancy among female family planning clients. *Contraception.* 2014;89(2):122-128. doi:10.1016/j.contraception. 2013.10.011.

113. Devries KM, Kishor S., Johnson H, Stöckl H, Bacchus LJ, Garcia-Morena, et al. Intimate partner violence during pregnancy: analysis of prevalence data from 19 countries. *Reprod Health Matters.* 2010;18(36):158-170.

114. Torres S, Campbell J, Campbell D, Ryan J, King C, Price P, et al. Abuse during and before pregnancy: prevalence and cultural correlated. *Violence Vict.* 2000;15:303-321.

115. Goodwin M, Gazmararian J, Johnson C, Gilbert B, Saltzman L. Pregnancy intendedness and physical abuse around the time of pregnancy: findings from the Pregnancy Risk Assessment Monitoring System, 1996-1997. *Matern Child Health J.* 2000;4(2):85-92.

116. Paluzzi P. The Relationship between Drug Use and the Experience of Physical Violence among Inner City Pregnant Women [Doctoral Thesis]. Baltimore, MD: Johns Hopkins School of Public Health; 2001.

117. Krulewitch CJ, Pierre-Louis ML, de Leon-Gomez R, Guy R, Green R. Hidden from view: violent deaths among pregnant women in the district of Columbia, 1988–1996. *J Midwifery Womens Health.* 2001;46(1):4-10.

118. Simkin P, Klaus P. *When Survivors Give Birth.* Seattle, WA: Classic Day Publishing; 2004.

119. Ramsay J, Carter Y, Davidson L, Dunne D, Eldrige S, Feder G, et al. Advocacy interventions to reduce or eliminate violence and promote the physical and psychosocial well-being of women who experience intimate partner abuse. *Cochrane Database Syst Rev.* 2009(3)CD005043.

120. Centers for Disease Control and Prevention. Elder Abuse: Definitions. Available at: http://www.cdc.gov/violenceprevention/elderabuse/definitions.html. Accessed March 17, 2016.

121. Acierno R, Hernandez MA, Amstadter AB, Resnick HS, Steve K, Muzzy W, et al. Prevalence and correlates of emotional, physical, sexual, and financial abuse and potential neglect in the United States: the national elder mistreatment study. *Am J Public Health*. 2010;100(2):292-297.

122. Johannesen M, LoGiudice D. Elder abuse: a systematic review of risk factors in community-dwelling elders. *Age Ageing*. 2013;42:292-298.

123. Lachs, MS, Pillemer K. Elder abuse. *Lancet*. 2004;364(9441):1263-1272.

124. Moyer VA, on behalf of the US Preventive Services Task Force. Screening for intimate partner violence and abuse of elderly and vulnerable adults: US Preventive Services Task Force Recommendation Statement. *Ann Intern Med*. 2013;158:478-486.

125. Collins KA. Elder maltreatment: a review. *Arch Pathol Lab Med*. 2006;130(9):1294.

126. Hoover RM, Polson M. Detecting elder abuse and neglect: assessment and intervention. *Am Fam Physician*. 2014;89(6):453-460.

127. American College of Obstetricians and Gynecologists. Elder abuse and women's health. Committee Opinion No. 568. *Obstet Gynecol*. 2013;122:187-191.

128. The Sentencing Project. Fact Sheet: Incarcerated Women. Washington DC: The Sentencing Project; 2013. Available at: http://www.sentencingproject.org/doc/publications/cc_Incarcerated_Women_Factsheet_Dec2012final.pdf. Accessed March 17, 2016.

129. Carson A. *Correctional Populations in the United States 2014*. Washington, DC: United States Department of Justice, Bureau of Justice Statistics; 2015.

130. Mauer M. The Changing Racial Dynamics of Women's Incarceration. The Sentencing Project; 2013. Available at: http://sentencingproject.org/doc/publications/rd_Changing%20Racial%20Dynamics%202013.pdf. Accessed March 17, 2016.

131. Bloom B, Owen B, Covington S. Gender-Responsive Strategies: Research, Practice, and Guiding Principles for Women Offenders. National Institute of Corrections, June 2003. Available at: https://s3.amazonaws.com/static.nicic.gov/Library/018017.pdf. Accessed March 17, 2016.

132. Guerino P, Beck JA. Prison Rape Elimination Act of 2003 (PREA): Sexual Victimization Reported by Adult Correctional Authorities, 2007–2008. United States Department of Justice, Bureau of Justice Statistics, January 2011.

133. Glaze LE, Maruschak LM. Parents in Prison and Their Minor Children. United States Department of Justice, Bureau of Justice Statistics, August 2008.

134. Fickenscher A, Lapidus J, Silk-Walker P, Becker T. Women behind bars: health needs of inmates in a county jail. *Public Health Rep*. 2001;116(3):191-196.

135. Kelly PJ, Cheng A-L, Spencer-Carver E, Ramaswamy M. A syndemic model of women incarcerated in community jails. *Public Health Nurs*. 2014;31(2):118-125. doi:10.1111/phn.12056.

136. Raj A, Rose J, Decker M, Rosengard C, Hebert M, Stein M, et al. Prevalence and patterns of sexual assault across the life span among incarcerated women. *Violence against Women*. 2008;14:528-541.

137. McDaniels-Wilson C1, Belknap J. The extensive sexual violation and sexual abuse histories of incarcerated women. *Violence Against Women*. 2008;14(10):1090-1127.

138. Tripodi SJ, Pettus-Davis C. Histories of childhood victimization and subsequent mental health problems, substance use, and sexual victimization for a sample of incarcerated women in the US. *Int J Law Psychiatry*. 2013;36(1):30-40.

139. James DJ, Glaze LE. Mental Health Problems of Prison and Jail Inmates. United States Department of Justice, Bureau of Justice Statistics, September 2006.

140. Drapalski AL, Youman K, Stuewig J, Tangney J. Gender differences in jail inmates' symptoms of mental illness, treatment history and treatment seeking. *Crim Behav Ment Health*. 2009;19(3):193-206. doi: 10.1002/cbm.733.

141. Fazel S, Bains P, Doll H. Substance abuse and dependence in prisoners: a systematic review. *Addiction*. 2006;101(2):181-191.

142. Mumola CJ, Karberg JC. Drug Use and Dependence, State and Federal Prisoners, 2004. United States Department of Justice, Bureau of Justice Statistics, October 2006.

143. Ramaswamy M, Diaz F, Pankey T, Hunt SL, Park A, Kelly PJ. Correlates of preincarceration health care use among women and men in jail. *J Correct Health Care*. 2015;21(3):286-297.

144. Binswanger IA, Merrill JO, Krueger PM, White MC, Booth RE, Elmore JG. Gender differences in chronic medical, psychiatric, and substance-dependence disorders among jail inmates. *Am J Public Health*. 2010;100(3):476-482.

145. Centers for Disease Control and Prevention. HIV Among Incarcerated Populations. Available at: http://www.cdc.gov/hiv/group/correctional.html. Accessed March 17, 2016.

146. Parvez F, Katyal M, Alper H, Leibowitz R, Venters H. Female sex workers incarcerated in New York City jails: prevalence of sexually transmitted infections and associated risk behaviors. *Sexually Transm Infect.* 2013;89(4):280-284.

147. Javanbakht M, Boudov M, Anderson LJ, Malek M, Smith LV, Chien M, et al. Sexually transmitted infections among incarcerated women: findings from a decade of screening in a Los Angeles County jail, 2002–2012. *Am J Public Health.* 2014; 104(11):e103-e109.

148. Wilper AP, Woolhandler S, Boyd JW, Lasser KE, McCormick D, Bor DH, et al. The health and health care of U.S. prisoners: results of a nationwide survey. *Am J Public Health.* 2009;99(4):666-672.

149. Federal Bureau of Prisons. Preventive Health Care: Federal Bureau of Prisons Clinical Practice Guidelines. 2013. Available at: http://www.bop.gov/resources/pdfs/phc.pdf. Accessed March 17, 2016.

150. Turney K, Wildeman C. Self-reported health among recently incarcerated mothers. *Am J Public Health.* 2015;105:2014-2020.

151. Binswanger IA, Blatchford PJ, Mueller SR, Stern MF. Mortality after prison release: opioid overdose and other causes of death, risk factors, and time trends from 1999 to 2009. *Ann Intern Med.* 2013; 159:592-600.

152. Sufrin CB, Creinin MD, Chang JC. Contraception services for incarcerated women: a national survey of correctional health providers. *Contraception.* 2009; 80(6):561-565.

153. Schonberg D, Bennett AH, Sufrin C, Karasz A, Gold M. What women want: a qualitative study of contraception in jail. *Am J Public Health.* 2015; 105(11):2269-2274.

154. Clarke JG, Rosengard C, Rose JS, Hebert MR, Peipert J, Stein MD. Improving birth control service utilization by offering services prerelease vs postincarceration. *Am J Public Health.* 2006;96:840-845.

155. Sufrin C, Oxnard T, Goldenson J, Simonson K, Jackson A. Long-acting reversible contraceptives for incarcerated women: feasibility and safety of on-site provision. 2015;47(4):203-211.

156. Nijhawan AE, Salloway R, Nunn AS, Poshkus M, Clarke JG. Preventive healthcare for underserved women: results of a prison survey. *J Womens Health.* 2010;19(1):17-22.

157. Binswanger IA, Mueller S, Clark CB, Cropsey KL. Risk factors for cervical cancer in criminal justice settings. *J Womens Health.* 2011;20(12): 1839-1845.

158. Binswanger JA, Krueger PM, Steiner JF. Prevalence of chronic medical conditions among jail and prison inmates in the United States compared with the general population. *J Epidemiol Community Health.* 2009;63:912-919.

159. Ramaswamy M, Simmons R, Kelly PJ. The development of a brief jail-based cervical health promotion intervention. *Health Promot Pract.* 2015; 16(3):432-442.

160. Dignam B, Adashi EY. Health rights in the balance: the case against perinatal shackling of women behind bars. *Health Hum Rights.* 2014;16(2):E13-E23.

161. Knight M, Plugge. The outcomes of pregnancy among imprisoned women: a systematic review. *BJOG.* 2005;112:1467-1474.

162. Bell JF, Zimmerman FJ, Cawthon ML, Huebner CE, Ward DH, Schroeder CA. Jail incarceration and birth outcomes. *J Urban Health.* 2004;81(4): 630-644.

163. Dumont DM, Wildeman C, Lee H, Gjelsvik A, Valera PA, Clarke JG. Incarceration, maternal hardship, and perinatal health behaviors. *Matern Child Health J.* 2014;18(9):2179-2187.

164. Beck CT, LoGiudice J, Gable RK. A mixed-methods study of secondary traumatic stress in certified nurse-midwives: shaken belief in the birth process. *J Midwifery Womens Health.* 2015;60:16-23.

CHAPTER 8

NEUROLOGY

Lynn C. Simko

Introduction

The central nervous system is the captain of all body systems. It regulates everything from the body's response to cold (piloerection) to stress (increased rate and depth of breathing, dilated pupils, and tachycardia seen with the fight-or-flight response) and regulates blood flow to vital organs through vasoconstriction and vasodilation. Additionally, the brain has endocrine organs, including the hypothalamus and the pituitary gland, which can affect metabolism and the release of a host of hormones including growth hormone, luteinizing hormone, follicle-stimulating hormone, prolactin, melanocyte-stimulating hormone, vasopressin, and oxytocin.[1] The central nervous system is a complex organ. Successful treatment of neurologic disorders requires that an astute history and physical assessment be done in order to make a correct differential diagnosis and treatment plan. This chapter will equip women's health providers with the knowledge necessary to diagnosis, treat, and, if needed, refer a woman for specialty care for a neurologic problem.

Common Symptoms

Symptoms suggestive of an underlying neurologic disorder include *headaches, vertigo, dizziness, numbness, weakness, tingling,* and *paresthesias.* The most common of these are headaches. As a symptom, headaches are nonspecific and most are benign. In addition to the primary headache disorders, they are associated with a wide range of conditions such as fever, sinus congestion, and hypoglycemia, among other conditions. **Table 8-1** describes the most common symptoms of benign headache disorders.[2] Clues elicited through a thorough history and physical examination can help distinguish among the possibilities. The new onset of a severe headache can be associated with a number of critical neurologic disorders such as brain tumor, meningitis, or a hemorrhagic cerebral vascular accident.

Vertigo and dizziness account for about 5–6% of all visits to healthcare providers. It can be difficult to differentiate dizziness and vertigo and often women use these terms interchangeably; however, they are not the same sensation. *Dizziness* is an

Table 8-1 Symptoms of Common Headaches

Characteristics	Tension-Type	Cluster	Migraine Without Aura	Migraine with Aura
Quality of Pain				
Severe		X	X	X
Dull	X			
Throbbing			X	X
Nonthrobbing	X			
Sharp or jab-like		X		
Tightness	X			
Location of Pain				
Unilateral		X	X	X
Bilateral	X			
Temporal		X	X	X
Frontal	X		X	X
Occipital	X		X	X
Cervical spine	X			
Ocular		X		
Duration of Pain	30 minutes–7 days	15 minutes–3 hours	4–72 hours	5–60 minutes

Data from Cox B. The principles of neurological assessment. *Pract Nurs*. 2008;36(7):45-50; Hainer BL, Matheson EM. Approach to acute headache in adults. *Am Fam Physician*. 2013 May 15;87(10):682-687.

imprecise term that includes feelings of faintness, lightheadedness, and unsteadiness. *Vertigo* is defined as an illusion of movement of self or the environment. Vertigo is often described as a spinning or wheeling sensation; women complain that they feel like the room is circling around them. Symptoms are usually associated with changes in head position.[4]

Vertigo is closely associated with problems in the inner ear (vestibular disorders). The labyrinth, an inner ear neurosensory organ, is made up of two components: the cochlea, used for hearing, and the semicircular canals, used for balance. Usually, vertigo is initiated by an inequity of sensory inputs into the two vestibular nuclei from more, or less, activity of either or both parts of the labyrinth. Any disorders of the labyrinth, visual-vestibular interaction nuclei in the brain stem and cerebellum, and sensory pathways to or from the thalamus can cause vertigo.[5] Conditions associated with vertigo are listed in **Table 8-2**.

Numbness can be described as a loss of sensation or feeling in a particular part of the body. Other sensations such as feeling "pins and needles" are also present.[7] The underlying cause is usually due to transient compression or prolonged neurologic damage and neuropathy. In the first case, complete resolution of symptoms occurs with position change. In the second case, neuropathy is caused by a chronic disease such as diabetes, and the symptoms are permanent.[7]

Table 8-2 Causes of Vertigo

Disorder	Description of the Disorder
Benign paroxysmal positional vertigo (BPPV)	BPPV causes intense, short episodes of vertigo instantaneously following a change in the position of the patient's head. It often occurs when the patient turns over in bed or sits up in the morning. BPPV is the most common etiology of vertigo.
Inflammation in the inner ear (known as acute vestibular neuritis)	Signs and symptoms of inflammation in the inner ear include sudden onset of extreme constant vertigo that may last for several days, along with nausea and vomiting and trouble with balance. When linked with sudden hearing loss, it is called labyrinthitis. The condition will clear spontaneously, although medical care may speed recovery.
Meniere's disease	Excessive buildup of fluid in the patient's inner ear leads to abrupt episodes of vertigo persisting as long as several hours accompanied by variable hearing loss, ringing in the ear, and a sensation of fullness in the involved ear.
Vestibular migraine	Some patients who have migraine with aura may have an vertigo or dizziness. Such vertigo incidents can last hours to days and can be linked with a migraine headache to noise and light sensitivity.
Acoustic neuroma	A benign tumor on the vestibular nerve, acoustic neuroma produces gradual hearing loss and tinnitus on one side accompanied by dizziness or imbalance.
Other causes	Rarely, vertigo can be a symptom of a serious neurologic problem such as a stroke, multiple sclerosis, or brain hemorrhage. Other neurologic abnormalities typically are present including diplopia, slurred speech, limb incoordination, and facial weakness or numbness.

Data from Tusa R. Dizziness. *Med Clin North Am.* 2009;93:263; Wipperman J. Dizziness and vertigo. *Prim Care.* 2014 Mar;41(1): 115-131. doi: 10.1016/j.pop.2013.10.004.

Paresthesia is a sensation of tickling, tingling, burning, or pricking of the skin with no apparent long-term physical effect.[8] The underlying pathophysiology is the same as that leading to numbness: compression or neuropathy. Like numbness, it is almost always a transient feeling, but may become permanent if significant neurologic damage has occurred.[8]

Weakness is reduced strength in one or more muscles/muscle groups. Weakness may be all over the body or occur only on one side of the body, in one muscle, or along one limb. Weakness is more notable when it is concentrated in one area versus being more widespread. Weakness in one area

may occur due to a stroke, during a flare-up of multiple sclerosis (MS), or after injury to a nerve. Weakness can be a subjective or objective finding. It is subjective when a woman reports she is weak even though there is no real loss of strength (e.g., as a result of the flu) or objective if found during a physical exam by a medical practitioner.[9] True weakness or neuromuscular weakness describes a condition where the force exerted by the muscles is less than would be expected.[10]

Weakness can be due to central or local disruptions in neural pathways governing muscle contraction and/or the release of calcium at the local level. These processes impede the 'flow' of electrical impulses from the brain, which signals them to contract through the release of calcium by the sarcoplasmic reticulum. Fatigue (reduced ability to generate force) may occur due to malfunctions in the nerve or within the muscle cells themselves. Research suggests that muscle fatigue is caused by calcium leaking out of the muscle cell.[10] This makes less calcium available for the muscle cell. Enzymes activated by this released calcium are theorized to erode muscle fibers.

Substrates within the muscle generally serve to power muscular contractions. They include molecules such as adenosine triphosphate (ATP), creatine phosphate, and glycogen. ATP binds to the myosin head and causes the "ratcheting" that results in contraction according to the sliding filament model. Creatine phosphate stores energy so ATP can be rapidly regenerated within the muscle cells from adenosine diphosphate (ADP) and inorganic phosphate ions, allowing for sustained powerful contractions that last between 5 and 7 seconds. Glycogen is the intramuscular storage form of glucose used to generate energy quickly.[10] Exercise depletes substrates and energy stores. Without sufficient energy, muscles cannot contract.

Syncope is defined as a transient and abrupt loss of consciousness with complete return to preexisting neurologic function.[9-11] Syncope is not a diagnosis in and of itself, but a symptom of an underlying cause. Syncope has multiple etiologies, with most carrying a benign prognosis, but a few less common causes can carry a risk of serious morbidity or death.[12] The pathophysiologic process that prompts syncope is hypoperfusion to the brain.[13] Prior classifications of syncope have been based on etiologic grounds, but a more recent proposal suggests that this classification should be replaced by a mechanistic approach.[14] Syncope is now classified as neurally mediated (i.e., situational, vasovagal, or carotid sinus hypersensitivity), orthostatic, neurogenic, or cardiac.[11]

General Approach to Investigating Neurologic Problems

History

The resolution of common neurologic problems first requires an accurate diagnosis. Often a careful assessment of a woman's symptoms will make the diagnosis clear without the need to order adjunctive laboratory or imaging studies. Understanding the timeline of symptoms, when they occurred, and how they initially presented and then evolved over time; the frequency and characteristics of symptoms; whether symptoms are episodic or continuous; and the degree to which symptoms interfere with daily living or sleep can help pinpoint the possibilities and direct the focus of the physical exam.[3]

Abbreviated Neurologic Exam

A basic neurologic assessment should be done in general practice, because it can uncover neurologic abnormalities, which may then require referral and further investigation.[15] Standard components of a neurologic examination include an evaluation of mental status, coordination, and reflexes, as well as testing of the cranial, sensory, and motor nerves.[15,16] *Mental status exam* is often referred to as higher cortical functioning assessment. This part of the neurologic assessment examines the woman's orientation to person, place and time, general information, short and long-term memory, and the use of numbers and spelling.[16] In the process of history taking, the woman's memory and intelligence are revealed; in completion of the forms, spelling and orientation to person (listing and checking their name), and time (with the date) can be assessed; the fact that the woman came to the appropriate office building demonstrates orientation to place; answering questions about a woman's health history helps indicate short- and long-term memory; and payment of the visit's copay does assess the use of numbers.[16] In summary, level of consciousness (LOC) is assessed during the history taking.[15]

The Glasgow Coma Scale (GCS) also assists with assessing a woman's LOC for women who are more neurologically debilitated. It measures eye opening, motor response, and verbal response. The highest possible score is a 15, with a score of 7 or lower representing a comatose state. The lower the GCS score, the lower the LOC.[17] See **Table 8-3** for GCS scoring.

Motor functioning assesses power and tone of the body. When examining the arms and legs, one should look for any asymmetry, muscle wasting, or floppiness. By going through passive range of motion (ROM) of the extremities, one can assess muscle tone and range of movement. Muscular strength can be assessed by asking the woman to push against the examiner's resistance. As an initial basic neurologic examination, ask the woman to squeeze both of your hands and to push back against pressure with both arms and legs.[15] **Table 8-4** presents the grading of muscle strength. Muscle strength is charted as the muscle strength over 5, such as 3/5 indicating fair muscle strength or a 5/5 for normal muscle strength assessment.

Additional *sensory testing* that should be done includes testing vibration, joint position sense, and pinprick sensation. Sensation can be assessed by dermatomes, which correspond with the sensory nerve root responsible for the symptoms. Sensory testing can be assessed by testing responsiveness to hot and cold, pain and vibration, or sharp and dull. A 128 Hz tuning fork is used to determine awareness of vibrations. Sensory perception of pain can be tested using a sharp object, such as a safety pin or toothpick. Distinguishing sharpness from dullness can be elicited by comparing the sensation produced from being touched by the sharp end of the pin/toothpick to the sensation produced by being touched by

the rounded end of the pin/toothpick. A cotton ball can be used to assess the ability to distinguish a soft touch.[15] Testing joint position sense should be performed on the great toe and index finger. The examiner should hold the digits by the lateral and medial sides during testing. The woman opens her eyes while the examiner moves

Table 8-3 Glasgow Coma Scale

Components	Score
Eye Opening	
Spontaneous	4
To sound	3
To pain	2
Never	1
Motor Response	
Obeys commands	6
Localizes pain	5
Normal flexion (withdrawal)	4
Abnormal flexion	3
Extension	2
No response	1
Verbal Response	
Oriented	5
Confused conversation	4
Inappropriate words	3
Incomprehensible sounds	2
No response	1

Scores range from a low of 3 to a high of 15.

If the patient is intubated and cannot talk, record the score with a "t" after the number. The best possible score for an intubated patient is 11t (eye opening of 4t, motor response 6t, verbal response 1t).

Reproduced from Teasdale G, Jennett B. Assessment of coma and impaired consciousness. A practical scale. *Lancet.* 1974;2(7872): 81-4. © 1974 with permission from Elsevier; Croft A. The practical neurological examination. *Dyn Chiropract.* 2011;29(4):14,37.

Table 8-4 Grading Muscle Strength

Rating	Description
0	Zero: no evidence of muscle contractility
1	Trace: no joint motion and slight evidence of muscle contractility
2	Poor: can complete ROM with gravity eliminated
3	Fair: can complete ROM against gravity
4	Good: can complete ROM against gravity with some resistance
5	Normal: ROM unimpaired against gravity with full resistance

ROM = range of motion

the toe up or down; then the woman closes her eyes and is asked whether the digit is up or down. All of the assessments of sensory perception must be completed with the woman's eyes closed. The most critical area to assess is at the distal end of the extremity, because this indicates that the entire dermatome is neurologically intact.[17]

Reflexes, which transform sensory messages into motor actions, are carried by way of the spinal cord nerves. Reflexes depend on functioning sensory and motor neurons. *Deep tendon reflexes* include the biceps, triceps, brachioradial, patella, and Achilles. See **Figure 8-1** for an illustration of eliciting each reflex. Stimulation of all of these deep reflexes should cause a jerk if the spinal nerve is intact. If no jerk is assessed, then there is a problem with the passage of the message toward (sensory nerve) or away (motor nerve) from the spinal cord.[16] If one has difficulty in eliciting a positive reflex response, one can always have the woman consciously contract muscles in order to stimulate the deep tendon reflex. For example, if the provider is having difficulty eliciting a patellar or Achilles reflex, the woman can be asked to cross her arms and forcibly cause resistance from one arm to the other. Similarly, if the provider is having difficulty eliciting an upper body deep tendon reflex, the woman should be asked to consciously push one leg against the other from the hip to the knees. These maneuvers will enhance the reflex response so it can be assessed. The grading of reflexes is summarized in **Table 8-5**.

Cranial nerve assessment of the 12 cranial nerves is easily done. **Table 8-6** explains the testing of the 12 cranial nerves along with their classification as sensory, motor, or both. Cranial nerve assessment should be done if a problem affecting the cranial nerve is suspected such as in the presence of symptoms suggestive of stroke, a new-onset headache, or vague complaints of weakness or syncope.

Assessment of *coordination, joint position sense, proprioception,* and *cerebellar function* can be done with the woman sitting on an exam table and with the woman standing. To assess proprioception, have the woman stand upright and stay still for 20 seconds. Then ask the woman to close her eyes but remain standing still. Stand near the woman in the event she falls; a normal response is to sway only slightly and to be able to hold this position with the eyes closed. If the woman is unable to stand with her eyes closed, this is considered to be a positive Romberg test. Most often this is due to proprioceptive problems and is likely to be cerebellar in origin.[16] Heel-to-toe walking may help to distinguish gait disturbance; one may also have the woman walk on tiptoes and heels. Test the pronator drift by asking the woman to keep her arms out in front, palms facing upward, with eyes open and then closed. Any drifting of either arm downward is an abnormal/positive pronator drift.

Figure 8-1 Demonstration of deep tendon reflex responses.

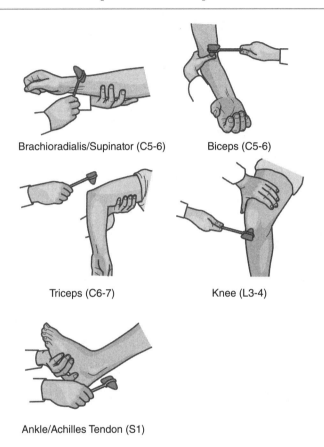

Brachioradialis/Supinator (C5-6)   Biceps (C5-6)

Triceps (C6-7)   Knee (L3-4)

Ankle/Achilles Tendon (S1)

Table 8-5 Scale for Recording Reflex Activity

Numerical Scale/+ Scale	Scale for Recording Reflex Activity
0	Absent, no response
1(+)	Slightly present
2(++)	Normal
3(+++)	Stronger, more brisk than average
4(++++)	Hyperactive
	1 and 3 may be normal for some patients

Table 8-6 Assessment of the Cranial Nerves

Cranial Nerve	Sensory	Motor	How to Assess
CN I	CN I		Check air movement and scent in each nostril separately. Ask for recognition of a familiar scent such as coffee, soap, or peppermint with eyes closed (not usually assessed).
CN II, CN III	CN II	CN III	Visual acuity: A Snellen chart or written text is used. Ability to read, using glasses or contacts if worn regularly. Check both distance and near vision.
			Visual fields: With each eye covered in turn, the location at which one can see a finger held at the outer edge of each quadrant and moved inward until seen.
			Perform fundoscopy as indicated by symptoms.
CN III, CN IV, CN VI		CN III, CN IV, CN VI	Pupils should be *equal* in size, *round* and *regular* in shape, and react to *light* and *accommodation* (PERRLA). Shine a bright light into one eye at a time; the pupils should constrict rapidly. Have the patient focus on your index finger and then slowly move it to the patient's nose; the pupils should constrict and eyes should converge. To assess eye movements, ask the patient to follow finger movement downward, upward, to each side, and diagonally. Hold a finger at the extremes of the lateral gazes and assess for nystagmus (flickering of the eyes). Observe for drooping of eyelid (ptosis).
CN V	CN V	CN V	Observe for facial atrophy or tremors. Ask whether she has pain or numbness when chewing, then have her move her jaw against resistance. Assess for perception of soft touch along the jaw and cheek, using a cotton ball. Evaluate corneal reflex by touching a piece of sterile gauze to the cornea; the patient should blink. The corneal reflex may be blunted in contact lens wearers.
CN VII	CN VII	CN VII	Observe for facial symmetry. Have the patient smile, frown, puff out both cheeks, raise her eyebrows, and close her eyes tightly and resist any attempt to open them.
CN VIII	CN VIII		Whisper a phrase or word into the patient's ear and ask her to repeat it.
CN IX, CN X	CN IX CN X	CN IX, CN X	Use a tongue depressor to test the gag reflex. Observe the movement of the uvula and soft palate for any abnormalities of movement during swallowing.
CN X	CN X	CN X	Listen for evidence of hoarseness during speech.
CN XI		CN XI	Have the patient move her head from side to side against resistance. Ask her to shrug shoulders while you apply downward pressure.
CN XII		CN XII	Have the woman project her tongue out of the mouth and move it side to side. Observe for atrophy or tremor. Apply pressure against tongue movement with a tongue depressor.

Data from Cox B. The principles of neurological assessment. *Pract Nurs.* 2008;36(7):45-50; Ball JW, Dains JE, Flynn JA, Solomon BS, Stewart RW. Neurologic system. In *Seidel's Guide to Physical Examination*. St. Louis, MO: Mosby; 2015. 544-580.

Healthcare providers may also assess tremors while doing the pronator drift testing. Another test for vestibular and cerebellar function is to have the woman touch the examiner's index finger and then her nose with her eyes open. An abnormal response is if the woman is unable to do so despite several attempts; this response suggests an underlying neurologic disorder.[18] Other tasks that can indicate cerebellar problems are to have the woman place her palms up and then palms down on each thigh with eyes closed (this can be done rapidly if a normal response is found; this is called rapid alternating movement). Another maneuver used to assess cerebellar function is to ask the woman to run her heel and foot down the shin of the other leg and then repeat this maneuver on the opposite side with her eyes closed. A woman should be able to perform this maneuver smoothly and keep the heel on the shin. If she is unable to do this, a cerebellar problem should be suspected.[19]

Neurologic and Laboratory Testing

Several tests may be needed to identify the underlying etiologies precipitating neurologic symptoms; choosing the correct test is essential to obtain useful information, while minimizing unnecessary testing and costs. Laboratory tests which may be helpful in evaluating neurologic symptoms are listed in **Table 8-7**. Other tests are helpful in evaluating

Table 8-7 Lab Data Needed in the Evaluation of a Neurologic Problem

Neurologic Abnormality	Broad Disease Process	Specific Serum Lab Tests
Numbness or paresthesia	Metabolic disturbances	Basic metabolic panel
	Diabetes mellitus	Glycosylated hemoglobin A1C (HbA1C) Fasting plasma glucose
	Renal impairment	Blood urea nitrogen Creatinine GFR Albumin Pre-albumin Hematocrit & hemoglobin
	Thyroid Disorders	Thyroid-stimulating hormone (TSH) T_3 T_4
	Vitamin Deficiency	Vitamin B_6 Vitamin B_{12} Vitamin D Folic acid Iron
	Alcoholism	Liver function tests
Syncope & Loss of Consciousness	Cardiovascular conduction disorders	Potassium Calcium Magnesium Troponin CPK-MB
	Acute blood loss/hemorrhage	Complete blood count (CBC)

symptoms but are commonly ordered by specialist. In this case, the role of women's health providers is to help interpret the results to women and improve their understanding of the utility of the various tests and the meaning of their results. For example, magnetic resonance imaging (MRI) uses nonionizing forms of radiation (magnetic fields) to produce computerized cross-sectional images in the same fashion as a computed tomography (CT) scan. However, MRI provides more finely detailed pictures that look remarkably like anatomical slices of the body. MRI is superior to CT scan in the early diagnosis of demyelinating disorders such as MS and the detection of cerebral infarction. It is also helpful in identifying small lesions, such as hemorrhages and tumors, that may not appear on a CT scan.[20] If function is key to a diagnosis, as opposed to a structural deficit, positron emission tomography (PET) is superior to the CT and MRI scans in that it provides knowledge about oxygen (O_2) and glucose metabolism and cerebral blood flow. Some tests are contraindicated in women who are pregnant or lactating. Single-photon emission computed tomography (SPECT) is useful in studying cerebral blood flow, head trauma, brain death, amnesia, neoplasms, or persistent vegetative state. However, this test is contraindicated in pregnant women and those who are breastfeeding, because the radioactive tracer may be passed to the developing fetus or the nursing baby. Table 8-8 summarizes the tests that may need to be performed in order to help diagnose a neurologic problem. Table 8-9 describes the significance of cerebrospinal fluid (CSF) examination.[19]

Headache

Essential History, Physical, and Laboratory Assessment

HISTORY

A targeted headache history frequently leads to an accurate diagnosis and distinguishes between headaches that can be categorized as benign or threatening. Although most headaches are benign, those which are not represent critical findings that must be quickly identified. Being able to distinguish between these two categories can help ensure that clinicians develop a safe and cost-effective treatment plan with a high probability of success. Headaches that have been present for 20 to 30 years are in and of themselves not likely to be progressive or be indicative of a life-threatening neurologic disease; rather these headaches represent a pain syndrome that should not be associated with loss of life. Table 8-10 lists "red flags" that can be elicited during the history, which may indicate that a "sick" or pathologic headache is a possibility.[2,21]

A suggested framework for the targeted history can be found in Table 8-11.[2] Headaches that begin early in life, from childhood up until the second decade of life, are often vascular in nature. Headaches that begin later in life are most commonly *tension-type headaches* or are due to medication overuse. The duration and frequency of the headache may seem at first indiscriminate or erratic, but further questioning often reveals an identifiable pattern. *Vascular headaches* tend to occur in an episodic fashion, with the duration of pain ranging from minutes (cluster headache) to hours (migraine). Headaches with an organic origin, such as sinus disease, brain tumor, or ocular disease, tend to be continuous; an acute exacerbation can be precipitated by engaging in a Valsalva maneuver, changing position, or exercising. These headache syndromes will exacerbate over time if the fundamental organic disease is not appropriately diagnosed and treated or if the disease does not resolve spontaneously.[2]

Both the quality and location of pain can provide clues to the underlying etiology of headache. Unilateral or occipital pain that then becomes diffuse over the head during a Valsalva maneuver may indicate increased intracranial pressure or the presence of other intracranial problems. Poorly localized pain is of concern, because pain from tumors

Table 8-8 Tests Utilized in Making a Definitive Neurologic Diagnosis

Test	Description	Results
Cerebral angiography	Visualizes cerebral blood flow. Contrast dye is inserted through a catheter, usually placed in the femoral artery.	Detects blockages in the arteries or veins in the brain, head, or neck. This test is less common, because newer options are safer for the patient.
Computed tomography (CT)	Accurate, noninvasive, painless, and least expensive method of diagnosing neurologic disorders. Contrast media may be used to enhance the images.	Identifies bone, soft tissue, blood, and cerebrospinal fluid (CSF). Tumors, hemorrhage, bone malformations, and hydrocephalus can be distinguished.
3-dimensional CT scan	Same as CT scan; produces 3-dimensional images by computer modeling.	Same as CT scan.
CT angiography	Utilizes contrast dye IV before the CT scan.	Used to locate blockages or narrowing of blood vessels, aneurysms, and other blood vessel abnormalities such as arterial-venous malformation (AVM).
Xenon CT	CT study during which patient inhales xenon.	Gas diffusion into tissue demonstrates degree of blood flow to brain tissue.
Intrathecal contrast-enhanced CT	Intrathecal injection of a contrast medium.	Diagnoses problems of the spine and spinal nerve roots.
Positron emission tomography (PET)	Injects radioisotope intravascularly prior to imaging.	Supplies information about the function of the brain, specifically cerebral blood flow, and oxygen and glucose metabolism.
Single-photon emission computed tomography (SPECT)	Utilizes an IV radiopharmaceutical agent that lets radioisotopes cross the blood–brain barrier.	Useful in diagnosing cerebral blood flow, neoplasms, persistent vegetative state, amnesia, or brain death. *This test is contraindicated in women who are pregnant or breastfeeding.*
Magnetic resonance imaging (MRI)	Uses magnetic fields rather than ionizing radiation. If one needs enhanced images, the use of gadolinium, which is a non-iodine-based contrast medium, is used.	Visualizes all neurologic structures.

(continues)

Table 8-8 Tests Utilized in Making a Definitive Neurologic Diagnosis *(continued)*

Test	Description	Results
Magnetic resonance angiography (MRA)	Same as with MRI except in this test non-iodine-based contrast medium is always used.	Evaluates blood flow and blood vessel abnormalities such as intracranial aneurysms, AVM, or arterial blockage.
Magnetic resonance spectroscopy (MRS)	While MRI uses the signal from hydrogen protons to form anatomic images, proton MRS uses this information to determine the concentration of brain metabolites such as N-acetyl aspartate (NAA), choline (Cho), creatine (Cr), and lactate in the tissue examined.	Diagnoses abnormalities in the brain's biochemical process, which can occur with Alzheimer's disease, epilepsy, or stroke.
Electroencephalograph (EEG)	Records the electrical activity in the cerebral hemispheres.	Used to diagnose seizure activity. The EEG can be normal even when a pathological condition is present.
Electromyography (EMG)	Detects the electrical potential generated by skeletal muscle cells.	Identifies nerve and muscle problems as well as spinal cord disorders.
Evoked potentials	Measures the electrical signals to the brain generated by touch, sight, or hearing.	Assesses sensory nerve problems and confirms neurologic problems such as multiple sclerosis, brain tumor, spinal cord injury, or acoustic neuroma.
Lumbar puncture	Insertion of a needle between the 3rd and 4th lumbar vertebrae to withdraw CSF.	Contraindicated in patients with signs or symptoms of increased intracranial pressure. Used to obtain CSF pressure readings, CSF for lab analysis, and to inject spinal anesthetics and medications.

Reproduced from Plieri R. Assessment of the nervous system. In: Ignatavicius D, Workman M, eds., *Medical-Surgical Nursing: Patient-Centered Collaborative Care.* 7th ed. St. Louis, MO: Elsevier; 2013. © 2013 Elsevier.

Table 8-9 Findings and Significance of Cerebrospinal Fluid

Finding	Significance
Color/Appearance	
• Clear, colorless	• Within normal limits (WNL)
• Pink-red to orange	• Red blood cells present
• Yellow	• Bilirubin present due to hemolysis of red blood cells; possible causes: jaundice, hypercarotenemia, increased cerebrospinal fluid (CSF) protein, subarachnoid hemorrhage, or hemoglobinemia
• Unclear or cloudy	• Cell count is raised
• Brown	• Methemoglobin present, indicating a prior meningeal hemorrhage
Glucose	
• 50–70 mg/dL or 60–70% of serum glucose level	• WNL
• Less than 50 mg/dL	• Usually associated with infection with a pathological organism; bacterial, viral or fungal meningitis; leukemia of the central nervous system (CNS); or cancer
Cells	
• 0–5 small lymphocytes/mm^3	• WNL
• > 5 lymphocytes/mm^3	• Reaction to tumor, blood, chemical substance, or infection
Proteins Total	
• 15–45 mg/dL	• WNL; for the elderly WNL is up to 70 mg/dL
• 45–100 mg/dL	• Paraventricular tumor
• 50–200 mg/dL	• Viral infection
• > 500 mg/dL	• Bacterial infection, Guillain-Barré syndrome
• < 15 mg/dL	• Pseudotumor cerebri, hyperthyroidism, meningismus, and a normal finding after lumbar puncture
Albumin:Globulin Ratio	
• 8:1	• WNL
Immune Gamma Globulin (IgG)	
• 3–12% of total protein	• WNL
• More than 12% of total protein	• Viral infection, multiple sclerosis, neurosyphilis
Pressure	
• > 20 cm H$_2$O	• Increased spinal pressure, most often from tumors, infection within the CNS, or from bleeding

of the hypopharynx and posterior fossa can be diffuse, making them easy to miss.[18] Rapid onset-to-peak time (seconds to minutes) suggests the presence of organic disease, especially if the headache worsens with activities such as the Valsalva maneuver, exercise, and bending forward. Cluster headaches are an exception to this rule; they are vascular but have a fast onset-to-peak time.

The history should contain questions about other symptoms. Nausea, vomiting, photophobia,

Table 8-10 Red Flags in the Headache History and Physical Examination

Red Flag	Possible Conditions
No prior history of headache or change in symptoms from prior headaches	Cancer, stroke, infection, aneurysm, cerebral sinus thrombosis
Papilledema	Idiopathic intracranial hypertension, cerebral sinus thrombosis
Onset at > 50 years of age	Stroke, giant cell arteritis, mass lesion
New headache of unusual severity ("the worst"), "thunderclap" headache	Ruptured aneurysm
Headache associated with neurologic symptoms	Mass lesion, encephalitis
Headache associated with Valsalva maneuver or change in head position	Spontaneous CSF leak or Chiari malformation
Headache associated with systemic illness, such as cancer, autoimmune disease, or HIV	Mass lesion, autoimmune meningitis, thrombosis, brain metastasis
Signs or symptoms of systemic illness (e.g., chills, weight loss, fever)	Meningitis, encephalitis, cancer
Headache associated with exertion	Aneurysm rupture
Headache with mental confusion, seizures, weakness, numbness, or speaking difficulties	Stroke/CVA

CSF = cerebrospinal fluid, CVA = cerebrovascular accident

Data from Latimer K. Chronic headache: stop the pain before it starts. *J Fam Pract.* 2013;62(3):126-133; Waldman S. Targeted headache history. *Med Clin North Am.* 2013;97:185-195.

Table 8-11 Targeted Headache History

- Age of onset
- Duration of headaches
- Chronicity of headaches
- Frequency of headaches
- Location
- Character of pain
- Severity of pain
- Onset-to-peak time
- Associated symptoms
- Environmental factors
- Premonitory symptoms and aura
- Family history
- Past surgical and medical history
- Past treatments and diagnostic tests
- Pregnancy and menstruation

and aversion to strong odors are associated with migraine headaches. Cluster headache is frequently accompanied by symptoms of heavy rhinorrhea, blanching of the face on the affected side, lacrimation, and Horner syndrome (decreased pupil size, drooping eyelid, and decreased sweating on the affected side of the face). Meningeal signs (e.g., nuchal rigidity) will occur quickly after onset of subarachnoid hemorrhage, as will focal neurologic changes related to stroke.[2]

Environmental factors have also been associated with headache pain. Contact with any vasodilating substances in the diet (e.g., polyphenols of plant origin)[22] or absorption through the skin (e.g., topical nitroglycerine) or respiratory tract (e.g., aminophylline) may precipitate vascular headaches. Pressure or stress in the workplace, high altitude, airborne contaminants carried by heating and cooling systems, carbon monoxide, and industrial fumes are other factors that have been reported to trigger vascular headaches. Premonitory symptoms and aura are usually linked with vascular headaches, especially migraine, and generally precede the migraine by 2 to 48 hours. Common premonitory symptoms are depression, changes in libido, abnormal hunger, craving certain foods, elation, and fatigue. These premonitory symptoms can occur before an attack of migraine without aura; they also can occur with migraine with aura but generally precede the aura. The symptoms of a migraine with aura mostly originate in the visual cortex of the occipital lobe. They are probably caused by localized ischemia in this area of the brain. Other examples of aura are disturbances of feeling, smell, or motor function. Tumors in the occipital lobe may produce signs and symptoms similar to migrainous aura. These symptoms are more persistent than those associated with migraine with aura, and careful questioning may help recognize symptoms that indicate a structural lesion.[2]

Numerous conditions are associated with headaches. The provider should ask about infections; previous malignancies; trauma; previous cranial surgery; diseases of the eye, ear, nose, throat, and cervical spine; thyroid disease; changes in sleep, diet, or workplace; recent lumbar puncture or myelogram; use of medications that can cause headaches (e.g., topical nitroglycerin); travel outside of the country; anemia; and any environmental stress.[2] Inquiries should also be made about headaches among other family members. Migraine is a familial disorder. If one parent has the disease, the incidence in offspring is 45%; if both parents suffer from migraines, the child has a 70–75% chance of suffering from migraines.[2]

Past treatments of headache are common in women seeking professional help to cope with headache pain. Often these individuals have engaged in multiple strategies in the past in an effort to relieve the pain. The provider must be careful to avoid common pitfalls when exploring this part of history; specifically, the provider must assess whether an individual has received an adequate trial of a given treatment in terms of dosage, length of treatment, and compliance; whether the patient has resorted to drug-seeking behavior because of failure of past treatment regimens in relieving pain; and whether medication overuse has contributed to the headache. Medication overuse headache (MOH) can distort the classic symptoms of all types of headache, making diagnosis perplexing and treatment difficult. Any prior diagnostic tests should be reviewed. Factors that would prompt additional testing include an onset of a new headache, change in a previously stable headache pattern, the discovery of a new systemic illness that may be contributing to or causing the headache, or the need to investigate a new neurologic finding.[2]

Migraine headaches may be precipitated by hormonal events. They commonly occur with the start of menses or the initiation of oral contraceptives and lessen in frequency in mid-to-late pregnancy and after menopause. MacGregor and Hackshaw found that migraines occur 1.7 times more frequently immediately before menstruation and up to 2.5 times more frequently within the first 3 days of the cycle, and that migraines associated with the menses were more likely to be rated severe than at other times of the month.[23] A common problem is that providers may assume that any headache associated with menses is vascular in nature, yet many women also experience tension-type headaches during menses.

PHYSICAL

A comprehensive examination should be performed when a woman reports experiencing headaches. Because headaches are associated with fever, sinus infections, allergies, dental abscesses, and eyestrain, among many other problems, a thorough examination of the head, neck, eyes, ears, nose, throat, lungs, and heart is necessary. An abbreviated neurologic exam, as described earlier, should also be performed. In particular, the provider should determine that no abnormal physical findings as outlined in Table 8-10 are present.

LABORATORY/IMAGING ASSESSMENT

Many women worry that their headache is a symptom of brain cancer. However, cancer is extremely rare, and no additional laboratory or imaging tests are needed in the evaluation of a headache unless "red flags" are present in the history or found on the physical examination. A prospective study in the United Kingdom demonstrated that among middle-aged women reporting either undefined headaches or migraines, there was no increase in the incidence of brain cancers.[24] If imaging is needed, then referral to a neurologist for either a CT or MRI is indicated to help eliminate the possibility that a headache is due to a serious neurologic condition.[2,21,25] If a cluster headache is suspected, MRI is the preferred imaging modality in order to rule out secondary causes, particularly in the pituitary gland in new-onset headaches.[26]

Tension Headache

Tension headaches are the most common type of headache, suffered by approximately 90% of the population at some time in their lifetimes.[27] The female to male ratio is 1:1. Tension headaches are characterized by a mild to moderate bilateral headache, and usually present with bilateral dull, nonthrobbing pain and tightness or sensation of a band around the head pressing in. The onset is usually gradual, and headaches can persist from several hours to several days.[8] The pain occurs at the frontal or occipital areas of the head and/or at the cervical spine.[2] Affected individuals can report either, but not both, photophobia or phonophobia. Stress is the most commonly reported trigger for tension headaches. Some individuals who suffer tension headaches also suffer from migraine headaches.[8] Unlike migraine, tension headaches are not affected by physical activity.

The pathophysiology of the tension headache has both a central and a peripheral mechanism. The central mechanism is thought to involve hypersensitivity of pain fibers from the trigeminal nerve. Although the exact pathway is still unknown, the peripheral mechanism is thought to involve contraction of the jaw and neck muscles. The tension headache sufferer tends to have more localized tenderness and pain of the pericranial muscles.[8]

MEDICATIONS

Most women are able to manage tension headache using over-the-counter (OTC) pain relievers. However, others need prescription products. An unfortunate few have more frequent and bothersome symptoms. How to manage chronic headaches is discussed later in this chapter. **Table 8-12** describes common medications used in the treatment of neurologic disorders covered in this chapter. The following medications are used for tension headaches:[9]

Table 8-12 Common Medications for Neurologic Disorders

Disorder	Generic	Brand Name	Dose	Pregnancy Category
Tension Headache	Ibuprofen	Advil	200–800 mg tid	B in 1st and 2nd trimester
	Naproxen	Apo-Naproxen	500 mg followed by 200–500 mg q 6–8 h	D in 3rd trimester
	Amitriptyline	Amitril	50–100 mg once daily	C
	Topiramate	Topamax	Initiate with 25 mg bid, increase by 25 mg/wk to 200 mg/day or max total dose	C
Migraine	Acetaminophen	Tylenol	PO: 325–650 mg q 4–6 h PR: 650 mg q 4–6 h	B
	Indomethacin	Indocin	PO: 25–50 mg tid or qid (max 200 mg/day) or 75 mg sustained release once or twice daily	B 1st and 2nd trimesters D 3rd trimester
	Sumatriptan	Imitrex	subQ: 6 mg, may repeat at least 1 h after injection PO 25 mg × 1 dose, may repeat once after 2 h Intranasal 5, 10, or 20 mg, may repeat after 2 h	C
	Dihydroergotamine	D.H.E. 45	IV/IM/subQ: 1 mg, may be repeated at 1 h intervals to a total of 3 mg IM or 2 mg IV/subQ (max 6 mg/wk) Intranasal: 1 spray (0.5 mg) in each nostril, may repeat with additional spray in 15 min if no relief (max 4 sprays per attack); wait 6–8 h before treating another attack (max 8 sprays per 24 h, 24 sprays/wk)	X
	Propranolol	Inderal	80 mg/day in divided doses, may need 160–240 mg/day	C
	Verapamil hydrochloride	Calan	80 mg q 6–8 h, may increase up to 320–480 mg/day in divided doses	C
	Lisinopril	Prinivil	5–40 mg/day	C 1st trimester, D 2nd & 3rd trimesters
	Valproic acid	Depakote	250 mg bid (max 1000 mg/day)	D

(continues)

Table 8-12 Common Medications for Neurologic Disorders *(continued)*

Disorder	Generic	Brand Name	Dose	Pregnancy Category
Cluster Headaches	Octreotide acetate	Sandostatin	subQ: 100–600 mcg/day in 2–4 divided doses, titrate to response IM: May switch to depot injection after 2 wk at 20 mg q 4 wk × 3 months	B
	Lithium carbonate	Lithane	300 mg tid or qid	C 1st trimester, D 2nd & 3rd trimesters
	Ergotamine tartrate	Ergostat	SL: 1–2 mg followed by 1–2 mg q 30 min until headache abates or until max of 6 mg/24 h or 10 mg/wk	X
	Melatonin		10 mg at bedtime	C
Numbness/ Tingling/ Paresthesia	Gabapentin	Neurontin	Start 300 mg on day 1, 300 mg bid on day 2, 300 mg tid on day 3, and continue to increase over a week to an initial total dose of 400 mg tid; may increase to 1800–2400 mg/day	C
Syncope	Midodrine hydrochloride	Orvaten	10 mg tid during the daytime hours, dosed at less than 3 h apart, with last dose at least 4 h before bedtime (max 20 mg/dose)	C
	Mexiletine	Mexitil	200–300 mg q 8 h (max 1200 mg/day)	C

X = for, bid = twice daily, h = hour(s), IM = intramuscular, IV = intravenous, PO = per os ("by mouth"), q = every, qid = 4 times per day, SL = sublingual, subQ = subcutaneous, tid = 3 times per day, wk = week(s)

- Pain medications: OTC pain medications are usually the first line of defense for a tension headache. These include acetaminophen, aspirin, ibuprofen, and naproxen. Higher doses may require prescriptions.

- Combination medications: Aspirin or acetaminophen or both are often combined with caffeine or a sedative drug in a single medication. Drug combinations may be more effective than single-ingredient pain relievers. Many combination drugs are also available OTC. Women should be cautioned not to mix medications to avoid accidental overdoses.

- Triptans: These medications are usually reserved for those who suffer from migraine headaches. Because not all migraines present with classical features, some women with tension headaches may actually be suffering from atypical migraines. Use of a triptan can help in this circumstance.

- Narcotics: Opiates are rarely used due to their side effects and potential for dependency. They should be avoided in the general practice when a diagnosis of tension headache has been made. Clinicians should be aware of the risk of narcotic seeking when a report of tension headache leads to patient request for narcotics as "most effective."

- Preventive medication may be helpful for women with frequent or severe tension headaches. See the section on chronic headaches.

COMPLEMENTARY/ ALTERNATIVE THERAPIES

Rest, ice packs, or a long hot shower may be all a woman has to do to relieve a tension headache. However, some women may require more aggressive treatment, particularly those with frequent episodes. In these circumstances, the following strategies may be helpful:

- *Reduce stress.* Women can reduce stress by trying to plan ahead, setting aside time to consciously relax, and, if caught in a stressful situation, step back from the situation to regroup if needed.

- *Use hot or cold therapy.* Applying heat or ice to sore muscles may lessen a tension headache. When using heat, women can use a heating pad set on low, a warm compress, a hot-water bottle, or a hot towel. A hot shower or bath may also help. For cold therapy, women can use ice, frozen vegetables, or an ice pack in a cloth to protect the skin.

- *Maintain perfect posture.* Good posture can help keep muscles from tensing. When standing, the shoulders should be back, the head level, and the buttocks pulled in. When sitting, the thighs should be parallel to the ground and the head upright.

- *Use massage.* Massage can help reduce stress and relieve tension. Massage is especially effective for relieving tight, tender muscles in the back or the neck, head, and shoulders.

- *Practice deep breathing, biofeedback, and behavior therapies.* These techniques can promote relaxation and provide relief from a tension headache.[25] Biofeedback training teaches an individual ways to control certain body responses that help reduce pain. During a session, the affected individual is connected to a device that monitors and gives feedback on body functions such as muscle tension, heart rate, and blood pressure (BP). The woman then learns how to reduce muscle tension and slow the heart rate and breathing. Cognitive behavioral therapy is another effective method that can help individuals manage stress and thus have fewer and less severe tension headaches.

- *Perform other relaxation techniques such as deep breathing, yoga, meditation, and progressive muscle relaxation techniques.* These techniques can be learned in a class or at home using books or videos. Using medication in conjunction with stress management techniques may be more efficient than using either treatment alone in reducing tension headache.[25]

PATIENT INSTRUCTIONS

Managing tension headaches is often a balance between fostering healthy lifestyle habits, finding effective nondrug treatments, and using medications appropriately. Following healthy lifestyle practices such as getting enough, but not too much, sleep; refraining from smoking; exercising regularly; limiting alcohol, sugar, and caffeine; drinking plenty of water; and eating regular, balanced meals may help prevent headaches.[25]

Understanding how to manage tension headache is another critical component of patient teaching. Women should be knowledgeable about:

- How to complete a headache diary/history[28]; doing so can help identify triggers (see **Table 8-13**).
- The availability and use of preventive medications. See the section on chronic headaches.
- The possibility of developing MOH. Overuse of pain relievers can interfere with the preventive medications and reduce their effectiveness.

PREGNANCY AND LACTATION

In general, women try to avoid using medications in pregnancy whenever possible; therefore, starting with the measures described earlier on lifestyle and the use of complementary and alternative therapies is appropriate, particularly because headaches generally lessen in pregnancy. If needed, acetaminophen can be used; it is safe throughout pregnancy, whereas aspirin or any of the nonsteroidal anti-inflammatory drugs (NSAIDs; e.g., ibuprofen and naproxen) are best avoided in the third trimester. Use of these products late in pregnancy is associated with premature closure of the ductus arteriosus.

Several medications that are used to prevent headaches can be considered for use in pregnancy, although generally few women need to continue their use. Both topiramate, an anticonvulsant,

Table 8-13 Headache Diary

Information

Date and time

Duration

Intensity

Location of pain

Description of pain

Triggers (e.g., foods, physical activities, stress, smoke, bright lights, changes in weather, and noise)

Symptoms/warning signs

Rest/activity

Food eaten today

Medications taken for relief

Level of relief

Data from American Headache Society, Committee for Headache Education. Headache Diaries. Available at: http://www.achenet.org/resources/headache_diaries/. 2011. Accessed March 22, 2016; Fumal A, Schoenen J. Tension-type headache: current research and clinical management. *Lancet Neurol.* 2008;7(1):70-83.

and amitriptyline hydrochloride, an antidepressant, are commonly used as preventive medications in nonpregnant women; they are classified as category C medications in pregnancy.

Migraine Headache

Migraines present with unilateral, pulsating, moderate to severe pain, which is accompanied by nausea and/or vomiting or photophobia and phonophobia. Migraine is a benign chronic headache often activated by a triggering factor and may be accompanied by neurologic dysfunction. Triggering factors can include noise, jet lag, weather changes, hunger, stress, sunlight, exertion, and foods such as chocolate, cheese, and red wine.

These headaches are rare in children and occur most commonly in 25- to 55-year-old individuals. Migraine headaches are more frequent among women, with a 2:1 female-to-male ratio.[29] The most recent assessment of 3-month prevalence for migraine among women is 19.1%.[29] Hormonal factors account for the majority of the gender differences in migraines. Those individuals with a positive family history of migraine headaches have an increased risk of developing migraines. As with tension headaches, overuse of medications used to treat migraines can also cause MOH.[21,30]

The pathology in a migraine headache involves neurologic, vascular, hormonal, and neurotransmitter components and is somewhat different among the various types of migraine headaches. Vascular changes in migraines with aura are more pronounced, whereas migraine without aura is not associated with a reduction in blood flow.[8] Regardless, the endpoint is a condition of regional hypoperfusion. The ensuing perivascular inflammation leads to the typical headache. Disturbances in the blood–brain barrier in the area postrema cause nausea and vomiting.[8]

Due to hormonal changes, migraines are more frequent before and during menstruation and are decreased during menopause and pregnancy. The cyclic withdrawal of estrogens can trigger migraine attacks. Cyclic changes in estrogen are absent in pregnancy and after menopause; thus migraine attacks are less common in these situations.

Menstrual migraines affect two-thirds of the women who complain of migraine headaches. Menstrual migraines have two subtypes: menstrual-related migraines and menstrual headache. In order to meet the definition of having menstrual-related migraines without aura, headaches must begin during the perimenstrual time period (2 days before to 3 days after the onset of menstruation) and occur in two-thirds of menstrual cycles. A pure menstrual migraine without aura meets similar criteria to these except that migraine headaches occur only in the perimenstrual time period and do not happen at other times of the month.[31]

The decline in serum estradiol levels that occurs shortly before and during the perimenstrual time period is thought to be the underlying trigger that can precipitate menstrual migraines in vulnerable women. Estrogen may modulate activity of vasoactive substances at the neurovascular junction, act directly on vascular smooth muscle, and activate vasoregulatory responses in the hypothalamus. However, there is no direct evidence that these fluctuations in estrogen are associated with the frequency and severity of migraines.[8] Other theories posit that the physiologic triggers of menstrual migraines are either 1) declines in serum magnesium levels, 2) changes in the inhibitory neurotransmitter systems that regulate neuronal firing times inside second-order neurons of the trigeminal nervous system, or 3) the release of prostaglandins from a shedding endometrium that sensitizes peripheral nociceptors.[31]

Migraine headaches are composed of several stages: the prodrome phase, in which the woman has specific signs and symptoms such as mood changes or food cravings; headache phase, in which the headache can last a few hours or days; termination phase, when the headache intensity decreases; and the postprodrome phase, in which the woman has muscle pain, fatigue, and irritability.[32] Some individuals also experience an aura. The aura phase occurs after the prodrome and generally involves visual changes, flashing lights, or diplopia.[33]

The International Headache Society has classified migraine headaches into five clinical subtypes: migraine without aura, migraine with aura, ophthalmoplegic migraine, retinal migraine, and complicated migraine.[34,35] Individuals with migraine with or without aura may have subtle changes in behavior, mood, and level of alertness noted during their neurologic assessment. Specific neurologic changes seen with different types of migraines include oculomotor CN III palsy (ophthalmoplegic migraine), hemiparesis (hemiplegic migraine), ataxia (basilar migraine), and visual loss (retinal migraine), making these variants easy to diagnose due to their objective neurologic findings.[32,35]

Migraine without aura is the most common subtype. These headaches last from 4 to 72 hours. Classic symptoms of migraine headache without aura include throbbing and unilateral pain that is often worse behind one eye or ear. The pain is described as moderate to severe and is aggravated by activity. The woman may also experience a sensitive scalp, anorexia, phonophobia, photophobia, and nausea with or without vomiting. Affected individuals tend to have the same clinical signs and symptoms each time they have a migraine headache. Migraine headaches can seriously disrupt an individual's ability to function in his or her work and personal life if pain is not controlled or relieved in its early stages.[33,35]

About 1 in 5 women who experience migraines have auras. An aura is a feeling or series of sensations that occur about 10 to 30 minutes before a migraine headache and remits within 60 minutes after the headache begins. Common signs and symptoms of an aura include seeing blind spots, flashing lights, or zigzag lines; feeling numbness or tingling in the hands or face; having an unusual sense of taste, smell, or touch; or sensing mental "fuzziness." The aura is usually followed by some or all of the symptoms of a migraine without aura.[36] Aphasia or sensory deficits may also be present. Other symptoms of the migraine include vomiting, nausea, scalp tenderness, and photophobia. Ten percent of patients experience diarrhea.

Medication

There are two major classifications of medications used for migraine headaches: pain-relieving medications and preventive medications. Pain-relieving medications, also known as acute or abortive treatment, are used during a migraine

headache and are designed to arrest symptoms. Preventive medications are taken daily to reduce the frequency or severity of migraine headaches. The use of preventive medications is discussed in the section on chronic headaches.

Pain-Relieving Medications Pain-relieving medications should be taken as soon as the woman recognizes that a migraine headache will soon be or is already occurring. It is often helpful if the woman can rest or sleep in a dark room after taking these medications. Care must be taken to monitor their use; if taken too often or for long periods of time, pain-relieving drugs can cause ulcers, gastrointestinal bleeding, and MOH.

Choice of a specific medication is based on the severity of the migraine. If the headache is mild, then use of aspirin, NSAIDs, or acetaminophen may provide needed relief. A combination of acetaminophen, aspirin, and caffeine is another alternative for moderate migraine pain. However, few women have mild or moderate migraine headaches, so most require stronger treatment. Triptans are commonly prescribed, because they are effective in relieving moderate to severe migraine headache pain and can also relieve the nausea that commonly accompanies migraine. Anti-nausea medications may be prescribed as adjunctive therapy for women who experience significant nausea unrelieved with the use of triptans. Frequently prescribed medications include metoclopramide (Reglan) and prochlorperazine (Compro). Chlorpromazine is often given intravenously in the emergency room for headaches unresponsive to triptans.

Triptans work by promoting constriction of blood vessels and blocking pain pathways in the brain. Among commonly used medications in this class are sumatriptan (Imitrex) and rizatriptan (Maxalt). Some triptans are available as injections, nasal sprays, or oral tablets. Side effects include nausea, drowsiness, muscle weakness, and dizziness. Triptans are not advised to be given to women at risk for strokes and heart attacks. A single-tablet combination of sumatriptan and naproxen sodium (Treximet) is more effective in relieving migraine symptoms than either medication alone.

Ergots, ergotamine, and caffeine combination medications (Migergot) are not as effective as triptans, but are used in the treatment of refractory pain. They are more effective than triptans in patients whose migraine headache lasts more than 48 hours. Use of ergotamine is associated with MOH. Dihydroergotamine (D.H.E. 45, Migranal) is an ergot that has fewer side effects and is more effective than ergotamine. It is also available as an injection and nasal spray and is less likely to lead to MOH. See the section on the management of chronic headaches, which discusses the management of more persistent forms of migraine headaches. Ergot-containing medications are contraindicated in pregnancy.

Complementary/ Alternative Therapies

The American Headache Society and the American Academy of Neurology recently reviewed the state of the science on the use of herbs, minerals, and vitamins in the management of migraines.[37] Based on an analysis of the evidence, preventive therapies were classified as being effective, possibly effective, ineffective, or having insufficient evidence to determine effectiveness. The following products were deemed effective (butterbur), probably effective (feverfew, riboflavin, magnesium), and possibly effective (coenzyme Q10).[37] Other nonmedication-based strategies that may help in the management of migraines include:

- Relaxation techniques such as meditation, yoga, or progressive muscle relaxation techniques, which may help prevent or ease the pain of a migraine headache
- Acupuncture, biofeedback, massage therapy, and cognitive behavioral therapy (as discussed in the section on tension headaches), which can be used in addition to medical therapy

Contraception

Another issue is how best to manage reproductive-aged women with migraine headaches who desire a reliable contraceptive method. Use of estrogen-containing contraceptives can increase the risk of complications for some women, but provide relief from attacks in others, particularly in those with menstrual migraine. Although the underlying mechanism is unknown, women who have migraines are more likely to experience stroke than women with migraines who do not use estrogen-containing contraception; risk of stroke increases with age and type of migraine. The Centers for Disease Control and Prevention Medical Eligibility Criteria grade the safety of contraception as follows: 1 (no restriction), 2 (advantages generally outweigh theoretical or proven risks), 3 (theoretical or proven risks generally outweigh advantages), or 4 (unacceptable risk). In general, use of estrogen-containing contraceptives for women with migraines is discouraged. Ratings range from a high of 2 to 3 for women younger than 35 years of age who have migraines without aura to a 4 for women who experience migraine with aura, regardless of age.[38]

Research indicates that the use of a progestogen-only contraceptive may promote a stable estrogen level when given in ovulation-inhibiting dosages. In a study of headache diaries kept by women experiencing migraine who took desogestrel 75 mcg, there was a positive effect on migraine with and without aura, reducing symptoms and length and frequency of headaches.[39]

Patient Instructions

Women with migraines should understand that particular lifestyle practices can trigger migraines. Common triggers include caffeine, alcohol, certain foods and odors, and tobacco; limiting exposures to these substances may minimize the frequency and severity of migraine headaches. Other supportive measures include developing a daily routine with regular sleep and meal patterns, getting an adequate amount of sleep each night, minimizing stress, and exercising regularly. Using stress management techniques such as meditation can be helpful. Exercise should begin with a slow warm-up, because intense exercise can cause headaches, especially if the onset of exercise is sudden. Obesity is thought to be a factor in migraine headaches; regular exercise has been promoted to help the woman lose weight and may prevent migraines.[40]

If estrogen appears to trigger or worsen migraine headaches, then avoiding estrogen-containing medications completely, or alternatively lowering the dose, may afford relief. Other options include switching to a lower dose combined oral contraceptive formulation, prescribing progestin-only contraceptives, or switching from an oral to a topical estrogen-replacement product.[40]

The woman should rest in a dark, quiet room from the moment she recognizes that a migraine headache is coming on. Ice wrapped in a small towel and applied to the back of the neck or applying gentle force to the painful areas of the scalp may help relieve symptoms. Keeping a headache diary will help the woman learn more about her specific triggers and what treatments are most effective.[40]

Many strategies are successful in minimizing pain associated with headache no matter what specific type of headache an individual is experiencing. See the discussion on measures described earlier regarding patient instructions for tension headaches for other ideas on how to manage headaches.

During Pregnancy, Lactation, and Menstruation

Pregnancy   Most women experience fewer headaches during pregnancy, making the use of abortive medication less common in pregnancy. Based on an analysis of data from registries of women using triptans, triptans appear to pose little or no risk in pregnancy.[41] Dihydroergotamine is associated with an increase in premature births, but not with an increase in risk for spontaneous abortions or birth defects.[11] Preventive medications are best avoided during pregnancy whenever possible. First-line agents include magnesium, beta blockers such as propranolol or metoprolol, and, if no improvement is seen, amitriptyline or nortriptyline.[42] Women on valproate medications before pregnancy should stop as soon as they decide to conceive, because these medications are associated with birth defects.

Lactation   Advice for the management of migraine headaches while breastfeeding is essentially the same as the management recommended during pregnancy. Preventive medications should also be avoided during breastfeeding, but if necessary the choices are the same as those considered safe in pregnancy; magnesium, propranolol, metoprolol, and nadolol are the preferred agents, although amitriptyline and nortriptyline can also be used safely.[42] Products with a low concentration in breast milk including ibuprofen, eletriptan, and diclofenac can be used during lactation. Information on the safety of many products during lactation is poor. Few data are available on the triptans. Use of aspirin may be associated with the development of Reye's syndrome in the infant. Use of opioids poses a risk of sedation and apnea in the infant at high doses.[43]

Menstruation   The medication management of menstrual-related and menstrual migraines is the same as that for migraines in general, with the exception that short-term prophylactic therapies can be offered as the timing of the headache can be predicted based on the patterns of a woman's menstrual cycle.[31] Medications can be administered 1 to 2 days before the start of the anticipated menstrual period and continued for 4 to 7 days. These medications include NSAIDs, triptans, and estrogen transdermal patches/gel. Commonly used triptans (e.g., frovatriptan 2.5 mg daily or bid, naratriptan 1 mg bid, and zolmitriptan 2.5 mg bid and 2.5 mg tid) are effective at preventing migraines when administered for 4 to 5 days during the perimenstrual time period. Naproxen sodium 550 mg bid given 6 days before to 7 days after menses has also been shown to be successful in preventing menstrual migraine. The use of 100 mcg estradiol transdermal patches is another effective alternative.[31]

Continuous prophylactic therapy is another option. Women with irregular cycles who have difficulty predicting their next cycle may benefit most from this option.[31] With continuous therapy, medications are taken every day of the month and can be used to prevent both menstrual-related and unrelated headaches. These medications are the same as those discussed earlier in the section of the prevention of tension and migraine headaches and include beta-blockers, tricyclic antidepressants, calcium channel blockers, and anticonvulsants.

Hormonal therapies can also be offered and are used specifically for the management of menstrual migraine. The most commonly used regimen is the use of oral contraceptives, particularly long-duration combined oral contraceptives given as a daily combination of estrogen and progestogen for 3 months followed by a placebo week to allow a withdrawal bleed. Use of progestin-only contraception that decreases or prevents ovulation and menstrual cycling may also be effective. Another rarely used alternative is treatment with gonadotropin-releasing hormone agonists. Hormonal treatments prevent menstrual migraine because they reduce hormonal fluctuation.[31]

Chronic Headache

The term *chronic headache* encompasses many different diagnoses; chronic tension headaches,

chronic migraine headaches, and MOHs are typical. The presentation of chronic tension and migraine headaches is similar to that of episodic tension and migraine headaches. A diagnosis of chronic tension headache is made when headaches occur at least 15 days per month.[21] Women with chronic tension headaches or more problematic migraines (defined as experiencing three or more migraine headaches a month, headaches that fail to respond to abortive medications, or headaches lasting more than 12 hours) may benefit from being prescribed a preventive regimen.[44]

Overuse of headache medication can cause chronic headaches. This phenomenon is referred to as MOH, and sometimes as drug-induced headache or rebound headache. Headaches related to medication overuse have erratic intensity. Women with MOH often awaken from sleep with neck pain and/or a headache.[22] MOH often complicates chronic presentations of migraine and tension headaches, because women often use higher and more frequent doses of OTC medications in an attempt to self-manage their headache pain. The International Classification of Headache Disorders (ICHS-II), defines overuse as using a single abortive headache drug $\geq$ 10 times per month or using 2 or more such drugs together $\geq$ 15 times a month.[35] Triptans are particularly problematic, because they are frequently used as abortive medications in the treatment of migraines and cluster headaches, and of all the medications used in the management of acute headaches, they are the most likely to cause MOH. In addition, MOH occurs more quickly and in lower doses with these products compared to other acute headache drugs. Other analgesics, especially combination products such as butalbital/acetaminophen/caffeine (Fioricet), are also commonly associated with the development of MOH. NSAIDs are less likely to cause MOH.[21]

Management of Chronic Headaches

Because the management of chronic headaches can be quite complex, affected individuals may benefit from a consultation with a neurologist. Preventive drugs often are used and can reduce the severity, length, and frequency of headaches, as well as increase the effectiveness of symptom-relieving medications used during acute attacks.[40] Preventive regimens can be used indefinitely, but at minimum for at least 2 months, by women with frequent severe headaches or for those whose headaches are not relieved by abortive medications. Women should expect headaches to reduce in severity and frequency after several weeks of use. After a reasonable trial, women can stop these medications to see if their headaches remain infrequent. Some women, whose headaches were debilitating before using a preventive regimen or whose headaches increase in frequency after stopping their preventive regimen, may choose to remain on preventive medications long term.

The choice of preventive medications is directed primarily by the presence of comorbid conditions and the tolerability of the various products rather than the type of chronic headache. Commonly used products include the following:

- *Cardiovascular medications* such as beta blockers (e.g., propranolol and metoprolol), calcium channel blockers (e.g., verapamil), or angiotensin-converting enzyme inhibitors (e.g., lisinopril) are used for all types of chronic headaches.
- *Antidepressants* may be effective in reducing the number of migraine and tension headaches. These medications increase the amount of serotonin and other brain chemicals. Nortriptyline and amitriptyline are the most commonly used products. Side effects may include weight gain, drowsiness, and dry mouth. Amitriptyline is the only tricyclic antidepressant proven to effectively prevent migraine headaches. Venlafaxine (Effexor XR), a serotonin

and norepinephrine reuptake inhibitor, has shown efficacy both for chronic tension-type headaches and chronic migraines. Other antidepressants, such as mirtazapine, have been suggested for use. These products can be highly effective in women without depression and can be offered freely to nondepressed women.

- *Anti-seizure drugs* such as valproate sodium (Depacon) and topiramate (Topamax) have been shown to decrease the frequency of headaches.[25] Valproate medications should not be used in pregnant women, because their use is associated with birth defects in the exposed infant.
- Indomethacin may help prevent migraine headaches and is available in suppository form, which is helpful if the woman is nauseated.
- Glucocorticoids and opioid medications are used as therapies of last resort. Care must be taken to prevent steroid toxicity. Opioid medications containing codeine are sometimes used to treat migraine headaches for women who cannot take triptans or ergot, but they can be habit forming.[40]

Nonpharmacologic treatments may also be effective. All of the strategies discussed under the sections on migraine and tension headaches should be employed. Some women also find counseling helpful in the management of pain.[25] On occasion, OnabotulinumtoxinA (Botox) is used in treating chronic headaches in adults. Injections are made into muscles of the neck and forehead. This treatment, if helpful, must be repeated every 12 weeks. Acupuncture may also provide temporary relief, particularly from chronic tension headache pain.[25]

Cluster Headache

Cluster headache is a primary headache syndrome diagnosed by its distinct clinical history. Cluster headaches affect approximately 1/1000 Americans, with a prevalence calculated at

53/100,000 per year.[45] It is more common in individuals between 20 and 40 years of age; the female-to-male ratio is 1:4.[27] While the evidence is limited, the severity and character of cluster headaches appear to be the same in women regardless of their reproductive status. A cluster headache presents with unilateral severe pain, often described as being steady, burning, and sharp, accompanied by tearing of the eyes and a stuffy nose. These latter symptoms, along with rhinorrhea, facial sweating, eyelid edema, ptosis, and pupillary constriction (miosis) occur on the same side as the headache. Ptosis can become permanent. The pain may arise in, behind, and around one eye and may radiate to the temple, forehead or cheek, ear, or neck. Pain involves one side of the face from neck to temples, can quickly get worse, peaking within 5 to 10 minutes. The strongest pain may last 30 minutes to 2 hours.[46] Like migraine headaches, cluster headaches can also cause sensitivity to light and sound, an aura, and nausea and vomiting. Unlike other types of headaches, the affected individual is restless and often walks, paces, or sits and rocks during an attack.[33]

Cluster headaches are triggered by environmental factors such as alcohol and cigarette smoking, bright light, high altitudes, heat, exertion, certain medications, cocaine, and foods high in nitrates, such as bacon and preserved meats.[27] They also have a familial tendency similar to migraine headaches. The pathophysiology appears to be related to the body's sudden release of histamine or serotonin secondary to problems with the hypothalamus. The evidence suggests dysregulation of cortisol or melatonin levels as a component of the problem.[47]

Several physical findings are associated with cluster headaches. A hallmark finding on the physical exam is Horner syndrome. Other physical signs that may be evident during an attack include bradycardia, pallor or flushing of the face, increased skin temperature, increased intraocular pressure, and tenderness over the temporal artery. No other neurologic changes will be observed.[27]

Cluster headaches have a distinctive pattern. While cluster headaches may occur any time during the day or night, typically they present 2 to 3 hours after falling asleep and are associated with the rapid eye movement portion of sleep. They are also more likely to occur at other times associated with relaxation, such as when napping. Cluster headaches tend to occur at the same time of the day. Attacks occur repeatedly over a week or longer and then remit, with long pain-free periods of at least a month between attacks.[48] This episodic pattern is the most common presentation; however, some individuals have a more chronic, intractable form in which there may not be a remission for more than 1 year.[33,48] Although psychiatric comorbidities are not well studied in cluster headache, depression, aggressive behavior, and increased potential for suicide have been identified as concerns. Rates of depression and anxiety vary depending on study approach and may be lower or higher than in other headache syndromes.[49]

MEDICATIONS

Cluster headache, if suspected, should be referred to a specialist for care. There is no cure for cluster headaches; the goal of therapy is to shorten the duration and limit the severity of attack—and to prevent attacks if possible. Cluster headaches are difficult to treat, because the pain comes on suddenly and often subsides within a short period of time. Because onset is rapid, pain is extreme, and the duration of each episode can be as short as 10 minutes, fast-acting drugs are needed for treatment to be effective.[46]

- Acute treatments:
  - *Oxygen.* Inhaling 100% O_2 through a mask at a flow rate of 12 liters per minute can provide impressive relief for most individuals.[46] The use of O_2 is thought to decrease cerebral

blood flow and inhibit activity of the carotid bodies, which are sensitive to O_2 levels in the body.[33] This harmless, low-cost procedure can be effective within 15 to 30 minutes, and can be discontinued once the headache is relieved. The disadvantages of using O_2 include the inconvenience of a portable O_2 tank and potential to be inaccessible when needed.

- *Triptans.* The subcutaneous injection of sumatriptan (Imitrex) can also be an effective medication for acute cluster headaches. Sumatriptan is contraindicated in women with uncontrolled hypertension or heart disease. Sumatriptan also comes as a nasal spray, but it appears to be less effective than when administered as a subcutaneous injection and takes longer to work. Zolmitriptan (Zomig) is another triptan medication, which can be administered via a nasal spray or a pill form for relief from cluster headache pain.

- *Octreotide.* Octreotide (Sandostatin) is an injectable synthetic version of the brain hormone somatostatin and has been shown to be a successful treatment for cluster headaches.

- *Local anesthetics.* The numbing effect of lidocaine (Xylocaine) can be successful against cluster headache pain when given intranasally for some individuals.

- *Dihydroergotamine.* The intravenous (IV) form D.H.E. 45 is another option. The IV administration of D.H.E. 45 must be administered in the office setting or emergency room. The intranasal form (Migranal) has not been proven to be effective against cluster headache pain.[46]

- Preventive treatments for cluster headaches should be initiated at the onset of the cluster episode with the goal of suppressing attacks. The selection of which medicine to use often depends on the length and regularity of the headache episodes. Medications can be tapered off once the expected time of the cluster episode ends.

- *Calcium channel blockers.* Verapamil (Calan, Verelan) is the first choice of the calcium channel blockers for women with cluster headaches. Verapamil is usually used in combination with other prophylactic medications such as lithium carbonate or methysergide for maximum effect. At times, long-term use of verapamil is needed to manage chronic cluster headaches.

- *Corticosteroids.* Corticosteroids, such as prednisone and dexamethasone, are inflammation-suppressing drugs. They are fast-acting preventive medications that are effective in 70–80% of women with cluster headaches.[46] Corticosteroids are generally used only if they can be started at the onset of the attack or if the woman has a pattern of brief cluster periods and long remissions. Corticosteroids have serious side effects such as diabetes, cataracts, and hypertension, so they are good for short-term administration and inappropriate for long-term use. The usual dosing of prednisone is 60–100 mg, which should be given once daily for 5 days; then the dose should be decreased by 10 mg daily.

- *Lithium carbonate.* Lithium carbonate is used to treat bipolar disease, but may be successful in avoiding chronic cluster headache if other medications have not helped. Lithium carbonate has side effects such as increased thirst, diarrhea, and tremor that can be minimized by adjusting the dose. Because lithium carbonate is nephrotoxic, its use requires periodic blood testing to monitor renal health and to detect potential iatrogenic morbidities.

- *Nerve block.* Injecting a combination of an anesthetic and a corticosteroid into the area around the occipital nerve may help relieve chronic cluster headache pain. This injection is made at the back of the head where the occipital nerve is located. Occipital nerve blocks may be valuable for short-term relief until long-term medications can take effect.

- *Ergots.* Ergotamine, sublingual (SL), can be taken before bed to prevent nighttime cluster headache attacks. Subcutaneous D.H.E. 45 may also be helpful. Ergot drugs may be effective if taken early in the woman's cluster headache attacks, but they cannot be given concomitantly with triptans and can be used only for short periods of time.
- *Melatonin.* The data on melatonin as a preventive or adjunct for cluster headache are inconsistent, although 10 mg at bedtime may be of assistance.[49]
- *Depakote.* Other preventive drugs used for cluster headaches include anti-seizure drugs such as divalproex (Depakote) and topiramate (Topamax).[46]

Surgery may be indicated for those individuals who do not obtain relief with aggressive treatment or who cannot tolerate medications or their side effects. Because surgery may be associated with permanent brain or nerve damage, these procedures are done as a last resort. The goal of surgery is to impair the nerve pathways thought to be accountable for pain, most commonly the trigeminal nerve that innervates the area behind and around the eye.[46] This procedure is called percutaneous stereotactic rhizotomy (PSR). It is performed on an outpatient basis under general anesthesia. The surgeon passes a hollow needle through the inside of the cheek into the trigeminal nerve fibers and transmits a hot current that goes through the needle to destroy some of the nerve fibers. Individuals treated by PSR may report muscle weakness in the jaw or permanent insensitivity to pain on the treated side.[33]

Occipital nerve stimulation requires a surgeon to insert electrodes and attach them to a small pacemaker-like generator. The electrodes send impulses to stimulate the area of the occipital nerve, which is thought to block pain signals. Small research studies have found that this procedure helps decrease the pain in some individuals with chronic cluster headache pain.[6]

Deep brain stimulation is another alternative. Long-term, high-frequency electrical stimulation is released by an implanted stimulator in the posterior hypothalamus (similar to the pulse generator of an implanted permanent pacemaker). Because the hypothalamus is the area of the brain thought to affect the timing and frequency of cluster headache attacks, this treatment may reduce or eliminate chronic cluster headache pain.[33,46]

COMPLEMENTARY/ ALTERNATIVE THERAPIES

Little evidence is available about the effectiveness of complementary therapies for the prevention or treatment of cluster headaches. In an extensive review of the literature, Bilchik concluded that the evidence was insufficient to recommend any specific product or method.[50] One study that surveyed 100 cluster headache patients reported that only 10% of individuals reported any relief with the use of acupuncture, therapeutic touch, homeopathy, or chiropractic treatment.[51] However, several modalities have been studied to a greater extent than others. Extract from kudzu, a vine species originally found in Asian countries, was shown to reduce the frequency, intensity, and duration of cluster headache pain. However, kudzu did not decrease the length of the cluster cycle.[52] Melatonin, previously discussed under medications, has shown a modest helpfulness in handling nighttime attacks.[46,50]

PATIENT INSTRUCTIONS

Several self-care practices may minimize symptoms. Having a regular sleep pattern can prevent attacks, because irregular or disrupted sleep cycles can trigger cluster headaches. Because alcohol and cigarette smoke are other known triggers, avoiding these substances may also help.[46] Techniques to prevent cluster headaches can help reduce the risk of MOH from overuse of abortive medications. Use of preventive medications can also help potentiate the effects of acute medications.

If a cluster headache occurs, women can engage in practices to ameliorate the attack. Wearing sunglasses and sitting away from windows can minimize glare and exposure to light.[33] Cluster headaches can be frightening and unbearable and can trigger anxiety or depression. The emotional distress and pain associated with cluster headaches can negatively impact relationships with family and friends, productivity at work, and diminish quality of life. Talking to a counselor or therapist may be helpful. Support groups are another alternative, because they are a good place to share experiences and learn from others coping with similar problems.

DURING PREGNANCY AND LACTATION

Little is known about cluster headaches during pregnancy and lactation. The drugs of first choice in the treatment of cluster headaches are high-flow O_2 (7–15 L/min), intranasal sumatriptan, and intranasal lidocaine. All three of these medications can be given to pregnant and lactating females who are experiencing an acute cluster headache attack.[53] Due to the rarity of cluster headaches in the pregnant female, it is suggested that providers refer these women to a neurologist for treatment and follow up.

Syncope

Syncope is a transient event caused by cerebral hypoperfusion, which resolves completely, with no long-term change in neurologic function.[11-13] Very rarely syncope is associated with significant medical problems.[13] Differential diagnosis includes epileptic seizures and functional/psychogenic syndromes such as pseudo-epileptic or pseudo-syncopal.[12]

Syncope can be classified as being neurally mediated, orthostatic, neurologic, or cardiac in origin.[11] *Neurally mediated* syncope is the most frequent type of syncope and is seen primarily in young adults. A reflex response to noxious stimuli produces bradycardia, vasodilation, and systemic hypotension leading to diminished cerebral blood flow. It can be vasovagal (which occurs when the body overreacts to triggers such as stress, fear, heat, extreme emotional distress, or the sight of blood) or situational (i.e., micturition, gastrointestinal stimulation, cough, or phobias), or the result of carotid sinus hypersensitivity (caused by pressure on the carotid sinus from rotating the head, shaving, or wearing a too-tight collar).[11,54] *Orthostatic* syncope is caused by a fall in BP, which can be due to drug-induced orthostatic hypotension, primary autonomic failure from Parkinson disease or MS, secondary autonomic failure from diabetes mellitus or spinal cord injury, or volume depletion from vomiting, diarrhea, or acute blood loss.[11] *Neurologic* syncope is classified into three categories. In cerebrovascular syncope, or subclavian steal syndrome, the proximal part of the left subclavian artery is blocked so there is no blood flow into the left vertebral artery and onward to the left arm. To compensate, blood from the right vertebral artery enters the left vertebral artery and flows back to supply blood to the left arm. Neurogenic syncope occurs preceding a transient ischemic attack (TIA) or cerebrovascular accident (CVA). Psychogenic syncope is produced by anxiety, depression, panic disorders, and somatization disorders.

Cardiac causes of syncope disrupt blood flow and are caused by numerous conditions such as pulmonary embolus, acute aortic dissection, pulmonary hypertension, aortic stenosis, pulmonary stenosis, or acute myocardial infarction/ischemia.

Other causes of cardiac syncope are obstructive cardiomyopathy and arrhythmias.[9] Cardiac-related syncope is associated with a twofold increase in the risk of death when compared with those without a history of syncope. The 5-year survival rate after a cardiac-related syncopal event is approximately 50%.[18] Previously undetected structural cardiac disease or ventricular arrhythmias can be life threatening.[18,55] These include the various presentations of sinus node dysfunction, atrioventricular node dysfunction, ventricular tachyarrhythmias, and decreased stroke volume, further delineated in **Table 8-14**.

Some conditions, such as psychogenic transient loss of consciousness (TLOC), can be mistaken for syncope. With psychogenic TLOC there is an "apparent" but not a "real" loss of consciousness. One type is psychogenic nonepileptic seizures in which attacks appear to resemble epileptic seizures because of the presence of motor aberrations such as stiff posture or myoclonic jerks. In the second type, known as psychogenic pseudosyncope, the attacks resemble syncope or coma as they comprise sleeplike immobile state with eyes closed.[12] These presentations are not life threatening, but may be indicative of underlying psychologic problems. While not usual, epileptic seizures can be mistaken for syncope.[56] **Table 8-15** describes the clinical features that distinguish syncope and epilepsy.

History

Because syncope can be caused by such a broad array of conditions, a comprehensive history is necessary. The history should focus on whether common triggers for syncopal episodes were present before the episode occurred. Some of these triggers include prolonged standing, having blood drawn or seeing blood, straining such as when

Table 8-14 Life-Threatening Cardiac Causes of Syncope

- Sinus node dysfunction (syncope is a common presentation, but there is little worry regarding sudden death; sinus node dysfunction is usually not life threatening)
  - Sick sinus syndrome
  - Marked sinus bradycardia
  - Sinus arrest
  - Sinoatrial block
  - Conversion pauses
- Atrioventricular node dysfunction
  - Infranodal atrioventricular block (Mobitz II second-degree block)
  - Complete heart block
  - Alternating bundle branch block
- Ventricular tachyarrhythmias
  - Polymorphic ventricular tachycardia secondary to ischemia
  - Scar-related monomorphic ventricular tachycardia
  - Ventricular fibrillation
- Reduction in stroke volume from structural complications
  - Cardiac perforation and/or pericardial tamponade
  - Ventricular septal rupture
  - Papillary muscle rupture

Table 8-15 Clinical Findings: Epilepsy Versus Syncope

Clinical Results	Syncope	Seizure
Symptoms prior to event	• Nausea, vomiting, hot/cold sensation, abdominal discomfort • Perspiring (neurally mediated) • Distress, feeling cold	• Blue face • Aura (e.g., unusual smell) • Parasthesia, numbness
Eye-witness observations	• Jerky movements start after loss of consciousness • Duration is brief • No automatisms	• Tonic-clonic movements occur with loss of consciousness • Relatively lengthy duration • Automatisms such as lip-smacking or chewing
Post-episode signs and symptoms	• Fatigue of unpredictable duration	• Lengthy confusion

Modified from Benditt D, Adkisson W. Approach to the patient with syncope: venues, presentations, diagnosis. *Cardiol Clin.* 2013;31:9-25.

having a bowel movement, fear of bodily injury, and heat exposure.

It is also critical to get a full description of the syncopal episode. Some women may feel lightheaded prior to losing consciousness and can then later describe the pre-syncope period. Some of the symptoms that occur with syncope, especially vasovagal syncope, are nausea, yawning, blurred vision, feeling warmth or experiencing a cold clammy sweat, tunnel vision, or lightheadedness. Inquiries should be made to determine if the woman experienced only a short loss of consciousness and then had a prompt return to a normal neurologic state. A family member, if present during the syncopal episode, can usually describe what really happened when, and if, the woman lost consciousness. Vasovagal syncope symptoms that a bystander may notice include skin paleness, slow weak pulse, dilated pupils, and jerky abnormal movements.[54] Understanding the context in which a syncopal episode occurred can help determine if it was induced by situations known to be associated with syncope. A family history of sudden cardiac death or

sudden infant death syndrome is a red flag and requires a thorough investigation. A more comprehensive evaluation is warranted as some cardiac causes of syncope are genetically inherited and can be fatal.[18,54]

Physical Examination

By the time a woman is seen in the office with a complaint of syncope, she will have fully recovered and few, if any, abnormalities will be seen on the physical examination. An orthostatic BP measurement should be obtained but is frequently normal. Orthostatic hypotension usually occurs immediately before a syncopal event but is transient in nature and resolved by the time the individual is seen in the office. More persistent orthostatic hypotension can be diagnosed by a decline in systolic BP of at least 20 mmHg within 3 to 5 minutes of standing. If this finding is seen, non-neurogenic causes of orthostatic hypotension, such as dehydration, medication effects, and comorbidities (e.g., ethanol, diabetes, and adrenal insufficiency), should be suspected.[19]

Particular attention should be given to the cardiac exam. While rare, unrecognized and untreated cardiac conditions can lead to sudden death; therefore, an astute provider should always pay close attention to signs of these conditions. Cardiac conduction abnormalities and mechanical cardiac disorders such as ventricular septal defect, cardiac perforation, and outlet syndromes can cause syncope. Careful auscultation of cardiac heart sounds can help diagnose some of these structural cardiovascular abnormalities, such as a systolic murmur compatible with severe aortic stenosis or left ventricular outflow obstruction.[18] The presence of cardiac bruits or an abnormal reaction to carotid massage should also be assessed. A positive carotid sinus massage suggests that the syncopal event is vasovagal in origin, but it is contraindicated in a woman with a carotid bruit or previous history of CVA or TIA within the previous 3 months. When performing a carotid sinus massage, the provider applies pressure over the carotid bifurcation while the woman is being monitored by an electrocardiography monitor and automatic BP monitor. A positive response is associated with bradycardia and a fall in BP of 50 mmHg or more.[11]

Signs of new focal neurologic lesions, such as dysarthria, diplopia, hemiparesis, and vertigo, may suggest that a reported collapse was not true syncope, but rather a primary neurologic problem; however, this is not a concrete rule. For example, signs of severe autonomic disease or Parkinsonism may suggest a possible orthostatic syncopal episode.[19] If the underlying etiology is not clear after a comprehensive history and physical is completed, further evaluation by a neurologist should be considered.

Laboratory

An electrocardiogram (ECG) can identify cardiac conduction problems. Particular attention should be paid to the QT interval, because both shorter and longer QT intervals are associated with poorer outcomes. A QT interval greater than 450 milliseconds for males and greater than 470 milliseconds in females is abnormal and possibly indicative of long QT syndrome (LQTS). LQTS is an inherited ion channelopathy associated with familial syncope and sudden cardiac death. A short QT syndrome (SQTS) can also be problematic. A QT interval of less than 300 to 320 milliseconds is associated with syncope and sudden cardiac death.[18]

Other commonly used tests in the evaluation of syncope include an echocardiogram, blood work, and a stress test.[55] Echocardiograms can help identify a structural mechanical cause of syncope. Blood work such as a hemoglobin and hematocrit may be ordered to rule out anemia as a cause of the woman's symptoms. If a cardiac etiology is suspected, a brain natriuretic peptide (BNP) serum level has been found to help make this diagnosis. This assay is usually elevated in a woman with congestive heart failure, and if it is 300 pg/mL or greater may indicate an underlying cardiac cause of syncope.[19] A stress test is used to evaluate prognosis and to establish functional capacity. A stress test involves checking physiologic parameters, such as ECG at rest and again when the heart has been stressed either by a pharmacologic agent or exercise. Other parameters followed are BP and respiratory rate.[57]

A tilt-table test may also be ordered to rule out orthostatic causes of syncope. There are three types of tilt-table tests: passive tilt, pharmacologic provocation, and passive tilt testing with lower body negative pressure. In the passive tilt-table test, a woman lies flat on the exam table and then the head is raised by 60°–70° for 20–60 minutes. If no orthostatic or presyncopal event is induced, then pharmacologic provocation is used to increase the orthostatic challenge. Usually IV isoproterenol or IV/SL nitroglycerin is used, with a high response rate seen immediately after administration. One of the disadvantages of the pharmacologic method is that it is associated with a higher false-positive rate than other methods. Tilt testing using a lower body negative pressure technique combines the passive tilt-table test with lower body negative pressure supplied by a chamber that fits over the patient from the waist down. This creates a stronger orthostatic stress without invasive procedures or drug side effects. This technique provokes pre-syncope in almost all subjects, which allows for symptom recognition in women with syncope. This test is considered to be the "gold standard" and has a high specificity (92%) and sensitivity (85%).[11,58]

Management of Syncope

MEDICATION

Table 8-12 described common medications used in the treatment of neurologic disorders. The specific medications used in the treatment of syncope depend on the cause of the syncope:

- Vasovagal syncope:
  - Midodrine (Orvaten) may be ordered for the woman with vasovagal syncope caused by low BP.
  - IV atropine may be ordered for a woman in the emergency room or as an inpatient in the hospital to increase heart rate.
  - Although not a medication, a permanent pacemaker may be needed to prevent the heart rate from dropping below a preset rate in the pacemaker.
  - All medications that cause a drop in heart rate and BP should be discontinued.
- Cardiac syncope:
  - Mexiletine is an antiarrhythmic used for ventricular arrhythmias that produce syncope.

Complementary/Alternative Therapies

There has been no research conducted on complementary or alternative choices for use with syncope.

Patient Instructions

Women should be advised to:

- Drink plenty of water daily (as long as they do not have underlying congestive heart failure).
- Avoid any known triggers.
- Eat a well-balanced diet and avoid alcohol.
- Use compression stockings to help with venous return to the heart. Compression stockings are most helpful in those whose syncope is due to a vasovagal cause.
- Do foot exercises and tense up leg muscles when standing to promote good circulation.
- Increase salt in the diet to help increase water retention, although not all women should be advised to increase their salt intake. This advice will depend on whether other underlying medical conditions are present that would preclude added salt use.
- Avoid prolonged standing, especially in crowded and hot places.
- Lie down and lift their legs if they suspect they may faint. If they cannot safely lie down, they should sit down and put their head down between the knees until the feeling of syncope has passed. These techniques increase venous return to the heart and to the brain.
- Take special care after placement of a cardiac pacemaker. Women with pacemakers may be at greater risk of syncopal events. These individuals should take their radial pulse every morning to check that they are not developing borderline bradycardia. They should also avoid lifting their affected arm above the shoulder level for 1 week after the pacemaker is implanted.

During Pregnancy and Lactation

Syncope is common in pregnancy. It usually occurs from orthostatic hypotension. Pregnant women have increased fluid demands due to the developing fetus and have greater fluid loss due to increased perspiration. Prolonged standing can lead to cerebral hypoperfusion because blood remains trapped in the lower extremities from vascular compression by the enlarging uterus. Abrupt changes in position can also cause feelings of dizziness for similar reasons. Treatment is supportive and focuses on encouraging adequate hydration, consumption of small frequent meals to maintain normal glucose levels, and strategies such as pacing or assuming a recumbent position to minimize prolonged sitting or standing. Medications are not used in pregnancy.

Vertigo and Dizziness

Dizziness is a catchall phrase used to describe a multitude of symptoms. Dizziness may be more accurately defined as one of the following sensations: vertigo (false sense of motion or spinning), lightheadedness (the feeling of near fainting), disequilibrium (unsteadiness or loss of balance), and dizziness (floating, heavy-headedness, or swimming). During a "dizzy spell," the brain receives signals from one or more sensory systems in the body, which can become disrupted or confused.

Key inputs from the eyes, which help the patient to determine where her body is in space and how it is moving; the sensory nerves, which transmit messages to the woman's brain about body movements and positions; and the inner ear, which contains sensors that help sense gravity and back-and-forth motion, must be coordinated together in order to avoid the sensation of dizziness.[5,6] Disruptions along any of these pathways can induce dizziness. While this sensation can be disturbing, it is rarely a signal of a serious or life-threatening sensation.

Women who report vertigo or dizziness often have difficulty describing their symptoms. They may use the word "dizziness" to describe any of the symptoms listed in the previous paragraph, but also use this word to describe nausea, gait instability, anxiety, or generalized weakness. In whatever fashion the woman describes her symptoms, it is vital to ask questions in an effort to clarify her complaint. Individuals who cannot describe their sensations clearly may be more likely to be affected by one of the nonspecific causes of dizziness or vertigo.[6,59] Causes of disequilibrium are shown in **Table 8-16**.

Table 8-16 Causes of Disequilibrium

Disorder	Description of the Disorder
Vestibular (inner ear) problems	Anomalies in the inner ear can cause the patient to feel like she is unsteady while walking, particularly in the dark.
Sensory disorders	Nerve damage in the legs and worsening vision are commonplace in older adults and can cause difficulty maintaining balance.
Joint and muscle problems	Osteoarthritis and muscle weakness can cause loss of balance in weight-bearing joints.
Neurologic conditions	Parkinson's disease and cerebellar ataxia can lead to progressive loss of balance
Medications	Sedatives, tranquilizers, and anti-seizure medications can have a side effect that will cause loss of balance.

Data from American Academy of Neurology. Headache. https://www.aan.com/Guidelines/Home/ByTopic?topicId=16. April 2012. Accessed March 23, 2016.

Numbness and Paresthesia— Peripheral Neuropathy

Numbness can be described as a loss of sensation or feeling in a part of the body. Numbness may occur along a single nerve, or bilaterally in a symmetrical pattern. Numbness is usually associated with damage, compression, or irritation of several nerves or a single branch of a nerve, most commonly located in the periphery of the body. Diseases affecting the peripheral nerves, such as diabetes and hypothyroidism, can cause loss of sensation, as can vitamin deficiencies, exposure to heavy metals, toxins, infections, and numerous medications. Rarely, numbness can be caused by problems in the brain or spinal cord.[60] Causes of peripheral neuropathy are presented in **Table 8-17**.

Incomplete loss of sensation—often described as a "pins and needles" or burning sensation—is paresthesia. It has no apparent long-term physical effect. It may occur if, for example, the woman has lain or sat in a position for a period of time with resultant prolonged pressure on nerve roots. This sensation is a safety mechanism that prompts an individual to change position so that irreversible nerve damage does not occur.

More constant and nonremitting symptoms are usually due to a neuropathy rather than compression. The symptoms of peripheral neuropathy depend on which nerves—sensory, motor, or autonomic—are damaged. Peripheral neuropathy may affect one nerve (mononeuropathy), two or more nerves in different areas (multiple mononeuropathy), or many nerves (polyneuropathy).[60] The incidence of peripheral neuropathy is estimated at 2.4% in the general population,[61] and 10 times as much (26.4%) among diabetics.[62]

More than 100 types of peripheral neuropathies have been identified, each with their own distinctive set of symptoms, pattern of development, and prognosis. For example, peripheral neuropathy associated with diabetes presents with numbness and tingling in the feet; the numbness and tingling then spread upward into the legs.

Carpal tunnel syndrome is a common presentation of peripheral neuropathy in reproductive-aged women. Overall incidence is between 1% and 7%, with a prevalence in women approximately 3 times that in men.[63] Compression of the median nerve, where it travels through the wrist bones, causes loss of sensation in the central portion of the hand (thumb, index and middle fingers). The injury may be unilateral (often in the dominant hand) or bilateral. Overuse, pregnancy, obesity, and hypothyroidism have all been associated with increased risk.

History

As in vertigo, symptoms of numbness, tingling, or paresthesia can also encompass a number of etiologies. Transient feelings are of less concern, because they are more likely to be due to positional changes and are unlikely to be associated with significant disease. Screening for signs and symptoms of chronic diseases is essential if prolonged symptoms are present, as is an evaluation for symptoms that suggest a central rather than peripheral origin, such as difficulty with speech, impaired vision, ataxia, or loss of bladder and bowel control.[60] Treatable causes should be considered and excluded. See Table 8-17.

Physical

A comprehensive physical is needed to investigate symptoms of numbness and paresthesias. It should include a complete head, eyes, ears, nose, and throat (HEENT) exam; respiratory, cardiac, and neurologic examination; and assessment of normal radial, posterior tibial, and pedal pulses. The presence of pedal edema, or lower leg discoloration, may be signs of vascular insufficiency. During the clinical examination, evaluation for

Table 8-17 Potential Causes of Peripheral Neuropathies

Cause	Comments	Laboratory Tests
Diseases		
Acquired immunodeficiency syndrome	Mainly sensory	Human immunodeficiency virus test
Carcinoma (paraneoplastic syndrome)	Usually sensory	Paraneoplastic panel (anti-Hu, anti-Yo, anti-Ri, anti-Tr, anti-Ma, and anti-CV2 antibodies)
Chronic liver disease	Mainly demyelinating, especially in viral hepatitis	Hepatic transaminase, bilirubin, albumin, and alkaline phosphatase levels
Critical illness neuropathy	Usually acute or subacute	No specific laboratory test
Diabetes mellitus	Chronic; axonal may predominate	Fasting blood glucose level, glucose tolerance test, A1C level
End-stage renal disease	—	Serum creatinine and blood urea nitrogen levels
Hypothyroidism	Usually acute or subacute, but can be chronic	Thyroid-stimulating hormone level
Leprosy	Usually sensory	Phenolic glycolipid-1 antibody, skin biopsy
Lyme disease	—	Lyme titers
Lymphoma	Mainly axonal	CBC, imaging
Monoclonal gammopathy	Usually chronic	Urine and serum protein electrophoresis with immunofixation
Amyloidosis	Usually sensory	
Multiple myeloma	Axonal damage predominates after treatment	
Plasmacytoma (osteosclerotic myeloma)	May have some axonal damage	
Monoclonal gammopathy of undetermined significance		
IgM	Most common; may have some axonal damage	
IgG or IgA	Demyelinating features often predominate	

(continues)

337

Table 8-17 Potential Causes of Peripheral Neuropathies *(continued)*

Cause	Comments	Laboratory Tests
Porphyria	Acute	Porphyrin titers
Syphilis	—	Rapid plasma reagin, VDRL, cerebrospinal fluid analysis
Vitamin B_6 deficiency	Sensory more than motor	Vitamin B_6 level
Vitamin B_{12} deficiency	Peripheral neuropathy is intermixed with upper motor neuron signs	CBC, vitamin B_{12} and homocysteine levels, methylmalonic acid test
Drugs*		
Amiodarone (Cordarone)	Mainly axonal with sensorimotor	No specific tests
Chloroquine (Aralen)	May have some axonal damage	
Digoxin	Mainly sensory	
Heroin	Sensorimotor	
Hydralazine	Mainly sensory	
Isoniazid	Mainly sensory	
Lithium	Sensorimotor	
Metronidazole (Flagyl)	Mainly sensory	
Misoprostol (Cytotec)	Motor	
Nitrofurantoin (Furadantin)	Sensorimotor	
Phenytoin (Dilantin)	Mainly sensory	
Procainamide (Pronestyl)	May have some axonal damage	
Statins	Mainly sensory	
Vincristine (Oncovin)	Sensorimotor	
Vitamin B_6 excess	Mainly sensory	

Genetic Disorders †

Charcot-Marie-Tooth disease		Genetic testing
Type 1	Also called HMSN-I	
Type 2	Also called HMSN-II	
Metachromatic leukodystrophy	—	
Neuropathy with liability to pressure palsies	—	
Refsum disease	Also called HMSN-IV	

Toxins*

Diphtheria toxin	Acute presentation	Histopathology
Ethanol (alcohol)	Sensorimotor	No specific or practical laboratory test
Heavy metals (e.g., arsenic, lead, mercury, gold)	Lead and mercury mainly cause motor neuropathy	24-hour urine collection for heavy metal titers
	Arsenic causes sensorimotor neuropathy	
	Gold may cause some demyelination	
Organophosphates	Sensorimotor	No specific or practical laboratory test
Tetanus	Motor; acute presentation	No specific or practical laboratory test
Tic paralysis	Motor; acute presentation	No specific or practical laboratory test

Other

Idiopathic polyneuropathy	Diagnosis of exclusion; usually chronic	No laboratory test

CBC = complete blood count, HMSN = hereditary motor-sensory neuropathy, Ig = immunoglobulin, VDRL = venereal disease research laboratory.

*Usually acute or subacute, but can be chronic.

†Usually chronic.

Modified from Azhary H, Farooq MU, Bhanushali M, Majid A, Kassab MY. Peripheral neuropathy: differential diagnosis and management. *Am Fam Physician.* 2010;81(7):887-892.

suspected causes of neuropathy, such as the evaluation of Tinel's sign for carpal tunnel, the use of a tuning fork to evaluate sensory perception, and the joint position test are included.

Laboratory and Clinical Testing

Basic laboratory testing includes complete blood count, metabolic panel, erythrocyte sedimentation rate, fasting blood glucose and hemoglobin A1C, thyroid-stimulating hormone, and vitamin B_{12}, based on suspected cause. Further tests would be chosen based on the history. Nerve conduction studies or electromyography (EMG) testing can be used as adjunctive evaluation.[60]

Management of Numbness/ Tingling/Paresthesia

Paresthesia is managed by treating the underlying cause of the neuropathy. For example, carpal tunnel syndrome may be managed with wrist braces to position the wrist in a neutral position, the use of steroid injections, or as a final treatment, surgical release.[63,64] If the underlying cause is corrected, the neuropathy often improves on its own. Another treatment goal is to manage the pain associated with peripheral neuropathy. Persistent peripheral neuropathy should be managed by a specialist, although the initial evaluation can be completed in the women's health office, if the clinician is prepared.

MEDICATIONS FOR NUMBNESS OR PARESTHESIA

The following medications can be used in the treatment of numbness or paresthesia:

- *Pain relievers*. Mild symptoms may be relieved by OTC pain drugs. For severe pain, prescription medications may be needed. Drugs containing opiates can lead to constipation, dependence, and sedation. These should be prescribed only when other treatments fail.

- *Anti-seizure medications*. Medications such as gabapentin (Neurontin), pregabalin (Lyrica), topiramate (Topamax), and phenytoin (Dilantin) can also be prescribed for nerve pain.
- *Capsaicin*. Capsaicin is a cream that contains a naturally occurring substance found in hot peppers. One of its side effects is that it creates a sensation of heat at the site of application. Relief from paresthesia does not occur immediately. Unfortunately, not all women can tolerate the sensation of heat long enough for the cream to reduce symptoms of numbness and/ or paresthesia.
- *Lidocaine patch*. The patch is applied to the site where the pain is most severe. The use of up to four patches per day may be needed to relieve the pain.
- *Antidepressants*. Tricyclic antidepressant drugs such as amitriptyline and nortriptyline (Aventyl, Pamelor) have been found to help relieve pain by interfering with pain pathways in the brain and spinal cord. Serotonin and norepinephrine reuptake inhibitors such as duloxetine (Cymbalta) have been found to be effective in treating peripheral neuropathy caused by diabetes.

COMPLEMENTARY/ ALTERNATIVE THERAPIES

The following complementary and alternative therapies can be used in the treatment of numbness or paresthesia:

- Transcutaneous electrical nerve stimulation (TENS) may help relieve symptoms. Electrodes are placed on the skin, and a light electric current is delivered through the electrodes at variable frequencies. TENS must be used regularly to be effective.
- Acupuncture may afford some relief, although it may require multiple sessions before noticeable improvement occurs. Acupuncture is believed to be safe when performed by a certified practitioner using sterile needles.

- Alpha-lipoic acid is an antioxidant that can help the symptoms of peripheral neuropathy. Alpha-lipoic acid may affect blood sugar levels and may cause stomach upset and a skin rash.
- Biofeedback will help lessen the reaction through specific techniques such as guided imagery or relaxation.

PATIENT INSTRUCTIONS

The following strategies can help control or improve peripheral neuropathy and decrease nerve damage:

- Quit smoking. Smoking can affect circulation, increasing the risk of foot problems and possibly amputation—particularly in those whose vascular or neurologic system is already compromised.
- Maintain euglycemia. Controlling a woman's blood sugar level can prevent or minimize the progression of neuropathy in women with diabetes.
- Eat a healthy diet. Healthy eating is especially important to ensure the woman will get essential vitamins and minerals. Eating a healthy diet that is rich in fruits, vegetables, whole grains, and lean protein is important for everyone, but is critical in those with vitamin deficiencies. For example, consuming foods high in vitamin B_{12} such as fish, eggs, meats, low-fat dairy foods, and fortified cereals can minimize damage associated with vitamin B_{12} deficiency.
- Exercise. Exercising regularly at least 30 minutes to 1 hour at minimum 3 times a week promotes healthy vascular circulation, decreases neuropathy, and helps control blood sugar levels.
- Avoid activities and exposures that produce or worsen symptoms, such as being in a cramped position, crossing knees, leaning on elbows, or engaging in repetitive movements for a prolonged period of time.
- Using a thermometer to check the temperature of water before washing or bathing may be needed to prevent burns related to loss of hot/cold sensation.

- Affected women should practice good foot care. They should check their feet daily for signs of cuts, calluses, or blisters and wear soft, loose cotton socks and padded shoes. Because women with neuropathies are at risk for poor healing, the prevention and early detection of skin damage can minimize the chance of developing more serious infections.

Weakness

A feeling of weakness is a result of reduced muscular strength, occurring either in isolated muscle groups or more systemically. Many suspected causes of weakness require referral to a neurologist in order to complete the assessment.

History

As when investigating any health problem, an understanding of the initial presentation and its evolution over time is important. Asking about the location of the weakness, whether it affects only one extremity or is unilateral or bilateral can help uncover neurologic problems such as stroke or isolated nerve injury. Generalized weakness may indicate systemic problems such as thyroid disorders, vitamin deficiencies, or depression. If weakness is worse later in the day or with activity, then muscular problems may be more likely. Knowing the degree it affects an individual in her performance of activities of daily living can help gauge the severity of the underlying disease.

Physical

Investigation of a report of weakness requires a thorough neurologic exam and a targeted history. A complete physical examination including assessment of the cranial nerves, reflexes, muscle strength and atrophy, and balance is needed to focus the evaluation of symptoms.[65] See the section earlier in this chapter on how to conduct an abbreviated neurologic exam. A suspected stroke, while rarely seen in the women's health setting, requires ongoing assessment, because findings can change rapidly in the presence of an evolving stroke. If a stroke is suspected, then immediate referral to a stroke center is warranted.

Laboratory

The specific laboratory and imaging studies ordered in a particular case will depend on the findings elicited in the history and physical. A basic panel of tests as outlined in Table 8-7 should be obtained. Unilateral weakness may be indicative of CVA or stroke. Usually one of the first tests ordered if a stroke is suspected is a CT scan without contrast to help determine if the stroke is hemorrhagic or ischemic in nature. If it is ischemic, the usual treatment is recombinant tissue plasminogen activator to be given within 3 to 4.5 hours of the start of symptoms.[56] Prompt treatment can prevent or minimize further damage.

Management

Weakness is a symptom and not a diagnosis of a disease pattern and can be caused by many neurologic disorders such as muscular dystrophy, Guillain-Barré syndrome, myasthenia gravis, stroke, and Parkinson disease, to name a few. Among reproductive-aged women, the most likely diagnosis is MS.[66] MS is usually diagnosed between the ages of 20 and 40 years and is one of the leading causes of disability in young adults.[56] It is twice as common in females than males. Currently, approximately 500,000 people in the United States are affected by MS.[66]

Multiple Sclerosis

MS is a chronic immune-mediated neurodegenerative disease that affects the myelin sheath and conduction pathway of the central nervous system. It is characterized by an inflammatory response in which the myelin sheath is damaged and thinned, resulting in impeded conduction of nerve impulses from the central nervous system to the spinal cord and the rest of the body. Areas of the nervous system that are most commonly affected are the optic nerve, pyramidal tracts, brainstem nuclei, posterior columns, and the periventricular region of the brain. Symptoms associated with neurologic damage wax and wane but become more severe and persistent as the disease progresses. While the rate of progression can vary widely, progression is associated with the development of permanent neurologic deficits. Table 8-18 describes the major types of MS.[66]

History

Often a woman with MS will report that she had symptoms of fatigue, difficulty with gait or balance, or clumsiness on and off for a number of years, but did not seek medical attention. Because symptoms are nonspecific and can remit for long periods of time, particularly early in the course of the disease, women may delay health care and as symptoms worsen may need to consult several healthcare professionals before a diagnosis is made. If MS is suspected, then inquiries should be made about the presence of any precipitating factors, because overexertion, fatigue, stress, or temperature extremes may prompt an exacerbation. Environmental risk factors for MS include smoking, Epstein-Barr virus infection, and low vitamin D levels.[67] There is also a genetic component to MS; if siblings are affected, then the risk of developing MS is substantially higher.

Occasionally MS will present with neurologic changes that may not be evident to the affected individual. The provider should ask if the family has noticed personality change such as poor judgment, loss of attention, or euphoria.[66] Neurologic damage from MS can affect sensation, as well as cognition. Women with MS may experience facial pain, hypalgesia, decreased temperature perception, numbness, and sensations of burning or crawling on the skin. The woman may also report

Table 8-18 Major Types of Multiple Sclerosis

Type of Multiple Sclerosis	Description
Relapsing-Remitting MS (RRMS)	Most common variant, encompassing 80% or more of new diagnoses. The course of the illness can be mild or moderate. Symptoms progress and resolve in a few weeks or months.
Primary Progressive MS (PPMS)	Steady neurologic deterioration without remission of symptoms. Patient has gradual disability without acute attacks.
Secondary Progressive MS (SPMS)	Initially presents in a relapsing and remitting pattern before becoming steadily progressive. Functioning continues to deteriorate with no clear-cut times of remission. Over time, most RRMS patient will convert to this pattern.
Progressive-Relapsing MS (PRMS)	Numerous relapses demonstrating only partial recovery with or without return to baseline function. Cumulative symptoms become more frequent and severe.

Data from Milo R, Miller A. Revised diagnostic criteria of multiple sclerosis. *Autoimmun Rev.* 2014 Apr-May;13(4-5):518-524; Palmieri R, Ignatavicius D. Care of critically ill patients with neurologic problems. In: Ignatavicius D, Workman M, eds. *Medical-Surgical Nursing: Patient-Centered Collaborative Care.* 7th ed. St. Louis, MO: Elsevier; 2013.

fecal and/or urinary incontinence, as well as alterations in sexuality. Cognitive changes appear for most affected individuals late in the course of the disease. Women may be distressed by declines in short-term memory, impaired concentration and judgment, and difficulty in performing calculations. Women with MS are often depressed, anxious, apathetic, or emotionally labile. Some of the medications that are used to treat MS can cause the woman to be giddy or euphoric; occasionally, these same symptoms can be due to the disease itself. **Table 8-19** lists the most common findings seen in individuals with MS.

If the history is suggestive of MS, or findings on the initial physical examination are concerning, the woman should be referred to a neurologist for further evaluation and management.

Physical Examination

Because MS affects all myelinated fibers, numerous abnormalities may be found on the physical exam. Particular attention should be paid to findings elicited on a complete neurologic and musculoskeletal assessment. Stiffness, especially of the lower extremities, and night-time flexor spasms are common. On the musculoskeletal examination, the provider may see hyperactive reflexes, a positive Babinski reflex, or absent abdominal reflexes. The gait may be unsteady due to muscle fatigue, spasticity, and weakness. Cerebellar problems will be evident in intention tremors, dysmetria, and dysdiadochokinesia (the inability to stop one motor movement and start another one). The woman may show signs of imbalance, clumsy movements, and poor coordination.

Laboratory Evaluation

No single test is diagnostic of MS; rather, several tests are needed to arrive at a diagnosis. Results can vary depending on whether the woman is in remission or currently experiencing an exacerbation. For example, during an exacerbation white blood cells (WBCs) and protein may be elevated in the CSF. In addition, results on

Table 8-19 Common Features of MS

Feature
Paresthesia
Intention tremors
Dysmetria (inability to direct or limit movement)
Ataxia
Hypalgesia (decreased sensitivity to pain)
Heat intolerance
Dysphagia
Dysarthria (slurred speech)
Scotoma (area of decreased vision in the field)
Decreased hearing and visual acuity
Bowel and bladder dysfunction
Alterations in sexual function
Tinnitus, vertigo
Fatigue
Muscle weakness and spasticity
Diplopia
Nystagmus
Cognitive changes

Data from Milo R, Miller A. Revised diagnostic criteria of multiple sclerosis. *Autoimmun Rev.* 2014 Apr-May; 13(4-5): 518-524; Palmieri R, Ignatavicius D. Care of critically ill patients with neurologic problems. In: Ignatavicius D, Workman M, eds. *Medical-Surgical Nursing: Patient-Centered Collaborative Care.* 7th ed. St. Louis, MO: Elsevier; 2013.

a CSF electrophoresis may reveal an increase in myelin basic protein and the presence of oligoclonal bands (IgG bands). Findings on evoked potential studies for auditory, visual, and brainstem function are often abnormal. Plaques seen on an MRI are considered diagnostic for MS. Increase in white matter and the presence of plaques seen on a CT scan also strongly support the diagnosis of MS. EMG changes may not be seen until later in the course of the disease, but generally are grossly abnormal in women with advanced MS. Arriving at a diagnosis depends on the results of a combination of these tests. According to the MacDonald criteria, the following results are needed to confirm the diagnosis: two events separated in time and space, positive CSF findings, MRI evidence of MS, and confirmation that a second attack has occurred based on an analysis of the results of a test for evoked potentials.[66]

Medications

The following drugs are recommended to be used as early as possible in the course of the disease, because continuous use is thought to minimize progression of the disease:

- Natalizumab (Tysabri) is the first monoclonal antibody approved for MS that binds to WBCs to thwart further damage to the myelin sheath. This medication has been associated with significant liver damage; use requires obtaining liver enzymes on a regular schedule.
- Interferon beta (Avonex) is an immunomodulator that modifies the course of MS and has an antiviral effect.
- Glatiramer acetate (Copaxone) is a synthetic protein that is similar to myelin-based protein.
- Mitoxantrone (Novantrone) is a chemotherapeutic drug and has been associated with decreasing exacerbations and neurologic disabilities.
- Immunosuppressive therapy with a combination of methylprednisolone (Solu-Medrol) and cyclophosphamide (Cytoxan) may be used during an exacerbation period to stabilize MS.
- Baclofen (Lioresal), diazepam (Valium), or dantrolene sodium (Dantrium) may be prescribed to alleviate muscle spasticity. Severe spasticity may be treated with an intrathecal baclofen surgically implanted pump.
- Carbamazepine (Tegretol) or tricyclic antidepressants are used to treat paresthesia.
- Propranolol hydrochloride (Inderal) and clonazepam (Klonopin) may be used to treat cerebellar ataxia.
- Amantadine hydrochloride (Symmetrel) may be used to treat fatigue if the use of nonpharmacologic measures is not effective.

- Anticholinergic agents are used to treat bladder dysfunction (detrusor hyperreflexia).
- Antiepileptic drugs, analgesics, NSAIDs, antispasmodics, or antidepressants may be used for pain, which often accompanies MS.[66,68]

Complementary/ Alternative Therapies

Complementary and alternative therapies have been used by women with MS and have been effective in decreasing symptoms. To increase their comfort, many women with MS use the following modalities: moist, moderate heat; massage; electrical stimulation; and exercise to boost muscle strength. Guided imagery and acupuncture are also used to decrease pain. Marijuana appears to be particularly helpful in relieving pain from muscle spasm. Although the research is not conclusive, bee venom may help and being stung is a strategy that some women purposely employ. Nutritional supplements, such as Osmolite or Glucerna, are another strategy some women use, although the research on their effectiveness is limited.[66]

Pregnancy/Lactation

For most women with MS, pregnancy appears to be protective at least in the short term, possibly due to changes in the immune system in pregnancy. The frequency of relapse declines in pregnancy but increases in the first 3 to 6 months after birth before returning to baseline.[69-71] Neither lactation nor contraceptive use appears to affect the rate of relapse or the progression of the disease.[69]

Care must be taken if a woman is considering a pregnancy. Some healthcare professionals advise women with MS to discontinue disease-modifying therapy (DMT) prior to attempting conception. For example, the immunosuppressant mitoxantrone is a known teratogen and should not be used unless a woman is also using highly reliable contraception. However, more commonly used products appear to be safer, although information is extremely limited. Data from pregnancy registries for glatiramer acetate (GA), interferon beta-1a, and natalizumab have not shown identifiable patterns of malformation suggesting teratogenicity.[70]

During lactation, IV immunoglobulin and corticosteroids are generally safe and may be associated with a reduction in postpartum relapses. However, women who require high-dose IV corticosteroids should avoid breastfeeding and should "pump and dump" until 24 to 48 hours after the completion of their IV treatment. There appears to be little to no transfer of interferon beta-1a, glatiramer acetate, and natalizumab into breast milk, but data on their safety are limited. The use of mitoxantrone and fingolimod is not recommended during lactation.[70]

References

1. Workman M. Assessment of the endocrine system. In: Ignatavicius D, Workman M, eds. *Medical-Surgical Nursing: Patient-Centered Collaborative Care*. 7th ed. St. Louis, MO: Elsevier; 2013.
2. Waldman S. Targeted headache history. *Med Clin North Am*. 2013;97:185-195.
3. Cox B. The principles of neurological assessment. *Pract Nurs*. 2008;36(7):45-50.
4. Beneck H, Agus S, Kuessner D, Goodall G, Strupp M. The burden and impact of vertigo: findings from the REVERT patient registry. *Front Neurol*. 2013; 4:136.
5. Furman M, Rizzolo D. Evaluating the patient with vertigo: a complex complaint made simple. *JAAPA*. 2011;24(10):52-58.
6. Tusa R. Dizziness. *Med Clin North Am*. 2009; 93(2):263-271.
7. Ferri F. *Ferri's Clinical Advisor 2013: 5 Books in 1*. Philadelphia, PA: Mosby Elsevier; 2012.
8. Boss B. Disorders of the central and peripheral nervous systems and the neuromuscular junction. In: McCance KL, Huether SE, Brashers VL, Rote NS, eds. *Pathophysiology: The Biologic Basis for Disease in Adults and Children*. 6th ed. St. Louis, MO: Elsevier; 2013.

9. Griggs R, Jozefowicz R, Aminoff M. Approach to the patient with neurologic disease. In: Goldman L, Ausiello D, eds. *Goldman's Cecil Medicine.* 24th ed. Philadelphia, PA: Saunders Elsevier; 2011.

10. Noakes T. Physiological models to understand exercise fatigue and the adaptations that predict or enhance athletic performance. *Scand J Med Sci Sports.* 2000;10(3):123-145.

11. Gauer R. Evaluation of syncope. *Am Fam Physician.* 2011;84(6):640-650.

12. Sheldon R. Syncope diagnostic scores. *Prog Cardiovasc Dis.* 2013;55:390-395.

13. Van Dijk J, Wieling W. Pathophysiological basis of syncope and neurological conditions that mimic syncope. *Prog Cardiovasc Dis.* 2013;55:345-356.

14. Sutton R. Clinical classification of syncope. *Prog Cardiovasc Dis.* 2013;55:339-344.

15. Miller K. The practical neurological examination: part 5: assessment of sensory function. *Dyn Chiropract.* 2011;29(19):36.

16. Croft A. The practical neurological examination. *Dyn Chiropract.* 2011;29(4):14,37.

17. Plieri R. Assessment of the nervous system. In: Ignataviciuss D, Workman M, eds. *Medical-Surgical Nursing: Patient-Centered Collaborative Care.* 7th ed. St. Louis, MO: Elsevier; 2013.

18. Khoo C, Chakrabarti S, Arbour L, Krahn A. Recognizing life-threatening causes of syncope. *Cardiol Clin.* 2013;31:51-66.

19. Benditt D, Adkisson W. Approach to the patient with syncope: venues, presentations, diagnosis. *Cardiol Clin.* 2013;31:9-25.

20. Hilton G. Patient assessment: nervous system. In: Morton P, Fontaine D, eds. *Critical Care Nursing.* 10th ed. Philadelphia, PA: Lippincott Williams & Wilkins; 2013.

21. Latimer K. Chronic headache: stop the pain before it starts. *J Fam Pract.* 2013;62(3):126-133.

22. Landete J. Updated knowledge about polyphenols: function, bioavailability, metabolism, and health. *Crit Rev Food Sci Nutr.* 2012;52(10):936-948.

23. MacGregor EA, Hackshaw A. Prevalence of migraine on each day of the natural menstrual cycle. *Neurology.* 2004;63(2):351.

24. Kurth T, Buring JE, Rist PM. Headache, migraine and risk of brain tumors in women: prospective cohort study. *J Headache Pain.* 2015;16(1):501. doi: 10.1186/s10194-015-0501-0.

25. Fumal A, Schoenen J. Tension-type headache: current research and clinical management. *Lancet Neurol.* 2008;7(1):70-83.

26. Weaver-Agostino J. Cluster headache. *Am Fam Physician.* 2013;88(2):122-128.

27. Hindiyeh N, Krusz J, Cowan R. Does exercise make migraines worse and tension type headaches better? *Curr Pain Headache Rep.* 2013;17(12):380.

28. American Headache Society, Committee for Headache Education. Headache Diaries. Available at: http://www.achenet.org/resources/headache_diaries/. Accessed March 22, 2016.

29. Burch RC, Loder S, Loder E, Smitherman TA. The prevalence and burden of migraine and severe headache in the United States: Updated statistics From government health surveillance studies. *Headache.* 2015;55: 21-34. doi: 10.1111/head.12482.

30. Diener H. Headache: insight, understanding, treatment and patient management. *Int J Clin Pract.* 2013;67(Suppl 178):33-36.

31. Martin, VT. Menstrual migraine: New approaches to diagnosis and treatment. American Headache Society. Available at: http://www.americanheadachesociety.org/assets/1/7/Vincent_Martin_-_Menstrual_Martin.pdf. Accessed March 23, 2016.

32. Donohoe C. The role of the physical examination in the evaluation of headache. *Med Clin North Am.* 2013;97:197-216.

33. Palmieri R. Care of patients with problems of the central nervous system: the brain. In: Ignatavicius D, Workman M, eds. *Medical-Surgical Nursing: Patient-Centered Collaborative Care.* 7th ed. St. Louis, MO: Elsevier; 2013.

34. Abstracts of the 2013 International Headache Congress, 27–30 June 2013, John B. Hynes Veterans Memorial, Convention Center, Boston, MA, USA. *Cephalalgia.* 2013(33):1-309.

35. International Headache Society. *International Classification of Headache Disorders.* 2nd ed. Oxford, UK: Blackwell Publishing. *Cephalgia.* 2003;24(Suppl 1). Available at: http://ihs-classification.org/_downloads/mixed/ihc_II_main_no_print.pdf. Accessed March 23, 2016.

36. Lipton R, Buse D, Serrano D, Holland S, Reed ML. Examination of unmet treatment needs among persons with episodic migraine: results of the American Migraine Prevalence and Prevention (AMMPP) study. *Headache.* 2013;53(8):1300-1311.

37. Holland S, Silberstein S, Freitag F, Dodick D, Argoff C. Evidence-based guideline update: NSAIDs and other complementary treatments for episodic migraine prevention in adults. *Neurology.* 2012;78(17):1346-1353.

38. Curtis KM. U.S. Medical Eligibility Criteria for contraceptive use, 2010: adapted from the World Health Organization Medical Eligibility Criteria

for contraceptive use, 4th edition. *MMWR.* 2010; 59(RR04):1-6.

39. Nappi RE, Merki-Feld GS, Terreno E, Pellegrinelli A, Viana M. Hormonal contraception in women with migraine: is progestogen-only contraception a better choice? *J Headache Pain.* 2013;14:66. doi: 10.1186/1129-2377-14-66.

40. American Academy of Neurology. Headache. April 2012. Available at: https://www.aan.com/Guidelines/Home/ByTopic?topicId=16. Accessed March 23, 2016.

41. Digre K. Headaches during pregnancy. *Clin Obstet Gynecol.* 2013;56(2):317-329.

42. Pringsheim T. Canadian Headache Society guideline for migraine prophylaxis. *Can J Neurol Sci.* 2012;39(Suppl 2):S1-59.

43. Hutchinson S, Marmura MJ, Calhoun A, Lucas S, Silberstein S, Peterlin B. Use of common migraine treatments in breast-feeding women: a summary of recommendations. *Headache.* 2013;53:614-627.

44. Beithon J, Gallenberg M, Johnson K, Kildahl P, Krenik J, Liebow M, et al. *Diagnosis and Treatment of Headache.* Bloomington, MN: Institute for Clinical Systems Improvement (ICSI); 2013:90. Available at: https://www.icsi.org/_asset/qwrznq/Headache.pdf. Accessed March 23, 2016.

45. Fischera M, Marziniak M, Gralow I, Evers S. The incidence and prevalence of cluster headache: a meta-analysis of population-based studies. *Cephalalgia.* 2008;28(6):614-618.

46. Tfelt-Hansen P, Jensen R. Management of cluster headache. *CNS Drugs.* 2012;26(7):571-580.

47. May A, Leone M. Update on cluster headache. *Curr Opin Neurol.* 2003;16(3):333-340.

48. van Kleef M, Lataster A, Narouze S, Mekhail N, Geurts JW, van Zundert J. Evidence-based interventional pain medicine according to clinical diagnoses. 2. Cluster headache. *Pain Pract.* 2009;9(6):435-442.

49. Robbins MS. The psychiatric comorbidities of cluster headache. *Curr Pain Headache Rep.* 2013;17:313.

50. Bilchik T. A review of nonvalidated and complementary therapies for cluster headache. *Curr Pain Headache Rep.* 2004;82(2):157-161.

51. Rossi P. Use of complementary and alternative medicine by patients with cluster headache: results of a multi-centre headache clinic survey. *Complement Ther Med.* 2008;16(4):220-227.

52. Sewell R. Response of cluster headache to kudzu. *Headache.* 2009;49:98.

53. Calhoun A, Peterlin B. Treatment of cluster headache in pregnancy and lactation. *Curr Pain Headache Rep.* 2010;14:164-173.

54. Misiri J, Candler S, Kusumoto F. Evaluation of syncope and palpitations in women. *J Womens Health.* 2011;20(10):1505-1515.

55. Brignole M, Hamdan M. New concepts in the assessment of syncope. *J Am Coll Cardio.* 2012;59(18):1583-1591.

56. Palmieri R, Ignatavicius D. Care of critically ill patients with neurologic problems. In: Ignatavicius D, Workman M, eds. *Medical-Surgical Nursing: Patient-Centered Collaborative Care.* 7th ed. St. Louis, MO: Elsevier; 2013.

57. Morton P, Reck K, Hamel J, Walther A, VonRueden K, Headley J. Patient assessment: cardiovascular system. I. In: Morton P, Fontaine D, eds. *Critical Care Nursing: A Holistic Approach.* 10th ed. New York, NY: Lippincott Williams & Wilkins; 2013.

58. Protheroe C, Ravensbergen H, Inskip J, Claydon V. Tilt testing with combined lower body negative pressure: a "gold standard" for measuring orthostatic tolerance. *J Vis Exp.* 2013;73:e4315-e4325.

59. Kutz J. The dizzy patient. *Med Clin North Am.* 2010;94:989.

60. Azhary H, Farooq MU, Bhanushali M, Majid A, Kassab MY. Peripheral neuropathy: differential diagnosis and management. *Am Fam Physician.* 2010;81(7):887-892.

61. Hughes RA. Peripheral neuropathy. *BMJ.* 2002; 324(7335):466-469.

62. Davies M, Brophy S, Williams R, Taylor A. The prevalence, severity, and impact of painful diabetic peripheral neuropathy in type 2 diabetes. *Diabetes Care.* 2006;29(7):1518-1522.

63. Middleton SD, Anakwe RE. Carpal tunnel syndrome. *BMJ.* 2014;349:g6437.

64. Gerritsen AA, de Vet HC, Scholten RJ, Bertelsmann FW, de Krom MC, Bouter LM. Splinting vs surgery in the treatment of carpal tunnel syndrome: a randomized controlled trial. *JAMA.* 2002;288: 1245-1251.

65. Ignatavicius D. Assessment of the musculoskeletal system. In: Ignatavicius D, Workman M, eds. *Medical-Surgical Nursing: Patient-Centered Collaborative Care.* 7th ed. St. Louis, MO: Elsevier; 2013.

66. Palmiere R, Ignataviciud D. Care of patients with problems of the central nervous system: the spinal cord. In: Ignatavicius D, Workman M, eds. *Medical-Surgical Nursing: Patient-Centered Collaborative Care.* 7th ed. St. Louis, MO: Elsevier; 2013.

67. Nicholas J, Boster A, Racke M. Multiple sclerosis: five new things. *Neurology.* 2013;3(5):404-412.

68. Costello K. Multiple sclerosis research: diagnostic, disease-modifying treatments, and emerging therapies. *J Neurosci Nurs.* 2013;45(6S):S14-S23.

69. McCombe P, Greer J. Female reproductive issues in multiple sclerosis. *Mult Scler.* 2012;19(4):392-402.

70. Houtchens M, Kolb C. Multiple sclerosis and pregnancy: therapeutic considerations. *J Neurol.* 2013;260:1201-1214.

71. Fragoso Y, Adoni T, Alves-Leon SV, Azambuja ND Jr, Barreira AA, Brooks JB, et al. Long-term effects of exposure to disease-modifying drugs in the offspring of mothers with multiple sclerosis: a retrospective chart review. *CNS Drugs.* 2013;27(11):955-961.

CHAPTER 9

COMMON CONDITIONS OF THE EYE

Melanie Cheung | Derek Hoare

Numerous conditions of the eye present in the primary care setting. Conditions may be focal and simple to treat, more serious and require urgent medical attention, or be part of a syndrome associated with a systemic disease. Some conditions are immediately obvious to the practitioner and the woman, while others may go unnoticed unless specifically sought during a thorough physical exam.

This chapter introduces basic anatomy, physiology, and pathology of the eye and provides a basic guide to history taking and examination of the eye with an overview of the presentation, diagnosis, and management of commonly encountered eye conditions. The reader is referred to *Grant's Atlas of Anatomy*[1] for further reading on eye anatomy. This approach should equip providers to recognize and appropriately manage or refer women who have eye complaints.

Anatomy and Function

The eye is a complex structure responsible for delivering visual information from the surrounding world to the brain. Conditions of the eye can be caused by problems in the accessory structures of the eye, within the eyeball, or in the portion of the eye that is visible to others.

The accessory structures consist of the eyelids, eyelashes, eyebrows, and the lacrimal apparatus. The eyelids are responsible for protecting the eye from injury, controlling the amount of light that enters the eye, and spreading lubricating secretions over the eyeball. The layers of the eyelid from anterior to posterior consist of the epidermis and dermis, subcutaneous tissue, muscle fibers, the tarsal plate, tarsal glands, and the conjunctiva. Meibomian glands secrete a fluid that prevents the eyelids from sticking together, and these are found in the tarsal plate. Eyelashes project from the border of the eyelid. Sebaceous glands that secrete a lubricating fluid are found at the base of the eyelash hair follicles. The lacrimal glands are responsible for tear production. Excess tears drain into the lacrimal canals and then into the lacrimal sac and nasolacrimal duct.

The eyeball consists of three separate chambers (**Figure 9-1**). The anterior chamber is found behind the cornea and anterior to the iris. The posterior chamber is situated behind the iris and

Figure 9-1 Anatomy of the eye.

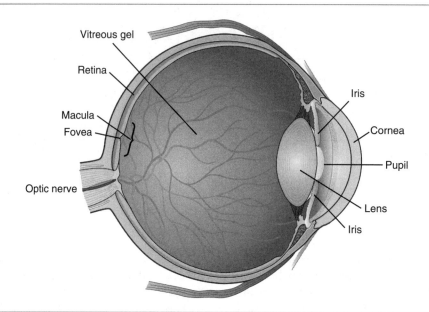

anterior to the lens. The anterior and posterior chambers contain aqueous humour. The vitreous chamber is found behind the lens and contains vitreous humour.

At the front of the eyeball is the cornea, a transparent layer covering the iris, pupil, and the anterior chamber. It acts as a barrier preventing harmful substances from entering the eye. It is transparent to allow light to enter, and curved to play a role in refracting (bending) light to focus it onto the retina.

The iris is the colored part of the eye. It contains smooth muscle fibers that contract and relax to change the diameter of the pupil. This controls the amount of light that enters the eye.

Behind the iris and pupil is the lens. These biconvex, transparent, flexible structures function to refract light and focus it onto the retina and facilitate clear vision (**Figure 9-2**).

At the back of the eye, the retina is responsible for converting visual information into electrical impulses that are carried as information to the brain via the optic nerve. The retina is made up of millions of photoreceptor cells known as rods and cones. Rods are responsible for peripheral vision and vision in dim lighting. Cones are responsible for color vision and vision in bright light. Cones are found in greater numbers around the macula and fovea. The macula is an area near the center of the retina and is responsible for central vision. The fovea is a pit found within the macula that contains a very high concentration of cones and no rods. The fovea is the area with the highest visual acuity (sharpness of vision). The outer layer of the retina is known as the retinal pigment epithelium, and this layer acts to nourish photoreceptor cells.

The sclera (white of the eye) is a layer of connective tissue that surrounds the eyeball except

Figure 9-2 Successive levels of refraction to focus light onto the retina.

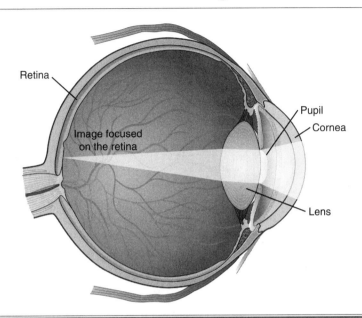

for the area covered by the cornea. At the junction of the cornea and the sclera is the scleral venous sinus (trabecular meshwork). This sinus is responsible for draining away aqueous humour, which is continually replenished by the ciliary bodies located behind the iris, in the posterior chamber of the eye (**Figure 9-3**).

Essential History and Physical

A wide range of signs and symptoms can indicate eye pathology. Whatever the presenting feature, a systematic approach to taking a history and examining the eye supported by knowledge of eye anatomy, physiology, and common eye pathologies will help the health provider recognize and diagnose common eye conditions. This will allow the health provider to reassure the woman, treat minor conditions, and prompt timely referral of more serious conditions to the relevant clinical specialists. For a summary of differential diagnoses by symptom see **Table 9-1**.

History

Taking a good history will provide vital clues to finding the cause of the presenting problem. Health providers should be aware of demographics such as age, ethnicity, and occupation, all of which may be relevant to the presenting problem or influence management. Critical components of the history include determining how long the problem has been an issue and whether it developed acutely (e.g., sudden loss of vision found in

Figure 9-3 Aqueous humour, a clear fluid, flows continuously in and out of the anterior chamber of the eye and nourishes nearby tissues. The fluid leaves the chamber at the open angle where the cornea and iris meet. When the fluid reaches the angle, it flows through a spongy meshwork and leaves the eye.

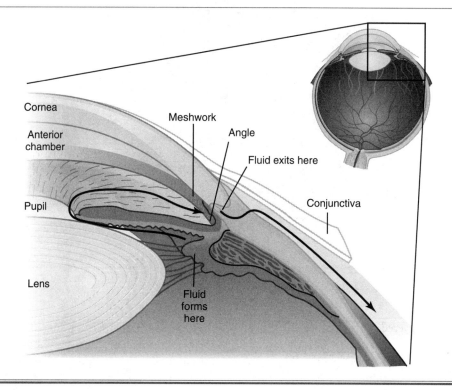

Modified from National Eye Institute, National Institutes of Health.

retinal detachment) or over a longer period (e.g., infection). The woman should be asked specifically about her symptoms, such as redness or swelling, pain, itching, or the presence of watery or purulent discharge. Specific symptoms can suggest a specific diagnosis. For example, symptoms that can help differentiate bacterial from viral infections include whether the eyelashes are glued down upon waking in the morning. The presence of other associated symptoms should also be ascertained—in particular whether there

are vision changes, headache, nausea/vomiting, or photophobia. Knowing which symptoms are present can help direct diagnostic testing and is useful in helping determine which diagnoses should be under consideration.

Other critical questions include whether there has been any trauma or injury to the eye, the presence or absence of any other underlying conditions, recent illnesses, exposures to infections, and whether the affected individual is experiencing any other symptoms potentially related to the eye problem. It should also be ascertained whether the woman may be or is pregnant, and whether she wears glasses or uses contact lenses. The presence of previous or existing medical problems can suggest particular etiologies. Diabetes, hypertension, thyroid disease, and autoimmune or immune-compromising illnesses are risk factors for a number of common eye conditions, discussed

Table 9-1 Differential Diagnoses by Symptom

Symptom and Condition	History and Associated Symptoms	Features	Indications for Referral
Flaky Skin and Irritation Along Eyelid Margins			
Blepharitis	Allergy, seborrhea, or other dermatologic condition	• Normal vision • Normal fundoscopic exam • Conjunctival inflammation • Erythema and edema of eyelid • May have crusting of lid from discharge • Eyelash loss or pointing in opposite directions of other eyelashes	Condition unresponsive to treatment or initial presentation is severe.
Eye Papule (solid raised lesion up to 10 mm diameter)			
Chalazion	Nonabrupt onset May have history of previous occurrence	• Normal vision unless vision blurred by cyst on upper lid • Nontender cyst • Normal fundoscopic exam	Persists despite soaking. Surgical incision and drainage may be needed. Multiple recurrences, or evaluation findings suggest sebaceous gland neoplasia.
Stye	Nonabrupt onset	• Normal vision • Red, tender eyelid • Boil-like lesion on eyelid • May have conjunctival erythema • Normal fundoscopic exam	No resolution after 10–14 days.
Eye Discharge			
Bacterial conjunctivitis	Exposure to others with similar complaints	• Sudden onset • Diffuse redness • Purulent discharge • Edema of the conjunctiva • Normal vision • Normal fundoscopic exam	Unresponsive to treatment, suspect chlamydia or gonorrheal infection, or accompanied by a sensation of foreign body (to rule out keratitis).

(continues)

Table 9-1 Differential Diagnoses by Symptom (*continued*)

Symptom and Condition	History and Associated Symptoms	Features	Indications for Referral
Viral conjunctivitis	Concomitant URI Exposure to others with similar complaint	• Diffuse redness • Edema of the conjunctiva • Blurry vision due to clear watery discharge, otherwise normal vision • Edema of the eyelid • Normal vision • Normal fundoscopic exam • May start in one eye and spread to other eye • Possible pre-auricular lymph node edema	No improvement in 14 days.
Allergic conjunctivitis	Exposure to known trigger including environmental, medication, cosmetics	• Diffuse redness • Eyelid edema • Itching • Tearing • Stringy, white discharge • Nasal congestion • Normal vision • Normal fundoscopy	No response to treatment.
Redness of the Eye			
Subconjunctival hemorrhage	History of coughing, or vigorous physical activity or Valsalva maneuver such as pushing in labor	• Erythema • Painless • Normal vision • Normal fundoscopy	No spontaneous healing seen within ~2 weeks
Pain			
Scleritis, iritis, uveitis	History of chronic disease such as inflammatory bowel disease, autoimmune disorders, or infections such as CMV or toxoplasmosis	• Irritation or itchiness • Erythema of sclera, iris • Painful orbit to palpation • Photophobia	Condition suspected or present. Warrants evaluation by an ophthalmologist.
Trauma	History of injury to eye ("black eye")	• Bruising of eyelid • Otherwise normal eye and fundoscopy • Normal vision	Injury accompanied by blurred vision or vision loss, possible infection, painful orbit, headache, bleeding, unequal pupils, suspected injury to surrounding tissue, flashing lights, bleeding, or injury to sclera.

Table 9-1 Differential Diagnoses by Symptom (*continued*)

Symptom and Condition	History and Associated Symptoms	Features	Indications for Referral
Foreign body	History of sudden onset of symptoms with or without exposure to known substance	• Redness • Excessive tearing • Sense of presence of irritant • Photophobia • Fundoscopy normal, but may be difficult to perform	Condition suspected or present. Warrants evaluation by ophthalmologist.
Chemical splash	History of splash	• Eye pain • Erythema • May have ulcers or blisters	Condition suspected or present. Warrants evaluation by an ophthalmologist.
Corneal abrasion	History of trauma or prolonged contact lens use	• Redness concentrated around limbus • Photophobia • Exam with penlight across cornea may demonstrate abrasion • Fluorescein exam may be necessary to see abrasion: refer	Condition suspected or present. Warrants evaluation by an ophthalmologist.
Herpes zoster and herpes simplex	History of varicella or herpes simplex	• Painful lesions noted on face, eyelid, nose	Condition suspected or present. Warrants evaluation by an ophthalmologist.
Acute angle-closure glaucoma	Symptoms often occur in evening; usually in older person. May report history of anticholinergic or sympathomimetic agents (some antidepressants, nasal decongestants). Precipitated by incident of pupillary dilation such as in darkened room.	• Eye redness • Moderate to severe pain • Symptoms usually occur in one eye • Reports halos around lights • Dilated pupil • Cornea appears "steamy" • Eye feels hard to palpation due to increased intraocular pressure • Possible headache, nausea, and vomiting	Condition suspected or present. Warrants evaluation by an ophthalmologist.
Visual Disturbance			
Refractive error	Slow onset Blurry or double vision Headache	• Painless • Decrease of visual acuity • Normal fundoscopy	Condition suspected as corrective lenses are needed.

(*continues*)

Table 9-1 Differential Diagnoses by Symptom (*continued*)

Symptom and Condition	History and Associated Symptoms	Features	Indications for Referral
Retinal detachment	Spots before the eyes Flashes of light Sudden loss of vision Sudden or progressively blurry vision No pain or redness	• Loss of portion or whole visual field • "Hanging" retina or irregular retinal surface	Condition suspected or present. Warrants evaluation by an ophthalmologist.
Glaucoma	Occurs most frequently in older population History of ophthalmic or systemic corticosteroid medication use for several weeks	• May be symptom free • Usually found on routine ophthalmic examination • Fundoscopy: cupping of disc	Condition suspected or present. Warrants evaluation by an ophthalmologist.
Age-related macular degeneration	Gradual loss of vision, blurry vision, or "holes in vision"	• Unilateral • Distortion of vision using the Amsler grid	Condition suspected or present. Warrants evaluation by an ophthalmologist. Requires urgent referral if sudden onset.
Cataracts	Slow onset Most frequently occurs in older population and persons with a history of diabetes mellitus	• Painless • Decreased visual acuity • Lens over pupil appears hazy or cloudy when examined with penlight • In late disease, unable to do fundoscopy due to cloudy lens • May be unilateral	Condition suspected or present. Warrants evaluation by an ophthalmologist.

CMV = cytomegalovirus, URI = upper respiratory infection

later. Because the risk of developing these conditions is often greater in individuals whose families members also suffer from them, determining if family members are affected by diabetes, congenital glaucoma, or refractive errors may help direct the investigation of symptoms.

All healthcare providers should also be aware if a woman has any allergies or is currently using any medications. Environmental allergies may present with eye irritation and redness or increased tearing. Medications of particular concern are steroids and anticoagulant medications such as warfarin. Subconjunctival hemorrhage may look quite severe in a woman who takes anticoagulant medication due to a prolonged clotting time. Cataracts have been associated with the long-term use of systemic corticosteroids.[2]

A thorough social history is also helpful. Smoking, alcohol, and diet all affect eye health. The woman's work and personal life and daily routine should be taken into consideration, because they are factors that can influence management. For example, extended use of a computer screen may cause eyestrain. Declining dexterity with age may makes it difficult for some women to administer eyedrops.

Physical

The physical examination starts with a general inspection. Is the woman sitting comfortably, or is she holding her head in pain? Is there any obvious swelling/bruising to the eye or surrounding structures? Then the woman is examined more closely. Any asymmetry between the two eyes is noted. Then each part of the eye is inspected carefully for redness or a rash on the skin around the eye. Inspect the eyelids for redness, obvious swelling, or a lump. Look at the position of the eyelashes: Are they growing inward? Is there any discharge from the eye, either watery or purulent? Examine the conjunctiva for redness, injection, or inflammation. Look at the sclera for redness. Examine the iris and pupil for their size and shape. The combination of features identified through this examination will help determine a diagnosis or inform further examination.

In the primary care setting, several tests can provide diagnostic clues. Visual acuity can be assessed using a Snellen chart. Visual fields are assessed by covering one of the woman's eyes, and using a digit or more classically a bright-colored pin to examine the visual fields of the other eye. This may identify peripheral vision loss such as in glaucoma. Normal eye movements are evaluated by simply asking her to follow the examiner's moving finger. Pupillary response can be assessed using a simple light. Abnormal eye movements may indicate underlying nerve/muscle pathology. If the health provider is trained to use an ophthalmoscope, and is confident to do so, fundoscopic examination will provide valuable information on the health of the back of the eye. The ophthalmoscope can also be used to test for a "red reflex" from the eye, which may be

lost when a cataract or, in very rare cases, a tumor is present. Loss of the red reflex indicates a need for ophthalmologist assessment.

Depending on the requirements indicated by the initial examination, a more detailed examination and investigation may require referral to an ophthalmologist. Examples of specialized equipment include a slit lamp, which is an instrument that provides a magnified view of the anterior structures of the eye. Retinal photography produces images of the retina and allows assessment of the optic disc and retinal arteries and veins. Tonometry can be performed to measure the pressure within the eye, important in testing for glaucoma.

Eye Conditions

Minor/Self-Limiting Conditions

Blepharitis

Blepharitis is a chronic inflammatory condition affecting the eyelid margins. The woman may present with burning or itching of the eyes/eyelids. There may be flaking or crusting, erythema, and/or edema seen along the eyelid margin. In severe cases, *trichiasis* (misdirection of eyelash growth toward the eye) and *madarosis* (loss of eyelashes) may be seen.[3] Symptoms may be worse in the morning with sticking down of the eyelids.

Blepharitis is usually associated with a bacterial (staphylococcal) infection, or with skin conditions such as seborrheic keratosis and rosacea. There is no specific diagnostic test to confirm blepharitis; the diagnosis is usually based on clinical history and examination. However, the health provider may refer the woman to ophthalmology if there is doubt about the diagnosis or if the symptoms are recurrent or troublesome.

The mainstay of treatment is good eye hygiene. This consists of a daily routine of applying warmth, massage, and cleansing of the eyelids. In some instances, women are treated with topical or systemic antibiotics. Topical corticosteroids may also be prescribed. The use of such interventions has been questioned, and a recent review on the effects of antibiotics and corticosteroids in the treatment of blepharitis was inconclusive.[4] Management is therefore focused on symptoms.

CHALAZION

A chalazion, also known as a meibomian cyst, is a fluid-filled sac that usually affects the upper eyelid. It is caused by blockage of a meibomian gland, a sebaceous gland that produces sebum to lubricate the eye. Blockage is thought to be caused by thickened secretions, but it is not always clear why this occurs. It may be associated with inflammation or infection. If the gland cannot drain, fluid builds up, and the resulting inflammation leads to formation of a hard nodular lump (granuloma) on the eyelid. A chalazion is usually not infected and is not painful. The woman may present with an irritated or unsightly lump on the eyelid. Diagnosis is confirmed by history of the pathology and examination.

Often a chalazion is self-limited and does not require any treatment. The woman may benefit from good eye hygiene including a warm compress and daily massage to the eye area. If the chalazion is particularly bothersome, the woman may opt for a minor procedure to have the cyst incised and drained by an ophthalmologist. Corticosteroid injection has more recently been proposed as a treatment option but is yet to be proven more beneficial than incision and drainage as a first-line management.[5]

STYE

A stye, also known as a *hordeolum*, is an infection of the eyelash root (follicle). It presents as an erythematous, tender, pus-filled swelling at the edge of the eyelid. A stye usually affects one eye, but it can be seen bilaterally. It is sometimes associated with chronic blepharitis. Stye infections are usually caused by *Staphylococcus* bacteria. Diagnosis

is made by clinical history and examination of the eye structures.

In most instances, the stye will rupture and drain without any treatment. A warm compress can be applied to encourage rupture. Antibiotics are not usually recommended for the treatment of a stye but may help to prevent the spread of infection.[6] If a stye persists or is recurrent, then an ophthalmologist's advice should be sought. In rare cases, surgical lancing of the stye may be required.

CONJUNCTIVITIS

Conjunctivitis is inflammation of the conjunctiva and is commonly encountered in the primary care setting. Infective forms can easily spread from one eye to the other, so it often affects both eyes. The causes of conjunctivitis are classified as either infective or noninfective. The diagnosis of conjunctivitis is determined by the history and clinical examination of the woman. Treatment depends on the pathogen.

Infectious Conjunctivitis
Bacterial Conjunctivitis   Bacterial conjunctivitis is most commonly caused by *Staphylococcus aureus, Streptococcus pneumonia,* or *Haemophilus influenzae*.[7] In some cases, the causative infection can be the sexually transmitted diseases chlamydia or gonorrhea, and the risk of a woman having these infections should be considered while taking the medical history. The woman may complain of gritty, irritated, red eyes. There is often a purulent discharge and crusting on the eyelids; the eyelids may be stuck down upon waking in the morning. Diagnosis is determined by the clinical history and examination of the eyes.

Treatment of bacterial conjunctivitis is slightly controversial. It is thought that many cases of bacterial conjunctivitis will resolve without treatment.[8] In their systematic review, Sheikh and colleagues concluded that acute bacterial conjunctivitis is frequently a self-limiting condition (resolving in 5 to 10 days when using eyedrops containing no antibiotics), but the use of antibiotics is associated with significantly improved rates of early clinical remission, and early and late microbiologic remission.[6] Similarly, in a randomized controlled trial involving 30 general practitioner centers in the United Kingdom, Everitt and colleagues compared management involving 1) no antibiotics, 2) immediate antibiotics, or 3) delayed antibiotics.[8] They concluded that a delayed prescribing approach is best and led to reduced drug use (near 50%), symptom control comparable to immediate use of antibiotics, and reduced reattendance for eye infections.[8] Table 9-2 includes common antibiotics used in eye infections.

Viral Conjunctivitis Viral conjunctivitis is commonly caused by adenovirus. Adenovirus causes respiratory infections and the common cold; thus women may present with a recent history of such symptoms. At presentation, she may complain of eye discomfort, and her eye will be red. Swelling of the eyelids and conjunctiva may be present. There may be haziness of vision. A clear, watery discharge is often present. As with all viral illnesses, management is supportive with treatment of the symptoms.[9] Cool compresses and simple analgesics may be beneficial.

All forms of infective conjunctivitis are extremely contagious, so the affected individual should practice good hygiene practices to prevent transmission to others. Contact lens use should be avoided and hands washed regularly, particularly before and after touching the eyes. Women should avoid sharing towels and pillows to avoid transmission of the causative agent to others.

Noninfectious Conjunctivitis

Allergic Conjunctivitis Allergic conjunctivitis is an intense itching of the eyes that is caused by an immune response to an allergen, such as

Table 9-2 Medications Commonly Used to Treat the Eye

Medication Type	Common Examples	Conditions
Antibacterial eyedrops and ointments	• Trimethoprim/polymyxin B • Bacitracin/polymyxin B • Sulfacetamide • Erythromycin • Ciprofloxacin	Bacterial eye infections Prophylaxis in corneal abrasions
Antihistamine/ anti-inflammatory eyedrops	• Antazoline • Sodium cromoglycate	Inflammation
Beta blockers	• Timolol • Betaxolol	Glaucoma
Prostaglandin analogues	• Bimatoprost • Latanoprost • Travoprost	Glaucoma
Carbonic anhydrase inhibitors	• Acetazolamide • Brinzolamide	Glaucoma
Sympathomimetics	• Brimonidine	Glaucoma

dust mites or pollen. The eyes may also be red. Clinical history might reveal a personal or family history of atopy, asthma, eczema, or hay fever. There may be other associated symptoms such as sneezing or throat irritation. A specific allergen may be identifiable by the woman.

Treatment of allergic conjunctivitis consists of oral or topical antihistamines and mast cell stabilizers. The woman should try to identify the source of allergen and avoid it where possible. Sublingual immunotherapy (SLIT) is a treatment offered by allergists where small doses of an allergen are placed under the woman's tongue. The perceived outcome is increased tolerance to the allergen. Trials have shown this method of treatment to be moderately effective in reducing ocular symptoms.[10] However, further trials are needed to assess the long-term effectiveness and cost-effectiveness of SLIT. Although SLIT is used throughout Europe, it has yet to receive Food and Drug Administration approval in the United States.[11] In the United States, similar treatments with subcutaneous injections are offered by allergists and are effective in reducing symptoms.

Subconjunctival Hemorrhage Subconjunctival hemorrhage is caused by rupture of a blood vessel resulting in a small bleed between the conjunctiva and the sclera. It is often associated with physical strain such as coughing, vomiting, or eye trauma, and is sometimes seen in women who take anticoagulant medication such as warfarin. The appearance can be quite alarming with redness covering a large part of the sclera, but the woman suffers no other symptoms and is often unaware of the bleed until she looks in the mirror. Diagnosis is reached in accordance with the woman's history and presence of a red/blood-stained sclera. A subconjunctival hemorrhage requires no treatment and should resolve within 2 weeks.[12]

Urgent and/or Chronic Ophthalmic Conditions

Rarely, eye conditions occur that require more urgent evaluation or ongoing management by a specialist.

EPISCLERITIS

Episcleritis is inflammation of the thin layer of tissue found between the conjunctiva and the sclera, the episclera. It can affect both eyes and is more commonly found in women than in men. Symptoms of episcleritis include the acute onset of red painful eyes, a watery discharge, and photophobia. The exact cause is unknown, but it has been associated with health conditions including rheumatoid arthritis, ankylosing spondylitis, systemic lupus erythematous, Crohn's disease, ulcerative colitis, syphilis, and shingles.[13] Diagnosis is determined by history and examination. The presence of an underlying systemic disease should always be considered, and a corresponding workup conducted, if episcleritis is suspected to be the cause of the symptoms. In this case, a woman should be referred to an appropriate specialist for further investigation. Episcleritis itself is a self-limiting condition and usually resolves within 10 days. Simple analgesics may be beneficial. In more severe or persistent disease, corticosteroids have been used.

SCLERITIS

Scleritis is inflammation of the sclera. It affects the entire thickness of the sclera and is a much more severe condition than episcleritis. It is also much rarer but important to include in the differential list, because without prompt management permanent damage to vision may ensue. An exact cause is not always known.

Symptoms of scleritis are more gradual in onset than with episcleritis, and include eye redness, photophobia, watery discharge, pain on eye movements, and pain that may radiate to the forehead, temple, or jaw. Changes in vision may also be evident. As with episcleritis, scleritis may be associated with local or systemic infection, or associated with an immune condition.[14] Women with suspected scleritis should be given urgent referral to an ophthalmologist for further investigation and treatment.

Treatment depends on the type of scleritis (diffuse anterior, nodular, and necrotizing are the most common) and may include immunosuppressive medication and/or biologic agents (e.g., tumor necrosis factor inhibitors).[14] Any underlying disease process should also be addressed.

Uveitis and Iritis

Uveitis is inflammation of the uveal tract, which consists of the iris, the ciliary body, and the choroid. When only the iris is inflamed, this is known as anterior uveitis or iritis. Inflammation can affect the entire uveal tract and surrounding structures (panuveitis). Presenting symptoms may include pain affecting one or both eyes, redness, photophobia, blurring of vision, and, in certain cases, floaters (moving shadows in the visual field).

In half of all cases of uveitis, no cause is identified. The remaining cases are associated with autoimmune or inflammatory conditions, infections, trauma, and, in rare cases, cancers such as lymphoma. If uveitis is a possible diagnosis, the woman should be seen by an ophthalmologist within 24 hours for a confirmation exam. Treatment with corticosteroids may be started after the diagnosis is confirmed. Immunosuppressant therapy and/or surgical intervention may play a role in treatment. If left untreated or if treated inadequately, uveitis can be a sight-threatening disease.[15]

Eye Injury

Trauma to the eye can range from a trivial injury requiring no treatment to extremely serious trauma posing a threat to the woman's eyesight. Careful examination is needed to identify cases that need referral to an ophthalmic specialist. Important assessments include close inspection of the eye (including looking under the eyelid) to identify foreign bodies, penetrating injuries, or scratches on the cornea. Injuries requiring immediate referral to the emergency department include high-velocity or penetrating injuries, severe eye pain, any visual loss/changes, and hyphemia (blood in the anterior chamber of the eye).

Healthcare providers may attempt to remove a nonpenetrating foreign body such as a lost contact lens, dirt, or small wood/steel chips (e.g., as in an occupation-related injury) from the eye with a cotton bud if they are confident that they can remove it and are trained to do so. Topical anesthetic may be used to relieve pain. The eye must be examined thoroughly, including everting the upper eyelid to look for a subtarsal foreign body.[16] All penetrating injuries and foreign bodies that prove difficult to remove should be referred to the emergency department/specialist eye unit.

Chemical splash refers to the entry of an irritant substance into the eye. Women may present with pain, irritation, redness, inability to open the eye due to discomfort, or blurred vision. Immediate management of a chemical splash involves irrigation of the eye and conjunctival sac until the tear surface is neutralized (i.e., returns to a pH of about 7). Early irrigation is associated with better outcome. Litmus or pH testing paper can be used to assess the acidity of the tear surface to help determine the end point of irrigation, but measurement errors can occur. If this method is used, it is recommended that a control litmus pH test be performed at the same time.[17] The eye can be irrigated with normal saline if the irritant is a mild chemical such as shampoo. If the chemical splash involves substances more harmful to the eye such as strongly acidic or alkylating agents, the woman should be referred immediately to the emergency department. En route to the emergency department, the eye can be irrigated with water or saline.

Corneal abrasion is a scratch to the cornea of the eye that may result from scratching or vigorous rubbing of the eye, contact lens use, foreign body, or chemical injury. The woman may complain of feeling grit in the eye, a watery discharge, pain, redness, or blurring of vision. The woman should be referred for a thorough ophthalmic examination using a slit lamp and fluorescein staining to confirm the diagnosis and to determine the treatment course. Usually a corneal abrasion is treated only with topical prophylactic antibiotics (see Table 9-2 for a summary of commonly used medications). However, simple analgesics and an eye patch are sometimes indicated.

Cellulitis

Periorbital cellulitis is a bacterial infection that affects the eyelid. The infection may be initiated by a simple scratch or insect bite that allows the entry of bacteria into the body, or it may have spread from an infection of the respiratory tract. The woman may present with fever and swelling and tenderness of the eyelids that are warm to the touch. Further examination of chest sounds and the appearance of the throat may be required to identify potential origins of infection if this is not clear on the initial history and examination. Women with cellulitis affecting the eye will need specialty care and treatment with antibiotics. Recent studies have also suggested that oral corticosteroids may be beneficial as an anti-inflammatory adjunct to antibiotics in the treatment of periorbital cellulitis.[18]

Periorbital cellulitis is not to be confused with orbital cellulitis, which is a potentially life-threatening but uncommon ophthalmic emergency.

It refers to the acute spread of infection into the eye socket. Women with orbital cellulitis will need urgent hospital admission and treatment with intravenous antibiotics.

Herpes Infections

Herpes Simplex

Herpes simplex virus 1 (HSV-1) is a viral infection usually contracted during childhood. For the most part, the virus remains dormant at the root of a nerve. In cases of eye infection, this is the trigeminal nerve (cranial nerve V5), which is responsible for sensation to the face and supplies muscles of mastication. When HSV-1 is active, viral particles can travel along the nerve to the eye and cause inflammation of the retina, iris, cornea, conjunctiva, eyelids, and surrounding skin.[19] Superficial infection of the cornea is known as epithelial keratitis and is the most common ocular manifestation of HSV infection, accounting for 70–80% of cases.[20] Stromal keratitis is an infection affecting the deeper layers of the cornea, which can result in scarring of the cornea. Corneal scarring can lead to permanent loss of vision; prompt treatment is essential.

At presentation the woman may complain of pain around her eye, watery discharge, blurred vision, or photophobia. The eyelids, sclera, and/or the conjunctiva may appear red. If HSV infection is suspected, she should be seen by an ophthalmologist who can treat the infection and monitor the progression or resolution of the infection. Superficial HSV infection is treated with antiviral eyedrops. In the case of stromal keratitis, corticosteroid eyedrops may be used in addition.

Herpes Zoster

Herpes zoster (commonly known as shingles) is a virus that infects a nerve and the area of skin supplied by that nerve (the dermatome). As is the case for HSV-1, herpes zoster can lie dormant in a nerve root for many years. Herpes zoster ophthalmicus occurs when the virus travels along the optic division of the trigeminal nerve and affects the eye. The woman may initially complain of pain, burning, tingling, or numbness of the skin around the eye. Two to 3 days after the first onset of symptoms, a blistering rash will develop in the same area. The rash is well localized to a specific dermatome. When the eye is involved, there may be redness and cloudiness or swelling of the cornea affecting vision. Diagnosis is made on clinical grounds. Management is best achieved by the woman's primary care provider in consultation with an ophthalmologist.

Treatment varies depending on the severity of the presentation. Antiviral eyedrops and in some cases corticosteroids are prescribed for the treatment of herpes zoster ophthalmicus.[21,22] However, ocular conditions that require oral or topical corticosteroids are serious conditions requiring management on the part of the specialist. Therefore, the decision for the need for these agents should be under the purview of a specialist.

Glaucoma

Glaucoma refers to a group of conditions that cause high pressure within the eye. High pressure is the result of abnormal drainage of aqueous humour, which can be acute or progressive, as discussed later. In the healthy eye, the ciliary bodies continuously produce aqueous humour that flows from the posterior chamber of the eye, through the pupil to the anterior chamber before draining into the scleral venous sinus (trabecular meshwork), which is found at the junction of the sclera and cornea. If the aqueous humour is unable to drain away, it builds up inside the eye chambers and causes an increase in pressure. This increased intraocular pressure can damage the optic nerve and lead to blindness.

Glaucoma is the second most common cause of blindness in the world, and the most common cause of irreversible blindness.[23] Cases of glaucoma can be divided according to four different forms. The more commonly encountered forms are primary open-angle glaucoma and angle-closure glaucoma. Two rarer forms are congenital glaucoma and secondary glaucoma, which may be caused by inflammatory conditions, eye injuries, or long-term use of medications such as corticosteroids.

PRIMARY OPEN-ANGLE GLAUCOMA

Primary open-angle glaucoma is by far the most common type. It is a chronic, slowly progressive condition caused by gradual blockage of the scleral venous sinuses (trabecular meshwork). The reason for this blockage is often unknown. The risk factors for open-angle glaucoma include increasing age, African origin, family history, shortsightedness, and diabetes mellitus.[24,25] As a slowly progressing disease, open-angle glaucoma rarely has few symptoms until the disease is quite extensive. Open-angle glaucoma is usually detected with screening eye tests carried out by the optometrist.

When glaucoma is suspected in the primary care setting, patients should be referred to an ophthalmologist. A visual acuity test is carried out, and the peripheral visual fields are examined. A tonometry test can be performed by a specialist to test the pressure within the eye, and the back of the eye is examined with a slit lamp or an ophthalmoscope to look for cupping of the optic disc (where the head of the optic nerve takes on a disc-shaped appearance at the back of the eye). This change in appearance is caused by loss of optic nerve fibers secondary to increased intraocular pressure.

Damage to the eye that occurs due to glaucoma cannot be reversed, so the mainstay of treatment is to reduce the intraocular pressure and prevent any further damage from occurring. A number of medications (delivered as eyedrops) with different mechanisms of action are used in the treatment of open-angle glaucoma, including the following:

- Prostaglandin analogues increase the flow of fluid out of the eye.
- Beta-blockers and carbonic anhydrase inhibitors reduce the production of fluid within the eye, thereby reducing pressure.
- Sympathomimetics (drugs that mimic the effects of transmitter substances such as catecholamines or epinephrine on the sympathetic nervous system) are thought to reduce fluid production and increase drainage, leading to an overall reduced pressure.

In some cases, it is possible to treat open-angle glaucoma with laser therapy that targets the trabecular meshwork. A trabeculectomy is a surgical procedure that creates an opening in the wall of the eye to release fluid, reducing intraocular pressure. A recent review compared the outcome of treatment with medication with that of surgery and concluded there was insufficient evidence to suggest that either method was superior as a first line of treatment.[26]

Angle-Closure Glaucoma

Angle-closure glaucoma is less common than open-angle glaucoma but is more likely to result in blindness.[27,28] As such, it is an ophthalmic emergency. It is thought to occur when the iris is shifted to be more anterior than normal, reducing the angle between the iris and the sclera where the trabecular meshwork is found. If this angle is reduced or closed, it inhibits the drainage of aqueous humour and leads to increased intraocular pressure. Causes may include pulling forward of the iris in inflammatory conditions or pushing forward of the iris by a thickened lens that blocks the pupil and therefore the passage of aqueous humour.

The woman presents with an acute onset of painful eye and blurred vision, and in some cases patients report seeing a "halo" around lights, or redness. She may complain of headache, nausea, and/or vomiting. Women with suspected closed-angle glaucoma should be referred urgently to the emergency eye department where treatment may consist of medications, laser, or surgery.

Refractive Error

Refractive error is a common condition that causes blurring of the vision. As light rays pass through the eye, they are refracted (bent) at the cornea and the lens, and are then focused on the retina (Figure 9-2). There are four types of refractive error:[29]

- Myopia: difficulty in seeing distant objects clearly
- Hyperopia: difficulty in seeing near objects clearly
- Astigmatism: distorted vision resulting from changes in the curvature of the cornea
- Presbyopia: age-related eye condition where the lens is unable to change shape enough to allow sufficient focus

Women with a refractive error should be under the care of an eye specialist and managed with the appropriate glasses or contact lenses to correct the error. Laser eye surgery is now a commonly selected option to treat refractive error. Refractive laser eye surgery involves either a procedure where a partial-thickness flap is cut in the cornea to allow ablation of the stromal bed beneath (laser assisted in situ keratomileusis) or a surface laser technique (photorefractive keratotomy and laser epithelial keratomileusis) where the epithelium is removed exposing the corneal stroma that is then ablated. The procedure recommended is based on the condition and morphology of the cornea and eye socket, as well as the available expertise and equipment.[30] Potential candidates for either approach are typically over 21 years of age, with a prescription for glasses that has been stable for 12 months, up to severe myopia or hyperopia, or moderate astigmatism.

Success in terms of improved visual acuity and satisfaction is generally high with laser eye surgery.[31,32] However, the results are less predictable where there is a higher baseline refractive error, and about 4% of patients will require retreatment due to under- or over-correction or regression.[31] Potential complications of laser eye surgery include dry eyes and hazy vision. More serious complications are rare but include infectious or diffuse lamellar keratitis, or a loss of corneal stability due to excessive ablation (corneal ectasia), which is a serious threat to sight.[30]

Retinal Detachment

Retinal detachment is defined as a tearing away/ separation of the sensory retina from the retinal pigment epithelium, with an accumulation of fluid in the potential space between them.[33] It is most commonly associated with weakness of the retina due to age-related degeneration, short-sightedness, and in women who have had eye surgery, such as cataract removal. The woman may present with changes in vision, flashing lights, or floaters (dots or shadows in their field of vision). Vision may become blurred or cloudy, or there may be visual loss often described as "a curtain coming down."

Retinal detachment is a medical emergency and must be referred to an ophthalmologist immediately. The ophthalmologist can examine the back of the woman's eye with an ophthalmoscope. Retinal detachment requires surgery to reattach the retina, and there are three techniques that may be used:

- Scleral buckling is a technique used to cause an indentation of the sclera (eye wall) over the area of detachment to bring it back into contact with the retina.
- Pneumatic retinopexy involves the injection of a gas or silicone bubble into the vitreous humour of the eye. The bubble presses the retina back into place.

- Vitrectomy refers to the removal of the vitreous humour from the eye and injecting gas or silicone, which holds the retina in place while it heals.

Delays in treatment can lead to extended areas of the retina becoming detached, up to involvement of the macula, which if left untreated can lead to permanent blindness.[34] Delayed surgery (duration of detachment) is also associated with poorer visual outcome. A retrospective analysis of surgical patients by Akhtar and colleagues found that 92% of patients who underwent surgery within 1 week showed some improvement, with visual acuity improving on average by 43% from baseline; of those patients presenting for surgery more than 1 month after retinal detachment, 65% showed improvement but the average improvement in visual acuity was only 13%.[35]

Patients are routinely prescribed topical antibiotics and corticosteroids postoperatively, and cycloplegics or ocular hypotensive drugs may also be indicated.[36] Postoperative pain, worsening vision, or an increasingly red eye requires immediate follow up. Headaches and nausea, possibly indicating increased intraocular pressure, should also be reported. The most common complication of any form of retinal detachment surgery is re-detachment of the retina. New tears in the retina can develop after surgery, sometimes due to scar tissue, starting the detachment process again.

Common Health Conditions Associated with Visual Problems

Aging

Eye conditions that are more common with increasing age include refractive error and glaucoma, discussed earlier in this chapter. Additional eye conditions more typically seen in older adults include macular degeneration and cataracts.

Macular Degeneration

Macular degeneration is a condition that causes visual impairment and affects individuals over age 50. In the United States, it is thought that up to 1.6 million people age 50 years and older have evidence of late macular degeneration; and with a growing aging population, this figure is set to rise.[37]

The macula is a small area at the back of the eye (retina) responsible for high-resolution visual acuity in central vision. The central visual field is used looking directly at an object such as when reading. Macular degeneration leads to a gradual blurring of central vision and can eventually leave a blank patch in the center of the woman's vision. It can affect both eyes, often progressing at different rates. There are two types of macular degeneration, dry and wet. The dry type is more common and is caused by cellular atrophy of the retina. Progression of the disease is slow, and it may be several years before a woman's vision is severely affected.

Wet macular degeneration involves the growth of new, abnormal blood vessels in the area of the macula. These vessels can leak blood and damage the retina, leading to visual impairment. This process can develop very quickly and can severely affect the woman's vision within months. In addition to aging, macular degeneration is associated with smoking, high blood pressure, and family history.

Women with suspected macular degeneration should be referred to an ophthalmologist who can examine vision, assess the back of the eye using a fundoscope and slit lamp, and perform digital imaging of the retina. Angiography may also be performed to assess the blood vessels at the back of the eye. Treatment for dry macular degeneration is limited to improving lifestyle choices through smoking cessation, a healthy diet, and treatment of high blood pressure if present. Visual aids such as a magnifying glass or large-print books may be beneficial. In wet macular degeneration, medications are used to prevent the growth of new blood vessels. These medications, known as antivascular endothelial growth factors, are administered by injection into the eye. In the past, steroids with anti-angiogenic properties have been used to treat wet macular degeneration, but recent studies have judged this therapy to be unsuccessful at preventing visual loss. It has been superseded by treatment involving antivascular endothelial growth factors.[38] Photodynamic therapy and laser photocoagulation are further methods of treatment but are not always appropriate treatments. An ophthalmologist's opinion is required.

Cataract

Cataract is the term used to describe a clouding of the lens. When the lens is cloudy, it reduces the ability of light to pass through it and focus onto the retina, which leads to visual impairment. Cataracts are more commonly found in older adults but can be found in younger people. They are associated with smoking, family history, trauma to the eye, and long-term use of certain medications, such as steroids. Cataracts can be diagnosed by an eye examination with an ophthalmoscope. Treatment involves a surgical procedure under local anesthetic to remove the cloudy lens and insert an artificial one.

Diabetes

Diabetes is associated with complications of the eye such as glaucoma and cataracts, both discussed in this chapter. By far the most common form of diabetic eye disease is diabetic retinopathy. This results from poor blood sugar control where persistently high blood glucose levels cause damage to the microvasculature. This leads to blockage or leaking of small vessels throughout the body, including those that supply the back of the eye. Damage to these vessels can interfere with the blood supply to the retina and in the long term can lead to blindness.

All women with diabetes should be offered an annual retinal screening examination by an ophthalmologist that includes dilated retinal photography.[39] In the primary care setting, the healthcare provider can preserve vision by promoting good blood glucose control and healthy lifestyle choices to reduce the risk of hypertension and high cholesterol.

Thyroid Disease

Thyroid disease results from the production of autoantibodies that attack the thyroid tissue. These same antibodies can attack tissue around the eyes and cause thyroid eye disease. If the lacrimal glands (tear-producing glands) are involved, symptoms can include dry, irritated eyes. The eyelids may be reddened and swollen. Muscles and fat surrounding the eye may be affected, causing retraction of the eyelid and bulging (protrusion) of the eyes from the orbit, a feature known as exophthalmos. The woman may also complain of diplopia (double vision). The diagnosis may be suspected if the history contains other evidence of thyroid disease. The hyperthyroid woman may describe symptoms of anxiety, palpitations, and sweating, and there may be notable weight loss or a palpable goiter. If thyroid disease is suspected, then thyroid function tests should be obtained, and, if confirmed, treated. Treatment of eye symptoms may include artificial tears to sooth dry eyes or steroids to reduce inflammation. The woman may opt to have surgery to correct persisting eye anomalies such as exophthalmos, lid retraction, and diplopia (double vision) if these symptoms persist despite treatment of the underlying condition. Radiotherapy is sometimes used in the management of thyroid eye disease and plays a role in the reduction of tissue swelling.

Pregnancy

Eye changes in pregnancy should be taken seriously and investigated thoroughly so that eyesight is protected from permanent damage. Changes to the eyes that can occur during pregnancy are categorized as either *physiologic changes* or *pregnancy-specific eye disease*.

Physiologic changes relate to changes in the body's fluid status, leading to conjunctival injection, for example, or change in hormonal status, which can lead to increased pigmented areas (chloasma), usually on the face, but occasionally on the skin around the eyes. The cornea may become thicker with changes in curvature. This can cause temporary alterations in refraction and/or blurred vision. The woman may complain of uncomfortable, irritated dry eyes that can be easily treated with artificial tears. All of these changes should resolve within weeks of giving birth or cessation of breastfeeding.

Pregnancy-specific eye diseases are most frequently associated with pre-eclampsia/eclampsia and gestational diabetes. Pre-eclampsia/eclampsia is a condition associated with high blood pressure and proteinuria that if untreated can lead to life-threatening illness of both mother and baby.[40] Changes in vision caused by pre-eclampsia include blurred or decreased vision, photophobia, diplopia, visual field defects, and blindness.[41]

Gestational diabetes arises during pregnancy and resolves after delivery. Poor blood glucose control can lead to damage of the microvasculature, which in turn can affect the retina. Management includes use of dietary changes and, if needed, medication to restore blood glucose control. Women with pre-existing diabetes should already be on an annual vision screening program. These women may require additional screening throughout their pregnancy.

References

1. Agur A, Dalley A. *Grant's Atlas of Anatomy.* 13th ed. Baltimore, MD: Lippincott Williams & Wilkins; 2013.

2. American Academy of Ophthalmology Retina Panel. *Preferred Practice Pattern® Guidelines.* Available at: http://www.aao.org/ppp. Accessed May 8, 2014.

3. Lindsley K, Matsumura S, Hatef E, Akpek EK. Interventions for chronic blepharitis. *Cochrane Database Syst Rev.* 2012;5:CD005556.

4. Ben SGJ, Rosen N, Rosner M, Spierer A. Intralesional triamcinolone acetonide injection versus incision and curettage for primary chalazia: a prospective, randomized study. *Am J Ophthalmol.* 2011;151(4):714-718.

5. Sethuraman U, Kamat D. The red eye: evaluation and management. *Clin Pediatr.* 2009;48(6):588-600.

6. Sheikh A, Hurwitz B, van Schayck CP, McLean S, Nurmatov U. Antibiotics versus placebo for acute bacterial conjunctivitis. *Cochrane Database Syst Rev.* 2012;9:CD001211.

7. Høvding G. Acute bacterial conjunctivitis. *Acta Ophthalmol.* 2008;86(1):5-17.

8. Everitt HA, Little PS, Smith PW. A randomised controlled trial of management strategies for acute infective conjunctivitis in general practice. *BMJ.* 2006;333(7563):321.

9. Azari A, Barney N. Conjunctivitis, a systematic review of diagnosis and treatment. *JAMA.* 2013; 310(16):1721-1729.

10. Calderon MA, Penagos M, Sheikh A, Canonica GW, Durham S. Sublingual immunotherapy for treating allergic conjunctivitis. *Cochrane Database Syst Rev.* 2011;7:CD007685.

11. Park D, Daher N, Blaiss MS. Adult and pediatric clinical trials of sublingual immunotherapy in the USA. *Expert Rev Clin Immunol.* 2012;8(6):557-564.

12. Vorvick L, Reinhardt R. A differential guide to 5 common eye complaints. *J Fam Pract.* 2013;62(7): 345-355.

13. Roy FH. *Ocular Differential Diagnosis. Vol 1.* 7th ed. Baltimore, MD: Williams & Wilkins; 2002.

14. Wakefield D, Di Girolamo N, Thurau S, Wildner G, McCluskey P. Scleritis: challenges in immunopathogenesis and treatment. *Discov Med.* 2013; 16(88):153-157.

15. Gupta R, Murray PI. Chronic non-infectious uveitis in the elderly: epidemiology, pathophysiology and management. *Drugs Aging.* 2006;23(7):535-558.

16. Khaw PT, Shah P, Elkington AR. Injury to the eye. *BMJ.* 2004;328:36-38.

17. Connor AJ, Severn P. Use of a control test to aid pH assessment of chemical eye injuries. *Emerg Med J.* 2009;26(11):811-812.

18. Pushker N, Tejwani LK, Bajaj MS, Khurana S, Velpandian T, Chandra M. Role of oral corticosteroids in orbital cellulitis. *Am J Ophthalmol.* 2013;156(1):178-183.

19. Barker NH. *Ocular herpes simplex.* Available at: http://clinicalevidence.bmj.com/x/systematic-review /0707/overview.html. Accessed March 29, 2016.

20. Wilhelmus KR. Antiviral treatment and other therapeutic interventions for herpes simplex virus epithelial keratitis. *Cochrane Database Syst Rev.* 2010; 12:CD002898.

21. Muir P. Management of herpes simplex and varicella-zoster infections. *Prescriber.* 2014;25(3): 14-23.

22. Sanjay S, Huang P, Lavanya R. Herpes zoster ophthalmicus. *Curr Treat Options Neurol.* 2011; 13(1):79-91.

23. Khaw T, Shah P, Elkington AR. ABC of eyes. Glaucoma 2: treatment. *BMJ.* 2004;328:156-158.

24. Burr JM, Mowatt G, Hernandez R, Siddiqui MA, Cook J, Lourenco T, et al. The clinical effectiveness and cost effectiveness of screening for open angle glaucoma: a systematic review and economic evaluation. *Health Technol Assess.* 2007;11(41):iii-iv, ix-x, 1-190.

25. Rudnicka AR, Mt-Isa S, Owen CG, Cook DG, Ashby D. Variations in primary open-angle glaucoma prevalence by age, gender, and race: a Bayesian meta-analysis. *IOVS.* 2006;47(10):4254-4261.

26. Burr J, Azuara-Blanco A, Avenell A, Tuulonen A. Medical versus surgical interventions for open angle glaucoma. *Cochrane Database Syst Rev.* 2012;9: CD004399.

27. Quigley HA. Number of people with glaucoma worldwide. *Br J Ophthalmol.* 1996;80(5):389-393.

28. Resnikoff S, Pascolini D, Etya'ale D, Kocur I, Pararajasegaram R, Pokharel GP, et al. Global data on visual impairment in the year 2002. *Bull World Health Organ.* 2002;82(11):844-851.

29. Cochrane G, du Toit R, Le Mesurier R. Management of refractive errors. *BMJ.* 2010;340:c1711.

30. Bastawrous A, Silvester A, Batterbury M. Laser refractive eye surgery. *BMJ.* 2011;342:2-11.

31. Yuen LH, Chan WK, Koh J, Mehta JS, Tan DT. A 10-year prospective audit of LASIK outcomes for myopia in 37932 eyes at a single institution in Asia. *Ophthalmology.* 2010;117(6):1236-1244.

32. Pasquali TA, Smadja D, Savetsky MJ, Reggiani Mello GH, Alkhawaldeh F, Krueger RR. Long-term follow-up after laser vision correction in physicians: quality of life and patient satisfaction. *J Cataract Refract Surg.* 2014;40(3):395-402.

33. Wilkinson CP. Interventions for asymptomatic retinal breaks and lattice degeneration for preventing retinal detachment. *Cochrane Database Syst Rev.* 2012;3:CD003170.

34. Koch KR, Hermann MM, Kirchhof B, Fauser S. Success rates of retinal detachment surgery: routine versus emergency setting. *Graefe's Arch Clin Exp Ophthalmol.* 2012;250(12):1731-1736.

35. Akhtar N, Waris A, Ayra R, Yusuf F. Duration of retinal detachment and its effect on visual outcome. *JK-Practitioner.* 2012;17(4):24-25.

36. Kang HK, Luff AJ. Management of retinal detachment: a guide for non-ophthalmologists. *BMJ.* 2008;336:1235-1240.

37. Tielsch JM, Friedman DS, Congdon N, Kempen J. *Vision Problems in the U.S. Prevalence of adult vision impairment and age-related eye disease in America.* Chicago, IL: Prevent Blindness America; 2002.

38. Geltzer A, Turalba A, Vedula SS. Surgical implantation of steroids with antiangiogenic characteristics for treating neovascular age-related macular degeneration. *Cochrane Database Syst Rev.* 2013;1: CD005022.

39. Ockrim Z, Yorston D. Managing diabetic retinopathy. *BMJ.* 2010;25:341:c5400.

40. American College of Obstetricians and Gynecologists. *Diagnosis and Management of Preeclampsia and Eclampsia. ACOG Practice Bulletin 33.* Washington, DC: American College of Obstetricians and Gynecologists; 2010.

41. Vigil-De Gracia P, Ortega-Paz L. Retinal detachment in association with pre-eclampsia, eclampsia, and HELLP syndrome. *Int J Gynaecol Obstet.* 2011; 114(3):223-225.

CHAPTER 10

THE EAR

Holly Thomas | Deborah A. Hall | Matija Daniel

Introduction

The ear is the organ that detects sound (auditory system) and aids in body position and balance (vestibular system). Often the entire organ is considered the "ear," but it can be classified according to four distinct subdivisions: the outer ear, middle ear, inner ear, and vestibulocochlear nerve (**Table 10-1**, **Figure 10-1**). This chapter is organized around those four subdivisions of the ear. Each subdivision can be affected in different ways by infections, disease, and degenerative conditions. This first section provides an introduction to the structure and primary functions of the different subdivisions. The remainder of the chapter considers the range of otologic symptoms and conditions relating to the different subdivisions. While descriptions of the various otologic conditions are general, recommended healthcare

approaches to assessment and management can differ across countries. For example, a survey of subjective tinnitus conducted with general practitioners (GPs) and ear, nose, and throat (ENT) specialists in six developed countries indicated that multidisciplinary teams often engaged neurology professionals in Germany, Italy, and Spain, while in the United Kingdom and United States, audiologists played a primary role.[1]

Physiology

Outer Ear

The pinna is the visible part of the outer ear. It is composed of a thin plate of yellow elastic cartilage and connected to the surrounding parts by ligaments, muscles, and fibrous tissue. The pinna gathers vibrations caused by tiny movements of

Disclaimers: *The authors are funded by the National Institute for Health Research (NIHR). The views expressed are those of the author(s) and not necessarily those of the National Health Service (NHS), the NIHR, or the Department of Health (United Kingdom). The authors have made all reasonable efforts to ensure that the information provided in this review is based on available scientific evidence.*

Table 10-1 Parts of the Ear: Structure and Function

Structure	Description	Primary Function
Outer ear	Visible (external) part of the ear	Captures sound vibration energy and sends it down the ear canal to the eardrum
Middle ear	Subdivision of the ear that is internal to the eardrum and external to the oval window of the cochlea	Efficiently transfers sound vibration energy in the air to energy waves within the fluid of the cochlea
Inner ear	The cochlea and semicircular canals form fluid-filled compartments of the inner ear.	The cochlea encodes sound information. The vestibular system encodes balance and motion information.
Vestibulocochlear nerve	The 8th cranial nerve containing the auditory (cochlear) nerve and the vestibular nerve	Carries nerve impulses from the inner ear to the brain

Figure 10-1 Structural components of the ear.

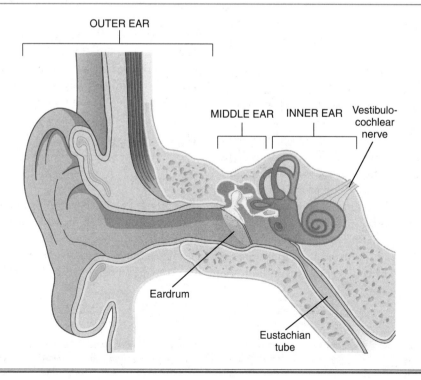

OUTER EAR

MIDDLE EAR   INNER EAR   Vestibulo-cochlear nerve

Eardrum

Eustachian tube

air and focuses them down the ear canal (external auditory meatus). The canal is a simple tube running to the middle ear, and it ends at the eardrum (tympanic membrane). The folds and channels of the pinna determine the precise journey of the sound waves to the eardrum, providing spatial cues to the elevation of the sound in the external environment. Two working ears are necessary to provide binaural hearing. The signals from a sound source arrive at each ear at slightly different times, and the brain is able to decode this information to work out the horizontal position of the sound in the external environment.

Middle Ear

The middle ear is a hollow space (*tympanic cavity*) that is internal to the eardrum and external to the oval window of the cochlea. The mammalian middle ear has three tiny bones (ossicles), which mechanically transmit vibrations of the eardrum to the oval window at the entrance to the cochlea. The *ossicles* are called the malleus, incus, and stapes. They act to amplify the vibrations and optimize the frequencies and sound pressure on their way to the inner ear so that they efficiently transfer the energy into pressure waves within the fluid of the cochlea. By the time sound waves reach the organ of Corti, their pressure amplitude is 22 times that of the air impinging on the pinna. The Eustachian tube joins the tympanic cavity with the nasal cavity, allowing pressure to equalize with the external environment. If the air pressure is not equal, then the ear may feel blocked.

Inner Ear

The *cochlea* and *semicircular canals* are fluid-filled (perilymph and endolymph) compartments that make up the inner ear. The cochlea contains the *organ of Corti*, a highly specialized structure that converts the mechanical signals into electrochemical impulses and then onto nerve impulses,

which are transmitted to the brain. The organ of Corti contains between 15,000 and 20,000 auditory nerve receptors arranged in orderly rows of hair-like cells (stereocilia) on the surface of the basilar membrane. When the basilar membrane vibrates in response to sound-evoked pressure waves in the fluid, the stereocilia bend in response to such vibrations. This flexing of the stereocilia opens ion channels that are permeable to potassium and calcium, leading to cell depolarization. The result of a chain of neurochemical events is the electrical signaling to brain via spiral ganglion neurons and the auditory nerve.

The vestibular system uses the same processes of perilymphatic pressure waves and receptor cells (hair cells), as does the cochlea. The type of spatial orientation or motion detected by a hair cell depends on its associated mechanical structures, such as the curved tube of one of the three semicircular canals or the calcium carbonate crystals (otoliths or otoconia) contained within the saccule and utricle. Information about the orientation of the head and any rotations or linear motion is sent to the brain via vestibular ganglion neurons and the vestibular nerve.

Vestibulocochlear Nerve

The auditory (cochlear) nerve and the vestibular nerve together form a cranial nerve known as the vestibulocochlear nerve. The auditory nerve carries sound signals from the cochlea to the brain via the ascending auditory pathways. In humans the vestibular nerve carries orientation and balance information from the semicircular canals and the otoliths. Balance is the result of several body systems working together—the visual system (eyes), vestibular system (ears), and *proprioception* (the body's sense of where it is in space)—thus the brain integrates vestibular information with information from other senses. In practice, retrocochlear disorders usually refer to a disorder involving either the 8th cranial nerve or the cerebellopontine angle.

Otologic Symptoms

Pain

Pain experienced in the ear is known as *otalgia*, and causes can be categorized into primary or secondary. Primary causes of otalgia relate to swelling, inflammation, or infection of the ear itself. The origin of pain can be external ear, middle ear, or mastoid and Eustachian. External causes are usually obvious on examination. Middle ear causes may require more investigation, but could be noticed upon examination of the tympanic member (eardrum). **Table 10-2** presents information about the common causes of ear pain.

If no evidence for primary pain is found, secondary causes should be considered. Secondary causes of otalgia are those referring pain to the ear as a result of shared nerve supply. The ear is innervated by a number of cranial nerves and two spinal elements. Sensory innervations of the ear include: 1) pinna (upper cervical spine C2 and cervical spine C3), 2) external ear (cranial nerves V, VII, and X), 3) temporomandibular region (cranial nerves VII, V), 4) middle ear (V, VII, IX), and 5) temporomandibular joint and surrounding skin (upper cervical spine C2 and cervical spine C3).

Table 10-2 Common Causes of Ear Pain

Primary	External	Foreign body
		Otitis externa
		Eczema
		Furuncle (abscess)
		Wax impaction
		Malignancy (e.g., basal cell carcinoma, a.k.a. rodent ulcer)
	Middle	Acute otitis media
		Traumatic perforation
		Otitic barotrauma
		Cholesteatoma
	Mastoid and Eustachian tube	Acute mastoiditis
		Complications of cholesteatoma
	Inner	Pain is only a symptom of pathology
Secondary	Oral cavity	Dental, ulceration, malignancy
	Temporomandibular joint	Arthritis, trauma, infection
	Pharynx and tonsil area	Acute tonsillitis/postop pain, peritonsillar abscess, malignancy
	Larynx	Laryngitis, supraglottic carcinoma
	Mumps and parotitis	Mumps, viral infection of parotid, bacterial parotitis (common in immunosuppressed patients), stones
	Miscellaneous	Heart attack, thyroid problems
	Neural	Herpes zoster

Thus, it is not surprising that in 50% of the cases pain is due to secondary causes. The most common source for referred pain is dental abnormalities, followed by temporomandibular joint pathology. Ear pain can also be caused by tumors of the tonsil area and the base of tongue, so an otorhinolaryngology opinion may be warranted.

Auditory Symptoms of Hearing Loss

Hearing loss can be classified as conductive, sensorineural, or mixed.[2] Conductive hearing loss results from abnormalities in the structures conveying sound energy to the inner ear (i.e., external ear, tympanic membrane, or middle ear). Sensorineural hearing loss results from inner ear and vestibulocochlear nerve dysfunction or other abnormalities in the hearing pathway from the cochlea to the brain.

Clinical presentation of hearing loss can be sudden, gradual, or fluctuating and differ in sensitivity from a mild loss to profound. Sudden onset hearing loss requires prompt investigation, because it could be a symptom of a serious underlying condition and may require medication to offer the best prognosis. While hearing loss is more prevalent with increased age, and is more common in men than women, one particular disorder is rather more prevalent among young females. This condition is otosclerosis, a conductive hearing loss caused by excess bony growth in the middle ear. This commonly manifests itself during hormonal changes such as pregnancy, so it is especially relevant in the women's healthcare setting.[3] However, hearing loss in pregnancy is an uncommon problem. Some patients with conductive hearing loss will also report autophony, the feeling that their own speech sounds louder "in the head"; this is thought to occur because environmental sounds are not reaching the inner ear due to the conductive loss, yet inner ear function is normal and remains sensitive.

Vestibular Symptoms

Dizziness is among the most common complaints in medicine, affecting approximately 20% to 30% of persons in the general population.[4] Dizziness is a nonspecific term often used by patients to describe a number of qualitatively different symptoms. These include four broad categories of balance dysfunction: vertigo, disequilibrium, presyncope, and nonspecific dizziness (see **Table 10-3**).

Table 10-3 Categories of Dizziness Relating to Balance Dysfunction

Vestibular Problem	Description
Vertigo	An illusion of movement often with a rotary element typically thought to arise from an abnormality in the vestibular system or central vestibular pathway; patient description: "room is spinning"
Disequilibrium	A feeling of unsteadiness or of being off balance
Presyncope	A sensation of being about to lose consciousness, usually caused by a decrease in global cerebral blood flow; fainting feeling
Nonspecific dizziness (lightheadedness)	Dizziness reported without any of the above symptoms

The balance system is a sophisticated network constantly acting to maintain equilibrium. Equilibrium is maintained by the integration of three key inputs: vision and vestibular and proprioception, which integrate in the brain stem. Not all dizziness is vertigo, even though patients often describe their experiences as vertigo. Two significant physiologic pathways produce symptoms of dizziness. These are orthostatic hypotension, often a result of hypovolemia, and decreased cardiac output, whether related to decreased venous return or cardiomyopathy.[5] Other nonspecific causes of dizziness are summarized in **Table 10-4**. History is key in determining the diagnosis, with the three most useful questions being the nature of the dizziness, its duration, and accompanying features.

The etiology of dizziness varies from vestibular to neurologic to cardiovascular pathology.[6-8] Rarely, vertigo can be a symptom of a serious neurologic problem such as a stroke, multiple sclerosis, or brain hemorrhage. With these neurologic problems, there are usually other neurologic abnormalities such as diplopia, slurred speech, limb incoordination, and facial weakness or numbness. Central and peripheral vertigo may be distinguished by their associated symptoms, described in **Table 10-5**.

An intense spinning sensation lasting a few seconds precipitated by rolling over in bed or by head position changes is typical of benign paroxysmal positional vertigo (BPPV). This is the most common cause of vertigo, and occurs when the calcium carbonate crystals in the vestibular system become dislodged. The crystals can usually be repositioned by a set of body-positioning maneuvers carried out by the audiologist or the otorhinolaryngologist in clinic. Spinning lasting a few hours, associated with unilateral aural fullness, sensorineural hearing loss, and worsening tinnitus, is typical of Meniere's disease. The etiology of this condition is poorly understood, and it often has a significant impact on the quality of life due to its chronic relapsing nature. An abnormal amount or quality of the fluid filling the inner ear is thought to underlie the problem. A variety

Table 10-4   Causes of Nonspecific Dizziness

Disorder	Description of the Disorder
Medications	Hypertensive medications can lower the blood pressure (BP) too far and cause nonspecific dizziness and faintness. Other medications may have a side effect of decreasing the BP, thus causing nonspecific dizziness that resolves once the medication is stopped.
Inner ear disorders	Certain inner ear abnormalities may cause unrelenting, non-vertigo-type dizziness.
Anxiety disorders	Panic attacks and goraphobia (a fear of leaving the home or being in large, open spaces) can cause dizziness.
Anemia	Anemia can cause dizziness along with pale skin, fatigue, and weakness.
Hypoglycemia	Dizziness can be accompanied by sweating and confusion in the insulin-dependent patient.
Ear infections	Ear infections can cause dizziness that will clear up once the infection goes away.

Data from Tusa R. Dizziness. *Med Clin North Am.* 2009;93:263; Kutz J. The dizzy patient. *Med Clin North Am.* 2010;94:989.

Table 10-5 Symptoms and Signs of Central and Peripheral Vertigo

Central Vertigo		Peripheral Vertigo	
Symptoms	Examples	Symptoms	Examples
Gradual onset	• Migraine headache	Sudden onset	• Meniere's disease
Unaffected by head position and movement	• Neoplasm • Vertebral artery dissection	Affected by head position and movement	• Benign paroxysmal positional vertigo (BPPV)
Motor function, gait instability, and loss of coordination frequent	• Cerebellar hemorrhage and infarct • Multiple sclerosis	Motor function, gait, and coordination typically intact	• Ototoxicity • Superior canal dehiscence syndrome
Constant with milder symptoms	• Mal de debarquement syndrome • Vertebrobasilar insufficiency	Intermittent with severe symptoms	• Labyrinthitis
Nausea and vomiting less predictable		Nausea and vomiting more frequent and severe	

Data from Kutz J. The dizzy patient. *Med Clin North Am.* 2010;94:989; Khoo C, Chakrabarti S, Arbour L, Krahn A. Recognizing life-threatening causes of syncope. *Cardiol Clin.* 2013;31:51-66; Furman M, Rizzolo D. Evaluating the patient with vertigo: a complex complaint made simple. *JAAPA.* 2011;24(10):52-58.

of treatments are available, from salt avoidance through medical treatment to more invasive strategies such as injection of gentamycin into the middle ear with the intention of ablating vestibular function. Vestibular neuritis (sometimes also called labyrinthitis, especially if hearing loss is associated) is a common cause of dizziness in young adults, presenting with an acute onset, persistent spinning sensation, and difficulty with balance associated with nausea and vomiting and lasting several days to a week, often in association with a viral upper respiratory tract infection. Treatment is supportive, and may include vestibular sedatives such as prochlorperazine.

Another common cause of dizziness is migrainous vertigo. The duration of spinning can be variable, and often there is a family or personal history of migraine headaches. Dietary modification helps many, but pharmacotherapy may also be required. It is important to note that any use of drugs in the treatment of vertigo during pregnancy should be carefully balanced between the therapeutic benefits and the potential impact on the development of the fetus, mandating a discussion between the obstetric and otorhinolaryngology teams.

During pregnancy, vertigo and dizziness are some of the most common complaints within primary care,[9] but little is known about the link. Potential causes include the normal decrease in blood pressure seen as pregnancy advances and lack of adequate fluid intake. Postpartum vertigo is also reported.[3] In many cases, its cause is non-otologic, but some case reports indicate abrupt changes in middle ear and intracranial pressure.

Tinnitus

Tinnitus refers to the perception of sound within the ear or head, in the absence of external sound stimulation. The reported prevalence is between 10% and 15% of the adult population.[10] It is a symptom, rather than a disease itself; thus it usually points to some other otologic condition. Tinnitus can be subjective, when the experience is of the individual alone, or, less commonly, objective, when an observer can hear the tinnitus. Clinical presentation of tinnitus can be sudden, but in most cases is gradual. The sensation is generally described as a hissing, sizzling, whistling, or ringing, although, in some cases, more complex sounds such as voices or music are perceived. When voices or music, or both, are heard as a form of tinnitus, the perceptions are indistinct and convey no meaning, in contrast with the auditory hallucinations that can occur with psychotic illness. Tinnitus can sometimes be a rhythmical or pulsatile sound. If pulsatile tinnitus appears to be synchronous with the heartbeat, then a vascular origin is likely, particularly if the tinnitus is unilateral (e.g., arteriovenous malformation, glomus tumor). Pulsatile tinnitus experienced all over the head is a feature of a hyperdynamic circulation, and thus not unusual in pregnancy, but blood pressure measurement is mandatory. Pulsatile tinnitus can sometimes appear asynchronous with the heartbeat, in which case myoclonus (rhythmic spasming) of the middle ear or palatal muscles is probable. Tinnitus can be constant or intermittent, and many patients experience more than one sound.

Tinnitus is more common with increasing age. It is also associated with trauma; exposure to excessive noise; medical conditions such as hypertension, rheumatoid arthritis, systemic lupus, and diabetes; various otologic problems; and ototoxic medications.[10] Pregnancy has been reported to increase the incidence of tinnitus, but further research to confirm a causal link is warranted.[3] However, in most pregnant women, symptoms reflect a benign complaint that resolves with delivery. The interested reader is referred to a *Lancet* "seminar," which provides a broad-ranging overview of tinnitus, covering epidemiology, pathogenesis, diagnosis, treatment, and prevention.[10]

Essential History, Physical Examination, and Laboratory Data

The following is a brief guide to the important assessments and history taking that aid the identification of relevant otologic symptoms requiring further investigation, thus ensuring the best possible prognosis for patients. Audiology is a profession that abides by clinical protocols and guidelines, published by the relevant professional bodies (e.g., the American Speech-Language-Hearing Association [ASHA] and the American Academy of Audiology [AAA]). Audiologists are required to practice within their scope of competency, education, and experience and abide by ethical standards of their professional organization.

History

When a woman presents with otologic symptoms, a full medical history should be obtained, including prior occurrences of the symptom, hospitalizations, and medication use; previous surgery or injury to the head or neck; pregnancy; or other medical problems such as cardiovascular disorders or diabetes that could impact the presentation or management of ear-related problems. For example, if a patient has recently undergone ear surgery and presents with symptoms of dizziness and hearing loss, there is a high possibility she has incurred a perilymph fistula; this can also occur following parturition.

In addition to a general history, it is essential to elicit a history of the complaint itself, any associated symptoms, and progression of the problem to help limit the possibilities under consideration. For each symptom, the patient should be asked when and where the symptom originated; characteristics of the symptom and changes over time; and whether the onset was associated with a specific precipitating event such as trauma, illness, or allergic exacerbation. See **Table 10-6**

Table 10-6 Symptom-Specific History and Differential Diagnosis

Symptom	History Checklist	Differential Diagnosis	Referral Indicators
Ear discharge	Onset, course, duration, color, odor, blood, other otologic symptoms, facial palsy, use of foreign bodies in ear canal.	*Outer*: Otitis externa. *Middle*: Tympanic membrane perforation associated with acute otitis media, chronic suppurative otitis media, trauma.	• Persistent ear discharge > 6 weeks. • History of discharge other than wax in last 90 days. • Presence of complications such as facial palsy or dizziness should prompt urgent referral.
Ear pain	Onset, course, duration, localization, other otologic symptoms, dental problems, fullness. Inquiry is made for exposure to extreme cold, barotraumas from flying and diving, or excessive noise; jaw problems and recent dental work or toothache; use of cotton-tipped applicators.	*Outer*: Otitis externa, cerumen impaction, foreign body, furunculosis, trauma. *Middle*: Acute otitis media, bullous myringitis, traumatic perforation of tympanic membrane, acute mastoiditis. *Neural*: Herpes zoster.	• Persistent pain lasting > 7 days in last 90 days. • Neurologic findings (e.g., facial palsy).
Hearing loss	Onset, course, duration, fluctuation, laterality, other otologic symptoms, facial palsy, family history, noise exposure, medication (be aware of ototoxic drugs).	*Outer*: Cerumen impaction, otitis externa, foreign body. *Middle*: Otitis media with effusion, acute otitis media, chronic suppurative otitis media, cholesteatoma, otosclerosis, Eustachian tube dysfunction. *Inner*: Presbycusis, Meniere's disease, noise-induced, drug-induced (ototoxicity), genetic. *Retrocochlear*: Vestibular schwannoma.	• Sudden-onset hearing loss (i.e., within 1 week). • Rapid deterioration (i.e., 90 days or less). • Fluctuating, other than associated with common cold. • Unilateral hearing loss. • Unilateral hearing loss with neurologic findings (e.g., facial palsy, dysarthria, nystagmus).

(continues)

Table 10-6 Symptom-Specific History and Differential Diagnosis *(continued)*

Symptom	History Checklist	Differential Diagnosis	Referral Indicators
Dizziness	Onset, course, duration, fluctuation, characteristics (e.g., rotatory or unsteadiness), other otologic symptoms, facial palsy, sickness, loss of consciousness, family history, medication (be aware of ototoxic drugs), blood pressure, surgery, diabetes, cardiovascular.	*Otologic*: Benign paroxysmal positional vertigo, labyrinthitis, Meniere's disease, vertebrobasilar insufficiency, ischemia. *Neural*: Multiple sclerosis, intracranial lesions or tumors, vestibular neuritis, migraine, clinical depression or anxiety, psychogenic. *Medical*: Cardiovascular disease, orthostatic hypertension, dysrhythmia. *Metabolic*: Hypoglycemia, hyperventilation syndrome, diabetes mellitus. *Iatrogenic*: Complication of ear surgery, drug induced.	• Dizziness post-surgery. • Dizziness with accompanying headaches and sickness. • Swaying/floating sensation. • Hallucination of movement. • Vertigo following parturition (possible perilymph fistula).
Tinnitus	Onset, course, duration, laterality, characteristics (e.g., pulsatile or constant), other otologic symptoms, facial palsy, family history, noise exposure, medication (be aware of ototoxic drugs).	*Extra-auditory*: Temporomandibular joint disorder, carotid atherosclerosis. *Outer*: Cerumen impaction, otitis externa. *Middle*: Conductive hearing loss, otosclerosis, Eustachian tube dysfunction. *Inner*: Presbycusis, noise-induced hearing loss, Meniere's disease, vestibular schwannoma.	• Unilateral, pulsatile, or distressing tinnitus lasting > 5 mins per incidence. • Troublesome tinnitus leading to associated psychologic problems.

for further symptom-specific history taking and potential differential diagnosis.

Physical Examination

Following the history, physical examination is undertaken with the aim of determining origin of symptoms. The pinna is inspected from the front and from the back, particularly looking for surgical scars, redness, swelling, or tenderness. The pinna is then pulled up and back while the otoscope is used to inspect the ear canal and the tympanic membrane. The otoscope is held like a pen in the hand opposite to the ear being examined.

The largest speculum that can be accommodated in the ear canal should be used; remember to move the otoscope so that the full extent of the ear is seen. It is important to be gentle as the ear canal may be sensitive.

One should note the presence of canal narrowing, wax, edema, discharge, and tympanic membrane abnormalities including perforation, redness, presence of bubbles, ventilation tubes, bulging, and scarring (myringosclerosis/tympanosclerosis can be seen as chalk-like patches on the tympanic membrane due to scarring). During pregnancy increased vascularity is often seen as redness in the ear canal or on the tympanic membrane.

Wax or discharge in the ear canal may have to be removed to allow full examination. Pneumatic otoscopy can also be helpful to look at eardrum mobility as an adjunct to diagnosing otitis media, in which typically the eardrum will be immobile. The technique involves the placement of a soft speculum into the ear canal to obtain an airtight seal, with the pressure in the ear canal then varied with an insufflation bulb; practice is required to ensure validity and reliability of the technique.

In the case of dizziness, a full neurologic examination is also performed looking for possible central causes of dizziness, with a specific focus on nystagmus and balance. For example, spontaneous horizontal nystagmus, with or without rotary nystagmus, is diagnostic of vestibular neuronitis. Central vertigo will present as nystagmus that is vertical, horizontal, or rotational and does not lessen when the woman focuses her gaze. Balance should be assessed by checking tandem gait, normal gait, heel and toe walking, and balance in a fixed position. Women with peripheral vertigo have decreased balance but are capable of walking; however, women with central vertigo have a more acute imbalance that limits their capability to stand on their own.[8]

Specialist diagnostic tests of balance function include Romberg's test (standing still with eyes closed, feet together, and hands outstretched, looking for instability), Unterberger's stepping test (marching on spot with eyes closed, looking for instability and rotation), and the Dix-Hallpike test (patient lying down with head hanging off the edge of the bed and rotated to one side, looking for torsional nystagmus typical of BPPV). Further details of specialist diagnostic testing for vestibular conditions are provided in **Table 10-7**.

In addition to the ears, examination may also include other parts of the head and neck (e.g., looking for enlarged lymph glands that might indicate infection or a tumor). The nose and postnasal space are inspected for problems that might lead to middle ear disease. The mouth is checked for cleft palate, also associated with middle ear disease. The cardiovascular system is evaluated, particularly blood pressure, as well as carotid and cranial bruits.

Laboratory studies will vary based on history and physical findings, but common studies performed include glucose testing, complete blood counts, electrolytes, and thyroid function.

While a basic assessment should always be carried out in the primary care setting, the investigation of many symptoms, particularly those that are severe or persistent, requires the expertise of a specialist. Table 10-7 describes some of the tests that are conducted by a specialist practitioner to assess hearing loss, while **Table 10-8** describes some of the common hearing test findings that can be expected.

Referral Criteria

Where any findings indicate possible need for further specialist assessment (e.g., audiologic, otologic, neurologic, or neuro-otologic), most patients are referred to audiology, otorhinolaryngology, or audiovestibular medicine.[11] Examples of situations requiring further specialty evaluation include symptoms suggestive of middle ear or vestibular disease or a suspicion that tumors such as a vestibular schwannoma are present.

A comprehensive list of referral indicators is given in Table 10-6. While some otologic symptoms may be common and nonspecific, others can be indicative of severe underlying disease and require immediate investigation to achieve the best possible prognosis. For example, idiopathic sudden sensorineural hearing loss is often reported as a full or blocked ear, which some people may mistake for a buildup of cerumen and thus may not value as warranting urgent medical attention. Sudden sensorineural hearing loss is in fact one of the only types of hearing loss that can be treated medically, but recovery is dependent on a number of factors including early intervention.[12] Although in 85–90% of cases the etiology

Table 10-7 Diagnostic Testing for Vestibular Conditions

Vestibular Diagnostic Test	Description	Purpose
Caloric test	Hot and cold air or water is instilled into the ear, and any resulting nystagmus is examined (not a reliable diagnostic test).	Identifies canal paresis
Clinical test of sensory interaction on balance (CTSIB)	A set of verbal instructions for patients to perform specific bodily movements (some with eyes open, some with eyes closed).	Assesses vestibular function by removing visual input and proprioception
Computerized dynamic posturography (CDP)	Patient stands on a movable, dual force plate support surface within a movable surround (enclosure). The patient experiences various motion effects, during which her postural stability and motor reactions are recorded.	Assesses complex interplay between balance, visual input, and proprioception
Dix-Hallpike maneuver	Positional test to assess nystagmus characteristics.	Identifies benign paroxysmal positional vertigo
Electronystagmography/videonystagmography	A vestibular test to look for nystagmus and smooth eye tracking.	Identifies peripheral or central lesions that give rise to nystagmus or poor eye movement tracking
Eye movement/nystagmus testing	Patient follows a moving finger with her eyes.	Identifies peripheral or central lesions that give rise to nystagmus or poor eye movement tracking
Fukuda stepping test (Unterberger's test)	Patient's ability to march in place with eyes closed.	Assesses for an imbalance between two vestibular systems that leads to patient rotating.
Romberg's test	Patient's ability to stand with feet together and eyes closed, and to walk heel-to-toe in a straight line.	Assesses vestibular function by removing visual input

Auditory Diagnostic Test	Description	Purpose
Audiometry	Quantitative measurement of air conduction and bone conduction hearing thresholds.	Determines type and degree of hearing loss
Auditory brainstem response	Recording of electrical events in response to auditory stimulus.	Estimates auditory threshold in difficult-to-test individuals (e.g., babies or cognitively impaired), enables intra-operative monitoring, and detects auditory nerve and brainstem lesions
Computerized tomography (CT)	Produces cross-sectional digital image of target tissue.	Permits study of bony structures in auditory system (e.g., ossicular chain or cochlear abnormalities)
Electrocochleography	Recording of the electrical events of the co-chlea (specifically the cochlear summating potential and the action potential, independently or in combination).	Objectively identifies Meniere's disease, enables intraoperative monitoring
Magnetic resonance image (MRI)	Spatial characterization of soft tissue in digital format.	Permits highly detailed study of soft tissue in the auditory system (e.g., investigation of vestibular schwannoma/cerebellopontine angle lesions)
Otoacoustic emissions	Objective measure of cochlear function, specifically outer hair cell function.	Screens to determine amplification function of cochlea
Otoscopy	Magnified examination of the ear using an otoscope.	Inspects abnormalities in the external ear and tympanic membrane
Rinne's test	Comparison of air conduction with tuning fork held by the pinna with bone conduction with tuning fork placed on the mastoid process.	Screens for unilateral conductive and sensorineural hearing loss
Stapedial reflexes	Measure of the integrity of the stapedial reflex arc.	Detects retrocochlear pathology
Tone decay	Assessment of auditory fatigue.	Indicates a defect in retrocochlear transmission of sound (e.g., cerebellopontine lesions)
Tympanometry	Measure of the compliance and impedance of the tympanic membrane and middle ear space.	Determines physical properties of the middle ear
Weber's test	Patient report of her perception of a vibrating tuning fork placed in the middle of the forehead.	Screens for unilateral conductive and sensorineural hearing loss
Whisper test	Tester whispers a combination of letters and numbers from a distance of 2 feet (standing to the patient's side so lip reading does not occur), while rubbing the opposite ear to provide masking.	Crudely tests hearing (A normal-hearing person should hear the whisper.)

Table 10-8 Some Common Hearing Test Findings

Type of Hearing Loss	Rinne's Test	Weber's Test	Whisper Test
Conductive: Wax impaction, foreign body, otitis externa, all types of otitis media, tympanic membrane perforation, otosclerosis	Bone conduction louder than air conduction	Heard on affected side	Diminished or absent
Sensorineural: Idiopathic sensorineural hearing loss, presbycusis, Meniere's disease, ototoxic medication, congenital, genetic	Air conduction louder than bone conduction	Heard on the good side	Diminished or absent

Note that tuning fork tests are less reliable when mixed or bilateral hearing loss is present. In cases of severe sensorineural hearing loss, false-negative Rinne's findings may also occur. Bone conduction is louder than air conduction suggesting conductive loss, but in fact the bone conduction is perceived on the normal-hearing side.

of sudden sensorineural hearing loss is not known at the time of presentation, 10–15% of patients reporting sudden sensorineural hearing loss experience it as part of a rare life-threatening condition.[12] Sudden-onset hearing loss during pregnancy is rare and has been described in several case reports, but whether there is a relationship between hearing loss and pregnancy is unknown.[3]

Other symptoms should prompt investigation of a possible underlying cause. For example, persistent unilateral tinnitus might be an initial presenting feature of a vestibular schwannoma. If a vestibular schwannoma is suspected, the otorhinolaryngologist will arrange for magnetic resonance imaging (MRI) screening. Noncontrast MRI as an initial imaging screen in the investigation of acoustic neuroma is less costly than, and likely to be as sensitive as, contrast MRI.[13] While current treatment for vestibular schwannoma is conservative, based upon primary observation of small tumors,[13] it is still essential that these patients are closely monitored. MRI scans of the lesion are imperative to monitor the size and position of the tumor when it is suspected to be close to the nerves and brain stem.

MRI is also the study of choice to detect central causes of vestibular dysfunction, acute cerebellar ischemia, and acute or chronic hemorrhagic cerebral vascular accident (CVA). MRI is used if a woman presents with asymmetric hearing loss, sudden onset of symptoms, vertical nystagmus, or focal neurologic deficits.[8]

Diagnostic Clues

Many clinical presentations of reported auditory and vestibular symptoms may not lead to a single confirmed diagnosis. Different conditions may share some of the same presenting clinical features. In these circumstances, the healthcare practitioner should remain aware of the range of diagnostic possibilities and refer to the appropriate specialist if the diagnosis is unclear, the presentation is complicated, or if further investigations are required.

In some cases, the healthcare practitioner can become more confident about a specific diagnosis by drawing on convergent evidence from a range of diagnostic tests. For example, worsening conductive hearing loss during pregnancy with a family history of otosclerosis and characteristic audiometric features would strongly suggest otosclerosis. Otosclerosis is a progressive disorder in which bony material grows around the stapes of the middle ear causing gradual hearing loss. Symptoms can include hearing loss and tinnitus. The etiology is complex, with both a genetic predisposition and environmental influences likely. The condition typically affects young women, and many authors have reported its initial presentation during pregnancy or a worsening of symptoms during pregnancy in almost two-thirds of women with otosclerosis,[10] possibly due to hormonal influence. Hearing can improve, and distress from tinnitus can lessen after delivery.[14] Audiometry shows a conductive hearing loss that is typically worst at the 2 kHz frequency.

Some conditions consist of a combination of several clinically recognizable features. Meniere's syndrome—a progressive disorder of the inner ear—is one example. The syndrome is characterized by recurrent acute episodes of a triad of symptoms: vertigo, hearing loss, and tinnitus. An associated symptom is a sensation of pressure in the ear (aural fullness). Vertigo (causing dizziness, nausea, and vomiting) is often the most prominent symptom. Even when the condition is more advanced, the three major symptoms can fluctuate unpredictably over time. As a consequence, Meniere's syndrome is a complex and difficult illness to manage for the individual person, the family, and the doctor.

Meniere's syndrome can often be misdiagnosed, especially in primary care. A reliable diagnosis is made on clinical history, detailed physical, vestibular examination (particularly to exclude other causes), and audiologic tests. In the early stages of the condition, hearing between attacks is often normal, with low-frequency sensorineural hearing loss present during or before attacks. As the disease progresses, the sensorineural hearing loss becomes more permanent and also affects middle and high frequencies resulting in a typically "flat" audiometric profile. Other investigations may be required to exclude other conditions that share some of the same symptomatology, with MRI particularly useful to exclude a vestibular schwannoma, which could present in a similar manner. Potential differential diagnosis includes a number of other causes. For example, vestibular migraine ("migraine-associated dizziness"/"migraine-associated vertigo") may present in a similar manner, and a degree of overlap with Meniere's syndrome is thought to occur. Vestibular neuronitis can present with severe vertigo, nausea, and vomiting, typically in a young patient, but usually this is a unique episode and dizziness lasts a week or so rather than the several hours typical of Meniere's syndrome.

The true epidemiology of Meniere's syndrome is not known, because the inconsistent diagnostic criteria may lead to reporting biases. A recent review indicated that reported prevalence rates range from 3.5 per 100,000 to 513 per 100,000, rising with age;[15] one US study estimated its prevalence at 190 per 100,000, rising to as high as 440 per 100,000 for patients age 65 or older.[16] The precise etiology of the condition is difficult to establish. For up-to-date information, several good online resources are provided in the reference section.[17,18]

A case report suggests that pre-existing Meniere's syndrome may be exacerbated during pregnancy, especially vertigo attacks in the early phase (weeks 5–16) of pregnancy.[19] The authors highlight an association between symptom severity and serum osmolality (thinning of the blood by ≤ 10 mOsm/kg), with this possibly causing an increase in the volume (and thereby pressure) of endolymphatic fluid in the inner ear.

Specific Conditions

This final section presents a number of otologic conditions in more specific detail. Some of the most common conditions affecting each of the

Table 10-9 Medications Commonly Used to Manage Otologic Conditions

Indication	Drug	Dose	Safety Pregnancy	Breastfeeding
Otitis externa	Acetic acid (vinegar)	3 drops tid	B	Unknown
	Ciprofloxacin/dexamethasone	3 drops bid	C	Unknown
	Clotrimazole solution (for fungal infections)	3 drops bid	C	Unknown
	Cortisporin (neomycin, poly-mixin, hydrocortisone mix)	3 drops tid	C	Unknown
Acute otitis media	Amoxicillin (preferred)	500 mg tid	B	Safe
	Amoxicillin/clavulanate	500 mg tid	B	Safe
	Azithromycin (use if allergy to penicillin)	1 g once daily	B	Unknown
	Cefdinir	600 mg once daily	B	Safe
Dizziness	Prochlorperazine	5 mg tid	C	Unknown
	Meclizine	25 mg qid	B	Unknown

The use of any medication during pregnancy and when breastfeeding should take place only if the benefits outweigh the risk to the mother and child. In general, topical administration is unlikely to be absorbed to any significant extent. FDA labeling for safety during pregnancy and lactation should be verified before prescribing any medication with which the practitioner is not familiar.

bid = 2 times per day, qid = 4 times per day, tid = 3 times per day.

four subdivisions of the ear (outer, middle, inner, and retrocochlear) are covered here. **Table 10-9** reports some of the commonly used medications to manage otologic conditions.

Outer Ear Conditions: Otitis Externa, Foreign Bodies, and Earwax

CLINICAL PRESENTATION

Otitis externa refers to inflammation or infection of the ear canal. It is characterized by severe pain (especially if the pinna is pulled on), discharge, hearing loss, and itching. The ear canal appears swollen and red or eczematous, and is filled with discharge. Other clinical features may include tenderness on moving the jaw, tender regional lymphadenopathy, lack of wax in the ear canal, and dry hypertrophic skin, which often results in partial narrowing of the ear canal.

Otitis externa is extremely common, leading to an estimated 2.4 million healthcare visits per year in the United States (8.1 visits per 1000 population).[20] Otitis externa is uncommon in young children, in whom ear pain and discharge are much more likely to be due to acute otitis media. A particularly aggressive form is necrotizing (also called malignant) otitis externa, which is a skull base osteomyelitis occurring in immunocompromised patients; this condition, while rare, is associated with significant morbidity and even mortality. It should be suspected if pain and headache persist despite adequate treatment, particularly in immunosuppressed individuals.[21] Effective treatment of necrotizing otitis externa requires specialist input, with strict glucose control, topical cleaning and debridement, topical and systemic antibiotics, and in some cases surgery or hyperbaric oxygen. In some patients, a localized small boil, or furuncle, in the ear canal may be responsible for the symptoms. The furuncle presents with severe ear pain and can be identified as a localized swelling in the ear canal. It can be treated with systemic antibiotics, but surgical drainage may also be required.

Foreign bodies are also a common cause of otitis externa. A typical cause would be the use of cotton-tipped applicators by the patient in an attempt to clean the ears, with the cotton becoming dislodged and stuck in the ear canal. There may be no symptoms, but conductive hearing loss may result. Inorganic foreign bodies generally cause fewer symptoms than organic ones. Insects can occasionally also enter the ear canal; pain can be intense as the insect scratches in its attempts to exit the ear canal.

Ear cerumen occurs naturally in the ear and usually does not create any clinical problem unless impacted; at that time, it can cause conductive hearing loss. Earwax that completely blocks the ear canal is associated with a sensation of fullness and discomfort in the ear and diminished hearing.

ETIOLOGY AND RISK FACTORS

Otitis externa commonly results from bacterial infection, usually *Pseudomonas aeruginosa* or *Staphylococcus aureus*. Chronic infections are also often caused by fungi such as *Candida* and *Aspergillus* and are typically associated with severe itching. Otitis externa is sometimes known as "swimmer's ear," because acute symptoms tend to be associated with water exposure (e.g., recreational water activities, bathing, and excessive sweating) and warm, humid environments.[20] Other factors predisposing otitis externa are local allergens or irritants, eczema, psoriasis or other skin conditions, frequent use of earbuds and headphones, and hearing aid use.

A common risk factor for all three outer ear conditions—otitis externa, foreign body, and wax impaction—is ear instrumentation. This is typically done by patients using cotton-tipped applicators in an attempt to clean the ears. In reality, the ear canal possesses a natural transport mechanism whereby cerumen is transported from deep in the ear canal to the outside. Cerumen serves a protective function, yet patient attempts to remove it generally lead to more problems. Wax impaction can become a problem with hearing aid use that prevents the wax from being transported outward and can also occur in patients with very narrow or hairy ear canals. However, for most people, wax serves a beneficial and protective function.

CLINICAL HISTORY AND EXAMINATION

History taking should consider the nature of the clinical presentation, as well as the nature of any discharge or bleeding. Notes should include information about the duration and onset of the symptoms, any recurrence of symptoms, and whether the condition is unilateral or bilateral. Examination should include physical examination with otoscopy. The healthcare practitioner should be looking for signs of tenderness when pulling on the outer ear or moving the jaw, inflamed skin of the ear canal, tender regional lymph nodes, signs of dermatitis around the pinna, and serous or purulent discharge in the ear canal. Clinical history and examination are usually sufficient to make a diagnosis of otitis externa, with microbiology swabs not warranted in most cases.

MANAGEMENT AND REFERRAL

Otitis externa is a painful condition, and appropriate oral analgesia is required, taking into account any pregnancy-related contraindications. Patients should be advised to avoid water exposure and not to instrument the ears in any way. In mild cases, ear canal acidification with acetic acid drops may be all that is required. Otherwise, first-line treatment should be with topical antibiotic/steroid drops or sprays. A systematic review of the evidence indicates that topical treatments alone are effective for uncomplicated acute otitis externa.[22] If the ear canal is full of discharge or very swollen, topical drops will be unable to access the deep parts of the ear canal, and so the recommendation would be aural toilet in the otorhinolaryngology clinic, possibly combined with placement of a wick. Systemic antibiotics are not warranted in most cases, unless infection has spread beyond the ear canal or the patient is systemically unwell; suitable choices would be floxacillin, amoxicillin/clavulanic acid, or a macrolide.[21]

The use of some antibiotics in pregnancy may be more concerning than others. Commonly prescribed antibiotic drops used in the treatment of ear infections include the aminoglycosides, and sometimes, the quinolones. While significant systemic absorption of these antibiotics is unlikely, acetic acid drops would be an alternative, as would frequent aural toilet.

Fungal infections are less common than bacterial ones. They are generally more difficult to treat and therefore may best be managed in consultation with a specialist. Fungal infections should be suspected if an individual reports pruritus or ear discharge, typically characterized as being white and fluffy, although the color may vary. Treatment generally consists of aspiration of the ear canal and the use of acetic acid drops. Because fungal infections can be difficult to eradicate, post-treatment follow up is recommended.[21]

Management of a foreign body is best accomplished by a specialist. Objects of particular concern are insects, which can cause significant pain, and batteries, which require urgent removal because leakage of corrosive material from the battery can lead to severe and permanent damage. The equipment needed to remove a foreign body is not readily available in most office settings. Unskilled attempts to remove a foreign body may result in lodging the object even deeper into the ear canal, and attempting to flush the object out may also worsen the situation, particularly if the object is rice, which can swell upon exposure to water. However, distilling a drop or two of oil, if available, may be helpful if an insect is thought to be inside the ear canal. Oil will drown the insect, prevent further movement, and provide welcome relief from the pain resulting from a moving insect trying to escape the ear canal. This can afford some relief until the patient can be seen by an expert in the audiology office or in the emergency room for further management.

The management of excessive earwax is more straightforward. In most cases the use of earwax solution will soften or dissolve the earwax. These products are available without a prescription. However, to be effective, they must be used properly. After distilling the drops, the patient should tilt the head back toward the shoulder; this will allow the dissolved wax to exit the ear canal rather than pool deeper in the ear closer to the eardrum. If earwax solution alone is not effective in dissolving the wax, it will at least soften it, making ear lavage easier. Using an ear curette or lavage to remove earwax must be carefully done to prevent injury to the ear; neither should be performed if a perforation of the eardrum is suspected. Lavaging the ear can be done using a 10-mL syringe filled with normal saline solution attached to an 18-gauge intravenous (IV) catheter with the needle removed. Gentle and slow distillation of the normal saline via the IV catheter can soften and flush out the earwax. Use of an ear curette may also facilitate removal of excessive earwax.

Middle Ear Condition: Otitis Media with Effusion

A variety of middle ear inflammatory conditions exist, with somewhat confusing terminology.

Broadly speaking, middle ear inflammation (otitis media) can be acute or chronic. Acute otitis media is typically a childhood condition, characterized by preceding upper respiratory tract infection, fever, and otalgia, possibly leading to tympanic membrane rupture and then ear discharge. It is the most common specific diagnosis in a febrile child, and accounts for $2.88 billion in added healthcare expenses annually in the United States.[23] Viruses, bacteria, and barotrauma can lead to acute otitis media.

Chronic inflammation of the middle ear can broadly be split into three categories. Otitis media with effusion (OME) is characterized by the presence of middle ear fluid behind an intact eardrum in the absence of symptoms and signs of acute infection. Chronic suppurative otitis media refers to suppurative middle ear inflammation usually associated with tympanic membrane perforation. Cholesteatoma is characterized by the presence of squamous epithelium—skin—in the middle ear (usually middle ear contains respiratory-type epithelium). Both cholesteatoma and chronic suppurative otitis media present with persistent offensive ear discharge, whereas discharge is not a feature of OME.

OME typically presents with hearing difficulties. It affects children more frequently than adults and is the most common cause of hearing loss in children in the developed world. For many children and adults, OME is a temporary and self-resolving problem. Rarely, it may persist and be symptomatic; in this case, treatment via insertion of ventilation tubes (tympanostomy tubes, grommet) may be necessary.[24,25]

CLINICAL PRESENTATION

OME is characterized by the presence of an effusion (thick, glue-like fluid) behind the tympanic membrane in the middle ear in the absence of symptoms or signs of acute inflammation. Unlike acute infections that present with pain, OME presents with hearing loss, pressure, blocked ear feeling, or a popping sensation. If a young child is affected, he or she may not be able to articulate these clearly, but effects on communication, schooling, or speech development may be noted.

ETIOLOGY AND RISK FACTORS

The etiology of OME is only just being elucidated. OME is much more complex than just dysfunction of the Eustachian tube, with genetic factors and infection particularly important. The role of bacteria has long been debated, with recent evidence suggesting that bacterial biofilms are important in the pathogenesis of OME.[26] Biofilms are structured communities of bacteria attached to a surface; they exert a low-grade chronic inflammatory stimulus that causes the middle ear to produce the thick fluid that then accumulates as glue. It is likely that a complex interplay between genetic and environmental factors, particularly infection, determines whether a person develops OME. The presence of unilateral OME in an adult should be treated with caution, because a tumor of the postnasal space may be responsible; thus, examination of the postnasal space in an adult with unilateral OME is mandatory.

Many OME risk factors relate to factors that increase exposure or undermine the immune response. Overcrowding, passive smoking, and wintertime are known risk factors. The condition is more common among men than women. Patients with specific comorbidities such as cleft palate, craniofacial abnormality, immunodeficiency, ciliary dyskinesia, or Down syndrome are also more at risk. Professionals working with mothers are in a great position to provide parental education regarding risk factors for middle ear disease in children. Parents should be informed that breastfeeding has a beneficial protective effect, while pacifier use and passive smoking should be avoided.

CLINICAL HISTORY AND EXAMINATION

History taking should cover duration and fluctuation of symptoms and the effects that hearing loss has on daily functioning, especially employment or education, communication, and social participation. Acute otitis media also frequently coexists. Otoscopy can accurately diagnose OME in experienced hands, but is typically much less reliable when performed by a less-experienced clinician.[27] Audiometry and tympanometry are key diagnostic tests to confirm conductive hearing loss and the presence of an immobile tympanic membrane or negative middle ear pressure. Patients with Down syndrome present particular problems in diagnosis because of small ear canals, wax accumulation, and difficulties in conducting audiologic testing. Clinical practice guidelines on the management of OME exist in the United States[24] and in the United Kingdom,[25] but as with other guidelines these may not be followed in clinical practice.[28] Further, these guidelines are directed at children, not adults, making the management of OME in clinical practice even less consistent for adults than for children.

MANAGEMENT AND REFERRAL

Patients with suspected OME-associated hearing loss should be referred for audiometric assessment. Adults with unilateral OME should also have examination of the nose and postnasal space to exclude coexistent pathology. Although rarely needed, insertion of ventilation tubes is a treatment option for persistent, symptomatic OME. This surgical procedure can often be carried out under local anesthesia in adults, but in children a general anesthetic is usually needed. The eardrum is incised, and the ventilation tube placed into the eardrum with the intention of ventilating the middle ear space. Ventilation tubes extrude, typically 6 or 9 months later, but in many patients the symptoms unfortunately then recur.

Hearing aids are an alternative treatment for OME when surgery is contraindicated or not acceptable—for example, when OME persists despite surgical intervention. Auto-inflation of the Eustachian tube may also be tried; this involves repeated attempts at the Valsalva maneuver, with the intention of forcing air into the Eustachian tube and "popping" the ears. If a specific underlying cause for OME is identified (e.g., nasal polyps), then treatment can be focused on the underlying cause. However, although a large range of medical treatments (antibiotics, steroids, nose sprays) have been tried for OME, none are particularly effective.[25]

OME is not expected to lead to any urgent complications, but OME is common and may coexist with other middle ear disease. Thus, urgent referral to otorhinolaryngology should be prompted by pinna protrusion and tenderness or swelling over the mastoid and postauricular area, because these may signify mastoiditis (infection of the mastoid air cells that communicate with the middle ear), which may require systemic antibiotics or surgery. Routine referral should be prompted by persistent offensive discharge, because this may signify cholesteatoma or chronic suppurative otitis media.

The presence of persistent tympanic membrane perforation will also generally require referral. Perforation typically follows an episode of acute otitis media, and although the drum heals in most cases, sometimes perforation persists. Direct trauma can also lead to perforation, and again most heal spontaneously. Short-term advice for tympanic perforation would include avoidance of water, but if a perforation persists and causes ear discharge or hearing difficulties, then surgical repair may be required. Perforation or a bleeding ear can also occur as a result of skull base fracture. Health professionals working with women need to be cognizant of the possibility of major head injury occurring as a result of physical abuse.

Inner Ear Conditions: Sensorineural Hearing Loss and Vertigo

Age-related hearing loss (presbycusis) is a common form of sensorineural hearing loss. It is ranked as the third most prevalent chronic condition in elderly people after hypertension and arthritis. Its prevalence and severity increase with age, rising from about 30–35% of adults ages 65 and older to an estimated 40–50% of adults ages 75 and older.[29]

CLINICAL PRESENTATION

Sensorineural hearing loss has many different presentations. Its onset can be gradual or immediate; its severity can be mild, moderate, severe, or profound; it can be present in one or both ears, and be accompanied by tinnitus or dizziness; and it may be preceded by fluctuating hearing loss in cases of Meniere's or autoimmune disease.[30] Hearing loss causes increased communication difficulties, which often result in reduced activity and participation in everyday life, leading to social withdrawal, depression, and reduced quality of life.

ETIOLOGY AND RISK FACTORS

Sensorineural hearing loss is the underlying cause in the majority of individuals with hearing loss and is due to a loss of transduction of sound in the inner ear, vestibulocochlear nerve, or central auditory system. The main cause of sensorineural hearing loss is damage to the inner ear hair cells in the organ of Corti, but causes can occur anywhere in the neural pathway from the cochlea to the brain.

Sensorineural hearing loss can be congenital or acquired. Most areas in the developed world now offer universal newborn hearing screening, and the health practitioner working with pregnant women will be in the ideal position to facilitate screening. Hearing loss is common, and may affect as many as 4 per 1000 newborns;[31] underlying causes of congenital hearing loss can be

environmental or genetic. Environmental factors include bacterial or viral infections such as maternal rubella[32] and cytomegalovirus,[33] ototoxic antibiotics such as gentamycin, or situations such as birth asphyxia and severe neonatal jaundice, which restrict blood flow to the brain.[34] Care must be taken when prescribing medications to expectant mothers so as to avoid the harmful effect of these drugs on the unborn child. Genetic causes can be nonsyndromic (70%) or syndromic (30%).[35] It is possible for genetic counseling to determine the likelihood of passing on deafness to offspring. Genetic hearing loss can manifest itself later in childhood but would usually be picked up by routine hearing screening and observations made at school and home.

Acquired sensorineural hearing loss includes age-related hearing loss (presbycusis) and noise-induced hearing loss. Presbycusis reflects a natural deterioration of hearing over the lifespan as a result of cumulative noise exposure and the unintended side effects of medications that cause damage to the hair cells in the inner ear.[36] For example, some aminoglycosides and macrolides have well-known ototoxic properties. These effects are permanent. Other risk factors for hearing loss that have been explored by researchers include cardiovascular health, smoking, and diet (e.g., high serum cholesterol levels).

Noise-induced hearing loss can occur as a result of either sudden, intense bursts of loud and puncturing sound such as gun blast or intense, prolonged exposure to excessively loud sound such as factory noise or listening to personal music players. In some cases, the acute hearing loss is temporary (e.g., temporary threshold shift). However, there is emerging evidence that when hearing function recovers, there can be permanent damage to the synapses between the sensory hair cells and the auditory nerve.[37] As a general rule, the louder a sound, the less time one can safely listen to it without causing damage to the inner ear.

CLINICAL HISTORY AND EXAMINATION

History taking should consider the nature of the clinical presentation, as well as the nature of any associated otologic symptoms such as tinnitus and dizziness. Particular attention should be paid to the duration and onset of the symptoms and whether they are unilateral or bilateral. Where sudden hearing loss is suspected, the patient should be referred urgently for further investigation (see Table 10-6 for red flags indicating a need for urgent referral). Otherwise, following the initial examination by the nonspecialist, a referral to audiology or otorhinolaryngology should be made.

MANAGEMENT AND REFERRAL

Noise-induced hearing loss can be prevented with the use of adequate hearing protection, such as that provided by the use of circumaural ear defenders or earplugs. Patients presenting with noise-induced hearing loss—typically recognizable from a 4-kHz "notch" in the audiogram—should be advised to use hearing protection and minimize noise exposure with the goal of preventing further damage to the inner ear. The primary intervention to remediate the symptoms of sensorineural hearing loss is the provision of hearing aids to amplify sound and audiologic counseling to aid rehabilitation. Although an estimated 17% of American adults report having hearing loss, only 20% of those who could benefit from hearing aids actually use them.[38] Factors that typically lead to nonuse of hearing aids are the lack of patient confidence in them, they are perceived as not helpful, or they are too complicated to use. Audiologic counseling is essential to help the patient explore and remediate barriers to nonuse of hearing aids and thus improve hearing aid use and benefit.

Hearing loss symptoms should be fully evaluated to identify any causes that require medical or surgical treatment, such as syphilis in the latent or congenital form, immune-mediated sensorineural hearing loss, vestibular schwannoma, sudden sensorineural hearing loss, and perilymphatic fistula. In patients presenting with idiopathic sudden sensorineural hearing loss, treatment with steroids can potentially maximize the possibility of hearing recovery.[39] Typically, this would be prednisolone 60 mg once daily for a week. If it is determined that oral prednisolone should be avoided, an alternative would be steroid injection into the middle ear under local anesthetic. Particularly in pregnancy, this alternative can be considered, because it is associated with treatment success and would minimize transplacental transfer of prednisolone to the fetus. When there is no treatable cause and hearing loss is too profound for the use of a hearing aid, surgical intervention (cochlea implant or brainstem implant) may be considered to bypass the mechanical functioning of the cochlea.

OFFICE MANAGEMENT OF THE WOMAN WITH VERTIGO

Although the symptoms, etiology, and general evaluation of dizziness and vertigo have been discussed in previous sections, the management of women with BPPV—possibly with medication or lifestyle counseling—and referral criteria are reviewed here.

The most common cause of peripheral vertigo is BPPV, which can generally be easily and successfully managed in the office setting. It results from displacement of calcium carbonate crystals, called otoconia, from the utricle into the semicircular canals. Typically, women with BPPV will be able to reproduce their symptoms by lying down or moving the head, because these trapped otoconia continue to move within the semicircular canals during position change.[40]

Treatment for BPPV is usually through canalith repositioning (see **Figure 10-2**). This procedure can be performed in the office or at an outpatient physical therapy center. During the canalith repositioning procedure, a woman is asked to make

Figure 10-2 Epley canalith repositioning procedure (CRP). Pause 1 minute between each position.

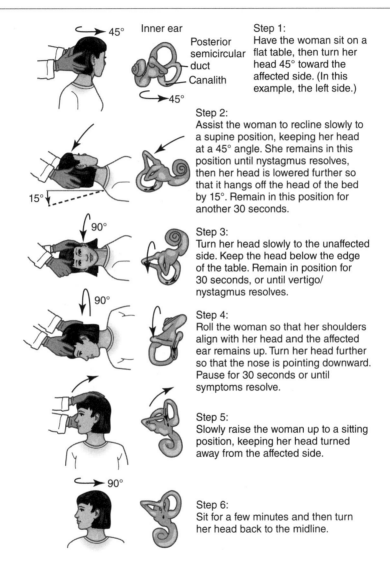

Step 1:
Have the woman sit on a flat table, then turn her head 45° toward the affected side. (In this example, the left side.)

Step 2:
Assist the woman to recline slowly to a supine position, keeping her head at a 45° angle. She remains in this position until nystagmus resolves, then her head is lowered further so that it hangs off the head of the bed by 15°. Remain in this position for another 30 seconds.

Step 3:
Turn her head slowly to the unaffected side. Keep the head below the edge of the table. Remain in position for 30 seconds, or until vertigo/nystagmus resolves.

Step 4:
Roll the woman so that her shoulders align with her head and the affected ear remains up. Turn her head further so that the nose is pointing downward. Pause for 30 seconds or until symptoms resolve.

Step 5:
Slowly raise the woman up to a sitting position, keeping her head turned away from the affected side.

Step 6:
Sit for a few minutes and then turn her head back to the midline.

Modified from Hornibrook J. Benign paroxysmal positional vertigo (BPPV): history, pathophysiology, office treatment and future directions. *Int J Otolaryngol.* 2011;2011:835671. doi: 10.1155/2011/835671. CCC license available at http://creativecommons.org/licenses/by/3.0/.

numerous simple and slow maneuvers to reposition her head. The goal is to move free-floating otoconia from the fluid-filled semicircular canals of the inner ear into a tiny bag-like open area (vestibule) that houses one of the otolith organs (utricle); once these particles are trapped, they can be resorbed. Each position is held for about 30 seconds after any symptoms or abnormal eye movement stop. This treatment is usually effective after one or two sessions. After the procedure, the woman must avoid lying flat or placing the treated ear below shoulder level for the rest of that day. For the first night following the procedure, the woman should elevate her head on a few pillows when she goes to sleep. This allows time for the otoconia floating in the labyrinth to settle into the vestibule and be resorbed by the fluids in the inner ear. On the morning after the procedure, the woman's restrictions will be lifted and she can resume her normal activities.[40]

MEDICATIONS

The use of medication for vertigo/dizziness is limited to managing problematic symptoms:

- Women with severe nausea and vomiting may benefit from IV fluid and antiemetic medications such as ondansetron (Zofran) or prochlorperazine (Compazine).
- Diazepam, midazolam, or other benzodiazepines may be helpful as a vestibular suppressant for women with severe vertigo.[41]

PATIENT INSTRUCTIONS FOR VERTIGO

Women should avoid known triggers such as caffeine, alcohol, and tobacco.[7,42] Standing up slowly may minimize symptoms. If symptoms occur, the woman should sit or lie down immediately.

Women with persistent vertigo or dizziness must be aware that dizziness can make them lose their balance and increases the risk of falling and being seriously injured. Consequently, the woman should fall-proof her home by removing tripping hazards such as exposed electrical cords or area rugs. Nonslip mats should be used on the bathroom floor and shower floor. The woman should also use good lighting on stairs and hallways, especially if she gets out of bed at night. Walking with a cane or walker may be needed for stability.[42] Care is also needed when driving. Woman who experience frequent dizziness should avoid driving a car or operating heavy machinery.

INDICATIONS FOR REFERRAL

Care in the emergency department is needed if a woman has never experienced an episode of vertigo before or if the woman has had prior episodes but is currently experiencing severe dizziness or vertigo and is also experiencing any of the following: a new, different, or severe headache; significant head injury; trouble speaking; a stiff neck; blurred vision; leg or arm weakness; falling or difficulty walking; chest pain; loss of consciousness; or sudden hearing loss. Women should be advised to call 911 if they experience any of these symptoms. Women with these symptoms who are being seen in the office setting need emergency transport to the hospital, because these symptoms may be due to severe/life-threatening neurologic disorders.[41]

Retrocochlear Condition: Vestibular Schwannoma

The technically preferred term for this condition is *vestibular schwannoma*, but the term *acoustic neuroma* is more commonly used.

CLINICAL PRESENTATION

Vestibular schwannoma refers to a benign tumor that can occur along the course of the 8th cranial nerve (vestibulocochlear nerve), either within the auditory meatus or medial to it in the cerebellopontine angle. Most such tumors are unilateral, and thus patients usually present with a unilateral sensorineural hearing loss and tinnitus.

Tumors inside the auditory meatus erode the bony walls of the canal as they grow and often expand medially into the cerebellopontine angle, as this is the path of least resistance. The presenting complaints vary widely depending on the size and location of the tumor. Very small tumors may be asymptomatic. But as the tumor grows, it compresses, deforms, and displaces the nerve. Pressure from the tumor can also interfere with the blood supply to the cochlea. As tumor size increases, pressure can also be exerted on other cranial nerves (especially the facial and trigeminal nerves) and can even displace the brain stem in late stages when other symptoms would normally have been picked up.[43]

Symptoms of a more extensive vestibular schwannoma that is impacting the brain stem (e.g., headaches, vomiting, tinnitus) may be exacerbated by hormonal changes associated with pregnancy.[9] One possible explanation is that the tumor undergoes selective fluid accumulation in late pregnancy, contributing to increased intracranial pressure and subsequent tinnitus. Although rare, vestibular schwannoma will always be included in the differential diagnosis when a woman with tinnitus is assessed by an otorhinolaryngologist.

ETIOLOGY AND RISK FACTORS

This type of tumor represents about 6% of all intracranial tumors and 70–80% of all cerebellopontine angle tumors. The annual incidence of vestibular schwannoma is 1 to 2 out of 100,000, with a 3:2 female-to-male ratio.[44] In recent years, incidence has increased because of a rise in the detection of smaller tumors following better availability of MRI.

Most growths are sporadic without any known cause. Tumor suppressor gene abnormalities on chromosome p22 (merlin or schwannomin protein) are thought to explain some tumor growth. There is a familial autosomal dominant form in which patients have bilateral tumors in addition to other intracranial tumors (neurofibromatosis type 2). Otherwise, there are no known specific risk factors.

CLINICAL HISTORY AND EXAMINATION

Any asymmetric sensorineural hearing loss could point to a retrocochlear pathology and indicates a need for an audiology assessment. Onset is usually gradual, but may occur suddenly. Other key diagnostic factors include facial numbness in the tongue and jaw, which is generally a late symptom that occurs in larger tumors. Another possible feature is a nystagmus on a lateral gaze that is often associated with progressive episodes of dizziness. A gadolinium-enhanced magnetic resonance scan is the standard confirmatory test.

MANAGEMENT AND REFERRAL

A suspected vestibular schwannoma requires immediate referral to the appropriate specialist. Danger signs include 1) a recent sudden onset sensorineural hearing loss, with or without tinnitus, and 2) unexplained neurologic symptoms or signs that are suggestive of brainstem compression or raised intracranial pressure. Evaluation by otolaryngology and/or neurology is warranted in this situation.

Most tumors, when identified, are small. Interval scanning to monitor growth is frequently used as the first-line management option. Active treatments include a variety of surgical approaches or gamma knife stereotactic radiosurgery. In pregnancy, unless the symptoms are severe or suggest intracranial compromise, it would be reasonable to delay any MRI scanning until after delivery (in discussion with patient), although MRI is generally considered safe in pregnancy. Any surgical intervention is also best delayed, unless the benefits of treatment outweigh the risks of major surgery under general anesthesia in pregnancy.

References

1. Hall DA, Láinez MJA, Newman CW, Sanchez TG, Egler M, Tennigkeit F, et al. Treatment options for subjective tinnitus: self reports from a sample of general practitioners and ENT physicians within Europe and the USA. *BMC Health Serv Res.* 2011;11:302.
2. Royal College of Physicians. *Hearing and Balance Disorders: Achieving Excellence in Diagnosis and Management.* London, UK: Royal College of Physicians; 2007.
3. Kumar R, Hayhurst KL, Robson AK. Ear, nose and throat manifestations during pregnancy. *Otolaryngol Head Neck Surg.* 2011;145(2):188-198.
4. Karatas M. Central vertigo and dizziness: epidemiology, differential diagnosis, and common causes. *Neurologist.* 2008;14(6):355-364.
5. Tusa R. Dizziness. *Med Clin North Am.* 2009;93:263.
6. Kutz J. The dizzy patient. *Med Clin North Am.* 2010;94:989.
7. Khoo C, Chakrabarti S, Arbour L, Krahn A. Recognizing life-threatening causes of syncope. *Cardiol Clin.* 2013;31:51-66.
8. Furman M, Rizzolo D. Evaluating the patient with vertigo: a complex complaint made simple. *JAAPA.* 2011;24(10):52-58.
9. Black FO. Maternal susceptibility to nausea and vomiting of pregnancy: is the vestibular system involved? *Am J Obstet Gynecol.* 2002;186 (5 suppl):S184-S189.
10. Baguley D, McFerran D, Hall DA. Seminar. Tinnitus. *Lancet.* 2013;382(9904):1600-1607.
11. British Academy of Audiology. Guidelines for referral to audiology of adults with hearing difficulty. 2009. Available at: http://www.baaudiology.org/files/3513/5898/2984/BAA_Direct_Referral_Criteria_0909_amended1.pdf. Accessed March 31, 2016.
12. Fetterman BL, Saunders JE, Luxford WM. Prognosis and treatment of sudden sensorineural hearing loss. *Otol Neurotol.* 1996;17(4):529-536.
13. Fortnum H, O'Neill C, Taylor R, Lenthall R, Nikolopoulos T, Lightfoot G, et al. The role of magnetic resonance imaging in the identification of suspected acoustic neuroma: a systematic review of clinical and cost-effectiveness and natural history. *Health Technol Assess.* 2009;13(18):iii–iv, ix–xi, 1-154.
14. Smith S, Hoare DJ. Ringing in my ears: tinnitus in pregnancy. *Pract Midwife.* 2012;15(8):20-23.
15. Alexander TH, Harris JP. Current epidemiology of Meniere's syndrome. *Otolaryngol Clin North Am.* 2010;43(5):965-970.
16. Harris JP, Alexander TH. Current-day prevalence of Ménière's syndrome. *Audiol Neurootol.* 2010;15(5):318-322.
17. National Institute for Health and Care Excellence, NICE. Clinical Knowledge Summaries—Ménière's disease. 2012. Available at: http://cks.nice.org.uk/menieres-disease#!topicsummary. Accessed October 3, 2013.
18. *BMJ Best Practice.* Best Practice—Ménière's disease. BMJ Publishing Group Ltd.; 2013. Available at: http://bestpractice.bmj.com/best-practice/monograph/155.html. Accessed October 3, 2013.
19. Uchide K, Suzuki N, Takiguchi T, Terada S, Inoue M. The possible effect of pregnancy on Ménière's disease. *ORL J Otorhinolaryngol Relat Spec.* 1997;59(5):292-295.
20. Centers for Disease Control and Prevention. Estimated burden of acute otitis externa—United States, 2003–2007. *MMWR.* 2011;60(19):605-609.
21. Sander R. Otitis externa: a practical guide to treatment and prevention. *Am Fam Physician.* 2001;63(5):927-937.
22. Kaushik V, Malik T, Saeed SR. Interventions for acute otitis externa (review). *Cochrane Database Syst Rev.* 2010;1:CD004740.
23. Ahmed S, Shapiro NL, Bhattacharyya N. Incremental health care utilization and costs for acute otitis media in children. *Laryngoscope.* 2014;124(1):301-305.
24. Rosenfeld RM, Schwartz SR, Pynnonen MA, Tunkel DE, Hussey HM, Fichera JS, et al. Clinical practice guideline: tympanostomy tubes in children. *Otolaryngol Head Neck Surg.* 2013;149(1 Suppl):S1-S35.
25. National Institute for Health and Clinical Excellence. Surgical management of Otitis Media with Effusion in children. Clinical guidance 60. London, UK: NICE; 2008. Available at: http://www.nice.org.uk/nicemedia/pdf/cg60niceguideline.pdf. Accessed March 31, 2016.
26. Daniel M, Imtiaz-Umer S, Fergie N, Birchall J, Bayston R. Bacterial involvement in otitis media with effusion. *Int J Pediatr Otorhinolaryngol.* 2012;76(10):1416-1422.
27. Browning GG. *Clinical Otology and Audiology.* Oxford, UK: Butterworth-Heinemann Ltd; 1986.
28. Daniel M, Kamani T, El-Shunnar S, Jaberoo MC, Harrison A, Yalamanchili S, et al. National Institute for Clinical Excellence guidelines on the surgical management of otitis media with effusion: are they

being followed and have they changed practice? *Int J Pediatr Otorhinolaryngol.* 2013;77:54-58.

29. Cruickshanks KJ, Wiley TL, Tweed TS, Klein BE, Klein R, Mares-Perlman JA, et al. Prevalence of hearing loss in older adults in Beaver Dam, Wisconsin. The Epidemiology of Hearing Loss Study. *Am J Epidemiol.* 1998;148(9):879-886.

30. Stachler RJ, Chandrasekhar SS, Archer SM, Rosenfeld RM, Schwartz SR, Barrs DM, et al. Clinical practice Guideline: sudden hearing loss. *Otolaryngol Head Neck Surg.* 2012;146:S1-S35.

31. National Center for Hearing Assessment and Management. Universal newborn hearing screening: issues and evidence. Available at: http://www.infanthearing.org/summary. Accessed March 31, 2016.

32. Hardy JB. Clinical and developmental aspects of congenital rubella. *Arch Otolaryngol.* 1973;98:230-236.

33. Ross DS, Fowler KB. Cytomegalovirus: a major cause of hearing loss in children. *ASHA Leader.* 2008;13:14-17.

34. Olusanya BO1, Somefun AO. Sensorineural hearing loss in infants with neonatal jaundice in Lagos: a community-based study. *Ann Trop Paediatr.* 2009;29(2):119-128.

35. Katz J, Burkard RF, Medwetsky L. *Handbook of Clinical Audiology.* Wolters Kluwer Health/Lippincott Williams & Wilkins; 2009:547.

36. Schmiedt RA. The physiology of cochlear presbycusis. In: Gordon-Salant S, Frisina RD, Poeppel AN, Fry RR, eds. *The Aging Auditory System. Springer Handbook of Auditory Research.* New York, NY: Springer Science and Business Media; 2010:9-37.

37. Kujawa SG, Liberman MC. Adding insult to injury: cochlear nerve degeneration after "temporary" noise-induced hearing loss. *J Neurosci.* 2009;29:14077-14085.

38. National Institutes of Health. Hearing aids. Available at: https://report.nih.gov/nihfactsheets/viewfactsheet.aspx?csid=95. Accessed March 31, 2016.

39. Wei BP, Stathopoulos D, O'Leary S. Steroids for idiopathic sudden sensorineural hearing loss. *Cochrane Database Syst Rev.* 2013;7:CD003998.

40. Hornibrook J. Benign paroxysmal positional vertigo (BPPV): history, pathophysiology, office treatment and future directions. *Int J Otolaryngol.* 2011;2011:835671.

41. Nguyen-Huynh A. Evidence-based practice: management of vertigo. *Otolaryngol Clin North Am.* 2012;45:925-940.

42. Snyder S, Kivlehan S, Collopy K. The patient with vertigo: evaluation of the dizzy patient can pose challenges in the prehospital setting. *EMSWorld.* 2011;40(10):45-50.

43. Gelfand SA. *Essentials of Audiology.* New York, NY: Thieme Medical Publishers; 1997.

44. Tos M, Charabi S, Thomsen J. Clinical experience with vestibular schwannomas: epidemiology, symptomatology, diagnosis, and surgical results. *Eur Arch Otorhinolaryngol.* 1998;255(1):1-6.

CHAPTER 11

ORAL HEALTH

Barbara K. Hackley

Disparities in oral health are among the worst health inequities in the nation. More than 75% of adults have lost at least 1 tooth, and 25% have lost all of their natural teeth, to dental disease.[1] The use of dental services such as dental sealants and treatment of caries is highest among Non-Hispanic White individuals and those above the poverty line; consequently, this population has lower rates of periodontal disease, and people in this group are more likely to retain their teeth than minority populations.[2] Periodontal disease is highest among lower-income individuals, African Americans, and those with less than a high school education or who smoke cigarettes.[3] Untreated dental decay is twice as high among African Americans and Hispanics than among White individuals.[3]

The impact of untreated dental disease on the quality of life is considerable. Untreated disease leads to swollen gums, bleeding, abscesses, and loss of teeth; all of these problems are associated with significant pain, which in turn is associated with high rates of school and work absenteeism.[4] Inflammation associated with untreated dental disease appears to exacerbate chronic diseases.[5]

After controlling for age, sex, race/ethnicity, obesity, education, and dental care utilization in a cross-sectional study (N = 275,424), individuals missing all of their teeth compared to those missing none were significantly more likely to have cardiovascular disease (adjusted odds ratio [AOR] 1.85, 95% confidence interval [CI], 1.71, 2.01).[5] Better oral hygiene and treatment of oral disease are associated with better diabetic control and lower rates of cardiovascular disease.[4] Prevention of poor oral health can help ensure that individuals can consume a healthier diet. Loss of teeth reduces chewing efficacy and increases the likelihood that affected adults will choose to consume softer, more processed foods, which are typically higher in calories and fats and lower in vitamins and fiber. The cosmetic impact can be just as devastating as the physical consequences of poor dental health. In fact, embarrassment and self-consciousness were among the strongest motivators for seeking dental care in one cross-sectional study of adults (N = 364).[6]

While primary care providers play a limited role in the treatment of oral disease, they can contribute to the national goal of reducing poor oral health by promoting good hygienic practices among their patients, as well as by recognizing dental health problems and facilitating early entry to appropriate care for those individuals affected by dental disease. Utilization of dental health services by adults has fallen over recent years; this trend appears to be related to declining rates of private insurance coverage and increasing rates of public insurance or lack of insurance coverage.[7] Insurance coverage varies widely from state to state.[8] Services are generally more limited in rural than urban areas.[9] Therefore, primary care clinicians need to work to develop linkages to local community resources to improve healthcare access.

Preventive Health Care

Public health policies that promote fluoridation of water, comprehensive dental health insurance, and access to competent dental practitioners provide the foundation for good oral health on a national level. On an individual level, preventive health care for adults focuses on two primary strategies: 1) following good personal dental health practices and 2) receiving regular screening and early treatment of dental disease by dental health professionals.

Personal Dental Health Practices

Individuals who consume a healthy diet and engage in good oral hygiene practices can prevent or minimize dental disease. Epidemiologic studies link greater consumption of fruits and vegetables and lower consumption of meat with lower rates of oral cancer.[10] Higher intakes of vitamins and minerals, specifically vitamin A, vitamin B complex, vitamin C, and calcium, are associated with lower rates of gingivitis or periodontal disease and higher numbers of retained teeth.[11] Consuming more dietary fiber is also thought to contribute to better oral health. Chewing more fibrous foods scrubs the surface of the teeth and stimulates the

release of saliva by the parotid salivary gland, which can decrease the volume of bacteria in the mouth.[11] Both mechanisms can reduce the development of plaque. Higher intakes of sugars and higher consumption of low-fiber carbohydrates have been associated with increased plaque in cross-sectional studies.[11] Good oral hygiene practices can counter the plaque-producing impact of consuming an unhealthy diet.[11]

Dental plaque is a yellowish biofilm composed of bacteria that adhere to the teeth. Biofilms are composed of numerous bacteria. Some biofilms are more healthy, others less so. Changes in the pH of the oral cavity and an increase in the presence of unhealthy nutrients such as sugar can promote the development of less healthy biofilms.[12] The microcommunity becomes unbalanced, resulting in a relative increase in the prevalence of bacteria such as *Porphyromonas gingivalis*, *Treponema denticola*, and *Tannerella forsythia*, *which are* associated with dental disease.[12] Pathologic biofilms are associated with aggressive destruction of tooth enamel, greater numbers of cavities, and more aggressive forms of periodontal disease. Failure to remove plaque promptly leads to a hardening of the biofilm and the development of tartar.

Strategies that can effectively remove plaque include regular tooth brushing and the adjunctive use of toothpaste, mouthwashes, and techniques to cleanse the interdental surfaces. By far the most effective is tooth brushing, although its effectiveness is determined by the length of time an individual brushes and whether the person brushes over all surfaces.[13] It is unclear which specific design of a manual toothbrush, as well as the manner in which a particular design is used, is most effective in removing plaque; however, double- or triple-headed brushes, compared to flat ones, appear to remove more plaque. Electric toothbrushes, compared to manual ones, appear to be more effective at removing plaque.[13]

No matter what method or type of toothbrush is used, plaque often remains in the interdental spaces. Therefore, use of dental floss or tape may be necessary to remove plaque lodged in areas not reached by brushing.[13] Overall, the evidence does not support the universal use of flossing, because the evidence has not consistently found significant reductions in plaque formation or gingivitis when flossing was added to a regimen including daily tooth brushing.[14] However, the evidence supporting the use of interdental brushes is stronger and more consistent, justifying the recommendation for use of these products as an alternative to flossing.[14] Toothpaste aids in the mechanical removal of plaque, and those that contain fluoride can reduce the incidence of caries.[14] Adjunctive use of mouthwashes also appears to be effective; individuals using those containing chlorhexidine twice daily experience less plaque, gingivitis, and caries.[13,14]

Other healthcare practices can undermine oral health. Higher consumption of alcohol is associated with greater prevalence of gingivitis, periodontal disease, and oral cancer.[11,15] Likewise, the use of tobacco products increases these same risks.[15] Engaging in both of these practices increases the risk of cancer exponentially.[15] One meta-analysis of 45 studies reported that the relative risk (RR) for oral cancer increased from 1.21 (95% CI, 1.10-1.33) for < 1 drink per day to 5.24 (95% CI, 4.36-6.30) for heavy alcohol drinking (≥ 4 drinks per day).[16] Cigarette smoking is associated with a similar magnitude of increased RR of developing oral cancers, reported to range from an RR of 1.4 to 5 in 12 studies included in a systematic review of the literature.[17] It is also associated with increased risk of dental caries, implant failure, and tooth loss.[17]

Poor oral hygiene, cigarette smoking, and alcohol consumption are associated with changes in the flora of the oral cavity.[15] Changes in microbial profiles, an increase in the prevalence of more pathologic bacteria, and resultant chronic inflammation are theorized to be underlying triggers promoting the development of oral cancer.[10,15]

Further, those who smoke are also exposed to inhaled carcinogens. Cessation of cigarette smoking and the use of smokeless tobacco are associated with declining risks of oral cancer.[17] Therefore, screening for alcohol and tobacco use and helping those who use these substances quit are critical elements of providing good dental health care. These services are in the purview of primary care providers and as such should be incorporated into care provided in the outpatient setting.

Screening and Early Treatment of Dental Health Conditions

Regular care with a dental professional can minimize the impact of dental disease on an individual. Daily dental hygiene is insufficient at removing all plaque. However, regular professional dental cleaning by a dentist or hygienist can remove much of the residual plaque and provide an opportunity for dental professionals to make recommendations specific to the needs of individual clients. Further, regular dental care is associated with loss of fewer teeth[18] and earlier detection of oral cancers.[19] Currently, the American Dental Association (ADA) recommends that adults be seen at minimum once a year and more frequently for those at risk for or currently affected by dental disease.

Routine dental care consists of periodic examinations to detect the presence and extent of tooth decay, gingivitis, and other oral diseases; cleaning and polishing; use of adjunctive dental x-rays; and treatment of identified concerns. Dental x-rays are most commonly used in adults to detect and monitor progression of caries and periodontal disease. Dental x-rays are associated with an increased risk of developing meningiomas, salivary gland tumors, and thyroid cancer. For example, although the exact risk varies by procedure, dose, and equipment used, one excess cancer death is estimated to occur for every 47,620 full-mouth examinations made with D-speed film and round collimation.[20] Using low-dose techniques and having patients wear radiopaque aprons with collars during dental x-ray procedures can protect radiosensitive tissue such as the thyroid, salivary glands, bone marrow, and brain.

Recognizing Dental Disease

Women's health professionals can be instrumental in recognizing when individuals need dental health care, and then motivating them to seek it out. Fear of dentists' offices appears to be learned—either directly from a person's own traumatic dental experience, usually in childhood, or indirectly from a family member. More than 50% of adults with dental anxiety or fear have a close family member who is also afraid of receiving dental care.[21] Unfortunately, fear triggers a vicious cycle—with fear leading to delayed care, delayed care resulting in progression of disease, and progression of disease leading to the use of more invasive and painful procedures.[21] Part of helping a woman receive services is ascertaining her level of comfort in receiving care and discussing strategies used by dental professionals in helping individuals cope with fear and anxiety.

Clinical Presentation

The presentation of dental disease is not always straightforward. While toothache is a common complaint in those with dental problems, other symptoms are also common. Headache, malaise, and occasionally fever may be reported first, with an underlying dental problem only being determined after closer inquiry. Particularly if women have longstanding neglected dental health care needs, they may not recognize that their symptoms are originating from a dental problem. A thorough history and examination are necessary to uncover the etiology of the complaint. The underlying physiology of headache due to

dental conditions includes referred pain to the jaw and head from infections in the mouth or from muscle spasms. Muscle spasms in the head and neck can result from the pressure of grinding teeth or from the changes in normal mastication and swallowing, which occur when an individual has misaligned or missing teeth. Women who report that their headache is present upon waking or that their head and neck are sensitive to touch or that they have noticed clicking in their jaws should be suspected of having an underlying dental condition or an unstable temporomandibular joint (TMJ). Malaise and fever are common symptoms of infection and may indicate the presence of an abscess. Other common symptoms indicating the possible presence of underlying dental disease include sensitivity, with discomfort arising with ingestion of hot or cold substances, bleeding gums, or the presence of a painful, discolored, or raised lesion in the mouth. While bleeding gums most likely indicate underlying gingivitis, they may also be symptomatic of systemic diseases. Lesions of the mouth may be indicative of localized infections, plugged salivary ducts, oral cancers, or systemic diseases. Therefore, the astute provider should always consider a wide range of possible etiologies before determining that a woman's symptoms are of dental origin.

Essential History, Physical, and Laboratory Evaluation

A careful and focused history and physical is essential to providing good primary dental health care. It can help determine if specialty services are necessary and if so, which specialty could best meet the needs of a particular individual. Because many systemic medical conditions also have oral symptoms, a thorough evaluation may uncover other previously unsuspected conditions that require treatment. See **Table 11-1** for diagnostic clues that can be elicited on the history

Table 11-1 Dental Conditions

Symptom	Disease Entity	History	Physical
Toothache	Caries	Poor oral hygiene Asymptomatic until lesion large	Initial lesion appears as a white spot on the surface of the tooth and progresses to deeper cavitation.
	Gingivitis	Usually painless Bleeding with brushing or eating Halitosis	Swollen gums bleed on contact.
	Periodontal disease	Increased risk with diabetes	Bleeding, swollen gums Gingivitis with progressive loss of supportive connective tissue
	Abscess	Painful gums	Pockets of pus Red, swollen gums
	Impacted teeth	Painful, tender gums	
Sensitive teeth	No obvious disease	Painful with ingestion of hot and cold substances	No obvious damage
Painless lesion	Oral cancer	Use of tobacco products and/or alcohol Lump on lips or in oral cavity	Lesions on ventral and lateral aspects of tongue, floor of the mouth, soft palate Ulcerated white, red, or red/white lesions with nodular, irregular appearance

and physical exam that may suggest specific dental conditions. **Table 11-2** describes other local and systemic conditions whose symptomatology can be similar to those seen in many dental conditions. These diseases should be considered as part of the differential diagnosis when investigating common symptoms suggestive of oral health problems.

History

The history should ascertain whether the woman has had any previously identified dental health problems, her utilization of dental care services in the past, and her personal dental hygiene practices. The provider should inquire about initial symptoms, progression of symptomatology, and accompanying symptoms. The extent of her use of alcohol and tobacco products should also be determined as these are risk factors for cancer and dental disease. Asking about the use of new medication is also beneficial, because some medications, such as beta-blockers and hypoglycemics, are known to be associated with the development of oral lesions.[22]

Oral symptoms are not always related to local disease. Questions that might uncover systemic diseases should focus particularly on symptoms suggestive of liver or kidney disease, bone marrow conditions, autoimmune diseases, or of infections such as sinusitis.[23] Infections of the oral cavity that occur without a recognized predisposing factor may

Table 11-2 Diagnostic Clues Distinguishing Systematic Versus Oral Dental Conditions

Symptom	Disease Entity	History	Physical
Painful lesions	Aphthous stomatitis	Highly prevalent Recurrent lesions Heal within 14 days Triggered by stress, infections, and food hypersensitivities Usually benign but is also a nonspecific finding seen with chronic blood loss, inflammatory bowel disease, autoimmune disorders, and other conditions	Superficial ulcerations commonly found on buccal and labial mucosa and occasionally seen on the roof of the mouth
	Herpes	Personal history of herpes in self or in partners Recurrent, usually with prodrome triggered by stress, fever, or exposure to sun	Initial vesicles rupture and can become painful ulcers.
Painless lesion	Lupus	Fatigue Alopecia Arthralgia Skin rashes	Nonspecific lesions, can be ulcerated or lichenified on soft or hard palate or buccal mucosa Discoid lesion on lips
	Crohn's disease	Oral lesions may be initial sign of disease and present before onset of GI symptoms. Fatigue and fever. Prolonged diarrhea and weight loss.	Nonspecific lesions, can be deep granulomatous Cobblestone mucosa Oral and perioral swelling
Pain in neck and jaw	TMJ	Grinding teeth Clicking in the jaw felt with movement Jaws "lock" Jaw muscle stiffness Referred pain to head and ear	Clicking elicited over the TMJ on palpation Reproduced pain on exam
White patch	Fungal infection	More common if recent antibiotic or steroid use Commonly seen in those with underlying pathology	Nonadherent, patch can be wiped off
	Lichen planus	Uncommon presentation Usual presentation of itchy purple papules and plaques, most commonly found on extremities and trunk; can affect nails Erosive lesions can make eating painful	White keratotic striations on buccal mucosa Can be atrophic, erosive, and plaque like May involve the tongue or gingivae

Table 11-2 Diagnostic Clues Distinguishing Systematic Versus
Oral Dental Conditions (*continued*)

Symptom	Disease Entity	History	Physical
Pigmentation changes	Addison's disease	Fatigue, malaise, arthralgia Anorexia, weight loss, GI symptoms	Diffuse brown macular hyperpigmentation most commonly of buccal mucosa
	Kaposi's sarcoma	Brownish, purplish macules of skin. Nodular lesions may ulcerate and bleed. Lesions most commonly occur on feet and extremities.	Hyperpigmentation of hard palate or gingival margin
	Melanoma	Mucosal melanomas rare compared to cutaneous versions	Area of irregular hyperpigmentation, bleeding mass, or ulceration of mucosa, often of hard palate
	Lead poisoning	Asymptomatic until levels very high History suggestive of lead exposure	Bluish black discoloration of the gums along the edge of the teeth and gums
Enamel erosion	Bulimia	Inappropriate dietary behaviors	Erosions seen on palatal surfaces of the teeth if woman purges by self-induced vomiting
	GERD	Heartburn, regurgitation, dysphagia	Upper teeth more affected Discolored teeth
Difficulty in mastication	Malocclusion	No treatment for malocclusion	Poorly fitting bite
	Neurologic disease	Stroke	Inability to chew and swallow effectively
Dry mouth	Sjögren syndrome	Difficulty swallowing Dysphagia	Thick, ropey saliva Parotid enlargement Bald tongue, cracked and fissured tongue
Bleeding gums	Platelet disorders	Associated with a multitude of problems: liver disease, cancer, immune thrombocytopenia, HIV, certain drugs, malnutrition	Prolonged bleeding after minor cuts
	Coagulopathies	Inherited blooding disorders Von Willebrand disease Use of anticoagulant medication	Heavier bleeding or resumed bleeding after tooth extraction
Tongue	Benign migratory glossitis	Asymptomatic inflammatory condition	Loss of filiform papillae resulting in erythematous patches with whitish border on dorsal aspect of the tongue Location and size of patches can change over time.
	Fissured tongue	Usually normal variant Occasionally seen in certain syndromes	Grooves on the dorsum of tongue

GI = gastrointestinal, TMJ = temporomandibular joint

be a sign of underlying pathology. For example, fungal infections that occur in the absence of dentures, recent use of antibiotics, or xerostomia might indicate the presence of immunosuppression.[23] Rarely, patients will report changes in sensation of the mouth such as burning; these symptoms may result from nerve damage, Lyme disease, pernicious anemia, or polyneuropathy from diabetes.[23,24] See Table 11-2 for further details.

PHYSICAL

A complete examination of the head, neck, mouth, and respiratory tract should be performed. A careful examination of the mouth, mucosa, palate, and the repair of the teeth is mandatory. Looking for signs of infection such as localized swelling and erythema is also important. Palpation of the sinuses may uncover sinus infections. An examination of the ear can help rule in or out the presence of otitis media, externa, or serous, which may be contributing to a woman's symptoms. Additional evaluation of the abdomen, skin, and cardiac systems may be necessary depending on the finding elicited on the initial history and physical examination.

Localized changes in pigmentation of the oral cavity suggest localized disease.[23] For example, erythema of the gums suggests localized infection such as gingivitis or periodontal disease. Conversely, more generalized color changes may suggest systemic disease. For example, jaundice associated with liver problems may present with a pervasive generalized yellow hue of the oral mucosa. Similarly, anemia may present with generalized pale mucosa. Rarely, changes in pigmentation or ulcerations can be indicative of celiac disease, Crohn's disease, psoriasis, renal failure, and lupus.[23] In some cases, such as with Crohn's disease, oral lesions may present years before the onset of symptoms commonly thought to be primary symptoms of the disease in question; in the case of Crohn's disease, these are gastrointestinal symptoms.[24]

LABORATORY

The use of laboratory testing in the primary care setting is minimal with the exception of swabbing lesions to obtain a herpes culture if the etiology of the lesion is unclear by visual inspection alone. The need for other testing, including imaging studies, will be determined by the specialist, if additional care is warranted.

Management of Common Conditions

This section gives an overview of the management of common dental conditions seen in adults. Fear of pain is one of the most common reasons why adults delay treatment. Effective approaches are rooted in the development of trust between patient and provider; therefore, referral to a known empathic dental professional is critical. Providing realistic information and promoting the use of distraction and relaxation, as well as a referral to a psychologist if needed for desensitization, cognitive restructuring, or hypnosis, may be helpful. Examples of techniques employed during the procedure itself include discussion with the dentist before the procedure about agreed-upon rest breaks and emergency signals indicating that she has reached the limit of her ability to cope and needs to stop the procedure.[25] Giving anxious individuals some control over the progression of a procedure can improve their ability to cope. Pharmaceutic options also include the use of intravenous sedation, conscious sedation, or general anesthesia for those for whom behavioral techniques provide insufficient relief from dental anxiety and fear.[25]

Caries

Caries develop along a continuum from preclinical disease, where damage is occurring but not yet detectable, to obvious cavitation and exposure of the pulp. Tooth enamel is not uniform. Caries start in the most acid-soluble sites on the tooth, creating defects and increasing the porosity of the tooth, which then allows biofilm acids to diffuse below the surface and demineralize the more soluble subsurface of the tooth.[26] Caries are first visible as a white spot on the surface of the tooth after the surface is dried for a few seconds. As caries progress, more and more enamel is affected. Then the surface of the dentin begins to be involved, forming deeper and more extensive microcavitations.[26] Eventually, the cavitation becomes so large that the enamel surface collapses and exposes the dentin. If untreated, damage can extend to the pulp, increasing the risk of infection and the need for more extensive repair. See **Figure 11-1**.

Dental x-rays cannot detect caries at the earliest stages of development and are most useful in detecting extensive lesions or those with greater cavitation. Newer techniques are being developed using optical technologies that can detect the changes in opacity of the tooth caused by demineralization. These techniques, which include fluorescence-based systems, transillumination, and impedance spectroscopy, appear to detect caries at earlier stages and on more surfaces of the tooth than do dental x-rays.[26] However, these techniques are not yet in widespread clinical use.

Treatment options depend on the stage of the caries. Using fluoride-containing toothpaste and mouthwash on a daily basis can arrest the progression of early-stage caries. The defect can be remineralized and converted into an inactive lesion.[27] However, restoration is needed in the following situations: when a cavity is visually detected, pain or discomfort is elicited from exposure to cold water or food impaction, or a lesion penetrating more than one-third of the dentin is seen on x-ray.[27] Generally, the tooth is drilled to remove debris and infected pulp and then filled with a resin compound or amalgam. Porcelain and gold are alternative materials used for fillings. If the cavity is in a visible spot in the mouth, resin is generally used because it is white in color and less noticeable than amalgam. Amalgam is composed of silver, mercury, tin, and sometimes zinc; it is also called "silver fillings" due to its coloration. Although amalgam contains mercury, it is still commonly used because it is inexpensive,

Figure 11-1 Stages of tooth decay.

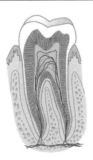 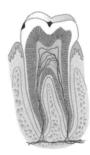 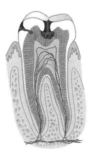 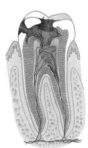

| Healthy tooth | Decay in enamel | Decay in dentin | Decay in pulp |

durable, and capable of forming a tight seal with large cavities.[28] Despite the controversy over the safety of this filling, the ADA states that the amount of mercury contained within amalgam is too little to be of clinical concern.[29] According to a recent Cochrane review, insufficient evidence is available to determine the comparative safety of resin versus amalgam.[30] Use of dental amalgam is likely to decline as the tenets of the 2013 global accord, the Minamata Convention on Mercury, on phasing out mercury-containing substances are implemented and the quality of resin products continues to improve.[31]

If treatment of caries is delayed and the structure of the tooth is severely undermined by extensive decay, then use of fillings may not be feasible. In this case, a crown or cap is placed over the affected tooth. The crown is designed to match the color, size, and shape of an individual's natural teeth.

Another treatment option is performance of a root canal if damage has extended into the pulp of the tooth. A root canal removes inflamed or infected dental pulp. Once the pulp is removed, the space is cleansed, filled with a biocompatible compound, and then sealed to protect the roots of the tooth. Once the root canal is complete, the tooth will need to be restored (with a filling, crown, or post and crown) to regain full function of the tooth.

Abscess

Tooth abscesses can result from untreated decay, trauma, deep fillings, failed root canal, or a cracked tooth. However the pulp is damaged, the result is the same. Colonization of the root canal with diverse bacteriologic agents occurs and leads to the development of a biofilm and infection. The resulting infection is polymicrobial, composed of a mix of strict anaerobes and facultative anaerobes.[32] Symptoms include fever, pain, swelling, and erythema usually localized to the affected tooth, although the infection can spread to surrounding tissue. Rarely, a tooth abscess can be fatal if the infection spreads to the adjacent structures within the neck. Sometimes the abscess may need to be drained. Antibiotic coverage before and after the procedure can hasten recovery. Amoxicillin is the antimicrobial of first choice.[32] If there is a high prevalence of resistance to amoxicillin in the local community, then the use of either metronidazole or amoxicillin in combination with clavulanic acid is an alternative.[32] Clindamycin can be used in individuals who are allergic to the penicillins.[32] If infection is widespread, the tooth may not be able to be saved. In this case, the only treatment option may be to remove the affected tooth and consider placement of an implant after the infection is resolved.

Gingivitis and Periodontal Disease

The same process that leads to caries also can lead to gingivitis and periodontal disease. Plaque can build up under the gum line and cause inflammation, swelling, and bleeding of the gums. Other conditions such as pregnancy or immune suppression, infections such as oral herpes, and medications such as some of the calcium channel blockers can contribute to the development of gingivitis. With gingivitis, the gum starts to pull away from the neck of the tooth, creating a gap that allows bacteria to enter, worsening the inflammation. Deposits can form in the gap between the tooth and gum. These deposits worsen the inflammatory process and can be difficult to remove. Eventually, the gums recede and expose the nerve root. Once this occurs, infection and inflammation can spread into the supporting structures of the tooth and increase the risk of tooth loss.

Signs that gingivitis has advanced to cause periodontal disease include teeth that have sensitive necks, bad breath, decay in the tooth at the gum line, gum recession, and/or loose teeth.[33] Treatment involves good personal oral hygiene, cessation of smoking, and professional cleaning to remove as much plaque as possible. Particular attention is paid to scaling along the gum line to remove as much plaque as possible near the gums. Sometimes subgingival debridement of inflamed gum tissue under local anesthesia is needed and is likely to be successful if the gum pockets are < 5 mm in depth.[33] Successful treatment will result in gum-probing depths that are stable or decline over time. Occasionally, more aggressive treatment is needed if periodontal disease is progressive, severe, or chronic. "Open" surgery is more likely to be performed if gum pocket depths are 6 mm or more. In open surgery, the nerve root is exposed either through gingivectomy or flap procedure to allow for the removal of calculus and biofilm.[33] Gingival grafts, which cover the exposed nerve root, are another option that can relieve root sensitivity and minimize cervical root caries.[34]

Individuals with periodontal disease are also at higher risk of abscesses. Abscess can occur if food or debris becomes lodged in the gaps in the gum or if insufficient scale is removed at the time of treatment. Abscesses result in bone destruction and increase the likelihood of tooth loss. Treatment includes drainage of pus, scaling of the affected tooth, debridement of soft tissue, and irrigation of the site with sterile saline.[35] Patients should be seen 24 to 48 hours after treatment to assess whether the infection is resolving. Antibiotics are often also used and may be given as a pretreatment to allow some resolution of the infection before performing surgical treatment.[35]

Tooth Loss

Unfortunately, it is not always possible to save a tooth if damage is widespread. Teeth may also need to be removed if the mouth is overcrowded. Tooth extractions are usually performed under local anesthesia, but general anesthesia may be used if several teeth need to be removed at the same time. Recovery is generally straightforward. Compression with gauze pads will minimize bleeding. A blood clot will form in the socket and will stop the bleeding. Patients should avoid doing activities that could dislodge the clot such as vigorous rinsing and spitting, use of a straw, and vigorous activity for the first 24 hours postoperatively. Postoperative pain can usually be managed with over-the-counter pain medications or a mild narcotic. Follow up with the oral surgeon is needed within a few days to confirm healing and to detect any complications.

In the event that a tooth is removed, function can be restored with placement of a denture, bridge, or implant. Each option has distinct advantages and disadvantages. The implant sits in the original tooth socket and, over time, becomes integrated into the bony structure of the mouth. This prevents future bone loss, which can occur with other options. The implant is then capped with a crown to match the color and shape of the surrounding teeth. Placement can be done at the time the original tooth was removed or delayed until healing is complete. Insufficient evidence exists to determine the most appropriate timing of placement of an implant, although concern has been expressed by some that early placement may be associated with a greater risk of implant failure.[36]

Bridges can be permanently installed, can span the gap caused by several missing teeth, and are cosmetically pleasing. However, a bridge must be attached to healthy teeth. Attaching the bridge to the supporting teeth requires that the teeth be filed to allow the bridge to be installed. This can compromise the integrity of the supporting teeth and make them more vulnerable to the development of plaque and caries. Further, if the dental implant damages the supporting teeth, the follow-up treatment involves treating more teeth—the original missing teeth and the newly problematic ones.

Dentures are one of the least expensive options, but they require a good fit to be comfortable, may require modifications in a person's diet to prevent them becoming loose while eating, and do not protect against bone loss. While implants are generally considered to be the best option from a dental health perspective, they are the most expensive option and require repeated visits over an extended time. Further, implants require that the gums and bony structure of the teeth be healthy. Failure rates are higher in those with underlying periodontitis, chronic conditions such as diabetes, and those with bruxism.

Temporomandibular Disorders

TMJ disorders are more common in women than men and in individuals between the ages of 20 and 40 years.[37] Problems with the TMJ or masticatory muscles can present as pain in the mouth, jaw, neck, or shoulders when speaking, chewing, or opening the mouth. Opening the mouth wide can be difficult, because it can elicit a clicking or popping feeling in the jaw. In more severe presentations, TMJ disorders limit the degree to which the mouth can be opened. The underlying etiology of these symptoms is musculoskeletal—due to malfunction of the TMJ or spasms in the muscles used in chewing. Common causes include injury, dislocation of the disc in the TMJ, arthritis, grinding or clenching the teeth, or stress, which causes a person to tighten the facial muscles or clench the teeth.[37] Having a crossbite or poor posture, particularly during sleep, is thought to increase the risk of developing a misalignment of the TMJ.

To be effective, treatment should target the underlying cause. Often, several modalities are used together to maximize relief from symptoms.[37] Physical therapy is used to regain and maintain full range of motion in the jaw. Stretching the facial muscles, which can be done by making various facial expressions, can provide relief. Another way to stretch affected muscles is to open the mouth as wide as comfortably possible, apply slight pressure on the joint, and then open the mouth completely. Use of heat or cold packs and eating soft food can prevent the problem from worsening. Splints are used for those individuals who grind or clench their teeth. Splints protect the teeth and compensate or correct bite defects, which lessen the pain associated with TMJ disorders.[37] Surgery is the treatment of last resort. Surgical options range from a relatively simple procedure such as rinsing out the joint with sterile fluids to complex surgeries such as joint replacement.[37]

Dental Trauma

Injuries can inflict extensive damage. Consequently, women presenting with oral-facial trauma are best referred for immediate evaluation and treatment in the emergency department. Even what appears to be simple, such as an avulsed tooth, may be associated with fractures of the head and jaw or injuries to the cervical spine.[38] During the course of an injury, individuals have been known to inhale fragments of tooth, making a chest x-ray mandatory if not all teeth are accounted for during the physical exam.[39] Therefore, the primary role in the outpatient setting is to stabilize the patient and facilitate rapid transport to a facility capable of managing oral-facial injuries.

Intact avulsed permanent teeth can be replaced in adults and are usually reintegrated into the bony structure of the mouth. Rapid replacement is necessary, because a delay of more than 2 hours is associated with loss of periodontal ligament cells, which attach the tooth to the bone.[39] Ideally, the tooth should be replaced within 5 minutes. Contact with the root of the tooth should be avoided. The tooth is washed in saline, replaced in the socket, and held firmly in place. Any clot should be left intact, not wiped away. If replacement of the tooth is not possible, the tooth is brought with the woman to the emergency department. Transport in saliva in the buccal sulcus of the mouth can help preserve the periodontal ligament cells until the tooth can be replaced, as they will begin to die out if allowed to dry. In the event of an avulsed tooth, an oral antibiotic (either metronidazole[39] or tetracycline[38]) and analgesia should be prescribed and the woman advised to use chlorhexidine mouthwash.[39] Vaccination for tetanus may also be needed depending on the woman's immunization history.

Care of the Pregnant and Breastfeeding Woman

Dental care is essentially unchanged by pregnancy. The American College of Obstetricians and Gynecologists and the ADA recommend that women continue to receive oral healthcare services in pregnancy and after birth.[40] Yet fewer than 50% of women do so.[41] Women younger than 24 years of age and those receiving Medicaid insurance have the greatest need but are the least likely to receive care.[41] Barriers to care include lack of insurance coverage, not being encouraged by obstetric providers to seek care, and uncertainty about the safety of dental services in pregnancy.[41]

No evidence exists that dental care is unsafe in pregnancy.[42] A meta-analysis of 11 randomized clinical control studies evaluated the relationships between receipt of dental care and preterm birth, low birth weight, and spontaneous abortion. Overall, no differences were noted in the incidence of preterm birth $\leq$ 37 weeks' gestation (OR 0.93, 0.79 to 1.10; P = 0.39), low birth weight < 2500 g (OR 0.85, 0.70 to 1.04; P = 0.11), or spontaneous abortion (OR 0.84, 0.58 to 1.22; P = 0.37) in those who received scaling treatments or root planning and those

who did not.[42] It should be noted that differences were noted between lower and higher quality studies, with lower quality studies showing that dental care was associated with lower rates of preterm birth.[42] The receipt of dental services has been thought previously to improve outcomes.[43] However, three meta-analyses do not support this conclusion, but do offer reassurance that dental care has no deleterious impact on pregnancy outcomes.[42,44,45]

Recommended dental practices include using older antibiotics (penicillin, amoxicillin, and clindamycin), antifungals (nystatin), anesthetics (lidocaine 2% with 1:100,000 epinephrine), and analgesics (acetaminophen with codeine), because the safety record for these products is more robust.[46] Use of dental x-rays is also acceptable as long as an abdominal shield is used.[46] No contraindications exist for routine care such as cleaning or treating caries or even for more invasive procedures such as tooth extraction or root canals.[46] In fact, the emphasis should be on prompt treatment of identified disease to prevent progression.

Unfortunately, dental health can be undermined by physiologic changes accompanying pregnancy. Higher colonization with *Prevotella intermedia,* which is associated with more rapid progression of periodontal disease, is fueled by rising levels of progesterone and estrogen in pregnancy.[46] Changes in the hormonal milieu and immune system in pregnancy can encourage the development of gingivitis, exacerbate preexisting disease, and encourage disease progression.[46] Some women, particularly those with underlying gingivitis, develop epulis gravidarum, which is a benign tumor of the gingival tissue. This condition affects 0.2-9.6% of pregnant women, most commonly in the second or third trimester.[46] Generally, it regresses after the birth but may require surgical removal if it becomes too large or too uncomfortable.[46] Therefore, women should perform regular oral hygiene and receive ongoing dental care in pregnancy.

References

1. Healthy People. Oral Health, Healthy People 2020 Objectives. 2013. Available at: http://www.healthy people.gov/2020/topicsobjectives2020/objective slist.aspx?topicId=32. Accessed April 1, 2016.
2. Dye BA, Li X, Thornton-Evans G. Oral health disparities as determined by selected Healthy People 2020 Oral Health Objectives for the United States, 2009-2010. 2012. Available at: http://www.cdc.gov /nchs/data/databriefs/db104.htm. Accessed April 1, 2016.
3. Centers for Disease Control and Prevention. Oral Health Strategic Plan for 2011-2014. 2013. Available at: http://www.cdc.gov/OralHealth/strategic_ planning/plan4.htm. Accessed April 1, 2016.
4. Griffin SO, Jones JA, Brunson D, Griffin PM, Bailey WD. Burden of oral disease among older adults and implications for public health priorities. *Am J Public Health.* 2012;102(3):411-418.
5. Wiener RC, Sambamoorthi U. Cross-sectional association between the number of missing teeth and cardiovascular disease among adults aged 50 or older: BRFSS 2010. *Int J Vasc Med.* 2014;2014:6.
6. Hassan AH, Amin HES. Association of orthodontic treatment needs and oral health-related quality of life in young adults. *Am J Orthod Dentofacial Orthop.* 2010;137(1):42-47.
7. Wall TP, Vujicic M, Nasseh K. Recent trends in the utilization of dental care in the United States. *J Dental Educ.* 2012;76(8):1020-1027.
8. Choi MK. The impact of Medicaid insurance coverage on dental service use. *J Health Econ.* 2011; 30(5):1020-1031.
9. Ahn S, Burdine JN, Smith ML, Ory MG, Phillips CD. Residential rurality and oral health disparities: Influences of contextual and individual factors. *J Prim Prev.* 2011;32(1):29-41.
10. Meurman JH. Infectious and dietary risk factors of oral cancer. *Oral Oncol.* 2010;46(6):411-413.
11. Quiles J, Varela-López A. The role of nutrition in periodontal diseases. In: D. Ekuni, et al. eds. *Studies on Periodontal Disease.* New York, NY: Springer; 2014: 251-278.
12. Marsh PD, Moter A, Devine DA. Dental plaque biofilms: communities, conflict and control. *Periodontol 2000.* 2011;55(1):16-35.
13. Löe H. Oral hygiene in the prevention of caries and periodontal disease. *Int Dent J.* 2000;50(3): 129-139.
14. Van Der Weijden F, Slot DE. Oral hygiene in the prevention of periodontal diseases: the evidence. *Periodontol 2000.* 2011;55(1):104-123.
15. Hooper SJ, Wilson MJ. Crean SJ. Exploring the link between microorganisms and oral cancer: a systematic review of the literature. *Head Neck.* 2009;31(9): 1228-1239.
16. Tramacere I, Negri E, Bagnardi V, Garavello W, Rota M, Scotti L, et al. A meta-analysis of alcohol drinking and oral and pharyngeal cancers. Part 1: overall results and dose-risk relation. *Oral Oncol.* 2010;46(7):497-503.
17. Warnakulasuriya S, Dietrich T, Bornstein MM, Casals Peidró E, Preshaw PM, Walter C, et al. Oral health risks of tobacco use and effects of cessation. *Int Dent J.* 2010;60(1):7-30.
18. Renvert S, Persson RE, Persson GR. A history of frequent dental care reduces the risk of tooth loss but not periodontitis in older subjects. *Swed Dent J.* 2011; 35(2):69-75.
19. Langevin S, Michaud DS, Eliot M, Peters ES, McClean MD, Kelsey KT. Regular dental visits are associated with earlier stage at diagnosis for oral and pharyngeal cancer. *Cancer Causes Control.* 2012; 23(11):1821-1829.
20. White SC, Mallya SM. Update on the biological effects of ionizing radiation, relative dose factors and radiation hygiene. *Aust Dent J.* 2012;57:2-8.
21. Beaton L, Freeman R, Humphris G. Why are people afraid of the dentist? Observations and explanations. *Med Princ Pract.* 2014;23(4):295-301.
22. Escudier M, Nunes C, Sanderson JD. Disorders of the mouth. *Medicine.* 2011;39(3):127-131.
23. Lockhart PB, Hong CHL, Diermen DE. The influence of systemic diseases on the diagnosis of oral diseases: a problem-based approach. *Dent Clin North Am.* 2011;55:15-28.
24. Islam NM, Bhattacharyya I, Cohen DM. Common oral manifestations of systemic disease. *Otolaryngol Clin North Am.* 2011;44(1):161-182.
25. Armfield JM, Heaton LJ. Management of fear and anxiety in the dental clinic: a review. *Aust Dent J.* 2013;58(4):390-407.
26. Zero DT, Zandona AF, Vail MM, Spolnik KJ. Dental caries and pulpal disease. *Dent Clin North Am.* 2011; 55:29-46.
27. Momoi Y, Hayashi M, Fujitani M, Fukushima M, Imazato S, Kubo S, et al. Clinical guidelines for treating caries in adults following a minimal intervention policy—Evidence and consensus based report. *J Dent.* 2012;40(2):95-105.
28. Rathore M, Singh A, Pant VA. The dental amalgam toxicity fear: a myth or actuality. *Toxicol Int.* 2012; 19(2):81-88.

29. American Dental Association. Statement on Dental Amalgam. 2009. Available at: http://www.ada.org/en/about-the-ada/ada-positions-policies-and-statements/statement-on-dental-amalgam. Accessed April 1, 2016.

30. Alcaraz R, Graciela M. Direct composite resin fillings versus amalgam fillings for permanent or adult posterior teeth. *Cochrane Database Syst Rev.* 2014; 3:CD005620.

31. Mackey TK. The Minamata Convention on Mercury: attempting to address the global controversy of dental amalgam use and mercury waste disposal. *Sci Total Environ.* 2013;472:125-129.

32. Shweta S, Prakash SK. Dental abscess: a microbiological review. *Dent Res J.* 2013;10(5):585-591.

33. Gjermo PE, Grytten J. Cost-effectiveness of various treatment modalities for adult chronic periodontitis. *Periodontol 2000.* 2009;51:269-275.

34. Kassab MM, Badawi H, Dentino AR. Treatment of gingival recession. *Dent Clin North Am.* 2010;54(1): 129-140.

35. Herrera D, Roldán S, Sanz M. The periodontal abscess: a review. *J Clin Periodontol.* 2000;27:377-386.

36. Esposito M, Grusovin MG, Polyzos IP, Felice P, Worthington HV. Timing of implant placement after tooth extraction: immediate, immediate-delayed or delayed implants? A Cochrane systematic review. *Eur J Oral Implantol.* 2010;3(3):189-205.

37. Ingawalé S, Goswami T. Temporomandibular joint: disorders, treatments, and biomechanics. *Ann Biomed Eng.* 2009;37(5):976-996.

38. MacLeod S, Rudd TC. Update on the management of dentoalveolar trauma. *Curr Opin Otolaryngol Head Neck Surg.* 2012;20(4):318-324.

39. Ceallaigh PÓ, Ekanaykaee K, Beirne CJ, Patton DW. Diagnosis and management of common maxillofacial injuries in the emergency department. Part 5: dentoalveolar injuries. *Emerg Med J.* 2007; 24(6):429-430.

40. Oral Health Care During Pregnancy Expert Workgroup. Oral health care during pregnancy: a national consensus statement of an expert workgroup meeting. 2012. Available at: http://www.mchoralhealth.org/PDFs/OralHealthPregnancyConsensus.pdf. Accessed April 1, 2016.

41. Iida H, Kumar JV, Radigan AM. Oral health during perinatal period in New York State. Evaluation of 2005 Pregnancy Risk Assessment Monitoring System data. *N Y State Dent J.* 2009;75(6):43-47.

42. Polyzos NP, Polyzos IP, Zavos A, Valachis A, Mauri D, Papanikolaou EG, et al. Obstetric outcomes after treatment of periodontal disease during pregnancy: systematic review and meta-analysis. *BMJ.* 2010; 341:C7017.

43. Polyzos NP, Polyzos IP, Mauri D, Tzioras S, Tsappi M, Cortinovis I, et al. Effect of periodontal disease treatment during pregnancy on preterm birth incidence: a metaanalysis of randomized trials. *Am J Obstet Gynecol.* 2009;200(3):225-232.

44. Fogacci MF, Vettore MV, Thomé Leão AT. The effect of periodontal therapy on preterm low birth weight: a meta-analysis. *Obstet Gynecol.* 2011;117(1):153-165. doi:10.1097/AOG.0b013e3181fdebc0.

45. Uppal A, Uppal S, Pinto A, Dutta M, Shrivatsa S, Dandolu V, et al. The effectiveness of periodontal disease treatment during pregnancy in reducing the risk of experiencing preterm birth and low birth weight: a meta-analysis. *J Am Dent Assoc.* 2010; 141(12):1423-1434.

46. Steinberg, BJ, Hilton IV, Iida H, Samelson R. Oral health and dental care during pregnancy. *Dent Clin North Am.* 2013;57(2):195-210.

CHAPTER 12

DIABETES

Allison A. Vorderstrasse

Diabetes is one of the most commonly seen endocrine diseases in the primary care setting, primarily because the prevalence of obesity, one of the primary risk factors for diabetes, is rapidly increasing. An overwhelming 65.2% of US adults are now overweight or obese.[1] Rates of being overweight or obese have increased by 50% per decade since 1976. Recognizing and counseling women at risk for diabetes should be a major focus of preventive education in the primary care setting. Women's healthcare practitioners must be prepared to appropriately screen, diagnose, and consult or refer new cases of diabetes for management as appropriate.

Epidemiology

At least 29.1 million individuals in the United States are estimated to have diabetes, including approximately 8 million undiagnosed cases.[2] Most (90-95%) of the cases of diabetes in the United States are type 2 diabetes; the remaining cases are primarily type 1 diabetes. Genetic mutations, autoimmune diseases, chemical reactions, and damage to the pancreas from injury or disease are less common causes. If current trends continue, one in three US adults will have diabetes by 2050. The

prevalence is approximately the same for men and women, but differs by race and ethnicity. Diabetes occurs more frequently in African American, American Indian, Alaskan Native, Hispanic, and Asian populations than in non-Hispanic whites. The incidence also increases among persons with dyslipidemia, hypertension, previously recognized prediabetes, a family history of diabetes, and in women with previous gestational diabetes mellitus (GDM) and polycystic ovarian syndrome (PCOS).[2,3]

Diabetes is broadly defined as a disorder that leads to hyperglycemia due to either inadequate insulin production, inadequate insulin secretion, or a combination of the two.[4] Of the four primary types of diabetes, this chapter focuses on the two most common types of diabetes: type 1 and type 2. Secondary diabetes (1–5% of all cases) can be triggered by genetic disorders including genetic defects of the pancreatic beta cell and genetic abnormalities of the insulin receptor, pancreatic diseases, drug and chemical exposures, and infections.[5] A fourth category, GDM, is defined as the onset or first recognition of diabetes during pregnancy. Women with GDM should be retested after 6 weeks postpartum to determine whether the condition has resolved. Women who develop GDM are at a significantly increased risk of developing overt diabetes later in life and should be screened at 1- to 3-year intervals depending on postpartum blood glucose testing results.[3,6]

Course of Disease

Diabetes is a complex, multifactorial disease, resulting from interactions among genetics, lifestyle choices, and environmental factors. Types 1 and 2 diabetes represent different pathophysiologic mechanisms that result in a similar phenotypic picture of hyperglycemia. In normal physiology, insulin is synthesized in and secreted by the pancreatic beta cells. Insulin is secreted at a steady basal level and in response to a meal; it is important in the metabolism of carbohydrates, fat, and protein. However, the ability of insulin to enable glucose utilization by the target tissues of skeletal muscle, the liver, and adipose tissue is its primary post-meal function. Insulin allows energy use by binding to receptors on cell membranes in target tissues and allowing glucose transport into the cells. Excess energy is stored as glycogen in muscle and as fat in adipose tissue.

Type 1 diabetes is characterized by destruction of the pancreatic beta cells resulting in an inability to produce and secrete insulin. Autoimmune destruction has a genetic component and may also be triggered by viral infections. Some individuals have a genetic tendency toward beta cell destruction even in the absence of an autoimmune process.[4,7] Destruction can occur slowly over months or years, or very quickly over several weeks. Symptoms of hyperglycemia typically appear when 80% of the beta cells have been destroyed.

Individuals who have a first-degree relative with type 1 diabetes are at increased risk of developing diabetes themselves. In general, the risk is less than 10%, although it is higher in those who have 2 parents or a twin with type 1 diabetes.[4] Type 1 diabetes occurs more commonly in children and adolescents but is also diagnosed in adults of all ages. Since about 2005, additional autoimmune types of diabetes, such as maturity-onset diabetes of the young (MODY) and latent autoimmune diabetes in adults, have been diagnosed in adults, particularly young adults.[5,8,9] Although rare, identifying late-onset autoimmune diabetes in the diagnostic process is critically important, because treatment differs significantly from the treatment of type 2 diabetes.

The classic symptoms of significant hyperglycemia are polydipsia, polyuria, and unexplained weight loss, and sometimes polyphagia. These symptoms are seen more often in type 1 diabetes when acute pancreatic beta cell destruction occurs. Rarely, if the onset of type 1 diabetes is fairly rapid, ketoacidosis rather than the classic symptoms of diabetes may lead to the initial diagnosis.

Type 2 diabetes represents insulin resistance and/or a relative insulin deficiency or an insulin secretory defect.[4,5] Genetics and lifestyle both play a large role in type 2 diabetes,[3,4,9] and many individuals with type 2 diabetes have a positive family history of diabetes; factors such as obesity and lack of physical activity are also common.

In type 2 diabetes, the target tissues (muscle, liver, and adipose) gradually lose their sensitivity to insulin over time, preventing efficient use of glucose in most tissues. The brain is an exception, because it does not require insulin for glucose utilization. This loss of tissue sensitivity is referred to as insulin resistance.[4,7] As insulin resistance increases, insulin secretion increases, initially resulting in a mild hyperinsulinemic state. Over time, inflammatory beta cell damage in the pancreas causes the organ to lose ability to secrete enough insulin to maintain euglycemia, resulting in hyperglycemia. Abnormalities in carbohydrate, protein, and fat metabolism occur that are related to the inability of insulin to act at the target tissue level in many body systems.[7]

Symptoms may not be as evident at the onset of type 2 diabetes as with type 1 diabetes, although fatigue, blurred vision, and increased susceptibility to infections may occur.[4] Type 2 diabetes is a progressive disease with increasing loss of function of the pancreatic beta cells over time and decreasing effectiveness of oral medications.[3,4,10]

The chronic hyperglycemia that accompanies poorly controlled diabetes causes injury to multiple organ systems. Diabetic individuals have a twofold risk of cardiovascular complications compared to nondiabetic adults, making cardiovascular disease (CVD) the leading cause of death among diabetics.[11] Morbidity and mortality from complications of diabetes extend to nonvascular conditions as well, including cancer, digestive diseases, and infection.[12] Other complications include peripheral vascular disease, retinopathy, neuropathy, and nephropathy. Diabetes represents the leading cause of end-stage renal disease, nontraumatic amputation of the lower extremities, and adult blindness.[3,4]

Evaluation for Diabetes

History and Physical

Providers should have a high index of suspicion for diabetes, as the symptoms of type 2 diabetes rarely cause patients to seek care, making careful attention to the identification and investigation of risk factors critically important to early detection and treatment. **Table 12-1** provides a summary of risk factors and clinical findings that are indicative of a need for testing or screening for diabetes.[3,13]

Once a high risk of diabetes or a diagnosis of diabetes has been identified, a thorough investigation is required to confirm the diagnosis, identify possible complications, and develop a plan for immediate and ongoing treatment. This evaluation should begin with a complete medical history including past medical and family medical history; current review of systems particularly related to symptoms and complications of diabetes; patterns of dietary intake and physical activity; risk factors

for CVD; contraceptive and reproductive history; use of tobacco, alcohol, or other substances; current medication use including over-the-counter medications and herbal or other supplements; and any cultural or other lifestyle factors that might influence the management of diabetes. **Table 12-2** summarizes the additional personal history related to diabetes, physical examination, laboratory tests, and referrals necessary. These baseline laboratory tests are needed to establish the degree of glucose dysregulation and the presence of comorbidities.

Laboratory Testing

Diagnostic testing for diabetes can be performed using several methods. Each must be confirmed by a repeat test on a different day unless there is unequivocal hyperglycemia. A random plasma glucose ≥ 200 mg/dl in the presence of the classic symptoms of hyperglycemia (polydipsia, polyuria, and weight loss) is diagnostic. Fasting plasma glucose ≥ 126 mg/dl following an 8-hour fast and a two-hour postprandial plasma glucose ≥ 200 mg/dl taken 2 hours after consumption of 75 grams of a standard oral glucose solution are diagnostic in individuals who are asymptomatic. The hemoglobin A1C can also be measured; a level of 6.5 or higher confirms the diagnosis. Individuals with impaired fasting glucose (IFG) or impaired glucose tolerance (IGT) (fasting plasma glucose 100 to 125 mg/dL; 2-hour post-75 g oral glucose tolerance test [OGTT] plasma glucose 140 to 199 mg/dL; hemoglobin A1c [HbA1c] 5.7 to 6.4%) are referred to as having prediabetes, reflecting their increased level of risk for developing overt diabetes in the future.[3]

Approximately 8 million Americans are believed to have undiagnosed type 2 diabetes.[2] An estimated 86 million Americans have prediabetes and may benefit from programs designed to prevent the development of type 2 diabetes, yet only about 11.1% of those with prediabetes have been

Table 12-1 Criteria for Testing for Diabetes in Asymptomatic Adult Individuals

	Authoritative Organization	
American Diabetes Association	**USPSTF**	**AACE/ACE**
Low Risk Individuals		
Begin at age 45 years	Begin between ages 40 and 70 years in women with a BMI ≥ 25 kg/m^2	Begin at age 45 years
High Risk Individuals		
Screen younger adults with a BMI ≥ 25 kg/m^2* who have ≥ 1 risk factors • Physical inactivity • First-degree relative with diabetes • High-risk race/ethnicity • Women who delivered a baby > 9 pounds or were diagnosed with GDM • Hypertension • HDL cholesterol level < 35 mg/dL (0.90 mmol/L) and/or a triglyceride level >250 mg/dL (2.82 mmol/L) • A1c ≥ 5.7%, IGT, or IFG on previous testing • Other clinical conditions associated with insulin resistance (e.g., severe obesity, acanthosis nigricans) • History of CVD	Consider screening at < 40 years in women who have ≥ 1 risk factors • Family history of diabetes • High risk race/ethnicity • History of GDM or PCOS	Consider screening in younger adults with ≥ 1 risk factors • CVD • Family history of diabetes • Sedentary lifestyle • High risk race/ethnicity • HDL cholesterol level < 35 mg/dL (0.90 mmol/L) and/or a triglyceride level >250 mg/dL (2.82 mmol/L) • IGT, IFG, or metabolic syndrome • PCOS, acanthosis nigricans, NAFLD • Hypertension • Women who delivered a baby > 9 pounds or were diagnosed with GDM • Antipsychotic therapy for schizophrenia or bipolar • Chronic corticosteroid exposure
Frequency of Testing		
If the results are normal, testing should be repeated at least at 3-year intervals, with consideration of more frequent testing depending on initial results (e.g., those with prediabetes should be tested yearly) and risk status.	Does not address	If testing is normal, repeat in 3 years. Consider screening in 2 years in individuals with 2 or more risk factors

AACE = American Association of Clinical Endocrinologists, ACE = American College of Endocrinology, BMI = body mass index, CVD = cardiovascular disease, GDM = gestational diabetes mellitus, HDL = high-density lipoprotein, IFG = impaired fasting glucose, IGT = impaired glucose tolerance, high-risk race/ethnicity (e.g. African- Americans, American Indians or Alaskan Natives, Asian Americans, Hispanics or Latinos, or Native Hawaiians or Pacific Islanders), NAFLD = nonalcoholic fatty liver disease, PCOS = polycystic ovarian syndrome.

*At-risk BMI may be lower in some ethnic groups.

Data from American Diabetes Association. Standards of medical care in diabetes—2014. *Diabetes Care.* 2014;37(Suppl 1):S14-80; U.S. Preventative Services Task Force. Final recommendation statement: abnormal blood glucose and type 2 diabetes mellitus: screening. http://www.uspreventiveservicestaskforce.org/Page/Document/RecommendationStatementFinal/screening-for-abnormal-blood-glucose-and-type-2-diabetes. April 2016. Accessed June 23, 2016; Handelsman Y, Bloomgarden Z, Grunberger G, et al. American Association of Clinical Endocrinologists and American College of Endocrinology-Clinical Practice Guidelines for developing a diabetes mellitus comprehensive care plan, 2015. Endocr Pract. 2015;21(suppl 1):1-87.doi:10.4158/EP15672.GLSUPPL.

Table 12-2 Comprehensive Diabetes Evaluation

Medical history related to diabetes:
- Age and characteristics of onset of diabetes (e.g., asymptomatic laboratory finding, symptoms)
- Dietary history, physical activity, weight history
- Diabetes education history/knowledge of diabetes
- Results of glucose monitoring (if applicable)
- Hypoglycemic episodes—awareness and severity, cause, treatment
- History of or symptoms of diabetes-related complications:
  - Microvascular: retinopathy, nephropathy, neuropathy
  - Macrovascular: CHD, CVD, PAD
  - Other: dental problems, psychosocial issues

Physical examination:
- Height, weight, BMI
- Blood pressure
- Fundoscopic examination
- Thyroid palpation
- Skin examination
- Foot examination (including inspection, palpation of pulses, reflexes, and sensory testing—proprioception, vibration, monofilament sensation)

Laboratory evaluation:
- A1c, if not done within the last 2–3 months
- If not performed within the last year:
  - Fasting lipid profile (total cholesterol, LDL, HDL, triglycerides)
  - Liver function tests
  - Test for urine albumin excretion with spot urine albumin-to-creatinine ratio
  - Serum creatinine and calculated GFR
  - TSH (in type 1 diabetes, dyslipidemia, or women over age 50 years)

Referrals:
- Eyecare professional for annual dilated eye exam
- Registered dietician for medical nutrition therapy
- Diabetes self-management education
- Dentist for periodontal examination
- Mental health professional, if needed

Family planning for women of reproductive age

BMI = body mass index, CHD = coronary heart disease, CVD = cardiovascular disease, GFR = glomerular filtration rate, HDL = high-density lipoprotein, LDL = low-density lipoprotein, PAD = peripheral artery disease, TSH = thyroid-stimulating hormone.

Modified from American Diabetes Association. Standards of medical care in diabetes—2014. *Diabetes Care*. 2014;37(Suppl 1): S14-80. *Diabetes Care* by American Diabetes Association. Reproduced with permission of American Diabetes Association.

told that they have it.[2] As many as 50% or more of individuals may have developed a complication by the time of diagnosis.[3]

Although there are no randomized controlled trials demonstrating benefits of earlier diagnosis and treatment of diabetes, the American Diabetes Association (ADA) has made recommendations based on expert opinion for screening for type 2 diabetes. Screening of adults starting at age 30 (with risk factors as indicated in Table 12-1) or age 45 (without risk factors) every 3 to 5 years has been modeled to be cost effective.[14] Women with previous GDM, who have given birth to an infant weighing over nine pounds or who have PCOS, are also at increased risk and should be screened at least every 3 years.[3,6] It should be noted that the US Preventive Services Task Force (USPSTF) recommends screening only asymptomatic adults with hypertension (blood pressure [BP] > 135/80 mmHg).[13]

Screening laboratory evaluations should also include fasting lipids, urinalysis for microalbuminuria, ketones, protein and sediment, thyroid-stimulating hormone (TSH), serum creatinine, and electrocardiogram to assess related metabolic indicators or presence of diabetes-related complications.

Differential Diagnosis

Individuals presenting with classic symptoms of diabetes should be carefully screened for diabetes and other possible conditions. Classic symptoms are much more likely to present in individuals with type 1 diabetes than type 2. Because type 2 diabetes is much more prevalent and may exist for several years prior to diagnosis, the clinician should be alert to risk factors for diabetes related to age, obesity, and ethnicity as well as symptoms of diabetes complications (Table 12-3).

Diabetes should be managed by a healthcare provider who is experienced in the care of diabetic individuals. A multidisciplinary team approach to diabetes treatment, including nurses, registered dieticians, and behavioral health professionals as well as the primary care provider has been associated with improved outcomes and is preferred. If laboratory values cannot be brought into the range of recommended ADA guidelines, or a patient requires more complex medication therapies for diabetes management, then referral to an endocrinologist for more intensive management is warranted.[3]

Table 12-3 Differential Diagnosis for Diabetes by Signs and Symptoms

Polydypsia/polyuria
    Diabetes mellitus type 1
    Diabetes mellitus type 2
    Diabetes insipidus
Obesity
    Excessive caloric intake
    Diabetes type 2
    Hypothyroidism
    Cushing disease
    Fluid retention
    Smoking cessation
    Drug effects
        Steroids
        NSAIDs
        Oral contraceptives
        Some antidepressants
Weight loss
    Diabetes type 1
    Hyperthyroidism
    Cancer
    Depression
    Anorexia
    Drug effects
        Sedatives
        Antidepressants
        NSAIDs
        Antibiotics
Idiopathic
Gastrointestinal causes (malabsorption and sprue)

Management

The primary objectives of diabetes treatment are to bring blood glucose within or close to normal limits and to prevent or delay the development of complications. The Diabetes Control and Complications Trial (DCCT) demonstrated a reduction in microvascular complications with tight control of type 1 diabetes, although tight control of blood glucose was shown to increase the risk of hypoglycemia and weight gain.[15] Similarly, the United Kingdom Prospective Diabetes Study (UKPDS) demonstrated that tight control (goal of fasting plasma glucose 6 mmol/L, equivalent to approximately 108 mg/dL, and pre-meal blood glucose of 4 to 7 mmol/L, equivalent to approximately 72 to 126 mg/dL, for those on insulin) reduced microvascular complications in individuals with type 2 diabetes.[16] More recently, the ACCORD, VADT, and ORIGIN trials have demonstrated that management of glycemic control, blood pressure, and lipids may reduce microvascular complications; the data also indicate that some participants experienced higher rates of macrovascular-related (CVD) mortality, possibly due to weight gain and hypoglycemia.[17-20] It does appear that controlling blood pressure is important in reducing cardiovascular morality and that intensive glucose control (HbA1c < 6.0%) may be effective and safe for some patients.[10,19-21]

For individuals with either type 1 or type 2 diabetes, based on the results of these trials, the ADA recommends a general goal for nonpregnant adults of HbA1c below 7%.[3] This measurement represents an assessment of blood glucose levels over the previous 2- to 3-month period. HbA1c levels should be checked at least twice annually for individuals meeting the target goals, and quarterly for those outside the target. More stringent HbA1c goals of < 6.5% may be appropriate for some patients if hypoglycemia and adverse treatment effects can be avoided, particularly in those with more recent onset of diabetes, those who are younger, and those without CVD.[3] In those who are older, have advanced microvascular or macrovascular complications, have a history of severe hypoglycemia, or have other comorbid conditions, a less stringent goal of < 8% for example, may be appropriate.[3,10,19,21] Setting personalized metabolic control goals based on the patient and her clinical status is therefore important.

Because CVD is a major cause of death for individuals with diabetes, and because diabetes, hypertension, and dyslipidemia are all independent risk factors for CVD, management of blood pressure and lipids is essential in the treatment of diabetes. **Table 12-4** shows ADA-recommended blood glucose treatment goals and accompanying recommendations for blood pressure and lipid treatment goals.[3] Information included in ADA publications and other sources provides data for clinicians on the management of lipids and blood pressure that is beyond the scope of this chapter.[3,22,23]

Type 1 Diabetes

Individuals with type 1 diabetes are managed with insulin therapy to replace what the pancreatic beta cells can no longer produce in sufficient quantity, and a dietary plan of meals and snacks spaced throughout the day, so that euglycemia is maintained. To minimize the formation of antibodies, human insulin is used. Insulin is manufactured in rapid-, short-, intermediate-, and long-acting forms. It can be given by multiple subcutaneous injections or continuous infusion via an insulin pump.[3,24] **Table 12-5** outlines the major types of insulin and their duration of action and peak effect.

Short- and longer-acting (basal) insulin are used together to control fasting blood glucose levels and to minimize postprandial excursions (increase and subsequent decrease) in blood glucose. Basal insulin (via injection or insulin pump) is used to maintain steady insulin availability, mimicking the normal action of the pancreas. Preprandial insulin needs are determined based on carbohydrate intake.[25] Most individuals with type 1 diabetes require at least 3 insulin injections daily or use an insulin pump that provides a basal level of insulin infusion along with boluses taken before each meal. Determination of the exact dosing regimen is based on individual parameters that include insulin sensitivity, diet, physical activity level, blood glucose levels, and types of insulin used.[3]

Table 12-4 Summary of Recommendations for Glycemic, Blood Pressure, and Lipid Control for Most Adults with Diabetes

Hemoglobin A1C level	< 7.0%*
Preprandial capillary plasma glucose	70–130 mg/dL* (3.9–7.2 mmol/L)
Peak postprandial capillary plasma glucose (1–2 hours after beginning of meal)	< 180 mg/dL* (< 10.0 mmol/L)
Blood pressure	< 140/80 mmHg**
Lipids LDL cholesterol	< 100 mg/dL (2.6 mmol/L)† Statin therapy for those with history of MI or age over 40 years with other cardiovascular risk factors

CVD = cardiovascular disease, LDL = low-density lipoprotein, MI = myocardial infarction, SBP = systolic blood pressure

*More or less stringent glycemic goals may be appropriate based on individual patient characteristics including duration of diabetes, age/life expectancy, comorbid conditions, known CVD or advanced microvascular complications, hypoglycemia unawareness, and other individual considerations.

**Based on patient characteristics and response to therapy, lower SBP targets may be appropriate.

†In those with CVD, a lower LDL cholesterol goal of < 70 mg/dL (1.8 mmol/L) using a high dose of statin is an option.

Data from American Diabetes Association. Standards of medical care in diabetes—2014. *Diabetes Care.* 2014;37 (Suppl 1):S14-80.

Table 12-5 Types and Action of Insulin

Type of Insulin	Onset (Minutes/Hours)	Peak (Hours)	Duration (Hours)
Rapid Acting			
Insulin lispro (Humalog)	5–15 minutes	½–1	3–4
Insulin aspart (NovoLog)	10–20 minutes	¾–1	3–5
Glulisine	20 minutes	1	4
Short Acting			
Regular Human (Humulin R, Novolin R)	30 minutes	1–2	6–8
Intermediate Acting			
NPH human (Humulin N, Novolin N)	1–2 hours	3–8	12–15
Long Acting			
Insulin glargine (Lantus) insulin analog	1–2 hours	Flat	24
Detemir	1.6 hours	Flat	Up to 24 hours

NPH = neutral protamine Hagedorn

Note: Estimates only, may vary in individual patients. All values are for subcutaneous administration of insulin.

Data from Morello CM. Pharmacokinetics and pharmacodynamics of insulin analogs in special populations with type 2 diabetes mellitus. *Int J Gen Med.* 2011;4:827-835.

A regular meal and snack plan is equally important for patients managing type 1 diabetes to avoid glucose excursions. This means that dietary patterns should be as routine as possible, and consistent amounts of carbohydrates, protein, and fats at each meal or snack are helpful in maintaining a normal glucose level. Regular exercise is important for those with type 1 diabetes and is one of the variables considered when calculating dietary and insulin needs. Exercise and athletic participation are not restricted in diabetes; however, important considerations include monitoring blood glucose before and after exercise, using carbohydrates as needed to prevent hypoglycemia, staying hydrated, and avoiding exercise if fasting blood glucose is > 250 with ketosis or > 300 without ketosis.[3,10]

Type 2 Diabetes

Dietary management, also referred to as medical nutrition therapy (MNT), and exercise are important cornerstones of both the initial and ongoing management of type 2 diabetes. The goals are weight reduction (if appropriate) and a reduction in insulin resistance as well as reduction of cardiovascular risk factors by controlling lipids and blood pressure. MNT may be provided by a registered dietician or nutritionist who works as a part of the diabetes care team. Goals include prevention of large excursions in blood glucose level and encouraging carbohydrate intake that incorporates dietary fiber from whole grains, fruit, and vegetables. There is not a recommended combination of macronutrients for those with diabetes; a balanced diet of all food groups that is based on individual health goals and preferences and meets the dietary recommendations for the general public is appropriate.[25] Recommendations should be personalized to accommodate individual preferences and lifestyle and should be culturally appropriate.[25]

Including regular exercise to improve cardiovascular fitness is important to diabetes management. A minimum of 30 minutes of exercise 3 times weekly is suggested. Studies have demonstrated improvements in carbohydrate metabolism and insulin sensitivity using regimens of 30 to 60 minutes of aerobic activity 3 to 4 times weekly.[3] Results are more impressive in individuals with milder diabetes and those with greater degrees of insulin resistance. Initial self-monitoring of exercise sessions and regular follow up and ongoing support from diabetes team members are likely to improve adherence to the exercise program.[26] Depending on the age of the individual, length of time since diagnosis of diabetes, and possible diabetes complications, careful evaluation of cardiovascular status may be warranted prior to initiating an exercise program. When MNT and exercise do not result in meeting the desired blood glucose goals, medication is added to the therapeutic regimen. **Figure 12-1** provides an algorithm with timelines for stepwise treatment of type 2 diabetes as recommended by the European Association for the Study of Diabetes (EASD) and ADA.[10] **Table 12-6** describes the major classes of hypoglycemic medications, their mechanism of action, side effects, and dosing schedules. Metformin (Glucophage) is often the first drug of choice when adding medication to the MNT and exercise plan.[10] Metformin may also have a positive effect on blood lipids, which can result in less weight gain or even weight loss when compared to other medications. Metformin is contraindicated for individuals with kidney disease, alcoholism or binge drinking behavior, and hepatic dysfunction.

Multidrug regimens may be necessary to lower blood glucose to an acceptable level. Sulfonylureas are often added to metformin if two-drug combinations are needed to attain metabolic control goals. They are generally effective and low in cost but do carry a moderate risk of hypoglycemia and weight gain.[3,10] Thiazolidinediones may also

Figure 12-1 European Association for the Study of Diabetes (EASD)/American Diabetes Association (ADA) algorithm for stepwise treatment of type 2 diabetes.

STEP 1	STEP 2	STEP 3	STEP 4
Initial drug monotherapy	Two-drug combinations	Three-drug combinations	More complex insulin strategies

Metformin Efficacy: High Hypoglycemia Risk: Low Weight: Neutral/loss Major SEs: GI/lactic acidosis Cost: Low *To avoid GI side effects at initiation, consider starting at 500mg QD or BID and increasing by 500mg/wk (Maximum total daily dose is 2,000–2,500 mg). Take with meals.*	**Metformin +**		**Insulin** (multiple daily doses often in combination with one or two non-insulin agents)
	Sulfonylurea (SU) Efficacy: High Hypoglycemia Risk: Moderate Weight: Gain Major SEs: Hypoglycemia Cost: Low	**Sulfonylurea +** TZD or DPP-4-i or GLP-1-RA or Insulin (usually basal)	
	OR **Thiazolidinedione (TZD)** Efficacy: High Hypoglycemia Risk: Low Weight: Gain Major SEs: Edema, HF, Fx's Cost: High	OR **Thiazolidinedione +** SU or DPP-4-i or GLP-1-RA or Insulin (usually basal)	
	OR **DPP-4 Inhibitor (DPP-4-i)** Efficacy: Intermediate Hypoglycemia Risk: Low Weight: Neutral Major SEs: Rare Cost: High	OR **DPP-4 Inhibitor +** SU or TZD or Insulin (usually basal)	
	OR **GLP-1 Receptor agonist (GLP-1-RA)** Efficacy: High Hypoglycemia Risk: Low Weight: Loss Major SEs: GI Cost: High	OR **GLP-1 Receptor agonist +** SU or TZD or Insulin (usually basal)	
	OR **Insulin (usually basal)** Efficacy: Highest Hypoglycemia Risk: High Weight: Gain Major SEs: Hypoglycemia Cost: Variable	OR **Insulin (usually basal) +** TZD or DPP-4-i or GLP-1-RA	

IF INDIVIDUAL GOALS NOT REACHED AFTER 3 MONTHS →

IF INDIVIDUAL GOALS NOT REACHED AFTER 3 MONTHS →

IF INDIVIDUAL GOALS NOT REACHED AFTER 3–6 MONTHS →

Data from Inzucchi SE, Bergenstal RM, Buse JB, et al. Management of hyperglycemia in type 2 diabetes: a patient-centered approach: position statement of the American Diabetes Association (ADA) and the European Association for the Study of Diabetes (EASD). Diabetes Care. Jun 2012;35(6):1364-1379.

Table 12-6 Pharmacotherapeutic Agents For Treating Type 2 Diabetes

Name Generic/Brand	Dose	Maximum Daily Dose	Side Effects and Considerations	Effect on Weight
Sulfonylureas				
Glimepiride (Amaryl)	1-2 mg once/daily with first meal of the day.	8 mg	Sulfonylureas may cause hypoglycemia. Dizziness, headaches and sun sensitivity have been reported in approximately 2% of users	Weight gain
Glyburide (DiaBeta)	1.25–5 mg once/daily with first meal	20 mg in divided doses		Weight gain
Glyburide (Glynase)	0.75 mg once/daily	12 mg in divided doses	Allergic skin rashes and GI disturbances include nausea, diarrhea and constipation.	Weight gain
Glipizide (Glucotrol)	5 mg once/daily before first meal	40 mg	Side effects be dose dependent and disappear after lowering and/or dividing daily dose	Weight gain
Glipizide (Glucotrol XL)	5 mg once/daily at first meal	20 mg		Weight gain
Meglitinides				
Repaglinide (Prandin)	0.5 mg–2 mg before each meal	Up to 4 mg before each meal	Hypoglycemia in approximately 31% of users. Upper respiratory infections, headaches, nausea, diarrhea, sinusitis, joint pain found in 6% or less.	Weight gain
Nateglinide (Starlix)	120 mg 3 times/daily before meals	360 mg a day		Weight gain
Biguanides				
Metformin (Glucophage)	500 mg twice/daily or 850 mg qd	2,500-2,550 mg a day	GI symptoms such as diarrhea, nausea, vomiting, abdominal bloating and flatulence found in up to 1/3 of people. Some need to decrease or discontinue either temporarily or permanently due to these effects. Hypoglycemia almost unknown.	Weight neutral or loss

Table 12-6 Pharmacotherapeutic Agents For Treating Type 2 Diabetes (*continued*)

Name Generic/Brand	Dose	Maximum Daily Dose	Side Effects and Considerations	Effect on Weight
Alpha-glucosidase Inhibitors				
Acarbose (Precose)	25 mg tid with meals	50 mg tid for women <133 lbs and 100 mg tid for women >133 lbs	Abdominal pain, diarrhea, flatulence, all reduced with time.	Weight neutral
Miglitol (Glyset)	25-50 mg with dinner	100 mg q meal		Weight neutral
Thiazolidinediones				
Rosiglitazone (Avandia)	4 mg qd -bid	8 mg	Increase in LDL and HDL in clinical trials. Increased risk of hypoglycemia when taken with insulin.	Weight gain
Pioglitazone (Actos)	15 mg daily; can be taken in combination with insulin, metformin and sulfonylureas	45 mg	No effects on lipids. Increased risk of hypoglycemia when taken with insulin.	Weight gain
DPP-4 Inhibitors				
Sitagliptin phosphate (Januvia)	100 mg qd with or without food	100 mg qd	Stuffy nose, sore throat, upper respiratory infection and headache. Lower doses may be needed for persons with renal compromise.	Weight neutral
SGLP-2				
Canagliflozin (Invokana)	100-300 mg daily before food	100 mg tablets	Urinary tract infections, vulvovaginal mycotic infections Contraindicated with renal impairment	Weight neutral

Incretin Mimetics GLP-1			
Exenatide (Byetta)	5 mcg pre-filled pen SQ bid prior to meal	5-10 mcg SQ bid prior to meal	Hypoglycemia possible if used in combination with sulfonylureas. If occurs, dose of sulfonylurea can be decreased. Nausea, vomiting diarrhea, headache, anorexia and acid stomach. SE mostly decrease over time.	Weight loss
Albiglutide (Tanzeum)	30 mg SQ once a week may be increased to 50 mg	30 mg or 50 mg single dose pen	Hypoglycemia possible if use with insulin or sulfonylureas. Black Box warning of risk of thyroid c-cell tumors	Weight loss
Amylin Mimetics			
Pramlintide (Symlin)	60-120 mcg before meals	Injector kit with various doses available	Contraindicated for individual on potassium Hypoglycemia possible if use with insulin. Black Box warning about hypoglycemia with insulin	Weight neutral
Bile Acid Sequestrants			
Colesevelam (Welchol)	3750 mg PO once/daily or 1875 mg PO twice/daily Taken before meals	Multiple dose tablets and powders	Must be taken 4 hours after or before other medications	Weight neutral or loss

* Contraindicated for new diagnosis and initial treatment

be used as adjunct therapy with other medications. Individuals taking this class of medication should be observed for hepatic changes, edema or other signs of heart failure, and bone fractures.[10] Dipeptidyl peptidase 4 (DPP-4) inhibitors block the DPP-4 enzyme that breaks down incretins. Therefore, more incretins are available to help stimulate insulin release and block release of glucagon, resulting in a lowering of blood glucose levels. They have been found to be effective in lowering HbA1c with low risk of hypoglycemia and very rare incidence of any major side effects.[10] Glucagon-like peptide 1 (GLP-1) receptor agonists act in a similar way to incretins, stimulating the release of insulin and decreasing the release of glucagon, thereby lowering glucose levels. They are effective in lowering HbA1c and carry a low risk of hypoglycemia, have mostly gastrointestinal side effects, and may result in weight loss.[10]

Insulin therapy (Table 12-6), particularly basal insulin, may be used initially in type 2 diabetes, but is often reserved until blood glucose goals cannot be met with other medications. Often patients prefer to start oral medications initially and reserve insulin, which must be taken by injection, until later. Nearly half of individuals with type 2 diabetes in the UKPDS study required insulin within 6 years of their diagnosis.[27] Monotherapy, whether it is diet and exercise, oral medication, or insulin, will not be sufficient for the majority of patients with type 2 diabetes over time.[10] A study that examined metabolic control and clinical management of type 2 diabetes found that there was a high degree of clinical inertia, leading to many years of poor metabolic control for most patients. Ultimately, at least 90% of individuals enrolled in this study required insulin therapy.[28] Despite the lack of early initiation of insulin therapy in clinical practice, there are data to support that it improves metabolic control earlier, reduces the burden on beta cells from hyperglycemia and resulting hyperinsulinemia, and delays microvascular complications.[29] Initiation of insulin therapy should be overseen by a healthcare provider skilled in the management of diabetes. Referral to a diabetologist may be helpful at any point but is required if good control cannot be achieved or maintained.

The most recent studies of intensive therapies with more aggressive metabolic goals (i.e., HbA1c < 6.0%) have demonstrated some improvement in microvascular complications, yet some studies reported an increase in macrovascular complications and mortality.[19] Because of the epidemic of type 2 diabetes and the diagnosis of diabetes in younger individuals who will require therapy for many years, experts in the field have recommended that the progression from diet and exercise, to drug monotherapy, to combined therapy and insulin use, including consideration of earlier insulin use in some cases, should be more rapid in order to achieve blood glucose goals more quickly and slow the development of diabetes complications.[10,19] Intensive treatment using metformin as the initial medication has been shown to reduce costs in the long term by reducing the costs of hospitalization associated with the development of diabetes complications.[3,10]

Patient Education

Patient education is critical for effective management of both type 1 and type 2 diabetes. Goals for blood glucose, lipids, and blood pressure can be met only if the individual with diabetes is educated about all aspects of diabetes management and understands how to work with other members of the diabetes care team to maximize desired outcomes. The ADA has developed national standards for diabetes self-management education for use by healthcare entities in developing their local diabetes education programs.[30]

Self-monitoring of blood glucose (SMBG) is a key component of diabetes management. All individuals with diabetes should be counseled in this method, because it provides critical information needed to develop an effective self-care plan. This information can then be shared with other members of the team and used to develop strategies specific to the needs of individual patients. SMBG and regular HbA1c measurements are used to adjust diet, activity, and medication recommendations.

In addition, a good understanding of general dietary principles and ways to adapt dietary recommendations to accommodate individual food preferences, changing activity levels, and the presence of illness is critical. Nutrition education should ideally be provided by a registered dietician or nutritionist who is experienced in working with individuals with diabetes.[25] Ongoing access to a dietician is also helpful. In particular, individuals with type 1 diabetes need to learn principles related to insulin adjustment in order to develop individual plans. Use of an intensive management regimen assumes that the individual will be sufficiently knowledgeable about how to make adjustments in insulin dosages according to daily blood glucose levels as well. ADA standards include the recommendation that diabetes education is provided by a team representing various professions, and that this team includes experts in providing diabetes education.[30]

Prevention of Type 2 Diabetes

Several seminal studies have demonstrated that type 2 diabetes can be prevented or delayed.[31-34] The most impressive was a randomized controlled trial of lifestyle intervention, metformin, and placebo.[31] The Diabetes Prevention Program Research Group randomized more than 3000 nondiabetic individuals at 27 centers into each of the 3 treatment groups. The sample included obese individuals age 25 and older; 68% were women, and 45% were minorities. The lifestyle group received an intensive intervention program with goals of a 7% reduction in initial body weight through a healthy low-fat diet and moderate-intensity exercise for 150 minutes per week. The metformin group was

prescribed 850 mg twice daily; both metformin and placebo groups received written information and a single visit recommending standard healthy lifestyle advice. After an average follow-up period of nearly 3 years, the lifestyle group had a reduced incidence of diabetes of 59% and the metformin group of 31% compared to controls. Both interventions were significantly more effective than placebo, and lifestyle was more effective than metformin, even after taking into account genetic risk for type 2 diabetes.[31,35]

Based on the evidence, the ADA has established recommendations for the delay or prevention of type 2 diabetes.[3] The rationale for prevention efforts includes the following:

- Diabetes is known to be a serious health problem with significant public burden.
- The early course of the disease and significant risk factors are known.
- Tests to detect the pre-disease state exist.
- There are safe and cost-effective methods to delay or prevent the disease.

The ADA recommendations include:

- Referral to an effective ongoing support program that targets a weight loss of 7% body weight and meeting physical activity goals of at least 150 minutes/week of moderate activity
- Follow-up counseling in regard to these goals
- Recommended coverage by third-party payers for prevention programs
- Consideration of metformin especially in those who are obese, younger than 60 years of age, or women with prior GDM
- Screening for and treatment of cardiovascular risk factors[3]

In addition to prediabetes, another area of concern for preventive strategies is the group of individuals with a constellation of physical and laboratory measurements known as metabolic syndrome. This condition was defined in the Third Report of the National Cholesterol Education Program Expert Panel on Detection, Evaluation, and

Treatment of High Blood Cholesterol in Adults (Adult Treatment Panel III) and includes abdominal obesity, hypertriglyceridemia, low high-density lipoprotein (HDL) cholesterol, hypertension, and high fasting blood glucose.[36] Under the most stringent current diagnostic criteria for metabolic syndrome and data from National Health and Nutrition Examination Survey (NHANES), an estimated 34% of US adults have the metabolic syndrome.[37]

Impact of Pregnancy and Breastfeeding

A preconception care program is essential for women with type 1 or type 2 diabetes who desire to become pregnant.[3,38,39] Preconception care is complicated, because more than half of pregnancies in the United States are unplanned or unintended. However, as part of overall diabetes management, women of childbearing age should be counseled on appropriate contraceptive methods, and the importance of preconception care should be stressed at all healthcare visits. Despite the fairly well-documented benefits, only about 30% of women with diabetes receive preconception care.[39]

Preconception care should be provided by an interdisciplinary team with an overall goal to bring HbA1c levels to under 7% in order to reduce the occurrence of anomalies and other complications.[3,38,39] Major malformations in the fetus, such as cardiovascular, central nervous system, skeletal, and genitourinary anomalies, are known to occur more frequently in women with diabetes, and occur at higher rates with increasing HbA1c levels.[38,39] Malformations are believed to be the result of maternal hyperglycemia during the sensitive period of organogenesis. Near-normal blood glucose control prior to conception is essential in the prevention of these abnormalities. Additional risks for women with preexisting diabetes include spontaneous abortion, stillbirth, preterm labor, and fetal macrosomia.[38-40] Because of the association between diabetes and autoimmune thyroid disease, women with diabetes should undergo thyroid testing prior to pregnancy.[3,38,39] Initiation of 1 mg of folic acid daily is recommended for 3 months prior to conception to reduce the incidence of neural tube defects.[3,34,35] Women should also be screened for diabetic retinopathy, nephropathy, neuropathy, and CVD when they are considering pregnancy.[3,38,39]

Once a woman with type 1 or 2 diabetes has become pregnant, care should be coordinated by a healthcare provider skilled in the management of diabetes in pregnancy. Midwives may certainly be involved as a member of the care team. Care of a patient with diabetes will be similar to care provided during the preconception period. The focus is on keeping blood glucose levels close to the normal range in order to provide a healthy environment for fetal growth and development.[3,38,40] It is also important to quickly recognize and treat hypoglycemia. Hypoglycemia is common during pregnancy in women with preexisting diabetes following overnight fasting, and this may occur even before a pregnancy diagnosis is confirmed. Although the major focus of care is preventing hyperglycemia,[3,38,40] strict control of blood glucose is associated with episodes of severe hypoglycemia (requiring assistance from another person and possibly including coma). Although studies have not demonstrated an association between maternal hypoglycemia and fetal anomalies, the safest course is to reduce both hyper- and hypoglycemia, particularly severe episodes.[3,38,40]

The ADA and the American College of Obstetricians and Gynecologists agree on the basics of how to care for women with diabetes when they become pregnant.[38,40,41] Evaluations for retinopathy and nephropathy should occur early in pregnancy. Because of a higher rate of thyroid disease during pregnancy and the postpartum period for women with diabetes, thyroid function testing is recommended.[3,41] Diabetic nephropathy occurs in 5–10% of pregnancies and contributes to increased risk for hypertensive complications and preterm labor.[3] An ultrasound to evaluate for the presence of anomalies should occur at about 18 to 20 weeks' gestation.[40] Where earlier evaluation for fetal anomalies is available, this should be offered to the mother. Nutrition and exercise continue to be important in the management of diabetes during pregnancy. Women of normal prepregnant weight are encouraged to

consume a dietary intake of 30 to 35 kcal/kg of body weight. Recommendations are highly individualized based on prepregnancy weight, glycemic control, and other personal and cultural factors. A woman should develop individualized goals with a registered dietician to consume adequate calories and a distribution of carbohydrates (particularly complex carbohydrates and fiber), protein, and healthy fats to support her pregnancy and her weight goals.[3,40,41] **Table 12-7**

Table 12-7 Evaluation and Monitoring for Women with Pregestational Diabetes

Initial Pregnancy Evaluation	Frequency of Evaluation During Pregnancy
A1c	Every 1–3 months
Blood pressure	Every visit and as indicated. May experience worsening of preexisting hypertension or onset of pregnancy-induced hypertension starting in second trimester.
Fasting lipid profile (if not recently performed)	As indicated
TSH and thyroid peroxidase antibodies; TSH-receptor antibodies if TSH is less than 0.03 mIU/L	To monitor treatment if necessary
Hemoglobin, serum ferritin	To monitor treatment if necessary
ALT/AST; possible liver ultrasound based on lab findings	As indicated
Random urine albumin creatinine ratio (ACR) or 24-hour urine collection for microalbuminuria and creatinine clearance (if urine in dipstick is positive for albumin or protein, then measure 24-hour protein excretion)	Every 1–3 months if abnormal
Dilated retinal exam (if not performed recently prepregnancy)	Every 1–6 months depending on risk of progression of retinopathy
Assess CHD risk factors. Resting ECG if asymptomatic and age 35 or older (if not performed recently). Cardiology consultation if suspected angina, atypical chest pain, dyspnea, abnormal ECG, or other reasons to suspect CHD.	As indicated
Consider testing for cardiac autonomic neuropathy, diabetic cardiomyopathy or heart failure, or peripheral arteriosclerotic disease if high risk or shows any signs of these issues.	As indicated

ALT = alanine transaminase, AST = aspartate transaminase, CHD = coronary heart disease, ECG = electrocardiogram, TSH = thyroid-stimulating hormone

Data from Kitzmiller JL, Block JM, Brown FM, Catalano PM, Conway DL, Coustan DR, et al. Managing preexisting diabetes for pregnancy: summary of evidence and consensus recommendations for care. *Diabetes Care.* 2008;31(5):1060-1079; Ali S, Dornhorst A. Diabetes in pregnancy: health risks and management. *Postgrad Med J.* 2011;87(1028):417-427.

summarizes the recommendations for ongoing evaluation and monitoring of pregestational diabetes in pregnancy.

Insulin, which does not cross the placenta, has historically been the medication of choice for treating hyperglycemia in pregnancy. Recent reviews have examined the use of oral hypoglycemic medications in pregnancy for pregestational diabetes and GDM. Several studies recommend the use of metformin for GDM, a condition diagnosed after organogenesis has occurred.[3,40,41] Metformin, a pregnancy category B drug, has also been studied during pregnancy in the treatment of women with PCOS. Most other oral diabetes medications are category C or higher and are not considered to be first-line agents.[3]

In general, insulin dosages are reduced in the first trimester to prevent hypoglycemia resulting from increased insulin sensitivity in the first trimester, as well as decreased intake due to nausea and vomiting. Insulin needs are generally the highest between 28 and 32 weeks' gestation.[41] Use of both a long-acting and short-acting insulin such as lispro (Humalog) or aspart (NovoLog) may provide the best metabolic control and reduce postprandial hyperglycemia, episodes of hypoglycemia between meals, and HbA1c.[41] A plan for continuing dietary and blood glucose monitoring, increased fetal surveillance, and timing of delivery should be developed among members of the care team, including the pregnant woman and her family.

Care during the third trimester focuses on preventing stillbirth, promoting intrauterine fetal growth and oxygenation, and planning the appropriate time for the birth. Planning is important in order to maximize fetal/neonatal health and minimize maternal morbidity related to birth. Continued blood glucose monitoring and fetal surveillance provide the information for developing this plan. Twice-weekly fetal assessment using the biophysical profile and/or nonstress test has been recommended beginning at 32 weeks' gestation. If test results remain normal and blood glucose control is good, the woman may be allowed to progress to her due date. Cesarean section is considered for those with specific complications (i.e., proliferative retinopathy with risk of hemorrhage) or macrosomia (< 4000 grams) based on provider recommendations.[41] If labor and a vaginal birth are planned, the goal is to maintain the blood glucose approximately 80 to 110 mg/dL during labor, typically through the use of an intravenous insulin drip.[42] Controlling hyperglycemia during labor reduces the likelihood of neonatal hypoglycemia.

Goals for care during pregnancy, in addition to improving pregnancy outcomes, include establishing a healthy lifestyle that can be maintained.[41] The postpartum care of women with diabetes is similar to that for women without diabetes. Women with type 1 or 2 diabetes should continue to be managed by a multidisciplinary team with the goal of continued glycemic control. Insulin needs decrease rapidly after the birth and may be reduced by approximately half of the antepartum dose as meals are initiated.[38,40,42] Recovery is determined as for any other woman and includes appropriate recommendations for family planning methods. Provision of an appropriate and effective contraceptive is an important step in preconception care for a possible next pregnancy. Because of evidence that the incidence of childhood diabetes is lower among those who were breastfed, breastfeeding should be encouraged and supported. Breastfeeding may also promote improved glycemic and lipid profiles in women with diabetes.[38,40,42]

References

1. Wyatt SB, Winters KP, Dubbert PM. Overweight and obesity: prevalence, consequences, and causes of a growing public health problem. *Am J Med Sci.* 2006;331(4):166-174.
2. American Diabetes Association. Fast Facts: Data and statistics about diabetes. 2013. Available at: http://professional.diabetes.org/facts. Accessed April 17, 2016.
3. American Diabetes Association. Standards of medical care in diabetes—2014. *Diabetes Care.* 2014; 37(Suppl 1):S14-S80.
4. McCance KL, Huether SE. *Pathophysiology: The Biologic Basis for Disease in Adults and Children.* 6th ed. Maryland Heights, MO: Mosby Elsevier; 2010.
5. American Diabetes Association. Diagnosis and classification of diabetes mellitus. *Diabetes Care.* 2014; 37(Suppl 1):S81-S90.
6. Ratner RE. Prevention of type 2 diabetes in women with previous gestational diabetes. *Diabetes Care.* 2007;30(Suppl 2):S242-S245.
7. Hall JE, Guyton AC. *Guyton and Hall Textbook of Medical Physiology.* 12th ed. Philadelphia, PA: Saunders/Elsevier; 2011.
8. Brophy S, Davies H, Mannan S, Brunt H, Williams R. Interventions for latent autoimmune diabetes (LADA) in adults. *Cochrane Database Syst Rev.* 2011(9): CD006165.
9. Kota SK, Meher LK, Jammula S, Kota SK, Modi KD. Genetics of type 2 diabetes mellitus and other specific types of diabetes; its role in treatment modalities. *Diabetes Metab Syndr.* 2012;6(1):54-58.
10. Inzucchi SE, Bergenstal RM, Buse JB, Diamant M, Ferrannini E, Nauck M, et al. Management of hyperglycemia in type 2 diabetes: a patient-centered approach: position statement of the American Diabetes Association (ADA) and the European Association for the Study of Diabetes (EASD). *Diabetes Care.* 2012;35(6):1364-1379.
11. The Emerging Risk Factors Collaboration. Diabetes mellitus, fasting blood glucose concentration, and risk of vascular disease: a collaborative meta-analysis of 102 prospective studies. *Lancet.* 2010; 375:2215-2222.
12. The Emerging Risk Factors Collaboration. Diabetes mellitus, fasting glucose, and risk of cause-specific death. *N Engl J Med.* 2011;364:829-884.
13. US Preventive Services Task Force. Screening for Type 2 Diabetes Mellitus in Adults: Clinical Summary of U.S. Preventive Services Task Force Recommendation. 2008. Available at: http://www.uspreventiveservicestaskforce.org/uspstf08/type2/type2summ.htm. Accessed April 5, 2016.
14. Kahn R, Alperin P, Eddy D, Borch-Johnsen K, Buse J, Feigelman J, et al. Age at initiation and frequency of screening to detect type 2 diabetes: a cost-effectiveness analysis. *Lancet.* 2010;375(9723): 1365-1374.
15. The Diabetes Control and Complications Trial Research Group. The effect of intensive treatment of diabetes on the development and progression of long-term complications in insulin-dependent diabetes mellitus. *N Engl J Med.* 1993;329(14):977-986.
16. UK Prospective Diabetes Study (UKPDS) Group. Intensive blood-glucose control with sulphonylureas or insulin compared with conventional treatment and risk of complications in patients with type 2 diabetes (UKPDS 33). *Lancet.* 1998;352(9131):837-853.
17. Duckworth W, Abraira C, Moritz T, Reda D, Emanuele N, Reaven PD, et al. Glucose control and vascular complications in veterans with type 2 diabetes. *N Engl J Med.* 2009;360:129-139.
18. The ORIGIN Trial Investigators. Basal insulin and cardiovascular and other outcomes in dysglycemia. *N Engl J Med.* 2012;367:319-328.
19. Konig M, Lamos EM, Stein SA, Davis SN. An insight into the recent diabetes trials: what is the best approach to prevent macrovascular and microvascular complications? *Curr Diabetes Rev.* 2013; 9(5):371-381.
20. Margolis KL, O'Connor PJ, Morgan TM, Buse JB, Cohen RM, Cushman WC, et al. Outcomes of combined cardiovascular risk factor management strategies in type 2 diabetes: the ACCORD randomized trial. *Diabetes Care.* 2014;37(6):1721-1728.
21. Fullerton B, Jeitler K, Seitz M, Horvath K, Berghold A, Siebenhofer A. Intensive glucose control versus conventional glucose control for type 1 diabetes mellitus. *Cochrane Database Syst Rev.* 2014;2:CD009122.
22. Lastra G, Syed S, Kurukulasuriya LR, Manrique C, Sowers JR. Type 2 diabetes mellitus and hypertension: an update. *Endocrinol Metab Clin North Am.* 2014;43(1):103-122.
23. Martin SS, Metkus TS, Horne A, Blaha MJ, Hasan R, Campbell CY, et al. Waiting for the National Cholesterol Education Program Adult Treatment Panel IV Guidelines, and in the meantime, some challenges and recommendations. *Am J Cardiol.* 2012; 110(2):307-313.

24. Morello CM. Pharmacokinetics and pharmacodynamics of insulin analogs in special populations with type 2 diabetes mellitus. *Int J Gen Med*. 2011; 4:827-835.

25. Evert AB, Boucher JL, Cypress M, Dunbar SA, Franz MJ, Mayer-Davis EJ, et al. Nutrition therapy recommendations for the management of adults with diabetes. *Diabetes Care*. 2013;36(11):3821-3842.

26. Matthews L, Kirk A, Macmillan F, Mutrie N. Can physical activity interventions for adults with type 2 diabetes be translated into practice settings? A systematic review using the RE-AIM framework. *Transl Behav Med*. 2014;4(1):60-78.

27. Wright A, Burden AC, Paisey RB, Cull CA, Holman RR, Group UKPDS. Sulfonylurea inadequacy: efficacy of addition of insulin over 6 years in patients with type 2 diabetes in the U.K. Prospective Diabetes Study (UKPDS 57). *Diabetes Care*. 2002;25(2):330-336.

28. Brown JB, Nichols GA, Perry A. The burden of treatment failure in type 2 diabetes. *Diabetes Care*. 2004;27(7):1535-1540.

29. Owens DR. Clinical evidence for the earlier initiation of insulin therapy in type 2 diabetes. *Diabetes Technol Ther*. 2013;15(9):776-785.

30. Haas L, Maryniuk M, Beck J, Cox CE, Duker P, Edwards L, et al. National standards for diabetes self-management education and support. *Diabetes Care*. 2014;37(Suppl 1):S144-S153.

31. Diabetes Prevention Program Research Group, Knowler WC, Fowler SE, Hamman RF, Christophi CA, Hoffman HJ, et al. 10-year follow-up of diabetes incidence and weight loss in the Diabetes Prevention Program Outcomes Study. *Lancet*. 2009; 374(9702):1677-1686.

32. DREAM (Diabetes REduction Assessment with ramipril and rosiglitazone Medication) Trial Investigators, Gerstein HC, Yusuf S, Bosch J, Pogue J, Sheridan P, et al. Effect of rosiglitazone on the frequency of diabetes in patients with impaired glucose tolerance or impaired fasting glucose: a randomised controlled trial. *Lancet*. 2006;368(9541):1096-1105.

33. Pan XR, Li GW, Hu YH, Wang JX, Yang WY, An ZX, et al. Effects of diet and exercise in preventing NIDDM in people with impaired glucose tolerance. The Da Qing IGT and Diabetes Study. *Diabetes Care*. 1997;20(4):537-544.

34. Tuomilehto J, Lindstrom J, Eriksson JG, Valle TT, Hämäläinen H, Ilanne-Parikka P, et al. Prevention of type 2 diabetes mellitus by changes in lifestyle among subjects with impaired glucose tolerance. *N Engl J Med*. 2001;344(18):1343-1350.

35. Florez JC, Jablonski KA, Bayley N, Pollin TI, de Bakker PI, Shuldiner AR, et al. TCF7L2 polymorphisms and progression to diabetes in the Diabetes Prevention Program. *N Engl J Med*. 2006;355(3): 241-250.

36. National Cholesterol Education Program Expert Panel on Detection, Evaluation, and Treatment of High Blood Cholesterol in Adults. Third Report of the National Cholesterol Education Program (NCEP) Expert Panel on Detection, Evaluation, and Treatment of High Blood Cholesterol in Adults (Adult Treatment Panel III) final report. *Circulation*. 2002;106(25):3143-3421.

37. Ramphal L, Zhang J, Suzuki S. Ethnic disparities in the prevalence of the metabolic syndrome in American adults: data from the Examination of National Health and Nutrition Examination Survey 1999–2010. *Proceedings*. 2014;27(2):92-95.

38. Ringholm L, Mathiesen ER, Kelstrup L, Damm P. Managing type 1 diabetes mellitus in pregnancy— from planning to breastfeeding. Nature reviews. *Endocrinology*. 2012;8(11):659-667.

39. Wahabi HA, Alzeidan RA, Esmaeil SA. Pre-pregnancy care for women with pre-gestational diabetes mellitus: a systematic review and meta-analysis. *BMC Public Health*. 2012;12:792.

40. McCance DR. Pregnancy and diabetes. *Best Pract Res Clin Endocrinol Metab*. 2011;25(6):945-958.

41. Kitzmiller JL, Block JM, Brown FM, Catalano PM, Conway DL, Coustan DR, et al. Managing preexisting diabetes for pregnancy: summary of evidence and consensus recommendations for care. *Diabetes Care*. 2008;31(5):1060-1079.

42. Ali S, Dornhorst A. Diabetes in pregnancy: health risks and management. *Postgrad Med J*. 2011; 87(1028):417-427.

CHAPTER 13

THYROID AND OTHER ENDOCRINE DISORDERS

Barbara K. Hackley | Jan M. Kriebs

Hypothyroidism and hyperthyroidism are 10 times more common in women than in men[1] and are the second most common endocrine disorder affecting women of reproductive age, behind diabetes mellitus.[2] While less common, hyperparathyroidism is a significant primary care concern in women.

Thyroid Disease

Thyroid disease is a general term that refers to both under- and overactivity of the thyroid gland and has multiple causes. The discussion of clinical conditions addresses hypothyroid conditions, hyperthyroidism, and thyroid nodules.

Screening Recommendations

Authorities disagree about whether screening for thyroid dysfunction in asymptomatic adults is warranted. The American Thyroid Association (ATA) recommends screening women over the age of 35 every 5 years, and the American Association of Clinical Endocrinologists (AACE) recommends screening "older women."[3] However, the US Preventive Services Task Force and the American Academy of Family Physicians conclude that the evidence is insufficient to recommend for or against routine screening.[3,4] Similarly, there is insufficient evidence to recommend for or against screening for thyroid dysfunction in pregnancy.[3,5] Rather, the AACE and ATA recommend aggressive case finding based on an individual's risk profile.[3]

Thyroid Physiology

The thyroid gland produces three hormones: calcitonin, thyroxine (T_4), and triiodothyronine (T_3). Calcitonin regulates calcium metabolism. T_3 and T_4 are considered to be the "thyroid hormones"; both are synthesized within thyroglobulin, a glycoprotein in the thyroid gland. Uptake of iodine (a substrate essential for the production of both T_3 and T_4) into thyroglobulin is facilitated by the enzyme thyroperoxidase. The production of T_3 is also dependent on synthesis by tissue outside of the thyroid gland. Approximately 80% of T_3 is formed by deionization of T_4 in the kidney, liver, muscle, brain, and other tissues in the body.[6] Both T_4 and T_3 are stored

Figure 13-1 Thyroid physiology.

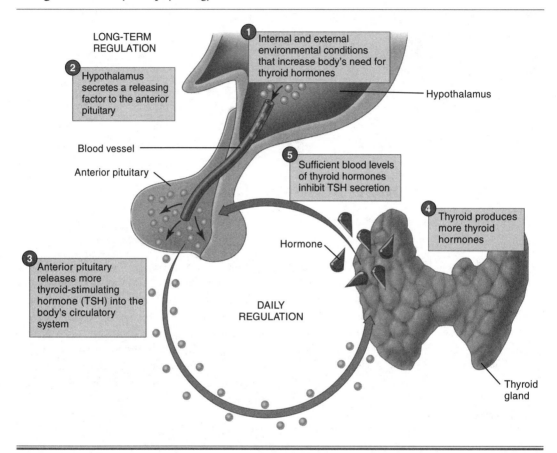

in thyroglobulin and released as needed into the peripheral circulation.

Once in the serum, T_3 and T_4 are bound by three proteins; about 75% to T_4-binding globulin. Unbound thyroid hormones, freely floating in the bloodstream, are the portion of the hormones that have clinical impact. Because greater than 99% of T_3 and T_4 are bound to these proteins, this system ensures that there is always a sufficient amount of hormone in reserve to meet the changing metabolic needs of the body.

The production of T_3 and T_4 is regulated by a finely tuned feedback loop.[6] Thyrotropin-releasing hormone (TRH) is produced in the hypothalamus and stimulates the release of thyroid-stimulating hormone (TSH) from the anterior pituitary. TSH in turn stimulates the production and release of T_3 and T_4. Higher levels of circulating T_3 and T_4 suppress the release of TSH from the pituitary both directly and indirectly, by decreasing the release of TRH from the hypothalamus. **Figure 13-1** depicts the interrelationships between key hormones involved in the feedback loop regulating the production and release of thyroid hormones.

Clinical Presentation

Unfortunately, thyroid dysfunction is easily missed. Thyroid hormones influence physiologic function throughout the body; symptoms can be numerous and nonspecific. Women with thyroid dysfunction may notice changes in their skin, bowel function, energy level, mood, appetite, sleep cycle, and menstruation. Similarly, on examination, the provider may notice changes in the skin and nails, tachycardia, enlarged or asymmetrical thyroid gland, exophthalmos, or diplopia, among other findings. Further, while most cases of thyroid dysfunction are due to autoimmune processes, changes in thyroid function can be caused by underlying systemic diseases, as an aftermath of surgery, or precipitated by the use of certain medications. Consequently, a comprehensive evaluation is needed to distinguish among the possibilities.

History, Physical, and Laboratory Evaluation

The nonspecific nature of most signs and symptoms associated with thyroid dysfunction requires a comprehensive evaluation for accurate diagnosis. See **Table 13-1** for a description of common symptoms, physical findings, and laboratory findings associated with hypothyroidism and hyperthyroidism.

History

The history should focus on the evolution of symptoms and, even more importantly, the presence or absence of risk factors associated with thyroid disease. Greater risk for developing hypothyroidism is associated with being elderly, having

another autoimmune disorder such as diabetes, having a family member with the disease, or being female. Use of certain medications, treatment with radiation, or surgical treatment for hyperthyroidism, thyroid cancer, or thyroid nodule can damage the thyroid and disrupt normal function. The presence or absence of risk factors and data elicited through the history focus the physical examination and laboratory assessment.

Physical

A comprehensive head-to-toe examination is needed, because all bodily systems are affected by thyroid dysfunction. Physical changes associated with thyroid disease, particularly with hypothyroidism, are usually absent unless thyroid function is severely impaired. Physical changes due to hyperthyroidism are more obvious and include tachycardia, widened pulse pressure, weight loss, and changes in the appearance of the eyes. An enlarged or asymmetric thyroid gland, the presence of a nodule, or thyroid tenderness may be detected on physical examination. However, in many cases thyroid dysfunction occurs in the presence of a normal physical examination.

Laboratory/Imaging

The specific tests used to evaluate thyroid conditions depend on the underlying reason for testing. A TSH level is all that is necessary for screening for either hypothyroidism or hyperthyroidism. Using a full thyroid panel is expensive and does not increase the likelihood of detecting disease in asymptomatic individuals. Neither is testing for antithyroid antibodies necessary, because serum antibodies are found in nearly 20% of all women over the age of 50 and are not indicative of active disease.[7] Consequently, authorities recommend choosing the fewest and least expensive testing options for screening and advise reserving the use of more extensive testing for evaluating abnormal TSH levels. **Table 13-2** describes patterns

Table 13-1 Signs and Symptoms of Hypothyroidism and Hyperthyroidism

Condition	History	Physical	Laboratory
Hypothyroidism	Fatigue	Goiter	EKG: Prolonged QT interval
	Cold intolerance	Weight gain	Anemia
	Hoarse voice	Slowed reflexes	
	Dry skin and hair	Macroglossia	
	Weight gain	Bruising	
	Sleep apnea	Bradycardia	
	Infertility	Mild hypertension	
	Miscarriage	Narrow pulse pressure	
	Impaired memory	Yellow hue to skin	
	Constipation	Nonpitting edema	
	Depression	Coarse hair and skin	
	Myalgia/arthralgia	Thin, brittle nails	
	Irregular menses		
Hyperthyroidism	Weight loss	Tachycardia	Anemia
	Diarrhea	Atrial fibrillation	Hypokalemia
	Dysphagia	Widened pulse pressure	
	Muscle weakness	Enlarged thyroid	
	Depression	Thyroid nodule	
	Anxiety	Thyroid thrill/bruit	
	Insomnia	Hyperreflexia	
		Osteoporosis	
		Proptosis	
		Exophthalmos	
		Warm, moist, smooth skin	

of thyroid function tests associated with different thyroid conditions.

If the TSH is abnormal on screening, further evaluation is needed. The first tests to order are a free T_4 level and a repeat TSH. A low free T_4 and a high TSH indicate overt hypothyroidism. Normal free T_4 and an elevated TSH are seen with subclinical hypothyroidism. The opposite pattern is seen in hyperthyroidism. Overt hyperthyroidism is present when the free T_4 is high and the TSH is low. In subclinical hyperthyroidism, the free T_4 is normal and the TSH is low.

Some authorities also recommend testing for thyroid antibodies based on the results of the free T_4 and TSH. The thyroid antibodies include antithyroglobulin antibodies (TgAb),

Table 13-2 Expected Laboratory Findings with the Major Categories
of Thyroid Disease

Diagnosis	TSH	Free T$_4$	Free T$_3$
Central hypothyroidism	Low*	Low	Low/normal
Overt hypothyroidism	Elevated	Low	Low to high
Subclinical hypothyroidism	Elevated	Normal	Normal
Euthyroid	Normal	Normal	Normal
Subclinical hyperthyroidism	Low	Normal	Normal
Overt hyperthyroidism	Low	High	High

*May also be normal or slightly elevated

antimicrosomal/thyroid peroxidase antibodies (TPOAb), and TSH receptor antibodies (TSHRAb). Both TgAb and TPOAb attack thyroglobulin and destroy thyroid tissue, reducing the ability of the thyroid to release a sufficient amount of thyroid hormones. TSHRAb can be either a TSH agonist or antagonist.[3] Both TSHRAb and TPOAb can be elevated in autoimmune causes of hypo- and hyperthyroidism. However, TPOAb levels are more consistently present and higher in autoimmune hypothyroidism (i.e., Hashimoto's disease) than in autoimmune hyperthyroidism (i.e., Graves' disease). In contrast, TSHRAb is more likely to be present and at higher levels in Graves' disease than in Hashimoto's.[8] Consequently, TSHRAb may be ordered if hyperthyroidism is suspected, whereas TPOAb is ordered if hypothyroidism is suspected.[3,8] In overt hypothyroidism, elevated TPOAb values confirm that the underlying cause is Hashimoto's disease.[3] Elevated levels of TPOAb in individuals with subclinical hypothyroidism indicate a significantly higher risk of future progression to clinical disease. Higher levels of TPOAb are also associated with higher risk of infertility and recurrent miscarriage even if TSH and free T$_4$ are normal.

Some, but not all authorities, recommend testing for elevated TPOAb in these situations.[3]

If the underlying cause of thyroid dysfunction is unclear, then ordering total T$_3$ and T$_4$ tests to obtain a T$_4$/T$_3$ ratio may be helpful. Because more T$_3$ is synthesized than T$_4$ in a hyperactive gland, the ratio (ng/mcg) is usually > 20 in Graves' disease and toxic nodular goiter, and < 20 in painless or postpartum thyroiditis.[9] Rarely, hyperthyroidism is due to T$_3$ toxicosis, a condition in which free T$_3$ levels are high, but free T$_4$ levels are normal.[10] Subclinical hyperthyroidism can be confirmed if both free T$_3$ and free T$_4$ values are normal when TSH values are high.

Results on thyroid function tests may also suggest central hypothyroidism, which is a very rare cause. Central hypothyroidism should be considered if a woman has a history of known pituitary or hypothalamus disease, a mass in the pituitary, or symptoms of other hormonal imbalances. In central hypothyroidism, the free T$_4$ is low or low to normal, but the TSH result can be variable. A low free T$_4$ and low TSH are strongly associated with central hypothyroidism, but in some cases the TSH can be normal or slightly elevated (up to 10 mIU/L). Additional testing may clarify the presentation. Because central hypothyroidism is associated with hypothalamic or pituitary conditions, low levels of gonadotropins and other pituitary hormones suggest central hypothyroidism. In addition, the absence of TPOAb rules out autoimmune causes of hypothyroidism.

Other tests may be needed to evaluate hyperthyroidism, goiter, or thyroid nodule; the specific test(s) needed will depend on the findings of the physical exam and the results of thyroid function tests. These additional tests may include a radioiodine uptake scan, an ultrasound of the thyroid, or a fine-needle aspiration.

Findings on a radioiodine uptake scan can be used to distinguish between the two underlying pathways leading to hyperthyroidism: 1) increased production of thyroid hormones seen with such conditions as Graves' disease, toxic adenoma, toxic multinodular goiter, or cancer and 2) damage to the thyroid from infection or inflammation, which results in the excessive release of preformed thyroid hormones. Specific findings suggest different etiologies: 1) focal areas of increased and decreased uptake are associated with toxic multinodular goiter, 2) focal increased uptake is seen in toxic adenoma, 3) diffuse increased uptake is seen in Graves' disease, and 4) low or nearly absent uptake suggests conditions like thyroiditis or excess intake of thyroid replacement medication. The use of radioiodine uptake scan is contraindicated in pregnant and breastfeeding women.[9] A safer option in these situations is to measure TSHRAb levels, which have a sensitivity of 90% in the detection of Graves' disease.[8] Alternatively, the ratio of total T_4 to T_3 is another safe option in pregnant and breastfeeding women.[11]

Sonograms are particularly helpful in the evaluation of suspected structural changes in the thyroid such as a goiter or nodule. Suspicious findings for cancer seen on ultrasound include nodule size > 2 cm, microcalcifications, and solid composition.[12] If suspicious findings are seen on a sonogram, tissue samples are obtained via fine-needle

aspiration. Results are used to determine if cancer is present and to direct the treatment course.[12]

Hypothyroidism

Prevalence

The exact prevalence of hypothyroidism has been difficult to quantify for several reasons. First, rates vary significantly among populations. In one study carried out in Colorado (N = 25,862), 9.5% of subjects at a state fair were found to have elevated TSH levels[13] compared to 7.5% of women and 2.8% of men in a longitudinal study in England.[14] Variations in the prevalence do not appear to be fully explained by iodine intake. For instance, one area of endemic iodine deficiency reported rates of hypothyroidism as high as 17%,[15] while another noted a rate of only 2.1%.[16] TSH values also appear to vary by age and race/ethnicity, with TSH levels found to be higher in older individuals and in non-Hispanic White compared to Black adults.[3,17] Secondly, the sensitivity of the assays used to detect disease has improved significantly over time. Lastly, the definition of normal thyroid function has also differed among studies. Various studies have used upper limits ranging from 4.1 mIU/L[18,19] to 4.5 mIU/L,[20] 5.1 mIU/L,[13] and 6 mIU/L.[14] Current guidelines from the ATA and AACE place the upper limit of normal of TSH at 4.1 mIU/L.[3]

Etiology

Hypothyroidism can be classified as primary or secondary (also called central hypothyroidism). **Table 13-3** provides the differential diagnoses for hypothyroidism. Primary hypothyroidism is the result of conditions that impair the thyroid's ability to synthesize or release thyroid hormones. These conditions include insufficient iodine intake, chronic autoimmune thyroiditis

Table 13-3 Differential Diagnosis of Hypothyroidism

Primary Hypothyroidism
Chronic autoimmune thyroiditis
  Goitrous
  Atrophic
Transient hypothyroidism
  Subacute lymphocytic thyroiditis
  Subacute granulomatous thyroiditis
  Postpartum thyroiditis
  Subtotal thyroidectomy
  Post-radiation therapy for Graves' disease
  Post-viral subacute thyroiditis
Iatrogenic
  Post-thyroidectomy
  Radioiodine therapy or external radiation
Iodine deficiency or excess
Infiltrative diseases
  Fibrous thyroiditis
  Hemochromatosis
  Sarcoidosis
Drugs
  Lithium
  Amiodarone
  Interferon-alpha
  Perchlorate
  Antiretroviral therapy

Secondary Hypothyroidism
Pituitary disease
Hypothalamic disease
Other causes
  Generalized thyroid hormone resistance
  Recovery from severe illness
  Untreated primary adrenal insufficiency
  Depression
  Amyloidosis
  Assay error due to interfering substances
  Overtreatment of overt hyperthyroidism

(Hashimoto's disease), postpartum thyroiditis, iatrogenic causes such as thyroidectomy, anticancer treatments or medication use, and congenital hypothyroidism. Insufficient iodine intake is unlikely in the US population, where the 2007–2008 National Health and Nutrition Examination Survey (NHANES) found average urinary iodine levels to be adequate across all populations (> 150 mg/L), except among pregnant women, whose iodine requirement is higher (> 220 mg/L).[21] Some medications can decrease TSH secretion (i.e., dopamine, glucocorticoids, metformin, and opiates), decrease thyroid hormone secretion (i.e., lithium), or increase thyroid hormone metabolism (i.e., phenobarbital, rifampin, or phenytoin).[6] Congenital hypothyroidism is seen in infants born with thyroid aplasia or hypoplasia or other disorders associated with defective synthesis of thyroid hormones. By far the most common causes of hypothyroidism in the United States are autoimmune processes. Therefore, it is not surprising that rates of hypothyroidism are higher among women with diabetes, pernicious anemia, rheumatoid arthritis, and lupus as well as other autoimmune disorders.[3]

Both overt and subclinical autoimmune hypothyroidism are commonly seen in women, especially as they age. Of the two, overt hypothyroidism is less common, occurring in approximately 0.3% to 0.4% of the general population, compared to subclinical hypothyroidism, which affects 4% to 8.5% of the US population without known thyroid diseases.[3,13,20] Subclinical hypothyroidism may progress to overt hypothyroidism over time, but rates of progression are debated and vary from 2% to 5% per year. Risk of progression to overt disease is highest in those with thyroid antibodies and higher TSH values.[22] While the designation of normal thyroid values can vary slightly by laboratory and authority, the generally accepted definition of overt hypothyroidism is having a subnormal free T_4 and a TSH value of greater than 10 mIU/L.[3] Subclinical hypothyroidism is defined as having an elevated serum TSH and a normal free T_4 concentration.[3]

Hypothyroidism can also be a result of secondary causes, conditions that affect the pituitary gland and hypothalamus itself.[3] Damage to the pituitary reduces its ability to produce TRH, which results in a downstream effect of limiting the release of TSH from the hypothalamus. Likewise, direct damage to the hypothalamus also results in lower levels of TSH. Lower TSH levels, from whatever cause, result in less stimulation to the thyroid gland, lower levels of thyroid hormones, and the development of hypothyroidism. Examples of conditions associated with secondary or central causes of hypothyroidism include: pituitary adenoma, surgery or radiation treatment of tumors in the pituitary or hypothalamus, sarcoidosis and other autoimmune diseases, subarachnoid hemorrhage, and Sheehan's syndrome, which results in necrosis in the pituitary gland from severe postpartum hemorrhage.[23] A careful history should focus on identifying risk factors for hypothalamic-pituitary dysfunction, because laboratory findings can be similar in central and subclinical hypothyroidism. Central hypothyroidism is confirmed if free T_4 and TSH values are both low. However, central hypothyroidism can also be present if free T_4 levels are low and TSH values are normal or mildly elevated.[3]

Presentation

Symptoms of hypothyroidism correspond to disease severity. Because serum free T_4 is normal in subclinical hypothyroidism, individuals with subclinical hypothyroidism are generally asymptomatic and feel clinically well. Overt hypothyroidism is associated with a wide variety of symptoms. Symptoms are less obvious when the loss of thyroid hormone occurs gradually, but can be severe and numerous in those with profound or acute loss of thyroid function such as after thyroidectomy or radioiodine therapy. For example, carpal tunnel syndrome, sleep apnea, pituitary hyperplasia (with or without hyperprolactinemia and galactorrhea), and hyponatremia are rarely seen in insidious forms of hypothyroidism, but can be seen within a few weeks in individuals with an abrupt and profound loss of thyroid function.[3]

The most severe presentation of hypothyroidism is myxedema coma, which presents with hypothermia, hypotension, hypoglycemia, and mental confusion or coma. It can be life threatening, with associated mortality rates of 30% to 60%, and therefore requires timely recognition and treatment.[6] Myxedema has been reported to be associated with prolongation of the QT interval and torsades de pointes and gastrointestinal bleeding from coagulopathy. Precipitants of myxedema include infection or sepsis, strokes, congestive heart failure, trauma, some medications, metabolic disturbances, and exposure to cold ambient air. While extremely rare, it is more likely to occur in older women over the age of 60.[6]

Treatment

On the whole, treatment for overt hypothyroidism is quite effective and safe; the mainstay of treatment remains levothyroxine sodium (Synthroid). Treatment with thyroid replacement is usually lifelong. There is no agreement as to the ideal method for initiating treatment for overt hypothyroidism. Some specialists have advocated that women with newly diagnosed hypothyroidism should be started on a daily dose of 25 to 50 mcg of levothyroxine, while others have recommended that a higher replacement dose be initiated, especially if the patient is young and without heart disease.[7] Adverse effects of replacement with levothyroxine include nervousness, atrial fibrillation, and, in about one-fifth of patients with angina pectoris, exacerbation of chest pain. Generally, those with ischemic cardiovascular disease and those over the age of 60 should be started at a lower dose to prevent these side effects.[6]

Use of levothyroxine requires periodic monitoring. Doses should be slowly increased until the patient is euthyroid by laboratory standards. The reference range for a normal TSH level should be based on a third-generation TSH assay. If this is not available, the normal TSH range is considered to be between 0.45 mIU/L and 4.12 mIU/L.[3] TSH levels take about 4 weeks to adjust after a dose change, so in general it is not useful to test more frequently than every 4 to 8 weeks.[7] Once euthyroidism is achieved, TSH levels only need to be repeated annually.[3] Of note is that there can be variations in the bioavailability of the drug in different products produced by different manufacturers. Over- or undertreatment can result if levothyroxine formulations made by different manufacturers are interchanged.[6] This problem can be minimized if the patient understands that pharmacies may stock products from different companies and fills her prescription only at her primary pharmacy, requesting that a single product be provided.

The advisability of treating subclinical hypothyroidism has been debated over the past several years without consensus being reached.[24] Subclinical hypothyroidism with TSH levels greater than 10 mIU/L is associated with cardiovascular morbidity and mortality, but treatment does not appear to reduce morbidity or overall mortality. Unfortunately, the quality of the research is poor, making it difficult to reach reliable conclusions. Therefore, most authorities recommend repeating thyroid function tests periodically and withholding treatment if TSH levels are less than 10 mIU/L.[24,25] However, the AACE and ATA recommend more aggressive treatment for women planning a pregnancy or currently pregnant. Untreated subclinical hypothyroidism can be monitored in nonpregnant women by screening with a free T_4 and TSH every 6 months for the first 2 years and yearly thereafter if lab values indicate no disease progression.[24] Periodic monitoring with TPOAb is unnecessary, because it has no clinical utility other than being indicative of higher risk for disease progression.[24]

Hyperthyroidism

Like hypothyroidism, hyperthyroidism is also divided into two types: overt and subclinical.

Subclinical hyperthyroidism is the more common condition, affecting approximately 0.7% to 1.8% of the US population.[26] Both types present with low TSH levels. However, in overt hyperthyroidism, the free T_4 level is elevated, and in subclinical hyperthyroidism it is normal.

Etiology

Multiple physiologic pathways can result in excessive circulating thyroid hormones; these include 1) inappropriate stimulation of the thyroid gland; 2) activation of thyroid synthesis and secretion; 3) excessive release of preformed hormones due to autoimmune, infectious, chemical, or mechanical damage; and 4) exposure to excess thyroid hormones from endogenous or exogenous sources.[9] By far, the most common cause of hyperthyroidism is Graves' disease. Graves' disease is an autoimmune disorder in which TSHRAb binds with the TSH receptor leading to increased production of thyroid hormones and increased growth and vascularity of the thyroid gland.[10] Noncancerous nodules found in toxic adenomas or in toxic multinodular goiters can produce excess hormones. Pituitary adenomas can also lead to high TSH levels and greater production of thyroid hormones. Inflammation or infection such as seen in thyroiditis can damage the thyroid and release preformed thyroid hormones. Lastly, some medications such as amiodarone, lithium, interferon alpha, and interleukin-2 affect the thyroid and are associated with higher levels of thyroid hormones. **Table 13-4** lists causes of hyperthyroidism.

Presentation

Like hypothyroidism, subclinical hyperthyroidism is usually asymptomatic. Overt hyperthyroidism can present with few or no symptoms, but it can also be life threatening if thyrotoxicosis is severe, as in thyroid storm. Symptoms such as

Table 13-4 Differential Diagnosis
of Hyperthyroidism

Primary Hyperthyroidism
    Hyperthyroid goiter (Graves' disease)
    Multinodular hyperthyroid goiter (toxic multi-
        nodular goiter)
    Autonomous hyperfunctioning nodule (Plum-
        mer's disease)

Secondary Hyperthyroidism
    Transient hyperthyroidism (e.g., critical illness)
    Pregnancy
        High human chorionic gonadotropin
            (hCG) levels (first 4 months' pregnancy)
        Molar pregnancy
        Transient hyperthyroidism of hyperemesis
            gravidarum (THHG)
    Postpartum thyroiditis (particularly in patients
        with diabetes mellitus)
    Struma ovarii (thyroid tissue within dermoid
        tumors and teratomas)
    TSH-induced hyperthyroidism
        TSH-secreting pituitary adenomas
        Partial resistance to feedback (defect in T_3
            receptor)

Other Causes
    Medications inhibiting T_4 to T_3 conversion
        (i.e., amiodarone)
    Iodine-induced hyperthyroidism
    Recovery from hyperthyroidism
    Drugs
        Dopamine and glucocorticoids
    Thyrotoxicosis factitia
        Over-replacement/overuse of thyroid
            hormone
        Consumption of beef contaminated with
            bovine thyroid gland (rare)

anxiety and tachycardia are more pronounced in those with severe disease and in those with a larger goiter or who are of younger age.[9]

Physical examination findings can suggest specific etiologies. For example, a tender thyroid can suggest subacute thyroiditis. Subacute thyroiditis often develops after a viral infection and appears to be associated with adenovirus, echovirus, influenza, coxsackie virus, and mumps virus.[10] Patients may also report pain that radiates to the neck or jaw, sore throat, or dysphagia. Usually, this condition resolves in 6 to 12 months. A single nodule may be seen in thyroid adenoma, whereas multiple nodules are found in multinodular goiter. The presence of any nodule, whether single or multiple, must raise the suspicion of thyroid cancer. Thyroid storm should be suspected if hyperthyroidism is affecting multiple systems. Symptoms can affect the cardiovascular (tachycardia, arrhythmias, hypotension), neurologic (agitation, delirium, stupor, coma), and gastrointestinal (nausea, diarrhea) systems. Fever and hepatic failure can also occur. The greater the number of symptoms, the greater the likelihood that thyroid storm is occurring. Prompt treatment is needed to prevent morbidity and mortality. Thyroid storm can be triggered by an abrupt cessation of antithyroid medication, infections, and following treatment of hyperthyroidism with radioiodine iodine therapy.[9]

Treatment

Untreated hyperthyroidism is associated with weight loss, osteoporosis, atrial fibrillation, embolism, and rarely with cardiac collapse and death.[9] Consequently, hyperthyroidism is nearly always treated or closely monitored if treatment is not thought to be immediately necessary. Like hypothyroidism, hyperthyroidism can be due to multiple etiologies; therefore, the exact treatment will depend on the underlying cause. While treatment may vary, some individuals with more extreme symptoms, no matter what the underlying cause, may need supportive care to manage symptoms until thyroid hormone levels decline with treatment. Beta-adrenergic medications should be offered to those with symptomatic thyrotoxicosis and those with underlying cardiac disease or resting heart rate above 90 beats per minute.[9]

By far, the most common cause of overt hypothyroidism is Graves' disease. The treatment options for Graves' disease in nonpregnant women includes medications, usually propylthiouracil (PTU) or methimazole (MMI) (Tapazole); surgery; or radioablation. Both PTU and MMI inhibit the production of T_4 and T_3. PTU inhibits iodine and peroxidase from interacting with thyroglobulin and forming T_4 and T_3. MMI blocks oxidation of iodine in the thyroid and blocks iodine incorporation into tyrosine to form T_4 and T_3.[10] Unfortunately, relapse can occur. Radioiodine, administered orally, usually results in euthyroidism in 6 to 18 weeks. Surgery should be reserved for the rare patient who is allergic to both PTU and MMI, is poorly compliant with medications, or who has large goiters causing difficulty swallowing.[10] There are two general options: subtotal or total thyroidectomy. Hypothyroidism can develop after any of these treatments for hyperthyroidism, necessitating ongoing assessment with thyroid function tests.

Some of these same treatments are also used in the management of other conditions resulting in hyperthyroidism. Thyroid adenoma and multinodular goiter can be treated with radioactive iodine ablation of the thyroid or thyroidectomy. Antithyroid medications are not an option in the treatment of these conditions, because relapse is almost certain once the medications are discontinued.[10] Subacute and postpartum thyroiditis generally resolve over time; treatment for these conditions is supportive.

Thyroid Nodule

Women who present with a thyroid nodule need prompt evaluation, because 5% or more of nodules are due to thyroid cancer.[12,27] Risk factors associated with thyroid cancer include a family history of thyroid cancer, history of radiation to the head and neck, and being younger than 30 or older than 60 years. Benign causes of thyroid nodules include multinodular goiter, cysts, and adenomas. The workup commonly includes a TSH and thyroid ultrasound. Depending on the results of the initial workup, either a radionuclide thyroid scan or a fine-needle aspiration may be performed.[27] Referral to an endocrinologist or ear nose, and throat (ENT) specialist is warranted for the management and follow up of a known or suspected thyroid nodule.

Pregnancy

The definitions used to categorize thyroid disease are similar, but not identical, in pregnant and nonpregnant women. Because of hormonal changes in pregnancy, the free T_4 is slightly less reliable, and normal TSH levels decline to a small degree. The AACE and ATA recommend defining thyroid disease in pregnancy based on trimester-specific values. These trimester-specific cutoffs for TSH levels are slightly lower than those used in nonpregnant women (first trimester: 0.1–2.5 mIU/L; second trimester, 0.2–3.0 mIU/L; third trimester, 0.3–3.0 mIU/L).[11] As in nonpregnant women, an elevated TSH and low free T_4 indicate the presence of hypothyroidism. However, hypothyroidism can also be present even with apparently normal free T_4 values during pregnancy. Therefore, the AACE and the ATA consider pregnant women with a normal free T_4 and a TSH level between 2.5 and 10 mIU/L as having subclinical hypothyroidism and those with a TSH value of greater than 10 mIU/L as having overt hypothyroidism in pregnancy. Other experts maintain that the free T_4 levels must be low in pregnancy to be diagnosed with overt hypothyroidism (defined by these authors as having a low free T_4 and a TSH value of $\geq$ 3 mIU/L).[28]

Treatment of subclinical hypothyroidism in pregnancy is controversial. The AACE and ATA recommend more aggressive treatment in pregnancy than do other authorities; specifically, they recommend *treating* women with subclinical hypothyroidism who test positive for TPOAbs.[11] They also suggest *considering* treatment in women whose TSH level exceeds trimester-specific recommendations as outlined earlier,[3] as well as to *consider* treatment in women with normal TSH levels who test positive for TPOAbs, particularly if they have a history of miscarriage.[3] However, the American College of Obstetricians and Gynecologists (ACOG) does not recommend treatment under these conditions, even for those with hyperemesis or mildly enlarged thyroid glands.[29] These different interpretations result from the lack of good evidence to determine the best approach to care.[28] Unfortunately, the evidence is inconsistent. Some studies, but not all, demonstrate associations between subclinical hypothyroidism and poorer perinatal outcomes. In addition, it has not yet been demonstrated that treating subclinical hypothyroidism results in better outcomes. However, all authorities agree that women with untreated subclinical hypothyroidism should be monitored periodically throughout pregnancy and treated in the rare event that subclinical disease progresses to overt disease.[3,28]

Overt hypothyroidism is always treated during pregnancy, because untreated or undertreated disease is associated with increased risk of miscarriage, intrauterine demise, low birth weight, and placental abruption.[7,11] Women with known hypothyroidism should remain on their usual dose, at least in early pregnancy. Dosage of levothyroxine often needs to be increased as the pregnancy continues, making it important to check thyroid function tests regularly throughout pregnancy. During pregnancy, T_4-binding globulin (TBG) levels increase, as do total T_4 and T_3 levels. The TSH level remains relatively unaffected and is used to monitor whether the dose of levothyroxine is adequate in both pregnant and nonpregnant women. Both the AACE and ATA recommend checking TSH levels every 4 weeks in early

pregnancy and then obtaining another TSH between 26 and 32 weeks of pregnancy. The goal is to keep free T_4 values normal and the upper limit of the TSH value < 2.5mIU/L in the first trimester, < 3.0 mIU/L in the second trimester, and < 3.5 mIU/L in the third trimester.[3] These experts also recommend measuring TSHRAb levels using a sensitive assay in hypothyroid pregnant patients with a history of Graves' disease who were treated with radioactive iodine or thyroidectomy prior to pregnancy, initially in the first trimester and repeated between 20 and 26 weeks' gestation if the TSHRAb was elevated initially. Elevated TSHRAbs are associated with increased risk of developing fetal or neonatal Graves' disease.[3]

The treatment of subclinical hyperthyroidism is not recommended in pregnancy. There is clear evidence that antithyroid medications can cause harm and no evidence that treatment provides any benefits. Further, many women have transient elevations of thyroid hormones due to the surge in human chorionic gonadotropin (hCG) seen in the first trimester; these changes generally resolve by mid-pregnancy. Gestational hyperthyroidism occurs in 1% to 3% of all pregnancies and is more common in women with conditions associated with higher than average hCG levels such as hyperemesis gravidarum, hydatidiform mole, and multiple pregnancies.[11]

Overt hyperthyroidism is associated with increased risk of miscarriage, prematurity, low birth weight, intrauterine growth restriction, stillbirth, thyroid storm, and maternal congestive heart failure.[11] Because of these complications, overt hyperthyroidism is almost always treated in pregnancy, although the exact treatment chosen for a particular woman will depend on the severity of the presentation and underlying cause. Graves' disease is by far the most common etiology of overt hyperthyroidism in pregnancy and occurs in 0.1% to 1% of pregnancies.[11] Rarely, hyperthyroidism is due to toxic multinodular goiter, toxic adenoma, or factitious thyrotoxicosis.

Graves' disease can be newly diagnosed in pregnancy or be a recurrence of previous disease. The preferred treatment approach in pregnancy is the use of antithyroid medications: PTU and MMI. The use of MMI is associated with a greater risk of aplasia cutis and "MMI embryopathy" that includes choanal or esophageal atresia and dysmorphic facies. While these effects have not been seen with the use of PTU, PTU carries a higher risk of developing hepatotoxicity. Recommended treatments are trimester specific, with PTU being the preferred choice in the first trimester and MMI being preferred for use in the second and third trimesters of pregnancy.[11] Adjunctive use of beta-adrenergic blocking agents, such as propranolol, may provide relief from the most distressing symptoms of hyperthyroidism: increased heart rate, elevated systolic blood pressure, muscle weakness, tremor, and irritability. In most cases, the drug can be stopped in 2 to 6 weeks as thyroid hormone levels become normalized.[11] Both MMI and PTU cross through the placenta to the fetus. To lessen the possibility that fetal hypothyroidism might develop from exposure to these drugs, the goal in therapy is to maintain the maternal free T_4 at or just above the upper limit of the normal range.[11] Maternal free T_4 and TSH should be monitored every 2 weeks when therapy is initiated and every 4 to 6 weeks once target laboratory values are achieved to ensure that the mother is not being overtreated. For some women, TSH values will remain undetectable throughout pregnancy despite treatment.

The fetus exposed to maternal hyperthyroidism in pregnancy is also at risk for thyroid problems during and after pregnancy. Risks include the development of hypothyroidism from exposure to maternal antithyroid medications, transient central hypothyroidism from exposure to high levels of maternal thyroid hormones, or hyperthyroidism, particularly if the mother has high levels of serum TSHRAbs. TSHRAb levels should be measured between 20 and 24 weeks. A value of $\geq$ 3 times normal indicates that the fetus is at high risk of developing hyperthyroidism. Fetal hyperthyroidism affects 1% to 5% of infants whose mothers have Graves' disease in pregnancy and is associated with higher rates of fetal and neonatal morbidity and mortality if untreated. Fetal hyperthyroidism should be suspected if any of the following findings are noted during fetal surveillance: sustained fetal tachycardia > 170 beats per minute, intrauterine growth restriction, fetal goiter, signs of congestive heart failure, or fetal hydrops. Because hyperthyroidism poses significant risks for the fetus, ongoing consultation with a fetal medicine physician is mandatory.[11]

Thyroid nodules are uncommon in pregnancy but, if found, require careful evaluation. Rarely, they are associated with thyroid cancer. Findings that increase the suspicion of cancer include a personal or family history of thyroid cancer, radiation treatment to the head or neck during childhood, persistent cough, or dysphonia. A thyroid ultrasound is the most accurate test for detecting thyroid nodules and monitoring their growth and size. Several findings on ultrasound can suggest cancer; these include hypoechoic pattern, irregular margins, chaotic intranodular vascular spots, nodules that are taller than they are wide, and microcalcifications.[11] Nodules that are large or with suspicious ultrasound findings require further evaluation with a fine-needle aspiration. Radioiodine imaging, which is commonly used in evaluating thyroid nodules, is contraindicated in pregnancy, although use prior to 12 weeks' gestation does not appear to damage the fetal thyroid. If thyroid cancer is found, surgical treatment during pregnancy may or may not be recommended depending on the size, aggressiveness, and type of thyroid cancer. Generally, if treatment is needed for benign thyroid nodules, it is held off until after pregnancy, unless the nodule grows rapidly or compresses the adjacent tissue to such a degree to cause symptoms.

Postpartum

While Graves' disease is more common in pregnancy, postpartum thyroiditis is the most common cause of hyperthyroidism after childbirth.[11] It is an autoimmune disorder and is triggered by the immune changes associated with pregnancy. It is more common in women who test positive for TPOAbs and who have other autoimmune disorders. Postpartum thyroiditis is generally not treated because the course of the disease waxes and wanes. It presents initially with hyperthyroidism, followed by a period of hypothyroidism, before resolving within 1 year after the birth. Women are followed with thyroid function tests every 4 to 8 weeks in the first year and annually thereafter.[11] If women become symptomatic, beta-blockers can be used during the hyperthyroid phase and thyroid replacement during the hypothyroid phase. Consultation with an endocrinologist or other expert in the treatment of thyroid disease is recommended before treatment is initiated.

Postpartum thyroiditis can be confused with Graves' disease, which is the second most common cause of postpartum hyperthyroidism. Relapse rates in postpartum women who have recovered from Graves' disease have been reported to be greater than 80%, making the diagnosis a strong possibility in this group.[11] Several diagnostic clues can help distinguish these two entities. Specific physical findings such as goiter, exophthalmos, and bruit also suggest Graves' disease rather than postpartum thyroiditis. TSHRAb is almost always present in Graves' disease but not with postpartum thyroiditis. In addition, the radioiodine uptake results are either normal or elevated in Graves' disease and low in postpartum thyroiditis.[11] If Graves' disease is detected, then treatment with antithyroid medications is the preferred treatment option. There appears to be little risk that the infant will develop hypothyroidism from exposure to medications through breast milk, although the infant should be monitored periodically. Mothers should also take their antithyroid medications in divided doses immediately after breastfeeding.[11]

Parathyroid Disease

The four small parathyroid glands rest along the posterior aspect of the thyroid and function to regulate calcium metabolism. Calcium levels in the blood need to remain between 8.5 and 10.5 mg/dL for proper bone development and muscle and nerve function. Parathyroid hormone (PTH) acts as a continuous regulator of calcium concentration. When serum calcium concentrations decrease, PTH secretion increases with effects on bone resorption, calcium absorption from the intestines, and increased reabsorption in the kidney. Any abnormality in the feedback loop that maintains calcium-PTH homeostasis leads to hyperparathyroidism. This condition is the third most common of the endocrine disorders, following diabetes and thyroid disease. The incidence is highest among postmenopausal women, although in younger adults, there is gender parity.[30] Yeh and colleagues reported rates of 12–24 per 100,000 in a racially mixed population for all adults under age 50, with rates rising among women to 196/100,000 for those over 70 years.[31] Their study also reported rates higher among blacks or African Americans compared to Caucasians, and lower rates for Asians and Hispanics.[31]

Primary hyperparathyroidism is most commonly a result of a single adenoma (75–89%), hyperplasia (~6%), or carcinoma (1%).[30,32] Calcium deficiency, vitamin D deficiency, kidney failure and rare genetic disorders can also play a role in parathyroid disease, as can medications such as lithium and thiazide diuretics and radiation exposure to the head and neck.

Clinical Presentation

Primary hyperparathyroidism is commonly found on screening, when an elevated serum calcium is identified. An elevated or normal PTH level, coupled with elevated calcium (> 1 mg/dL above the normal limit), is diagnostic.[33] Most cases in the developed world are asymptomatic or exhibit only mild, nonspecific symptoms, such as fatigue, muscle weakness, mild cognitive impairment, or anxiety.[34] Kidney stones are associated with 4–15% of cases.[35] More severe disease is associated with progressive cardiac disease and higher cardiac mortality, and with recurrent nephrolithiasis.[36] Asymptomatic, mild hyperparathyroidism may remain stable for many years.

Included in the differential diagnosis, particularly for young adults, is familial benign hypocalciuric hypercalcemia, an autosomal dominant mutation. A careful family history for hypercalcemia and failed neck surgery suggests this diagnosis. Skeletal changes and nephrolithiasis are uncommon. Laboratory findings include decreased renal calcium/creatinine clearance ratio and normal or near normal PTH levels.[30]

Management

Evaluation of parathyroid disease includes assessment of serum calcium, renal function with 24-hour urine calcium and creatinine clearance, and vitamin D, as well as bone mineral density screening and renal ultrasound for stones. Ultrasound of the gland itself is not required for evaluation, but is important for localization of lesions prior to surgery.

All women diagnosed with or suspected of hyperparathyroidism should be referred to an endocrinologist; this is not an appropriate condition for management by women's health providers alone.

While there is no medical therapy that is curative, use of estrogen replacement, bisphosphonates, vitamin D and calcium replacement, and regular surveillance can be recommended for those with mild disease or who are not surgical candidates. Cinacalcet can be used for treatment of elevated calcium levels when bone density is normal. The definitive treatment when significant disease is present is removal of the affected gland or glands. Young age at onset, serum calcium > 1 mg/dL above normal, decreased creatinine glomerular filtration rate, and osteoporosis are indications for surgery. Cure rates of > 95% are reported, and complications are relatively rare.[33]

Adrenal Gland Disorders

The adrenal glands sit on top of each kidney and are composed of the cortex and medulla. The outer portion, or cortex, produces the corticosteroids: the glucocorticoids cortisol (hydrocortisone) and corticosterone, and the mineralocorticoid aldosterone. Glucocorticoid production is stimulated from the hypothalamus and pituitary, while the kidneys trigger mineralocorticoid release. The circadian cycle of cortisol synthesis in the adrenal cortex requires stimulation of adrenocorticotrophic hormone (ACTH) by corticotrophin-releasing hormone (CRH) in the hypothalamus, leading to stimulation of the adrenal by ACTH. Cortisol is responsible for maintaining blood pressure and cardiovascular function, slowing inflammatory responses and supporting metabolism. It is a key component in the human response to stress. Aldosterone regulates the sodium/potassium balance in the blood, which also supports blood pressure control. Small amounts of sex steroids are also secreted in the adrenal cortex. The inner medulla is responsible for production of epinephrine and norepinephrine in response to stress signals from the sympathetic nervous system. Among the significant diseases caused by malfunction of the adrenal glands, two are reviewed here, Addison's disease and Cushing's disease. Whenever either of these two conditions is diagnosed or suspected, immediate referral to an endocrinologist is necessary, as lifelong therapy will be required.

Adrenal Insufficiency

Addison's disease is the result of primary adrenal insufficiency, leading to decreased cortisol production. It occurs rarely, in about 4/100,000 individuals, with equal distribution between the sexes. Typically, it is the result of an auto-immune response that destroys adrenal function; it can occur as a single entity or as part of a more complex auto-immune syndrome.[37] A similar presentation occurs when the hypothalamic/pituitary stimulation of cortisol production fails, called secondary adrenal insufficiency. However, in Addison's disease aldosterone production is also decreased. Among the rarer causes of primary adrenal insufficiency are congenital adrenal hyperplasia, infection, and damage to or removal of the adrenal glands. Causes of secondary insufficiency include pituitary or hypothalamic tumors, infection, or injury. These will also produce other symptoms of damage to the hypothalamic-pituitary-adrenal (HPA) axis.[37]

Symptoms of adrenal insufficiency include: fatigue, weakness, anorexia, weight loss, nausea, vomiting, abdominal pain, diarrhea alternating with constipation, orthostatic hypotension, salt craving, hyponatremia, hyperkalemia, metabolic acidosis, depression, decreased cold tolerance, and (in primary insufficiency) hyperpigmentation or vitiligo. Women may experience ovarian insufficiency, with irregular menses and decreased libido.[37-39]

Diagnosis of Addison's disease is often delayed, as the symptoms, except for salt craving, are nonspecific. It is often not until a crisis occurs that a diagnosis is made.[40] Adrenal crisis is characterized by profound weakness, severe vomiting and diarrhea leading to dehydration; severe pain in the abdomen, lower back, or legs; peripheral vascular collapse; and kidney failure.[37,38]

When adrenal insufficiency is suspected based on clinical signs and symptoms, testing may include early morning serum ACTH, cortisol and electrolyte levels, or an ACTH stimulation test. When adrenal crisis is suspected, emergency treatment is initiated without delay for testing.[37] Pregnant women with unexplained nausea, fatigue, and hypotension should also be considered for screening.[41] The Endocrine Society Guidelines recommend the corticotropin stimulation test (CSH) as the definitive test, since it provides the most accurate diagnosis. However, it is typically ordered by an endocrinologist rather than as the first line.[41]

Management of adrenal insufficiency includes glucocorticoid treatment, usually with hydrocortisone, and for primary insufficiency, fludrocortisone. Dosing and dietary recommendations are required for those with shift work, strenuous exercise or other medical conditions that would be affected by steroid therapy, such as diabetes or hypertension. Illness or physical stress will affect dose requirements. Women with adrenal insufficiency should be educated regarding dosing alterations and should carry an emergency alert at all times (e.g., bracelet, card) regarding the possible need for stress dosing. Management is always directed by an endocrinologist or other professional experienced in the management of adrenal disease.[37]

Cushing's Syndrome

In contrast to Addison's disease, Cushing's syndrome results from excess glucocorticoid circulation, caused by loss of the daily circadian cycle of cortisol release. The cause may be endogenous, from injury to the HPA axis, or exogenous, from the administration of large and ongoing doses of steroids (e.g., for asthma or rheumatoid arthritis).[42] The latter cause is more commonly seen in clinical practice.[43] Pituitary adenomas are the cause of 70% of endogenous disease.[44] They are most common in women between the ages of 25 and 40.[42] Cushing's syndrome is classified as a rare disease, with an incidence of 1-1.5/100,000 individuals in the United States. However, the incidence appears to be rising, and the disease has been found to be more common than previously anticipated in some groups, including those with type 2 diabetes, hypertension, and osteoporosis.[44] Any case of hypercortisolism can be referred to as Cushing's syndrome; only those cases with pituitary abnormalities are properly called Cushing's disease.

Common symptoms on initial presentation include fatigue, depression, weight gain with central obesity, dyslipidemia, hypertension, and menstrual irregularity. The skin may thin and develop wide red-purple striae, particularly on the trunk and abdomen. In more advanced disease, facial rounding, limb wasting, hirsutism accompanied by male pattern baldness, diabetes, spontaneous bruising, fractures, and muscle weakness may be seen.[42,45]

Before screening for endogenous Cushing's disease, a medical history to exclude chronic steroid use as the cause of hypercortisolism is necessary. The Endocrine Society recommends screening only for individuals with less specific features such as hypertension or osteoporosis that are unexplained and for those with progressive symptoms. Diagnosis of endogenous disease is based on overnight urinary and salivary cortisol levels and dexamethasone suppression testing.[46] The Endocrine Society recommends selecting one of the three as the initial test, and referring those with positive findings, or those with negative findings and progressive symptoms, to be followed by an endocrinologist. Pregnant women should not have the dexamethasone suppression test as the initial screen.[46]

When Cushing's syndrome is diagnosed, immediate referral to an endocrinologist is indicated. Surgery and/or medication will be necessary. Effective treatment can at least partially reverse loss of bone mineral density and cognitive loss, but decreased quality of life and increased cardiovascular risk generally persist.[46]

References

1. Vanderpump MPJ. The epidemiology of thyroid disease. *Br Med Bull.* 2011;99(1):39-51.
2. American College of Obstetricians and Gynecologists. ACOG Practice Bulletin. Clinical management guidelines for obstetrician-gynecologists. Number 37. Thyroid disease in pregnancy. *Obstet Gynecol.* 2002;100(2):387-396.
3. Garber J, Garber R, Cobin H, Gharib J, Hennessey I, Klein J, et al. Clinical practice guidelines for hypothyroidism in adults: cosponsored by the American Association of Clinical Endocrinologists and the American Thyroid Association. *Thyroid.* 2012;22(12):1200-1235.
4. American Academy of Family Physicians (AAFP). Summary of recommendations for clinical preventive services. National Guideline Clearinghouse: 2013. Available at: https://www.guidelinecentral.com/summaries/summary-of-recommendations-for-clinical-preventive-services/. Accessed February 26, 2015.
5. Negro R, Schwartz A, Gismondi R, Tinelli A, Mangieri T, Stagnaro-Green A. Universal screening versus case finding for detection and treatment of thyroid hormonal dysfunction during pregnancy. *J Clin Endocrinol Metab.* 2010;95(4):1699-1707.
6. Dubbs SB, Spangler R. Hypothyroidism: causes, killers, and life-saving treatments. *Emerg Med Clin North Am.* 2014;32(2):303-317.
7. Almandoz JP, Gharib H. Hypothyroidism: etiology, diagnosis, and management. *Med Clin North Am.* 2012;96(2):203-221.
8. Galofré JC, Davies TF. Thyroid antibody measurements are becoming increasingly important in the evaluation and diagnosis of thyroid conditions. 2008. Available at: http://bmctoday.net/reviewofendo/2008/04/article.asp?f=review0408_08.php. Accessed April 6, 2016.
9. Bahn RS, Burch HB, Cooper DS, Garber JR, Greenlee MC, Klein I, et al. Hyperthyroidism and other causes of thyrotoxicosis: Management guidelines of the American Thyroid Association and American Association of Clinical Endocrinologists. *Thyroid.* 2011;21(6):593-646.

10. Nayak B, Hodak SP. Hyperthyroidism. *Endocrinol Metab Clin North Am.* 2007;36(3):617-656.

11. Stagnaro-Green A, Abalovich M, Alexander E, Azizi F, Mestman J, Negro R, et al. Guidelines of the American Thyroid Association for the diagnosis and management of thyroid disease during pregnancy and postpartum. *Thyroid.* 2011;21(10):1081-1125.

12. Smith-Bindman R, Lebda P, Feldstein VA, Sellami D, Goldstein RB, Brasic N, et al. Risk of thyroid cancer based on thyroid ultrasound imaging characteristics results of a population-based study. *JAMA Intern Med.* 2013;173(19):1788-1795.

13. Canaris G, Manowitz N, Mayor G, Ridgway E. The Colorado thyroid disease prevalence study. *Arch Intern Med.* 2000;160(4):526-534.

14. Tunbridge W, Evered D, Hall R, Appleton D, Brewis M, Clark F, et al. The spectrum of thyroid disease in a community: the Whickham survey. *Clin Endocrinol.* 1977;7:481-493.

15. Bara IN, Lamsal M, Koner B, Koirala S. Thyroid dysfunction in eastern Nepal. *Southeast Asian J Trop Med Public Health.* 2002;33(3):638-641.

16. Knudsen N, Jorgensen T, Rasmussen S, Christiansen E, Perrild H. The prevalence of thyroid dysfunction in a population with borderline iodine deficiency. *Clin Endocrinol.* 1999;51(3):361-367.

17. Yutaka A, Belin RM, Clickner R, Jeffries R, Phillips L, Mahaffey KR. Serum TSH and total T4 in the United States population and their association with participant characteristics: National Health and Nutrition Examination Survey (NHANES 1999–2002). *Thyroid.* 2007;17(12):1211-1223.

18. Lincoln S, Ke R, Kutteh W. Screening for hypothyroidism in infertile women. *J Reprod Med.* 1999;44(5):455-457.

19. Bjoro T, Holmen J, Kruger O, Midthjell K, Hunstad K, Schreiner T, et al. Prevalence of thyroid disease, thyroid dysfunction and thyroid peroxidase antibodies in a large, unselected population. The Health Study of Nord-Trondelag (HUNT). *Eur J Endocrinol.* 2000;143(5):639-647.

20. Hollowell JG, Staehling NW, Flanders WD, Hannon WH, Gunter EW, Spencer CA, et al. Serum TSH, T4, and thyroid antibodies in the United States population (1988 to 1994): National Health and Nutrition Examination Survey (NHANES III). *J Clin Endocrinol Metab.* 2002;87(2):489-499.

21. Caldwell KL, Makhmudov A, Ely E, Jones RL, Wang RY. Iodine status of the U.S. population, National Health and Nutrition Examination Survey, 2005–2006 and 2007-2008. *Thyroid.* 2011;21(4):419-427.

22. Surks MI, Ortiz E, Daniels GH, Sawin CT, Col NF, Cobin RH, et al. Subclinical thyroid disease: scientific review and guidelines for diagnosis and management. *JAMA.* 2004;291(2):228-238.

23. Persani, L. Clinical review: central hypothyroidism: pathogenic, diagnostic, and therapeutic challenges. *J Clin Endocrinol Metab.* 2012;97(9):3068-3078.

24. Karmisholt J, Andersen S, Laurberg P. Variation in thyroid function in subclinical hypothyroidism: importance of clinical follow-up and therapy. *Eur J Endocrinol.* 2011;164(3):317-323.

25. Franklyn JA. Hypothyroidism. *Medicine.* 2009; 37(8):426-429.

26. Cooper DS, Biondi B. Subclinical thyroid disease. *Lancet.* 2012;379(9821):1142-1154.

27. Cooper DS, Doherty GM, Haugen BR, Kloos RT, Lee SL, Mandel SJ, et al. Revised American Thyroid Association management guidelines for patients with thyroid nodules and differentiated thyroid cancer. *Thyroid.* 2009;19(11):1-48.

28. Fitzpatrick DL, Russell MA. Diagnosis and management of thyroid disease in pregnancy. *Obstet Gynecol Clin North Am.* 2010;37(2):173-193.

29. American College of Obstetrics and Gynecology. ACOG Committee Opinion. Number 381. Subclinical hypothyroidism in pregnancy. *Obstet Gynecol.* 2002;100:387-396.

30. Fraser WD. Hyperparathyroidism. *Lancet.* 2009; 374:145-158.

31. Yeh MW, Ituarte PH, Zhou HC, Nishimoto S, Liu IL, Harari A, et al. Incidence and prevalence of primary hyperparathyroidism in a racially mixed population. *J Clin Endocrinol Metab.* 2013;98(3):1122-1129.

32. Ruda JM, Hollenbeak CS, Stack BC Jr. A systematic review of the diagnosis and treatment of primary hyperparathyroidism from 1995 to 2003. *Otolaryngol Head Neck Surg.* 2005;132(3):359-372.

33. Marcocci C, Cetani F. Clinical practice. Primary hyperparathyroidism. *N Engl J Med.* 2011;365(25): 2389-2397.

34. Silverberg SJ, Lewiecki EM, Mosekilde L, Peacock M, Rubin MR. Presentation of asymptomatic primary hyperparathyroidism: proceedings of the Third International Workshop. *J Clin Endocrinol Metab.* 2009;94:351-365.

35. Rejnmark L, Vestergaard P, Mosekilde L. Nephrolithiasis and renal calcifications in primary hyperparathyroidism. *J Clin Endocrinol Metab.* 2011; 96:2377-2385.

36. Walker MD, Silverberg SJ. Cardiovascular aspects of primary hyperparathyroidism. *J Endocrinol Invest.* 2008;31:925-931.

37. Bancos I, Hahner S, Tomlinson J, Arlt W. Diagnosis and management of adrenal insufficiency. *Lancet Diabetes Endocrinol.* 2015 Mar;3(3):216-226. doi: 10.1016/S2213-8587(14)70142-1. Epub 2014 Aug 3.

38. Grossman AB. Adrenal disorders. Merck Manuals. Available at: http://www.merckmanuals.com/professional/endocrine-and-metabolic-disorders/adrenal-disorders/overview-of-adrenal-function. Accessed April 17, 2016.

39. Nicolaides NC, Chrousos G, Charmandari E. Adrenal insufficiency. In: De Groot LJ, Beck-Peccoz P, Chrousos G, et al., eds. *Endotext* [Internet]. South Dartmouth (MA): MDText.com, Inc.; 2000-2014 Aug 18. Available at: http://www.ncbi.nlm.nih.gov/books/NBK279083/. Accessed April 17, 2016.

40. Bleicken B, Hahner S, Ventz M, Quinkler M. Delayed diagnosis of adrenal insufficiency is common: a cross-sectional study in 216 patients. *Am J Med Sci.* 2010;339:525-531.

41. Bornstein SR, Allolio B, Arlt W, Barthel A, Don-Wauchope A, Hammer GD, et al. Diagnosis and treatment of primary adrenal insufficiency: An Endocrine Society Clinical Practice Guideline. *J Clin Endocrinol Metab.* 2016;101:364-389.

42. Sulentic P, Morris DG, Grossman A. Cushing's Disease. In: De Groot LJ, Beck-Peccoz P, Chrousos G, et al., eds. *Endotext* [Internet]. South Dartmouth (MA): MDText.com, Inc.; 2000-2014 Aug 18. Available at: http://www.ncbi.nlm.nih.gov/books/NBK279083/. Accessed April 17, 2016.

43. Raff H, Carroll T. Cushing's syndrome: from physiological principles to diagnosis and clinical care. *J Physiol.* 2015;593(Pt 3):493-506. doi:10.1113/jphysiol.2014.282871.

44. Nieman LK, Ilias I. Evaluation and treatment of Cushing's syndrome. *Am J Med.* 2005;118(12):1340-1346.

45. Findling JW. Raff H. Screening and diagnosis of Cushing's syndrome. *Endocrinol Metab Clin North Am.* 2005;34:385-402.

46. Nieman LK, Biller BMK, Findling JW, et al. The diagnosis of Cushing's Syndrome: An Endocrine Society Clinical Practice Guideline. *J Clin Endocrinol Metab.* 2008;93(5): 1526-1540. doi:10.1210/jc.2008-0125.

CHAPTER 14

HEMATOLOGY

Barbara K. Hackley

Hematologic testing is a frequent component of office evaluation. During the course of a routine healthcare visit, women may report fatigue or heavy menstruation. They may present with fever and malaise. Rarely, women may have symptoms of more serious conditions such as thromboembolic disease. One of the first tests ordered in each of these situations is a complete blood count (CBC). This chapter is organized around the principal components of the CBC that are used in the evaluation of suspected infection, anemia, and vascular disease.

White Blood Cells

The white blood cells (WBCs) arise in the stem cells of the bone marrow, but evolve into different lineages. The pluripotent stem cells in the bone marrow give rise to mixed myeloid stem cells and lymphoid stem cells. The lymphoid stem cell creates progenitor cells, which result in the development of natural killer (NK) cells, T lymphocytes, and B lymphocytes.[1] The mixed myeloid stem cells create separate progenitor cells that lead to the development of the monocytes, neutrophils, eosinophils, and basophils, as well

as red blood cells (RBCs) and platelets as shown in **Figure 14-1**. Specifically for the WBCs, one progenitor leads to the development of two of the granulocytes (neutrophils and monocytes), a second leads to the development of the eosinophils, and a third leads to the development of the basophils (the third type of granulocyte).

The WBCs are categorized into two groups: granulocytes (neutrophils, eosinophils, and basophils) and agranulocytes (lymphocytes and monocytes). This division is based on whether granules appear to be present in the cytoplasm of the WBC under microscopy after staining. If stained granules are visible in the cell, the WBC is called a granulocyte and if it is not visible, it is an agranulocyte.

Granulocytes

Granulocytes are also called *polymorphonuclear leukocytes* (PMN or PML); the different titles reflect the granular sacs in the cytoplasm of the cell and varying nuclear shapes. Because they are nonspecific, they play a key role in the innate immune system. Their ability to react quickly upon exposure to a pathogen prevents spread of infection. The term *band cell* is used to describe an

Figure 14-1 Development of blood cell lines.

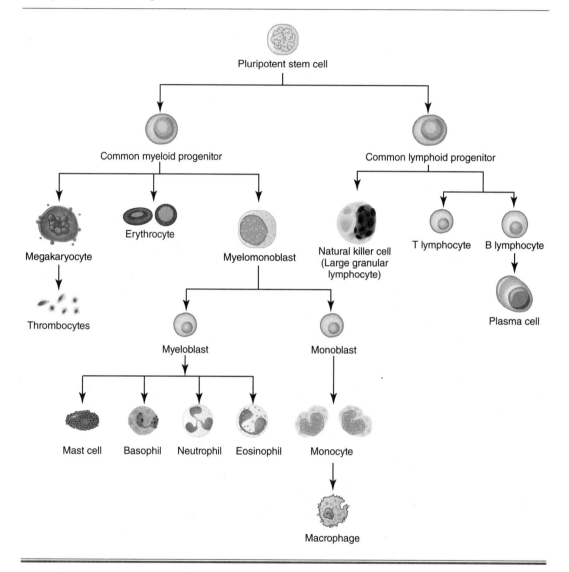

immature granulocyte (and usually refers to an immature neutrophil).

Neutrophils comprise 50% to 70% of circulating WBCs.[2] They are short lived, although recent data suggest that they can survive either in the bloodstream or in the marrow, liver, lungs, or spleen in a marginated or supplemental pool of cells, available to increase the supply during acute infection and extend their life during episodes of inflammation. In addition to their role in direct phagocytosis of invading microorganisms, they also release antibacterial proteins from the granular sacs in their cytoplasm that act both during phagocytosis and extracellularly.[3] Neutrophils interact with other white cell types including B and T lymphocytes and may serve to modulate immune responses and resolve inflammation as healing progresses.[4]

The eosinophils and basophils compose a much smaller percentage of WBCs, with *eosinophils* comprising 1–6% of circulating cells, and *basophils* usually < 0.5%.[5] The eosinophils are present in particularly high numbers in the mucosa of the respiratory and gastrointestinal (GI) tracts and are thought to play a role in mucosal immunity. They help regulate immediate hypersensitivity response through the release of leukotriene C4, and are present in particularly high numbers in individuals with allergies. They are also present in elevated numbers in individuals affected by parasites; one of the functions of eosinophils is to remove parasites, which are too large for phagocytes to manage.[1,5]

Basophils serve a similar function in allergic responses. Once activated, they release inflammatory mediators such as histamine, leukotrienes, and proteases, producing an immediate hypersensitivity response.[1,5] They are active in parasitic and viral infections.[2] In addition, basophils release a small amount of heparin when activated, delaying blood clotting.[1] Mast cells are tissue cells, also produced in the bone marrow and having similar properties to basophils.[5]

Agranulocytes

The *agranulocytes* include the monocytes and lymphocytes. *Monocytes* compose between 2% and 10% of the WBCs and circulate through the bloodstream for up to 72 hours before entering tissue spaces to become macrophages. The macrophages ingest foreign material, cellular debris, and bacteria. A small number of macrophages

develop into specialized dendritic cells, whose function is to "mark" an antigen so that T lymphocytes can recognize and attack it.[1,5]

The *lymphocytes* comprise 20–40% of circulating cells.[5] Based on function, they are divided into three subtypes. B cells represent 60–70% of circulating lymphocytes, T cells 20–30%, and NK cells 10–15%.[1] After differentiation in the bone marrow, lymphocytes undergo further transformation. For T cells, this occurs in the thymus, while B and NK cells migrate directly to the lymphatic system. *B cells* underlie humoral, antibody-specific immunity and are keyed to release antibodies to specific antigens in the blood and lymph systems. In their mature form, T cells reside in the bone marrow and peripheral tissue, as well as in the lymph nodes.[2] B cells are part of the humoral immunity system.

The *T cells* are part of the cellular immunity system. Unlike B cells that can bind directly to antigen, T cells need the assistance of other proteins to bind to viruses or bacteria. They can be classified into two categories with various subtypes: CD4 cells (helper cells and memory cells) and CD8 cells (cytotoxic cells and suppressor cells).[1] Once the virus or bacterium is "marked" by special proteins, T helper cells recognize and bind with the protein-antigen complex. This activates the helper cell, which then releases cytokines (particularly interferon) and leads to the proliferation of other T cells, including memory and cytotoxic T cells. B cells that are bound to antigen can also activate T helper cells that stimulate B cells to develop into specific antibody-secreting plasma cells. Cytotoxic cells release substances that lyse and kill the infected cell. Suppressor cells are released more slowly and switch off the cytotoxic and helper cells when the infection is no longer present. Memory T cells can recognize the antigen in the future and develop into specific cytotoxic cells that match the antigen on re-exposure.

The *natural killer cells* function similarly to the cytotoxic T cells and destroy cells that are cancerous or infected. They are not specific to a particular antigen and therefore can respond quickly, but not specifically, at the first sign of infection. The NK cells, along with the neutrophils, act indiscriminately and are activated immediately when viral or bacterial or chemical agents enter the body, forming the first line of defense against infection.[1]

Interpretation of WBC Abnormalities

Abnormalities in the numbers of WBCs, either elevated (leukocytosis) or decreased (leukopenia) should first direct the provider to examine the peripheral smear to determine which type(s) of WBCs are affected, the morphology of the cells themselves, and accompanying patterns in RBCs or platelets. Each type of WBC serves a specific role; therefore, elevations in a particular type of WBC may give a clue to the underlying etiology. In addition, because the WBCs, RBCs, and platelets all originate from pluripotent stem cells, abnormalities in all three lines may indicate a bone marrow problem. Abnormalities specific to one lineage may indicate problems in the downstream production or maturation of those cells or an increase in the demand due to a stress such as infection or massive hemorrhage. Increase in demand or damage to the bone marrow may lead to an early release of cells from the bone marrow, and immature cells may be noted on the peripheral smear. A careful review of findings available on the CBC can then be used to direct the history and physical exam to find constellations of symptoms and physical/laboratory findings that suggest a specific diagnosis.

LEUKOCYTOSIS

Leukocytosis is defined as an elevation in WBCs on the CBC. While the upper limits of normal vary slightly from laboratory to laboratory, the generally accepted definition in nonpregnant adults is an increase in WBCs > 11,000 mcL.[2]

Leukocytosis can be the result of a normal physiologic response to infection or inflammation, but can also be due to a primary bone marrow problem such as leukemia or lymphoma. The underlying pathways leading to an increase in WBCs include increased production, release of WBCs from storage in the bone marrow, processes that reduce the adhesion of WBCs to the vascular endothelium making more available in the peripheral circulation, and decreased migration into the peripheral tissue.[2]

Specific patterns of elevations of the WBCs suggest certain etiologies.[2] Myeloid leukocytoses are those that present with elevations in the granulocytes or monocytes.[6] Causes of leukocytosis are shown in **Table 14-1**. Neutrophilia is the most common cause of leukocytosis and is most frequently associated with bacterial infections.[7] In infection, the WBCs are mildly to moderately elevated (11,000 to 30,000 mcL) and are primarily composed of mature neutrophils and bands. Other findings include a "left shift" to less mature forms of WBCs and the presence of toxic granulations or Döhle bodies. On occasion, sepsis may be associated with leukopenia early in the course of infection before the WBCs rebound in number as the infection progresses. Viral infections do not generally cause neutrophilia, other than as an early response to inflammation. Other causes of leukocytosis associated with a neutrophilic response include malignancy, inflammation, certain medications, hemorrhage, and splenectomy.[6]

Most eosinophilias are reactive. Commonly associated with asthma, allergies, and drug hypersensitivities, other potential causes include parasitic infections, connective tissue diseases, sarcoidosis, lymphomas, and adrenal insufficiency. Any systemic disorder producing inflammation (cardiac, GI) may also result in eosinophilia.[8,9] Isolated basophilia is rare, except in chronic myeloid leukemia. More benignly, it is associated with chronic sinus infections and viral infections such as varicella.[8,9]

Monocytosis, although rare as an isolated finding, is found in chronic infection, following splenectomy, and with autoimmune disorders. Persistent monocytosis is suspicious for a malignancy.[8]

Lymphocytosis is absolutely elevated (above the normal range) with the acute phase of some viral infections and with chronic infections such as tuberculosis, as well as with acute and chronic lymphocytic leukemia. Relative increases in the WBC may also be seen in thyrotoxicosis, Addison's disease, and connective tissue disorders.[9]

Leukocytosis also occurs post-splenectomy or with sequestration of white cells in splenomegaly, as the spleen is one of the largest storage compartments of WBCs in the body.

Table 14-1 Causes of Leukocytosis and Leukopenia

Type	Etiology	Examples
Leukocytosis		
Neutrophilia	Infection	Bacterial
	Chronic inflammation	Rheumatic disease
		Inflammatory disease
		Chronic hepatitis
		Tissue necrosis
		Arthritis
	Stress	Exercise
		Anxiety
	Trauma	Spleen damage
	Tobacco use	
	Pregnancy	
	Medications	Corticosteroids
		Beta-agonist
		Lithium
	Cancer	Leukemia
	Marrow stimulation	Hemolytic anemia
		Immune thrombocytopenia
	Congenital	Hereditary neutrophil
		Down syndrome
Monocytosis	Infection	Tuberculosis
		Endocarditis
		Syphilis
	Autoimmune	Systemic lupus erythematosis
		Inflammatory bowel disease
	Cancer	Leukemia
		Lymphoma
		Solid tumors
	Post-splenectomy	

(continues)

Table 14-1 Causes of Leukocytosis and Leukopenia (*continued*)

Type	Etiology	Examples
Lymphocytosis	Viral infections	Epstein-Barr
		Cytomegalovirus
	Bacterial/parasitic infections	Hepatitis
		Pertussis
		Tuberculosis
		Toxoplasmosis
	Cancer	Leukemia
		Lymphoma
	Infections	Sepsis
		Parasitic
		Viral or bacterial
	Medications	Antibiotics including minocycline, metronidazole
		Anticonvulsants including lamotrigine, valproic acid
		Chemotherapy
	Other	Hypo- or hyperthyroidism
		Vitamin B_{12} deficiency
		Folic acid deficiency
		Splenomegaly
		Radiation

LEUKOPENIA

Leukopenia is defined as having too few WBCs (< 4500 mcL).[7] It occurs as a result of a decrease in the production of or an increase in the destruction of WBCs. Because the neutrophils compose the greatest number of the WBCs, leukopenia is most commonly associated with insufficient production or increased destruction of the neutrophils. High demand for neutrophils, as seen with severe infection, can exhaust the supply of neutrophils and result in neutropenia. Excess destruction, as seen with splenomegaly, is also associated with neutropenia. Drugs associated with neutropenia include antimicrobials, nonsteroidal anti-inflammatory medications, antidepressants, and anticonvulsants, among others.[7]

Reductions in the numbers of other types of WBCs rarely lead to leukopenia, because they make up a smaller proportion of the total population of WBCs. Monocytopenia is associated with aplastic anemia, leukemia, and use of corticosteroid medications.[7] Lymphopenia occurs naturally with age, but is also seen with human immunodeficiency virus (HIV) infection.[7] Whatever the cause, severe leukopenia is of grave concern, because individuals with leukopenia no longer have the ability to mount a defense against infection.

Clinical Presentation

Abnormalities in the WBC count have a nonspecific presentation, because changes in the numbers of WBCs are associated with a myriad of conditions. Because numerous etiologies are associated with abnormalities in the WBCs, a careful and thorough assessment is essential to uncover the underlying cause.

Essential History, Physical, and Laboratory Data

HISTORY AND PHYSICAL EXAMINATION

The history should cover symptomatology, the presence of comorbid conditions, medication use, and the use of alcohol, drugs, and cigarettes. Cigarette smoking, stress, medications, chronic conditions, and exercise are associated with leukocytosis. Fever and malaise of short duration suggest viral or bacterial infection. Recent surgery, trauma, exercise, or blood loss may be associated with transient elevations of WBCs. Swelling of the joints and generalized fatigue might suggest an autoimmune disorder. Weight loss and fatigue accompanied by abnormalities in the platelets or RBCs suggest cancer.

Similarly, the physical examination should be as comprehensive as the history. Elevated temperature and heart rate are seen with infection. Swollen, tender joints are seen with lupus and in autoimmune arthritis. Swollen lymph nodes suggest an infection, while the additional findings of an enlarged liver and/or splenomegaly and the presence of anemia and easy bruising suggest leukemia.

LABORATORY

What additional testing is needed in investigating abnormalities in the WBCs depends on the data elicited through the history, physical, and initial laboratory assessment. If leukocytosis is noted, a repeat CBC is often performed to document the duration of leukocytosis, to determine if the total numbers of WBCs are rising or falling, and to see if there is a shift in the proportions of the granulocytes, monocytes, or lymphocytes. An automated differential can be difficult to interpret in certain situations such as when nucleated immature RBCs, small fibrin clots, clumped platelets, or incompletely broken down red cells are noted on the peripheral smear.[8] A manual differential may be necessary to accurately distinguish the types of WBCs present. Short duration of leukocytosis suggests an acute event such as infection or acute leukemia; however, persistent leukocytosis may indicate chronic inflammation or cancer.[2] A left shift in the WBCs often accompanies infection, but can also be seen with cancer.[10]

Infection may be suspected based on symptoms and clinical findings. If an infection is suspected, then a culture of the affected site (e.g., urine, blood, stool, sputum) should be obtained. A stool sample for ova and parasites should be considered if the eosinophils are elevated. Testing with Monospot, Epstein-Barr virus (EBV), or cytomegalovirus (CMV) titers may be helpful in evaluating possible mononucleosis. Liver function tests can be ordered if viral and bacterial infections are suspected. Imaging tests may be ordered to evaluate potential abscesses, tumors, or bone marrow problems. Rarely, a bone marrow sample may need to be obtained if cancer or other bone marrow problem is suspected. If clinical findings point to a possible autoimmune disorder, an antinuclear antibody (ANA) test for lupus and rheumatic factor test for rheumatoid arthritis should be added to the panel.

Findings suspicious for leukemia include the presence of myeloblasts, promyelocytes, and myelocytes on the peripheral smear.[2] A WBC level of greater than 100,000 mcL is strongly suspicious of leukemia or a myeloproliferative disorder. Supporting evidence of the presence of leukemia or lymphoma includes having elevated levels of uric acid and lactate dehydrogenases.

Many of these same tests are needed in the evaluation of leukopenia. As with leukocytosis, a complete workup should include a repeat CBC with differential and peripheral smear, reticulocyte, erythrocyte sedimentation rate (ESR), and tests for autoimmune disorders (ANA, rheumatoid factor) and HIV. However, leukopenia is also associated with nutritional deficiencies and thyroid disorders. Additional tests should include thyroid-stimulating hormone (TSH), folic acid level, and vitamin B$_{12.}$[11]

Management of Conditions Affecting the WBCs

Prompt recognition of the underlying cause(s) of abnormalities in the WBCs will lead to timely treatment and better outcomes. It is beyond the scope of this chapter to describe the treatment of these conditions here. The reader is referred to the appropriate chapters for treatment of infections related to the respiratory, GI, and genitourinary systems. Suspected chronic conditions, autoimmune disorders, and/or cancer require evaluation by a primary care physician or specialist.

Red Blood Cells (RBCs)

Abnormalities of the RBC are classified as polycythemia, where the numbers of RBCs are increased, and anemia, where the numbers of RBCs are decreased. The most common causes of *polycythemia* are due to compensatory mechanisms triggered by low oxygen levels. Low oxygen stimulates erythropoietin, resulting in the production of a greater number of RBCs. Conditions associated with lower serum oxygen levels include congestive heart failure, chronic obstructive pulmonary disease, and living at a high altitude. Dehydration can also appear to cause polycythemia; however, in this case, RBC levels return to normal with adequate fluid intake. Rarely, an increase in the number of RBCs is due to polycythemia vera, a myeloproliferative disease of the bone marrow.[7]

Anemia is defined as a lower than normal number of RBCs in the blood, usually measured

as a decrease in the concentration of hemoglobin (the iron-rich protein in the blood that carries oxygen to all cells) and hematocrit (Hct) (the relative concentration of the solid constituents of the blood). Anemia is not a diagnosis in and of itself, but a symptom of an underlying condition. The finding of lower than expected hemoglobin or Hct should lead the healthcare provider to explore the possible diagnoses responsible for the abnormal laboratory values.

Anemia is common in the United States, affecting 9% of women between the ages of 12 and 50 years.[12] Although anemia is found in all populations, underlying etiologies vary by race/ethnicity. Certain inherited red cell disorders occur more frequently in specific populations, such as sickle cell disease in African Americans, beta thalassemia in persons of Mediterranean ethnicity, and alpha thalassemia in Asians and African Americans. Women's health providers need to be comfortable identifying and treating anemia, especially those that occur most frequently. This section covers the pathophysiology, clinical presentation, diagnostic methods, and management of the most common Hct and hemoglobin disorders.

Physiology

The *erythrocyte*, or RBC, is manufactured in the bone marrow. Erythrocytes function to carry oxygen to tissues. A normal mature RBC is a biconcave disk. Erythropoiesis, or RBC formation, is controlled via complex feedback loops. In general, an increased supply of RBCs in circulating body fluids inhibits production; anemia stimulates it. Erythropoietin, which is produced in the adult kidneys and liver in response to hypoxia, stimulates the bone marrow to manufacture RBCs.[7] The RBCs derive from the same pluripotent stem cells in the bone marrow that evolve to form the progenitors of the WBCs and platelets. In the case of the RBCs, the pluripotent stem cells go through a series of transformations to mixed myeloid stem cells to erythroid progenitor cells to pronormoblasts to erythrocytes.[1] Nucleated, immature RBC should not be seen as part of the circulating blood volume.[13] The erythrocytes are released as *reticulocytes,* an immature form of RBCs. RBCs continue to mature for 1 to 2 days after release into the circulation.[7]

RBCs contain hemoglobin, which binds with oxygen. Certain minerals and vitamins, including iron, folate, and vitamin B_{12}, are necessary for the production and maturation of RBCs. Inadequate dietary intake, depleted physiologic stores, or inflammation that blocks the release of iron from the reticuloendothelial system can lead to inadequate levels of critical RBC-building materials and result in anemia. Normal RBC production depends on having a functioning bone marrow, adequate erythropoietin levels (which are dependent on functioning kidneys in the adult), and the availability of all essential substrates needed for the formation of RBCs.[1] Hemoglobin is formed only during the early stages of RBC maturation; mature RBCs lack the necessary protein synthesizers. Because of this, if hemoglobin is damaged during production or maturation of an RBC, it cannot be repaired later. Mature RBCs also lack a nucleus, which make them incapable of repairing damage from aging or trauma. **Figure 14-2** depicts the RBC life cycle.

Hemoglobin (Hb or Hgb) is composed of two sections: the heme and the globin. The heme portion is made up of an iron atom in the center of a protoporphyrin ring. Each hemoglobin contains four heme groups. They are responsible for giving the blood its red color and for carrying oxygen. The globin portion of hemoglobin is composed of protein and contains four polypeptide chains. **Figure 14-3** depicts the hemoglobin molecule. Differences among types of hemoglobin lie in the sequencing and kinds of amino acids that make up the chains. Normal adult RBCs contain approximately 97.5%

Figure 14-2 RBC life cycle.

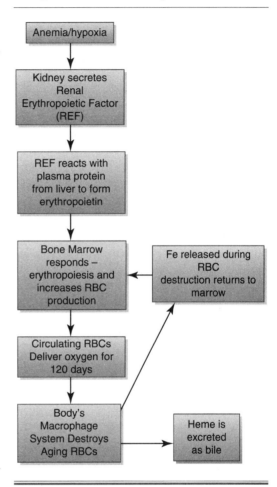

hemoglobin A_1, which is composed of two alpha and two beta chains. The remainder of the hemoglobin in normal adult erythrocytes is hemoglobin A_2, which is made up of different polypeptides than hemoglobin A_1. Hemoglobin A_2 has two alpha and two delta chains. The alpha chains remain the same, but delta chains are substituted for beta chains. A normal variant, fetal hemoglobin, or HbF, is found in large amounts in the human fetus. Its structure is similar to

Figure 14-3 Hemoglobin molecule and RBC.

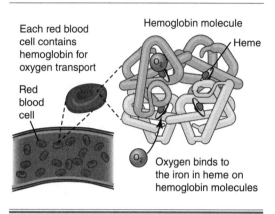

Each red blood cell contains hemoglobin for oxygen transport

Red blood cell

Hemoglobin molecule

Heme

O_2

O_2 Oxygen binds to the iron in heme on hemoglobin molecules

hemoglobin A_1 with two exceptions: The beta chains are replaced by gamma chains, and it has a higher affinity for oxygen, facilitating movement of oxygen from maternal circulation to the fetus. The majority of HbF is replaced by hemoglobin A (HbA) within 6 to 8 months after birth, although a small percentage of HbF remains throughout adulthood.[1] **Table 14-2** describes the normal hemoglobin variants.

RBCs live on average for 100–120 days. At the end of their lifespan, macrophages of the reticulo-endothelial system in the liver, spleen, and lymph nodes destroy the aging RBCs and split apart the globin and heme portions of the hemoglobin

molecule. Globin is further digested down to amino acids, which are utilized by the phagocytes for protein synthesis or released into the blood. The heme is first converted to biliverdin (green pigment), and then to bilirubin (yellow pigment), which is excreted in bile. The iron from the heme is returned to the bone marrow and reused in the production of new RBCs. Recycled iron from hemoglobin catabolism is essential to hemoglobin synthesis.[14]

Hemoglobinopathies

Inherited disorders can affect either the globin portion of the hemoglobin, as in the hemoglobinopathies, or the heme portion of the hemoglobin, as in the sideroblastic anemias and porphyrias. *Porphyrias*, such as erythropoietic protoporphyria, are a group of disorders in which abnormal genetic pathways lead to deficiencies in the production of essential enzymes needed for the synthesis of heme. Excessive levels of metabolic intermediates are produced and build up in the skin, urine, serum, or other tissues causing symptoms such as abdominal pain, neurologic changes, hyperbilirubinemia, photosensitivity, and other complications. Many sideroblastic anemias are caused by unknown genetic abnormalities that affect heme production. These conditions are relatively rare compared to the hemoglobinopathies.

Hemoglobinopathies are caused by genetic defects that result in abnormal hemoglobin

Table 14-2 Normal Hemoglobin

Variant		Composition	Percentage in Adults
HbA1	Normal adult	2 alpha chains, 2 beta chains	Up to 98% in adults
HbA2	Normal adult	2 alpha chains, 2 delta chains	Up to 3% in adults
HbF	Normal fetus and newborn	2 alpha chains, 2 gamma chains	May continue in small amounts throughout life

structure. These structural flaws fall into three categories:

- *Structural defects.* These can be present in the hemoglobin molecule. Alterations in the gene for one of the two hemoglobin subunit chains, alpha or beta, are called mutations. Often, mutations change a single amino acid building block in the subunit and are innocuous. Sometimes, as with sickle cell anemia, this single change produces a disease state.
- *Diminished production of one of the two hemoglobin subunit chains.* In normal hemoglobin, equal numbers of alpha and beta chains are necessary for normal function. Imbalances damage RBCs, making them vulnerable to destruction and causing anemia.
- *Abnormal associations of otherwise normal subunits.* Normally, one alpha subunit and one beta subunit combine to produce a normal hemoglobin dimer. With severe alpha thalassemia, for instance, the beta globin subunits begin to associate into groups of four (tetramers) due to diminished alpha chain partners. The tetramers are functionally inactive and are incapable of binding with oxygen. In severe beta thalassemia, alpha globin subunits rapidly degrade due to lack of a partner from the beta globin gene cluster.

In combination, these abnormalities lead to increased destruction of more fragile RBCs and, to a lesser extent, impaired production, resulting in significant anemia.

Abnormal hemoglobin chains, and the resulting *hemoglobinopathies*, are differentiated by letter. If an offspring inherits an abnormal gene for hemoglobin from only one parent, the individual is heterozygous, and half of the circulating hemoglobin is normal and half is abnormal. Sickle cell trait is an example of a heterozygous presentation. Individuals with sickle cell trait have inherited normal HbA from one parent and hemoglobin S (HbS) from the other. When identical abnormal genes are inherited from both parents, the offspring is homozygous, and all of the hemoglobin is abnormal, as is the case in those with sickle cell disease.

Not all hemoglobin abnormalities are harmful, and some may only cause mild to moderate anemia. However, some mutations can be so harmful that individuals cannot survive long enough to pass on these mutations to future generations. Consequently, harmful mutations tend to die out, but those that confer survival value persist and can become widespread in the population. The sickle cell gene is an example. HbS, which is found in those with sickle trait or disease, is insoluble at low oxygen tensions. Hypoxia changes the shape of the normally biconcave RBC to a sickle shape. These abnormal cells hemolyze, producing anemia, and cause stasis and chronic inflammation in the microcirculation leading to significant end-organ damage.[15] The sickle gene originated in African populations, conferring resistance to malaria in those with heterozygous presentations. While many individuals with sickle disease historically died before reaching reproductive age, those with the trait are commonly unaffected, live normal lives, and pass on the gene to their offspring. Offspring who inherit the trait benefit from the protective effect this gene carries against malaria and avoid the devastating consequences of sickle disease, which is the result of the homozygous expression of HbS. Nearly 100,000 individuals are thought to be affected by sickle disease in the United States.[16] See **Table 14-3** for other examples of clinically significant variant homozygous hemoglobins.

It is possible to inherit two different abnormal hemoglobin genes—one each from mother and father. The resulting anemia is known as a compound heterozygous variant anemia. Among the more common of these are hemoglobin SC disease, sickle/beta thalassemia, hemoglobin E/beta thalassemia, and alpha thalassemia/hemoglobin Constant Spring. Some of these anemias have

Table 14-3 Clinically Significant Variant Homozygous Hemoglobins

Type of Hb	Diagnosis	Clinical Implications	Notes
HbC	HbC disease	Mild hemolytic anemia/ splenomegaly	Trait is benign.
HbS	Sickle cell disease	Potentially life-threatening disease	Trait leads to mild anemia.
HbE	HbE disease	Mild microcytic anemia/ splenomegaly	Trait is benign.
Hb Constant Spring	Thalassemia disease	Severe anemia	Trait is benign.
HbH	Thalassemia disease	Moderately severe hemolytic anemia	Three alpha chains are deleted.
Hb Barts	Hb Barts disease or alpha thalassemia major	Incompatible with life	All 4 alpha chains are deleted; only gamma chains exist.

Table 14-4 Clinically Significant Variant Heterozygous Hemoglobins

Condition	Presentation
Hb SC disease	Similar to sickle cell disease, but milder
Sickle/beta thalassemia^0	Similar to sickle disease
Sickle/beta thalassemia$^+$	Milder presentation than with sickle/beta thalassemia^0
HbE/beta thalassemia	Variable, mild to severe

Note: ^{0} no beta globin production $^+$ reduced beta globin production

mild presentations; others are very disabling. The severity of the presentations of these conditions depends on which amino acid(s) are altered. See **Table 14-4** for a description of the most common heterozygous conditions.

Classification of Anemia

Two classification systems are used to describe anemia. One is based on the underlying cause of the anemia such as acute or chronic blood loss, RBC destruction, or malfunction in RBC production or maturation. The other system describes anemia by the size, shape, and color of the RBC. Both approaches can help focus the investigation of the cause of anemia for the individual patient.

ETIOLOGY

Three categories are used to describe the functional causes of anemia:

- *Proliferative disorders* include those in which production of RBCs is decreased. Examples of proliferative disorders include anemias due to bone marrow failure; reduced levels of hormones such as erythropoietin, thyroid, or androgens needed for RBC production; or insufficient levels of essential nutrients such as iron, folate, and vitamin B_{12}. Bone marrow failure can be the result of exposure to myelotoxic drugs, malignancies of the bone marrow, or chronic diseases. Erythropoietin production is reduced in the presence of renal disease and certain endocrine disorders. Iron may not be available due to presence of inflammation, which blocks the release of recycled iron removed by the reticuloendothelial system, or from inadequate dietary intake. Iron deficiency is the most common proliferative disorder found in women.

- *Maturational disorders* can also lead to anemia. In maturational disorders, the bone marrow is functioning normally and has all the essential ingredients needed to produce RBCs, but problems occur in the pathways that allow RBCs to develop normally. There are two processes that can lead to maturational disorders: Either an essential element, such as vitamin B_{12} or folate, needed for the maturation but not for initial production of RBCs is lacking, or there is a structural defect in the hemoglobin itself, such as in thalassemia, that adversely affects maturation. Anemia that results from genetic or acquired defects in iron metabolism, such as the sideroblastic anemias, also adversely affects RBC maturation.

- *Hemolytic disorders*, or increased RBC breakdown, may be due to abnormal phagocytic activity or increased fragmentation due to a number of autoimmune diseases such as warm or cold antibody hemolysis. In warm antibody hemolysis, also called immunoglobulin G (IgG)-mediated hemolysis, IgG binds RBCs and macrophages ingest the IgG-bound membrane. This kind of hemolytic activity can be seen with diseases such as non-Hodgkin's lymphoma, systemic lupus erythematosus, or chronic lymphocytic leukemia. Hemolysis also results from an increased breakdown

of the tissues directly resulting in enzymatic deficiencies on the cellular level such as in glucose-6-phosphate dehydrogenase (G6PD). Severe hemolysis can be accompanied by symptoms such as hepatomegaly, splenomegaly, hematuria, and jaundice.

Anemia can also result from acute or chronic blood loss. Chronic blood loss leads to the loss of recycled iron, depletion of iron stores, and anemia. Usually, symptoms are mild until anemia is severe. Acute blood loss is more obvious. Frank bleeding, jaundice, and tarry stools may be noted depending on the origin and cause of the blood loss.

MORPHOLOGY

Anemias can also be classified according to size of the RBC. *Macrocytic* anemias are those in which the mean corpuscle volume (MCV) is larger than normal. Conditions that are associated with macrocytic anemia include hypothyroidism; alcohol abuse; liver disease; anemias resulting in increased production of reticulocytes, which are normally bigger than fully mature RBCs; and vitamin B_{12} and folic acid deficiencies. *Microcytic* anemias, those with smaller than normal RBCs, include iron deficiency anemia, the thalassemias, hemoglobin E (HbE) disorders, sideroblastic anemia, and lead toxicity. *Normocytic* anemias are those in which cell size is normal, and can be caused by acute blood loss or by hemolytic disorders such as HbS disease, G6PD deficiency, and acquired hemolytic anemias. Anemia associated with chronic disease is usually normocytic, but may become microcytic.[17] The presence of nucleated RBCs in normocytic anemia suggests underlying damage to the bone marrow, as in lymphoma and some other cancers or chronic hypoxic stress.[13]

RBCs can also be described by their color. *Hypochromic* anemia, of which iron deficiency anemia is the most common variety, results from a reduction in red cell hemoglobin, making the RBCs appear pale in color. Thalassemia and sickle cell disease, like iron deficiency anemia, are both hypochromic and microcytic. *Normochromic* anemias are those in which the amount of hemoglobin in the cell is normal.[17] Normochromic anemias are most common in conditions causing acute blood loss or in the early stages of anemia before deficiencies are so low that production is impaired. However, normochromic normocytic anemias can herald more significant problems, albeit rarely. If a low WBC count or a low platelet count is noted, or if nucleated RBCs or immature WBCs are seen on the peripheral smear, more serious causes such as cancer should be considered and referral, and possible bone marrow biopsy, is warranted.

The shape of the RBC can also be quite distinctive in certain anemias and can indicate potential etiologies that should be considered. For example, spherocytes seen on a peripheral smear can indicate an autoimmune hemolytic anemia or an inherited condition called spherocytosis (also hemolytic in nature). See the Laboratory section in this chapter for further details on tests that describe the morphologic characteristics of anemia.

Routine Screening

Routine screening for anemia is not recommended for healthy asymptomatic nonpregnant women. Currently, authorities such as the US Preventive Services Task Force (USPSTF), the American Academy of Family Physicians, and the American College of Obstetricians and Gynecologists (ACOG) recommend routine screening for anemia only in asymptomatic women during pregnancy.[18-20] A 2006 Rand/UCLA review of the literature found it appropriate to screen every 5 years in asymptomatic nonpregnant women.[21] Measuring hemoglobin levels periodically in nonpregnant women at higher risk for anemia is reasonable; these include women with excessive menstrual flow, those at risk of anemia due to chronic diseases, and women with poor nutritional intake. Anemia screening requires the use of standard ranges for normal hemoglobin and/ or Hct. As shown in **Table 14-5**, these values are lower in pregnant women compared to nonpregnant women.

The US Congress first called for a sickle cell anemia national screening program in 1972, identifying women of childbearing age and children under the age of 7 years as high risk.[22] Screening of neonates was adopted in the United States after it became apparent that prophylactic administration of long-term antibiotics to well infants with sickle cell anemia could prevent or decrease the incidences of sepsis.[22] Since 2006, every state includes screening for sickle cell in their newborn screening program.[23] ACOG recommends screening in pregnancy, in particular for women of African or Mediterranean descent. The preferred screening test is the hemoglobin electrophoresis, which has the advantage of identifying other heterozygous conditions.[24]

Table 14-5 Normal Hemoglobin and Hematocrit Levels

Patient Profile	Hemoglobin Level (g/dL)	Hematocrit Level (%)
Nonpregnant, ≥ 18 years old	≥ 11.3	35.7
Pregnant, first trimester	11.0	33.0
Pregnant, second trimester	10.5	32.0
Pregnant, third trimester	11.0	33.0

Clinical Presentation

Symptoms associated with anemia may result from cellular hypoxia due to low hemoglobin and Hct levels, the compensatory mechanisms triggered by anemia, and/or the underlying cause of anemia. Hypoxia is caused by either a reduction in the amount of hemoglobin due to decreased production or increased destruction of RBCs or by a decrease in the overall volume of blood available for oxygen transport. A woman with anemic hypoxia may report a range of symptoms depending on the cause and severity of the anemia. These symptoms can include pallor and fatigue from low hemoglobin levels associated with chronic anemia, a racing heart rate and dizziness with hypovolemia from acute blood loss, or symptoms such as peripheral neuropathy due to vitamin B deficiency. Symptoms are most pronounced in those with lower hemoglobin and Hct levels, in anemia of acute onset, and in those with severe underlying disease.

Women associate fatigue with anemia. However, fatigue is uncommon unless anemia is severe or sudden. When anemia occurs suddenly, symptoms can be dramatic. With acute anemia the body does not have time for compensatory protective mechanisms to develop. Consequently, patients may report symptoms such as fainting from orthostatic changes related to hypovolemia. On physical exam, pulse rates of over 120 and significant flow murmurs may be detected. However, chronic anemia that develops slowly is often well tolerated until the red cell mass reaches critically low levels. With chronic anemia, the human body has time to compensate by:

- Increasing cardiac output
- Shunting blood to vital organs
- Decreasing the oxygen affinity of RBCs so that more oxygen is delivered to tissues
- Increasing erythropoietin levels in order to stimulate RBC production

Although these symptoms are more commonly a result of other conditions, subjective symptoms that may suggest severe anemia include fatigue, lethargy, dizziness, and anorexia. Women with moderate anemia may have pallor or sallow skin; colorless creases of the palms; and pale gums, nail beds, and eyelids. Decreased tolerance for exercise, dyspnea, and palpitations are all associated with moderate to severe anemia. As anemia worsens and compensatory mechanisms fail, more severe symptoms develop such as breathlessness, angina pectoris, headache, memory loss, inability to concentrate, insomnia, irregular heartbeat, anorexia, tachypnea, excessive sweating, swelling of hands or feet, thirst, tinnitus, and unexplained bleeding or bruising.

Another factor that can influence whether a woman experiences symptoms from anemia is her normal baseline hemoglobin and Hct levels. Patients with low but stable hemoglobin levels may be able to better tolerate a level of anemia that a woman with a higher baseline could not. For example, a woman with iron deficiency anemia whose Hct drops slowly to 28 may remain asymptomatic, but a woman whose Hct falls suddenly to this same level due to a postpartum hemorrhage may experience significant symptoms and require a blood transfusion.

Specific symptoms can suggest a particular underlying etiology. For instance, pernicious anemia is often diagnosed because of the onset of neurologic symptoms such as numbness or tingling in the extremities. Patients with sickle cell disease may report pain and swelling of the hands and feet, painful joints, or jaundiced eyes and skin due to the rapid breakdown of RBCs.

Essential History, Physical Examination, and Laboratory Data

Once anemia has been diagnosed by laboratory testing, further history, physical, and targeted laboratory evaluation can discern the underlying cause(s).

HISTORY

Because there are many different causes of anemia, the initial history will need to be broad in its coverage in order to elicit all possible etiologies. Clinicians should ask questions about dietary intake in order to uncover iron, folate, and vitamin B_{12} deficiencies. They should ask about environmental exposures to lead or other toxins as well as drugs that can trigger hemolysis. Symptoms such as tarry stools can suggest GI bleeding. Personal characteristics such as age, ethnic heritage, or pregnancy status may also help pinpoint a specific etiology. A positive family history may increase the suspicion that anemia may be due to any of the inherited disorders.

PHYSICAL EXAMINATION

Beginning with the head, the physical examination should include careful inspection of the skin and eyes for jaundice, examination of the mouth and throat for sores, and the tongue for redness, swelling, and shine (glossitis). Facial deformities such as bony prominences should be noted, because these findings are associated with chronic severe hemolytic anemias and thalassemia. Other physical indications of anemia include skin changes such as pallor, dryness, edema, and signs of bleeding such as petechiae or bruising, as well as brittle, ridged, or spoon-shaped nails. Patients with acute or severe anemia will appear in distress with tachycardia, a gallop rhythm, and tachypnea. Cardiomegaly and hepatomegaly may be present in very severe presentations.

Vital signs can help gauge the severity of the anemia. Orthostatic blood pressures are particularly helpful because they can provide objective measurements of the degree of hypovolemia commonly seen in anemia of acute onset. Orthostatic hypotension is defined as a decrease of at least 20 mmHg in systolic blood pressure when an individual moves from a supine to a standing position. To perform this assessment, blood pressure and heart rate should be measured in the supine, sitting, and standing positions following a few general principles:

- Obtain blood pressure ensuring that the brachial artery is at the level of the heart.
- Allow patient to rest supine for at least 5 minutes before obtaining baseline measurements.
- Allow patient to sit and stand for 2 to 3 minutes before obtaining vital signs in these positions.

In patients with intact autonomic nervous systems, the pulse will rise 5 to 12 beats per minute when standing after lying supine, and the blood pressure will remain stable. A substantial increase in the standing pulse rate suggests a contracted intravascular volume. A drop in systolic blood pressure of 20 mmHg or more, a drop in diastolic of 10 mmHg or more, or a rise in pulse rate of 20 beats or more would be considered an orthostatic response. In the rare event that there is a failure of the sympathetic component of the autonomic nervous system, the pulse rate will fail to rise even though the blood pressure falls.

LABORATORY DATA

Laboratory data are required in order to make the diagnosis of anemia and to determine the type of anemia. The most commonly used tests to screen and diagnose specific anemia are hemoglobin concentration and Hct. They are also used to determine if an already identified anemia is responding appropriately to treatment (Table 14-5).

Complete Blood Count   Second to hemoglobin and Hct, a CBC with differential and a reticulocyte count are most commonly used as screening tools. These tests are based on characteristics of RBCs and are generally more available and less expensive than biochemical tests for iron status (i.e., erythrocyte protoporphyrin concentration, serum ferritin concentration, and transferrin saturation), although they are a later indicator of changes in iron status.

The CBC yields a morphologic view of the RBC, describing the anemia by cell size, color, and shape. The size of an RBC determines the classification of the anemia as microcytic, normocytic, or macrocytic and is measured by MCV. The MCV is the average volume of RBCs, measured in femtoliters (fL). Low in cost and easily obtained, this is a particularly helpful test in classifying anemia. A low MCV (< 80) indicates microcytic anemia. An elevated MCV (> 100) suggests that macrocytic anemia such as folate/B_{12} deficiency or reactive reticulocytosis is present. Color and shape of the RBC provide further clues to the underlying cause of anemia.

Peripheral Smear   A peripheral smear examines the shape of RBCs and is helpful in suggesting specific etiologies that should be considered. Examples of abnormal findings found on the peripheral smear can be found in **Table 14-6**.

Reticulocyte   A reticulocyte count is helpful in two situations. First, it can help discern the underlying cause of anemia; second, once the etiology is identified, it can help reassure the clinician that the prescribed treatment is effective. A reticulocyte count measures how rapidly immature RBCs, known as reticulocytes, are made by the bone marrow and released into the bloodstream. Reticulocytes circulate in the blood for about 2 days before reaching maturity. Normally, about 1–2% of the circulating RBCs are reticulocytes. The reticulocyte count increases in response to rapid blood loss or in the presence of diseases in which RBCs are prematurely destroyed as the body attempts to rapidly replace lost RBCs. If the count is higher than normal, it suggests acute blood loss or hemolytic anemia and responsive bone marrow. If the count is low or normal in the presence of anemia, it is suggestive that the bone marrow is unable to respond to the body's feedback system. A reticulocyte count, for example, can be low in anemia due to hypoproliferation because of insufficient levels of critical elements,

Table 14-6   Peripheral Smear*

Findings on Peripheral Smear	Associated Anemia
Schistocytes or fragmented cells	Microangiopathic hemolytic anemia
Spherocytes	Hereditary spherocytosis Autoimmune hemolytic anemia Hemoglobinopathies Artifact
Ghost or bite cells	G6PD deficiency
Sickle-shaped cells	Sickle cell disease
Target cells	Hemoglobinopathies Iron deficiency
Stippled RBCs	Lead poisoning Thalassemia Alcoholism
Teardrop cells	Thalassemia major Severe iron deficiency
Howell-Jolly bodies	Hemolytic anemia Splenectomy
Heinz bodies	G6PD Alpha thalassemia Unstable forms of hemoglobin Congenital hemolytic anemia

*Not inclusive of all possibilities.

such as iron, which are necessary for the production of RBCs. Once iron supplementation begins, the bone marrow will respond and increase the production of reticulocytes. Therefore, a reticulocyte count is often ordered to monitor the effectiveness of treatment.

Red Blood Cell Distribution Width   An RBC distribution width (RDW) is a measurement of how uniform the RBCs are in size. The normal RDW level is 10.2% to 14.5%. A high RDW means the RBCs vary significantly in size. To determine why cell size is not uniform, the RDW is compared with the MCV, or average amount of space occupied by each RBC. Liver disease, hemolytic anemia, vitamin B_{12} deficiency, or folic acid deficiency must be considered if both the RDW and MCV are increased. Iron deficiency anemia is the main cause of a high RDW and low MCV, but thalassemia intermedia must also be considered. In addition, post-hemorrhagic anemias lead to high RDW readings with low MCV due to the release of immature RBCs from the bone marrow (leading to an increased variation in size). Early in the course of iron deficiency anemia, vitamin B_{12} deficiency, or folic acid deficiency, the RDW level may be increased but the MCV level is normal. A low RDW may be caused by macrocytic or microcytic anemia. In both of these cases, there is little variation in the size of the RBCs.

Erythrocyte Protoporphyrin or Free Erythrocyte Protoporphyrin   Erythrocyte protoporphyrin is the immediate precursor of hemoglobin. It increases when insufficient iron is available for the production of hemoglobin, because without an adequate amount of iron the body is unable to synthesize heme, and the protoporphyrin accumulates. A normal reading for this test is between 16 and 65 mcg/dL in adults. A concentration of greater than 70 mcg/dL of RBCs in adults often indicates iron deficiency. Other causes for it to be elevated include infection, inflammation, porphyria, and lead poisoning.

Ferritin   Ferritin is an intracellular protein that stores iron in the body. Serum ferritin concentration in the blood is directly proportional to the amount of stored iron in the body. Most of the iron that is not already bound by the heme portion of hemoglobin is stored as ferritin in the liver, bone marrow, and spleen; the remaining iron is found in transferrin in myoglobin, and a small amount in the enzyme systems active in energy metabolism. The average value in US women is

43 mcg/L. It is an early indicator of the compromised status of iron in the body; the body will deplete its stores of ferritin before iron deficiency becomes a problem. If a woman has a low hemoglobin or Hct, a serum ferritin concentration of less than or equal to 15 mcg/L confirms iron deficiency. Levels of ferritin greater than 15 mcg/L suggest that iron deficiency is not the cause of anemia, so other etiologies should be considered.

A normal or high serum ferritin level can be seen in the presence of other conditions such as chronic infection, inflammation, renal disease, iron overload, or other anemias (e.g., megaloblastic, hemolytic, and thalassemia).

Transferrin   *Transferrin* is manufactured in the liver and is the primary protein in blood to which iron binds. Transferrin levels increase when the serum iron concentration is low and decrease when it is high. The level can also be increased in the presence of liver damage and with the use of some medications such as birth control pills. The transferrin saturation indicates the degree to which there are available iron-binding sites on transferrin. This value is dependent on two laboratory measures—serum iron concentration and total iron-binding capacity (TIBC). Transferrin saturation is expressed as a percentage and is calculated by dividing serum iron concentration by TIBC and multiplying by 100. If the result is less than 16% in adults, it confirms iron deficiency. It is considered to be less sensitive than serum ferritin for reflecting iron stores in the body.

Serum Iron   Serum iron concentration is a measure of the total amount of iron in the blood bound to transferrin. Many factors alter this amount, including eating recently (raises level), infections and inflammation (decreases level), and time of day sample was drawn. As such, this test is not an accurate indicator of iron status alone, but together with serum ferritin and transferrin levels, it can help determine what type of anemia is present.

Total Iron-Binding Capacity (TIBC) The TIBC is a measure of the iron-binding capacity within the serum, or how much iron the blood would carry if the transferrin were fully saturated.

Hemoglobin Electrophoresis Hemoglobin electrophoresis measures the different types of hemoglobin in the blood. It is a test conducted when familial or ethnic history suggests an increased risk for an inherited abnormality such as sickle cell trait or thalassemia. As indicated in Table 14-2, normal adult hemoglobin consists mainly of HbA1, a small amount of HbA2, and a minor amount of HbF.

Other Tests Other tests should be considered when investigating anemia, depending on the suspected underlying cause. Folate and vitamin B$_{12}$ levels should be checked in the presence of macrocytic anemia. Suspicion of abnormal GI blood loss can be tested by a chemical hemoccult test of a rectal smear.

Management of Anemia

The treatment of anemia is dependent on its underlying cause and its severity. The discussion of the treatment of the various anemias is organized based on their morphology: microcytic, normocytic, or macrocytic.

MICROCYTIC ANEMIA

Only the commonly seen *microcytic* anemias are reviewed in this chapter. Often cues to the presence of one or more of these conditions can be gleaned from a careful review of the laboratory data. **Table 14-7** describes common laboratory findings seen in the various microcytic anemias.

Table 14-7 Laboratory Findings in Microcytic Anemia

Tests	Microcytic Anemia			
	Iron Deficiency Anemia	Alpha Trait Thalassemia	Beta Trait Thalassemia	Lead Poisoning
Ferritin	Low	Normal	Normal or high	Normal
TIBC	High	Normal	Normal	Normal
Reticulocyte	Low	Normal	Low	Low
RDW	High	Normal or high	Normal or high	
Hb electrophoresis	Normal	Normal, rarely low HbA2*	High HbA2, low HbA, sometimes high HbF	Normal
Other studies				High free erythrocyte protoporphyrin levels with prolonged exposure. Stippled erythrocytes on peripheral smear. Elevated lead levels.

*HbH or Hb Bart present in more severe presentations of alpha thalassemia (HbH disease).

Hb = hemoglobin, RDW = red blood cell distribution width, TIBC = total iron-binding capacity

Iron Deficiency Anemia

Iron deficiency anemia is the most common anemia in the world. In developing countries located in tropical climates, the most common cause is infestation of hookworm, which causes intestinal blood loss. This is rare in developed countries such as the United States, where anemia is often due to insufficient iron. Insufficient iron can occur during infancy, adolescence, or pregnancy when physiologic needs are greater than at other periods of life. It can also be due to inadequate iron intake, decreased iron absorption, or increased blood loss from heavy menses, bleeding of the GI tract, and other conditions. Causes of decreased iron absorption include gastrectomy, achlorhydria, or chronic diarrhea. It is rarely seen in teenage boys and young men, older children, or in adults over the age of 50.

Iron absorption is regulated by receptors predominantly in the duodenum and upper jejunum. Regulation of absorption is not completely understood, but it is clear that many factors can affect iron absorption. Factors can be categorized as those that *facilitate* absorption of iron such as ascorbate, citrate, and more soluble iron found in animal protein; *inhibit* absorption of iron such as tannins, iron overload, or antacids; or *compete* with iron for absorption such as lead, zinc, and other chemicals. All of these pathways result in the lack of sufficient iron to meet the needs of the body. An imbalance between iron needs and iron stores can not only be caused by failure to absorb enough iron, but also by the excessive loss of iron (e.g., hemorrhagic event, chronic blood loss).

Whatever the underlying cause, the onset of iron deficiency anemia is gradual. RBC production falls in response to declining iron reserves. Initially, the anemia is normochromic and normocytic, but as iron stores become further depleted, hypochromic microcytic anemia develops. Laboratory evaluation of iron deficiency anemia will show lower than normal hemoglobin, Hct, and reticulocyte levels, as well as low serum ferritin and saturation percentage and high transferrin and TIBC.[17] Hemoglobin levels fall before Hct in iron deficiency, but both are late indicators of the presence of iron deficiency. Because iron deficiency anemia is by far the most common cause of anemia in healthy women of reproductive age, low hemoglobin and Hct levels are often used to make a presumptive diagnosis of iron deficiency anemia without further testing. Low serum iron and ferritin levels in combination with an elevated TIBC are diagnostic of iron deficiency in well individuals. The Rand expert panel recommended against a trial of iron therapy in adult women over 40 with microcytic anemia based solely on the CBC.[21]

However, other diagnoses may need to be considered, because there are many causes of microcytic anemia besides iron deficiency. An examination of the peripheral smear can help narrow the list of possible diagnoses. For example, target cells can be present in thalassemia, hepatic disease, hemoglobin C disorders, and after splenectomy.[25] Deformed poikilocytes can be seen in sickle cell anemia, hemoglobin SC disease, and other hemoglobinopathies, but not with sickle cell trait.[25] Other tests may be needed to clarify the diagnosis. High ferritin levels in the presence of anemia should prompt the clinician to consider other diagnoses such as fever, cancer, or other inflammatory processes.

Management of iron deficiency anemia includes iron supplementation. Although a rate of 100–200 mg elemental iron is standard, there is evidence that lower doses may also be effective.[26] While there are many forms of iron supplements, some are absorbed more efficiently than others (see **Table 14-8**). All supplements are better absorbed if taken between meals, but the GI side effects can be a deterrent. Side effects include GI upset, such as nausea, diarrhea, heartburn or constipation, and black or tarry stools. Starting supplements with daily dosing and slowly increasing

Table 14-8 Common Types of Iron Supplementation

Iron Supplement	Absorption	Usual Dosage	Trade Names
Ferrous sulfate	High	325 mg PO × 1 to 3 daily	Slow Fe, Feratab
Ferrous gluconate	High	325 mg PO × 1 to 3 daily	Fergon
Ferrous fumarate	High	200 mg PO × 1 to 2 daily	Femiron, Feostat
Carbonyl iron	Low	45 mg PO × 1 daily	Feosol

to three times per day may be helpful in avoiding severe side effects. Taking smaller doses several times per day may also help alleviate these effects. Tolerance of iron supplementation is related to the level of elemental iron concentration. Ferrous gluconate, although more expensive than ferrous sulfate, has a lower elemental iron concentration and is therefore easier for patients to tolerate.

Some foods have ingredients that impair absorption and should not be consumed at the same time as an iron supplement. These include the calcium found in dairy products, tannins present in many teas, and phytic acid in legumes, cereal grains, and nuts. Absorption of both iron and folic acid is increased if taken with vitamin C; patients can be encouraged to take the supplement with citrus juice. Supplementation is more effective if enteric-coated and time-release products are avoided. Antacids, H2 blockers, and proton pump inhibitors also impair absorption.

Hemoglobin and Hct should be retested after 2 to 3 months of treatment. If the anemia does not respond to iron treatment (indicated by an increase in hemoglobin concentration of at least 1 g/dL or in Hct of at least 4%), compliance should be verified, and additional laboratory tests such as an MCV, RDW, and serum ferritin concentration are needed. If these tests confirm iron deficiency anemia, treatment should continue for an additional 2 months before rechecking Hct and hemoglobin.

THALASSEMIA

Thalassemias are an inherited form of hemolytic anemia in which the body produces defective hemoglobin. They are most commonly seen in individuals whose ancestry originates in the Mediterranean, the Middle East, India, and Southeast Asia, although they do also very rarely occur in individuals of Northern European or African descent.[27]

Genetic abnormalities limit the production of the hemoglobin chains and alter the rate of chain synthesis, making the chains imbalanced and more susceptible to hemolysis. The RBCs in persons with thalassemia are unusually small and fragile, microcytic in appearance. The thalassemias are categorized by whether the alpha or beta chain is affected.

Alpha Thalassemia Two functional genes are necessary for the production of each of the two alpha chains. Types of anemia resulting from problems within the alpha chains are designated the *alpha thalassemia* anemias; they include a broad spectrum of disease depending on how many, and to what degree, the four genes are affected. Loss of function of a gene can result from deletions within its specific gene cluster or from genetic changes within the gene cluster that result in absent or reduced synthesis of alpha chains. Most alpha thalassemias are due to deletions within the gene clusters, but some are due to genetic defects

Table 14-9   Classification of Alpha Thalassemia by Genotype

Genes Affected	Genotype	Description
4	- - / - -	H Barts, hydrops fetalis
3	- α/ - -	Hb H disease
	- α^{CS}/ - -	Constant Spring Hb H variant
2	αα/ - - OR	Homozygous alpha$^+$ α thalassemia trait
	- α/ - α	Heterozygous alpha^0 α thalassemia trait
1	αα/ - α	Silent carrier state

Note: Hemoglobin is made up of four genes. Normal hemoglobin would be shown as αα/αα.

CS = hemoglobin Constant Spring, - denotes missing gene.

that prompt the formation of longer, unstable chains. Hemoglobin Constant Spring is one of the most common nondeletional variants. In general, alpha thalassemia due to deletions has a milder course than the nondeletional alpha thalassemias.[27] Table 14-9 describes the genotype findings associated with the various variants.

Loss of function in three or four genes is associated with the most severe presentations. If all four genes are affected, the fetus will develop fetal hydrops and frequently dies in utero. The loss of function in three genes causes hemoglobin H disease, a moderately severe form of thalassemia. The abnormal RBCs have a high oxygen affinity, decreasing oxygen transport to tissue. It can be associated with hemolysis, which may be severe enough to require blood transfusion.[15] Individuals with a variant of hemoglobin H disease due to nondeletional causes such as hemoglobin Constant Spring are much more likely to experience hemolysis, require more blood transfusions, and are more likely to develop splenomegaly and other complications than individuals with deletional forms of hemoglobin H disease.[27,28]

Clinical symptoms are mild or absent if fewer genes are affected. The loss of two genes (alpha thalassemia minor, also known as alpha thalassemia trait) causes mild anemia resembling iron

deficiency anemia. Loss of function in one gene leads to a silent carrier state, which is clinically asymptomatic.

Laboratory findings differ depending on whether the alpha thalassemia is due to deletional or nondeletional etiologies. The amount of hemoglobin Barts found on hemoglobin electrophoresis can help indicate which form of deletional alpha thalassemia disease is present. Levels of hemoglobin Barts increase successively as the number of affected alpha chains increases. A low HbA$_2$ can sometimes be seen on the hemoglobin electrophoresis. Hemoglobin Constant Spring can be difficult to identify, because it is not seen on hemoglobin electrophoresis; therefore, the silent carrier state can be missed. Follow-up testing in suspected cases can detect the presence of hemoglobin Constant Spring or other nondeletional etiologies using polymerase chain reaction or genetic molecular tests.[28]

Beta Thalassemia   In normal adult hemoglobin, two alpha chains unite with two beta chains. Beta thalassemias are inherited disorders where there is an absence or reduction in the synthesis of the beta globin chains. Either one or both beta chains can be affected. In the homozygous state, beta globin synthesis is completely absent (beta −) or greatly

Table 14-10   Classification of Beta Thalassemia by Genotype

Genes Affected	Genotype	Description
2	b−/b−	Beta thalassemia major (Cooley's anemia)
	b−/b+	
	b+/b+	
1	b−/b+	Beta thalassemia intermedia
	b+/b+	
1	b−/bb	Silent carrier state
	bb/b+	

Note: − denotes limited to no production of beta chains, + denotes reduced production of beta chains.

reduced (beta +). The beta thalassemias are classified into three categories: 1) beta thalassemia major (which affects two genes leading to a severe decrease in beta globin synthesis), 2) beta thalassemia intermedia (which affects one gene leading to mild to moderate decrease in beta globin synthesis), and 3) beta thalassemia minor (which affects one gene in a limited way). Disease severity is inversely related to beta chain synthesis; higher production is associated with milder symptoms, and lower production is related to more distressing ones. Abnormal hemoglobin synthesis causes microcytosis, ineffective erythropoiesis, and hemolysis. **Table 14-10** describes the genotype variations seen in the various forms of beta thalassemia.

Beta thalassemia major, also known as Cooley's anemia, is the most severe form of the disease. Both beta globin chains are affected and beta globin synthesis is absent. It is fatal in childhood without transfusion. It becomes evident between 4 to 6 months after birth as protective levels of HbF decline and more adult hemoglobin begins to emerge.[15] Affected individuals may have characteristic mongoloid facies due to cranial and facial bone abnormalities. Ongoing blood transfusions can lead to iron overload, which then requires treatment with chelation to remove the excess iron.

Beta thalassemia intermedia is a mixture of genotypes that have variable presentations. HbF is more prevalent than usual, and HbA$_2$ is increased. Individuals with beta thalassemia intermedia at the milder end of the spectrum have minimal symptoms. Anemia can range from mild to severe but generally is not severe enough to require blood transfusions. Individuals with beta thalassemia intermedia can develop leg ulcers or gallstones and are at greater risk of thrombosis. More severe presentations may present similarly to beta thalassemia major; growth failure, bone deformities, and enlarged liver and spleen can occur but are less severe and less common than in beta thalassemia major.[29] Beta thalassemia minor is asymptomatic and will be detected only on laboratory evaluation.

If thalassemias are suspected, the laboratory evaluation should include a CBC with MCV and a hemoglobin electrophoresis. The MCV is always low in beta thalassemia and the RBC count is often elevated. With all the beta thalassemias, higher levels of HbF and HbA$_2$ can be seen on the hemoglobin electrophoresis. HbA$_1$ levels vary and can range from being reduced to absent depending on the severity of the beta thalassemia.[20] See **Table 14-11** for interpretation of hemoglobin electrophoresis results.

Table 14-11 Findings on the Hemoglobin Electrophoresis

	Normal Adult	Alpha Thalassemia Minor	Alpha Thalassemia Major	Beta Thalassemia Minor	Beta^O Thalassemia Major	Beta$^+$ Thalassemia Major	Sickle Cell Trait	Sickle Cell Disease	HgH Disease
HbA1	95–98%	90%		> 90%	0%	1–3%	60%	–	Up to 90%
HbA2	2–3%	4 – 5.8%		Slight increase	Up to 10%	Up to 9%	< 3.5%	< 3.5%	< 2%
HbF	0.8–2%	–		Up to 2.5%	Up to 90%	Up to 90%	< 2%	Up to 15%	< 5%
HbS	–	–	–	–	–	–	20–40%	70–98%	–
Hb Barts	–	5–10%	15–20%	–	–	–	–	–	2–10%
HbH	–	–		–	–	–	–	–	5–40%

*There are slight variations in references across labs; always check with the lab conducting the test.

Testing should be offered in pregnancy, particularly in women whose ancestors originated from the countries surrounding the Mediterranean or from Southeast Asia. Women should also be offered screening with hemoglobin electrophoresis if any of their family members have thalassemia, or if they have microcytosis with a normal or elevated RBC count. If a woman tests positive, screening of her partner is warranted. Genetic counseling should be offered to couples if both are carriers.

LEAD POISONING

Lead poisoning should be suspected in children who are anemic, although it can also affect adults. Women who engage in pica behavior, particularly of soil or paint chips, or who are from countries such as Mexico, Jamaica, and the Baltics where lead levels are known to be high, are at increased risk of having elevated lead levels. Supplementation with calcium and iron may be particularly helpful in these individuals and may prevent further absorption from the environment or release of stored lead in the bones.

MACROCYTIC ANEMIAS

The most common causes of *macrocytic* anemia are nutritional, specifically vitamin B_{12} deficiency and folic acid deficiency. Alcohol use is another common cause of macrocytic anemia and should not be overlooked in the differential. Less common causes include leukemia, myelofibrosis, multiple myeloma, drugs that affect DNA synthesis such as chemotherapeutic agents, and endocrine diseases such as hypothyroidism.[17] Laboratory findings commonly seen with macrocytic anemia include an increased MCV, a low reticulocyte count, and hypersegmented polymorph nuclear leukocytes on the peripheral smear. Markedly high MCV levels of > 110 fL are almost always indicative of a primary bone marrow problem.[10] **Table 14-12** describes laboratory findings seen in some of the common macrocytic anemias.

Folic Acid Deficiency Anemia Folic acid deficiency anemia is the most common of the megaloblastic anemias. Folic acid, a B vitamin, is used by the body to produce normal RBCs. Inadequate folic acid leads to the production of fewer macrocytic RBCs. Insufficient levels can be due to inadequate intake (infancy, elderly, alcoholics), malabsorption (gastric surgery), increased need (pregnancy, lactation), increased loss (hemolytic anemia, cancer, dialysis, inflammatory disease), and medications (methotrexate, trimethoprim, anticonvulsant drugs).[17] Foods high in folic acid should be eaten raw or cooked as little as possible, because light and heat destroy folic acid. Folic acid is found in foods such as cheese, eggs, green vegetables, meats, milk, mushrooms, and yeast; most breads are now fortified with folic acid. Folic acid depends on the presence of vitamin C for absorption. This disorder can be treated with supplementary folic acid at a dose of 1 mg per day for a minimum of 6 months with periodic blood tests to make certain that the deficiency is corrected.

Vitamin B_{12} Deficiency Insufficient levels of vitamin B_{12} can be due to inadequate intake (particularly among vegans), intrinsic factor deficiency (pernicious anemia, gastrectomy), and small intestine disease (Crohn's disease, tropical sprue, tapeworm, malabsorption). Vitamin B_{12} is necessary for the formation of RBCs and the maintenance of healthy nerve cells. Insufficient levels can lead to fatigue, shortness of breath, difficulty walking, and diarrhea. Peripheral neuropathy is bilateral. Pain and tingling often occur in a "glove and stocking-like" distribution. Neurologic symptoms are a frequent complaint leading to diagnosis.[17]

Pernicious anemia (also known as autoimmune gastritis) is among the most common types of vitamin B_{12} deficiency anemia. The onset of this disease tends to be slow, spanning decades. The average age at diagnosis is 60 years. It is

Table 14-12 Laboratory Findings in Macrocytic Anemia

Tests	Vitamin B_{12} Deficiency	Folate Deficiency	Alcohol Abuse	Hypothyroidism
Ferritin	Normal	Normal		
TIBC	Normal	Normal		
Reticulocyte	Low	Low	Normal	Low
RDW	High	High	Variable	Variable
Vitamin B_{12}	Low (If vitamin B_{12} results are equivocal, test for homocysteine and methylmalonic acid [MMA]. If elevated, the diagnosis is confirmed.)	Normal	Normal	Normal
Folate	Normal	Low (Confirmed if homocysteine level elevated)	Normal	Normal
Other studies	Hypersegmented neutrophils on peripheral smear	Hypersegmented neutrophils on peripheral smear	Abnormal liver tests Elevated γ-glutamyltransferase	Abnormal thyroid function tests

RDW = red blood cell distribution width, TIBC = total iron-binding capacity

caused by lack of intrinsic factor, a protein produced in the stomach that is needed to absorb vitamin B_{12} from the intestinal track. Laboratory findings seen in pernicious anemia include an elevated MCV, low Hct and hemoglobin levels, reduced amounts of serum B_{12}, and decreased WBCs, platelets, and reticulocytes. Methylmalonic acid, homocysteine, or both is used to confirm vitamin B_{12} deficiency in untreated patients; an elevated level of methylmalonic acid is more sensitive and specific for the diagnosis.[30] A positive result for intrinsic factor antibodies is diagnostic of pernicious anemia. An upper GI endoscopy should be considered, because gastric cancer is present in 5% of individuals with pernicious anemia, particularly if a woman has GI symptoms or coexisting iron deficiency anemia.[17]

Pernicious anemia requires lifelong treatment. Recommendations on the frequency, dosing, and type of supplementation include both parenteral and high-dose oral regimens. Initial treatment focuses on rebuilding body stores of B_{12} followed by maintenance doses thereafter. Either oral or intramuscular supplementation can be used. For example, 1000 to 2000 mcg per day can be given for 1 to 2 weeks followed by 1000 mcg per day for life.[31] Alternatively, 100 mcg to 1000 mcg of vitamin B_{12} can be given intramuscularly daily or every other day for 1 to 2 weeks followed by maintenance injections every 1 to 3 months.[31] An appropriate response to treatment is demonstrated by an increase in reticulocytes and correction of the anemia.[32] Treatment may also reverse any neurologic damage caused by vitamin B_{12} deficiency if therapy is instituted early in the course of the disease. However, paresthesias recur within months of stopping therapy.[30]

NORMOCYTIC ANEMIAS

The *normocytic* anemias are those anemias where MCV remains normal despite a drop in the hemoglobin and Hct. Unlike the micro- and macrocytic anemias that are frequently caused by structural defects in the hemoglobin, lack of sufficient substrates, or other production problems, the normocytic anemias are most commonly caused by blood loss or inflammation. Blood loss can be acute or chronic and can be due to covert or frank bleeding or hemolysis. Over time, many of the anemias due to blood loss will progress to becoming microcytic (due to a depletion of iron stores from loss of recycled iron) or macrocytic (due to the compensatory release of more immature RBCs, which are larger in size than mature RBCs). Another common cause of normocytic anemia is chronic diseases, which can progress to microcytic anemia because infection and inflammation interfere with bone marrow activity and erythropoietin production and/or function and are associated with a shortened RBC lifespan.[33,34] Table 14-13 outlines the associated laboratory findings that can help distinguish between the causes of normocytic anemia.

Acute Blood Loss   Acute hemorrhage leads to a precipitous drop in the numbers of RBCs. Hypoxia results from the ensuing reduction in the

Table 14-13 Laboratory Findings in Normocytic Anemia

	Normocytic Anemia				
Tests	Acute Blood Loss	Anemia Chronic Disease	Hemolysis	Renal Insufficiency	Iron Deficiency
Ferritin	Normal	Normal or high	Low	High	Low
TIBC	Normal	Low or normal	Variable		High
Reticulocyte	High	Low	Variable	Low	Low
RDW	Normal	Normal	Variable		High
Hb electrophoresis	Normal	Normal	HbF, HbA$_2$, HbS	Normal	Normal
Other studies		Low serum albumin High erythrocyte sedimentation rate (ESR)	Studies suggestive of hemolysis (Table 14-14)	Elevated serum creatinine Normal peripheral smear Normal bone marrow	

Hb = hemoglobin, RDW = red blood cell distribution width, TIBC = total iron-binding capacity

oxygen-carrying capacity of the blood. Decreased intravascular volume leads to hypovolemia and the development of hypotension. Symptoms progress from mild tachycardia and normal blood pressure to tachycardia, tachypnea, and decreased pulse pressure. Marked tachycardia and significantly decreased blood pressure are seen when 40% or more of the normal blood volume is lost. Extreme measures must be taken at this point in order to save the person's life.

In rare circumstances, a blood transfusion may be necessary to preserve life. Situations that warrant consideration of a blood transfusion include a hemorrhage of $\geq$ 1500 mL, a loss of $\geq$ 30% of blood volume, or hemoglobin levels that fall to $\leq$ 7 g per dL.[35] One unit of blood is equal to 250 mL and will raise the Hct by 3%. Other products such as plasma, platelets, and cryoprecipitate can also be used. Use of plasma is indicated with active bleeding and an international normalized ratio greater than 1.6.[35] The administration of platelets should be considered if bleeding is present with co-occurring thrombocytopenia and platelet dysfunction. Cryoprecipitate, which is created by abstracting the precipitate from fresh frozen plasma, has a high concentration of fibrogen and factor VIII and is used in the management of massive hemorrhage or consumptive coagulopathy.

Complications related to receiving a transfusion are rare. Infectious complications are much less common than noninfectious ones. Thanks to aggressive screening programs, the chance of contracting hepatitis B is 1 out of 350,000 transfusions and 1 out of 2.3 million transfusions for HIV.[35] Serious noninfectious reactions include acute hemolysis, allergic reaction, acute lung injury, fever, and circulatory overload.

The International Federation of Gynecology and Obstetrics (FIGO) has characterized abnormal bleeding among nonpregnant women of reproductive age along structural and non-structural lines. It defines acute abnormal uterine bleeding as "an episode of heavy bleeding that, in the opinion of the clinician, is of sufficient severity to require immediate intervention to prevent further blood loss."[36] ACOG has discussed management recommendations for the various causes of acute gynecologic bleeding, based on a history and physical examination following the FIGO guidelines.[37] These include but are not limited to coagulopathy, use of anticoagulant medications or nonsteroidal anti-inflammatory drugs, structural abnormalities, cancers, and the hormonal changes of menarche and menopause, when anovulatory bleeding is most common.[38]

The most common cause of acute blood loss in obstetric practice is postpartum hemorrhage, a potentially life-threatening complication of both vaginal and cesarean section deliveries. Although traditionally defined as a blood loss of greater than 500 mL, recognition that the normal blood loss from vaginal and cesarean delivery often exceeds this level has led to a broader definition of postpartum hemorrhage. Any bleeding that results in signs and symptoms of hemodynamic instability, or bleeding that could result in hemodynamic instability if untreated, is considered postpartum hemorrhage. Any bleeding resulting in a decrease in postpartum Hct of 10% from the prenatal Hct is also considered postpartum hemorrhage.

Hemolytic Anemia

Hemolytic anemias are those anemias in which there is an inadequate number of circulating RBCs caused by the premature destruction of RBCs. Whether inherited or acquired, hemolytic anemia occurs when the bone marrow is unable to compensate for the premature loss of RBCs by increasing their production, resulting in anemia.

Hemolytic anemia can be classified as intrinsic or extrinsic. Intrinsic hemolytic anemias are inherited disorders and include the thalassemias and sickle cell disease. Destruction of the RBCs is due to a defect in the cell itself, causing the RBCs to be more vulnerable and have a shorter lifespan. The underlying pathology associated with intrinsic cases can be related to the RBC cell membranes (e.g., hereditary spherocytosis), enzymes (e.g., G6PD), or the structure or synthesis of the hemoglobin (e.g., sickle cell disease, thalassemia).[17] Extrinsic hemolytic anemias can be due to immune-related causes (e.g., transfusion reactions), drugs (e.g., salazopyrine, dapsone, nitrates, penicillins, cephalosporins, erythromycin, acetaminophen), microangiopathies (e.g., thrombotic thrombocytopenia purpura, preeclampsia/HELLP [hemolysis, elevated liver enzyme, low platelet count], disseminated cancer, transplant rejection), infection (e.g., malaria, pneumoccal sepsis, Gram-negative organisms, HIV), or exposure to chemicals.[17,33,34] The RBCs are healthy and are produced normally. However, hemolysis occurs after RBCs are damaged by being pumped through a damaged microvasculature; exposed to substances, drugs, or infections; or sheared as they pass through a mechanical heart valve.[33] Some types of extrinsic hemolytic anemia are temporary, resolving spontaneously over several months. Others become chronic with periods of remission and recurrence.

General symptoms of hemolytic anemia include classic signs of anemia such as fatigue, pallor, shortness of breath, and tachypnea, and additional symptoms such as jaundice, dark urine, and enlarged spleen (which leads to further hemolysis when the spleen fails to filter out spherocytes and other abnormal RBCs). A hemolytic crisis, which is rare, presents with fever, chills, tachycardia, and hemoglobinuria (a potential cause of renal failure).

Specific laboratory findings are indicative of hemolysis. The hemoglobin and Hct levels will be low. Usually, the RBCs will be normochromic-normocytic, but may also be macrocytic or microcytic. The Coombs test will be positive. Additional findings listed in **Table 14-14** are indicative of hemolysis. Laboratory testing should also include an evaluation for iron and folate deficiency,

Table 14-14 Lab Values Associated with Hemolytic Anemia

Test	Expected Result
Hemoglobin/hematocrit	Low
Indirect bilirubin	High
Serum haptoglobin	Low
Urinalysis	Possible Hb, hemosiderin, urobilinogen
Reticulocyte count	High
RBC	Low
Serum LDH	High

LDH = lactate dehydrogenase, RBC = red blood cell

because RBC destruction can lead to depletion of iron and folic acid stores.[39]

Treatment depends on the specific type and cause of hemolytic anemia, as well as the patient's age, overall health, medical history, extent of disease, tolerance for specific treatment modalities, and expectations for the course of the disease. Treatment may include vitamin and mineral supplements, dietary changes, pharmacologic management, the avoidance of medications known to trigger hemolysis, or splenectomy.

Hereditary Hemolytic Anemia Inherited forms of hemolytic anemia are most often caused by hereditary *spherocytosis*, a congenital hemolytic icterus in which the RBCs are spherical in shape and drop their hemoglobin.[15] The spherical shape is caused by abnormalities in the protein network that maintains shape and flexibility of cell membrane. It is most commonly found in individuals of Northern European descent. The clinical presentation is variable, ranging from mild hemolysis occurring only during illness to more severe disease complicated by hemolysis, jaundice, splenomegaly, cholelithiasis, and crisis.[15]

Laboratory assessment may show anemia, reticulocytosis, high mean corpuscular hemoglobin concentration (MCHC), and spherocytes on peripheral smear. Diagnosis can be confirmed with a positive result on an eosin-5-maleimide (EMA) binding test. Hemolytic crisis is often triggered by infection and may require transfusion. Other rare RBC defects causing hereditary hemolytic anemia include hereditary elliptocytosis and hereditary stomatocytosis.

G6PD   Like HbS, G6PD is protective against malaria; therefore, it is not surprising that it too is most common in people from tropical Africa, subtropical Asia, the Mediterranean, and the Middle East.[8] G6PD is an X-linked genetic disease that affects the G6PD enzyme, which is responsible for blocking effects of oxidizing agents on RBCs. Without the protection provided by the G6PD enzyme, hemolysis occurs in response to illness, stress, and exposure to oxidant medications such as sulfas or nitrofurantoin (Macrodantin) and foods such as fava beans.

Diagnosis is commonly made during the neonatal period when persistent neonatal jaundice raises the suspicion that a neonate may have G6PD.[15] Males are more likely to be affected than females. Affected individuals can also be asymptomatic and may not be diagnosed until later in childhood when exposure to a precipitating event causes hemolysis. During an episode of hemolysis, laboratory findings will include anemia and reticulocytosis, and hemighost and bite cells may be present on the peripheral smear. Definitive diagnosis is made by testing for the G6PD enzyme. Management includes avoidance of precipitants, prompt diagnosis and treatment of all infections, genetic counseling, and prenatal diagnostic testing if a woman is G6PD deficient.[15]

Autoimmune Hemolytic Anemias   Autoimmune disease is rare, affecting 1 to 3 out of 100,000 individuals each year.[40] It is seen primarily in adults and is caused by autoantibodies that coat RBCs, causing them to be destroyed in the spleen, liver, or bone marrow. Autoimmune hemolytic anemias can be classified as cold-antibody hemolytic anemia, warm-antibody hemolytic anemia, or mixed anemia. Warm-antibody anemias are the most common and cause 75% of all cases of autoimmune hemolytic anemias, 15% of cases are due to cold-antibody anemia, and approximately 5% are due to cases of mixed cold- and warm-antibody anemia.[40]

Most, but not all, cases of autoimmune hemolytic anemia have an insidious onset with symptoms developing over several months. Symptoms are related to the degree of anemia; individuals with acute onset may present with pallor, jaundice, tachycardia, hepatosplenomegaly, tachycardia, and angina. In general, cold-antibody hemolytic anemia has a milder presentation with symptoms triggered by exposure to cold air. Within minutes to a few hours after exposure, an affected individual will report headache, abdominal cramps, and pain followed by chills and fever. Acrocyanosis can be noted in the fingers, toes, nose, and ears. Mixed-antibody anemias have a variable presentation.[40]

Diagnosis is based on an analysis of the clinical presentation and laboratory data. With autoimmune hemolytic anemia, the direct Coombs test will be high. More specific testing is needed to differentiate between warm-antibody hemolytic anemia (which is due to IgG autoantibodies) and cold-antibody disease (which is due to immunoglobulin M [IgM] autoantibodies).[40]

A hematology consult is warranted for patients with suspected autoimmune hemolytic anemia. Treatment for warm-antibody anemia generally consists of high-dose intravenous (IV) or oral corticosteroids. If medication is unsuccessful, the spleen is surgically removed. As a last resort, immune system suppressants are used.[17,40] Because individuals with cold-antibody hemolytic anemia have milder episodic symptoms, treatment is primarily preventive by reducing exposure to cold air. If symptoms develop, various medications such as rituximab, chlorambucil, and cyclophosphamide may be instituted.[40]

SICKLE CELL ANEMIA

The sickle cell anemias are hereditary conditions occurring when a sickle gene mutation on the beta chain of hemoglobin is inherited from one or both parents. Sickle cell disease occurs when the offspring receives sickle cell mutations from both parents; sickle cell trait occurs if only one parent passes on the mutation. Sickle cell anemia is seen predominately in Blacks and those of Mediterranean descent. Sickle cell disease affects 1 out of 500 African American infants and 1 out of 36,000 Hispanic American infants born each year in the United States.[41] Individuals with sickle cell anemia have a lifespan that is shortened by 25–30 years on average.

Symptoms of sickle cell disease are proportionate to the percentage of affected RBCs. Individuals with sickle trait have fewer affected RBCs and minimal symptoms, whereas individuals with sickle cell disease can develop significant complications. Other variant hemoglobinopathies are also possible such as HbS/E, HbS/C, HbS/beta thalassemia+, and HbS/beta thalssemia^0. Individuals with HbSS and HgS/beta thalssemia^0 have the most serious presentations.[42]

The underlying pathology leading to the morbidity and premature death associated with sickle cell anemia is complex. HbS polymerizes, or increases its molecular weight under low oxygen tension, forcing the hemoglobin-carrying RBCs to assume an abnormal crescent (or sickle) shape. Because of its abnormal shape, HbS is able to carry less oxygen and is more fragile compared to normal hemoglobin HbA_1. While a normal RBC lives for approximately 120 days, RBCs in sickle disease live only for 16–20 days.[15] RBC production cannot keep up, and chronic anemia and hypoxemia develop. Further, the deformed RBCs

easily adhere to vascular endothelium, reducing blood flow in the microvasculature and creating vascular obstruction. Cell injury leads to the release of inflammatory mediators and free radicals, resulting in chronic low-grade inflammation.[15] As a result, patients develop vasculopathy and tissue hypoxia, which damage the body's organs. Organ damage is often silent until well advanced.

No organ in the body is spared. Damage in the microvasculature can lead to frequent infections, particularly pneumonia, as well as cholelithiasis, retinopathy, hypertension, stroke, nephropathy, leg ulcers, decreased bone density, avascular necrosis, and thromboembolic events. One of the most ominous sequelae of sickle cell disease is acute chest syndrome, which is the most common cause of death in adults with sickle disease.[42] Acute chest syndrome is characterized by chest pain, fever, and new infiltrates seen on x-ray. It frequently accompanies sickle cell crisis, which can make acute chest syndrome more difficult to recognize and so delay treatment.

Symptoms associated with sickle cell are similar to those associated with other hemolytic anemias as described previously. However, the hallmark feature of the disease is painful sickle crises. During a sickle cell crisis, blood flow acutely diminishes, leading to stasis and vascular occlusion within the capillaries, decreasing oxygen and nutrition to the involved tissue, and causing tissue infarction, acute inflammation, and severe anoxic pain. The most commonly affected sites are the limbs and abdomen. Pain in joints or organs of the body can last for hours to weeks, sometimes requiring hospitalization for management. Careful evaluation is necessary, because many of the complications associated with sickle cell disease can mimic sickle cell crisis. Treatment for crisis is supportive—IV hydration, supplemental oxygen as needed, and pain management. Transfusions are avoided unless absolutely necessary because of the danger of iron overload, which can lead to iron deposition in the heart, the pancreas, the pituitary, and liver leading to end-organ damage. Sometimes chelation is required to reduce iron levels to a safer level. Use of the medication hydroxyurea can decrease the number of sickle cell crises an individual experiences, but is not helpful during an acute episode. One of its mechanisms of action is that it promotes the production of HbF; therefore, it is commonly used in individuals with recurrent crises to reduce the number of vasoocclusive episodes and prevent hospitalizations.[42]

Over time, pain becomes progressive for many individuals with sickle disease. Most children are pain-free between crises. However, 50% of adults report mild to moderate chronic pain that persists between crises—often requiring the frequent use of short-acting opioids to manage the pain.[43] Individuals with sickle cell disease can also develop neuropathies, which are described as numbness, tingling, shooting pain, or a pins-and-needles sensation. They are thought to be due to nerve injury and can be worsened by exposure to heat or cold.[44]

Management of the patient with sickle cell disease is collaborative, involving healthcare providers from several specialties (pain management, orthopedics, ophthalmology, neurology, nephrology, and mental health) and coordinated by a specialist experienced in treating individuals with sickle disease. Treatment plans are focused on the management of symptoms and comorbidities. The only definitive cure for sickle cell disease is hematopoietic stem cell transplantation. Cure rates in children are 85% or more if the transplant comes from a fully matched sibling donor. Unfortunately, hematopoietic stem cell transplantation is less frequently performed in adults because of less availability of well-matched donors and higher complication rates in adults compared to children.[42] Research in this area is ongoing.

Women with sickle cell disease are more likely to experience complications in pregnancy. Therefore, contraception counseling is critically important to ensure women only become pregnant when, and if, they desire pregnancy. All contraceptive options are suitable for those with sickle cell disease, including those that are hormonally based.[44]

Aplastic Anemia

Aplastic anemia is characterized by a markedly decreased production of all three types of blood cells by the bone marrow: RBCs, WBCs, and platelets.[45] It reflects a primary defect in, or damage to, stem cells or the marrow microenvironment. Aplastic anemia is categorized as being *idiopathic* where no cause can be detected; *hereditary* such as seen with Fanconi's anemia, Shwachman-Diamond syndrome, and dyskeratosis congenita; or *acquired* as a result of severe illness such as HIV, hepatitis, or EBV; long-term exposure to industrial chemicals; or use of anticancer drugs and other medications. Nearly 70% of all cases are idiopathic, 15% to 20% are inherited, and the remaining cases are due to exposure to a noxious agent.[46]

Symptoms that suggest aplastic anemia include unexplained bleeding (nosebleeds, easy bruising, or visual changes due to retinal hemorrhage), frequent infections, or severe fatigue.[46] Physical findings include general signs of anemia, such as pallor and tachycardia, and signs of thrombocytopenia, such as petechiae, purpura, or ecchymosis. No lymphadenopathy or hepatosplenomegaly is found on clinical examination. Short stature, microcephaly, hypogonadism, mental retardation, and skeletal anomalies may be seen in cases of inherited aplastic anemia. Collaborating laboratory findings include pancytopenia, reticulocytopenia, and macrocytosis. A bone marrow biopsy is required to confirm the disease.

Supportive care includes prophylactic antibiotic and/or antifungal coverage when neutrophils are low, transfusions with platelets to prevent hemorrhage once the platelet count drops below a particular threshold, and chelation if repeated transfusions result in iron overload.[46] Recognition and removal of exposure to any offending agents should also be done. Potential triggers include antibiotic, anti-inflammatory, anticonvulsant, antithyroid, and antimalarial medications, among others, as well as occupational and environmental exposures to benzenes and other solvents, pesticides, lubricating agents, and recreational drugs including methamphetamine.[46] Bone marrow transplant is the preferred treatment in individuals younger than 40 years with severe disease who have a human leukocyte antigen (HLA)-compatible sibling donor. Immunosuppressive therapy is recommended for individuals with severe disease who are older than 40 years, those who are transfusion dependent, and those who do not have an HLA-compatible sibling match.[46] Survival rates post-transplant with a compatible donor have risen to 80% in recent years, whereas the response rate with immunosuppressive therapy has been stable, remaining between 50% and 80%.[47]

ANEMIA OF CHRONIC DISEASE

Anemia of chronic disease is associated with a wide range of chronic malignant, autoimmune, leukemic, inflammatory, and infectious disease conditions.[33] The elderly are most at risk for this anemia, although anyone with a chronic disease may develop it.[32] This anemia develops slowly over time and is due to suppressed production of RBCs in the bone marrow. Symptoms depend on the underlying cause, but will be mild in most cases. A transfusion is sometimes necessary if severe. Chronic liver failure tends to produce the most severe symptoms.

Anemia of chronic disease can be difficult to distinguish from iron deficiency anemia. In both conditions, serum iron and saturation percentage will be low. However, unlike iron deficiency, in anemia of chronic disease, the ferritin level will be normal or increased and the TIBC will be decreased.[17] Therefore, ordering a ferritin level is very useful in helping to differentiate between the two conditions. The red cell indices will sometimes show microcytosis, but a normocytic anemia is much more common.[33] Other laboratory data may include:

- Low transferrin iron saturation percentage
- Low TIBC
- Low transferrin
- Normal serum transferring receptors

Anemia due to chronic disease may coexist with other anemias.[32] For example, an individual with rheumatoid arthritis may, in addition to an anemia of chronic disease, develop iron deficiency from chronic GI bleeding due to medication therapy. Treatment involves identification and eradication or treatment of the underlying cause. Supplementing with iron is not helpful until the underlying cause is addressed. It can delay the identification of serious underlying pathology such as cancer, which is more common among the elderly and is associated with anemia.

ANEMIA IN PREGNANCY

Pregnancy is a time of remarkable natural and expected changes in blood volume. Pregnancy is a state of relative hemodilution. Blood volume increases beginning in the first trimester, with the increase in circulating plasma occurring more rapidly than RBC production can match.[48] Thus, the cutoffs used to designate anemia are lower in pregnancy. Anemia is present if the hemoglobin is less than 11 g/dL in the first and third trimesters or less than 10.5 g/dL in the second trimester.

The newest recommendations from the USPSTF are that evidence does not support routine iron supplementation in nonanemic pregnant women.[49] Prenatal screening remains standard and should be accompanied by dietary counseling early in pregnancy. Anemia that is severe or unresponsive to iron supplementation requires prompt referral to a hematologist.

Pregnant women who are at higher risk of having a hemoglobinopathy should be screened, preferably with hemoglobin electrophoresis.[24] If a woman tests positive, her partner should also be tested. If this is not possible, then referral for counseling and possible amniocentesis is warranted. Women with sickle trait have a 25% risk of having an infant affected with sickle cell anemia if the father is also positive for sickle trait. Women who are carriers also are at a higher risk for asymptomatic bacteriuria and possibly pyelonephritis and require screening for cystitis with serial urine cultures.

Women with sickle disease or other hemoglobinopathies such as HbS/HbC disease and HbS/beta thalassemia may experience more frequent and severe complications during the pregnancy. They are at higher risk of miscarriage, preeclampsia, intrauterine growth restriction, and preterm birth, as well as disease-specific concerns such as sickle crisis.[48] Therefore, these women should be under the care of an obstetrician and hematologist skilled in the management of sickle disease.

Postpartum evaluation for anemia is warranted in certain circumstances. All women whose anemia continued throughout the third trimester, who experienced excessive blood loss during delivery, or who were pregnant with twins or multiples should be screened at their 6-week postpartum visit. Treatment and follow up during the postpartum period is the same for nonpregnant women.

Platelets

Like the RBCs and WBCs, platelets originate from the pluripotent stem cells in the bone marrow. The pluripotent stem cells give rise to a series of daughter cells that include the megakaryocytes and ultimately lead to the development of platelet cells. Platelets play an important role in hemostasis, as they form the initial plug in damaged endothelium. Injury exposes the underlying vascular endothelium to platelets, which then stimulates the platelets to release various substances. These substances have several important roles including triggering an initial response that leads to a rapid but unstable adherence of platelets at the site of injury; allowing the platelets to change shape, which increases their ability to adhere to damaged endothelium; activating other circulating platelets to ensure an effective and sufficient response to injury; and increasing the ability of platelets to bind together to form a larger clot. Damage to vascular endothelium releases von Willebrand factor, which assists in facilitating platelet adhesion by binding together platelets and collagen to create a platform where platelet adhesion can occur. It also stabilizes factor VIII (antihemophilic A factor), which in turn strengthens the developing fibrin meshwork in the platelet clot. Tissue factor is also released with vascular injury and triggers the coagulation cascade leading to the release of fibrin, which is woven into the platelet clot. The integration of fibrin strengthens and solidifies the platelet plug and prevents further bleeding.[50]

Essential History, Physical, and Laboratory Evaluation

The only test result on the CBC that offers an indication of the health of the coagulation system is the platelet count. A platelet count can be either too low (thrombocytopenia) or too high (thrombocytosis). Abnormal numbers of platelets can be spurious or a sign of a number of disparate entities. Therefore, an astute provider should inquire about the presence of infection, nutritional deficiencies, medication use, and alcohol and illegal substance use, as well as symptoms of platelet dysfunction or anemia.

A complete physical and laboratory evaluation are necessary to tease out the most likely diagnosis. Physical findings that may indicate platelet dysfunction include bleeding gums, easy bruising, epistaxis, and petechial rashes. Other signs of anemia may be present, such as increased heart rate, flow murmurs, and splenomegaly.

Laboratory testing should mirror the most likely diagnosis. With thrombocytopenia, a careful review of the peripheral smear is necessary to rule out laboratory error. A small percentage of the population will have "clumped" platelets, making it impossible for the automatic counters used in laboratory testing to provide an accurate assessment of the actual number of platelets. Rerunning the platelet count using an alternative anticoagulant such as citrate or heparin will demonstrate a higher platelet count. If thrombocytopenia is not thought to be a spurious laboratory finding, then at minimum, laboratory assessment should include a CBC with indices, differential, and reticulocyte count; clotting profile (prothrombin time [PT], activated partial thromboplastin time [APTT], and fibrinogen); kidney and liver tests; HIV testing; and thyroid function tests. Other tests to consider are an evaluation of nutritional deficiencies, tests for autoimmune disorders such as lupus or rheumatoid arthritis, workup for hemolytic anemia, and other coagulopathies depending on the specific differential list for a particular woman.

Follow-up testing for thrombocytosis should also include a CBC with indices, differential, and reticulocyte count. Nutritional deficiencies are more strongly associated with thrombocytosis and should be included in the panel. However, most cases of thrombocytosis are reactive in nature, so the platelet count should normalize as the underlying conditions resolve. Therefore, monitoring the platelet level is important in order not to miss more serious underlying conditions such as cancer.

Management of Common Conditions

The following section discusses the most common etiologies associated with thrombocytopenia and thrombocytosis. The reader is referred to a more comprehensive text on hematology for further details. **Table 14-15** lists conditions commonly associated with having lower or higher numbers of platelets.

THROMBOCYTOPENIA

The underlying etiologies leading to *thrombocytopenia* can be categorized as those related to increased destruction, underproduction, and sequestration. No matter the underlying cause, women are generally asymptomatic until platelet counts drop below 50,000 mcg/L.[51] At this level, more bleeding might be noted with minor trauma, but spontaneous bleeding does not generally occur until levels fall below 20,000 mcg/L.

Destruction of Platelets Destruction of platelets can occur from autoimmune causes or by damage to the platelets in the microvasculature. Pregnancy is associated with a benign thrombocytopenia that is caused by increased destruction of platelets. Some medications, such as sulfa antibiotics and some anticonvulsants, are also implicated in platelet destruction.

Immune Thrombocytopenia (ITP) *Immune thrombocytopenia* is a primary autoimmune disorder resulting in the destruction of platelets and impaired production of platelets, with a platelet count of less than 100,000 mcg/L in the absence of any known cause.[51] It can be either transient or persistent, and the degree of bleeding risk is variable. ITP is defined as "newly diagnosed" for the first 3 months. When ITP does not remit spontaneously, it is considered "persistent" until 12 months, then "chronic" if it is present beyond 12 months. It should be considered "severe" only if there is clinically significant bleeding.[52]

Table 14-15 Etiologies Associated with Abnormal Platelet Counts

Abnormality	Mechanism	Example
Thrombocytopenia	Decreased production	Bone marrow problems
		Folate deficiency
		Vitamin B_{12} deficiency
		Medications
		Aplastic anemia
		Radiation
		Alcohol/drug abuse
		Infections
		Congenital
	Increased destruction	Lupus
		Immune thrombocytopenic purpura
		Cancer
		Medications
		Infections
		Thrombotic thrombocytopenic purpura
		Disseminated intravascular coagulation
	Sequestration	Hypersplenism
Thrombocytosis	Physiologic	Exercise
		Stress
		Pregnancy
	Reactive	Acute blood loss
		Infection
		Hemolytic anemia
		Post-splenectomy
		Postoperative
		Trauma
	Other	Cancer
		Polycythemia vera

ITP is often first detected as an incidental finding on laboratory diagnosis; however, a viral infection may precede the findings. There is no correlation between symptoms of bleeding and platelet level. Laboratory testing reveals only thrombocytopenia and occasional large platelets on the peripheral smear. Bone marrow evaluation is generally not needed to arrive at a diagnosis.

Treatment is supportive unless platelet counts fall below 50,000 mcg/L. If needed, corticosteroids and IV immunoglobulins are the first line of therapy. Other medications may be needed if there is no response. The need to perform a splenectomy or bone marrow transplant is extremely rare.[53]

Secondary Causes of Immune Thrombocytopenia There are many secondary causes of ITP; many are associated with autoimmune disorders such as lupus and rheumatoid disorders. Nearly 50% of individuals with antiphospholipid antibody syndrome have thrombocytopenia, although it is generally episodic and mild. Infections such as HIV and hepatitis C are also associated with thrombocytopenia.[51]

Nonimmune Destruction Damage to platelets in the microvasculature can occur from exposure to thrombi associated with hemolytic uremic syndrome, thrombotic thrombocytopenic purpura, HELLP syndrome of pregnancy, disseminated intravascular coagulation (DIC), or exposure to structural abnormalities such as a poorly functioning heart valve, postcardiac bypass, or aneurysm.[51] DIC can be triggered by infection, trauma, or cancer and leads to activation of the coagulation system, consumption of clotting factors, and breakdown of fibrin. With DIC, laboratory findings will show a prolonged APTT with or without a prolonged PT and low fibrogen.[53]

Insufficient Production of Platelets Inadequate production of platelets is among the most common causes of thrombocytopenia in primary care. They are often of nutritional origin and are commonly associated with deficiencies in folic acid and vitamin B_{12} intake and occasionally with iron deficiency. Alcohol use is associated with both folic acid and vitamin B_{12} deficiencies. In addition, alcohol independently suppresses the bone marrow.[54]

Very rarely, thrombocytopenia can be due to congenital causes. The best-known congenital cause of thrombocytopenia is von Willebrand deficiency; in women it presents often after menarche, when excessive menstrual bleeding is noted. With this condition, women may report mucosal bleeding, heavy menstruation, and postpartum hemorrhage.[51] The peripheral smear may show platelet clumping and the presence of large platelets. Confirmation of the diagnosis can be done using immunoassays.

Sequestration In healthy individuals, 25% to 45% of platelets are stored in the spleen. Platelets can be mobilized as needed. However, with any of the conditions associated with splenomegaly, the spleen captures a greater percentage of available platelets and fails to release them in a timely fashion into the peripheral circulation. Consequently, conditions associated with splenomegaly can lead to thrombocytopenia. These conditions include hemolytic anemia, cirrhosis, infections, and cancer.

Thrombocytosis

The vast majority of cases associated with high levels of platelets are due to a reactive response of the body to a stressful situation. Up to 85% of cases of *thrombocytosis* are due to conditions such as infections, cancer, hemolytic anemia, kidney problems, and blood loss that result in elevated platelets from compensatory mechanisms dealing with the underlying pathology.[55] The thrombocytosis seen in reactive conditions is likely to resolve over time. Rarely, elevated levels of platelets are due to essential thrombocytosis or myeloproliferative states. Distinguishing between these possibilities is important, because thrombosis is more common in essential thrombocytosis than bleeding. Understanding the underlying pathophysiology can help elucidate risks, direct appropriate treatment, and determine if watchful waiting or aggressive management will lead to the best outcomes.[55]

Conclusion

Many of the conditions described in this chapter are amenable to diagnosis in the primary care setting. However, in some cases, additional evaluation by a specialist in hematologic disease will be required for definitive diagnosis and management. When the symptoms and clinical findings of a hematologic disorder are unclear or the management is complex, this is an area where consultation and referral are always appropriate.

References

1. Minors DS. Physiology of red and white blood cells. *Anaesth Intens Care Med.* 2004;5(5):174-178.
2. Cerny J, Rosmarin AG. Why does my patient have leukocytosis? *Hematol Oncol Clin North Am.* 2012;26(2):303-319.
3. Kolaczkowska E, Kubes P. Neutrophil recruitment and function in health and inflammation. *Nat Rev Immunol.* 2013;13(3):159-175.
4. Scapini P, Cassatella MA. Social networking of human neutrophils within the immune system. *Blood.* 2014;124(5):710-719.
5. Young B, O'Dowd G, Woodford P. *Wheater's Functional Histology: A Text and Colour Atlas.* 6th ed. Philadelphia, PA: Churchill Livingstone; 2013.
6. Chabot-Richards DS, George TI. Leukocytosis. *Int J Lab Hematol.* 2014;36:279-288.
7. George-Gay B, Parker K. Understanding the complete blood count with differential. *J Perianesth Nurs.* 2003;18(2):96-117.
8. George TI. Malignant or benign leukocytosis. *Hematol Am Soc Hematol Educ Program.* 2012;2012:475-484.
9. Abramson N, Melton B. Leukocytosis: basics of clinical assessment. *Am Fam Physician.* 2000;62(9):2053-2060.
10. Tefferi A, Hanson CA, Inwards DJ. How to interpret and pursue an abnormal complete blood cell count in adults. *Mayo Clin Proc.* 2005;80(7):923-936.
11. Reagan JL, Castillo JJ. Why is my patient neutropenic? *Hematol Oncol Clin North Am.* 2012;26(2):253-266.
12. Centers for Disease Control and Prevention. Fast Stats: Anemia or iron-deficiency 2015. Available at: http://www.cdc.gov/nchs/fastats/anemia.htm. Accessed April 7, 2016.
13. Constantino BT, Cogionis B. Nucleated RBCs—significance in the peripheral blood film. *Lab Med.* 2000;31(4):223-229.
14. Gordon-Smith T. Structure and function of red and white blood cells. *Medicine.* 2013;41:193-199.
15. Kesse-Adu R, Howard J. Inherited anaemias: sickle cell and thalassaemia. *Medicine.* 2013;41(4):219-224.
16. Hassell KL. Population estimates of sickle cell disease in the U.S. *Am J Prev Med.* 2010;38(4):S512–S521.
17. Parker-Williams EJ. Investigation and management of anaemia. *Medicine.* 2013;41(4):212-218.
18. American Academy of Family Physicians. Clinical Preventive Service Recommendation: Iron Deficiency Anemia. Available at: http://www.aafp.org/patient-care/clinical-recommendations/all/iron-deficiency-anemia.html. Accessed April 24, 2016.
19. American College of Obstetricians and Gynecologists. Anemia in pregnancy. Practice Bulletin no. 95. *Obstet Gynecol.* 2008;112(1):201-207.
20. U.S. Preventive Services Task Force. Screening for iron deficiency anemia—Including iron supplementation for children and pregnant women: Recommendation statement. 2006. Available at: http://www.uspreventiveservicestaskforce.org/Page/Document/RecommendationStatementFinal/iron-deficiency-anemia-screening. Accessed April 7, 2016.
21. Dubois RW, Goodnough LT, Ershler WB, Van Winkle L, Nissenson AR. Identification, diagnosis, and management of anemia in adult ambulatory patients treated by primary care physicians: evidence-based and consensus recommendations. *Curr Med Res Opin.* 2006;22(2):385-395.
22. Centers for Disease Control and Prevention. Update: Newborn screening for sickle cell disease—California, Illinois, and New York, 1998. *MMWR.* 2000;49(32):729-731.
23. Ojodu J, Hulihan MM, Pope SN, Grant AM. Incidence of sickle cell trait—United States, 2010. *MMWR.* 2014;63(49):1155-1158.
24. American College of Obstetricians and Gynecologists. Hemoglobinopathies in pregnancy. Practice Bulletin No. 78. *Obstet Gynecol.* 2007;109:229-237.

25. Lynch E. Peripheral blood smear. In: Walker HK, Hall WD, Hurst JW, eds. *Clinical Methods: The History, Physical, and Laboratory Examinations.* 3rd ed. Boston, MA: Butterworths; 1990. Available at: http://www.ncbi.nlm.nih.gov/books/NBK263/. Accessed April 7, 2016.

26. Liu K, Kaffes AJ. Iron deficiency anaemia: a review of diagnosis, investigation and management. *Eur J Gastroenterol Hepatol.* 2012;24(2):109-116.

27. Harteveld CL, Higgs DR. Alpha-thalassaemia. *Orphanet J Rare Dis.* 2010;5:13.

28. Vichinsky E. Advances in the treatment of alpha-thalassaemia. *Blood Rev.* 2012;26(Suppl 1):S31-S34.

29. Galanello R, Origa R. Beta-thalassemia. *Orphanet J Rare Dis.* 2010;5(1):11.

30. Stabler SP. Vitamin B12 deficiency. *N Engl J Med.* 2013;368:149-160.

31. Oh R, Brown D. Vitamin B12 deficiency. *Am Fam Physician* 2003;67(5):979-986.

32. Smith D. Anemia in the elderly. *Am Fam Physician.* 2000;62(7):1565-1572.

33. Tefferi A. Anemia in adults: a contemporary approach to diagnosis. *Mayo Clin Proc.* 2003; 78(10):1274-1280.

34. Brill JR, Baumgardner D. Normocytic anemia. *Am Fam Physician.* 2000;62(10):2255-2263.

35. Sharma S, Sharma P, Tyler L. Transfusion of blood and blood products: indications and complications. *Am Fam Physician.* 2011;83(6):719-724.

36. Munro MG, Critchley HO, Fraser IS; FIGO Menstrual Disorders Working Group. The FIGO classification of causes of abnormal uterine bleeding in the reproductive years. *Fertil Steril.* 2011;95(7): 2204-2208, 2208.e1-3.

37. American College of Obstetricians and Gynecologists. Committee Opinion No. 557. Management of acute abnormal uterine bleeding in nonpregnant reproductive-aged women. *Obstet Gynecol.* 2013;121:891-896.

38. American College of Obstetricians and Gynecologists. Practice Bulletin No. 128. Diagnosis of abnormal uterine bleeding in reproductive-aged women. *Obstet Gynecol.* 2012;120:197-206.

39. Bryan LJ, Zakai NA. Why is my patient anemic? *Hematol Oncol Clin North Am.* 2012;26(2):205-230.

40. Bass GF, Tuscano ET, Tuscano JM. Diagnosis and classification of autoimmune hemolytic anemia. *Autoimmun Rev.* 2014;13(4-5):560-564.

41. Centers for Disease Control and Prevention. Sickle cell disease. 2011. Available at: http://www.cdc.gov/ncbddd/sicklecell/data.html. Accessed April 7, 2016.

42. Kanter J, Kruse-Jarres R. Management of sickle cell disease from childhood through adulthood. *Blood Rev.* 2013;27(6):279-287.

43. Ballas SK, Gupta K, Adams-Graves P. Sickle cell pain: a critical reappraisal. *Blood.* 2012;120(18):3647-3656.

44. Haddad LB, Curtis KM, Legardy-Williams JK, Cwiak C, Jamieson DJ. Contraception for individuals with sickle cell disease: a systematic review of the literature. *Contraception.* 2012;85(6):527-537.

45. Hussein M, Haddad RY. Approach to anemia. *Disease-a-Month.* 2010;56(8):449-455.

46. Marsh J, Ball SE, Cavenag J, Darbyshire P, Dokal I, Gordon-Smith EC, et al. Guidelines for the diagnosis and management of aplastic anaemia. *Br J Haematol.* 2009;147(1):43-70.

47. Guinan EC. Diagnosis and management of aplastic anemia. *Hematology.* 2011;2011(1):76-81.

48. Rizack T, Rosene-Montella K. Special hematologic issues in the pregnant patient. *Hematol Oncol Clin North Am.* 2012;26(2):409-432.

49. Cantor AG, Bougatsos C, Dana T, Blazina I, McDonagh M. Routine iron supplementation and screening for iron deficiency anemia in pregnancy: a systematic review for the U.S. Preventive Services Task Force. *Ann Intern Med.* 2015;162(8): 566-576.

50. Austin SK. Haemostasis. *Medicine.* 2013;41(4): 208-211.

51. Wong EY, Rose MG. Why does my patient have thrombocytopenia? *Hematol Oncol Clin North Am.* 2012;26(2):231-252.

52. Radia D. Thrombocytopenia. *Medicine.* 2013; 41(4):225-227.

53. McDonald V. Acquired disorders of coagulation. *Medicine.* 2013;41(4):228-230.

54. Rodeghiero F, Stasi R, Gernsheimer T, Michel M, Provan D, Arnold DM, et al. Standardization of terminology, definitions and outcome criteria in immune thrombocytopenic purpura of adults and children: report from an international working group. *Blood.* 2009;113(11):2386-2393.

55. Sulai NH, Tefferi A. Why does my patient have thrombocytosis? *Hematol Oncol Clin North Am.* 2012;26(2):285-301.

CHAPTER 15

RESPIRATORY CONDITIONS

Karen Stemler | Barbara K. Hackley

Illnesses of the respiratory system present with myriad symptoms whether the etiologic source is viral, bacterial, or allergic. Symptoms affecting the upper and lower airway, cardiac, integumentary, and muscular systems are often reported. Similar symptoms can occur in many different conditions, making it difficult for the practitioner to determine the underlying cause(s). This chapter describes the possibilities and discusses the presentation, evaluation, and management of common respiratory illnesses in women.

Common Respiratory Symptoms

Some of the most common complaints reported by patients with respiratory illnesses include nasal congestion, fever, and cough (see **Table 15-1** for a more complete list). In pregnancy, rhinorrhea, nasal congestion, sinus congestion, and postnasal drip are particularly common. The same symptoms may be seen as a result of hormonal changes, with a viral or bacterial infection or as part of an allergic response, making the diagnosis of respiratory conditions more difficult in pregnancy. Some

symptoms often appear together and may suggest a specific diagnosis, but in general a practitioner must consider several etiologies. Additionally, the woman may have underlying problems or comorbid conditions that require a different or more aggressive management plan.

Table 15-1 Common Symptoms Seen in Respiratory Conditions

Difficulty sleeping
Ear pain or discomfort
Enlarged lymph nodes
General malaise, fever, chills
Itchy eyes/ears/nose/throat and sneezing
Loss of appetite
Myalgia
Nasal congestion and/or rhinorrhea
Sore throat
Shortness of breath, wheezing, chest tightness, and/or cough

Rhinitis

Rhinitis encompasses a constellation of symptoms: nasal congestion, rhinorrhea, and postnasal drip. The nose and the paranasal sinuses provide essential functions that help maintain a healthy respiratory tract by conditioning and purifying inspired air.[1] Coarse hairs line the distal nasal cavity and filter particles from the air. Mucous membranes, which cover the proximal nasal cavity, provide moisture to inspired air. If the secretions become thick or sticky, the mucous membranes may release mast cell mediators, resulting in mucosal inflammation and increased mucus production. This results in nasal congestion, a runny nose, or postnasal drip. Rhinorrhea is common with the common cold and after exposure to airborne allergens. With postnasal drip, patients usually complain of drainage in the back of the throat, resulting in a constant need to clear the throat. Nasal discharge, cobblestone appearance of the oropharyngeal mucosa, or mucus in the oropharynx may also be noted, but are not specific to postnasal drip.[2] The differential diagnosis of rhinitis includes allergies, infections such as the common cold and sinusitis, structural abnormalities (e.g., deviated septum, nasal polyps, and foreign body), hormonal (e.g., pregnancy, hypothyroidism), and drug-induced *rhinitis medicamentosa* (e.g., caused by oral contraceptives, aspirin or nonsteroidal anti-inflammatory drugs [NSAIDs], or cocaine abuse), among other causes.[3] Rhinitis can also be triggered by ingestion of foods such as hot red peppers, which contain capsaicin. Capsaicin stimulates sensory fibers releasing tachykinins and other neuropeptides.[4]

Fever

Microorganisms and bacterial exotoxins induce macrophages and endothelial cells to produce fever-producing chemical mediators or cytokines (e.g., interleukin-1, interleukin-6, and tumor necrosis factor). These cytokines induce the release of prostaglandin E from the hypothalamus, which increases the set point of the thermoregulatory center. Once the set point has increased, the hypothalamus responds with vasoconstriction and shivering to increase the core body temperature to this new set point and results in a fever.[1]

Noninfectious disorders can also stimulate the production of cytokines. Tissue injury from trauma or surgery can induce a fever, as can neoplasms such as leukemia or Hodgkin's disease. Fever can also occur if the hypothalamus is damaged by intracerebral bleeding, increased intracranial pressure, or trauma to the central nervous system. A fever due to hypothalamic damage will be unresponsive to antipyretic treatment.[1]

Several signs and symptoms occur from fever alone. Due to the inflammatory properties of interleukin-1, leukocytosis, anorexia, and malaise are often noted. The woman's heart rate will increase as the temperature increases. For every rise of 1°F, the heart rate will increase by 10 beats per minutes (BPM) or by 15 BPM for every increase of 1°C. Conditions such as inflammatory bowel disease, tuberculosis (TB) and Kawasaki disease need to be considered if the heart rate does not rise as expected or is out of proportion to the degree of fever.[5] Other common manifestations due to fever are myalgia, arthralgia, fatigue, and headache. An alteration in mental status (e.g., confusion, delirium, agitation, incoordination) can occur in the older adult with temperature elevations above 104°F (40°C) or with concurrent cerebral hypoxemia.[1]

Wheeze

Wheezing results from obstruction in the airway that precipitates shortness of breath and cough in some cases. Airway obstruction is a common feature of many respiratory conditions, but is also seen in other conditions such as vocal cord dysfunction and cardiac disease. Obstruction can occur from bronchospasm, blockage from masses

---

Table 15-2 Differential Diagnosis of Wheezing

Asthma

Bronchiectasis

Chronic obstructive pulmonary disease (COPD)

Congestive heart failure

Cystic fibrosis

Foreign body

Pulmonary edema

Pulmonary embolism

Tumor

Vocal cord dysfunction

---

or secretions, or compression. **Table 15-2** lists conditions associated with wheezing.

Cough

Pathogens can enter the lungs through inhalation, aspiration from the oropharynx, direct spread from the upper to lower respiratory tract via the mucosal membrane, or through the blood. The cough reflex is a defense mechanisms that helps prevent bacteria and other microorganisms from reaching the lower respiratory tract.[6] Each epithelial cell of the trachea and bronchus is lined with approximately 200 cilia, fluctuating several hundred times per minute, preventing stagnation of bacteria, and keeping the flow upward toward the larynx. The mucosal membrane, which lines the cilia, has antimicrobial compounds (i.e., lysozyme and secretory immunoglobulin A [IgA] antibodies) that target bacteria trapped by the cilia. If larger particles, secretions, or foreign bodies are aspirated, then the cough reflex is stimulated and forces these substances upward.[6]

The cough reflex is also needed in patients who smoke. In smokers, the cilia become damaged or paralyzed. As a result, smokers have

difficulty clearing respiratory secretions and have to rely on the cough reflex. If these mechanisms fail, the bacteria may still be inhibited by macrophages and neutrophils present in the alveoli.[6] When microorganisms remain in the lower respiratory tract, symptoms of infection may occur.

Cough can be a presenting symptom in many conditions. Relatively benign and self-limiting to serious, complicated conditions can cause an acute or chronic cough. Acute cough is defined as a cough lasting for less than 3 weeks and is often caused by infections, allergies, or an acute exacerbation of asthma or bronchitis. Subacute coughs are of intermediate duration but are generally assessed in the same way as chronic coughs. Chronic cough persists for longer than 8 weeks and generally reflects a more persistent condition.[7,8] The presentation may provide clues pointing to a specific etiology or etiologies. Inquiring about onset, progression, medications, and comorbidities generally pinpoints the underlying cause. A comprehensive history is needed, because the differential diagnosis list for cough is complex. Patients with gastroesophageal reflux disease (GERD) may or may not have gastrointestinal (GI) symptoms and might present only with a chronic cough.[9] Some medications such as angiotensin-converting enzyme inhibitors (ACEIs) may cause a chronic cough. **Table 15-3** and **Table 15-4** list various conditions associated with acute and chronic cough.

Postnasal drip should be suspected in individuals with a cough. Some patients will not have any upper respiratory signs or symptoms commonly found with postnasal drip, except for cough. These patients often respond well to first-generation antihistamine/decongestant therapy.[2,9] Second-generation, nonsedating antihistamines are not effective in treating an acute cough associated with the common cold. These agents also are not as effective as first-generation antihistamines in treating chronic, nonallergic coughs due to postnasal drip.[2,9]

Table 15-3 Differential Diagnosis of Acute Cough (< 3 weeks' duration)

Acute bacterial sinusitis (if postnasal drip)

Acute bronchitis

Allergic or environmental rhinitis (if postnasal drip)

Aspiration

Asthma

Chronic obstructive pulmonary disease (COPD) exacerbation

Common cold (most common)

Congestive heart failure

Pneumonia

Postnasal drip

Pertussis

Pulmonary embolism

Other viral syndrome

Table 15-4 Differential Diagnosis of Chronic Cough (≥ 3 to 8 weeks' duration)

Asthma

Bronchiectasis

Bronchogenic carcinoma (uncommon)

Chronic bronchitis (uncommon)

Chronic interstitial pulmonary disease

Chronic snoring or sleep apnea

Cystic fibrosis

Gastroesophageal reflux disease (GERD)

Medications: angiotensin-converting enzyme inhibitor (ACEI)

Pertussis

Postinfectious cough

Postnasal drip (*most common*):
- Seasonal allergic rhinitis
- Perennial allergic rhinitis
- Vasomotor rhinitis
- Postinfectious or postviral rhinitis
- Chronic bacterial sinusitis
- Allergic fungal sinusitis
- Nonallergic rhinitis

Psychogenic cough

Physiologic Changes in Pregnancy

Many of the physiologic changes that occur in pregnancy affect the presentation and course of respiratory conditions. Estrogen, progesterone, and placental growth hormone as well as non-hormonal factors such as inflammatory changes, immunologic changes, and parasympathetic up-regulation contribute to the development of nasal congestion in pregnancy.[10]

Other changes in pregnancy affect respiratory function. The pregnant woman's chest expands, the subcostal angles increase, and the diaphragm rises by approximately four centimeters. However, these changes do not affect inhalation and exhalation during pregnancy. Progesterone, derived from the placenta, stimulates the brain's respiratory center producing a hyperventilatory state. Hyperventilation decreases the alveolar carbon dioxide (CO_2) tension and the arterial Pa_{CO2}. The body compensates by decreasing the plasma bicarbonate level, resulting in a minimal change in PH. Given these natural changes, compensated respiratory alkalosis is noted in normal pregnancy. Some pregnant women have subjective symptoms from these changes and report breathlessness.[10] See **Table 15-5** for a description of respiratory changes seen in pregnant women.

During pregnancy, the T helper cells decrease in number and cellular immunity is impaired, leading to a mildly immunocompromised state,

Table 15-5 Normal Pulmonary Values in Nonpregnant and Pregnant Women

Term	Definition	Values Nonpregnant	Pregnant	Clinical Significance
Respiratory rate (RR)	Number of respirations per minute	16 per minute	Changes little	
Tidal volume (V_T)	The amount of air moved in one normal respiratory cycle	450 mL	600 mL (increases up to 40%)	
Residual volume (RV)	The amount of air that remains in the lung at the end of a maximal expiration	1000 mL	Decreases by approximately 200–400 mL	Improves gas transfer from alveoli to blood
Minute ventilation	The volume of air moved per minute; product of RR and V_T	7.2 L	9.6 L (increases up to 40% because of the increase in V_T)	Increased oxygen available for the fetus results in mild compensated respiratory alkalosis.
Forced vital capacity (FVC)	The maximum amount of air that can be moved from maximum inspiration to maximum expiration	3.5 L	Unchanged	If over 1 L, pregnancy is usually well tolerated.
FEV_1	Forced expiratory volume in 1 second	Approximately 80–85% of the vital capacity	Unchanged	
PEFR	Peak expiratory flow rate	Calculation depends on height, age, sex, and coexistent pulmonary condition	Unchanged	

Data from Hegewald MJ, Crapo RO. Respiratory physiology in pregnancy. *Clin Chest Med.* 2011;32(1):1-13.

making pregnant women more prone to infection. Infections such as community-acquired pneumonia (CAP), type A influenza, measles, TB, pneumocystis, and varicella pneumonia are more common and are often associated with more morbidity in pregnant than nonpregnant women.[11] The compensatory respiratory mechanisms triggered by pregnancy result in a reduced capacity for the respiratory system to compensate further if additional insults such as those caused by infection occur.

Management of Specific Respiratory Conditions

Correct management of respiratory conditions depends on an accurate diagnosis, based on a constellation of factors gleaned from the history, physical examination, and laboratory evaluation. Table 15-6 lists symptoms and signs that can help elucidate the underlying cause of respiratory symptoms. Table 15-7 is a quick reference for treatment of respiratory conditions covered in this chapter. Table 15-8 describes the safety of commonly used medications in the treatment of respiratory conditions in pregnancy.

Table 15-6 Key Historical, Physical, and Diagnostic Findings Suggestive of Common Respiratory Conditions

Diagnosis	Key History	Key Physical Findings	Diagnostic Testing
Allergies	Episodic or continuous itchiness of throat, nose, or eyes; skin rashes that occur repeatedly after exposure to an offending agent	Pale boggy turbinates; watery eyes Pale nasal mucosa or "allergic shiners"	Skin testing
Asthma	Episodic wheeze, cough, chest tightness, SOB that may be triggered or worsened by allergies, exercise, or exposure to cold air Symptoms worse at night and may awaken patient Associated with allergies, atopy, and nasal polyps	Expiratory wheeze Breathing easier in upright position Hyperinflated chest	Reversible airway obstruction Diurnal variation in peak flow measures of 20% or more
Bronchitis, acute	Symptoms present for < 3 weeks; cough, chest discomfort, low-grade fever, rhinorrhea, throat pain, fatigue, headache, postnasal drip	Wheezing or rhonchi	Peak flow meter readings-CXR rarely needed
Bronchitis, chronic	Persistent cough with an overproduction of sputum for ≥ 3 months in 2 consecutive years; symptoms: increased sputum, SOB, cough	Lowered FEV_1: If FEV_1 < 40%, hospitalization; if O_2 saturation < 92% and febrile, obtain CXR.	Spirometry Alpha$_1$ antitrypsin CBC: infection, erythrocythemia (Hct > 48% with chronic hypoxemia)
Common cold	Mild symptoms: rhinorrhea, sneezing, nasal congestion, postnasal drip Gradual onset; headache, nasal congestion, rhinorrhea; low energy	Thick, opaque nasal secretion Red and watery conjunctivae No to low-grade fever	No changes are seen in spirometry findings.

Diagnosis	Key History	Key Physical Findings	Diagnostic Testing
COPD	Exertional dyspnea Productive cough Associated with cigarette smoking Recurrent URIs Usually presents in midlife	Wheezing and rhonchi Hyperinflated chest Use of accessory muscles Decreased breath sounds	Spirometry findings demonstrate airway restriction < 70% of predicted value and more rapid loss of lung function than expected for age.
Influenza	Moderate to severe symptoms: nonproductive dry cough Abrupt onset; extreme fatigue Headache, nasal congestion, rhinorrhea	Toxic appearance Fever 100–104°F	None
Pneumonia	Severe symptoms: Acute cough, pleuritic chest pain, dyspnea, fever, fatigue, night sweats, malaise, myalgia, anorexia, toxic appearance	Tachycardia, tachypnea, fever, diminished or focal adventitious breath sounds, inspiratory crackles, and dullness to percussion	PA and lateral CXR show localized opacification from infiltrates.
Sinusitis, acute	Symptoms < 1 month. Major symptoms: may or may not have fever, purulent anterior or posterior discharge, nasal congestion or obstruction, facial fullness/pain Minor symptoms: headache, ear discomfort, tooth pain, halitosis, cough, fatigue	Mucopurulent nasal discharge, sinus tenderness with palpation or percussion	None
Sinusitis, chronic	Symptoms persistent for > 12 weeks. Allergies are often a trigger. Key symptoms: nasal congestion, postnasal drip, nasal discharge, headache, cough, facial pressure	Similar to acute sinusitis	Limited CT scan of the sinus (coronal plane) or if surgery planned, complete series of sinus films (generally ordered by specialist)
Tuberculosis, latent	Asymptomatic, exposure to tuberculosis	Positive TST, normal chest exam	CXR negative
Tuberculosis, active	Malaise, fatigue, night sweats, weight loss, fever, decreased appetite, cough > 2 weeks, productive sputum with or without hemoptysis	Positive TST; adventitious breath sounds may be auscultated	CXR—upper lobe infiltrates and unilateral hilar node enlargement; AFB, sputum culture

AFB = acid-fast bacillus, CBC = complete blood count, COPD = chronic obstructive pulmonary disease, CT = computed tomography, CXR = chest x-ray, FEV_1 = forced expiratory volume in 1 second, Hct = hematocrit, PA = post anterior, TST = Tuberculin skin test, (formerly known as PPD, purified protein derivative), SOB = shortness of breath, URI = upper respiratory infection

Table 15-7 Treatment of Common Respiratory Conditions

Diagnosis	Common Etiology	Preferred Rx	Comments
Common cold	Rhinovirus, parainfluenza, adenovirus, RSV, enterovirus, influenza A	Supportive measures: saline nasal spray, steam, fluids, and rest. Over-the-counter antihistamines, decongestants, anti-tussives, and analgesics may be used for symptomatic relief.	Antibiotics not recommended
Influenza	Influenza A and B	Supportive measures: saline nasal spray, steam, fluids, and rest. Antipyretics. Antiviral medications need to start within 2 days of symptoms onset.	Antibiotics not recommended
Sinusitis (acute)	Mostly commonly viral: rhinoviruses, influenza, parainfluenza. Rarely bacterial: *Streptococcus pneumoniae*, *Haemophilus influenza*, *Moraxella catarrhalis*, *Streptococcus pyogenes*.	Supportive therapy unless symptoms persist. Antibiotic choice depends on underlying pathogen, comorbidities, and community resistance patterns. Duration of antibiotic treatment: 7 to 10 days. See text for specific antibiotic choices.	Reserve antibiotics for use if symptoms continue for ≥ 10 days or increase despite supportive measures. May give antibiotics sooner with severe illness or if symptoms initially better and then worsened.
Sinusitis (chronic)	Most prominent: Staphylococci and respiratory anaerobes (i.e., *Prevotella*, *Porphyromonas*, *Fusobacterium*, *Peptostreptococcus* species).	Topical nasal decongestant (Afrin) Oxymetazoline HCl (0.05%) for 3–5 days maximum Oral decongestants (pseudoephedrine) Nasal corticosteroids Saline nasal spray and steam inhalants Warm compresses Analgesics 2nd-generation antihistamines with concurrent allergies (fexofenadine/loratadine) Mucolytics (Mucinex)	Consult ENT. Antibiotics are usually not effective.

Diagnosis	Common Etiology	Preferred Rx	Comments
Bronchitis (acute)	90% = viral 5–10% = related to mycoplasma pneumoniae, *Chlamydophila pneumoniae, Bordetella pertussis*; *S. pneumoniae, H. influenzae, M. catarrhalis* noted in underlying lung disease.	Bronchodilator (Ventolin) Antihistamine Antitussive agents	Antibiotics generally not recommended. Patients with comorbidities may need antibiotic coverage and treatment of exacerbations of underlying disease.
Bronchitis (chronic)	*H. influenzae, S. pneumoniae, M. catarrhalis* (50–60%)	Mucolytics (Mucinex) Oxygen supplementation Beta-adrenergic agonists (albuterol) Anticholinergic agents (ipratropium bromide) Oral corticosteroids Antibiotics if exacerbation (1st line: amoxicillin, trimethoprim-sulfamethoxazole [Bactrim], doxycycline; 2nd line: amoxicillin-clavulanate [Augmentin], 2nd-/3rd-gen cephalosporins, fluoroquinolone)	Referral to a pulmonologist.
Pneumonia	*S. pneumoniae* (most common)	Macrolides (azithromycin, clarithromycin) Fluoroquinolone (Levofloxacin) Alternative antibiotics: penicillins (Augmentin) and cephalosporins	Avoid ciprofloxacin (Cipro)
Tuberculosis (Latent)	*Mycobacterium tuberculosis*	Isoniazid 300 mg, daily for 9 months	

ENT = ear, nose, and throat; RSV = respiratory syncytial virus

Table 15-8 Use of Medications in Pregnancy and Lactation

Medication	Use	Mechanism of Action	Pregnancy Category	Lactation Category	Side Effects
Acetylcysteine (Mucomyst)	Mucolytic purposes		Compatible	Safety unknown	Bronchospasm, anaphylaxis, nausea, vomiting, rhinorrhea
Albuterol	Asthma or bronchitis	Stimulates beta 2-adrenergic receptors	Compatible	Probably safe	Tremor, nervousness, nausea, tachycardia, palpitations, insomnia
Amantadine	Influenza A	Antiviral	Limited data, risk in animal studies, avoid in 1st trimester	Limited data, potential toxicity	Nausea, dizziness, anxiety, irritability, dry mouth, headache, diarrhea, CHF arrhythmias
Amoxicillin (Amoxil)	Bacterial infections	Bactericidal	Potential risk in 1st and 3rd trimesters	Compatible	Contraindicated in penicillin allergy. Use with caution in cephalosporin allergy; nausea, vomiting, diarrhea, rash.
Amoxicillin-clavulanate potassium (Augmentin)	Bacterial infections	Bactericidal, inhibits beta-lactamases	Potential risk in 1st and 3rd trimesters	Compatible	Contraindicated with penicillin allergies; caution with liver/renal dysfunction. Diarrhea, nausea, vomiting, rash, mucocutaneous candidiasis.
Azithromycin	Bacterial infections	Bactericidal	Compatible	Compatible	Diarrhea, nausea, abdominal pain, dizziness, rash
Budesonide nasal spray (Rhinocort aqua)	Allergic rhinitis	Corticosteroid	Compatible	Limited data, probably compatible	Epistaxis, pharyngitis nasal irritation

Cefuroxime axetil (Ceftin)	Bacterial infections	Bactericidal	Compatible	Compatible	Caution with penicillin allergy, seizure disorder, renal dysfunction. Diarrhea, nausea, rash, abdominal cramps, elevated labs—BUN, creatinine, eosinophils, liver transaminases.
Cetirizine (Zyrtec)	Allergic rhinitis	Antihistamine	Limited data, suggest low risk	Unknown	Drowsiness, fatigue, dry mouth, pharyngitis, dizziness
Ciprofloxacin (Cipro)	Bacterial infections	Bactericidal	Probably low risk. Conflicting data, so best to avoid in pregnancy, especially in 1st trimester if possible.	Limited data, potential toxicity. American Academy of Pediatrics states compatible.	Caution in seizure disorder, renal or liver dysfunction, sun exposure; need to drink with plenty of water. Phototoxicity, nausea, diarrhea, vomiting, abdominal pain, headache, rash.
Clarithromycin (Biaxin)	Bacterial infections	Binds to P site of 50S ribosomal subunit, interfering with protein synthesis	Compatible	Compatible	Caution with liver or renal dysfunction. QT prolongation, pseudomembranous colitis, diarrhea, abdominal pain, taste changes, nausea, rash.
Cromolyn (Nasalcrom spray)	Allergic rhinitis	Mast cell stabilizer	Compatible	No human data, probably compatible	Sneezing, nasal burning, epistaxis, bad taste in mouth
Diphenhydramine (Benadryl)	Allergic rhinitis	1st-generation nonselective antihistamine	Compatible	Limited data, probably safe	Sedation, dry mouth, constipation, dizziness, tachycardia, wheezing, coordination problems, urinary retention, tinnitus

(*continues*)

Table 15-8 Use of Medications in Pregnancy and Lactation (*continued*)

Medication	Use	Mechanism of Action	Pregnancy Category	Lactation Category	Side Effects
Doxycycline	Bacterial infections	Bacteriostatic	Contraindicated in the 2nd and 3rd trimesters	Compatible	Headache, nausea, dyspepsia, diarrhea, rash, photosensitivity
Erythromycin	Bacterial infections	Bactericidal	Compatible (except estolate salt)	Compatible	Abdominal pain, abdominal cramps, stomatitis
Fexofenadine (Allegra)	Allergic rhinitis	2nd-generation selective antihistamine	No human data; animal data show risk.	Limited human data, probably compatible	Headache, dizziness, drowsiness
Fluticasone (Flonase)	Allergic rhinitis	Corticosteroid	Compatible	No human data, probably compatible	Pharyngitis, epistaxis, nasal burning, taste changes, sore throat, throat irritation, voice changes
Guaifenesin	Mucolytic uses	Increases volume and decreases viscosity of respiratory secretions	Compatible	No human data, probably compatible	Nausea, vomiting, GI irritation, headaches
Guaifenesin/ pseudoephedrine (Entex)	Antitussive/ decongestant		Avoid in 1st trimester	No human data, probably compatible	Nervousness, insomnia, headache, urinary retention, nausea, tachycardia, palpitations, tremor

Drug	Indication	Mechanism	Pregnancy	Lactation	Side Effects
Ipratropium nasal spray (Atrovent)	Rhinorrhea or rhinitis	Antagonizes acetylcholine receptors (anticholinergic); can decrease sputum production and cough	Limited data suggest low risk	No human data, probably compatible	Headache, URI, epistaxis, pharyngitis, nasal dryness/irritation
Isoniazid	Antituberculosis	Bactericidal	Compatible	Limited human data, probably compatible	Hepatotoxicity, agranulocytosis, thrombocytopenia, peripheral neuropathy, leucopenia, optic neuritis, nausea, vomiting, diarrhea, rash
Levofloxacin (Levaquin)	Bacterial infections	Bactericidal	Limited human data suggest low risk. However, due to conflicting reports, use should be avoided if possible in pregnancy, particularly in 1st trimester.	Limited human data, probably compatible	Caution with seizure disorder and renal dysfunction; photosensitivity. Nausea, diarrhea, vomiting, abdominal pain, headache, rash.
Loratadine (Claritin)	Allergic rhinitis	Selected antihistamine	Limited human data; animal data suggest low risk.	Limited human data, probably compatible	Headache, fatigue, dry mouth

(continues)

507

Table 15-8 Use of Medications in Pregnancy and Lactation (*continued*)

Medication	Use	Mechanism of Action	Pregnancy Category	Lactation Category	Side Effects
Naproxen	Pain and inflammation	Reduces prostaglandin synthesis	Human data suggest risk in 1st and 3rd trimesters	Limited human data, probably compatible	Anaphylaxis, GI bleed, bronchospasm, abdominal pain, constipation, headache, rash, drowsiness, tinnitus
Oseltamivir (Tamiflu)	Influenza A and B	Antiviral	Compatible	No human data, probably compatible	Nausea, vomiting, diarrhea, abdominal pain, headache
Oxymetazoline 0.05% (Afrin nasal spray)	Nasal congestion	Stimulates smooth muscle alpha-adrenergic receptors	Limited human and animal data	No human data, probably compatible	Nasal irritation, burning, dryness, rebound rhinitis if used for > 5 days
Pseudoephedrine (Sudafed)	Decongestant	Stimulates smooth muscle (sympathomimetic)	Avoid in 1st trimester. Potentially low risk of gastroschisis and small intestinal atresia in 1st trimester.	Limited human data, probably compatible	Insomnia, headache, dizziness, nervousness, excitability, agitation, anxiety, palpitations, tachycardia, tremor
Pyrazinamide	Antituberculosis	Unknown	Compatible	Limited human data, probably compatible	Anorexia, rash, arthralgia, photosensitivity, gout, hepatotoxicity, thrombocytopenia, interstitial nephritis
Rifampin	Antituberculosis	Antituberculosis	Compatible	Compatible	Renal failure, hepatotoxicity, thrombocytopenia, hemolytic anemia, leucopenia, interstitial nephritis, dizziness, abdominal pain, diarrhea, rash, stained contact lenses

Rimantadine	Influenza A	Inhibits viral replication	No human data; animal data suggest risk.	No human data, potential toxicity	Hallucinations, insomnia, nervousness, dizziness
Trimethoprim-sulfamethoxazole (Bactrim-DS, Septra-DS)	Bacterial infections	Bactericidal	Conflicting data. Sulfonamides should be avoided in 3rd trimester. Trimethoprim use associated with cardiovascular and neural tube defects.	Conflicting data. American Academy of Pediatrics classifies as compatible.	Contraindicated with allergy to Sulfa, G6PD-deficiency, folate deficiency, liver or renal dysfunction. Serious side effects: Stevens-Johnson syndrome, agranulocytosis, blood dyscrasias, rash, nausea, vomiting, diarrhea, dizziness, headache, GI upset.
Zanamivir (Relenza)	Influenza A and B	Antiviral	Limited human data, compatible	No human data, probably safe	Bronchospasm, nausea, dizziness, headache

BUN = blood urea nitrogen, CHF = congestive heart failure, G6PD = glucose-6-phosphate dehydrogenase, GI = gastrointestinal, URI = upper respiratory infection

Reproduced from Briggs GG, Freeman RK. *Drugs in Pregnancy and Lactation*. 10th ed. Philadelphia, PA: Wolters Kluwer; 2015.

Common Cold

The human rhinoviruses (HRV), which include more than 100 serotypes, are most commonly associated with upper respiratory infections (URIs).[12] Common causes include any of the following viruses: rhinovirus, influenza A/B/C, parainfluenza, respiratory syncytial virus, coronavirus, or adenovirus. They mostly occur in the fall and winter between September and March.[13]

The incubation period of the common cold is 1 to 3 days. The duration of cold symptoms varies from less than 7 days to a maximum of 14 days with a mean duration of 9.5 to 11 days.[12] Rhinorrhea, sneezing, nasal obstruction, and postnasal drip are commonly reported. In adults, nasal symptoms usually peak within 48 to 72 hours and then gradually subside. Other symptoms such as headache, facial pressure, sneezing, irritated throat, hoarseness, and cough may also be reported. Fever and malaise are less common.[13]

Essential History, Physical, and Laboratory Assessment

History

Generally, a patient with the common cold will present with mild symptoms. Inquiring about the progression and severity of symptoms will help distinguish the common cold from other more problematic conditions. Gradual onset, less acute symptoms, and no to low-grade fever are more indicative of the common cold than of other more serious infections such as influenza or pneumonia.

Physical

On examination, the conjunctiva will be clear, but there may be increased *lacrimation* (tearing). Clear fluid behind the tympanic membrane indicates a serous otitis. There should be no erythema, bulging, or displacement of the bony landmarks. The nasal turbinates usually are erythematous and edematous with clear discharge noted bilaterally. The posterior pharynx may be erythematous with minimal edema. If edema is present, it will be symmetrical. The tonsils should not exceed 1+ bilaterally (i.e., visible, but each tonsil is not encompassing more than 25% of posterior pharynx). Most likely, the oral pharynx is usually free of exudates. Lymphadenopathy is uncommon. If lymph nodes are palpable, they will be small in size (~0.5 cm) and only located in the anterior and/or posterior cervical chain. The heart rate and rhythm will be normal. Minor increases in heart rate may be due to a mild temperature or from insufficient fluid intake. The lungs will be clear without any crackles, rhonchi, or wheezing.

Laboratory Testing

No laboratory tests are helpful in evaluating the common cold. Rapid antigen detection or serologic tests have no clinical utility and are not cost effective or practical. Consequently, diagnostic testing is not recommended.

Management

Lifestyle

Regular health maintenance is important in maintaining proper immune function, which will help defend against the common cold. Key points to focus on are regular and thorough hand washing, adequate sleep, sufficient fluid with balanced nutrition, and the use of appropriate measures to manage stress.

Medication

Viral organisms are the cause of the common cold. In general, antibiotics are not needed. Bacterial coinfections are rare, and the overuse of antibiotics can result in side effects, allergic reactions, and the development of antibiotic resistance. Antibiotic therapy should be given only if a secondary bacterial infection (e.g., pneumonia, bacterial sinusitis) is strongly suspected. Other treatments such as dextromethorphan, intranasal ipratropium, and decongestants can be helpful.[14] Intranasal ipratropium reduces rhinorrhea but not nasal congestion.[15] Combination antihistamines/decongestants also may be helpful for cough and cold symptoms in adults, but unfavorable side effects (e.g., blurred vision, dizziness, dry mouth, tachycardia, urinary retention, agitation, hypertension, palpitations, dysrhythmia, and sleeplessness) have been reported.[14]

COMPLEMENTARY OR ALTERNATIVE CHOICES

Herbal and homeopathic treatments have been tested in vitro and in controlled studies; however, due to small sample sizes, study limitations, and variable outcome results, the effectiveness and safety of many of these treatments remain uncertain, especially in pregnant and lactating women. However, several meta-analyses support the use of specific products in select situations. A Cochrane review of the literature concluded that the evidence supports the regular use of vitamin C in the prevention of the common cold only in marathon runners and in skiers/soldiers exercising in Arctic environments. While regular use of vitamin C did not reduce the incidence of the common cold in the general population, it did shorten duration and lessen the severity of colds when they did occur.[16] Use of vitamin C as a therapeutic treatment of the common cold was found to be ineffective.[16] Initiating zinc lozenges at a dose of ≥ 75 mg/day within 24 hours of the onset of symptoms of the common cold has been found to be associated with a shorter duration of symptoms in a meta-analysis of 16 trials.[17] Insufficient evidence exists about the use of garlic to prevent the common cold. One recent Cochrane systematic review identified only one small study (N = 146) on the utility of garlic supplementation in the prevention of the common cold. This study reported 50%

fewer episodes of the common cold in the group taking a daily garlic supplement (with 180 mg of allicin).[18] Five out of six studies included in a systematic review of the literature on the effectiveness of *Echinacea purpurea* in the treatment of the common cold reported significantly shorter and less severe episodes of illness in those treated with *Echinacea purpurea*.[19] Of note is that more evidence is available for *Echinacea purpurea* than for *Echinacea angustifolia* or *pallida* and for aerial parts of the plant than the roots.[19] Other studies suggest that *Andrographis paniculata,* an herbal product branded as KalmCold, may reduce the severity and duration of symptoms associated with the common cold.[20,21] Taken together, the evidence suggests that vitamin C, zinc lozenges, echinacea, and KalmCold may be useful in mitigating the symptoms of the common cold, but more studies are needed to clarify which dosage and formulation are most effective.[19]

PATIENT INSTRUCTIONS

Transmission occurs with hand-to-nose or hand-to-eye contact after exposure to the nasal secretions of the infected individual. Good hand washing is the key to the prevention and control of the common cold. Adequate sleep and nutrition are essential in boosting the immune system's ability to combat and prevent further illness.

The following techniques may provide some relief from nasal or sinus congestion: 1) using a saline nasal solution two to four times per day, 2) humidified air, 3) steam treatments (e.g., breathing in steam from boiled water, steamy bath, or shower), and 4) drinking plenty of fluids. If a woman's symptoms worsen or no relief is noted in 1 to 2 weeks, she should return for a reevaluation.

MANAGEMENT DURING PREGNANCY AND LACTATION

The management of the common cold does not change in pregnancy or lactation. Medication use should be minimized but may be used as necessary to afford relief from moderate to severe symptoms. See Tables 15-6 and 15-7 for further information on appropriate treatments for the common cold.

Influenza

Pandemics due to influenza have occurred in 1918–1919 (Spanish flu—500,000 US deaths), 1957–1958 (Asian flu—69,800 US deaths), 1968–1969 (Hong Kong flu—33,800 US deaths), and 2009–2010 (novel virus, H1N1—8,870–18,300 deaths).[22] Individuals 65 years old and older are most affected by influenza, with higher numbers of hospitalizations and deaths than other age groups.[23,24] However, one of the features of the most recent pandemic in 2009–2010 was that up to one-third of patients admitted to intensive care units (ICUs) were previously healthy with no recognizable risk factors.[25] Excessive immune response is suspected in increased deaths among healthy individuals during a pandemic with a novel viral strain; lack of prior exposure to similar viruses is the underlying cause. While deaths are higher during pandemics, influenza causes significant morbidity and mortality every year. During 2012–2013, there were approximately 12,170 hospitalizations related to influenza.[24] Fatal outcomes have been cited in patients at highest risk, including newborns, pregnant women, older adults, immunosuppressed patients, and the chronically ill.

Essential History, Physical, and Laboratory Assessment

Symptoms are acute, often affecting the oropharyngeal and bronchial airways. These same symptoms are found with other viral illnesses such as the common cold, except the symptoms are more severe in influenza. Fever, malaise, myalgia, cough, and headache are commonly present with

Table 15-9 Complications Related to Influenza

Bronchitis
Dehydration
Exacerbation of comorbid medical problem (e.g., asthma, diabetes, congestive heart failure)
Otitis media
Pneumonia
Sinusitis

influenza.[13,25] Table 15-5 compares symptoms seen in individuals presenting with the common cold and influenza.

The approach to a patient suspected of having influenza is similar to that used in evaluating a common cold. However, complications are much more common with influenza infections than with other URIs. Patients may need to be evaluated for dehydration, pneumonia, or other problems outlined in **Table 15-9**.[25] High-risk individuals such as infants, children, and the elderly; pregnant women; and individuals with comorbidity or morbid obesity are particularly at risk for serious illness or bacterial coinfections. (**Table 15-10** describes individuals at high risk of influenza infection.) Bacterial coinfections usually occur within 6 days of influenza infection and are associated with increased mortality. A bacterial coinfection should be suspected if the patient demonstrates hypoxia, dyspnea, tachycardia, or signs of sepsis. A thorough history and physical exam are essential in order to confirm the diagnosis and to identify complications.

Providers should consider symptomatology, illness severity, and the presence of any comorbidity to determine if further diagnostic evaluation is needed.[26] Laboratory testing (i.e., complete blood count with differential [CBCD], electrolytes, and kidney function tests) or radiologic imaging (e.g., chest x-rays) may be necessary if complications

---

Table 15-10 High-Risk Factors
for Developing Influenza or
Complications Related to Influenza

Adults aged 65+

Children younger than 5 years, and especially those younger than 2 years old

Residents of a chronic-care facility, prison, or college dormitory

People with chronic medical disorders (e.g., neuro-muscular disorders, cerebral palsy, stroke, seizure disorders, dementia, cardiovascular disorders, diabetes, asthma or other respiratory disorders, chronic liver or renal disease, or sickle cell anemia)

People with immunosuppressive disorders (e.g., cancer, transplant recipients, use of immunosuppressive drugs, HIV/AIDS)

Pregnant women, up to 2 weeks postpartum, and pregnancy loss

Healthcare workers

Household contacts (including children) or caretakers of persons at high risk

---

are highly suspected. Further testing with a reverse transcription polymerase chain reaction (RT-PCR) assay or viral culture is rarely needed, but may be required to confirm a diagnosis of influenza in special situations. Laboratory tests are used when investigating a possible outbreak in an institutional setting and can be considered for use in the outpatient setting if test results will influence clinical management for the affected individual or for those in the general population.[27] During influenza season, outpatient testing should be conducted for immunocompetent persons who are at high risk of complications secondary to influenza, immunocompromised persons with febrile respiratory symptoms, elderly persons and infants with suspected sepsis or fever of unknown origin, and if test results will be

used by local community surveillance systems.[27] Specimens should be obtained within 5 days of symptom onset for immunocompetent individuals. Immunocompromised individuals can shed virus for weeks or months and may benefit from testing beyond 5 days.[27]

Several tests are available. Currently, the most sensitive and specific test is the RT-PCR.[27] It is more sensitive than a viral culture and can differentiate between influenza types and subtypes. Results are available in 4 to 6 hours. Another option is the direct fluorescent antibody or indirect fluorescent antibody staining.[27] Results are available within hours, but their accuracy depends on the quality of the specimen and laboratory expertise. Additionally, commercial rapid influenza diagnostic tests (RIDTs) are available. RIDTs are simple to use and results are available within 10 to 30 minutes, but their results should be interpreted with caution.[27] Although the specificity of RIDTs is usually greater than 90%, the sensitivity of these tests varies from 10% to 80%.[28] Negative test results should be followed by an RT-PCR or viral culture.[27] Viral cultures are generally not used for screening, but can be used on specimens collected from individuals suspected to have influenza when low influenza activity is present in the community, because the accuracy of RIDTs depends on the prevalence of infection in the surrounding community.[27] Viral cultures are also helpful in identifying the particular viral strains that are circulating in the surrounding community.

Management

LIFESTYLE

The influenza vaccination can prevent illness from influenza types A and B. Even if the vaccine fails and an individual becomes infected, the clinical course tends to be milder and is associated with less morbidity. Individuals 6 months and older, especially those at high risk, should receive the influenza vaccine annually.

MEDICATION

Antiviral medications, such as oseltamivir (Tamiflu), zanamivir (Relenza), and rimantadine hydrochloride (Flumadine), are used for prophylaxis or treatment of influenza. These medications should not be used as a substitute for vaccination.[27,29] Patients who have received the vaccine may still become symptomatic with influenza and may require treatment. Rimantadine is effective against influenza type A, not influenza type B. Due to increasing resistance, rimantadine is no longer recommended for the treatment or prevention of influenza.[29] Oseltamivir and zanamivir are active against influenza types A and B.[27] Both are approved for the prevention of influenza in adults and for the treatment of uncomplicated acute influenza A or B in adults who have been symptomatic for less than 48 hours. Due to reports of increasing resistance in some flu seasons, particularly to oseltamivir, providers should consult the Centers for Disease Control and Prevention (CDC) website annually to confirm recommendations regarding antiviral medications.

Antiviral medications are efficacious in shortening the duration of illness by 1 to 3 days in healthy adults if treatment is initiated within 48 hours of the onset of symptoms.[30] Antiviral medication use is most effective when taken within 48 hours of symptom onset.[23] Data are more limited about the efficacy of the use of antiviral medications to reduce the rates of complications related to influenza infections in high-risk individuals; however, a limited number of studies report lower rates of pneumonia, hospitalization, and mortality in high-risk individuals—even in those who initiated treatment with antiviral agents later than 48 hours after symptom onset.[30] See **Table 15-11** for more detailed information regarding antiviral medications for treatment and prophylaxis.

Increased mortality occurs in individuals coinfected with influenza and pneumonia.[27] If a bacterial coinfection is suspected or confirmed, antiviral and antibiotic treatments should be initiated early in the course of symptoms.[27] Common organisms that contribute to bacterial coinfections include *Staphylococcus aureus*, *Streptococcus pneumoniae*, and *Haemophilus influenzae*.[31] If a patient presents with abrupt respiratory distress or hemoptysis, referral for hospital admission and antibiotic coverage is necessary. A delay in antiviral treatment or necessary antibiotic coverage may result in worse clinical outcomes.[27]

Table 15-11 Antiviral Influenza Medications

Antiviral Agent		Dosage	Side Effects/Cautions
Oseltamivir	Chemoprophylaxis	75 mg once daily	• Preferred for use in pregnant women
	Treatment	75 mg twice daily	• Compatible with breastfeeding • Adjustments in dose may be necessary for those with impaired renal function • Nausea and vomiting common
Zanamivir	Chemoprophylaxis	10 mg (2 inhalations) once daily	• Not recommended for use in those with asthma or underlying pulmonary conditions
	Treatment	10 mg (2 inhalations) twice daily	• Compatible with breastfeeding

COMPLEMENTARY OR ALTERNATIVE CHOICES

Research on the use of complementary and alternative medications (CAMs) including vitamin C, zinc, echinacea, elderberry, garlic, ginseng, and oscillococcinum in the treatment of influenza is sparse. Methodologic flaws make it difficult to determine the effectiveness or safety of these products.[32] However, newer research on a Chinese medicine product, *Lianhuaqingwen,* suggests that the use of this product is better at relieving symptoms of the flu than oseltamivir.[33]

PATIENT INSTRUCTIONS

Adequate hydration is important. Those infected with influenza should be encouraged to consume two or more liters of water or other fluids. An easier gauge is to have the patient drink enough fluids to prevent thirst and to keep their urine a clear, light yellow. Caffeine and alcohol intake should be decreased or eliminated to prevent further fluid loss. Thorough, frequent hand washing should also be encouraged. Patients should remain out of school or work for 24 hours after fever or major symptoms have resolved.

Patient education regarding transmission and prevention should be given. Because adults can shed the influenza virus from 1 day before symptoms begin until 7 to 10 days later, individuals who have had close contact in this time period with someone with influenza may become infected.[29] Infected individuals should be instructed to avoid contact with pregnant women, children, older adults, and others who are immunocompromised or have a chronic illness. Frequent hand washing and adequate rest, fluid, and nutrition intake are the most important factors in preventing influenza. All individuals (i.e., older than 6 months of age) should receive the influenza vaccine annually, preferably as soon as it becomes available or during the influenza season, as long as no contraindications to vaccine receipt are present.

MANAGEMENT DURING PREGNANCY AND LACTATION

Physiologic changes associated with pregnancy, such as increased heart rate, stroke volume, and oxygen consumption; declining lung capacity; and alterations in immunologic function, put pregnant women and women within 2 weeks postpartum at increased risk for complications related to influenza.[29] The American College of Obstetricians and Gynecologists and the Advisory Committee on Immunization Practices recommend immunizing all women in pregnancy.[29,34]

The neuraminidase inhibitors are considered safe in pregnancy and during lactation. Antiviral postexposure chemoprophylaxis can be considered for asymptomatic pregnant women depending on the presence of underlying comorbidities and degree of exposure. Close contact is defined as having cared for or lived with a person with confirmed, probable, or suspected influenza. It also includes having been exposed to respiratory droplets or body fluids or being face to face with someone who likely has influenza.[35]

Treatment of influenza can be initiated with antiviral medications in pregnant women and postpartum women who have delivered within the last 2 weeks and who have symptoms suggestive of influenza. A woman may continue breastfeeding during the course of antiviral treatment with oseltamivir or zanamivir.[36,37] The preferred product, according to the CDC, in pregnant and lactating women is oseltamivir.[35]

Pneumonia

In the United States, CAP continues to be one of the leading causes of death, affecting disproportionally the young and the old.[38] The severity of illness and the prognosis depend on the patient's age, immune status, and the presence of comorbid conditions.

The most common causes of CAP are *S. pneumoniae, H. influenzae, Staphylococcus aureus,* and *Moraxella catarrhalis*.[39] Other common infective agents include *Mycoplasma pneumoniae* and *Chlamydophila pneumoniae*. Individuals with a prior history of methicillin-resistant *S. aureus* (MRSA) skin infections are at greater risk of developing pneumonia secondary to MRSA.[40] Viral infections, such as those due to influenza A virus, are other common causes of pneumonia. Fungal infections are rarely associated with pneumonia. In approximately 50% of cases, no causative agent can be identified.[41]

Essential History, Physical, and Laboratory Assessment

History

Pneumonia should be suspected if an individual has an acute cough (which may be productive or nonproductive) accompanied by shortness of breath, weakness, malaise, or a decline in mental status.[40] Oftentimes mental status changes or delirium are the only manifestation of pneumonia in the elderly.[42] Other symptoms, such as tachypnea, tachycardia, fatigue, malaise, night sweats, pleuritic chest pain, myalgia, and anorexia, may or may not be present. Occasionally, an individual with pneumonia may report abdominal pain due to compression from an infiltrate in the right lower lobe, which then stimulates the 10th and 11th thoracic nerves resulting in pain radiating to the right lower quadrant.

It is important to identify any preexisting medical problems. The differential diagnosis includes asthma exacerbation or reactive airway disease, congestive heart failure, chronic obstructive pulmonary disease (COPD), pulmonary embolism, lung cancer, empyema, lung abscess, pleurisy, and aspiration pneumonitis. If the patient is pregnant, pulmonary embolism or pulmonary edema associated with tocolytic treatment are other possibilities.[43]

The social history may help narrow down possible causes. Inquiring about travel history, occupation, animal exposures, and sexual history can suggest other etiologies. *Legionella* pneumonia has been associated with cruise ships and hotel stays.[40]

Physical

The most common objective findings suggestive of pneumonia are tachycardia greater than 100 BPM, tachypnea greater than 20 breaths per minute, fever of more than 100°F, diminished breath sounds, crackles on inspiration, or rhonchi. In the elderly, fever is often absent. Increased tactile fremitus may be found on examination in individuals with pneumonia. Other causes for increased tactile fremitus include the presence of a compressed lung or solid mass. Signs of consolidation may also be present with pneumonia. If consolidation is present, dullness will be heard over the affected lung zone during percussion, and increased vocal resonance, or *pectoriloquy* may be noted on auscultation. Both *egophony* (resonance over the lungs) and increased fremitus are highly specific for pneumonia but are helpful only when present. Pneumonia can still be present without these findings.[40]

Laboratory

Pulse oximetry is obtained if pneumonia is suspected or if dyspnea is present. If the pulse oximetry reading is less than 95% on room air with no underlying chronic lung disease or less than 92% with chronic lung disease, then further evaluation should be done. Laboratory testing is usually not needed in the outpatient setting, but may be useful if the diagnosis is unclear or if management is complicated by comorbidities. In these cases, the following lab tests may be ordered: a CBCD, basic metabolic panel, and human immunodeficiency virus (HIV). Leukocytosis (i.e., white blood cell count greater than

10,400 per mm^3) with a left shift on the CBCD is often seen with pneumonia.[40] A basic metabolic panel (i.e., glucose, electrolytes, and kidney function tests) is helpful in monitoring the risk status of an individual with pneumonia. Hypoglycemia has been associated with a higher mortality rate within the first 30 days after infection. The dosages of some medications such as antibiotics may need to be adjusted or an alternative treatment chosen if there is impaired kidney function. The electrolytes are needed to evaluate an individual's hydration status. Individuals with advanced HIV disease are at risk for CAP and opportunistic infections; thus an HIV test may be pertinent.

A chest radiograph with posteroanterior and lateral views can be obtained to confirm the diagnosis, check for the severity of the presentation, and to help narrow the diagnosis.[40] Other common diagnoses can mimic CAP, such as congestive heart failure or empyema, and if present, will impact treatment decisions. If the chest x-ray is negative, alternative diagnoses need to be reconsidered (e.g., influenza, bronchitis, pleurisy, asthma exacerbation, COPD, aspiration pneumonitis, or pulmonary embolism). If pneumonia is present, the chest x-ray will commonly show consolidation or infiltrates consistent with interstitial disease. In pregnancy, the chest radiograph is not ordered, unless the results will change patient management. Pregnancy should not prohibit the use of standard radiographic techniques.[43]

Cardiac evaluation is warranted in those with underlying comorbid conditions. A 12-lead electrocardiogram (ECG) should be considered in patients with preexisting cardiac disorders or arrhythmias. Also, if a patient is currently taking class Ia or class III antiarrhythmic agents, antibiotics, antipsychotics, antidepressants, and/or tricyclic antidepressants, measuring the QT interval on the ECG reading is recommended.[44,45] QT prolongation is associated with ECG changes,

cardiac arrhythmias, or syncope and can be precipitated by the use of certain drugs or combinations of drugs.[44,45] Checking for drug-to-drug interactions is key. The risk of QT prolongation is more likely to occur if multiple QT-prolongation drugs are taken concurrently. The presence of hypokalemia can also trigger cardiac changes; potassium replacement may be necessary to lower the risk for an arrhythmia.[45]

Management

The mainstay of treatment for pneumonia is antibiotic coverage. Complementary or alternative therapy plays no role in the management of pneumococcal infections.

LIFESTYLE

Receipt of pneumococcal vaccine is an important strategy for preventing pneumococcal infection in high-risk individuals. Individuals at higher risk of acquiring pneumonia or who have underlying conditions that increase their risk of experiencing severe presentations should receive the influenza and pneumococcal vaccines.

MEDICATION

Antibiotics are needed for the treatment of most cases of pneumonia. The provider should choose an antibiotic or a combination of two antibiotics that will empirically cover both typical and atypical pathogens.[46] In most cases, pneumonia is treated with a single agent, although a combined regimen may be necessary in those individuals with more complex presentations.

Determining whether monotherapy or combination therapy is more appropriate is based on an assessment of the patient's medical history and the contraindications and black-box warnings associated with the antibiotics under consideration. Choice of a particular antibiotic should also be based on an understanding of the epidemiology of antibiotic resistance, which is more common in individuals who are immunosuppressed or taking immunosuppressive therapy, who reside in a long-term care facility, who were treated with antibiotics in the past 90 days, and in those with comorbid illness (e.g., chronic heart, lung, liver, or renal disease; post-influenza; diabetes mellitus; cancer; asplenia; alcoholism; or intravenous drug use).[47]

First-line outpatient treatment of pneumonia in otherwise healthy patients includes the macrolides and doxycycline. Monotherapy with macrolides or doxycycline is recommended only for individuals with no prior antibiotic use in the past 90 days.[40] Macrolides (e.g., azithromycin, clarithromycin) are well tolerated and effective, placing them among the most commonly used agents. Doxycycline is contraindicated in pregnancy.[47]

Individuals with underlying comorbid conditions or recent antibiotic use should be treated more aggressively. The choice of which antibiotic agent to use is partially determined by which antibiotic(s) an individual has used in the prior 3 months. It is imperative to choose an alternative antibiotic from a different class than any antibiotic(s) taken in the past 3 months to decrease the incidence of antibiotic resistance.[40] Individuals who have been recently treated with antibiotics should be treated with a β-lactam (e.g., high-dose amoxicillin, amoxicillin-clavulanate, cefpodoxime, or cefprozil) plus a macrolide for improved outcomes with pneumococcal pneumonia.[40,48]

Since recommendations were released by the Infectious Diseases Society of America and the American Thoracic Society in 2007, changes in the epidemiology and prevalence of many of the causative organisms associated with pneumonia, changes in antibiotic resistance patterns, and the wider use of more effective pneumococcal vaccines have likely impacted the effectiveness of previously recommended antibiotic regimens.[39,41] In the absence of newer guidelines, some authorities recommend treatment based on the suspected causative agent: Bacterial infections should be treated with amoxicillin-clavulanate, influenza infections with oseltamivir, mycoplasma or chlamydial infections with doxycycline or azithromycin, and viral infections with supportive care.[41] Ongoing evaluation of the local epidemiology of infective agents and resistance patterns is critical in selecting appropriate antibiotics in a particular situation.

In the absence of high-risk factors, outpatient treatment with oral antibiotics can be initiated, but close follow up is critical. If no clinical improvement is noted within 72 hours or there is a continued progression or deterioration, pulmonary consult and/or hospital admission will be necessary for further workup and management. If there is no improvement or symptoms worsen despite antimicrobial coverage, the provider needs to consider other possibilities such as the need to change to a different antibiotic regimen, whether complications (e.g., empyema, or obstruction) are developing, or if another alternative or a concurrent diagnosis is present. Other conditions such as pulmonary embolism, congestive heart failure, sarcoidosis, aspiration, myocardial infarction, unstable angina, cardiac arrhythmias, or hypoxemia may mimic pneumonia in some situations.[42,49] The majority of cardiac complications secondary to pneumonia occur within 24 hours; risk declines rapidly over the first 7 days after illness onset.[49]

The decision for hospital admission depends on the patient's age, coexisting conditions, mental status, and vital signs. See **Table 15-12** for factors that increase the mortality risk. Patients who have underlying medical conditions, more severe presentations, or who are older must be evaluated for inpatient admission. Depending on the severity of symptoms, the patient may either be observed for 24 hours or admitted to the hospital for treatment. Individuals who are homeless, incarcerated, or living in a long-term care facility are more likely to be admitted than other patients with similar illness severity.[42]

Table 15-12 Risk Factors for Mortality Secondary to Community-Acquired Pneumonia

Age > 50 years

Coexisting conditions:

- Cancer (i.e., active/diagnosed within 1 year, excluding basal or squamous cell carcinoma)
- Chronic liver disease (i.e., cirrhosis, hepatitis)
- Congestive heart failure
- Stroke or transient ischemic attack
- Renal impairment (i.e., chronic renal disease or blood urea nitrogen > 30 mg per dL or elevated creatinine)
- Smoking

New-onset altered mental status

Abnormal vital signs:

- Temperature < 95°F (35°C) or >104°F (40°C)
- Systolic blood pressure < 90 mmHg
- Pulse > 124 beats per minute
- Respiratory rate > 29 beats per minute (i.e., older than 50 years old)
- Respiratory rate > 24 breaths per minute (i.e., younger than 50 years old)

Other diagnostic data:

- Radiographic finding: pleural effusion
- Random glucose > 249 mg per dL
- Hematocrit < 30 %
- Sodium < 130 mEq per L
- Arterial pH < 7.35
- Arterial partial pressure of oxygen < 60 mmHg

PATIENT INSTRUCTIONS

Careful instructions must be given to individuals about the symptoms of complications associated with pneumonia and when and where to access care if these symptoms develop. While most individuals can be managed on an outpatient basis with treatment with oral antibiotics, some will require hospitalization.

MANAGEMENT DURING PREGNANCY AND LACTATION

While the presentation is unchanged, CAP in pregnancy is more severe and more difficult to treat than CAP in nonpregnant women due to the anatomic and physiologic changes that occur in normal pregnancy.[50] Most cases of pneumonia are detected in the second and third trimesters, when these changes become more pronounced. A chest x-ray should be ordered in women suspected of having pneumonia. Lobar consolidation, cavitation, and pleural effusions are indicative of bacterial pneumonia, whereas viral pneumonia is more often associated with diffuse involvement with intestinal and alveolar patterns.[50] The most common etiologic agents are *S. pneumoniae*, *H. influenzae*, and *M. pneumoniae*.[50] Outpatient management is acceptable in otherwise healthy pregnant women if close follow up can be assured; if otherwise, pregnant women should be hospitalized for observation and treatment.[50]

Allergies

Allergic rhinitis occurs in approximately 10% to 20% of the general population in the United States and Europe.[51] The incidence is particularly high in individuals with asthma and atopy. Less than 2% of the general population experiences asthma without rhinitis, whereas 10% to 40% of individuals with asthma also have rhinitis.[51] Good control of allergy symptoms not only significantly improves asthma symptoms but may also delay or prevent the development of future asthma in individuals affected by allergic rhinitis.[52] Allergies also adversely affect patients' professional and personal lives.[51,53] Skillful management of these conditions not only may improve health, but also significantly improve the quality of life for those with allergies.

Exposure to allergens can lead to allergic rhinitis, food allergies, or contact dermatitis depending on which organ system is affected. Those with allergic rhinitis will report rhinorrhea, sneezing, nasal obstruction, itchy watery eyes, or sneezing. Those with food allergies may report oral irritation and tightness; some will report GI upset and diarrhea, and others will develop hives or contact dermatitis. Allergic contact dermatitis often presents as an itchy rash where exposure occurred. Many of these same symptoms are also present with other conditions. However, the hallmark finding with allergies is that symptoms develop after exposure to an offending trigger and remit once the trigger is removed. Diagnosis is easiest when the exposure to a trigger is episodic, such as in seasonal allergies, and is hardest when exposure is chronic, such as with indoor allergens, where it is difficult to remove the offending trigger. **Table 15-13** describes differential diagnoses for common allergy symptoms. GI and dermatologic disorders can sometimes mimic allergic disorders, especially in those who have persistent symptoms.

Despite the variety of ways that allergies can present, they all seem to be the result of similar impairments in the immune system.[54] In allergic rhinitis, exposure to allergens triggers CD4 T lymphocytes to release interleukin and other T helper 2 (Th2) cytokines. Cytokine release leads to inflammation through immunoglobulin E (IgE) production, mucosal infiltration, and the release of mediators caused by degranulation of mast cells. Like asthma, the chemical cascade in the early phase of allergic rhinitis leads to the release of mediators that damage blood vessels and stimulate the sensory nerves, leading to watery nasal discharge, mucosal edema, nasal congestion, and itching. During the late phase response, which occurs 6 to 8 hours after exposure, symptoms recur as the Th2 lymphocytes release cytokines, resulting in chronic nasal and sinus congestion.[54] While the pathophysiology of food allergies and allergic contact dermatitis is less well understood, they also seem to be at least partially a result of IgE production and mediator release similar to that in allergic rhinitis.

Essential History, Physical, and Laboratory Evaluation

HISTORY

Patients should be asked about the range of symptoms that may accompany allergies, because this will help identify all possible triggers and guide treatment choices. Environmental controls and medication management should be chosen to provide the greatest relief from the specific allergen(s) suspected of causing patients' symptoms.

Patients should be asked also about the timing of the onset of symptoms in relation to exposure to suspected triggers. Symptoms typically develop shortly after exposure to episodic triggers, making it easiest to identify these triggers. Questions focusing on whether symptoms occur year round or only in certain seasons can help pinpoint which specific allergens are problematic for an individual patient. Patients with symptoms only in the spring should be suspected of having allergies to pollen; those who experience symptoms only in the fall may have allergies to ragweed or mold. The onset and duration of allergies can also vary by geographic location depending on climate zones and elevations. For example, dust mite levels tend to be lower at higher elevations, and pollen counts tend to be higher earlier in the spring in the South.

Patients with year-round symptoms should be queried about exposure to animals, cockroaches, indoor molds, and house-dust mites. Asking a patient whether symptoms occur only in certain indoor living spaces (bedroom, basement) or times of day (nighttime or daytime) can help differentiate potential indoor triggers. For example, patients with dust mite allergies typically complain of symptoms upon arising in the morning because dust mite levels tend to be highest in pillows, mattresses, and bedding. Patients whose

Table 15-13 Differential Diagnosis for Common Allergy Symptoms

Symptom	Condition	History	Physical	Laboratory
Rhinorrhea	Allergic rhinitis	• Watery rhinorrhea, sneezing, nasal obstruction, nasal itching, conjunctivitis • Symptoms episodic or continuous depending on trigger • Itchy mouth and ears • History of other atopic conditions such as asthma and eczema	• Usually pale, boggy nasal mucosa; occasionally purple • Increased vascularity • Clear, watery nasal discharge • Edematous swollen turbinates • Significant congestion can lead to darkening of tissue below the eye (allergic shiners).	• Elevated serum eosinophils, although this is nonspecific and of little clinical utility • Positive skin testing for allergies
	Common cold	• Symptoms with identified onset and resolution within 10 to 14 days, including rhinorrhea, watery eyes • Possibly accompanied by myalgia, fever, and malaise	• Thick mucopurulent nasal discharge • Nasal mucosa normal or red and inflamed	• Not helpful
	Chronic sinusitis	• Rhinorrhea more likely to be posterior and result in postnasal drip • Painful sinuses	• Elicit pain over sinuses on exam	• Referral to ENT for possible CT scan
Watery eyes	Allergic conjunctivitis	• Red, watery eyes • Bilateral presentation • Itchy	• Red and watery conjunctiva	• Not helpful
	Bacterial conjunctivitis	• Usually unilateral onset, possibly spreading to other eye • Acute onset • Classic discharge with complaint of irritation and tearing	• Classically thick, yellow discharge/gluing the eye to the lower lid, most noticeable upon arising	• Culture and sensitivity not necessary unless diagnosis unclear or if symptoms are pronounced

(continues)

521

Table 15-13 Differential Diagnosis for Common Allergy Symptoms *(continued)*

Symptom	Condition	History	Physical	Laboratory
	Viral conjunctivitis	• Usually unilateral onset, possibly spreading to other eye	• Classically clear, watery discharge with conjunctival redness • Transient blurred vision, no photophobia	• Culture and sensitivity not necessary unless diagnosis not clear or if symptoms are pronounced
Skin rash	Allergic contact dermatitis	• Onset after exposure to offending trigger • Symptoms consistent upon re-exposure • If treated for eczema, may not respond as expected	• Acute exposure leads to erythematous macules, papules, or vesicles at site of exposure or adjacent areas • Chronic exposure leads to lichenification, scaling, or fissures	• Skin testing
	Atopic dermatitis	• Onset early in life • Chronic or relapsing pattern • Dry itchy skin • Worsens with stress • Family history of atopy	• Patchy lesions on hands, flexures (e.g., elbow), upper eyelid • Dry, thickened lesions	• Allergen specific IgE response
Diarrhea and stomach pain	Food allergies	• Symptoms occur after consumption of offending food • Symptoms consistent upon re-exposure • Predominantly GI tract symptoms, including oral itching, swelling of the airway, abdominal pain, and diarrhea	• Not helpful	• Not helpful
	Gastroenteritis	• Acute onset • Accompanied by diarrhea, headache, fever, muscle aches in viral conditions • Accompanied by explosive multiple stools with bacterial conditions		• Stool sample for bacterial causes

CT = computed tomography, ENT = ear, nose, and throat, GI = gastrointestinal

allergens may be triggered by chronic exposures should be asked whether eliminating these triggers (e.g., avoiding suspected foods or living in a home without pets for several weeks) has ever improved their symptoms. **Table 15-14** has further details on common allergy triggers.

Patients suspected of having food allergies or allergic contact dermatitis should be queried about timing of symptoms in relation to exposures. These conditions often mimic other GI and dermatologic disorders; this line of questioning is critical in uncovering potential allergens. Resolution of symptoms with food avoidance or with cessation of use of specific products supports

the diagnosis, as does a return of symptoms with resumption of use of these products or with consumption of offending foods.

PHYSICAL

Patients suspected of having allergies need a complete physical evaluation of the head, ear, eye, nose, throat, skin, and respiratory systems, because allergies commonly affect these systems. Patients suspected of having allergic contact dermatitis need a careful skin inspection, looking for rashes that originate at the exposure site. The physical exam is of little help when evaluating potential

Table 15-14 Allergy Triggers

Trigger	Indications	Environmental Controls
Cockroaches	More common in inner-city, multifamily dwellings	• Seal cracks in walls and floors. • Professionally exterminate. • Secure food waste. • Wash floors and walls.
Dust mites	Symptoms worse in the morning after sleeping all night in bed	• Wash all bedding in hot water every week and blankets/comforters at least 4 times a year. • Whether using polyester-filled pillows as opposed to feather or down is helpful is unclear, although this traditionally has been recommended. • Encase mattress and in particular pillows with allergy-proof covers. Use specially designed allergy covers, not "dust covers." Dust covers do not filter out dust mites, only larger dust particles. • Minimize use of soft materials by replacing carpets with linoleum or wood flooring, drapes with blinds or washable curtains, and upholstered furniture with leather furniture. • Hot wash or freeze soft toys. • Vacuum daily using a vacuum equipped with a high-efficiency particulate air (HEPA) filter or special allergen-proof vacuum cleaner bags or connected to a duct system. • Do not use humidifiers, because they increase the growth of dust mites. • Use of air conditioners can reduce summertime humidity.

(continues)

Table 15-14 Allergy Triggers *(continued)*

Trigger	Indications	Environmental Controls
Dust	Symptoms worsen with dusting and sweeping.	All of the measures listed under dust mites and also: • If forced air heat or air conditioning is used, cover the vents with a filter and wash or change this filter every month. • Where possible, have nonallergic household members be responsible for dusting and vacuuming. • Air filtration systems and ionizers are controversial and are not thought to significantly reduce symptoms for many individuals. • Keep dust-collecting items inside of cupboards.
Pet allergens	Symptoms begin or worsen after pet introduced into household and are relieved when away from household.	• Remove pet from household if possible. • If pet removal is not possible, try: ▪ Keep pet out of bedroom, especially off of the bed. ▪ Keep pet off furniture in all rooms and out of doors as much as possible. ▪ Wash pet weekly. ▪ Clean regularly with a vacuum equipped with HEPA filter or special allergy-proof bags.
Indoor molds	Symptoms worsen in areas of high humidity (basement, areas of water damage) or when area smells musty.	• Use dehumidifiers in damp areas of household. • Do not lay carpeting directly on concrete basement flooring. • Do not use humidifiers anywhere in the household.
Outdoor allergens	Suspect allergy to pollen and grasses if symptoms worse in the spring and early summer. Suspect allergies to ragweed and mold if symptoms worse in the fall. Fall allergies usually subside after the first hard frost.	• Use air conditioners even if not needed for cooling to filter outdoor air. Wash filters regularly. • Have air conditioners professionally cleaned to remove mold. • Avoid outdoor activities between 11:00 am and 3:00 pm when pollen counts are highest, or in early morning and late evening if mold allergies are a problem.

food allergies. However, individuals with food allergies or allergic contact dermatitis can infrequently experience symptoms of allergic rhinitis and need the same evaluation as those with primary allergic rhinitis. All patients with persistent allergic rhinitis symptoms need a thorough nasal exam to evaluate the nasal anatomy, the color of the mucosa, and the quality and quantity of the mucus. This exam is best facilitated with the use of a nasal speculum. Findings suggestive of allergies are outlined in Table 15-13.

LABORATORY

In general, laboratory testing is of limited value for allergies, with the exception of skin testing. Individuals with allergies may have elevated serum eosinophils, but this is a nonspecific finding also seen in some cancers, parasitic infections, skin disorders, and drug reactions, so it has little clinical utility in the diagnosis of allergies. A few authorities recommend nasal cytology, which can identify high levels of eosinophils in the nasal exudates of allergic individuals. In contrast, neutrophils tend to predominate in the nasal cytology of individuals with infection. Eosinophils can also be seen on cytology smears of individuals with asthma, nasal polyps, and aspirin sensitivity. The poor specificity of nasal smears limits their usefulness, although some clinicians use them to monitor the effectiveness of anti-inflammatory treatment.

Skin testing (also called puncture, prick, or epicutaneous skin testing) is considered to be the gold standard and is useful in identifying the specific allergens that produce symptoms.[55] Individuals being tested receive multiple small skin punctures; each one is inoculated with a different extract containing a single antigen of such common allergens such as dust mites, mold, and pollen. Allergic individuals develop a wheal to their specific offending allergens within 20 minutes of being inoculated. A positive test will result in a wheal 3 mm or greater in diameter than the negative control reaction and is accompanied by erythema. Women scheduled for skin testing should be advised to avoid the use of first-generation antihistamines for 3 days and the use of second-generation antihistamines for a minimum of 10 days before their skin testing appointments. These drugs can inhibit the wheal and flare reaction of these tests and lead to false-negative results.[55] Other medications such the phenothiazines or imipramine can also suppress wheal formation.[55]

Most skin panels test for 10 to 20 common allergens. Skin testing is particularly helpful in developing environmental control strategies designed to minimize exposure. They also can help determine whether or not treatment with allergen immunotherapy may be helpful in controlling symptoms. Serum tests are also available that can help identify problematic IgEs for allergic individuals but are of limited usefulness, because they are more expensive and less sensitive than skin testing.

Management

ALLERGIC RHINITIS

According to Allergic Rhinitis and its Impact on Asthma (ARIA), a nongovernmental organization working in collaboration with the World Health Organization (WHO), management of allergic rhinitis relies on three main principles: 1) instituting environmental controls to minimize exposure to offending allergens; 2) prescribing anti-inflammatory agents to halt the chemical cascade leading to IgE production, cytokine release, and mast cell activation; and 3) providing symptomatic relief through the use of decongestants and antihistamines.[4,56]

In 2001, the ARIA/WHO guidelines changed the classification system used to describe allergic rhinitis.[56] Traditionally, allergic rhinitis had been subdivided into seasonal and perennial categories. However, these categories do not adequately reflect the extent to which allergic rhinitis can negatively affect individuals. The new classification system subdivided allergic rhinitis into four categories based on the frequency of symptoms and the impacts these symptoms have on the lives of affected individuals. ARIA linked these classifications to recommended treatment guidelines based on a review of the evidence by a panel of international experts. Subsequently, ARIA has published a series of updated recommendations based on emerging evidence and expert consensus, in 2008 and most recently in 2010.[4,57]

The four categories of allergic rhinitis are:[4,56]

1. *Mild intermittent.* Symptoms occur fewer than 4 days per week or for fewer than 4 weeks at a time. Symptoms do not affect sleep or interfere with daily activities. Recommended treatments include oral antihistamines, intranasal antihistamines, intranasal decongestants, or

antileukotrienes. While the choice of treatment should be individualized, oral second-generation antihistamines are a well tolerated and effective first-line approach given their rapid onset of action and high efficacy.[4] Intranasal decongestants should be used sparingly due to the risk of developing rhinitis medicamentosa.[57]

2. *Severe intermittent.* Symptom frequency is categorized as for mild intermittent rhinitis (i.e., < 4 days/week or < 4 weeks at a time), but the severity is more pronounced. Symptoms are severe enough to lead to at least one of the following: disrupted sleep; troublesome symptoms; or impaired work, school, sport, or leisure time performance. Treatments include those recommended for *mild intermittent* with the additional option of intranasal *chromones* (e.g., cromolyn). Intranasal corticosteroids are highly effective and a good option when symptoms are severe.[4]

3. *Mild persistent.* Although symptoms occur more frequently (at least 4 days in a week lasting for more than 4 weeks at a time), they are mild and do not interfere with sleep or daily activities. Treatment options consist of all of those listed for *severe intermittent*; however, the patient should be reevaluated in 2 to 4 weeks and medications adjusted as needed. Those thought to have perennial symptoms may need to continue medications indefinitely. Those thought to have symptoms from exposure to episodic or seasonal triggers may be able to have their medication(s) titrated downward; usually intranasal corticosteroids doses are reduced by ½ until the patient is weaned off.

4. *Moderate to severe persistent.* Symptoms in this category are severe enough to disrupt sleep, are generally bothersome, or can interfere with an individual's ability to perform well in school or at work, as well as at home. They also occur frequently: at least 4 days a week and for more than 4 weeks at a time. Intranasal corticosteroids are considered to be first-line treatments. The patient should be reevaluated in 2–4 weeks. If symptoms have improved, treatment can be stepped down but continued for a minimum of 3 months or for the duration of the pollen season. Some patients may require continuous treatment with low-dose intranasal corticosteroids. If the initially prescribed regimen does not afford relief, the provider should check that the patient is using medications as directed, taking all prescribed doses using correct technique, and reconsider the initial diagnosis. If the initial diagnosis is correct, then the following treatment options may be helpful: Increase the intranasal corticosteroid dose, add an antihistamine if itchiness or sneezing is present, or prescribe adjunctive medications that target the most problematic symptom (intranasal ipratropium for rhinorrhea, oral decongestants for nasal congestion, or intraocular antihistamine, chromone, or saline for eye irritation). Immunotherapy should be strongly considered. If none of these approaches provide relief, referral may be warranted.

LIFESTYLE: ENVIRONMENTAL CONTROLS

The use of environmental controls has been an integral approach to the management of allergic rhinitis. ARIA's 2008 consensus opinion is that evidence supports the premise that environmental measures can reduce the amount of allergens in the environment, but that there is little evidence to suggest that reducing allergens improves the course of allergic rhinitis.[4,58] Best results are seen with a systematic approach to reducing allergen loads. For example, reducing allergic symptoms related to cockroach allergies requires implementing all known measures; these include professional extermination, securing food waste, washing walls and floors, and repairing cracks in walls and floors.[59] Recommendations for a specific patient on instituting environmental controls should be individualized based on the severity of symptoms, the specific allergen of concern, and the costs of implementing environmental measures.[4]

Which specific environmental control is recommended will vary according to the allergen(s) found to be problematic. One of the most difficult triggers to control is pet dander. Removing the pet from the home will result in the greatest clinical response. Families who give up their pet should be counseled that it may take 3 or more months of cleaning before enough pet allergens have been removed for symptoms to subside. However, pets are beloved family members in many households, and many families are reluctant to give them away. Other measures may provide some relief for families unwilling to give up their pets. Because pet allergens increase fivefold when the pet is in the room, the pet should be kept out of the bedroom and preferably stay outdoors as much as possible. Washing pets thoroughly also seems to reduce allergen levels, as does removing upholstered furniture and carpeting. Animal allergens accumulate to levels up to 100 times higher in carpets than on polished floors.[60]

Regular cleaning with a vacuum equipped with a high-efficiency particulate air (HEPA) filter or special allergen-proof bags or connected to a duct system can remove significant amounts of pet dander as well as dust-mite allergens, which are another common trigger. Women should be advised that use of vacuums without these special features may increase allergy symptoms; regular vacuums cannot filter out allergens, which tend to be of very small particle size. Using a vacuum without a HEPA filter will make allergens airborne when they are exhausted out of the vacuum. Individuals with dust-mite allergies also should avoid using indoor humidifiers. Because they are difficult to clean well, their use may increase the prevalence of indoor mold and dust mites that thrive in higher humidity environments. Dust mites are present in all households regardless of their cleanliness. Women should be reassured that measures needed to control dust mites or other allergens are not a reflection of any judgment made about their standards of cleanliness but are necessary to minimize exposure to triggers. Table 15-14 provides specific suggestions on control measures for common allergens.

MEDICATION CHOICES

Anti-inflammatory medications such as corticosteroids and mast cell stabilizers are commonly used in the treatment of allergic rhinitis. Other medications include decongestants and antihistamines. Which is best for an individual will depend on the severity and frequency of symptoms. In general, second-generation antihistamines are the preferred treatment for intermittent allergic rhinitis, and intranasal corticosteroids are preferred for those with more persistent symptoms.

Anti-Inflammatory Agents The two main categories of anti-inflammatory medications used in the treatment of allergic rhinitis are mast cell stabilizers and corticosteroids, both of which are available in topical formulations. Intranasal corticosteroids are more effective in relieving symptoms than intranasal mast cell stabilizers and have fewer systemic side effects than oral agents. A small percentage of women using intranasal corticosteroids report nasal dryness and irritation; even fewer report mild epistaxis.[58] Patients who experience these side effects may be able to minimize these problems if a saline nasal spray is used prior to using an intranasal corticosteroid or if the dose of corticosteroid is reduced. Nasal septal perforation has been reported with use of these drugs, so patients should be instructed in correct positioning of the device. Evidence of superficial erosions, significant crusting, or bleeding should prompt the patient to immediately discontinue use of these medications.

Patients with ocular symptoms may find relief with antihistamine or mast cell stabilizer eye drops or a combination of the two, or with the use of oral antihistamines. Saline eye drops may also provide relief. Steroidal eye drops should *never* be used in the treatment of ocular itching secondary to allergies because of the risks associated with ocular steroids and the availability of other safer alternatives (**Table 15-15**).

Table 15-15 Common Allergy Medications

Indication	Drug	Trade Name	Dose	Effective Against	Notes
Decongestants					
Allergic rhinitis	Pseudoephedrine (30 mg tab)	Sudafed	2 tabs PO qid	Nasal congestion and blockage, less effective against rhinorrhea	Good relief of nasal congestion but can develop insomnia, headache, dry mucous membranes, exacerbation of glaucoma, or thyrotoxicosis
Allergic rhinitis	Intranasal decongestants: oxymetazoline	Afrin	2 gtts each nostril bid	Nasal congestion	Rapid relief but rebound effect with prolonged use. Limit treatment to < 5 days; maximum length of treatment is 10 days. Do not repeat more than twice a month.
Antihistamines					
First Generation					
Allergic rhinitis	Diphenhydramine	Benadryl	25–50 mg PO tid or qid	Pruritus, rhinorrhea, eye symptoms. Less effective against nasal congestion.	More likely to be sedating, to potentiate alcohol, and to have anticholinergic side effects than second-generation antihistamines
	Clemastine	Tavist	1 mg PO bid		
	Chlorpheniramine	Chlor-Trimeton	4 mg PO qid		
	Hydroxyzine	Atarax, Vistaril	25 mg PO tid or qid		
	Cyproheptadine		4 mg PO tid		
Second Generation					
Allergic rhinitis	Azelastine nasal spray	Astelin 137 mcg/ spray	2 sprays each nostril bid	Nasal congestion and blockage	Less effective than intranasal corticosteroids. Has bitter taste.

Condition	Generic	Brand	Dosing	Symptoms	Comments
Allergic rhinitis	Cetirizine	Zyrtec	5 or 10 mg PO daily	Pruritus, rhinorrhea, eye symptoms. Little effect against nasal congestion.	First-line therapy. Should be used in combination with intranasal corticosteroids if symptoms are severe. Recommended over first-generation antihistamines because of less sedation and fewer side effects. More convenient because of once-daily dosing.
	Desloratadine	Clarinex	5 mg daily		
	Fexofenadine	Allegra	60 mg PO bid		
	Loratadine	Claritin	10 mg PO daily		

Intranasal Corticosteroids

Condition	Generic	Brand	Dosing	Symptoms	Comments
Allergic rhinitis	Beclomethasone nasal spray	Beconase AQ	1–2 sprays in each nostril bid	Pruritus, rhinorrhea, and nasal congestion. Partial relief from eye symptoms.	Intranasal corticosteroids recommended as first-line therapy for those with severe or persistent symptoms.
	Budesonide nasal spray	Rhinocort Aqua	Max 4 sprays each nostril daily		
	Fluticasone propionate nasal spray	Flonase	1 spray in each nostril bid initially, then daily		
	Mometasone furoate nasal spray	Nasonex	2 sprays in each nostril daily		
	Triamcinolone nasal spray	Nasacort AQ	2 sprays in each nostril daily		

Mast Cell Stabilizers

Condition	Generic	Brand	Dosing	Symptoms	Comments
Allergic conjunctivitis	Pemirolast potassium 0.1%	Alamast	1–2 gtts affected eye qid	Ocular itching	Provides effective relief with minor side effects
	Nedocromil sodium 2%	Alocril	1–2 gtts affected eye bid		
Allergic rhinitis	Cromolyn sodium 5.2 mg/spray	Nasalcrom	1 spray each nostril qid	Pruritus and rhinorrhea	Less effective than intranasal corticosteroids but excellent safety profile

(continues)

Table 15-15 Common Allergy Medications *(continued)*

Indication	Drug	Trade Name	Dose	Effective Against	Notes
Combined Medications					
Allergic conjunctivitis	Antihistamine/mast cell stabilizer Azelastine 0.05%/	Optivar	1 gtt affected eye bid	Ocular itching	Ocular stinging, bitter taste
	Antihistamine/mast cell stabilizer: olopatadine hydrochloride 0.1%	Patanol	1 gtt affected eye bid		
Allergic rhinitis	Antihistamine/decongestant Fexofenadine 60 mg/pseudoephedrine 120 mg	Allegra-D	1 tab PO bid	Pruritus, nasal congestion and blockage, rhinorrhea, eye symptoms	
	Antihistamine/decongestant Loratadine 10 mg/pseudoephedrine 240 mg	Claritin D	1 tab PO daily		
Topical Anticholinergics					
Allergic Rhinitis	Ipratropium bromide 0.03%	Atrovent Nasal Spray 0.03% 21 mcg per spray	2 sprays each nostril daily or up to tid	Rhinorrhea only	Use as adjunctive therapy if insufficient response with oral antihistamine or intranasal corticosteroid use.
Antileukotrienes					
Allergic Rhinitis	Montelukast Zafirlukast	Singulair Accolate	10 mg tab daily 20 mg tab twice daily	Rhinitis and asthma triggered by allergies, ocular symptoms	Most appropriate for use in those with seasonal allergies, unless patient also has asthma

bid = 2 times per day; grtts = drops; PO = per os (by mouth), qid = 4 times per day, tid = 3 times per day

Data from Bousquet J, Khaltaev N, Cruz AA, Denburg J, Fokkens WJ, Togias A, et al. Allergic rhinitis and its impact on asthma (ARIA) 2008. *Allergy.* 2008;63:8-160; Brożek JL, Bousquet J, Baena-Cagnani CE, Bonini S, Canonica GW, Casale TB, et al. Allergic rhinitis and its impact on asthma (ARIA) guidelines: 2010 revision. *J Allergy Clin Immunol.* 2010;126(3):466-476.

Medications for Symptomatic Relief Patients may choose various types of medications (nasal corticosteroids, antihistamines, or decongestants) and delivery routes (topical or systemic) for symptomatic relief, depending on their presentation and the product under consideration. In general, topical agents will have the fewest side effects, but patients who present with multiple symptoms, such as allergic conjunctivitis and rhinitis, may respond better to oral agents. *Decongestants* are best for those suffering primarily from nasal congestion; *antihistamines* are better for those with rhinorrhea and itchiness. Patients who have all of these symptoms may do best with combined products. These products can be used episodically for those with intermittent or seasonal allergies and daily for those with persistent symptoms. Intranasal decongestants should be used with caution, because overuse of these products can lead to a rebound effect and worsening of the patient's symptoms with extended use. The *antileukotrienes* play a limited role in the management of allergic rhinitis. They are less effective than the oral antihistamines and nasal corticosteroids. They may play a role for those with refractory allergies and in those who also have asthma or chronic rhinitis accompanied by nasal polyps.[61] In most situations, the nasal corticosteroids are considered to be first-line agents due to their superior effectiveness in relieving symptoms and low risk. Individuals should begin to experience relief in a few days; maximum benefit will be seen in several weeks. Given their high effectiveness and relatively fast onset of action, nasal corticosteroids are suitable for use in individuals with seasonal allergies, as well as in those with more persistent symptoms.[62] Table 15-15 describes common available medications.

Occasionally, patients with allergic rhinitis may also be prescribed intranasal ipratropium (Atrovent), a topical *anticholinergic*, as an adjunctive therapy. It is typically added to the medication regimen for those patients who, despite adequate treatment with intranasal corticosteroids and oral antihistamines, continue to have significant rhinorrhea or for those whose primary symptom is rhinorrhea.[54] It is ineffective against many other common symptoms, such as sneezing, congestion, or itching, that accompany allergic rhinitis. Common side effects include nasal irritation, crusting, and occasional mild epistaxis.

Immunotherapy Allergen immunotherapy is another treatment option. Immunotherapy has several benefits. It can reduce the dose of medication(s) needed to achieve control for asthmatic patients with allergies, may protect against the future development of asthma for those with allergic rhinitis, and may reduce the likelihood that allergic individuals will develop additional allergies.[4,54] It is indicated in the treatment of allergic rhinitis, allergic conjunctivitis, allergic asthma, and insect stings, but not for food allergies or atopic dermatitis. Immunotherapy is most effective if initiated early in the course of the disease in childhood or early adulthood.[4]

All patients receiving immunotherapy need skin testing in order to identify their particular allergens. Immunotherapy can be delivered via oral or subcutaneous routes. Some allergens, such as grasses, can be delivered through either route, but others can only be delivered subcutaneously.[63] During the course of immunotherapy, patients receive slowly increasing oral or subcutaneous doses of extracts to allergens that are particularly problematic for them. This desensitizes the patient and improves symptoms. However, immunotherapy involves a significant time commitment on the part of affected individuals, requiring long-term treatment to result in improved outcomes.[4]

Oral immunotherapy is much more common in Europe, where 80% of all patients initiating treatment are treated with sublingual administration.[63] Serious reactions appear to be lower with oral than subcutaneous treatment. However, in the United States, most individuals are still being treated with subcutaneous regimens. In order to be effective, subcutaneous doses needed to be increased to reach a target level and then repeated at weekly to monthly levels, usually for 3 years.[4] Failure to reach the target dose level or to receive doses as scheduled or for treatment to last a sufficient length of time reduces the effectiveness of immunotherapy. Serious side effects, such as severe asthma or anaphylaxis, are rare but do occur. One study reported that systemic reactions occurred in 0.1% of all injections, though none were fatal.[63] Because of the rare risk of serious reactions, subcutaneous immunotherapy is prescribed only by allergists and delivered in a setting where prompt emergency care is available.[4]

Management During Pregnancy and Lactation

Nasal congestion is common in pregnancy, and distinguishing this finding from allergic rhinitis can be difficult. Patients with nasal congestion due to estrogen increase during pregnancy will not have itchiness or rhinorrhea, only stuffiness. Treatment for allergic rhinitis will not afford relief.[4] In this case, the use of nasal saline, which has no side effects, may help.

Treatment of allergic rhinitis is essentially unchanged in pregnancy. Allergen avoidance is the primary treatment modality of allergic rhinitis in pregnancy. Medications should be prescribed if environmental measures fail to provide sufficient relief. Most authorities recommend the use of intranasal corticosteroids as the preferred treatment in pregnancy due to their low systemic absorption and high efficacy.[64,65] However, pregnant women who do not respond completely to these products may be offered other options. Studies of pregnancy safety of antihistamines are generally based on small, nonrandomized samples. Based on its evaluation of the evidence, the National Asthma

Education and Prevention Program (NAEPP) recommends using specific medications in the various classes; among the corticosteroids, more safety data are available on budesonide than other products, although none of the inhaled corticosteroids have been reported to be unsafe.[65] Pregnant women may remain on the intranasal corticosteroids they used before becoming pregnant, but women who are initiating therapy are best prescribed budesonide.[65] Second-generation antihistamines are preferred by some given their effectiveness and safety profile; more safety data are available for cetirizine and loratadine.[65] However, others recommend the use of chlorpheniramine, a first-generation antihistamine, because it has more extensive evidence documenting its safety in pregnancy.[64,66] Other alternatives include the use of nasal chromones, which have excellent safety data but lower efficacy, and the antileukotrienes, although few data are available on their safety in pregnancy.[66]

The use of oral decongestants is controversial. NAEPP recommends against their use, because exposure during the first trimester has been associated with gastroschisis, although the risks appear to be low.[67] Accumulating evidence indicates there may be a small increased risk of other defects among children exposed to some decongestants. A recent, large case-control study (n = 12,734 cases, n = 7606 controls) reported increased risks with the use of several decongestants in pregnancy: phenylephrine and endocardial cushion defect (odds ratio [OR] = 8.0; 95% confidence interval [CI] 2.5, 25.3), phenylpropanolamine and ear defects (OR = 7.8; 95% CI 2.2, 27.2), and phenylpropanolamine and pyloric stenosis (OR = 3.2; 95% CI 1.1, 8.8).[68]

Immunotherapy should not be started in pregnancy due to the risks of systemic reactions.[56,66] Women already on immunotherapy before the pregnancy may safely continue. The allergen extract doses should not be increased, in order to minimize the risk of anaphylaxis, although this risk is extremely rare during immunotherapy.

Many pregnant women with allergies also have asthma. Good control of allergic rhinitis may also reduce the need for asthma medications. These women should receive aggressive treatment of allergic rhinitis in pregnancy.[64]

FOOD ALLERGIES

In general, food allergies are thought to be more common in children than in adults. For adults, the most common triggers causing severe reactions are milk, eggs, fish, and shellfish, although nuts (peanuts, almonds, walnuts, pecans, hazelnuts), soya beans, some fruit such as apples and peaches, sesame, celery, and other foods also can cause problems.[4,69] Many individuals with food allergies also demonstrate cross-reactivity to allergens (ragweed and grass/banana; melon, birch pollen/apples; and latex/banana-kiwi-chestnut). Most of these reactions are mild, but occasionally severe cross-reactions do occur.[4]

The treatment for food allergies is avoidance. Patients exposed to food allergens may experience symptoms ranging from oral itching to GI upset to anaphylaxis.[70] **Table 15-16** lists symptoms of

---

Table 15-16 Symptoms of Anaphylaxis

Listed from most to least common:
- Hives
- Upper airway edema
- Wheezing/shortness of breath
- Flushing
- Dizziness
- Nausea, vomiting, diarrhea, cramping

Data from Arnold J, Williams PM. Anaphylaxis: recognition and management. *Am Fam Physician*. 2011;84(10): 1111-1118; Tang A. A practical guide to anaphylaxis. *Am Fam Physician*. 2003;68(7):1325-1332.

---

anaphylaxis. Patients at risk should wear an alert bracelet and carry diphenhydramine (Benadryl) and injectable epinephrine (EpiPen) for use in an emergency. The EpiPen comes in two strengths: adult (EpiPen) and pediatric (EpiPen Jr). Providers should order the adult dose (1:1000 dilution, 0.3 mg) and make sure the patient, and ideally another family member, is trained in its use.[70]

Management of food allergies is unchanged by pregnancy. The primary treatment modality is avoidance. All women, whether pregnant or not, need to be prepared in case of exposure by having ready access to appropriate emergency medications.

ALLERGIC CONTACT DERMATITIS

Allergic contact dermatitis is difficult to distinguish from other eczematous disorders. Initial exposure typically presents as erythematous macules, papules, or vesicles. Chronic exposure results in lichenification, scaling, or fissured dermatitis. These findings are not distinctive; consequently, the most important diagnostic clues are the location and evolution of the rash. For example, allergies to poison ivy often begin as linear lesions and occur on more exposed areas. Textile-related allergens tend to occur in areas covered by clothing. Skin testing can be particularly helpful in differentiating allergen-based from nonallergen-based dermatitis. Treatment is directed at avoidance and symptom management.[71-73] Weeping lesions are best treated with drying agents and lichenified lesions with emollients. Pruritus can be relieved with the use of topical antipruritics or oral antihistamines. Topical corticosteroid creams and lotions can also help.

Individuals with allergic contact dermatitis may also experience symptoms of allergic rhinitis and may therefore benefit from the treatment for their allergic rhinitis as well as their contact dermatitis.

Management of atopic dermatitis is also essentially unchanged by pregnancy.

Patient Instructions

Patients with allergies need to understand how to adapt their environment to meet their particular needs. Specific environmental strategies should be tailored to match the lifestyle needs of the individual woman. For example, asking a woman with limited financial resources to cover her bed and pillows with allergy-proof covers or invest in a HEPA vacuum will be ineffective, because it is unlikely that she can afford to comply with these suggestions. In this case, asking her to cover only the pillows on her bed in allergy-proof covers, to wash all of her bedding in hot water every week, and to ask another family member to wet mop her bedroom floor may provide enough environmental control to help minimize her symptoms and still be within her financial means. Similarly, asking a woman to give up a household pet may not be reasonable, but instituting other control measures (Table 15-14) may be effective.

Women also need to understand how to choose medications that are effective and easy to use. Individuals with intermittent symptoms with known triggers (e.g., exposure to animals, pollen, or mold) can institute therapy several days to weeks before the exposure and stop medications once exposure ceases. For example, women with ragweed allergies can start medications several weeks before the beginning of the ragweed season and stop with the first hard frost. Those with more persistent symptoms will need to choose products with dosing regimens or delivery systems that are acceptable to them. Some women find intranasal sprays to be uncomfortable and prefer oral medications. Others prefer topical agents with fewer systemic side effects. Because allergies are a chronic condition, it is critical to develop a partnership with patients and help women choose appropriate medication(s) and environmental control measures as their needs change.

Women with food allergies need to be taught how to read food packages to identify possible allergens, and to understand manufacturing processes that can lead to cross-contamination and potential exposure to problematic allergens.

Women who could experience anaphylactic reactions should be counseled to carry Benadryl, as well as an EpiPen and be skilled in its use. In addition, individuals who have severe reactions to various foods or insect bites should wear an ID band to alert others in the event of an anaphylactic episode.

Rhinosinusitis

Sinusitis is an inflammation of the paranasal mucosal sinuses. Usually, the nasal mucosa is also inflamed or obstructed and therefore, the term *rhinosinusitis* is more accurate.[74] Sinusitis is characterized by duration of symptoms, although authorities differ in the timeframes used to define subcategories of sinusitis. Acute sinusitis has been defined by some authorities as the presence of symptoms for less than 4 weeks, less than 8 weeks, or less than 12 weeks with complete resolution of symptoms.[75]

Similarly, chronic sinusitis has been described differently by different authorities; it has been described as symptoms that persist longer than 8 weeks by some authorities and longer than 12 weeks by others.[75] A few authorities also describe a middle category, subacute sinusitis, in which symptoms last from 4 weeks to either 8 weeks or 12 weeks. While authorities disagree on specific timeframes used to describe the various subcategories of sinusitis, all agree that assessing the severity of the presentation is critical in determining the most effective treatment modalities.[4,75]

Viral, bacterial, and fungal infections, as well as allergy or environmental irritants can cause acute sinus inflammatory reactions. Up to 30% of the cases of acute sinusitis and 80% of chronic sinusitis are associated with allergic rhinitis.[3]

Maxillary and ethmoid sinuses are predominantly affected. Rarely, bacterial pathogens invade the frontal or sphenoid sinuses, resulting in higher morbidity. Complications involving the orbit, the central nervous system, or both can occur with untreated acute bacterial sinusitis. Meningitis, subperiosteal abscess, orbital abscess, intraorbital or periorbital cellulitis, and brain abscess are rare complications.[76]

Acute rhinosinusitis is often associated with a viral upper respiratory tract infection, particularly the common cold. The transport of mucus is slowed by mucosal swelling and impaired cilia function resulting in a sufficient culture medium for viral and bacterial growth.[74] The most common viruses detected are rhinovirus, adenovirus, influenza virus, and parainfluenza virus.[74] Bacterial etiologies account for only 0.5% to 2% of acute rhinosinusitis, making antibiotic coverage unnecessary for most cases of sinusitis.[77] Bacteria isolated from infected maxillary sinuses include *S. pneumoniae, H. influenzae, M. catarrhalis, S. aureus,* and *Streptococcus pyogenes.* Fungal infections are rare and are mainly seen in immunocompromised patients (e.g., transplant recipients and those with diabetes, acquired immune deficiency syndrome [AIDS], or malignancies).[78]

Chronic sinusitis is associated with a number of diverse etiologies including vasomotor rhinitis, GERD, sarcoidosis, allergies, cystic fibrosis, anatomic abnormalities, and nasal polyps. Similar symptoms are seen in acute and chronic sinusitis (i.e., anterior or posterior mucopurulent drainage, nasal obstruction, and facial pain or pressure), but they are generally milder and more variable in chronic compared to acute presentations.[75] Differentiating chronic sinusitis from recurrent acute sinusitis, characterized by two to four episodes of acute infection with complete resolution between episodes, is essential in guiding decisions about testing and treatment.[75] Acute and recurrent infections require minimal, if any, testing and are treated similarly. Chronic presentations are more likely to require allergen testing, cultures, nasal

endoscopy with or without computed tomography (CT) to obtain nasal cultures and confirm the presence of polyps, and targeted treatment directed toward the underlying etiology.[75]

Essential History, Physical, and Laboratory Evaluation

HISTORY

A thorough history is needed; it is particularly important to focus on the evolution of symptoms over time. Unfortunately, it may be difficult for providers to distinguish between acute bacterial sinusitis, which may benefit from antibiotic coverage, and viral sinusitis, which will not. Hickner and colleagues reviewed seven studies that examined predictors of acute bacterial rhinosinusitis. In these studies, the following symptoms were commonly noted: unilateral or bilateral purulent rhinorrhea; mucopurulent nasal discharge on examination; and unilateral maxillary, facial, or tooth pain. The more symptoms present, the higher the probability of an infectious sinusitis.[79] Headache, postnasal drip, and cough are often noted with a URI, and these symptoms are not highly predictive of a bacterial sinusitis. However, the length of illness may provide clues to the underlying etiology. In most cases, symptoms associated with uncomplicated viral respiratory infection peak in 6 days and lessen by 10 days.[80] Bacterial sinus infections are most likely to occur as a secondary infection; therefore, symptoms that initially improve and then worsen or that persist for 10 or more days may be indicative of bacterial infection.[75] Most cases of sinusitis resolve with conservative management and appropriate antibiotic coverage if needed. Rarely an urgent ear, nose, and throat (ENT) or surgical consult is necessary. **Table 15-17** describes the signs and symptoms of bacterial and/or viral sinusitis. **Table 15-18** lists the symptoms that necessitate an urgent or emergent evaluation with an appropriate specialist.

Table 15-17 Common Signs and Symptoms Seen in Sinusitis

Bacterial Sinusitis	Both Viral and Bacterial Sinusitis: Nonspecific Symptoms
Mucopurulent nasal discharge	Fever
Unilateral maxillary pain/tooth pain	Headache
Unilateral facial pain	Generalized facial pain or tenderness
Unilateral sinus tenderness	Bilateral maxillary pain
Symptoms that initially improve then worsen	Bilateral toothache/pain
No improvement with decongestants	Postnasal drip
Symptoms last 10 or more days	Cough

Table 15-18 Referral Indications for Sinusitis

Symptoms Requiring Immediate Referral to an Appropriate Specialist*
Acutely ill with persistent fevers greater than 102°F
Severe headaches
Periorbital edema
Visual changes (decreased visual acuity, diplopia, disconjugate gaze, difficulty opening eye)
Exophthalmos (seen with cavernous sinus disease)
Changes in mental status or other central nervous system symptoms (may be seen with periorbital abscess, brain abscess, or meningitis)
Recalcitrant infection, with treatment failure with antimicrobial treatment
Immunosuppression
Comorbidities
Allergies to multiple antibiotic agents
Anatomic abnormalities causing obstruction, requiring surgical evaluation
3–4 episodes per year of acute bacterial rhinosinusitis
History of chronic rhinosinusitis with recurrent acute bacterial rhinosinusitis exacerbations
Immunotherapy for allergic rhinitis
Fungal sinusitis or granulomatous disease

*Allergist, ENT physician, infectious disease specialist, neurologist, ophthalmologist

Symptom presentation also provides clues that can help distinguish acute from chronic sinusitis. Two or more of the following symptoms need to be present for more than 8 to 12 weeks to meet the criteria of chronic sinusitis: 1) nasal congestion; 2) mucopurulent drainage; 3) facial pain, pressure, or fullness; and 4) a decreased sense of smell.[75] Other symptoms of chronic sinusitis include headache, cough, decreased ability to taste, and increased throat clearing. Loss of smell is more indicative of chronic than acute sinusitis.[75] Loss of smell may also indicate the presence of nasal polyps.[75]

Chronic or recurrent sinusitis often is related to allergic or environmental factors. If allergies are a triggering factor, symptoms such as itching of the nasal passages and sneezing are commonly reported. Other allergy symptoms include rhinorrhea; nasal congestion; itchiness of the eyes, ears, nose, mouth, and/or throat; repetitive sneezing; postnasal drip; and cough. Common asthma symptoms include chest tightness, shortness of breath, repetitive coughing, and/or wheezing. Both asthma and allergies are common comorbidities seen in patients with sinusitis. See the sections on asthma and allergies for further information.

PHYSICAL

When evaluating a possible rhinosinusitis, the ears, nose, throat, chest, and skin should be examined. The practitioner should note any eye discharge or darkening under the eyes. If both eyes have watery secretions with scant erythema to the conjunctiva, this suggests an allergic source. Allergic shiners, or darkening of the skin under the eyes, are also commonly seen. The ears should be examined for clear fluid behind the tympanic membrane, which may indicate serous otitis, or erythema, bulging to the tympanic membranes, and abnormal bony landmarks, which can be seen with otitis media. The nasal turbinates should be assessed for color and texture. Pallor and bogginess are seen with allergies; erythema and edema are seen in viral or bacterial infections. Also, the nasal passages should be checked for nasal discharge and polyps. The nose should be examined for a deviated septum, nasal polyps, foreign bodies, and tumors. The throat should be checked for postnasal drip, which can be clear or purulent,

as well as posterior pharyngeal erythema, edema, and inflammation of the gums. The neck should be examined for any cervical lymphadenopathy, which may indicate an inflammatory or infectious source in the head, eyes, sinuses, ear, or throat. The jaw should be palpated for any tenderness or misalignment. The lungs should be assessed with particular attention for any wheezing or rhonchi. The skin should be inspected for typical signs of atopic dermatitis. A neurologic exam, including a thorough eye examination, should be done if the patient complains of visual problems. If periorbital swelling, abnormal extraocular movements, or decreased visual acuity are noted, an urgent evaluation with an ENT specialist and/or ophthalmologist would be necessary.

The face, particularly over the maxillary sinuses, should be checked for any swelling or redness. The sinuses should be palpated for tenderness. See **Figure 15-1** for a picture of the normal landmarks for the sinuses. In acute sinusitis, marked discomfort is commonly elicited upon palpation of the sinuses; however, this finding is much less common in individuals with chronic sinusitis. The sinuses can be transilluminated to assess for blockage, although this test has a low diagnostic yield. If done, transillumination must be performed in a blackened room with an extremely bright source of light; otherwise, the exam will be inaccurate.

LABORATORY

Although impractical, aspiration of purulent secretions via a sinus puncture is considered the most accurate method of diagnosing acute bacterial sinusitis. Diagnosis is confirmed if the culture detects a minimum of 10^5 organisms per milliliter of a suspected pathogen. However, because this method is not commonly practiced, providers rely on the imperfect, but more practical, method of symptom review and clinical observations to diagnose acute rhinosinusitis.[75]

Figure 15-1 Bony landmarks of the sinuses.

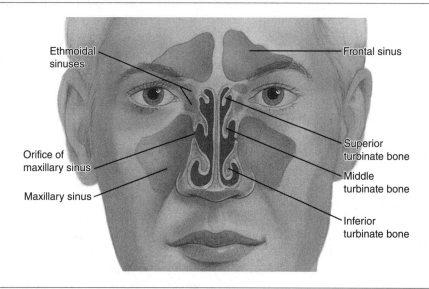

Ethmoidal sinuses

Frontal sinus

Orifice of maxillary sinus

Superior turbinate bone

Maxillary sinus

Middle turbinate bone

Inferior turbinate bone

Reproduced from Ghorayeb BY. Anatomy of the sinuses. ghorayeb.com.http://www.ghorayeb.com/AnatomySinuses.html. September 17, 2014. Accessed July 13, 2016.

Imaging is rarely needed in the evaluation of acute sinusitis. However, nasal endoscopy and nasal cultures may be useful tests in those with refractory cases. Nasal cultures can identify the causative organism leading to chronic infection. Nasal endoscopy leads to better visualization of the posterior nasal cavity, nasopharynx, and drainage patterns and facilitates obtaining nasal cultures.[75] Nasal endoscopy can also help identify a deviated nasal septum or nasal polyps.

If persistent symptoms are noted, consultation with an ENT specialist is warranted before diagnostic testing or treatment is ordered. Radiographs have no place in the diagnosis or treatment of either acute or chronic sinusitis.[75] If additional tests are needed, the best evaluation is an examination of the nasal airway by an expert, often via nasal endoscopy. Whether other imaging techniques are needed is debated among the various authoritative bodies, but authorities agree that if additional testing is needed, the CT scan is the preferred modality.[75] It is generally reserved for use in patients with recurrent or persistent sinus infections and may be helpful in detecting the presence of underlying anatomic abnormalities.[75] Magnetic resonance imaging (MRI) is rarely used but may be helpful in detecting tumors or fungal sinusitis.[74] Because MRI can evaluate nasal mucosa better than bony structures, it can help differentiate fungal infections from sinusitis caused by viral or bacterial organisms.[75]

Management

Rhinosinusitis is a common condition affecting one out of every seven adults in the United States.[76] Skillful management of this condition can reduce the social and economic burden associated with this disease. Management of acute sinusitis focuses on symptomatic relief and watchful waiting for complete resolution of symptoms.

LIFESTYLE

Many of the same measures that help in the relief of symptoms from other respiratory conditions such as the use of saline nose drops, management of nasal congestion, and control of allergic triggers are also helpful in the treatment of rhinosinusitis, because rhinosinusitis is often preceded by the common cold or allergic exacerbations. See the sections on the common cold and allergies for more details.

MEDICATIONS

If mild symptoms have been present for less than 10 days, symptomatic treatment with analgesics, decongestants, and intranasal corticosteroids may be effective.[75] If nasal decongestants are utilized, the patient needs to be warned of the possibility of worsening nasal congestion, especially if used for longer than 3 days. The use of steam, saline nasal spray, and saline irrigation is often also very helpful in relieving symptoms. Antihistamines are helpful only if the underlying cause of acute sinusitis is allergies.

Whether antibiotics are prescribed for rhinosinusitis depends on the underlying etiology. They are rarely needed, because bacterial pathogens are not a common cause of acute sinusitis. In general, antibiotics are avoided unless symptoms are persistent, severe, or worsening. Antibiotic coverage may be needed in the following clinical presentations, because they may indicate the presence of bacterial sinusitis: 1) symptoms of acute rhinosinusitis have persisted for 10 days or more without any clinical improvement; 2) onset with severe signs or symptoms of high fever (i.e., greater than 102°F) and facial pain or purulent nasal discharge, which have continued for a minimum of 3 consecutive days; or 3) worsening

symptoms (e.g., fever, headache, increase in nasal discharge) after a 5- to 6-day course of a URI that was initially improving.[80] In these cases, supportive treatments should be continued and an antibiotic may be prescribed.

In the United States, the usual pathogens associated with acute bacterial sinusitis are *S. pneumoniae, H. influenzae,* and *M. catarrhalis*.[13] Commonly used agents include amoxicillin-clavulanate and doxycycline.[76,81] Unfortunately, increasing antibiotic resistance to the cephalosporins, macrolides, and trimethoprim-sulfamethoxazole limit the usefulness of these agents in the treatment of acute bacterial sinusitis.[76] Azithromycin is the preferred product in pregnant women with penicillin allergy.[76] However, the choice of antibiotic coverage in a specific situation is dictated by personal circumstances and local antibiotic resistance patterns.[81]

The duration of antibiotic treatment depends on the risk of bacterial resistance, which is more prevalent in children younger than 2 years of age and in adults older than 65 years; in children enrolled in daycare; and in individuals who have received antibiotics in the past 30 days, were hospitalized in the past 5 days, have comorbidities, or are immunocompromised.[80] If a person has risk factors for bacterial resistance, 7 to 10 days of antibiotics are recommended as opposed to 5 to 7 days of antibiotics for individuals at low risk of antibiotic resistance.[80]

Further evaluation is needed if symptoms worsen after 3 days or if no improvement is noted after 3 to 5 days of antimicrobial coverage. Given the increasing level of antibiotic resistance seen in many communities, failure to respond in 2 to 3 days after initiating antibiotic coverage should raise the suspicion of antibiotic resistance.[81] Other possible reasons for treatment failure include noncompliance, viral or allergic etiology, or structural abnormality. Further evaluation by an otolaryngologist or allergist is recommended if a patient is immunosuppressed, demonstrates progressive symptoms despite prolonged antibiotic use, or if recurrent rhinosinusitis is noted.[80]

PATIENT INSTRUCTIONS

The woman should be educated about the causes and treatment(s) for acute sinusitis. Instructions regarding proper adherence to the nonprescriptive supportive treatments (steam treatments, normal saline nasal spray, and saline irrigations) are recommended. Patients should also be instructed to follow up immediately if their symptoms do not improve in 3 to 5 days, worsen, or they develop swelling, facial redness, visual disturbances, severe headaches, or high fevers.

MANAGEMENT IN PREGNANCY AND LACTATION

The evaluation of sinusitis is essentially the same for pregnant as for nonpregnant patients. However, providers need to be aware that some of the medications used in the management of sinusitis are not recommended during pregnancy or lactation (see Table 15-8).

Chronic Rhinosinusitis

Chronic rhinosinusitis (CRS), which is defined as sinusitis that persists for 8 or 12 weeks or more, is commonly seen in primary care, allergy and immunology, and ENT specialty offices. National survey data have found that CRS is frequently seen in ambulatory or hospital settings and remains a major health concern in the United States resulting in significant work absenteeism. Work absenteeism secondary to sinusitis is highest among minority populations, who have greater difficulties with access to care.[82]

CRS results from chronic inflammatory mucosal changes in the nose and paranasal sinuses. The underlying etiology of CRS can be noninfectious (i.e., characterized by the presence of eosinophilia and mononuclear cells) or infectious (i.e., bacterial or viral). Noninfectious causes are more commonly reported than infectious causes. Noninfectious CRS is strongly associated with allergy-related illness and chronic hyperplastic sinusitis with nasal polyposis (CHS/NP). The most common bacteria associated with the development of CRS are staphylococci and respiratory anaerobes; however, *H. influenzae, M. catarrhalis, Pseudomonas aeruginosa,* group A *Streptococcus,* and *S. pneumoniae* have also been detected. It is believed that anaerobes develop after an initial bacterial infection as a result of mucus stasis, sinus obstruction, and local hypoxia. CRS can also develop from the same bacteria that caused an acute sinusitis.

Management

Several factors can worsen chronic sinusitis, with one of the main contributors being ostial blockage. Management of chronic sinusitis focuses on controlling or eliminating the underlying triggers. The mucosa becomes thickened from inflammation despite antibiotic treatment. Mucosal inflammation inhibits normal mucociliary clearance and may further obstruct sinus ostia. Mucus immobility, sinus ostial obstruction, and hypoxia all contribute to the growth of anaerobic bacteria, of which some have been found to be resistant to antibiotics.[76] Cigarette smoking, including active or past exposure to secondhand smoke, can decrease mucociliary clearance and is directly related to an increased risk of sinus disease.[61] Allergy and eosinophilia also contribute to chronic sinusitis. Women with allergies have a higher risk for extensive sinus disease. In comparison to seasonal allergens, house dust mites, animal dander, cockroaches, and fungal spores from indoor/outdoor sites are common allergens that can be more persistent and detected at higher levels. These allergens are more likely to result in hypersensitivity in patients with CRS than seasonal allergens.[61] Air pollutants, such as carbon monoxide, nitrous dioxide, and particulate matter, have increased the prevalence of CRS. Sulfur dioxide is another air pollutant that can also adversely affect mucociliary clearance, along with ozone and formaldehyde.[61]

LIFESTYLE

Because a majority of patients with chronic sinusitis have an underlying allergic component, identifying and reducing exposure to allergens can help minimize symptoms.

MEDICATION

Topical nasal corticosteroids, which have been approved to treat rhinitis, are considered to be effective and safe in the treatment of CRS.[75] In conjunction with intranasal corticosteroids, saline nasal sprays and saline lavage are found to be helpful in reducing postnasal drip, liquefying secretions, and clearing away allergens in the nasal cavity. Regardless of severity of symptoms, both intranasal corticosteroids and nasal saline lavage should be recommended initially for the treatment of CRS. A trial of topical nasal decongestant may be recommended. Decongestants can be helpful in the short-term because these agents can decrease nasal swelling and edema for improved ostial patency, but this medication should be discontinued after 3 to 5 days to prevent rebound congestion. Second-generation antihistamines (e.g., loratadine, fexofenadine, cetirizine) are often recommended; however, these medications should be reserved for patients with known allergic rhinitis. First-generation antihistamines (e.g., diphenhydramine) should be avoided, because their anticholinergic effects are drying, preventing mucus drainage and clearance. If respiratory secretions are thickened, guaifenesin (600–1200 mg tablet twice a day) has been found to be beneficial in thinning the mucus and promoting drainage

from the sinuses. One tablet of guaifenesin 600 mg/pseudoephedrine 120 mg every 12 hours provides both systemic and mucolytic properties and can be used in CRS.[61,75]

Given the lack of sufficient clinical trials that demonstrate the effectiveness of antibiotics in the treatment of CRS, antibiotics need to be used cautiously.[81] Unfortunately, cultures to identify the offending organism are not available in general office practice. Presumptive treatment with an antimicrobial agent can be considered for those individuals who develop a sudden exacerbation of symptoms. Treatment choices are the same as those for acute sinusitis. Caution should be used when considering presumptive treatment in individuals with CRS whose symptoms are prolonged and who have had repeated courses of antibiotics; these individuals are unlikely to respond to another course of antibiotic therapy. Mucosal thickening from chronic inflammation impedes normal mucociliary clearance, which can directly obstruct the ostiomeatal unit. This process will continue despite antibiotic coverage.[4] A consultation with an otolaryngologist (ENT specialist) may be beneficial in cases where symptoms are persistent despite treatment and in those who have recurrent exacerbations.

COMPLEMENTARY OR ALTERNATIVE CHOICES

CAMs, such as dietary and vitamin supplements, herbs, acupuncture, and homeopathic remedies, have been used in the treatment of chronic sinusitis.[83] Two dietary supplements, ma huang and bromelain, have some evidence investigating their safety. Ma huang contains ephedra alkaloids, which have been used as a nasal decongestant; however, cardiovascular and neurologic side effects have been reported.[84] Bromelains, found in pineapple, exhibit proteolytic and anti-inflammatory effects, which modify tissue permeability and reduce edema. They have also been given to reduce nasal inflammation, nasal discharge, and headache. Unfortunately, there are few data about their safety. Therefore, the safety of the complementary or alternative choices is often uncertain or unknown, especially in pregnancy and during lactation.

Patient Instructions

Women should be educated about a comprehensive treatment plan that involves adequate fluids, steam inhalation, warm compresses to sinuses, analgesics, decongestants, corticosteroid nasal inhalants, saline nasal spray, and irrigation.

Patients should also be instructed to return to care if symptoms do not resolve, because referral to a specialist may be warranted for more in-depth evaluation. A referral to an ENT specialist is warranted when the woman is not responding to antibiotic treatment, symptoms have worsened, or the patient is experiencing a recurrent sinusitis. Table 15-18 lists the criteria for referral to an appropriate specialist. The presence of nasal polyps, copious nasal secretions, chronic otitis media, immunodeficiency, allergies to several antibiotics, antibiotic resistance, or other circumstances that complicate the course of treatment require a referral to an ENT specialist. The specialist will determine if a CT is necessary and if sinus surgery is warranted; chronic hyperplastic sinusitis with nasal polyposis often requires surgical intervention.

Referrals to other specialists may also be helpful. If an allergy is suspected and environmental controls and treatment have failed to prevent or improve the outcome, a referral to an allergist is appropriate. A referral to a dentist may be indicated in some situations, because a unilateral maxillary sinusitis infection from a maxillary dental infection is an often unrecognized cause of chronic sinusitis. Patients with this disorder will often report upper teeth pain and a persistent rotten smell. Treatment via extraction or root canal often resolves the problem.

Management During Pregnancy and Lactation

Nasal congestion and sinus complaints are common in pregnancy. The underlying etiology is unknown but may be related to increasing estrogen levels, other hormonal changes, and increasing blood supply in pregnancy. It begins in early pregnancy, peaks in late pregnancy, and resolves within a few weeks after birth and affects up to 40% of all pregnant women.[10] These changes can increase the risk of sinusitis in women with other underlying risk factors.

Management in pregnancy varies depending on the underlying cause and severity of chronic sinusitis and the stage of pregnancy. Self-care practices such as the use of saline nose drops and nasal lavage are unchanged in pregnancy. Treatment for allergy can be instituted if it is a precipitating factor of chronic sinusitis. See the section on allergies for more details.

Acute Bronchitis

More than 90% of cases of uncomplicated acute bronchitis are triggered by a viral infection. The remaining cases are most often due to atypical bacteria such as *Mycoplasma pneumoniae*, *Chlamydia pneumoniae* (TWAR strain), and *Bordetella pertussis*. However, detecting the actual organism is not needed in uncomplicated cases; rather, the diagnosis and management are based on clinical findings.[85]

Acute bronchitis results from inflammation or infection of the bronchial epithelium of the tracheobronchial tree. The alveoli are not affected. Inflammation results in airway hyper-responsiveness and production of mucus. Acute bronchitis often presents with wheezing, rhonchi, and low peak flow readings. These findings make it difficult for providers to distinguish whether the "reactive airway" is simply from bronchitis or from undiagnosed asthma. If the diagnosis of asthma has not already been established, it is generally recommended to forgo a diagnosis of asthma in patients with a cough until the symptoms have lasted longer than 3 weeks. Cough-variant asthma should be suspected in patients with nocturnal symptoms or if symptoms are triggered by exposure to cold or exercise. See the section on asthma for more information.

With acute bronchitis, symptoms are usually present for less than 3 weeks.[86] The dominant symptom is cough. Patients may also report chest discomfort, low-grade fever, and upper respiratory symptoms such as phlegm, rhinorrhea, throat pain, fatigue, and headache. These signs and symptoms are common and can be present with other respiratory problems. Other causes of cough such as allergic rhinitis, sinusitis, congestive heart failure, asthma, acute exacerbation of COPD, pertussis, and pneumonia should be ruled out.[86]

Essential History, Physical, and Laboratory Evaluation

The diagnosis of bronchitis is primarily made from the history and physical examination findings.

HISTORY

As when evaluating any respiratory condition, history focuses on the evolution of symptoms and the length of time that symptoms have been present. Eliciting a history of persistent cough, particularly with onset after a URI, is highly suggestive of bronchitis.

PHYSICAL

A physical examination can help confirm the diagnosis and exclude other possibilities. Fever, tachycardia, or tachypnea suggest more serious infection such as pneumonia, particularly if areas of focal consolidation are found during auscultation and percussion of the lung fields. Wheezing,

rales, and rhonchi may be indicative of asthma or other obstructive lung conditions.[86]

LABORATORY

In general, laboratory and diagnostic testing are of little value. Chest radiography is not usually needed. However, if the patient has underlying cardiac or pulmonary disease (e.g., congestive heart failure, prior myocardial infarction, COPD/emphysema, or chronic cough) or smokes, then further diagnostic testing may be warranted. In these cases, a chest x-ray and peak flow measurements may be helpful. Cultures are rarely taken because most cases are due to viral infections or inflammation. Consequently, antibiotics are not commonly used in the treatment of acute bronchitis except in selected cases, such as when bacterial infections are present.[86]

Management

LIFESTYLE

Many of the same measures that provide symptomatic relief from the common cold also help individuals with acute bronchitis. Rest and hydration are particularly helpful. See the section on common cold for further details.

MEDICATION

In uncomplicated acute bronchitis, management should be directed at the relief of cough. Different medication choices are available, such as the antitussives and expectorants. The decision regarding the choice of which specific drug to use depends on the underlying cause of the cough. For example, if a reactive airway or wheezing is noted, then an inhaled beta-agonist (i.e., bronchodilator) usually is helpful. If an asthma exacerbation is concurrently noted, the patient may benefit from oral corticosteroids to help control any wheezing, coughing, or dyspnea. However, the use of oral corticosteroids in the absence of asthma is unwarranted.[85] If the cough is due to allergic rhinitis, an antihistamine may be beneficial. Antitussive agents are used to help suppress or control coughing when excess coughing induces chest discomfort.[86] This is often helpful for a cough caused by cigarette smoking or postnasal drip. Coughing is one of the body's defense mechanisms and therefore antitussives should be used only if suppressing the cough will not delay the patient's recovery. In some cases, promoting a more productive cough helps clear the airways of mucus. In such cases, use of a protussive agent or expectorant would be beneficial.

Historically, antibiotics have been prescribed by practitioners for the treatment of uncomplicated acute bronchitis, but their use is not recommended. Providers have been most likely to prescribe antibiotics in the presence of purulent sputum or nasal discharge, wheezing, or rhonchi. However, with acute bronchitis, purulent nasal or pharyngeal secretions do not necessarily indicate that the infection is due to bacteria. The use of antibiotics in the treatment of acute uncomplicated bronchitis does not improve clinical outcomes and encourages the development of antibiotic resistance.[86] The use of unnecessary medications adds to healthcare costs. In addition, patients may experience side effects with the use of antibiotics; some of these risks are significant, particularly the risk of developing *Clostridium difficile* infection after antibiotic use.[86] Antibiotics are recommended in acute bronchitis only when an underlying bacterial infection is suspected.[86] If pertussis is suspected or confirmed, timely administration of erythromycin or trimethoprim-sulfamethoxazole if a macrolide is contraindicated can provide relief to the affected individual and minimize the spread of pertussis to others.[86]

Patient Instructions

Providers may feel pressure from patients to prescribe an antibiotic. However, patient satisfaction is related to the quality of the interaction between the woman and her provider, not from the number of prescriptions received. Therefore, education is vital. Patients need to be informed of the diagnosis, treatment, and clinical course of acute bronchitis. For some women, describing uncomplicated acute bronchitis as a "chest cold" or "viral upper respiratory infection" makes it easier to accept the idea that an antibiotic is not necessary.[85] Other techniques to reduce the pressure of prescribing antibiotics unnecessarily include: 1) providing realistic expectations on the course of symptoms (i.e., approximately 3 weeks); 2) educating patients that antibiotics do not significantly reduce the duration of symptoms; 3) informing patients of side effects associated with antibiotic use, especially the concern for *Clostridium difficile*, which results in chronic diarrhea; or 4) providing a prescription that patients can hold onto and fill only if symptoms do not resolve within a specific timeframe.[85] Careful documentation should be provided regarding any patient education and risks associated with antibiotic use.

Management During Pregnancy and Lactation

The evaluation and treatment of acute bronchitis do not change during pregnancy and lactation. However, the provider needs to confirm that prescribed medications are safe to use in pregnancy. Table 15-8 describes commonly used medications and their safety in pregnancy and during lactation.

Asthma

Asthma is a common chronic condition, estimated to affect 8% of all Americans.[87] It affects more children than adults, more women than men, and is more common among ethnic minority and economically disadvantaged individuals.[88] Asthma costs society more than $1 billion dollars each year in lost work and school productivity and results in more than 3,500 deaths annually.[89]

Asthma is characterized by episodes of inflammation and narrowing of the airways. Attacks vary in severity and commonly present with wheezing, cough, shortness of breath, or chest pain and tightness. These symptoms result from exposure to triggers such as allergens, exercise, infections, and airway irritants and are at least partially reversible. Evidence of reversibility is defined as an increase of > 12% or > 200 mL in forced expiratory volume in 1 second (FEV_1) on spirometry testing after treatment with a short-acting bronchodilator.[65,90] Exposure to triggers results in a cascade of events including denudation of airway epithelium,

collagen deposition, mast cell inflammation, and inflammatory cell infiltration, which lead to bronchospasm, mucosal edema, and increased mucus production, all of which narrow the airway and cause breathlessness and wheezing (**Figure 15-2**).[65]

Chronic inflammation leads to hyper-responsiveness to a variety of stimuli and, for some individuals, to airway remodeling. In general, for those with milder asthma, airway obstruction is completely reversible either spontaneously or with treatment. Those with more severe asthma may develop airway remodeling and have only partial resolution of airway obstruction. Chronic inflammation can result in fibrosis, hypertrophy, and hyperplasia of airway smooth muscle

Figure 15-2 Physiologic mechanisms underlying asthma.

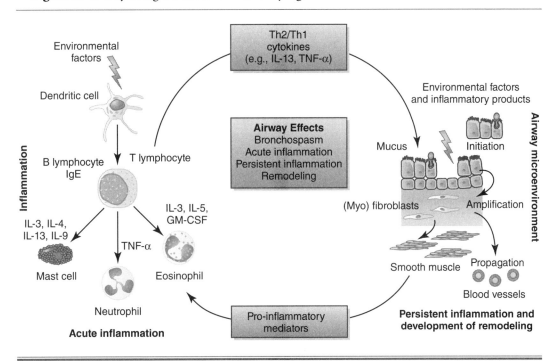

Modified and reprinted from Holgate ST, Polosa R. The mechanisms, diagnosis, and management of severe asthma in adults. *Lancet.* 2006;368(9537):780-93. Copyright 2006, with permission from Elsevier.

cells and increased mucous gland mass, making asthma difficult to distinguish from COPD. The underlying mechanisms of airway remodeling are poorly understood, nor is it clear to what extent treatment can prevent or limit the progression of airway remodeling.[91]

Patients complaining of persistent cough need to be evaluated for chronic respiratory conditions such as asthma and COPD, for conditions that cause postnasal drip such as allergies, sinusitis, and URI; underlying cardiac disorders that lead to pulmonary edema and dyspnea; and common coexisting conditions such as gastroesophageal reflux. Wheezing is also a symptom of obstructive respiratory tract disorders such as cystic fibrosis, vocal cord dysfunction, and mechanical obstruction from aspiration or tumors. Therefore, careful history, physical examination, and laboratory evaluation are necessary in order to differentiate asthma from other diagnostic possibilities. Table 15-6 provides diagnostic clues that can help distinguish asthma from other conditions.

Essential History, Physical, and Laboratory Evaluation

HISTORY

A thorough history is essential to diagnosis asthma, stage its severity, and monitor the effectiveness of treatment. Patients who present with recurrent episodes of wheezing, chest tightness, and shortness of breath and whose symptoms respond appropriately to treatment or to the removal of offending triggers can be assumed to have asthma. **Table 15-19** lists common asthma triggers.

Patients should be asked about the frequency of daytime and nighttime symptoms, because these questions allow the provider to stage asthma's severity and guide treatment choices. Treatment options vary according to the severity, frequency,

Table 15-19 Common Triggers for Asthma

- Airborne chemicals (e.g., cleaning products and perfumes)
- Allergens (e.g., mold, dust, pollen, animal dander)
- Cigarette smoke
- Cold air
- Exercise
- Food and food additives (e.g., sulfites)
- Laughing/crying
- Medications (e.g., aspirin, NSAIDs, beta-blockers, eye drops)
- Viral infections
- Weather changes

NSAIDs = nonsteroidal anti-inflammatory drugs

and impact symptoms have on a particular individual.[65,92] Providers should also determine what types of exposures trigger symptoms, note whether symptoms are sporadic or continual, and learn what approaches the patient has used in the past and whether these approaches were successful.

Appropriate asthma treatment allows a patient to maintain his or her normal activities with minimal or no symptoms. Providers should question patients on whether their symptoms cause them to limit their physical activity, miss school or work, or require the use of quick-relief medications. Providers also should routinely question patients about the frequency and consistency of use of all their asthma medications and monitor for common side effects. In addition, providers should determine whether or not their patients are at risk for severe exacerbations of asthma by asking about such risk factors as those listed in **Table 15-20**. Many of these individuals—particularly those with unstable asthma or who require high dosages to control

Table 15-20 Risk Factors for Asthma Exacerbations

- Prior intubations
- Prior admission to an intensive care unit
- Recent hospitalizations or emergency department visits
- Overuse of rescue inhalers
- Recent use of systemic corticosteroids
- Difficulty perceiving severity
- Presence of comorbid conditions: GERD, obesity, smoking, COPD

COPD = chronic obstructive pulmonary disease, GERD = gastroesophageal reflux disease

their symptoms—may require consultation with an asthma specialist.

PHYSICAL

The physical examination for an individual suspected of having asthma should not only look for data to confirm the diagnosis of asthma, but also for signs of other conditions that can mimic asthma and common comorbidities (**Table 15-21**).

LABORATORY

Chest x-rays, arterial blood gases, and other laboratory tests have only a limited role in the evaluation of asthma. Pulmonary function testing is the gold standard, useful in both diagnosis and management. Lung function in asthmatics tends to vary throughout the day and is usually poorest on arising in the morning and peaks midday. Asthma is reversible with treatment; therefore, whether an individual has been given treatment is important information when performing pulmonary function testing. A variation of more than 20% between early morning and midday measurements, or improvement in lung volumes of 12% after treatment, is indicative of asthma. The two most commonly used testing modalities

Table 15-21 Findings on Physical Examination Suggestive of Asthma and/or Asthma Comorbidities

Test	Description
Vital signs	P, RR, BP
	(Acute asthma symptoms can increase P, RR, and cause pulsus paradoxus.)
Pulse oximetry	Normal if > 95% SaO_2 on room air
Appearance	Observe posture patient assumes for comfortable breathing
Voice	Nasal quality
	Able to speak in full sentences with comfort
Skin	Cyanosis, diaphoresis, eczema
HEENT	Allergic shiners
	Sinus tenderness
	Presence of nasal polyps
	Pale, boggy nasal mucosa and nasal discharge
Respiratory	Wheezing
	Diminished breath sounds with the absence of wheezing in severe attacks
	Respiratory effort: use of accessory muscles, retractions
	Evidence of hyperinflation: barrel chest, hyperresonance
Cardiac	Heart sounds should be normal

BP = blood pressure; HEENT = head, ears, eyes, nose, and throat; P = pulse; RR = respiratory rate; SaO_2 = oxygen saturation

Data from National Asthma Education and Prevention Program. Expert Panel 2: Guidelines for the diagnosis and management of asthma. NIH Publication No. 97–4051. Bethesda, MD: National Institutes of Health; 1997.

are *spirometry*, most commonly used for diagnosis, and *peak flow meters*, usually used to monitor response to treatment.

Spirometry is generally performed in a dedicated laboratory, although office models are becoming increasingly common. Spirometry testing is not universal because of cost and access issues. Many providers do not order spirometry if the diagnosis is clear, if the patient is young with no other comorbidities, and if the patient responds as expected to treatment. However, spirometry always should be ordered for patients who do not

react appropriately to medications, whose course is atypical, or who have comorbidities that complicate the diagnosis or management of asthma.

Spirometry is helpful in distinguishing whether or not the patient has restrictive lung disease (where the patient has difficulty getting sufficient air into the respiratory tract) or obstructive lung disease (where the patient has difficulty getting air out of the respiratory tract). Measures used to differentiate restrictive and obstructive lung disease are: 1) forced vital capacity (FVC), 2) FEV_1 (in liters), and 3) the FEV_1/FVC ratio (**Table 15-22**).

Table 15-22 Pulmonary Function Tests

Measurement	Tool	Definition	Normal Value	Notes
Forced vital capacity (FVC)	Spirometry	The maximal volume of air exhaled using maximal effort, following maximal inspiration	> 80% of predicted value	Most useful measurement for diagnosing restrictive lung disease
Forced expiratory volume in 1 second (FEV_1)	Spirometry	Volume of air exhaled in the first second	> 80% of predicted value	Most important measurement for following obstructive lung disease; determines the severity of airway obstruction
FEV_1/FVC ratio	Spirometry	Expressed as a percentage and reflects how much of the total lung volume can be exhaled in the first second	Ratio < 70% indicates an obstructive disorder in middle-aged adults.	Ratio used to detect airway obstruction
Peak expiratory flow (PEF; measured in L/sec or L/min)	Peak flow meter	Largest expiratory flow achieved using maximal forced effort, following maximal inspiration	< 80% of personal best suggests obstruction.	Able to be obtained at home or in the office using a peak flow meter

Normal values for these tests vary by a patient's height, weight, age, and sex. Therefore, results are reported by the "expected value" for a specific patient. **Figure 15-3** shows measurements used to describe various lung volumes. **Figure 15-4** provides a pictorial example of a spirometry test.

Spirometry findings differ for patients with restrictive and obstructive lung disease (**Table 15-23**). Women with restrictive lung disease will have lower than expected lung volumes and so will have lower than expected FVC, because the airway will not allow normal filling to occur on inspiration. However, because exhalation is not impeded in women with restrictive disease, expiration can occur at a normal rate and their FEV_1 will be normal. Lung findings in patients with obstructive disease have the reverse pattern. The FVC will be normal because airway filling is not hindered, but these women will have lower than expected FEV_1 because obstruction delays the emptying of the lung with expiration.

Peak flow meters provide less data than spirometry but are easy to use. They are most useful in monitoring response to treatment in the office or at home. Individuals with more severe asthma have greater diurnal variation in lung function. Peak flow meters can be used to document this variation and can help stage the severity of the asthma and confirm treatment success. Appropriate treatment should minimize the diurnal pattern; measuring peak flows at various times throughout the day can help a provider decide whether the patient is on an appropriate preventive regimen. Peak flow measurements before and after treatment of an acute attack

Figure 15-3 Lung volumes.

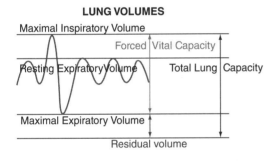

Figure 15-4 Sample spirometry volume time and flow volume times.

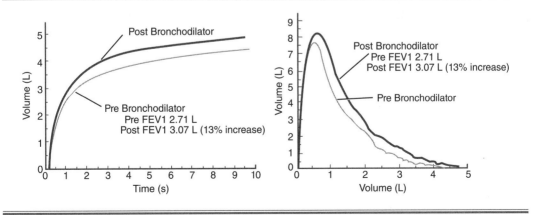

Reproduced from National Asthma Education and Prevention Program. *Expert Panel 2: Guidelines for the Diagnosis and Management of Asthma.* NIH Publication No. 97-4051. Bethesda, MD: National Institutes of Health; 1997.

Table 15-23 Obstructive and Restrictive Lung Disease

Test	Obstructive Disease		Restrictive Disease	
	Spirometry Findings	Examples	Spirometry Findings	Examples
FVC	Normal	Asthma	FVC Reduced	Obesity
FEV$_1$	Reduced	COPD	FEV$_1$ Normal	Fibrosis
FEV$_1$/FVC	Reduced	Cystic fibrosis	FEV$_1$/FVC Normal	Sarcoidosis
		Bronchiectasis		Pneumonia
		Bronchial		Congestive
		foreign body		heart disease
				Pleural
				effusions

COPD = chronic obstructive pulmonary disease, FEV$_1$ = forced expiratory volume in 1 second, FVC = forced vital capacity

Table 15-24 Correct Peak Flow Technique

Peak Flow Meter	Proper Technique
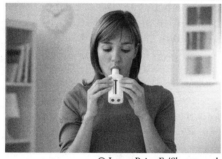 © Image Point Fr/Shutterstock	• Push indicator button to the bottom. • Stand up, and take a deep breath. • Blow out as hard and as fast as you can in a single blow. • Use the best measurement out of 3 tries.

also can document effectiveness of quick-relief measures.

Peak flow measurements differ from spirometry in several key ways. First, peak flow measurements do not give as complete a picture of pulmonary function. They do not provide information about vital capacity, nor do they measure the level of "obstruction" as well as spirometry does. There is no time element as there is with FEV$_1$ measurements, and peak flow meters only measure obstruction found in the large airways. Spirometry can measure obstruction in both large and small airways. Second, proper technique is vital in getting accurate pulmonary function tests. Spirometry has the capacity to confirm whether or not the patient used maximal effort, whereas peak flow meters do not. **Table 15-24** describes the proper technique to obtain accurate peak flow measurements.

Management

Since 1991, NAEPP has issued a series of Expert Panel Reports meant to improve the clinical management of asthma and to stimulate research.[65,90,93,94] These Expert Panel Reports have been seminal in setting standards for the diagnosis and management of asthma. The approach in these guidelines has been to: 1) classify the stages of asthma by severity, 2) link recommended pharmacologic therapies to these stages, and 3) advocate for active patient involvement in developing treatment plans and monitoring their effectiveness.

The stages of asthma are based on measurable objectives, such as the frequency and timing of symptoms, the degree of variation in pulmonary function throughout the day, and the degree of impairment patients experience from having asthma. Patients with infrequent symptoms are classified as having intermittent asthma. Those with more frequent symptoms are categorized as having persistent asthma by severity level (i.e., mild, moderate, or severe). An easy way to remember these stages is to focus on the "principle of two." The characteristics of the various stages of asthma are as follows:[92]

1. Intermittent asthma:
   - Daytime symptoms ≤ 2 days a week
   - Nighttime symptoms ≤ 2 nights a month
   - Use of short-acting beta-agonist inhaler ≤ 2 days a week
   - No interference with normal activity
   - FEV_1 > 80% predicted
   - Normal FEV_1/FVC ratio for age between exacerbations
   - 0 to 1 exacerbation requiring oral corticosteroids over the last year
2. Persistent mild asthma
   - Daytime symptoms > 2 days a week, but not daily
   - Nighttime symptoms 3 to 4 times a month
   - Use of short-acting beta-agonist for symptom relief > 2 days a week; no more than 1 time a day and not daily

   - Mild interference with normal activity
   - FEV_1 > 80% predicted
   - Normal FEV_1/FVC ratio for age between exacerbations
   - ≥ 2 exacerbation requiring oral corticosteroids over the last year
3. Persistent moderate asthma
   - Daily symptoms
   - Nighttime symptoms occurring more than once a week but not nightly
   - Daily use of short-acting beta-agonist for symptom control
   - Some limitation in performing normal activities
   - FEV_1 60% to 80% predicted
   - Normal FEV_1/FVC ratio for age reduced by 5%
   - ≥ 2 exacerbations requiring oral corticosteroids over the last year
4. Persistent severe asthma
   - Symptoms throughout each day
   - Often nightly symptoms
   - Use of short-acting beta-agonist throughout the day for symptom control
   - Major limitation in performing normal activities
   - FEV_1 < 60% predicted
   - Normal FEV_1/FVC ratio for age reduced by > 5%
   - ≥ 2 exacerbations requiring oral corticosteroids over the last year

Patients whose symptoms fall into two stages should be treated at the higher stage. For example, if a patient meets the criteria for intermittent asthma based on daytime symptoms, but meets the criteria for persistent mild asthma based on nighttime symptoms, she should receive treatment corresponding to persistent mild asthma.[65]

Guidelines released by NAEPP in 2007 emphasized the importance of evaluating the degree to which asthma is under control by adding on new criteria.[65] Specifically, providers should assess a patient's risk of experiencing an exacerbation and the degree to which they are symptom free. Over time, it has become clear that those individuals with the greatest variation in control are at higher risk of experiencing morbidity and mortality associated with asthma than those with more stable presentations. Those with higher risk of severe underlying disease have required unscheduled evaluation or treatment, hospitalization, or ICU admission for asthma symptoms. Risk assessment is operationalized in these guidelines as the frequency of having an exacerbation that required treatment with oral corticosteroids over the last year.[65] Individuals on daily controller medications should be in such good control that they meet the same criteria set for those with mild intermittent asthma, specifically minimal daytime and nighttime symptoms and little interference with normal activity.

The importance of this emphasis on control is underscored by the results of an observational study that investigated predictors of exacerbations in children (ages 6–11, n = 289) and adolescents/adults (ages 12 or older, n = 2094).[95] Failure to obtain data on impairment resulted in misclassifying asthma in 11% to 39% of patients. Adolescents and adults deemed not well or poorly controlled based on recent short-acting beta-agonist use were 50% more likely to experience an exacerbation than those who used short-acting beta-agonist inhalers less frequently.[95]

LIFESTYLE

The goal in asthma therapy is to allow the woman to be symptom free by using appropriate medications and environmental controls. Environmental control is particularly helpful in those women whose asthma is triggered by allergens. Several studies have documented increases in symptom-free days with control of environmental allergies.[90,96] Therefore, all asthmatics should be evaluated to determine to what extent allergens affect their asthma and if a link is found between asthma symptoms and allergens, environmental controls and appropriate medications should be recommended. See the section on allergies earlier in the chapter.

MEDICATIONS

The two principal categories of medications used in the management of asthma are quick-relief medications such as albuterol (Proventil, Ventolin) or another short-acting bronchodilator inhaler, and controller medications, usually steroidal inhalers. **Table 15-25** lists some common medications used for the relief of immediate symptoms and **Table 15-26** contains those used for long-term control needed to prevent symptoms from reoccurring. Women with intermittent asthma need only use short-acting beta-agonist inhalers as symptoms arise. Patients with more persistent asthma will need to continue to use short-acting bronchodilators, and add controller medication(s). The need to increase the use of quick-relief inhalers may indicate the need to add on or increase the dose of controller medications. Needing to use a short-acting beta-agonist two or more times in a week generally indicates poor control and should prompt a reevaluation of the patient's medication regimen.[65]

There are several categories of controller medications: systemic or inhaled steroids, long-acting inhaled β_2-agonists, leukotriene modifiers, nonsteroidal anti-inflammatory medications, and immunomodulators. Each type plays a role in asthma management, but the mainstay therapy in preventing asthma symptoms is inhaled corticosteroids.

Corticosteroids The inhaled corticosteroids minimize inflammation and may prevent long-term airway remodeling. They also provide the best control of all the maintenance medications and have fewer side effects than oral corticosteroids. Oral corticosteroids are avoided wherever

Table 15-25 Medications Used for Quick Relief of Asthma Symptoms

Drug	Trade Name/Form	Dose
Albuterol	Ventolin HFA MDI Proventil HFA MDI 200 puffs/canister	2 puffs 5 minutes before exercising. 2 puffs every 4 to 6 hours as needed. May double use for mild exacerbations. For acute exacerbation in home: Begin with MDI: 2–6 puffs every 20 minutes, up to 2 treatments. Patient should refer to instructions given by provider in this circumstance. Therapy individualized thereafter. For acute exacerbation in emergency department: Begin with MDI: 4–8 puffs every 20 min for 3 doses. Therapy individualized thereafter.
Albuterol nebulizer solution	0.63 mg/3 mL 1.25 mg/3 mL 2.5 mg/3 mL 5 mg/mL (0.5%)	For acute exacerbation: 2.5–5 mg every 20 min for 3 doses. Dilute with a minimum of 3 mL with oxygen flow of 6–8 L/min. Therapy individu- alized thereafter.
Levalbuterol nebulizer solution	Xopenex 0.31 mg/3 mL, 0.63 mg/3 mL, 1.25 mg/3 mL vial, single-use vials	For acute exacerbation: Nebulizer 1.25–2.5 mg every 4–8 h.

MDI = metered-dose inhaler

Data from National Heart Lung and Blood Institute. Asthma care: Quick reference. http://www.nhlbi.nih.gov/files/docs/guidelines/asthma_qrg.pdf. 2012. Accessed April 19, 2016; Sato K. Treatment of allergic rhinitis during pregnancy. *Clin Exp Allergy Rev.* 2012;12(1):31-36; National Heart Lung and Blood Institute. *Expert panel report 3: guidelines for the diagnosis and management of asthma.* NIH Publication No. 07-4051. Bethesda, MD: National Institutes of Health; 2007.

possible, because long-term exposure is associated with hypothalamic-pituitary-adrenal (HPA) suppression, osteoporosis, immunosuppression, and other adverse systemic effects.[65] Observational studies have documented slowed increases in bone mineral density and bone growth in children on daily inhaled corticosteroids[97] and higher risk of osteopenia and bone fracture in adults.[98] However, their use may be necessary for the management of more severe asthma and during exacerbations. The adverse effects of corticosteroid use are dose dependent and worsen as the total dose and length of exposure increase.[99] Inhaled corticosteroids may be safer than oral formulations, although the evidence is unclear.[98,99] Bone loss is less than with oral products, but may still occur. While the data are not conclusive, inhaled corticosteroids in the high-dose range may be associated with significant bone loss, prompting some authorities to recommend calcium/vitamin D supplementation for all adults on long-term oral or inhaled corticosteroids and in some situations screening for osteoporosis—particularly if other risk factors for osteoporosis are present.[65]

Table 15-26 Medications for Long-Term Control of Asthma Symptoms

Drug	Type/Trade Name/Dose	Low Dose: Daily Dose Number of Daily Inhalations	Medium Dose: Daily Dose Number of Daily Inhalations	High Dose: Daily Dose Number of Daily Inhalations
Inhaled corticosteroids				
Beclomethasone	MDI Qvar HFA (CFC free) 40 or 80 mcg/puff	MDI 80–240 mcg daily; 40 mcg: 1–3 puffs twice daily; 80 mcg: 1 puff am, 2 puffs pm	MDI 240–480 mcg daily; 40 mcg: 4–6 puffs twice daily; 80 mcg: 2–3 puffs twice daily	MDI > 480 mcg daily; 40 mcg: Use higher dose. 80 mcg: ≥ 4 puffs twice daily
Budesonide	DPI Pulmicort Turbuhaler 90 or 180 mcg/inhalation	DPI 180–540 mcg daily; 90 mcg: 1–3 inhalations twice daily; 180 mcg: 1 inhalation am, 2 inhalations pm	DPI 540–1080 mcg daily; 90 mcg: use higher dose; 180 mcg: 2–3 inhalations twice daily	DPI > 1080 mcg daily; 90 mcg: Use higher dose. 180 mcg: ≥ 4 inhalations twice daily
Ciclesonide	MDI Alvesco 80 or 160 mcg/puff	MDI 160–320 mcg daily; 80 mcg: 1–2 puffs twice daily	MDI 320–640 mcg daily; 80 mcg: 3–4 puffs twice daily; 160 mcg: 2 puffs twice daily	MDI > 640 mcg daily; 80 mcg: Use higher dose. 160 mcg: ≥ 3 puffs twice daily
Fluticasone	MDI Flovent 44, 110, or 220 mcg/puff	MDI 88–264 mcg daily; 44 mcg: 1–3 twice daily	MDI 264–440 mcg daily; 44 mcg: Use higher dose. 110 mcg: 2 puffs twice daily; 220 mcg: 1 puff twice daily	MDI > 440 mcg daily; 44 mcg: Use higher dose. 110 mcg: 3 puffs twice daily; 220 mcg: ≥ 2 puffs twice daily
	DPI Flovent Rotadisk 50, 100, or 250 mcg/inhalation	DPI 100–300 mcg daily; 50 mcg: 1–3 inhalations twice daily; 100 mcg: 2 inhalations twice daily; 250 mcg: 1 inhalation twice daily	DPI 300–500 mcg daily; 50 mcg: Use higher dose. 100 mcg: 2 inhalations twice daily; 250 mcg: 1 inhalation twice daily	DPI > 500 mcg daily; 50 mcg: Use higher dose. 100 mcg: ≥ 3 inhalations twice daily; 250 mcg: ≥ 2 inhalations twice daily
Mometasone	DPI Asmanex 110 or 220 mcg/inhalation	DPI 110–220 mcg daily; 110 mcg: 1–2 inhalations pm; 220 mcg: 1 inhalation pm	DPI 220–440 mcg daily; 110 mcg: 2 inhalations twice daily; 220 mcg: 1 inhalation twice daily	DPI > 440 mcg daily; 110 mcg: ≥ 3 inhalations twice daily; 220 mcg: ≥ 3 inhalations per day in divided doses

Long-Acting β₂-Agonist Inhalers

Drug	Form/Product	Dose		
Formoterol	DPI Foradil 12 mcg/ single-use capsule/18 or 60 capsules	DPI 1 capsule q 12 h		
Salmeterol	DPI Serevent Diskus 50 mcg/blister	DPI 1 blister q 12 h		

Nonsteroidal Anti-Inflammatory

Drug	Form/Product	Dose
Cromolyn	Nebulizer 20 mg/ ampule	Nebulizer 1 ampule 4 times per day

Leukotriene Modifiers

Drug	Form/Product	Dose
Montelukast sodium	Tablet Singular 10 mg	1 tab PO at bedtime
Zafirlukast	Tablet Accolate 10 mg and 20 mg	20 mg twice daily
Zileuton	Tablet Zyflo 600 mg	600 mg 4 times per day

Combination Products

Drug	Form/Product	Dose		
Salmeterol/ fluticasone	DPI Advair Diskus 100/50, 250/50, 500/50	Fluticasone 100 mcg/salmeterol 50 mcg per inhalation, 1 inhalation twice daily	Fluticasone 250 mcg/salmeterol 50 mcg per inhalation, 1 inhalation twice daily	Fluticasone 500 mcg/salmeterol 50 mcg per inhalation, 1 inhalation twice daily
Budesonide/ formoterol	MDI Symbicort 80 mcg/ 4.5 mcg 160 mcg/4.5 mcg	Dose depends on strength. Maximum 2 inhalations per day.		
Mometasone/ formoterol	MDI Dulera 100 mcg/ 5 mcg	2 inhalations twice daily		

CFC = chlorofluorocarbon, DPI = dry-powder inhaler, MDI = metered-dose inhaler, PO = per os (by mouth), q = every

Modified from National Heart Lung and Blood Institute. Asthma care: Quick reference. http://www.nhlbi.nih.gov/files/docs/guidelines/asthma_qrg.pdf. 2012. Accessed April 19, 2016.

Few data exist on the relative effectiveness and safety profiles of specific inhaled corticosteroids. Studies are needed to determine whether significant differences exist between the inhaled corticosteroids.

Long-Acting Inhaled β_2-Agonists   Patients who do not achieve adequate control on low-dose inhaled corticosteroids should add a long-acting inhaled β_2-agonist inhaler.[65] β_2-agonists relax smooth muscle and reduce bronchoconstriction. Long-acting inhaled β_2-agonists have a 12-hour duration of action after a single dose. They are *not* used for quick relief. Rather, they are used to control nighttime symptoms, to prevent exercise-induced asthma, and to enhance the effect of corticosteroid inhalers. Long-term use of the β_2-agonists as monotherapy is discouraged, because doing so can mask symptoms of worsening asthma and increases the risk of severe asthma exacerbations. Combining corticosteroid inhalers with long-acting β_2-agonist inhalers results in greater improvement in lung function and symptom control than the use of either agent alone. Not only does combination therapy lead to better control, because it allows lower doses of steroids to be used, it is less likely to lead to the development of sequelae associated with long-term steroid use. While long-acting inhaled β_2 agonists are not recommended as monotherapy, they are the preferred, first-line adjunctive option over the leukotriene modifiers.[65]

Leukotriene Modifiers   Leukotriene modifiers inhibit mediators released from mast cells, eosinophils, and basophils that contract airway smooth muscle, increase vascular permeability, increase mucus production, and activate inflammatory cells.[100] They are popular with patients because, as oral agents, they are much easier to use. They are less effective than inhaled corticosteroids or long-acting β_2-agonists inhalers, whether they

are prescribed as adjunctive or monotherapy. Adjunctive treatment with long-acting β_2-agonist inhalers results in better symptom control and lung function than adjunctive treatment with leukotriene modifiers. Similarly, patients on monotherapy with leukotriene modifiers are 60% more likely to suffer exacerbations requiring systemic corticosteroids, more likely to have poor FEV_1 measurements, and likely to have more nocturnal awakenings than patients treated with medium-dose inhaled corticosteroids.[101] Therefore, they are used primarily as adjunctive therapy and are particularly helpful for those individuals whose asthma has an allergic component.[65]

Nonsteroidal Anti-Inflammatory Medications Currently, the only agent in this class available in the United States for the treatment of asthma is cromolyn. Cromolyn affects mast cell mediator release and inhibits early and late asthmatic response triggered by allergens and exercise. It is administered via nebulization. Historically, it has been most commonly used as a metered-dose inhaler (MDI). However, asthma inhalers using chlorofluorocarbon (CFC)-containing propellants, including cromolyn, were discontinued several years ago, because CFC is known to deplete the ozone.

Immunomodulators   Immunomodulators are used as adjunctive therapy in individuals 12 years of age or older who have severe persistent asthma and who are also allergic to dust mites, cockroaches, cats, or dogs. They can trigger anaphylactic reactions and are generally prescribed only by specialists, such as allergists, in settings where prompt treatment of anaphylaxis is possible.[65] See the section on allergies earlier in the chapter for further details.

Other options are sometimes offered to those with severe asthma. Use of long-acting inhaled muscarinic antagonists such as tiotropium bromide (Spiriva, Respimat) can reduce symptoms and lessen exacerbations in those with poorly controlled asthma already on inhaled corticosteroids. Omalizumab is another product that has been shown to be effective in improving asthma control in selected individuals with severe asthma. Omalizumab inhibits the binding of IgE to receptors on mast cells and basophils, which limits the release of mediators of the allergic response. It is given as a subcutaneous injection. Its use is limited to individuals with moderate to severe asthma that is inadequately controlled on inhaled corticosteroids and who also have documented positive skin test to a perennial aeroallergen.[102]

MATCHING MEDICATIONS TO SYMPTOMS

All patients, regardless of stage, need to be prescribed a quick-relief medication. The drug of choice for the treatment of acute bronchospasm is a short-acting inhaled β_2-agonist. Systemic routes are not recommended, because they are less effective, have a longer onset of action, and are associated with more side effects. The most commonly prescribed agent is albuterol. Levalbuterol, which is a derivative of albuterol, is another alternative and may have a better side effect profile than albuterol. To date, controversy remains about whether the use of this more expensive medication is warranted. However, a randomized clinical trial (n = 112) reported comparable side effect profiles and clinical outcomes between the two products, but significantly higher costs associated with levalbuterol compared to albuterol use.[103] Other less selective β_2-agonists, such as isoproterenol, metaproterenol, isoetharine, and epinephrine, are not recommended; they can cause excessive cardiac stimulation, especially at high doses.[90]

The latest guidelines issued by the NAEPP recommend a systematic approach to prescribing medications for asthma control, which acknowledges the importance of using corticosteroids to reduce inflammation and potentially to prevent long-term airway remodeling.[65,104] At the same time, NAEPP recommendations support minimizing long-term exposure to high-dose corticosteroids; therefore, they recommend "stepping" up medications based on severity of symptoms and response to prescribed medications. **Table 15-27** describes the medications recommended for intermittent and persistent asthma.

Women on controller medications need regular surveillance to evaluate their current control. Overuse of quick-relief medications suggests the need to either add or increase the dose of controller medication(s). Use of a short-acting beta-agonist more than twice a week indicates less than optimal control. If women are not in good control, a step up in treatment may be warranted. However, before medications are changed, the provider should review inhaler technique, medication adherence, use of environmental controls, and treatment of comorbidities such as allergies.[65]

Individuals in poor control will present with one or more of the following signs or symptoms: daytime symptoms > 2 times a week, nighttime awakenings 1 to 3 times a week, and a peak flow or FEV_1 of 60% to 80% personal best. These individuals should have their medications stepped up 1 level and be reevaluated in 2 to 6 weeks. Individuals with worse control (defined as daily symptoms, nighttime awakenings $\geq$ 4 times a week, a peak flow or FEV_1 of < 60% personal best, and severe limitations of their physical activity) require more aggressive treatment. The NAEPP recommends that their medications be stepped up 1 to 2 levels. These individuals will also likely need to receive a short course of oral corticosteroids. Individuals with poor control should be reevaluated in 2 weeks.[104] Patients should remain at the higher step for a minimum of 3 months with good control before a step down in medication should be considered.[65] Immunotherapy can be considered for individuals who have an allergic component to their asthma.

Table 15-27 Step Approach to Prescribing Asthma Medications

Asthma Stages	Step	Preferred Treatment	Notes
Intermittent asthma	1	Short-acting beta-agonist	
Persistent asthma	2	Low-dose inhaled corticosteroids	Consider subcutaneous allergen immunotherapy if allergies.
	3	Low-dose inhaled corticosteroids plus a long-acting beta-agonist *or* Medium-dose inhaled corticosteroids	Consider subcutaneous allergen immunotherapy if allergies.
	4	Medium-dose inhaled corticosteroids plus a long-acting beta-agonist	Refer to asthma specialist. Consider subcutaneous allergen immunotherapy if allergies.
	5	High-dose inhaled corticosteroids plus a long-acting beta-agonist *and* consider omalizumab for patients with allergies	Consider subcutaneous allergen immunotherapy if allergies.
	6	High-dose inhaled corticosteroids plus a long-acting beta-agonist plus oral corticosteroids *and* consider omalizumab for patients with allergies	Consider subcutaneous allergen immunotherapy if allergies.

MEDICATION-DELIVERY SYSTEMS: INHALERS, SPACERS, AND NEBULIZERS

Inhalers   There are two types of inhalers in use: *dry-powder inhalers (DPIs)* and *metered-dose inhalers (MDIs)*. Most MDIs are pressurized and need a propellant to push the medication out of the attached canister. Historically, MDIs contained CFC propellants; however, when the United States signed the Montreal Protocol in 1987, it agreed to help protect the ozone layer by phasing out CFCs, which has stimulated the development of alternative propellants and new asthma products. The alternative propellant currently in use in MDIs is hydrofluoroalkane (HFA). The DPIs, which were introduced after the implementation of the Montreal Protocol, do not require the use of any propellant.

The DPIs contain individually packaged doses of dry-powder medication, which are loaded into a

reservoir. Each dose is dispensed into the breathing chamber just before use. Deposition of the medication into the lungs is triggered by inhalation for the majority of DPIs, although a few use another mechanism such as compressed air to activate the device. Most DPIs are *breath actuated*, meaning that a deep inhalation pulls the medication into the lungs. In contrast, most MDIs use a propellant to force medication into the lungs, although some are breath actuated like the DPI. The technique needed for the correct use of breath-actuated inhalers is very different from the technique needed for pressurized MDIs. Therefore, it is essential that the provider review with each patient the correct steps for how to use her particular medication (**Tables 15-28, 15-29,** and **15-30**).

Correct use of a DPI requires rapid, forceful inhalation as opposed to a coordinated slow breath with an MDI. Unlike the MDI, patients

Table 15-28 Correct Inhaler Technique

Inhaler	Correct Usage

Metered-dose inhaler (MDI)
 	
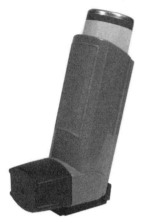
 	
© A. L. Carter/iStock/Thinkstock
	• Hold the inhaler upright and shake several times.
	• Hold the mouthpiece in either of the following two correct positions:
	  1. Seal your mouth around the mouthpiece.
	  2. Hold the mouthpiece 1 to 2 inches away from your lips (a spacer may also be used; see Table 15-29).
	• Do not block the inhaler opening with your tongue.
	• Press down on the inhaler as you start to breathe in.
	• Breathe in slowly and steadily over 3 to 5 seconds.
	• Remove the inhaler from your mouth.
	• Hold your breath for 10 seconds.
	• Breathe out slowly.
	• Rinse your mouth if using an inhaler containing corticosteroids.

Dry-powder inhaler (DPI) 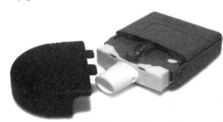 © Marjanneke de Jong/Shutterstock	• Store in dry place. • Hold the inhaler upright. • Load your inhaler. • Do *not* shake the inhaler or your medication will spill. • Seal your lips around the inhaler. • Do not block the inhaler opening with your tongue. • Breathe in quickly and forcefully to release the medication. • Remove the inhaler from your mouth. • Hold your breath afterward for 10 seconds. • Breathe out slowly. • Do not breathe out through the inhaler, because the humidity from your breath in combination with the dry-powder medication can clog the device. • In general, do not wash a DPI. Use a dry cloth to wipe out the device. • Do not use a DPI with a spacer. • Rinse your mouth if using an inhaler containing corticosteroids. • Each DPI is different; refer to the operating instructions for further details governing the patient's specific medication.

Table 15-29 Correct Spacer Technique

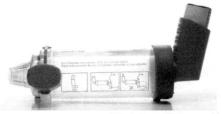

© Rob Byron/Shutterstock

- Use only with a metered-dose inhaler.
- Shake the inhaler.
- Attach the spacer to the mouthpiece of the inhaler.
- Press down on the inhaler and release one puff into the spacer.
- Place the mouthpiece into your mouth and inhale slowly.
- Hold your breath for 10 seconds and exhale.

Table 15-30 Correct Use of a Nebulizer

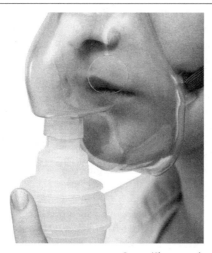

© vvoe/Shutterstock

- Measure the correct amount of normal saline and add to the cup.
- Measure the correct amount of medication and add to the cup.
- Fasten the mouthpiece to the T-shaped cylinder.
- Connect the T-shaped cylinder to the oxygen tank.
- Turn on the oxygen tank.
- Seal your mouth around the mouthpiece.
- Take slow, deep breaths.
- Hold each breath for 1 to 2 seconds.
- Continue until all of the medication is gone.
- Turn off the oxygen source.
- For home machines, disconnect the tubing.
- Rinse the mouthpiece and T-shaped cylinder in warm running water. Do not rinse the tubing.
- Reconnect the mouthpiece, T-shaped cylinder, and tubing.
- Run the oxygen for a few minutes to air dry the nebulizer.
- Disconnect and store in dry place.

should never shake a DPI before use, because this will cause the dose to be spilled and lost. In addition, patients using DPIs may not feel, smell, or taste the medication. Correct use of an MDI requires the patient to push down on the canister to dispense the medication at the very beginning of a slow, deep inhalation. DPIs are easier to use for those who find the coordination required by this technique too difficult. However, some patients may not be able to breathe in deeply or quickly enough as the correct use of a DPI requires. Correct technique is critical, because it is one of the major determinants of whether a patient receives the full, prescribed dose.[105] Therefore, the patient should be prescribed an inhaler type that she finds the easiest to use correctly.

Spacers *Spacers* are used with MDIs only. The MDI attaches to the spacer; medication is released into the spacer, and the patient inhales the medication through the spacer. Using an MDI in combination with a spacer provides many of the same advantages of DPIs. Like DPIs, they do not require a patient to inhale at the same moment that she pushes down on the canister to release the medication. Therefore, they are helpful for use by individuals who find that it is too difficult to coordinate the activation of an MDI and inhalation. In a literature review evaluating more than 50 studies on inhaler technique, Cochrane and colleagues reported that only about 7% to 23% of any drug delivered by an MDI reaches the lungs.[105] Use of a spacer can almost double the deposition of medication in the lungs and significantly reduces deposition into the oropharynx. Not only does a spacer improve medication delivery, but it can also minimize side effects of medications dispensed by MDIs. They help prevent the development of oral thrush, which is a common side effect of corticosteroid-containing inhalers, and minimize the systemic absorption of MDI-dispensed medications.[105] Table 15-29 describes proper spacer technique.

The major disadvantage of spacers is that they are bulky and awkward to carry. Therefore, they are best used with dosing patterns, such as daily or twice-daily dosing, which allow the patient to keep the spacer at home. Another approach is to prescribe several spacers so that the patient can leave one at home and another at school or work.

Nebulizers A *nebulizer* is a T-shaped cylinder with a mouthpiece at one end, a cup to hold medication in the middle, and a port at the other end. Tubing attaches to this port and connects to an oxygen tank. Medication and saline are added to the cup; oxygen bubbles through this solution and provides an aerosolized medicated mist to the patient. Nebulizers are popular with patients due to their ease of use. However, they are less practical than inhalers because they are not portable, nor do they provide any added benefit. Studies have shown that using an MDI with a spacer is as effective as a nebulizer

treatment, as long as the patient uses good inhaler technique.[65,106] Table 15-30 describes the proper nebulizer technique.

EXERCISE-INDUCED ASTHMA

Exercise-induced *bronchospasm* is common and thought to affect 10% of the population not known to have underlying asthma and up to 80% of individuals with asthma.[106] Typically, exercise-induced asthma presents with coughing, wheezing, chest tightness, or shortness of breath. Symptoms do not begin immediately; rather, they start later in the exercise session or soon after ceasing exercise. Symptoms tend to resolve in 20 to 30 minutes after exercise is stopped. A careful history is needed to determine the diagnosis, because the management of exercise-induced asthma versus chronic asthma worsened by exercise differs. Those with chronic asthma may require daily medications plus pretreatment before exercising, whereas those with exercise-induced asthma will need only pretreatment.[106] Other possible diagnoses, while rare, should be considered, including vocal cord dysfunction, GERD, and cardiac pathology. Because symptoms occur only on exertion, individuals with exercise-induced asthma are likely to have normal spirometry findings. Therefore, bronchoprovocation testing is recommended. A diagnosis of exercise-induced asthma can be made if the FEV_1 drops by $\geq 10\%$ from pre- to post-testing.[106]

The preferred pretreatment for exercise-induced asthma is the use of short-acting inhaled β_2-agonists 15 minutes before the onset of exercise. The effect of this pretreatment should last 2 to 3 hours. If this regimen provides only partial relief, then taking a long-acting inhaled β_2-agonist can provide relief for up to 12 hours.[65] The long-acting inhaled β_2-agonists may be particularly helpful for those who participate in marathons or other activities of long duration. Long-acting inhaled β_2-agonists should be taken a minimum of 30 minutes before exercising and will last 10 to 12 hours. However, long-term use of both the long- and short-term β_2-agonists as solo agents can result in tolerance to the medication and may mask the development of more persistent asthma. Therefore, many individuals with persistent exercise-induced asthma can benefit from using inhaled corticosteroids on a daily basis.[106]

Leukotriene modifiers are also sometimes used in the treatment of exercise-induced asthma. If used to prevent asthma, they should be taken 2 hours before exercising.[106] However, the same precautions exist—frequent use of these medications can mask symptoms and make it more difficult to recognize that an individual should step up her medication level.

Other nonpharmacologic approaches can help. Pre-exercise warm-ups are essential. Avoiding exposure to cold air by using a scarf outdoors or exercising indoors may help. Exercising indoors may also help those whose asthma is triggered by outdoor allergens or air pollution. The type of exercise also can make a difference. Sports such as long-distance running, cycling, basketball, soccer, ice hockey, ice skating, and cross-country skiing are more likely to trigger asthma than swimming, diving, sprinting, boxing, wrestling, karate, tennis, gymnastics, baseball, downhill skiing, isometrics, and water polo.

ACUTE EXACERBATIONS

All patients need to be educated on how to manage worsening asthma symptoms and when to come to the hospital or clinic for emergency management. The NAEPP strongly recommends that providers give all patients a written asthma action plan, which describes a specific individualized plan to follow based on changes in symptoms and/or pulmonary function.[65] A written action plan breaks down symptoms and peak flow measurements into three categories:

- *Red zone:* Requires immediate treatment and emergent evaluation by a healthcare provider

- *Yellow zone:* Requires immediate treatment and urgent evaluation by a healthcare provider if symptoms do not resolve with yellow zone management
- *Green zone:* Normal pulmonary function that requires continuation of maintenance medication

This "red-yellow-green stoplight" format presents a clear visual image for the patient to follow. **Figure 15-5** is an example of a written action plan. Action plans are based on the treatment recommendations made by the NAEPP.[65]

Exacerbations can be categorized by severity. Mild exacerbations usually can be managed at home using the predetermined action plan. Mild exacerbations are characterized by dyspnea with activity and peak flow measures > 70% of personal best. They resolve promptly with use of short-acting beta-agonists but may need a short course of oral corticosteroids to resolve completely. Moderate exacerbations usually require evaluation in the office or emergency department (ED). In these cases, dyspnea interferes with usual activities and peak flow measures range between 40% and 69% of personal best. Individuals with moderate exacerbations often require treatment with oral corticosteroids, particularly if these individuals do not respond promptly to short-acting beta-agonists or recently received a course of oral corticosteroids. Severe exacerbations are more concerning; individuals experiencing severe exacerbations present with dyspnea at rest and are breathless when speaking. Their peak flow measures are less than 40% of personal best. Treatment should be more aggressive. Nebulizer treatments with high-dose, short-acting beta-agonists plus ipratropium should be given in the ED. These individuals should also receive oral corticosteroids and may require hospitalization. Life-threatening presentations are characterized by the inability to speak; they require emergency transport to the hospital, nebulized short-acting beta-agonists and ipratropium, intravenous steroids, and possibly ICU admission.[65]

Figure 15-5 Written action plan.

Asthma Action Plan

GREEN ZONE

Doing Well
- No cough, wheeze, chest tightness, or shortness of breath during the day or night
- Can do usual activities

And, if a peak flow meter is used,

Peak flow: more than _____
(80 percent or more of my best peak flow)

My best peak flow is: _____

Take these long-term control medicines each day (include an anti-inflammatory).

Medicine	How much to take	When to take it

| Before exercise | ❏ _____ | ❏ 2 or ❏ 4 puffs _____ | 5 minutes before exercise |

YELLOW ZONE

Asthma Is Getting Worse
- Cough, wheeze, chest tightness, or shortness of breath, or
- Waking at night due to asthma, or
- Can do some, but not all, usual activities

-Or-

Peak flow: _____ to _____
(50 to 79 percent of my best peak flow)

First Add: quick-relief medicine—and keep taking your GREEN ZONE medicine.
_____ (short-acting beta₂-agonist) ❏ 2 or ❏ 4 puffs, every 20 minutes for up to 1 hour / ❏ Nebulizer, once

Second If your symptoms (and peak flow, if used) return to GREEN ZONE after 1 hour of above treatment:
❏ Continue monitoring to be sure you stay in the green zone.
-Or-
If your symptoms (and peak flow, if used) do not return to GREEN ZONE after 1 hour of above treatment:
❏ Take: _____ (short-acting beta₂-agonist) ❏ 2 or ❏ 4 puffs or ❏ Nebulizer
❏ Add: _____ (oral steroid) _____ mg per day For _____ (3–10) days
❏ Call the doctor ❏ before/ ❏ within _____ hours after taking the oral steroid.

RED ZONE

Medical Alert!
- Very short of breath, or
- Quick-relief medicines have not helped, or
- Cannot do usual activities, or
- Symptoms are same or get worse after 24 hours in Yellow Zone

-Or-

Peak flow: less than _____
(50 percent of my best peak flow)

Take this medicine:
❏ _____ (short-acting beta₂-agonist) ❏ 4 or ❏ 6 puffs or ❏ Nebulizer
❏ _____ (oral steroid) _____ mg

Then call your doctor NOW. Go to the hospital or call an ambulance if:
- You are still in the red zone after 15 minutes AND
- You have not reached your doctor.

DANGER SIGNS
- Trouble walking and talking due to shortness of breath
- Lips or fingernails are blue

- Take ❏ 4 or ❏ 6 puffs of your quick-relief medicine AND
- Go to the hospital or call for an ambulance _____ (phone) NOW!

See the reverse side for things you can do to avoid your asthma triggers.

For: _____ Doctor: _____ Date: _____
Doctor's Phone Number _____ Hospital/Emergency Department Phone Number _____

Reproduced from National Heart Lung and Blood Institute. Asthma action plan. http://www.nhlbi.nih.gov/health/resources/lung/asthma-action-plan. 2007. Accessed July 13, 2016.

Women experiencing acute asthma exacerbations require a prompt and focused evaluation to provide symptomatic relief and prevent worsening of the attack. In this situation, the history should focus primarily on asthma-related questions. It is essential to determine what medications the patient is currently prescribed, adherence to her prescribed regimen, recent use of any quick-relief medications at home, known triggers, and history of prior exacerbations requiring intubations or hospitalization. Critical elements of the physical exam include vital signs, pulse oximetry, and a peak flow if readily available. Observing the woman's comfort while talking and breathing can indicate the severity of the exacerbation. Pulse oximetry should be obtained on room air before giving the patient supplemental oxygen. Care should begin with immediate emergency treatment with a nebulizer using a short-acting β_2-agonist and consult for further management if needed with a provider skilled in asthma management. The goal is to administer medications without delay in order to prevent pulmonary deterioration; therefore, all providers must be skilled in the emergency management of asthma.

Patients with severe exacerbations may require oral or intravenous corticosteroids and a change in their maintenance medications in order to regain control. Patients are often given a steroid "burst" of 40 to 60 mg of oral prednisone for 3 to 10 days and are continued on a higher dose of their controller medication(s). After discharge, patients should be seen within 1 to 4 weeks by their primary asthma provider. The burst dose of steroids should continue until the patient is symptom free or the patient achieves 70% of her personal best peak flow.[65] Patients should remain on a higher level inhaled corticosteroid dose for 3 months and then can be slowly weaned down if the patient maintains good asthma control.

MANAGEMENT DURING PREGNANCY AND LACTATION

Debate exists about whether pregnancy improves or worsens asthma. Asthma has commonly been reported to remain unchanged in one-third of women, worsen in another one-third, and improve in the last one-third.[107] Studies based on asthma severity indicate that those women with milder disease experience little change in their asthma status in pregnancy, whereas those with more severe asthma do. For those who are affected, asthma symptoms appear to peak late in the second trimester and improve by delivery.[107]

Debate also exists about whether, and, if so, how, asthma affects fetal or maternal outcomes. There is some evidence to suggest that asthma may increase the risk of congenital anomalies, in particular anomalies of the respiratory tract, nervous system, or GI tract, in children born to asthmatic mothers. Asthma exacerbations in the first trimester requiring ED evaluation or oral corticosteroid

use are associated with a small increased risk of congenital anomalies.[108] Women with poorly controlled asthma as evidenced by the need for hospitalization or oral corticosteroids appear to be at higher risk of poor perinatal outcomes such as preterm birth and low birth weight than women in good control.[108] However, prospective case-matched studies indicate that women with actively managed asthma who achieve good control have rates of perinatal complications similar to women without asthma. For example, an observational study of more than 2000 pregnant and nonpregnant women reported that women using oral corticosteroids delivered 2 weeks earlier than women not using systemic corticosteroids. Asthma severity was not associated with preterm birth, but was associated with intrauterine growth restriction (IUGR). Each increased step of asthma severity was associated with a 24% increased risk of delivering an IUGR infant.[109]

The evidence on the safety of asthma medications in pregnancy is more robust for some medications than others. The short-acting beta-agonists have the most data documenting their safety, all of which have no reported associations between the use of short-acting beta-agonists and low birth weight, IUGR, or congenital anomalies.[108] A few studies have reported some associations between corticosteroid use and poor perinatal outcomes, although this evidence is significantly stronger for oral compared to inhaled products. In a review of the literature, Rocklin identified 12 studies investigating the relationships between inhaled corticosteroids and low birth weight, IUGR, and congenital anomalies; only two reported positive associations. Four of the eight studies investigating these same relationships with oral corticosteroid use reported positive associations. Little to no data are available on the safety of the leukotriene modifiers.[108]

Because uncontrolled asthma poses risk for the mother and fetus, all of the medications used in the treatment of asthma are recommended for use in pregnancy and lactation.[65,67] Treatment recommendations are unchanged by pregnancy. Any of the corticosteroid inhalers are acceptable, although budesonide (Pulmicort) is recommended by the NAEPP as the preferred treatment—not because budesonide is thought to be any safer than other corticosteroid inhaler choices, but because it has more extensive safety data.[65,67] Therefore, the NAEPP recommends beginning with budesonide for women initiating corticosteroid inhaler use in pregnancy, but does not advocate switching to budesonide for women already using other products. Oral corticosteroids can also be used in pregnancy. While the use of oral corticosteroids may be associated with some adverse outcomes, it is mandatory for severe asthma given the grave consequences of uncontrolled asthma. Of the other medications commonly used for asthma management, the leukotriene modifiers have the least available data, but are still thought to be safe.[67] Therefore, the approach to management of asthma is unchanged by pregnancy or lactation.

Unfortunately, pregnant women are often reluctant to use enough medication to achieve control. Providers also tend to underprescribe.[107] The end result is that pregnant women are much more likely to seek emergency care in pregnancy and to experience relapse after emergency treatment. In a study investigating the care received by pregnant and nonpregnant women with similar pretreatment asthma profiles, pregnant women received a similar number of nebulized β_2-agonist treatments in the ED, but were less likely to receive systemic corticosteroids or be prescribed steroids on discharge. At the 2-week follow-up interview, pregnant women were 3 times more likely to report ongoing exacerbation of their asthma.[110]

Acute asthma attacks are rare during labor and birth. Women should continue on their usual medications, but may require systemic corticosteroids if they are on an oral regimen before labor. The NAEPP recommends that women

---

Box 15-1 Stress Dose of Steroids

- Give if the woman has received oral steroids within previous 4 weeks.
- Start in labor and continue until 24 hours after delivery.
- Regimen: Hydrocortisone 100 mg IV every 8 hours.

---

receive a stress dose of corticosteroids during labor and the early postpartum period if oral steroids were used within the 4 weeks prior to admission (see **Box 15-1**).[67] Women with asthma should be asked about their sensitivity to aspirin or NSAIDs, which are commonly used for pain management postpartum. These pain relievers have been found to provoke exacerbations in a small subset of asthmatics.

PATIENT INSTRUCTIONS

Women need to know that asthma is a lifelong condition requiring ongoing care. Acceptance of this is a prerequisite for appropriate management of asthma. Even those women who recognize the need for treatment may have difficulty adhering to a daily medication regimen, particularly when they feel well. Studies have documented that 24% to 69% of patients fail to take all of their prescribed medications.[105] However, education, regular follow up, and use of adjunctive tools such as patient diaries and peak flow meters can significantly improve adherence. In one randomized study of 100 urban Latino and African American families, those families participating in an intervention using all of these techniques had significantly better adherence and fewer symptoms than the control group. Patients in the intervention group were more likely to take their medications regularly (82% intervention vs. 40% control group), refill their medications before they ran out (68% intervention vs. 48%

control group), and reported less activity restriction (20% decrease in the intervention group, 2% increase in control group).[111]

Women affected by asthma need to understand the physiology of asthma, how and when to take their medications, and what to do if their symptoms worsen. Written action plans can provide a structured approach for patients. These plans give patients guidance on how to monitor their symptoms, how to change their medications if symptoms worsen, and when to notify their provider (Figure 15-5).

Written action plans are recommended for use by the NAEPP with all asthmatics, regardless of the severity of their disease. According to the NAEPP, a written action plan should include[65]:

- Explicit patient-specific recommendations for environmental control and other preventive efforts that may be necessary to avoid or reduce exacerbations
- An algorithm of procedures that clearly describes how to use long-term control and rescue medication, given a set of specific circumstances and conditions, and clear instructions on how to make medicine adjustments when conditions change
- Steps the patient should take when medicines are ineffective or if an emergency arises
- Contacts for securing urgent care if needed

To be effective, written action plans require patient monitoring of their symptoms, which can be done subjectively based on patient perceptions or objectively based on peak flow measurements. The NAEPP does not recommend long-term daily use of peak flow measurements in those asthmatics with milder disease, although their use may be helpful during exacerbations.[65] Short-term monitoring over a 2- to 3-week period can be useful in determining control when maintenance medications are changed or when evaluating possible environmental triggers.

Short-term monitoring when a patient feels well can also establish a "personal best" measurement, which can be used as an objective basis for comparison during the treatment of any future exacerbations.

Women with moderate to severe disease who have a history of severe exacerbations or who cannot recognize worsening symptoms can benefit from more consistent use of peak flow meters. Daily peak flow monitoring in patients can be helpful in detecting early changes in disease status that require changes in medication management, evaluate the effectiveness of medication changes, provide objective measurements, and give guidance to those patients who cannot perceive air flow obstruction.[65]

COMPLEMENTARY AND ALTERNATIVE MEDICINE

Studies on the use of CAMs in asthma suffer from the same methodologic weaknesses found generally in the field, in particular small sample sizes, heterogeneous designs, and lack of randomization. Two large reviews concluded that the use of acupuncture and herbs cannot be recommended, based on the quality and quantity of available evidence.[112,113] A recent review of the literature suggested that although more research is needed, fish oil, pycnogenol, and possibly vitamin C may be effective as adjunctive therapy in the management of asthma.[114] Other studies suggest that there is a link between low vitamin D levels and poorer lung function in asthmatics. Supplementation should be considered in those with low serum levels.[115]

CONSULTATION

Asthma care needs to be provided in a system that allows for emergency evaluation and treatment. Therefore, the role of women's health providers in the care of asthmatic women will vary according to the system in which they practice as well as by the prevalence of this condition in their particular patient population and by their own particular interests. At a minimum, all providers should be able to evaluate whether women are receiving appropriate care, are using their medications correctly, and have an emergency plan in place if an exacerbation occurs. Providers should also be able to initiate care during an asthma attack, because prompt treatment is critical in preventing a severe episode. Providers who function in a system that can provide ready access to emergency care can independently manage women with mild intermittent, mild persistent, and well-controlled moderate persistent asthma. Consultation with an asthma specialist should be undertaken if a patient does not respond appropriately to care or if a patient requires numerous medication changes and/or high doses in order to achieve control. All women with persistent asthma who have received more than two courses of oral corticosteroids in the last year or who required hospitalization should be referred to an asthma specialist.[65]

Chronic Obstructive Pulmonary Disease

COPD results from chronic inflammation in the lungs, which limits airflow. The underlying pathophysiology is multifocal consisting of small airway disease (obstructive bronchiolitis) and parenchymal destruction (emphysema). Damage is progressive and results in structural changes, small airway fibrosis, loss of lung elasticity, and ultimately trapping of gas in the lungs.[116,117] The exact presentation depends on the type and extent of damage within the lung. Both chronic bronchitis and emphysema are conditions that fall under the rubric of COPD; however, individuals with chronic bronchitis present with chronic cough and excess mucus production but do not yet have airflow obstruction. Individuals with chronic bronchitis

are at risk of progression to emphysema, which is characterized by significant lung damage and obstruction resulting in hyperinflation of the lungs, hypoxemia and hypercapnia, and, in late-stage disease, pulmonary hypertension. Not all individuals with COPD will have mucus hypersecretion.[116]

Exacerbations of chronic bronchitis and COPD are common and hasten disease progression.[116] They are often triggered by infection or exposure to pollutants. Exacerbations of COPD can be described as mild (when symptoms prompt a change in inhaled medications), moderate (when symptoms necessitate a short course of antibiotics and/or oral corticosteroids), or severe (when hospitalization is required).[116] **Table 15-31** describes the spectrum of COPD presentations.

Chronic bronchitis presents with a persistent cough and an overproduction of sputum. To meet the definition of chronic bronchitis, symptoms must have been present for 3 or more months in 2 consecutive years. In addition, there must be no other explanation for the cause of chronic cough.[117] Symptoms are due to chronic airway inflammation that results in bronchial wall edema, increased sputum production, erythema, and mucosal friability of the bronchial airway. The walls of the alveoli lose their elasticity and become damaged or destroyed. Larger, fewer alveoli are present, resulting in a decline of CO_2–oxygen exchange. Air becomes trapped in the alveoli and breathing becomes labored.[118] These processes ultimately culminate in the development of COPD.

COPD is the fourth leading cause of death in the United States, and the prevalence is increasing worldwide.[119] The major factor contributing to the pathogenesis of chronic bronchitis and COPD is cigarette smoking. Besides acute exacerbations of chronic bronchitis, other contributors to the development or progression of COPD include infections; inhalation of dust, pollutants,

Table 15-31 COPD Presentations

Diagnosis	Symptoms
Asthma	• Recurrent episodes of wheezing, shortness of breath, chest tightness, or cough • Associated with atopic dermatitis and environmental allergies • Family history of asthma • Responds to treatment with bronchodilators and corticosteroids • May develop irreversible obstructive lung disease and progression to COPD in some individuals
Bronchiectasis	• Secondary to recurrent or persistent lung infections • Chronic productive cough with mucopurulent sputum
Chronic bronchitis (CB)	• Productive, expectorant cough for 3 or more months a year for a minimum of 2 consecutive years • Dyspnea
Chronic obstructive bronchitis/ COPD	• Meets CB definition *plus* has airflow obstruction and wheeze • Barrel chest, tripod positioning, nonexpectorant cough
Exacerbation of chronic obstructive bronchitis or COPD	• Meets definition of chronic bronchitis *plus* an increase in at least one of the following: purulent sputum, sputum volume, dyspnea, or cough

COPD = chronic obstructive pulmonary disease

Data from Engler RJM, With CM, Gregory PJ, Jellin JM. Complementary and alternative medicine for the allergist-immunologist: where do I start? *J Allergy Clin Immunol.* 2009;123(2):309-16.e4; Silvers WS, Bailey HK. Integrative approach to allergy and asthma using complementary and alternative medicine. *Ann Allergy Asthma Immunol.* 2014;112(4):280-285.

and biomass smoke; and occupational exposures.[119] Alpha-1 antitrypsin deficiency and prior TB also are associated with COPD but are less common.[118,120,121]

Essential History, Physical, and Laboratory Testing

HISTORY

A careful history and exam should guide practitioners in narrowing down the differential diagnosis of chronic bronchitis and COPD. Conditions listed in **Table 15-32** may present with similar symptoms. The hallmark findings of chronic bronchitis include the persistence of a productive cough and dyspnea. Individuals with an acute exacerbation of chronic bronchitis usually report an increase in cough; a change in the color (e.g., darker gray, green, or yellow), quantity, or consistency of sputum; or worsening dyspnea. In more advanced disease, patients may complain of a morning headache, which can occur with hypercapnia and hypoxia.[118]

Because most women with bronchitis or COPD have a history of smoking more than one pack of cigarettes per day for more than 20 years, it is important to document any past or present history of smoking. Inquiring about other factors such as occupation or environmental exposures to pollutants and exercise limitations or intolerances is essential. If the patient is having dyspnea without a history of smoking, she should be screened for a personal or family history of alpha-1 antitrypsin deficiency. Alpha-1 antitrypsin deficiency is a rare genetic disorder in which insufficient

Table 15-32 Differential Diagnosis of Acute Exacerbation of Chronic Bronchitis

Possible Diagnosis	History	Key Physical Exam	Laboratory Findings
Pneumonia	Fever > 101°F Cough Shortness of breath Malaise	Rales/crackles Focal fremitus Positive egophony Lowered peak flow readings	Infiltrate on chest x-ray
Congestive heart failure	Shortness of breath Cough	Rales or crackles on auscultation Lowered O_2 saturation	Chest x-ray findings: increased cardiothoracic ratio, pulmonary venous congestion, pulmonary venous hypertension and interstitial edema (i.e., superior pulmonary venous distention, large hila with indistinct borders, Kerley's B lines), severe pressure (i.e., pulmonary capillary wedge pressure > 25 mmHg), alveolar edema, and pleural effusions (biventricular failure)
Pulmonary embolism	Cough Shortness of breath Chest pain with inspiration Malaise	Tachycardia Hypotension Wheezing on auscultation	Chest x-ray: normal EKG changes Abnormal D-dimer, VQ scan, or Helical/spiral CT Pulmonary angiogram (confirmation)
Myocardial infarction	Midsternal, exertional chest pain Shortness of breath Dizziness Diaphoresis Nausea/vomiting Weakness Radiation to arm/chest/back/shoulder	Diaphoresis; cool, moist skin; anxious affect; tachycardia and hypertension (bradycardia and hypotension w/inferior wall MI); jugular vein distention; rales/crackles; and S3 heart sound if left ventricular heart failure present	ST wave elevation/inversion on EKG Positive stress test
Upper respiratory tract infection	Milder symptoms of rhinorrhea Nasal congestion Postnasal drip Afebrile or low-grade fever < 101°F	See section on common cold	Not helpful

(continues)

Table 15-32 Differential Diagnosis of Acute Exacerbation of Chronic Bronchitis (*continued*)

Possible Diagnosis	History	Key Physical Exam	Laboratory Findings
Noncompliance with medications	Patient reports missed medications.	Exacerbations of usual symptoms	Diagnosis of exclusion
Cough-variant asthma	Cough lasting longer than 3 weeks Allergy symptoms Chest tightness Shortness of breath and/or wheezing	Diminished breath sounds or wheezing Decreased peak flow readings Possible lowered O_2 saturation Possible clubbing/cyanosis	Reversible changes in pulmonary function tests

CT = computed tomography, EKG = electrocardiogram, MI = myocardial infarction

amounts of the alpha-1 antitrypsin protein are produced in the liver; this protein protects lung function, and its absence precipitates the eventual development of COPD.

PHYSICAL

Specific findings on physical exam may be suggestive of COPD. Signs of COPD include reduced or distant breath sounds, wheezing, prolonged exhalation, and an increase in the anteroposterior diameter (i.e., barrel chest). Women with advanced disease often have a low body mass index with muscle wasting. Other signs of severe COPD and respiratory compromise include low pulse oximetry reading, tachycardia, anxiety, pursed-lip breathing, use of accessory muscles, and cyanosis. If the patient is retaining CO_2, she will be lethargic.[118]

LABORATORY TESTING

Measures of respiratory function may be particularly helpful in the diagnosis and management of the disease. (See the section on pulmonary function tests [PFTs] earlier in the chapter.) Spirometry testing is the most useful test available to diagnose and monitor COPD. Reductions in the FEV_1, FVC, and the ratio of FEV_1/FVC can be seen in COPD. The FEV_1/FVC ratio can be used to objectively measure airway obstruction; a post-bronchodilator FEV_1/FVC ratio of less than 0.70 is the criterion used to diagnose COPD.[116] In patients whose FEV_1/FVC ratio meets the criterion for COPD, the FEV_1 level can help stage the severity of airflow limitation: mild ($FEV_1 \geq 80\%$ predicted), moderate (FEV_1 50% to 80% predicted), severe (FEV_1 30% to < 50% predicted), and very severe (FEV_1 < 30% predicted).[116] If the FEV_1 is less than 40%, the patient most likely needs to be hospitalized. Women with severe COPD usually have low oxygen saturation levels of 90% to 92% and require oxygen supplementation.

A complete blood count may be helpful to assess for chronic hypoxemia (evidenced by polycythemia (hematocrit > 55%), infection (leukocytosis), and anemia.[116] Anemia is not a consequence of COPD, but will result in worse dyspnea.[118]

Sputum cultures and Gram stains are not helpful in the diagnosis of acute exacerbation of chronic bronchitis due to their low sensitivity and specificity.[120] However, sputum cultures should be obtained in those at higher risk of having an underlying bacterial infection or of experiencing a more complicated course; these higher risk individuals include those with immunosuppression, those who are hospitalized or reside in an institutionalized setting, and those who have severe COPD—defined as having an FEV_1 less than 50%.[117] Sputum cultures should also be considered when symptoms do not improve after antibiotic therapy. In this case, the causative agent is likely to be either *Pseudomonas aeruginosa* or Enterobacteriaceae, both of which tend to be resistant to several antibiotics.[120]

Generally, radiographs are not helpful in chronic bronchitis except in the diagnosis of superimposed infection. Emphysema and COPD have classic radiographic findings—if airflow obstruction and air trapping are present—including a flattened diaphragm, hyperlucency, and hyperinflation of the lungs. Hyperinflation is present when lung tissue is visible on the x-ray beyond the 7th anterior rib, whereas with hyperlucency the lungs appear darker on a radiograph in comparison to a radiograph of healthy lung tissue. Other radiographic findings associated with COPD include an increased anteroposterior diameter and narrowing of the transverse diameter of the heart in the absence of cardiomegaly.

Radiographs are often ordered to rule out a complication of COPD such as a pneumothorax or a concurrent infection. Pneumonia should be suspected if the patient is febrile, oxygen saturation is less than 92%, or an infiltrate or effusion is found on the chest x-ray. See Table 15-32 for the differential diagnoses of acute exacerbation of chronic bronchitis and chronic bronchitis. **Figures 15-6** through 15-9 illustrate radiograph findings.

Figure 15-6 Normal chest radiograph of female.

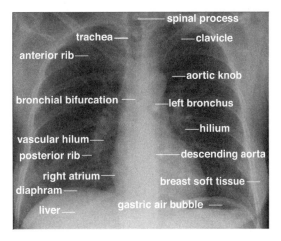

Figure 15-7 Chest radiograph of a female who has chronic bronchitis. Note infiltrate.

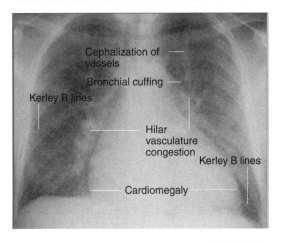

Figure 15-8 Congestive heart failure.

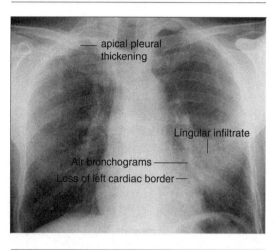

Figure 15-9 Chronic obstructive pulmonary disease—marked hyperinflation.

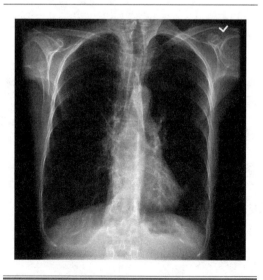

Management of Stable COPD

LIFESTYLE

Supportive treatments such as smoking cessation, adequate hydration, routine vaccinations, removal of environment irritants, appropriate utilization of oxygen, and pulmonary rehabilitation should be implemented. Smoking cessation, including cessation techniques, support groups, and medications, should be reviewed on an ongoing basis. Assessing the woman's home and work environment is also critical. Secondhand smoke, inhalants, pollutants, allergens, or social contact to an illness can all cause a relapse or recurrence of symptoms.[117] In order to prevent exacerbations, all individuals with chronic bronchitis should receive the influenza vaccine annually. Oxygen supplementation may be needed if hypoxia becomes severe. If respiratory failure occurs, noninvasive positive-pressure ventilation is used to increase ventilation.

MEDICATIONS

First-line agents for the treatment of all of the forms of COPD include the beta$_2$-adrenergic agonists, anticholinergic medications, and corticosteroids.[121] β_2-agonists and anticholinergic agents given as dual therapy maintain pulmonary function and, during an acute exacerbation, improve airflow, resulting in less wheezing and chest tightness. Oral corticosteroids are reserved for more severe or persistent respiratory symptoms and are used in conjunction with other prescription, adjunctive, and supportive treatments. See **Table 15-33** for common medications used in the treatment of COPD.

The Global Initiative for Chronic Obstructive Lung Disease (GOLD) recommends standardizing the approach to treatment based on the severity of the presentation of COPD.[116] The presentation of COPD is scored based on pulmonary lung function, number of exacerbations over the prior year, and exercise limitations using

Table 15-33 Common Medications Used in the Management of COPD

Medications	Form of Medication*	Medication Class	Reason Used
Bronchodilators			
Ipratropium bromide (Atrovent) Albuterol Levalbuterol (Xopenex) Metaproterenol (Alupent)	MDA/MDI (Atrovent) MDI (albuterol, Xopenex) Solution (albuterol, Alupent, Xopenex)	Anticholinergic Beta$_2$-adrenergic agonist (i.e., bronchodilator)	"Rescue inhaler" Immediate relief of acute respiratory symptoms
Tiotropium bromide (Spiriva)	Dry powder in capsules for oral inhalation	Long-acting anticholinergic	Primarily used in the treatment of COPD. Helps control symptoms and decreases use of short-acting beta$_2$-adrenergic agonists. Often used concurrently with inhaled corticosteroids and long-acting bronchodilator.
Corticosteroids			
Prednisone	Oral tablet	Systemic steroid	Acute exacerbations. Given for rapid onset and fast relief of persistent bronchospasm or wheezing. Gradual onset. Not recommended for treatment of acute exacerbations.
Fluticasone (Flovent) Beclomethasone (Qvar) Ciclesonide (Alvesco) Mometasone (Asmanex) Budesonide (Pulmicort)	MDI or DPI	Inhaled corticosteroids	May be prescribed with or shortly after the initiation of oral prednisone.
Combination Products			
Formoterol/mometasone (Dulera) Fluticasone/salmeterol (Advair) Budesonide/formoterol (Symbicort)	MDI	Combination of various inhaled corticosteroids and long-acting bronchodilator	Used in the control of moderate to severe asthma.
Ipratropium bromide with albuterol (Combivent)	MDI (Combivent) Solution (DuoNeb)	Combination bronchodilator with anticholinergic	Combination product preferred in treatment of acute exacerbation of COPD. Immediate relief of acute respiratory symptoms.

DPI = dry-powder inhaler, MDI = metered-dose inhaler.

Solution: Used in nebulizer.

Table 15-34 Recommended Medications by Severity of COPD

Stage	Signs and Symptoms	Treatment Recommendations
Low risk for exacerbation, fewer symptoms	• $FEV_1 \geq 50\%$ predicted • 0 to 1 exacerbation in the last year • No breathlessness except with strenuous exercise	Short-acting anticholinergic bronchodilator prn *or* short-acting bronchodilator prn
Low risk for exacerbation, more symptoms	• $FEV_1 > 50\%$ predicted • 0 to 1 exacerbation in the last year • Minimally: SOB when hurrying or when walking up a slight hill	Single long-acting bronchodilator, either anticholinergic or beta-agonist
High risk for exacerbations, fewer symptoms	• $FEV_1 \leq 50\%$ predicted • ≥ 2 exacerbations in the last year or 1 hospitalization • No breathlessness except with strenuous exercise	Inhaled corticosteroid and long-acting beta-agonist
High risk for exacerbations, more symptoms	• $FEV_1 \leq 50\%$ predicted • ≥ 2 exacerbations in the last year or 1 hospitalization • Minimally: SOB when hurrying or when walking up a slight hill	Inhaled corticosteroid and long-acting beta agonist

FEV_1 = forced expiratory volume in 1 second, prn = as needed, SOB = shortness of breath

Data from Vestbo J, Hurd SS, Agustí AG, Jones PW, Vogelmeier C, Anzueto A, et al. Global strategy for the diagnosis, management, and prevention of chronic obstructive pulmonary disease. *Am J Respir Crit Care Med.* 2013;187(4):347-365; Stenton C. The MRC breathlessness scale. *Occup Med.* 2008;58(3):226-227.

either the COPD Assessment Test or Medical Research Council (MRC) breathlessness scale. **Table 15-34** lists the four categories of COPD severity, describes signs and symptoms within these categories, and lists treatment recommendations.[116] Other medication choices are available, but the ones listed in this table are those considered by GOLD to be first-line options for individuals with stable presentations of COPD. The exercise limitations in this table are described according to the MRC breathlessness scale.[122]

Patient Instructions

To prevent or minimize progression of disease, patients must understand the etiology of their condition. Each individual with COPD will have a different risk profile. Focusing on avoiding environmental triggers such as cigarette smoke, occupational exposure, and pollution and minimizing exposure to infectious agents through vaccination and avoiding contact with individuals who are ill can prevent exacerbations. Prompt recognition and treatment of exacerbations can also minimize disease progression.

Referral

Given the complexity and seriousness of COPD, even individuals with stable presentations are best managed by pulmonologists or other experts in respiratory care.

Management of Exacerbations of Chronic Bronchitis and/or COPD

LIFESTYLE

Continued attention to lifestyle practices such as avoiding cigarette smoke, pollution, and occupational exposures is equally important during an exacerbation as when an individual has a stable presentation. See the previous section on lifestyle under stable COPD for details.

MEDICATIONS

To ensure optimal management of exacerbations, consideration of the patient's symptoms (e.g., increased sputum volume, increased purulence, increased dyspnea), comorbidities, underlying lung disease, severity of current illness, frequency of exacerbations, and age (older than 65 years old) helps determine whether the episode is "simple" or "complicated" and directs the course of treatment. Older patients or patients with neuromuscular disorders are at higher risk for respiratory tract infections due to dysphagia and risk of aspiration, poor nutritional status, decreased respiratory muscle function, and inability to effectively clear mucus.[117]

Acute exacerbations of chronic bronchitis and COPD are characterized by subjective worsening of one or more chronic symptoms (e.g., sputum production, purulence, or viscosity; shortness of breath; dyspnea; or cough). Providers should be aware that other conditions listed in Table 15-32 cause similar symptoms. However, up to 80% of acute exacerbations of chronic bronchitis are caused by bacterial pathogens such as *Klebsiella* species, *H. influenzae*, *Pseudomonas aeruginosa*, *S. pneumoniae*, and *M. catarrhalis*.[123,124] Pathogens can adhere to mucosal, oropharyngeal, and bronchial cells causing an inflammatory response and damaging the lower respiratory mucosa. This process inhibits the immune system, allowing increased bacterial replication and worsening inflammation.

Patients with complicated exacerbations of COPD have underlying risk factors that worsen their prognosis such as a history of antibiotic use in the past 3 months or another one of the risk factors listed in **Table 15-35**. Treatment of exacerbations employs skillful use of antibiotics, bronchodilators, and corticosteroids.[116]

Antibiotics are beneficial, because many exacerbations are triggered by infection.[117] Sputum purulence is a marker of airway inflammation

---

Table 15-35 Risk Factors for Complicated Acute Exacerbation of COPD

Purulent sputum, increased volume of sputum, and/or dyspnea (2 of the 3 symptoms)

Plus prior antibiotic use in the past 3 months

Or at least 1 of the following:

1. Comorbidity (e.g., ischemic or other cardiovascular disease, immunodeficiency, diabetes)

2. Supplemental oxygen therapy

3. Chronic corticosteroid use

4. $FEV_1 < 50\%$, signifying severe airway obstruction

5. > 2 or more recurrent exacerbations in the past 12 months

6. Adults > 65 years of age

Data from Albertson T, Louie S, Chan A. The diagnosis and treatment of elderly patients with acute exacerbation of chronic obstructive pulmonary disease and chronic bronchitis. *J Am Geriatr Soc.* 2010;58:570-579; Sethi S. Antibiotics in acute exacerbations of chronic bronchitis. *Expert Rev Anti Infect Ther.* 2010;8(4):405-417.

and may indicate the presence of a bacterial infection; this finding should prompt the provider to consider initiating antibiotic coverage.[120] Unfortunately, since 2000, antimicrobial resistance to *S. pneumoniae*, *H. influenzae*, and *M. catarrhalis* has emerged, and there is a lack of newer antibiotics being developed by the pharmaceutical industry.[120] Patients with complicated illness are often resistant to beta-lactam antibiotics.[120] To help prevent a surplus of bacterial resistance within the community setting, healthcare providers need to make a sustained effort to limit unnecessary antimicrobial therapy, mainly providing to those who have complicated exacerbations.[117,120]

When an antibiotic is necessary, high-dose, short-course antimicrobial coverage is as effective as lower dose, longer course therapy.[124] Choosing the appropriate antibiotic depends on prior health status, changes to pulmonary baseline, age, risk factors for resistance, and prior antibiotic use with or without failed treatment.[117] With less severe clinical presentations, one of the following narrow-spectrum antibiotics can be prescribed: azithromycin, clarithromycin, doxycycline, cefpodoxime, and cefdinir. If the patient is elderly, first-line antibiotics are amoxicillin, ampicillin, trimethoprim-sulfamethoxazole, and doxycycline.[117]

If the presentation is more severe or meets the criteria for complicated COPD, a broad-spectrum antibiotic, such as levofloxacin, moxifloxacin, amoxicillin-clavulanate, or second- or third-generation cephalosporins, is recommended. Currently, fluoroquinolones demonstrate the highest efficiency in eradicating bacterial pathogens in chronic bronchitis. Fluoroquinolones have a low level of bacterial resistance in comparison to other broad-spectrum antibiotics; however, overuse for insignificant infections will result in the emergence of bacterial resistance.[120]

Bronchodilators are also helpful. Short-acting bronchodilators, with or without a short-acting anticholinergic inhaler, are the preferred option.[116] Differences in outcomes have not been seen based on route of delivery; treatment via inhaler or nebulizer is equally effective. However, frail patients may find nebulizers easier to use.[116]

Corticosteroids are also often needed in the treatment of exacerbations. They have been found to shorten recovery time, improve lung function, and reduce hypoxemia. A dose of 30–40 mg prednisolone per day for 10 to 14 days is recommended by the GOLD consensus panel as the preferred approach.[116]

Expectorants, mucolytics, and antioxidants are adjunctive therapies that have shown some benefit. Expectorants (e.g., guaifenesin [Mucinex]) are only effective if given in higher doses (i.e., 600–1200 mg twice a day). Mucolytics (e.g., acetylcysteine) help decrease the viscosity of sputum; however, these medications often do not reach the distal airways where mucus plugging often is noted. Because cigarette smoke is a heavy oxidant and smoking is known to correlate with chronic bronchitis, the use of antioxidants has been postulated to be potentially beneficial.

Oxygen therapy may need to be initiated or adjusted to meet a minimal target oxygen saturation of 88% to 92%.[116] Failure to prevent hypoxemia below these levels would be an indication to consider hospitalization. Hospitalization may also need to be considered in those with significant comorbidities.

REFERRAL

Lung function deteriorates with each acute exacerbation of COPD.[117] Individuals with severe chronic bronchitis or COPD, those who have repeated exacerbations of chronic bronchitis or COPD, or who have minimal or no response to treatment should be referred to a pulmonologist promptly. Depending on the acuity level, they may need to be initially evaluated in the hospital setting. However, individuals with mental status changes, uncontrolled respiratory distress, or an abrupt decline in their pulmonary status need to be transferred immediately to the hospital for further evaluation, because these are red flags potentially signaling severe hypoxia.

Tuberculosis

The rate of TB infection has been declining in the United States since the mid-1990s. Still, approximately 10,500 cases were reported in 2010. Asians and Pacific Islander/native Hawaiians are disproportionally affected; African Americans less so. TB among foreign-born individuals accounts for 62% of all cases; almost half of these had been in the United States less than 5 years.[125] Poverty, lack of education, and HIV infection are associated with increased risk of acquiring the infection.

TB infections are categorized as being either latent or active. Latent tuberculosis infection (LTBI) is an inactive form of TB and indicates that the person has been exposed to TB. If a person is diagnosed with latent TB, there is no lung damage, the person is asymptomatic, and he or she is not contagious; however, he or she is at risk for developing the active form of TB. Progression from latent to active disease is common, occurring in 10% of individuals with latent infection.[126] The majority of cases of active TB are due to reactivation of latent TB, not from recent exposure to active infection.

Throughout the world, approximately 2 billion individuals have LTBI. Of those infected, an estimated 9.2 million people develop active TB each year, and 1.7 million die.[127] Individuals at highest risk for LTBI include immigrants from countries where TB is endemic.[128] The majority of cases occur in Asia, Africa, Eastern Europe, and Latin America.[128] Over time, 5% to 10% of those with latent TB will develop active disease. For people with a damaged immune system— for example, persons with diabetes—the risk is as much as three times higher. For HIV-positive women without viral suppression, the risk of active TB may be as much as 100 times higher than the overall rate.[129]

The causative agent, *Mycobacterium tuberculosis*, is spread from person to person through respiratory transmission of droplet nuclei.[130] In those with pulmonary or laryngeal TB, the bacterium is expelled through sneezing, coughing, talking, or singing. The bacterium can also be released into the environment during the performance of medical procedures such as bronchoscopy, the collection of samples via sputum induction, or the handling of tissue or bodily secretions.[131] The bacterium can remain in the air for several hours. If a susceptible individual inhales the bacterium, infection may result.

Contact with an untreated source patient (i.e., an individual with a positive sputum smear for acid-fast bacilli or an abnormal chest radiograph noting TB cavities) puts an individual at high risk for infection with *M. tuberculosis*. The following factors also impact the person's chances for infection: 1) the number of organisms released in the air, 2) the concentration of bacterium in relation to the space and the amount of ventilation (e.g., bedroom vs. nonenclosed backyard), 3) immune status of the exposed person, and 4) length of time of exposure to the infected environment.[131]

Because the bacterium is spread by droplet formation or aerosolization, casual contacts of individuals with active disease are at minimal risk. Close family members and those in close daily contact with the infected individual over a prolonged period of time are most likely to become infected. The droplets spread through the respiratory system before being neutralized by macrophage response. In some cases, the bacterium will also reach the lymph glands and spread through the body to other susceptible tissues. By traveling through the lymphatic system, the tubercle bacilli can reach the paratracheal area, which surround the trachea, and hilar lymph nodes, which are located near the mediastinum. This process forms the initial pulmonary lesion, or the Ghon focus. Some bacilli also enter the bloodstream and are transported to various organs, where they may later become activated.[131] The organs that are mainly affected are the lungs (particularly the upper lobes), brain, kidneys, and bones. The bacilli can also be found in the bone marrow, liver, and spleen; however, it is rarely detected in these locations, because these environments do not favor replication of the bacilli.

Within several days after the exposure, granulomata are formed. A *granuloma* is a nodule of inflammatory tissue formed when macrophages and T cells surround the TB bacterium. Clusters of granulomata form the tubercles, the nodular lesion of TB. The formation of granulomata prevents further replication and dissemination of disease. Once cell-mediated immunity develops in 2 to 12 weeks after infection, replication of *M. tuberculosis* ceases; a small amount of viable bacilli remains within the granuloma.[131] The granulomata and the Ghon focus may fibrose and calcify, leaving the TB infection dormant for several years.

The risk of reactivation and progression from latent to active TB depends on a number of factors, which are listed in **Table 15-36**.[128] In most individuals, the risk of reactivation is highest in the first 2 years after exposure. For

Table 15-36 Tuberculosis Screening

Individuals at Higher Risk of Exposure to Tuberculosis
Persons born in countries with high incidence or prevalence of TB (e.g., Africa, Asia, Latin America, Caribbean)
Persons who have had contact with a known or suspected case of TB
Persons who visit regularly (e.g., daily), work, or reside in residential facilities or group settings (e.g., nursing homes or other long-term care facilities, correctional facilities, homeless shelters, inpatient psychiatric institutions, hospitals)

Individuals at High Risk of Developing Active Tuberculosis
Untreated latent infection with *M. tuberculosis* in the past 2 years
Pulmonary fibrotic lesions on chest x-ray (evidence of TB without adequate treatment)
Immunosuppressive risk factors: • HIV or AIDS • Chronic corticosteroid use • Immunosuppressive therapy • Organ transplant recipient (particularly renal or cardiac) • Diabetes mellitus, poorly controlled • Silicosis • Head and neck cancers • Hematologic and reticuloendothelial diseases (e.g., leukemia, Hodgkin's disease) • End-stage renal disease or hemodialysis • Malnutrition • Alcohol abuse • Abuse of illegal drugs, particularly use of IV drugs, cocaine, or crack

Data from Gordin F, Masur H. Current approaches to tuberculosis in the United States. *JAMA.* 2012;308(3):283-289.

every 10 years post infection, the lifetime risk of reactivation of TB decreases by 10%. However, the risk of reactivation can vary widely. For example, untreated HIV infection holds the greatest risk for reactivation at 9.9%, while gastrectomy holds the lowest risk (1.3%). TB also increases HIV replication, accelerating the progression of HIV infection. The presentation of TB differs in those with acute HIV infection compared to healthy immunocompetent individuals. The most salient differences include 1) higher rates of false-negative purified protein derivative (PPD) results on the tuberculin skin test (TST), 2) higher incidence of extrapulmonary infection, 3) higher occurrence of hilar adenopathy, 4) normal chest radiograph despite the presence of pulmonary TB, 5) fewer focal infiltrates, and 6) more rapid progression and higher mortality.[130,132] Given these facts, it is imperative that all HIV-infected individuals be tested for TB, especially those who present with pulmonary symptoms. Equally important, all individuals with a positive TST result should be tested for HIV.[128] If positive, antiretroviral treatment should be initiated during the early weeks of latent TB treatment.[133]

Essential History, Physical, and Laboratory Testing

HISTORY

TB is often asymptomatic until significant lung damage has occurred. Individuals with active TB may expose others to the disease for years before a diagnosis is made. Having a high index of suspicion and inquiring about risk factors for exposure are essential to stopping the transmission of active disease. (See Table 15-36.) Individuals who have one or more risk factors should be queried further to determine if they have any symptoms of active infection. Patients with active TB may present with fatigue, malaise, night sweats, weight loss, decreased appetite, or persistent cough for longer than 2 weeks. Other symptoms may include fever, chills, sputum with or without hemoptysis, chest pain, or lymphadenopathy. Symptoms can be few and nonspecific.

PHYSICAL

Most LTBIs are asymptomatic, and no abnormalities are found on physical exam. However, some individuals with latent infection will present with unusual findings such as erythema nodosum or phlyctenular conjunctivitis. In erythema nodosum, mildly erythematous subcutaneous nodules are noted, usually on the lower extremities. Phlyctenular conjunctivitis causes the development of small grey or yellow nodules in the conjunctiva that result in discomfort, pain, and increased tearing of the affected eye. These findings are due to hypersensitivity reactions to the TB bacterium. Patients presenting with these symptoms may be infected and should initiate TB testing.

Active TB infection can occur anywhere in the body. However, physical findings are rare until the infection is advanced. Fever is common, affecting 37% to 80% of those infected with TB.[131] Cough, initially nonproductive and later becoming productive, is the most common symptom of pulmonary TB. Otherwise, physical exam findings are generally unremarkable.[131]

The most common site of infection is the lung, but infection also can occur in the larynx, kidneys, bone, soft tissue, lymphatic system, pericardium, and the brain.[130] See **Table 15-37** for a detailed description of the presentation of common extrapulmonary infections. Extrapulmonary TB is more common in HIV-positive patients because individuals with immunosuppression cannot mount an effective immune response to fight *M. tuberculosis*, thereby allowing the bacilli to travel to one or multiple nonpulmonary sites.[133] Invasive procedures are needed to establish a

Table 15-37 Tuberculosis Infections

Types	Key Diagnostic Findings
Pulmonary tuberculosis	• Reactivation of latent infection: infiltrate in upper lobes of 1 or both lungs, with cavitation • Recent infection: middle or lower lung zone infiltration, usually with ipsilateral hilar adenopathy • Old tuberculosis: nodular or fibrotic lesions (if TST+, treat) • Negative CXR: seen with HIV infection or other cause for immune suppression
Extrapulmonary tuberculosis	
• Tuberculosis lymphadenitis	• Painless enlargement of one or more lymph nodes (e.g., posterior/anterior cervical chain or supraclavicular fossa). Biopsy needed for diagnosis.
• Genitourinary tuberculosis	• Symptoms of dysuria, frequency, hematuria, flank pain; urinalysis with hematuria and pyuria. Urine culture will be negative. Culture urine for mycobacterium, fully evaluate for TB.
• Skeletal tuberculosis	• Swelling and decreased range of motion of affected site. Symptoms are subtle, therefore diagnosis often delayed. CT, MRI, or bone biopsy may be needed. Vertebral TB can lead to spinal cord compression and irreversible neurologic symptoms, including paraplegia.
• CNS tuberculosis, TB meningitis	• Symptoms of headache, neck stiffness, and loss of consciousness. CT of the head and lumbar puncture needed for diagnosis.
• Abdominal tuberculosis	• Clinical signs and symptoms depend on the site involved. Lesions can be found throughout GI tract (mouth to anus). Most common sites are terminal ileum and cecum. Laparoscopy or colonoscopy (with biopsy) is recommended for diagnosis.
• Pericardial tuberculosis	• Symptoms of chest pain (dull, aching, affected by position and inspiration), cough, dyspnea, orthopnea, edema; possible cardiac tamponade and hemodynamic changes.
Disseminated tuberculosis	• Seen with immunosuppression

CNS = central nervous system, CT = computed tomography, CXR = chest x-ray, GI = gastrointestinal, HIV = human immunodeficiency virus, MRI = magnetic resonance imaging, TST = tuberculin skin test, TB = tuberculosis.

Data from Gordin F, Masur H. Current approaches to tuberculosis in the United States. *JAMA.* 2012;308(3):283-289.

diagnosis.[131] Because TB can be a systemic infection, a thorough physical exam is needed in those suspected of having active TB.

Laboratory Testing

The purpose of screening for TB is to detect those individuals who have inactive disease and those who have recently been exposed and converted.

Screening should be performed only if there is a high level of suspicion. A decision to screen is also a decision to treat. Two screening options are available. The most commonly used test is the intradermal TST, formerly known as the PPD test for the material injected - tuberculin PPD. The newer option is the interferon-gamma release assay (IGRA), which is a blood test.[129,133] No matter what screening modality is chosen, screening for TB is recommended for two groups of individuals: 1) those at higher risk of exposure to *M. tuberculosis* compared to the general US population and 2) those who have a current medical condition that increases their risk for conversion from LTBI to active TB.[134,135]

IGRA Testing The IGRA has several advantages compared to the TST. It has comparable sensitivity and specificity to placement of the PPD using the Mantoux method (described in the following section). Second, it is more convenient, because the woman does not have to return for a reading 2 to 3 days later. Third, it is thought to be more accurate in those recently infected. Lastly, it will not cross-react with the bacillus Calmette–Guérin (BCG) vaccine, making the diagnosis of TB easier in individuals who received the BCG vaccine earlier in life.[134] However, IGRA is more expensive than performing the TST and requires transportation to the lab within 1 day.[128]

In 2010, the CDC updated recommendations.[136] Both the TST and IGRA can be used interchangeably in most situations. In general, only one screening test should be used. The IGRA is preferable for use in those less likely to return for care and in those who received the BCG test in the past, whereas the TST is preferred in the screening of children younger than 5 years of age. Rarely, it may be necessary to utilize both tests. This situation occurs when the index of suspicion is high that active infection is present or when the initial test result was indeterminate.[133]

TST (PPD) Testing Exposed individuals who have developed latent or active infection will develop an indurated area at the site of the PPD placement. Induration results from a type IV delayed hypersensitivity response and T lymphocyte function. The amount of induration determines whether or not a test is considered positive or negative. Low-risk individuals must have more induration than higher risk individuals in order for their tests to be considered positive. If a

person reports a positive TB test but no record is available or the size of the induration is not available, then a retest is recommended. In this case, an IGRA would be the preferred screening option. A TST could be considered as long as the patient did not have blistering from the last test and the test had not been done in recent years (e.g., past 5 years). All readings, whether they are positive or negative, should be recorded in millimeters and entered into the patient's chart.

Proper placement is essential. The Mantoux TST is administered by using 0.1 mL of PPD, which contains 5 tuberculin units (TU). Using a ¼- to ½-inch, 27-gauge needle of a tuberculin syringe, an intradermal injection is placed in the anterior or volar surface of the forearm to form a pale wheal that is approximately 6 mm to 10 mm in diameter. This wheal subsides approximately 20 minutes after placement. If a wheal does not develop from the injection, then the test was administered incorrectly and the test should be repeated. After the TST is administered correctly, the patient is to return in 48 to 72 hours for interpretation of the result.[130] The reading is based on the size of the *induration* (semi-firm to firm swelling), not erythema, at the site of skin testing. A two-step TST (i.e., administration of a second TST weeks following the first test) may be done if the initial test was negative, there is a high suspicion for TB, or in populations with moderate to high prevalence rates for TB. See **Table 15-38** for a description of how to correctly plant a TST and interpret the result. **Table 15-39** provides the criteria for a positive result when the TST is interpreted.

Several factors can lead to inaccurate results. Failing to elicit a wheal after placement indicates the TST was planted too deeply and may lead to a false-negative result. False-negative results can also occur in those with HIV infection, malignancies, corticosteroids or other immunosuppressive medications, and even advanced active TB.[130] The TST requires an intact immune system for the test to be accurate.[137] In addition, a false-negative

Table 15-38 Tuberculin Skin Test Administration

Correct TST placement
Dose: PPD 0.1 mL (5 TU)
Needle size: 27-gauge, ¼- to ½-inch tuberculin syringe
Type of injection: intradermal
Site: anterior or volar surface of forearm
Results: Pale wheal approximately 6–10 mm in diameter
If wheal does not develop, repeat test in opposite arm.

Correct interpretation of TST results
Read: 48–72 hours after placement by trained healthcare provider
Measure: induration (i.e., semi-firm to firm swelling) from left to right (i.e., perpendicular to long axis of arm)
Record: Chart all results (negative or positive). If no induration, indicate 0 mm.

PPD = purified protein derivative, TU = tuberculin unit

result can occur if the tuberculin skin testing is done near the time of administrating a live vaccine (i.e., measles, mumps, rubella, varicella, oral polio, yellow fever, oral typhoid, BCG, influenza nasal vaccine). Therefore, the skin testing should be done on either the same day as a live-virus vaccine is given or 4–6 weeks later; otherwise, the live vaccine can cause suppression of the TST response.[131]

There are only a few instances in which a TST should not be placed. The TST is contraindicated if a person has had an allergic or necrotic skin reaction from prior skin testing. A false-positive TST result can occur if the BCG vaccination was given recently or there was a cross-reaction with a nontuberculous mycobacterial infection.[131] However, receipt of the BCG vaccine is not a contraindication for testing.

The BCG vaccine is used only in countries with endemic TB.[131] The effectiveness of BCG ranges from 0% to 80%, and its protection diminishes over time. While the BCG vaccine does not consistently prevent pulmonary TB in most individuals, it does provide some protection from disseminated infection and meningitis in children.

Most individuals who received BCG vaccine in childhood will have a negative TST as adults; false positives are most common if the vaccine was given within the previous few months. A positive TST should be considered indicative of exposure to infection, regardless of whether the patient had been vaccinated with BCG.[135] A follow-up IGRA test can help determine if active infection is present.

Follow Up After Screening   Healthcare providers should ask about possible exposure to individuals with TB, even if screening is negative. A false-negative result may occur if exposure to TB occurred within the 2 weeks prior to placement of the TST or draw of an IGRA. In this situation, screening should be performed but also repeated later. The tubercle bacillus grows slowly over a period of 2 to 12 weeks.[131] Exposed individuals should be retested in 10 to 12 weeks to ensure adequate time has elapsed to detect an immune response if infection developed after exposure. If the follow-up test is also negative, the person does not have LTBI.

If screening is positive, the healthcare practitioner needs to rule out active TB. It is important to ask about symptoms related to active infection, as well as to obtain a chest x-ray. Chest x-ray results will be negative for individuals with latent infection; however, active infection is associated with distinctive chest x-ray findings. Upper lobe infiltrates and unilateral hilar node enlargement are highly specific for active TB.[135] Healed lesions appear as calcified parenchymal nodules, which may be associated with

Table 15-39 Criteria for Positive TST Result

Induration		
5 or more millimeters	**10 or more millimeters**	**15 or more millimeters**
HIV+	Foreign-born individuals native to high-prevalence areas, living in United States for less than 5 years	No known risk factors for TB
Recent close contact with an active TB patient	Injection drug users	
CXR with granulomatous changes consistent with history of TB	Residents and employees of high-risk settings	
Organ transplant patients or other immunosuppressed patients (receiving prednisone 15 mg/day or more for at least 1 month)	Microbacteriology laboratory personnel	
	Comorbid conditions such as diabetes mellitus, silicosis, end-stage renal disease, cancer, low body weight (less than 10% of ideal body weight)	
	Recipient of BCG vaccine	

BCG = bacillus Calmette–Guérin, CT = computed tomography, CXR = chest x-ray, HIV = human immunodeficiency virus, TB = tuberculosis.

Data from American Thoracic Society, Centers for Disease Control and Prevention. Diagnostic standards and classification of tuberculosis in adults and children. *Am J Respir Crit Care Med.* 2000;161(4):1376-1395; Centers for Disease Control and Prevention. Tuberculin skin testing. http://www.cdc.gov/tb/publications/factsheets/testing/skintesting.htm. May 11, 2016. Accessed May 2, 2016.

calcified hilar node enlargement. **Figure 15-10** depicts calcified nodules that can be seen with TB. All individuals with radiographic findings suggestive of TB require further evaluation. Follow-up testing with sputum microscopy with culture and sensitivity is currently the standard for diagnosing active TB.[133]

Management of Tuberculosis

Treatment of inactive disease is equally as important as treating active disease, because it is an important public health strategy to reduce the occurrence of TB disease in the United States. With successful treatment, the chance for conversion to active disease will significantly decrease and, with it, the chance of transmission to others.

Once the diagnosis of LTBI or active infection is confirmed and the risks and benefits of treatment are reviewed, appropriate treatment can begin. Many of the same medications are used in the treatment of latent and active infection. Active disease is treated more aggressively, requiring the use of multiple medications, higher

Figure 15-10 Calcified nodules in tuberculosis.

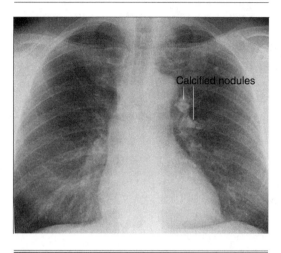

doses, and longer duration of treatment. Treatment for active disease must be continued until the affected individual is no longer infectious.

Latent Tuberculosis

Lifestyle   Because latent TB is not infectious, no changes need to be instituted to protect others from acquiring the infection. Encouraging general lifestyle practices that support the immune system should be part of the counseling given to individuals with latent infection.

Medication   The two most common medications used in the treatment of latent TB are isoniazid (INH) and rifampin. INH 300 mg once a day for 9 months is considered "first-line" treatment.[135] It is inexpensive and highly effective.[128] Six months of INH is acceptable for immunocompetent adults with new-onset latent TB; however, it is less effective than continuing treatment with INH for 9 months.[130] Rifampin is used for individuals intolerant or resistant to

INH. Practitioners need to be cautious of drug interactions with rifampin.[128] Rifampin reduces the effectiveness of oral contraceptives and some of the medications used in the treatment of HIV. Serious complications associated with its use include renal failure and interstitial nephritis. In addition, common side effects related to rifampin include, but are not limited to, headache, fatigue, pruritus, and a reddish-orange discoloration of body fluids. See **Table 15-40** regarding the current medications used to treat latent TB.

One of the major side effects from all the antituberculosis medications is hepatitis or hepatotoxicity. Hepatotoxicity is common with INH, which can range from mild elevations in transaminases to hepatic failure.[137] Other serious side effects are possible, including neuritis and blood dyscrasia (i.e., agranulocytosis, leukopenia, aplastic anemia, thrombocytopenia), seizures, optic neuritis, peripheral neuropathy, and paresthesias. Other common reactions to INH include GI complaints (i.e., nausea, vomiting, diarrhea, epigastric discomfort), dizziness, tinnitus, agitation, and rash.

If a person has a history of liver disease, alcohol overuse, or is currently using alcohol or other hepatotoxic agents (e.g., acetaminophen), then the person is more at risk for developing hepatotoxicity while on antituberculosis medications. The risk of hepatotoxicity also increases with age and is more likely to occur in individuals older than 35 years. A thorough clinical evaluation is needed to screen for other problems that may put the patient at risk for hepatic dysfunction. See **Table 15-41** for a list of conditions that place the patient at risk for hepatotoxicity while on antituberculosis medication.

Depending on the history and the antituberculosis medication under consideration, the following baseline and follow-up laboratory tests should be ordered: liver function tests (particularly aspartate aminotransferase [AST], alanine aminotransferase [ALT], bilirubin), complete blood count

Table 15-40 Medications Used to Treat Latent Tuberculosis

Medication	Dose	Duration	Comments
INH	300 mg	Daily for 6 to 9 months	HIV-negative: Treatment for 9 months is associated with higher effectiveness.
			HIV-positive: Need minimum of 9 months of treatment.
RIF	600 mg daily	4 months	Not first line; use as an alternative to INH; has better compliance but not tested as extensively as INH for 9 months.
			Used in patients with silicosis.
INH-RPT	INH 900 mg + RPT 900 mg weekly	3 months DOT	Not recommended for the following: HIV+ on antiretroviral treatment, pregnant (or expected pregnancy during treatment), or +INH/RIF resistance
INH, RIF	INH 300 mg + RIF 600 mg daily	3–4 months	Alternative for HIV+ patients
			Efficacy equal to INH for 6 months
INH, RIF	INH 900 mg + RIF 600 mg twice per week	3 months	Alternative for HIV+ patients

DOT = directly observed therapy, HIV = human immunodeficiency virus, INH = isoniazid, RIF = rifampin, RPT = rifapentine

Data from Centers for Disease Control and Prevention. The difference between latent TB infection and TB disease. http://www.cdc.gov/tb/publications/factsheets/general/LTBIandActiveTB.htm. 2014. Accessed April 20, 2016; Lobue P, Menzies D. Treatment of latent tuberculosis infection: an update. *Respirology.* 2010;15:603-622; LoBue P, Enarson DA, Thoen T. Tuberculosis in humans and its epidemiology, diagnosis and treatment in the United States. *Int J Tuberc Lung Dis.* 2010;14(10):1226-1232.

with platelet count (CBC/PLT), and kidney function tests (blood urea nitrogen [BUN] and creatinine [Cr]). If there is a risk of hepatitis or if there is an elevation of the AST/ALT, then hepatitis serologies (e.g., hepatitis A IgG/IgM, hepatitis B [i.e., HBsAg, HBsAb, HBcAb], and hepatitis C [i.e., HCV Ab]) may also be ordered to detect other possible causes of laboratory abnormalities and to detect conditions that may increase the likelihood of drug-induced hepatotoxicity.

During treatment, patients should receive monthly visits for a routine clinical assessment.[132] Baseline laboratory testing should be done, but the time intervals for follow-up laboratory testing depend on the medication and the patient's current health status. Monthly monitoring of liver function tests should be done for all patients who are pregnant or up to 3 months postpartum, have a history of liver disease (e.g., chronic hepatitis B or C, alcoholic hepatitis, cirrhosis), have a history of elevated liver function tests, drink alcohol regularly, are older than 35 years, or have other risks for liver disease. Otherwise, frequent laboratory tests are not necessary for the general population.[130,137]

If the patient has abnormal baseline liver function tests or if the patient develops symptoms while on treatment, strict follow up with clinical evaluation and laboratory testing is an absolute

Table 15-41 Risk Groups for Hepatotoxicity with Antituberculosis Medication

Age older than 35 years

Alcohol use/abuse

Cirrhosis

Hepatitis B or C

Hepatitis due to alcohol abuse

HIV-positive

Multiple medication use for other medical problems

Pregnant women

Postpartum period (less than 3 months)

Risk for chronic liver disease

necessity. Antituberculosis medication should be withheld if the transaminase levels are three times the upper limit of normal. In addition, consultation with an expert is necessary. Some specialists may recommend continued treatment as long as the patient remains asymptomatic, unless the transaminase levels exceed five times the upper limit of normal.[135] Frequency of follow-up testing depends on the patient's symptoms and the degree of abnormality of the test result (e.g., slightly abnormal vs. critical reading). If antituberculosis medications are discontinued, the signs and symptoms of hepatotoxicity will resolve.

Depending on whether the patient has any comorbidities, weekly to monthly visits are recommended to ensure tolerance to recommended therapy. Patients should be informed about the side effects associated with treatment and advised to stop their medication and return for reevaluation if symptoms occur.[135] The use of INH or pyrazinamide is contraindicated in patients with active hepatitis and end-stage liver disease.[135] If moderate to severe liver disease is present,

consultation with an infectious disease specialist, TB expert, or pulmonologist is recommended.

Not all women will want to comply with the treatment recommendations. While all patients with active disease require treatment, some with latent infection may decide against receiving prophylactic medication. They may not be willing or able to comply with medication regimes requiring daily long-term dosing or they may refuse because of the possible adverse effects. In this situation, a careful assessment of the risks is important. Patients at lower risk of progression, such as those who tested positive several years ago or who are at higher risk of developing hepatotoxicity may be less likely to benefit from prophylactic treatment.[129] Failure to complete the entire recommended course of treatment is associated with greater risk of developing drug resistance. Therefore, it may be better in some situations to defer or delay initiation of treatment for women who are unable to comply with treatment or who are at higher risk of treatment-associated complications.

Patient Instructions   Women must be educated about latent TB, their risk for developing active TB, treatment options, benefits related to the medication (e.g., cure of TB infection and prevention of active TB), risks associated with treatment, and major symptoms or side effects of the medication. If they develop symptoms of drug-induced hepatitis such as fever, jaundice, myalgia, excessive pruritus, fatigue, nausea, vomiting, loss of appetite, or abdominal pain, they should be instructed to discontinue the medication and contact their healthcare provider for further evaluation.

Management During Pregnancy and Lactation   Only high-risk individuals need to be tested in pregnancy. The decision to test should follow the same guidelines as for nonpregnant women.

Individuals who test positive usually require treatment in pregnancy to prevent transmission to the infant after birth. The risk of the infant developing infection in utero is low, but is associated with adverse outcomes. Mothers who develop active infection in pregnancy have double the risk of giving birth prematurely or delivering a growth-restricted infant than healthy women. Other complications associated with active infection include maternal hypertension and respiratory failure and fetal mortality.

In most cases, pregnancy or lactation should not delay initiation of therapy. Women with liver impairment, alcohol use, or chronic, heavy use of agents that can be hepatotoxic (e.g., acetaminophen) should not receive antituberculosis treatment during the antepartum period.[138] However, if women have risk factors for exposure or disease progression as outlined in Table 15-36, then the initiation of therapy should not be delayed on the basis of pregnancy, although strict laboratory and clinical monitoring is necessary.[135,139] Treatment of LTBI can be started as early as the first trimester in those at highest risk.[139] Regular visits are scheduled on a monthly to weekly basis during pregnancy. Incorporating the surveillance needed for those on TB prophylaxis into routine prenatal care makes follow up easier, because patients may be more compliant with appointments scheduled during pregnancy than in the postpartum period.[138]

INH for 9 months is the preferred medication for the treatment of LTBI in pregnant women.[135] Although rifampin is considered safe, there are insufficient data to support the use of rifampin in pregnancy. Some research has shown that INH and rifampin both cross the placenta, but teratogenic effects have not been reported.[139] Pyridoxine 25 to 50 mg is recommended to be given concurrently with INH to help prevent peripheral neuropathy, especially in individuals in whom the dietary intake of vitamin B6 is low (e.g.,

malnutrition, alcohol overuse, or pregnancy). Breastfeeding may be continued while on the antituberculosis agents (i.e., INH, rifampin).[139]

ACTIVE TUBERCULOSIS

The management of active TB should be overseen by an infectious disease expert. Consultation with public health experts is also needed in order to prevent transmission to others. However, primary care providers need to have a thorough understanding of the presentation and treatment of active disease.

Initially, individuals suspected or known to have active TB require the use of measures to prevent the spread of infection to others. These measures include having the patient wear a specially designed face mask when being transported within a medical facility, being evaluated or cared for in a healthcare facility only in negative-pressure rooms, and following standard respiratory precautions. Once the patient is hospitalized, samples will be collected and sent for an acid-fast bacilli (AFB) sputum smear and sputum culture.[131] If the sputum cultures are positive, the patient is treated for active TB and sputum cultures are collected monthly to monitor the effectiveness of treatment. If the sputum cultures remain positive after 4 months of treatment, medication noncompliance or malabsorption needs to be considered.[130] The Xpert MTB/RIF assay is another diagnostic test for active TB. It is currently being utilized in Europe as an effective and efficient method for identifying the *M. tuberculosis* complex, even in HIV-positive patients. This test is also being used to identify rifampin resistance. It is under review for utilization in the United States.[133]

Medications The transmission of TB can significantly decrease within days to weeks of initiating proper treatment.[130] The usual course of treatment includes the 4-drug combination of

INH, rifampin, ethambutol, and pyrazinamide for 2 months; then INH and rifampin are continued for an additional 4 months.[128] If the patient remains smear positive at 2 months, treatment should be extended for 6 to 9 months. Any type of extrapulmonary TB requires treatment for longer than 6 months.[128]

Multidrug-resistant tuberculosis (MDR-TB) is present if active TB is not responding favorably to INH and rifampin. In 2011, there were approximately 310,000 cases of MDR-TB.[133] MDR-TB can result from inappropriate treatment such as when active TB is inadvertently treated as latent TB, when aggressive treatment with new agents is not initiated in individuals with treatment failure, or when treatment is stopped earlier than recommended.[131-133] Consultation with an infectious disease expert is mandatory in these situations. Treatment of MDR-TB includes adding second-line medications to the regimen—usually for a minimum of 18 to 24 months. Unfortunately,

second-line treatment is less tolerable. Resistance is also possible. A fluoroquinolone can be added; however, if the organism(s) are also resistant to any fluoroquinolone and at least one second-line injectable drug (amikacin, kanamycin, capreomycin), the term extensively drug-resistant tuberculosis (XDR-TB) is given. XDR-TB has a significant mortality rate; the cure rate is as low as 30% to 40%.[130]

Patient Instructions Given the danger of spreading infection to others and the risk of developing multidrug resistance to available medications, it is essential that individuals with active TB understand the importance of adhering to their medication regimen. Some individuals may benefit from directly observed therapy.

Management During Pregnancy and Lactation Active TB in pregnancy should be managed by a team of physicians skilled in the management of high-risk pregnancy and TB.

References

1. Porth CM. *Pathophysiology: Concepts of Altered Health States*. 6th ed. Philadelphia, PA: Williams & Wilkins; 2002.
2. Pratter MR. Chronic upper airway cough syndrome secondary to rhinosinus diseases (previously referred to as postnasal drip syndrome): ACCP evidence-based clinical practice guidelines. *Chest.* 2006;129(Suppl 1):63S-671S.
3. Greiner AN, Hellings PW, Rotiroti G, Scadding GK. Allergic rhinitis. *Lancet.* 2011;378(9809):2112-2122.
4. Bousquet J, Khaltaev N, Cruz AA, Denburg J, Fokkens WJ, Togias A, et al. Allergic rhinitis and its impact on asthma (ARIA) 2008. *Allergy.* 2008;63:8-160.
5. Dalal S, Zhukovsky, D. Pathophysiology and management of fever. *J Support Oncol.* 2006;4:9-16.
6. Bloch KC. Infectious diseases. In: Ganong WF, ed. *Pathophysiology of Disease.* New York, NY: Lange/McGraw-Hill; 2003.
7. Canning BJ, Chang AB, Bolser DC, Smith JA, Mazzone SB, McGarvey L. Anatomy and neurophysiology of cough: CHEST Guideline and Expert Panel Report. *CHEST J.* 2014;146(6):1633-1648.
8. De Blasio F, Virchow JC, Polverino M, Zanasi A, Behrakis PK, Kilinç G, et al. Cough management: a practical approach. *Cough.* 2011;7(7):1-12.
9. Sylvester DC, Karkos PD, Vaughan C, Johnston J, Dwivedi R, Atkinson H, et al. Chronic cough, reflux, postnasal drip syndrome, and the otolaryngologist. *Int J Otolaryngol.* 2012;2012:5.
10. Hegewald MJ, Crapo RO. Respiratory physiology in pregnancy. *Clin Chest Med.* 2011;32(1):1-13.
11. Robinson DP, Klein SL. Pregnancy and pregnancy-associated hormones alter immune responses and disease pathogenesis. *Horm Behav.* 2012;62(3):263-271.
12. Fendrick AM. Viral respiratory infections due to rhinoviruses: current knowledge, new developments. *Am J Ther.* 2003;10(3):193-202.
13. Grief SN. Upper respiratory infections. *Prim Care.* 2013;40(3):757-770.
14. Fashner J, Ericson K, Werner S. Treatment of the common cold in children and adults. *Am Fam Physician.* 2012;86(2):153-159.
15. Albalawi Z, Othman S, Alfaleh K. Intranasal ipratropium bromide for the common cold. *Cochrane Database Syst Rev.* 2011;(7):CD008231.

16. Hemilä H, Chalker E. Vitamin C for preventing and treating the common cold. *Cochrane Database Syst Rev.* 2013;1:CD000980.
17. Singh M, Das RR. Zinc for the common cold. *Cochrane Database Syst Rev.* 2013;(2):CD001364 .
18. Lissiman E, Bhasale A, Cohen M. Garlic for the common cold. *Cochrane Database Syst Rev.* 2014;11:CD006206.
19. Nahas R, Balla A. Complementary and alternative medicine for prevention and treatment of the common cold. *Can Fam Physician.* 2011;57(1):31-36.
20. Poolsup N, Suthisisang C, Prathanturarug S, Asawamekin A, Chanchareon U. Andrographis paniculata in the symptomatic treatment of uncomplicated upper respiratory tract infection: systematic review of randomized controlled trials. *J Clin Pharm Ther.* 2004;29(1):37-45.
21. Saxena R, Singh R, Kumar P, Yadav SC, Negi MP, Saxena VS, et al. A randomized double blind placebo controlled clinical evaluation of extract of Andrographis paniculata (KalmCold) in patients with uncomplicated upper respiratory tract infection. *Phytomedicine.* 2010;17(3-4):178-185.
22. US Department of Health & Human Services. Pandemic flu history. Available at: http://www.flu.gov/pandemic/history/. Accessed April 20, 2016.
23. Bresee J, Hayden F. Epidemic influenza—responding to the expected but unpredictable. *N Engl J Med.* 2013;368(7):589-592.
24. Centers for Disease Control and Prevention. Weekly U.S. Influenza Surveillance Report. Available at: http://www.cdc.gov/flu/weekly. Accessed April 20, 2016.
25. Erlikh IV, Abraham S, Kondamudi VK. Management of influenza. *Am Fam Physician.* 2010;82(9):1087-1095.
26. Babin S, Hsieh Y, Rothman R, Gaydos C. A meta-analysis of point-of-care laboratory tests in the diagnosis of novel 2009 swine-lineage pandemic influenza A (H1N1). *Diagn Microbiol Infect Dis.* 2012:1-14.
27. Harper SA, Bradley JS, Englund JA, File TM, Gravenstein S, Hayden FG, et al. Seasonal influenza in adults and children—diagnosis, treatment, chemoprophylaxis, and institutional outbreak management: clinical practice guidelines of the Infectious Diseases Society of America. *Clin Infect Dis.* 2009;48(8):1003-1032.
28. Chartrand C, Leeflang M, Minion J, Brewer T, Pai M. Accuracy of rapid influenza diagnostic testing: a meta-analysis. *Ann Intern Med.* 2012;156(7):500-508.
29. Centers for Disease Control and Prevention. Influenza. In: Atkinson W, Wolfe S, Hamborsky J, eds. *Epidemiology and Prevention of Vaccine-Preventable Diseases.* 12th ed. Washington, DC: Public Health Foundation; 2012.
30. Fiore AE, Fry A, Shay D, Gubareva L, Bresee JS, Uyeki TM. Antiviral agents for the treatment and chemoprophylaxis of influenza: recommendations of the Advisory Committee on Immunization Practices (ACIP). *MMWR.* 2011;60(RR01):1-24.
31. Joseph C, Togawa Y, Shindo N. Bacterial and viral infections associated with influenza. *Influenza Other Respir Viruses.* 2013;7(Suppl 2):105-113.
32. Mathie R, Frye J, Fisher P. Homeopathic Oscillococcinum* for preventing and treating influenza and influenza-like illness. *Cochrane Database Syst Rev.* 2015;12:CD001957.
33. Zhao P, Yang H-z, Lv H-y, Wei Z-m. Efficacy of Lianhuaqingwen capsule compared with oseltamivir for influenza A virus infection: a meta-analysis of randomized, controlled trials. *Alt Ther.* 2014;20(2):25-30.
34. Walker D, Ball S, Black R, Izrael D, Ding H, Euler G. Influenza vaccination coverage among pregnant women—United States, 2010-2011 influenza season. *MMWR.* 2011;60(32):1078-1082.
35. Centers for Disease Control and Prevention. Recommendations for obstetric health care providers related to use of antiviral medications in the treatment and prevention of influenza. 2014. Available at: http://www.cdc.gov/flu/professionals/antivirals/avrec_ob.htm. Accessed April 20, 2016.
36. Bender M, Bernheisel C. Fever, cough, and hypoxia in a pregnant woman. *J Fam Pract.* 2010;59(4):E9-E11.
37. Tanaka T, Nakajima K, Murashima A, Garcia-Bournissen F, Koren G, Ito S. Safety of neuraminidase inhibitors against novel influenza A (H1N1) in pregnant and breastfeeding women. *Can Med Assoc J.* 2009;181(1-2):55-58.
38. Centers for Disease Control and Prevention. Leading causes of death. 2015. Available at: http://www.cdc.gov/nchs/fastats/leading-causes-of-death.htm. Accessed April 20, 2016.
39. Moran GJ, Rothman RE, Volturo GA. Emergency management of community-acquired bacterial pneumonia: what is new since the 2007 Infectious Diseases Society of America/American Thoracic Society guidelines. *Am J Emerg Med.* 2013;31(3):602-612.
40. Watkins R, Lemonovich T. Diagnosis and management of community-acquired pneumonia in adults. *Am Fam Physician.* 2011;83(11):1299-1306.
41. Musher DM, Thorner AR. Community-acquired pneumonia. *N Engl J Med.* 2014;371(17):1619-1628.
42. Butt S, Swiatlo E. Treatment of community-acquired pneumonia in an ambulatory setting. *Am J Med.* 2011;124:297-300.

43. Graves C. Pneumonia in pregnancy. *Clin Obstet Gynecol.* 2010;53(2):329-336.

44. Crouch M, Lumon L, Cassano A. Clinical relevance and management of drug-related QT interval prolongation. *Pharmacotherapy.* 2003;23(7):881-908.

45. Medication-induced QT interval prolongation and Torsades de Pointes. *US Pharm.* 2011;36(2):H5-2-8.

46. Mumoli N, Cei M. Community-acquired pneumonia. *CMAJ.* 2012;184(5):560.

47. Mandell LA, Wunderink RG, Anzueto A, Bartlett JG, Campbell GD, Dean NC, et al. Infectious Diseases Society of America/American Thoracic Society consensus guidelines on the management of community-acquired pneumonia in adults. *Clin Infect Dis.* 2007;44:S27-S72.

48. Musher D. New modalities in treating pneumococcal pneumonia. *Hosp Pract.* 2011;39(2):89-96.

49. Corrales-Medina V, Musher D, Shachkina S, Chirinos J. Acute pneumonia and the cardiovascular system. *Lancet.* 2013;381:496-505.

50. Sheffield JS, Cunningham FG. Community-acquired pneumonia in pregnancy. *Obstet Gynecol.* 2009;114(4):915-922.

51. Ozdoganoglu T, Songu M. The burden of allergic rhinitis and asthma. *Ther Adv Respir Dis.* 2012; 6(1):11-23.

52. Jacobsen L, Niggemann B, Dreborg S, Ferdousi HA, Halken S, Høst A, et al. Specific immunotherapy has long-term preventive effect of seasonal and perennial asthma: 10-year follow-up on the PAT study. *Allergy.* 2007;62:943-948.

53. Blaiss MS. Allergic rhinitis: direct and indirect costs. *Allergy Asthma Proc.* 2010;31(5):375-380.

54. Dykewicz MS, Hamilos DL. Rhinitis and sinusitis. *J Allergy Clin Immunol.* 2010;125(2, Suppl 2):S103-S115.

55. Bousquet J, Heinzerling L, Bachert C, Papadopoulos NG, Bousquet PJ, Burney PG, et al. Practical guide to skin prick tests in allergy to aeroallergens. *Allergy.* 2012;67(1):18-24.

56. Bousquet J, van Cauwenberge P, Khaltaev N, Organization WH. Allergic rhinitis and its impact on asthma. In collaboration with the World Health Organization. Executive summary of the workshop report. 7-10 December 1999, Geneva, Switzerland. *Allergy.* 2002;57(9):841-855.

57. Brożek JL, Bousquet J, Baena-Cagnani CE, Bonini S, Canonica GW, Casale TB, et al. Allergic rhinitis and its impact on asthma (ARIA) guidelines: 2010 revision. *J Allergy Clin Immunol.* 2010;126(3):466-476.

58. Wheatley LM, Togias A. Allergic rhinitis. *N Engl J Med.* 2015;372(5):456-463.

59. Peden D, Reed CE. Environmental and occupational allergies. *J Allergy Clin Immunol.* 2010;125(2, Suppl 2):S150-S160.

60. Custovic A, Simpson A, Chapman M, Woodcock A. Allergen avoidance in the treatment of asthma and atopic disorders. *Thorax.* 1998;53(1):63-72.

61. Hamilos DL. Chronic rhinosinusitis: Epidemiology and medical management. *J Allergy Clin Immunol.* 2011;128:693-707.

62. Brożek JL, Bousquet J, Baena-Cagnani CE, Bonini S, Canonica GW, Casale TB, et al. Allergic rhinitis and its impact on asthma (ARIA) guidelines: 2010 revision. *J Allergy Clin Immunol.* 2010;126(3):466-476.

63. Burks AW, Calderon MA, Casale T, Cox L, Demoly P, Jutel M, et al. Update on allergy immunotherapy: American Academy of Allergy, Asthma & Immunology/European Academy of Allergy and Clinical Immunology/PRACTALL consensus report. *J Allergy Clin Immunol.* 2013;131(5):1288-1296.e3.

64. Namazy JA, Schatz M. Asthma and rhinitis during pregnancy. *Mt Sinai J Med.* 2011;78(5):661-670.

65. National Heart Lung and Blood Institute, National Asthma Education and Prevention Program. Expert Panel Report 3: Guidelines for the Diagnosis and Management of Asthma. online 2007. Available at: http://www.nhlbi.nih.gov/guidelines/asthma/asthgdln.htm. Accessed April 20, 2016.

66. Sato K. Treatment of allergic rhinitis during pregnancy. *Clin Exp Allergy Rev.* 2012;12(1):31-36.

67. National Asthma Education and Prevention Program. Working Group Report on Managing Asthma During Pregnancy: Recommendations for Pharmacologic Treatment, Update 2004. Available at: https://www.nhlbi.nih.gov/files/docs/resources/lung/astpreg_full.pdf. Accessed April 20, 2016.

68. Yau W-P, Mitchell AA, Lin KJ, Werler MM, Hernández-Díaz S. Use of decongestants during pregnancy and the risk of birth defects. *Am J Epidemiol.* 2013;178(2):198-208.

69. Crespo J, Rodriquez J. Food allergy in adulthood. *Allergy.* 2003;58(2):98-113.

70. Arnold J, Williams PM. Anaphylaxis: recognition and management. *Am Fam Physician.* 2011;84(10):1111-1118.

71. Usatine R, Riojas M. Diagnosis and management of contact dermatitis. *Am Fam Physician.* 2010;82(3):249-255.

72. Tang A. A practical guide to anaphylaxis. *Am Fam Physician.* 2003;68(7):1325-1332.

73. Belsito D. The diagnostic evaluation, treatment, and prevention of allergic contact dermatitis in the new millennium. *J Allergy Clin Immunol.* 2000;105(3):409-420.

74. Aring A, Chan M. Acute rhinosinusitis in adults. *Am Fam Physician.* 2011;83(9):1057-1063.

75. Meltzer EO, Hamilos DL. Rhinosinusitis diagnosis and management for the clinician: a synopsis of recent consensus guidelines. *Mayo Clin Proc.* 2011;86(5):427-443.

76. DeCastro A, Mims L, Hueston WJ. Rhinosinusitis. *Prim Care.* 2014;41(1):47-61.

77. Lemiengre M, van Driel M, Merenstein D, Young J, De Sutter AI. Antibiotics for clinically diagnosed acute rhinosinusitis in adults. *Cochrane Database Syst Rev.* 2012;10:CD006089.

78. Brook I. Microbiology of sinusitis. *Proc Am Thorac Soc.* 2011;8(1):90-100.

79. Hickner JM, Bartlett JG, Besser RE, Gonzales R, Hoffman JR, Sande MA. Principles of appropriate antibiotic use for acute rhinosinusitis in adults: background. *Ann Intern Med.* 2001;134(6):498-505.

80. Chow A, Benninger M, Brook I, Brozek JL, Goldstein EJ, Hicks LA, et al. IDSA clinical practice guideline for acute bacterial rhinosinusitis in children and adults. *Clin Infect Dis.* 2012;54(8):1-67.

81. Mandal R, Patel N, Ferguson BJ. Role of antibiotics in sinusitis. *Curr Opin Infect Dis.* 2012;25:183-192.

82. Soler Z, Mace J, Litvack J, Smith T. Chronic rhinosinusitis, race, and ethnicity. *Am J Rhinol Allergy.* 2012;26:110-116.

83. Helms S, Miller A. Natural treatment of chronic rhinosinusitis. *Altern Med Rev.* 2006;11(3):196-207.

84. Asher BF, Seidman M, Snyderman C. Complementary and alternative medicine in otolaryngology. *Laryngoscope.* 2001;111:1383-1389.

85. Albert R. Diagnosis and treatment of acute bronchitis. *Am Fam Physician.* 2010;82(11):1345-1350.

86. Braman SS. Chronic cough due to acute bronchitis: ACCP evidence-based clinical practice guidelines. *CHEST J.* 2006;129(Suppl 1):95S-103S.

87. Blackwell D, Lucas J, Clarke T. Summary health statistics for U.S. adults: National Health Interview Survey, 2012. National Center for Health Statistics. *Vital Health Stat.* 2014;10(260). Available at: http://www.cdc.gov/nchs/data/series/sr_10/sr10_260.pdf. Accessed April 20, 2016.

88. Moorman JE, Zahran H, Truman BI, Molla MT. Current asthma prevalence—United States, 2006–2008. *MMWR.* 2011;60:84-6. Available at: http://www.cdc.gov/mmwr/preview/mmwrhtml/su6001a18.htm. Accessed April 20, 2016.

89. Barnett SBL, Nurmagambetov TA. Costs of asthma in the United States: 2002-2007. *J Allergy Clin Immunol.* 2011;127(1):145-152.

90. National Asthma Education and Prevention Program. Expert Panel 2: Guidelines for the diagnosis and management of asthma. Report No.: NIH Publication No. 97–4051. Bethesda, MD: National Institutes of Health; 1997.

91. Durrani SR, Viswanathan RK, Busse WW. What effect does asthma treatment have on airway remodeling? Current perspectives. *J Allergy Clin Immunol.* 2011;128(3):439-448.

92. National Heart Lung and Blood Institute. Asthma care: Quick reference: Diagnosing and Managing Asthma. 2012. Available at: http://www.nhlbi.nih.gov/files/docs/guidelines/asthma_qrg.pdf. Accessed April 20, 2016.

93. National Asthma Education and Prevention Program. Expert Panel Report: Guidelines for the diagnosis and management of asthma. Report No.: NIH Publication number 91-3642. Bethesda, MD: National Institutes of Health; 1991.

94. National Asthma Education and Prevention Program. Guidelines for the diagnosis and management of asthma update on selected topics 2002. Report No.: NIH Publication No. 02-5074. Bethesda, MD: National Institutes of Health; 2003.

95. Zeiger RS, Yegin A, Simons FER, Haselkorn T, Rasouliyan L, Szefler SJ, et al. Evaluation of the National Heart, Lung, and Blood Institute guidelines impairment domain for classifying asthma control and predicting asthma exacerbations. *Ann Allergy Asthma Immunol.* 2012;108(2):81-7.e3.

96. Dick S, Doust E, Cowie H, Ayres JG, Turner S. Associations between environmental exposures and asthma control and exacerbations in young children: a systematic review. *BMJ Open.* 2014;4(2):e003827.

97. Turpeinen M, Pelkonen AS, Nikander K, Sorva R, Selroos O, Juntunen-Backman K, et al. Bone mineral density in children treated with daily or periodical inhaled budesonide: the Helsinki Early Intervention Childhood Asthma Study. *Pediatr Res.* 2010;68(2):169-173.

98. Dam T, Harrison S, Fink HA, Ramsdell J, Barrett-Connor E. Bone mineral density and fractures in older men with chronic obstructive pulmonary disease or asthma. *Osteoporos Int.* 2010;21(8):1341-1349.

99. Leib ES, Saag KG, Adachi JD, Geusens PP, Binkley N, McCloskey EV, et al. Official positions for FRAX® clinical regarding glucocorticoids: the impact of the use of glucocorticoids on the estimate by FRAX® of the 10 year risk of fracture: from joint official positions development conference of the International Society for Clinical Densitometry and International Osteoporosis Foundation on FRAX®. *J Clin Densitom.* 2011;14(3):212-219.

100. Park H-W, Tantisira KG, Weiss ST. Pharmacogenomics in asthma therapy: where are we and

where do we go? *Annu Rev Pharmacol Toxicol.* 2015;55(1):129-147.

101. Ducharme F. Inhaled glucocorticoids versus leukotriene receptor antagonists as single agent asthma treatment: systematic review of the current evidence. *BMJ.* 2003;326(7390):621.

102. Chung KF. Managing severe asthma in adults: lessons from the ERS/ATS guidelines. *Curr Opin Pulm Med.* 2015;21(1):8-15.

103. Brunetti L, Poiani G, Dhanaliwala F, Poppiti K, Kang H, Suh DC. Clinical outcomes and treatment cost comparison of levalbuterol versus albuterol in hospitalized adults with chronic obstructive pulmonary disease or asthma. *Am J Health Syst Pharm.* 2015;72(12):1026-1035.

104. National Heart Lung and Blood Institute. Asthma care: Quick reference: Diagnosing and Managing Asthma. 2012. Available at: http://www.nhlbi.nih.gov/files/docs/guidelines/asthma_qrg.pdf. Accessed April 20, 2016.

105. Cochrane M, Bala M, Downs K, Mauskopf J, Ben-Joseph R. Inhaled corticosteroids for asthma therapy: patient compliance, devices, and inhalation technique. *Chest.* 2000;117(2):542-550.

106. Parsons JP. Exercise-induced bronchoconstriction. *Otolaryngol Clin North Am.* 2014;47(1):119-126.

107. McCallister J. Asthma in pregnancy: management strategies. *Curr Opin Pulm Med.* 2013;19(1):13-17.

108. Rocklin RE. Asthma, asthma medications and their effects on maternal/fetal outcomes during pregnancy. *Reprod Toxicol.* 2011;32(2):189-197.

109. Bracken M, Triche E, Belanger K, Saftlas A, Beckett W, Leaderer B. Asthma symptoms, severity, and drug therapy: a prospective study of effects on 2205 pregnancies. *Obstet Gynecol.* 2003;102(4):739-752.

110. Cydulka R, Emerman C, Schreiber D, Molander K, Woodruff P, Camargo CJ. Acute asthma among pregnant women presenting to the emergency department. *Am J Respir Crit Care Med.* 1999;160(3):887-892.

111. Bonner S, Zimmerman B, Evans D, Irigoyen M, Resnick D, Mellins R. An individualized intervention to improve asthma management among urban Latino and African American families. *J Asthma.* 2002;39(2):167-179.

112. George M, Topaz M. A systematic review of complementary and alternative medicine for asthma self-management. *Nurs Clin North Am.* 2013;48(1):10.

113. Clark C, Arnold E, Lasserson T, Wu T. Herbal interventions for chronic asthma in adults and children:

a systematic review and meta-analysis. *Prim Care Respir J.* 2010;19(4):307-314.

114. Engler RJM, With CM, Gregory PJ, Jellin JM. Complementary and alternative medicine for the allergist-immunologist: where do I start? *J Allergy Clin Immunol.* 2009;123(2):309-16.e4.

115. Silvers WS, Bailey HK. Integrative approach to allergy and asthma using complementary and alternative medicine. *Ann Allergy Asthma Immunol.* 2014;112(4):280-285.

116. Vestbo J, Hurd SS, Agustí AG, Jones PW, Vogelmeier C, Anzueto A, et al. Global strategy for the diagnosis, management, and prevention of chronic obstructive pulmonary disease. *Am J Respir Crit Care Med.* 2013;187(4):347-365.

117. Albertson T, Louie S, Chan A. The diagnosis and treatment of elderly patients with acute exacerbation of chronic obstructive pulmonary disease and chronic bronchitis. *J Am Geriatr Soc.* 2010;58:570-579.

118. Wise R. *Chronic Obstructive Pulmonary Disease. The Merck Manual for Health Care Professionals.* Whitehouse Station, NJ: Merck Sharp & Dohme Corp; 2012.

119. Diaz-Guzman E, Mannino DM. Epidemiology and prevalence of chronic obstructive pulmonary disease. *Clin Chest Med.* 2014;35(1):7-16.

120. Sethi S. Antibiotics in acute exacerbations of chronic bronchitis. *Expert Rev Anti-Infect Ther.* 2010;8(4):405-417.

121. Akgun K, Crothers K, Pisani M. Epidemiology and management of common pulmonary diseases in older persons. *J Gerontol A Biol Sci Med Sci.* 2012;67A(3):276-291.

122. Stenton C. The MRC breathlessness scale. *Occup Med.* 2008;58(3):226-227.

123. Gotfried M, Grossman R. Short-course fluoroquinolones in acute exacerbations of chronic bronchitis. *Expert Rev Respir Med.* 2010;4(5):661-672.

124. Hui D, Ling T, Chang S, Liao C, Yoo C, Kim D, et al. A multicentre surveillance study on the characteristics, bacterial aetiologies and in vitro antibiotic susceptibilities in patients with acute exacerbations of chronic bronchitis. *Respirology.* 2011;16(7):532-539.

125. Centers for Disease Control and Prevention. Reported Tuberculosis in the United States 2011. Atlanta, GA: U.S. Department of Health and Human Services, Centers for Disease Control and Prevention; 2012. Available at: http://www.cdc.gov/tb/statistics/reports/2011/pdf/report2011.pdf. Accessed April 20, 2016.

126. Centers for Disease Control and Prevention. The difference between latent TB infection and TB disease. 2012. Available at: http://www.cdc.gov/tb/publications/factsheets/general/LTBIandActiveTB.htm. Accessed April 20, 2016.

127. Aspler A, Long R, Trajman A, Dion M, Khan K, Schwartzman K, et al. Impact of treatment completion, intolerance and adverse events on health system costs in a randomized trial of 4 months rifampin or 9 months isoniazid for latent TB. *Thorax*. 2010;65:582-587.

128. Gordin F, Masur H. Current approaches to tuberculosis in the United States. *JAMA*. 2012;308(3):283-289.

129. Lobue P, Menzies D. Treatment of latent tuberculosis infection: an update. *Respirology*. 2010;15:603-622.

130. LoBue P, Enarson DA, Thoen T. Tuberculosis in humans and its epidemiology, diagnosis and treatment in the United States. *Int J Tuberc Lung Dis*. 2010;14(10):1226-1232.

131. American Thoracic Society, Centers for Disease Control and Prevention. Diagnostic standards and classification of tuberculosis in adults and children. *Am J Respir Crit Care Med*. 2000;161(4):1376-1395.

132. Jereb J, Goldberg S, Powell K, Villarino E, LoBue P. Recommendations for use of an isoniazid-rifapentine regimen with direct observation to treat latent *Mycobacterium tuberculosis* infection. *MMWR*. 2011;60(48):1650-1670.

133. Zumla A, Raviglione M, Hafner R, Fordham von Reyn C. Current concepts: tuberculosis. *N Engl J Med*. 2013;368:745-755.

134. Horsburgh CR, Rubin EJ. Latent tuberculosis infection in the United States. *N Engl J Med*. 2011;364(15):1441-1448.

135. American Thoracic Society, Centers for Disease Control and Prevention. Targeted tuberculin testing and treatment of latent tuberculosis infection. *Am J Respir Crit Care Med*. 2000;161(4):s221-s247.

136. Mazurek GH, Jereb J, Vernon A, LoBue P, Goldberg S, Castro K. Updated guidelines for using interferon gamma release assays to detect *Mycobacterium tuberculosis* infection—United States, 2010. *MMWR*. 2010;59(RR05):1-25.

137. Haroon M, Martin U, Devlin J. High incidence of intolerance to tuberculosis chemoprophylaxis. *Rheumatol Int*. 2010;32:33-37.

138. Boggess KA, Myers ER, Hamilton CD. Antepartum and postpartum isoniazid treatment of latent tuberculosis infection. *Obstet Gynecol*. 2000;96(5):757-762.

139. American Thoracic Society, Centers for Disease Control and Prevention. Treatment of tuberculosis. *MMWR*. 2003;52(RR 11):1-77.

CHAPTER 16

CARDIOVASCULAR HEALTH

Carolynn Bruno | Barbara K. Hackley

Cardiovascular disease (CVD) is the leading killer of women in the United States, accounting for 1 out of 4 deaths.[1] The rates of CVD-associated death are similar for black and white women.[1] The underlying causes of CVD begin early; lifestyle practices such as smoking, lack of exercise, and unhealthy diet choices increase one's risk of hypertension later in life. Increasing rates of obesity in children and adolescents have led to the development of cardiovascular problems at ever-earlier ages. While the full impact of CVD is not felt until women are in their 50s or later, risk factors in younger women need to be addressed to prevent progression to overt disease. Women's health providers must both be attuned to risks and actively promote healthy behaviors in all women and detect disease at the earliest possible stage. This chapter discusses how to evaluate signs and symptoms suggestive of cardiac disease, as well as how to recognize and manage common cardiovascular conditions in women such as hypertension, dyslipidemia, and thromboembolic disorders.

Clinical Presentation

CVD is known as a silent killer because symptoms do not manifest until the disease is well advanced. Myocardial infarction (MI) is one example. Women often experience symptoms that are not widely recognized as indicating an evolving MI. Symptoms more commonly reported by women than men include rapid onset of fatigue, poor sleep, shortness of breath, indigestion, body aches, and generally feeling unwell. Symptoms reported by both sexes include sensations of dizziness; pounding heart; change in heart rhythm; cold sweats; and pain, pressure, squeezing, or stabbing chest pain that may radiate to the neck, shoulder, back, arm, or jaw.[2] *Chest pain* is less common in women than in men, but still occurs in a significant percentage of women. In an observational study from the National Registry of Myocardial Infarction of more than 1 million patients, 42.0% of women reported no chest pain at hospitalization for MI compared to 30.7% of men.[3] As women age, symptoms of MI are increasingly likely to be composed of classic *angina* symptoms: heavy, gripping substernal chest pain that lasts a few minutes is provoked by stress or physical activity and is relieved with rest.[4] While chest pain should always prompt a clinician to investigate the possibility of the presence of an impending or acute MI, an astute clinician should also consider a range of other possibilities including gastrointestinal (GI), respiratory, hepatobiliary, or pleural/pericardial etiologies, as well as CVD. The presentation of these conditions may include chest pain along with other generally more prominent symptoms (**Table 16-1**).

Other symptoms such as dizziness, irregular heart rate, or palpitations may be indicative of an underlying cardiac condition. Dizziness is a nonspecific symptom commonly seen with orthostatic hypotension or emotional upset and may be associated with conditions of the ear or brain. It can be also reported by women experiencing arrhythmias or acute cardiac disease. Similarly, sensations of having an irregular heart rate or palpitations can also be due to a range of conditions including, but not limited to, an underlying cardiac condition (**Table 16-2**). One case series found that *palpitations* were identified as being cardiac in origin in 43% of cases. Other underlying causes of palpitations were anxiety or panic attack (31%), illicit or prescriptive drugs (6%), noncardiac causes (4%), and in 16% of the cases, no underlying etiology could be identified.[5] See the sections that follow for a fuller description of the workup of these symptoms.

Table 16-1 Differential Diagnosis of Chest Pain

System	Condition	Presenting Symptoms
Cardiovascular	Angina	Pain, pressure, or squeezing sensation spreading to arm, shoulder, jaw, or back.
	Myocardial infarction	Severe angina, shortness of breath, nausea, sweating, weakness
	Mitral valve prolapse	Palpitations, dizziness
	Aortic artery dissection	Often silent, sudden severe pain; tearing or ripping sensation during rupture
Respiratory	Pneumonia	Fever, chills, cough
	Pulmonary embolism	Shortness of breath, difficulty breathing, increased heart rate
	Asthma	Chest pain (rare symptom); wheezing, cough
Gastrointestinal	GERD	Heartburn, brash
Musculoskeletal	Costochondritis or muscle sprain	Pain elicited on palpation of affected area
Mental health	Anxiety	Variable complaints, including sharp, stabbing or persistent pain, muscle spasm, numbness

GERD = gastroesophageal reflux disease

Table 16-2 Differential Diagnoses for Palpitations

Disease	Examples	Associated Signs or Symptoms
Arrhythmia	Atrial fibrillation	Rapid, irregular rhythm
	Block or sinus node dysfunction	
	Sick sinus syndrome	
	Premature ventricular contractions	Pounding palpitations when resting, a sensation of skipped beats, can't catch breath
	Sinus tachycardia or arrhythmia	
	Supraventricular tachycardia	Syncope; rapid, regular pounding in neck
Emotional	Anxiety/panic	Associated with stress
Drugs	Alcohol	
	Caffeine	
	Cocaine	
	Tobacco	
	Beta-agonists	
	Theophylline	
Cardiac	AV septal defect	
	Cardiomyopathy	
	Congestive heart failure	
	Mitral value prolapse	Midsystolic click
Other	Anemia	
	Electrolyte imbalance	
	Fever	
	Hyperthyroidism	Nervousness, heat intolerance
	Hypovolemia	
	Hypoglycemia	

Essential History, Physical, and Laboratory Findings

A thorough history, physical, and laboratory assessment are needed to identify subclinical or overt disease. Identification of risk factors in well individuals and frank disease at its earliest stages allows time to intervene early enough to prevent end-organ damage.

History

In reviewing the history, key questions should focus on identifying risk factors such as unhealthy dietary intake, sedentary lifestyle, smoking, and being overweight or obese. Of all the modifiable risk factors, body mass index (BMI) poses the greatest risk for developing hypertension: Women with a BMI $\geq$ 30 kg/m^2 have a 4-fold, and those with a BMI $\geq$ 35 kg/m^2 have a 6-fold, increase in the risk of hypertension compared to normal-weight women.[6] These weight patterns are common, affecting 36.3% and 18.3% of women $\geq$ 20 years of age, respectively.[7] In addition, other risk factors specific to women increase the risk of developing CVD. These risks include menstrual irregularity due to polycystic ovarian syndrome (PCOS), history of preeclampsia, and age at menopause.[6] Women with PCOS are at higher risk for metabolic syndrome and diabetes, which puts them at risk for cardiovascular heart disease (CHD) in later years.[8] Women who experience early menopause lose the protection afforded by endogenous estrogen to the cardiac system and are at greater risk for more extensive atherosclerosis.[6] Other risk factors include having a family history of hypertension, CVD, or coagulopathies.

Pertinent personal history includes trends over time in weight, exercise level, and blood pressure (BP) readings, as well as whether the woman already has documented hypertension, CVD, diabetes, or renal disease. If a woman reports having varicose veins, then further inquiries are needed including age of onset; history of leg trauma, deep vein thrombosis (DVT), or lower extremity surgery; and prior pregnancies. Other women may report symptoms such as chest pain or palpitations that require an exploration of precipitating factors and a detailed description of symptom episodes.

Physical

A comprehensive physical examination is required when evaluating women with potential or overt CVD. The emphasis in the exam varies with the specific etiologies under consideration, but needs to be comprehensive enough to pinpoint underlying problem(s) and to detect sequelae of undetected or uncontrolled disease. All women should have BP, pulse rate, respiratory rate, BMI, and waist circumference performed when evaluating a potential cardiac condition.[4] Measured height and measured weight are necessary to correctly calculate BMI. Abdominal circumference > 35 inches in women is considered to be abdominal obesity and is associated with increased risk.

A head-to-toe assessment is the best approach. If a woman has risk factors for retinopathy such as hypertension, a full evaluation of the optic fundi by an ophthalmologist should be performed to assess for arteriolar narrowing, increased vascular tortuosity, arteriovenous (AV) nicking, hemorrhages, exudates, and disc edema. An ophthalmologist should also follow women at risk of retinopathy on a routine basis. The thyroid is palpated to evaluate for any nodules, irregularities, or enlargements. A cardiac examination includes evaluation for arrhythmias, murmurs, clicks, rubs, carotid bruit, or abnormal heart sounds. A pulmonary assessment is indicated, which includes inspection, percussion for consolidation, palpation for notable irregularities, and auscultation for the presence of adventitious sounds. The chest wall should be examined and palpated for pain, particularly at the costochondral junctions, to help rule out pain of musculoskeletal origin.

The abdomen is evaluated via inspection, auscultation, percussion, and palpation for the presence of bruits, pain, or masses. For example, epigastric and right upper quadrant tenderness suggest cholecystitis, while a pulsating abdominal mass found on palpation could indicate an abdominal aneurysm. Other signs of an abdominal aneurysm include discrepancies in bilateral measurements of BP and peripheral pulses and new focal deficits found on evaluation of cranial nerves.

The skin and peripheral vasculature should also be examined. Weak, thready pulses and pallor or cyanosis or edema in the extremities may indicate problems with perfusion. Venous thromboembolism (VTE), which includes DVT and pulmonary embolus (PE), results from inherited or acquired factors such as vessel wall damage, venous stasis, and hypercoagulable states. These are notable characteristics of conditions ranging from clotting factor deficiencies, to cancer, to combined hormonal contraception use. If varicosities are noted on the exam, veins should be mapped, noting the size and exact location after the woman has been standing for 5 to 10 minutes. The presence of unilateral leg edema is a sensitive indicator of DVT. Edema may be noted distal to the level of a clot. The involved area may be warm and tender to the touch and erythematous in color; a thrombosed vein may be palpable as a superficial cord. Pain may be elicited with compression of the knee. A positive Homan's sign, the presence of calf pain with dorsiflexion of the foot, may suggest DVT; however, it lacks specificity. Clinical diagnosis of DVT is confirmed with a high-sensitivity D-dimer and/or ultrasonography. In PE, additional diagnostic imaging, such as ventilation-perfusion scan, helical computed tomography (CT), or angiography is performed. Coagulation studies may be indicated for women with VTE.

Measurement of BP should be done at most visits, because hypertension is silent until the latter stages of the disease. An accurate diagnosis requires two elevated readings over several office visits using accurate equipment and measurement technique.[9] It is necessary to be sure that the sphygmomanometer is appropriately calibrated and that the inflatable portion of the cuff surrounds at least 80% of the circumference of the arm. The lower edge of the cuff should be placed 2 to 3 cm above the antecubital fossa. A false elevation in pressure will result from a cuff that is too small. BP readings should be taken after the individual has been resting for 5 or more minutes. Two or more readings separated by at least 2 minutes are averaged together and documented at each visit. BP should be checked in both arms.[10,11]

Hypertension is defined as having an elevated BP reading of $\geq 140/90$ mmHg. However, risk of cardiovascular events, kidney disease, and stroke is now known to occur on a continuum and increases as BP increases above the ideal level of 115/75 mmHg. Risk of adverse outcomes doubles with each 20-mmHg increase in systolic BP or each 10-mmHg increase in diastolic BP.[11] The recognition that risk increases along a continuum prompted the *Seventh Report of the Joint National Committee on Prevention, Detection, Evaluation, and Treatment of High Blood Pressure* (JNC 7), published in 2003, to create a new category in its guidelines: prehypertension, defined as a systolic BP levels of 120 to 139 mmHg and diastolic BP levels between 80 and 89 mmHg.[12] The importance of counseling individuals with prehypertension on adopting healthy lifestyle practices was stressed most recently by the American Society of Hypertension in 2014.[11]

The term *white coat hypertension (WCH)* is used to identify women who have elevated BP readings in a medical provider's office, but not in their own environment. This is not a benign condition; some of these women may be at risk for cardiovascular events. WCH can occur at any age but primarily affects people over the age of 65, with women more commonly affected than men. Some studies, but not all, have reported an increased risk of progression to frank hypertension and end-organ damage compared to normotensive individuals.[13] Unfortunately, few high-quality randomized studies have been conducted to date on WCH, making it difficult to determine whether, and to what extent, WCH can impact health.

Certainly, the presence of WCH makes it more difficult to establish a diagnosis of hypertension without additional monitoring. An ambulatory blood pressure monitor (ABPM) consists of an arm cuff attached to a device worn by an individual, usually for 24 hours. It continuously records BP readings and can help detect persistent elevations of BP. It can provide information about a patient's BP during daily activities as well as at rest. BP readings at night are expected to be lower than daytime readings. Optimal readings in the daytime are < 120–130/80 mmHg and at night time < 110–115/65 mmHg.[13] Values of 135/80–85 mmHg are classified as normal/high-normal daytime BPs. With WCH, both day- and nighttime readings are lower than office readings. However, in individuals with frank hypertension, BP levels remain elevated—with ABPM levels of ≥ 135/85 mmHg associated with office elevation of ≥ 140/90 mmHg.[13]

The utility of ABPM is debated. The most recent discussion of ABPM in federal guidelines was in the JNC 7, which concluded that ABPM was not cost effective enough to use in the routine evaluation of elevated BP. Rather, JNC 7 recommends that ABPM be used to diagnosis WCH or to monitor treatment of hypertension, particularly in those whose hypertension appears to be resistant to medication and in those who report hypotensive episodes while on medication.[9] The Task Force of the Eighth International Consensus Conference on Ambulatory Blood Pressure Monitoring recommends using ABPM in all individuals with 3 elevated office readings ≥ 140/90 mmHg who also have ≥ 2 home readings of < 140/90 mmHg and no evidence of end-organ damage.[14] However, other authorities recommend greater use of ABPM. The British National Institute for Health and Care Excellence (NICE) guidelines, published in 2011, recommend the liberal use of ABPM, recommending that all adults with elevated BP readings undergo ABPM, citing the substantial cost savings from the avoidance of unnecessary treatment in those without sustained elevations of BP.[15]

As an alternative, a woman can use a home BP machine to periodically record her BP. Home BP monitors have been shown to have diagnostic equivalency with ABPM and utility in the diagnosis and treatment of uncontrolled hypertension.[16]

Laboratory/Imaging Testing

Laboratory and imaging testing are done to detect or monitor end-organ damage, to assess the health and function of the heart itself, and to establish a diagnosis. The exact battery of tests ordered in an evaluation of a woman's symptoms will differ by risk profile and suspected condition(s).

The general laboratory assessment varies slightly depending on the presenting symptoms. For women with chest pain or hypertension, helpful laboratory tests include a complete blood count (CBC), urinalysis for the presence of albumin, serum electrolytes (potassium), thyroid-stimulating hormone (TSH), blood urea nitrogen (BUN), and chemistry for creatinine, fasting glucose, and lipid profiles.[11] A smaller panel of laboratory tests is needed for women with palpitations and includes a CBC, TSH, electrolytes, and potentially a drug screen.[17,18]

Other laboratory tests have been considered for use in screening for CVD, but the evidence is insufficient to recommend their routine use. These tests include C-reactive protein (CRP), homocysteine levels, and lipoprotein(a).[19] Lipoprotein(a) levels of > 30 mg/dL are associated with CVD as is an elevated CRP CVD. One meta-analysis of 10 studies reported an increased relative risk [RR] of 1.58 (95% confidence interval [CI] 1.37,1.83) for those with high CRP (> 3.0 mg/L) compared with those with low CRP (< 1.0 mg/L).[20] High homocysteine levels can also be seen with CVD; use of folic acid reduces these levels, but does not reduce cardiovascular death. Unfortunately, no studies have been conducted to determine how obtaining CRP, homocysteine, or lipoprotein(a) levels might add to risk stratification or change in management of CVD therefore, they are not recommended for screening in low-risk individuals.[19] Controversy exists about their role in evaluating and treating intermediate-risk individuals. A high level of CRP is associated with higher risk of future cardiovascular events for individuals at intermediate risk; this association has been used by some to justify more aggressive treatment for these individuals.[21]

COAGULATION STUDIES

Coagulation status is generally assessed using laboratory testing, and, in highly suspicious cases, specialized imaging and testing procedures. Prothrombin time (PT) measures the integrity of the *extrinsic* and common pathways of coagulation by adding calcium and an activator of the extrinsic pathway, thromboplastin, to a sample of blood. Deficiencies in these pathways results in a prolonged PT.[22] In contrast, activated partial thromboplastin time aPTT measures the integrity of the *intrinsic* and *common pathways of coagulation* by adding calcium and a trigger of the intrinsic pathway, phospholipid, to a sample of blood.[23] Deficiencies in these pathways lead to a prolonged partial prothrombin time (PTT). International normalized ratio (INR) improves the ability to interpret PT results. INR standardizes the results of the PT test by accounting for the variation in the sensitivities of various thromboplastin reagents, which differ by manufacturer.[22]

Prolonged PT and PTT results can be due to artifact, delay in processing, the use of anticoagulants, or the presence of systematic disease (such as liver disease, vitamin K deficiency, connective tissue disease), disseminated intravascular coagulation, or coagulation factor deficiencies.[22] If the results of a PT and PTT remain abnormal on a repeat draw, a mixing study of normal plasma

and/or other tests can help differentiate the possibilities. Consultation with a specialist can help determine the appropriate next step.

CARDIAC BIOMARKERS

Cardiac biomarkers of myocardial ischemia are used to evaluate a potential, evolving MI. Plasma creatine kinase (CK) is an enzyme that is released during muscle damage. As such, it is a nonspecific finding. The newer assays (i.e., CK-MB) have greater sensitivity and specificity for myocardial injury than earlier generations, but still can be elevated in a wide range of cardiac and noncardiac situations, such as in the presence of musculoskeletal trauma, rhabdomyolysis, myocarditis, severe hypothyroidism, seizures, cardioversion/defibrillation, post-cardiac catheterization, or renal failure.[24,25] The more accurate troponin biomarkers have largely replaced the use of CK-MB assays, although CK-MB does have specific utility. Relative to the troponin biomarkers that can remain elevated for 5 to 14 days, CK-MB has a shorter half-life. Consequently, serial measurements of CK-MB can be used to help determine if an individual is experiencing a series of MIs and has sustained additional cardiac damage beyond the initial insult.[26]

Troponin is one of the constituents of skeletal and cardiac muscle fibers and is composed of three subunits: troponin C, troponin I, and troponin T. The composition of troponin I and troponin T is such that they can be identified as being of cardiac or noncardiac origin. Consequently, troponins T or I are the preferred biomarkers when evaluating a potential acute coronary event; they have higher sensitivity and specificity than does CK-MB for myocardial necrosis.[27] However, troponin levels can also be elevated with nonischemic cardiac conditions, such as tachyarrhythmias, myocardial trauma, and heart failure, with pulmonary embolism and with other conditions.[24] Interpretation of troponin levels needs to be made with an understanding of the clinical context in which they were drawn.[27] Another limitation of troponin T is that it may not be elevated within the first 6 hours of cardiac injury, making it necessary to repeat the test later to determine if myocardial necrosis has occurred.[25,26]

CARDIAC STRUCTURE

Cardiac structure can be evaluated by sonography. A variety of testing options are available that allow a visual inspection of the cardiac chambers and valves. These tests are used to evaluate the structural integrity and hemodynamic function of the heart. One of the more sophisticated tests is Doppler imaging, which evaluates the direction, velocity, and amplitude of blood flow through the heart. Echocardiograms are used to identify shunting disorders such as septal defects, to describe the severity of stenotic and regurgitant valve diseases, to assess left ventricle filling pressures (helpful in determining the degree of heart failure, depending on ejection pressures), and the presence of obstruction associated with

cardiac myopathy.[28] Its major disadvantage is that it cannot evaluate extracardiac structures such as the aorta, aortic arch, pulmonary artery, and pulmonary veins, which can be better seen with CT or magnetic resonance imaging (MRI) scans.[28]

CARDIAC FUNCTION

Cardiac function can be assessed using one or more of the following modalities, depending on a woman's age and risk profile. The criteria used by the American Heart Association to categorize women as being of low, intermediate, or high risk for ischemic heart disease are listed in **Table 16-3**.[29] These categories are used to determine what baseline testing is recommended for evaluation of women presenting with chest pain or other symptoms suggestive of ischemic heart disease. The common tests used to evaluate cardiac complaints include:

- *12-lead electrocardiogram (EKG, or ECG)*: All women presenting with chest pain or palpitations should be evaluated with a 12-lead EKG. Findings indicative of an acute MI on an

Table 16-3 Risk Profiles for Women, Ischemic Heart Disease, American Heart Association*

Low Risk	Low to Intermediate Risk	Intermediate Risk	High Risk
Otherwise healthy premenopausal women	Symptomatic women in their 50s capable of performing routine activities of daily living	Symptomatic women in their 50s and 60s with functional limitations	Symptomatic women in their 70s Symptomatic women $\geq$ 40 years with peripheral artery disease or long-standing or poorly controlled diabetes

*Risk profiles used to determine appropriate testing for symptomatic women with chest pain or other equivalent ischemic symptom such as excessive dyspnea.

Data from Mieres JH, Gulati M, Bairey Merz N, Berman DS, Gerber TC, Hayes SN, et al. Role of noninvasive testing in the clinical evaluation of women with suspected ischemic heart disease: A consensus statement from the American Heart Association. *Circulation.* 2014;130(4):350-379.

ambulatory EKG include ST segment depression, ST elevation at the J point, or T wave inversions in two contiguous leads. Persistent Q waves or QS complexes are seen in those who had a previous MI.[23,29] Arrhythmias can also be noted on a 12-lead EKG and can help pinpoint the underlying etiology. However, if no explanation for a woman's symptoms are seen on a 12-lead EKG, follow-up testing with a 24-hour Holter or event monitor and/or stress test may be indicated depending on her risk profile and the differential diagnoses under consideration.

- *24-hour Holter monitor or event monitoring* can be useful in evaluating symptoms, such as palpitations, that are not occurring at the time a 12-lead EKG is ordered. A Holter monitor is worn for 24 to 48 hours, and cardiac activity is recorded continuously. When the woman experiences symptoms, she pushes a button to "mark" the EKG when symptoms are occurring. The EKG is then later reviewed to determine what cardiac changes are evident between, before, during, and after a symptomatic episode.

  If chest pain or palpitations occur frequently, but not daily, a more appropriate test to order is a 2-week event monitor. Like the Holter monitor, the women must wear the device continuously and record when symptoms are occurring. Unlike the Holter monitor, which records cardiac activity continuously, the event monitor marks cardiac activity just before, during, and after the perceived event. Some event monitors will also activate if an arrhythmia is detected.

  Newer, more sophisticated devices appear to increase diagnostic yield—likely due to higher compliance rates because of their wearability. The newer devices are significantly smaller in size, lead free, and less obtrusive to wear than conventional Holter and event monitors. Some devices transmit EKG readings via Bluetooth, others are mailed into the company and the results are supplied later after analysis.[30]

- An *exercise stress test* is one of the initial tests done to evaluate women with atypical or typical chest pain, shortness of breath, or extreme fatigue. It is the test of choice in low-risk women and in intermediate-risk women with normal baseline EKG who can tolerate exercise. Women who have functional limitations in their activities of daily living (equivalent to 5 metabolic equivalent of task) are better candidates for pharmacologic stress testing or other testing modalities as opposed to exercise stress testing.[29]

  A stress test can assess whether the body's response is healthy by monitoring for pain during the procedure, as well as by evaluating changes in heart rate, BP, and EKG readings over the course of the test. Exercise stress tests have lower sensitivity and specificity in women compared to men, but a negative test is useful in ruling out coronary artery disease.[4,29]

- *Stress echocardiography* combines ultrasound evaluation of the heart with stress testing.[29] Generally, this test is used as a follow-up test in those women who fail the exercise stress test or as an initial test in those with intermediate or high risk factors for obstructive coronary artery disease and either abnormal resting ST segment abnormalities or functional disability.[29] It has the advantage of being able to evaluate wall motion abnormalities, indicative of regional hypoxia in the cardiac muscle, making it a more sensitive test in women than the exercise stress test. Its sensitivity and specificity in detecting CVD are 81–89% and 86%, respectively.[23] Not only is stress echocardiography helpful in identifying ischemia, but it is also useful in the identification and evaluation of valvular abnormalities and cardiac myopathy.

- *Myocardial perfusion imaging (MPI)* is used in the evaluation of symptomatic women of intermediate to high risk who have abnormal resting ST segment changes, functional disability, or indeterminate- or intermediate-risk results on a stress EKG.[29] Two types of MPI are available: MPI with single-photon emission computed tomography (SPECT) or positron emission tomography (PET). MPI with PET appears to be produce higher quality images and better diagnostic yield, particularly for obese women, than MPI with SPECT.[29] In both techniques, a radioactive "tracer" is injected intravenously and emits gamma rays that are detected and converted by a computer into multiple images of the heart. These images are used to evaluate cardiac muscle perfusion and left ventricular function and can identify localized ischemia. It is equally sensitive in men and women with a sensitivity and specificity of 87% and 91%, respectively.[23]

- *Cardiac magnetic resonance imaging (CMR)* obtains images of the heart using a different technique from MPI. Rather than using radioactive tracers, a CMR uses radio waves to create an image of the heart. It historically has been used primarily in research, but is becoming more available and more widely used in clinical practice. It may be used in symptomatic intermediate- to high-risk women with resting ST segment abnormalities or in those with functional limitations.[29]
- *Coronary artery calcium (CAC) with CT* measures the degree of atherosclerosis burden by measuring the amount of calcium, found in plaque, in the heart. High values are associated with obstructive coronary artery disease. It is most useful in ruling out disease, because it has an almost 100% negative predictive value.[23] It is useful in detecting frank disease, but its utility in risk screening is currently under debate.[19] According to the 2014 American Heart Association recommendations, it can be used in symptomatic women at intermediate risk of ischemic disease with resting ST segment disabilities or functional disabilities or with indeterminate- or intermediate-risk stress EKG results.[29]

- *Cardiac catheterization* is the gold standard in evaluating cardiac disease, because the vessels and cardiac structures can be directly observed. A catheter is inserted through the groin, arm, or neck and then advanced to the heart; dye is injected and then a series of radiographs is taken that are used to evaluate the function of the cardiac muscles, valves, and arteries. One of the most important measurements obtained by cardiac catheterization is the left ventricle ejection fraction, which describes the percentage of blood that is pumped out of the chamber with each beat. Despite its accuracy, cardiac catheterization is not considered to be a first-line test, because it is an invasive procedure, except in specific circumstances.[24] In 2012, the American College of Cardiology Foundation, along with other professional organizations, released guidelines on the appropriate use of cardiac catheterization; appropriate indications include suspected or known acute coronary syndrome, high-risk results on prior testing, and the assessment of valvular disease, pericardial disease, and cardiomyopathies in selected situations.[31]

Cardiac Symptoms and Physical Findings

Symptoms that might suggest underlying cardiac pathology include chest pain and palpitations. Corroborating findings on physical exam may include an irregular or racing heart rate or heart murmur. This section discusses the evaluation of these common signs and symptoms.

Chest Pain

Chest pain is associated with many conditions, not all related to cardiac function. One of the most concerning is *acute coronary syndrome*, which is a broad category of conditions associated with cardiac ischemia. Acute coronary syndrome is categorized as 1) unstable angina, 2) non-ST segment elevation myocardial infarction (NSTEMI), and 3) ST segment elevation myocardial infarction (STEMI).[26] Having any of the following is suggestive of acute coronary syndrome: symptoms of ischemia; a rise in troponin and/or CK-MB (biomarkers of myocardial ischemia); ischemic EKG changes, specifically ST segment changes; pathologic Q waves on the EKG; or imaging evidence of new loss of viable myocardium.[24]

Distinguishing among the various entities associated with acute coronary syndrome is important, because the investigation and treatment vary by specific condition. Unstable angina and NSTEMI are similar in presentation but differ in degree of severity. Both conditions present with chest pain; neither will have ST segment elevations on EKG. Individuals with NSTEMI will have a positive cardiac biomarker result, whereas women with unstable angina will not. Treatment goals for unstable angina and NSTEMI are to provide relief from ischemia and prevent its recurrence, which can be achieved through a variety of treatment choices depending on an individual's age, risk status, and comorbidities. Treatment choices include cardiac catheterization and reperfusion vascular surgery, anti-ischemic therapy, and antithrombotic therapy.[26] However, reperfusion therapy is the preferred treatment option for women with STEMI. Ideally, reperfusion therapy is performed within 12 hours of symptom onset. Timeliness is critical, because mortality associated with STEMI increases significantly with delays in treatment.[32]

Other cardiac conditions associated with chest pain include mitral value prolapse (discussed later) and aortic dissection. *Aortic dissection,* while rare, is one of the most deadly cardiac conditions. It occurs more commonly in individuals with a history of hypertension, some genetic disorders (e.g., Marfan syndrome, Ehlers-Danlos syndrome), stimulant use, trauma, and family history of aortic disease.[33] It commonly presents with an acute onset of severe chest or interscapular pain, but if the woman experiences a slow leak through the intima (the innermost layer of the wall of an artery or vein), the presentation may be more occult. The pain may radiate to the extremities and abdomen. Neurologic deficits may be noted on the physical exam due to diminished blood supply to the central nervous system. Pulse discrepancy between extremities strongly suggests dissection, but this finding is not consistently present in aortic dissection. Urgent evaluation in a hospital equipped to deal with cardiothoracic emergencies is mandatory.[33]

The first step in evaluating chest pain is to determine whether the woman's complaints are indicative of acute coronary syndrome or other acute event and warrant emergent evaluation and hospitalization. Delays in receiving health care are a major predictor of poor outcome and are particularly prevalent among women, especially postmenopausal women. Patients should be screened for the presence of any coexisting cardiac risk factors. Younger women who present with ischemic-quality chest pain need to be questioned about cocaine use. When a woman reports chest pain and has known cardiac risk factors, prompt evaluation is needed in a setting that is equipped to provide urgent care. Transport should be by emergency medical services (EMS) rather than family members. EMS technicians can monitor a patient's condition on the way to the hospital and will transport the woman to a facility equipped to deal with cardiac emergencies.

In populations served by most women's health practices, chest pain is rarely associated with serious underlying pathology. Young reproductive-aged women are more likely to be healthy and to have few high-risk factors compared to older women. Therefore, while the differential diagnosis list for chest pain should always include cardiac disease, chest pain in younger women is more often due to underlying GI disease, pulmonary pathology, musculoskeletal causes, or psychologic distress. Treatment is specific to the underlying cause.

One of the most common noncardiac causes of chest pain is *gastroesophageal reflux disease* (GERD). It is described as a squeezing or burning sensation that may last from 1 minute to several hours. Conditions that decrease lower esophageal sphincter pressure, such as pregnancy, can predispose women to GERD. Other GI diseases such as cholecystitis, pancreatitis, and peptic ulcer disease are also sources of complaints of chest pain.

Causes of *pleuritic chest pain* include pericarditis, pneumonia, spontaneous pneumothorax, pulmonary embolism, and other conditions that lead to inflammation or distention of the pleura. Pleuritic pain is usually worsened by deep inspiration and coughing, but not affected by movement or palpation. The severity of pain is related to the degree of inflammation and is typically worse in infectious conditions. A spontaneous pneumothorax is characterized by a sudden onset of stabbing pleuritic chest pain. It occurs in younger people and women with known emphysema. Pulmonary embolism is characterized by the acute onset of dyspnea with pleuritic chest pain. Conditions that predispose to pulmonary embolism include:

- Current combined hormonal contraceptives or hormonal therapy
- Current pregnancy or recent childbirth
- History of thrombolytic events
- Recent air travel or high-altitude exposure
- Connective tissue disorders
- Antiphospholipid syndrome

See the section later in this chapter on thrombolytic conditions for further details.

Musculoskeletal chest pain is a frequent reason for ambulatory office visits; it may be attributed to overexertion or trauma. *Costochondritis* is an inflammatory condition causing localized swelling, erythema, warmth, and tenderness at the costochondral or chondrosternal junction. It is more common in women than men and in younger populations (children or adolescents). The pain may be sharp and localized to a specific area or diffuse and poorly localized. Movement, palpation, and deep breathing aggravate the pain. The symptoms may last for a variable amount of time with the intensity sharp to dull. Treatment is supportive; generally over-the-counter analgesics and application of heat are all that is needed.

Palpitations and chest pain often accompany a *panic disorder* and are more common in women than men. Women usually complain of chest tightness or heaviness in association with palpitations as well as dizziness from hyperventilation and dyspnea. Symptoms may be triggered by stress and can last for hours and occur over several days. Rest does not relieve the symptoms. Underlying cardiac disease must be ruled out prior to diagnosing a panic disorder.

Palpitations

The underlying mechanisms associated with palpitations include contractions of the heart that are too rapid, too slow, or irregular such as can occur with arrhythmia, systemic disease, medications, or illicit drugs; abnormal movements of the heart associated with structural problems such as mitral value prolapse or regurgitation; or increased perception of normal heartbeat and rhythm, which can occur in some women, particularly those with depression, anxiety, or somatization (Table 16-2).[34] The presentation may suggest a particular etiology. For example, tachyarrhythmias are associated with perceptions of breathlessness and having a heartbeat that it is too fast to count.[18] In contrast, women with ectopy may perceive skipped beats, fluttering, or extra beats and report a momentary feeling of their breath being taken away. Pulsation palpitations, which are felt as strong, regular heartbeats in the chest, can be reported by individuals with ventricular arrhythmias or structural heart problems, such as aortic regurgitation or systemic diseases associated with high stroke volume (i.e., fever, anemia).[34] Presyncopal symptoms and blackouts, as well as palpitations with exertion, are alarm symptoms and may indicate the presence of more serious arrhythmias.[18] Having a first-degree relative with sudden death, particularly under the age of 40 years, may indicate the possibility that palpitations are due to an inherited arrhythmia.[18]

All women with palpitations should have a thorough history and physical and baseline 12-lead EKG. The most common EKG changes seen in the evaluation of palpitations include normal sinus rhythm sometimes accompanied by atrial or ventricular ectopic beats, ventricular premature contractions, or brief episodes of ventricular tachycardia. These findings are not associated with significant underlying pathology or increased mortality. No further workup is needed for women with a benign EKG who have infrequent and tolerable symptoms. In these cases, woman can be reassured and advised to avoid caffeine, alcohol, and stressful situations.[17,34] However, palpitations are also associated with other more serious arrhythmias such as atrial fibrillation/flutter or paroxysmal supraventricular tachycardias.[34] Abnormal EKG changes that could indicate significant pathology include second- or third-degree atrioventricular (AV) block, left ventricular hypertrophy, left bundle branch block, abnormal T wave inversion and ST segment changes, short PR interval and delta waves, and abnormal QTc interval and T wave morphology.[18]

Consultation with a cardiologist should be considered in uncertain cases and in women without obvious disease who desire a second opinion and should be obtained for women with abnormal EKG findings, severe presentations, or who have high-risk profiles.[18,34] If referral is indicated,

preliminary testing may aid the specialist in more rapidly coming to a diagnosis. See the section earlier in this chapter on laboratory/imaging testing for tests used in the evaluation of cardiac symptoms.

Heart Murmur

Heart murmurs are prolonged extra sounds that can be heard during systole or diastole. Murmurs are caused by a disruption in the flow of blood into, through, or out of the heart. Many murmurs are benign; however, valvular disorders commonly produce murmurs. The role of the women's health provider is to help determine if the murmur is benign or pathologic, order baseline testing as indicated, and refer women whose presentation is unclear or indicative of pathology to a cardiologist.

The first task is to determine if heart sounds are normal. Heart sounds are normally low in pitch except in the presence of significant disease. There are four basic heart sounds: S_1, S_2, S_3, and S_4. S_1 and S_2 are the most distinct sounds. S_1 indicates the beginning of systole and results from the closure of the atrioventricular valves. It is best heard at the apex of the heart and is louder, lower in pitch, and longer than S_2. The S_1 sound is referred to as "lubb." S_2 indicates the end of systole and results from the closure of the semilunar valves. It is best heard at the base of the heart and has a higher pitch and shorter duration than S_1. The S_2 sound is referred to as "dubb." S_2 is actually two sounds. The closure of the aortic valve contributes to most of the sound of S_2, masking the sound of the pulmonic valve closing. The pulmonic valve closure occurs slightly later, giving S_2 two distinct components. When audible, this is referred to as split S_2. Split S_2 is physiologic if it occurs only during inspiration. Changing pressure in the cardiac chambers due to inspiration slightly delays the closure of the pulmonic valve. A split S_2 is considered pathologic if it is wider than usual (e.g., in pulmonic stenosis) or if it occurs during expiration (e.g., aortic stenosis) or during both expiration and inspiration (e.g., atrial septal defect).

S_3 and S_4 may or may not be present, and both are difficult to hear. S_3 is a low-pitched sound that resembles a gallop and occurs early in diastole. S_3 is more common in children and athletes and is not generally heard in individuals older than 40 years. If present in older individuals or in those with known cardiac risk factors, underlying cardiac disease—particularly heart failure or mitral or tricuspid regurgitation—should be suspected. It also is heard in women who are in high-output states such as severe anemia, thyrotoxicosis, and pregnancy. S_3 produces a cadence similar to "Kentucky," which is best heard using the bell of the stethoscope placed directly over the apical impulse with the women in the left lateral position. S_3 does not vary with respiration and persists when sitting upright. S_4 resembles the rhythm of "Tenn-es-see" or "A STIFF wall" and occurs late in diastole and is low pitched, best heard with the bell in a left lateral decubitus position. S_4 can be heard in women at any age and is often associated with cardiac pathology, particularly if loud. It is especially common among individuals, particularly the elderly, who have CHD, because CHD increases resistance to filling due to the loss of compliance of the ventricular walls.

Murmurs are classified according to their timing and duration, pitch, intensity, pattern, quality, location, radiation, and respiratory phase variations. Murmurs are most commonly referred to by their intensity. They are identified as grades I/VI to VI/VI (1 to 6) with intensity increasing as the grade gets higher. While it is beyond the scope of this chapter to review all types of murmurs, two conditions commonly seen in primary care are addressed: flow murmurs and mitral valve prolapse (MVP).

Flow murmurs are also referred to as *ejection* or innocent murmurs. They are systolic murmurs heard in the absence of any identifiable disease and are classified as benign. These murmurs are asymptomatic. They commonly occur in the setting of hyperdynamic or high-output conditions, such as fever, anemia, hyperthyroidism, and pregnancy. Flow murmurs are common in women under the age of 35. It is not uncommon for these murmurs to come and go when followed in serial exams. They are usually best heard at the base of the heart and have a crescendo–decrescendo pattern. Their intensity is usually grade III/VI or lower. Echocardiograms are not indicated in the evaluation of flow murmurs, because these murmurs are not pathologic and are considered to be normal variants.

Mitral valve prolapse is a cardiac valvular abnormality. Prevalence is approximately 2%, and it occurs equally in men and women.[35] It is the most common cause of severe mitral valve regurgitation in the United States.[35] It results from the systolic displacement of a redundant mitral leaflet (with or without thickening) into the left atrium during systole. In the "classic" presentation, the valves have 5-mm or greater thickening, and in the "nonclassic" presentation there is a lesser amount or complete absence of thickening.[35] Nonclassic presentations are thought to have a more benign course.

MVP is also referred to as click-murmur syndrome and should be suspected if a mid-systolic click is heard on examination. If it is accompanied by mitral valve regurgitation, a murmur may be heard at the apex. The murmur is often holosystolic and may have a high-pitched, blowing quality in a crescendo–decrescendo pattern.

Women with MVP are usually asymptomatic; symptoms depend on the underlying cause, the presence of other risk factors, and the degree of MVP. MVP is categorized as being a primary valvular disorder if no other identifiable disease is found, or a secondary disorder if it is due to conditions such as connective tissue disorders, congenital heart disease, rheumatic fever, or infective endocarditis.

Mitral valve regurgitation can occur when the valve is seriously damaged. Worsening of the prolapse occurs gradually for a small minority of women; women who were initially asymptomatic may become symptomatic over time. Generally, primary MVP has a benign course. However, morbidity is much more likely to occur with MVP in women with thickened valvular leaflets or moderate to severe regurgitation, those whose MVP is associated with reduced left ventricular ejection fraction or atrial fibrillation, and those older than 50 years.[35,36] For some, the degree of prolapse will require valvular surgery.

Two-dimensional echocardiography is the diagnostic test of choice, because cardiac auscultation has a low sensitivity.[35] This test will show the degree of mitral regurgitation or thickening of the valvular leaves. More sophisticated testing, such as three-dimensional echocardiography or Doppler imaging, may be ordered by a cardiologist if the degree of regurgitation is moderate or severe or if surgery is being contemplated.

Recommendations governing antibiotic coverage and appropriate medication(s) have changed dramatically in recent years. Due to a lack of scientific evidence that antibiotic coverage is useful in the prevention of infective endocarditis, two major authoritative bodies no longer recommend antibiotic coverage for GI, genitourinary (GU), or dental procedures except for those at highest risk.[37,38] High-risk individuals are those with prosthetic valves, a prior history of endocarditis, some types of congenital cardiac abnormalities, cardiac transplantation recipients who develop cardiac valvulopathy, and those with prosthetic cardiac valves or who have had valvular repair using prosthetic material.[38]

The rationale behind the change in recommendations by the American College of Cardiology and the American Heart Association is threefold. First, most cases of infective endocarditis are due to freely circulating pathogens and are unrelated to dental, GI, or GU procedures. Second, the risks of antibiotic coverage outweigh the theoretical benefit of antibiotics. Third, emphasis should be on the promotion of dental hygiene that can prevent infections of the oral cavity.[37,38]

Antibiotic coverage should be given to high-risk individuals undergoing dental procedures that involve manipulation of gingival tissue or periapical region of the teeth or perforation of the oral mucosa and to those undergoing respiratory tract procedures that involve incision or biopsy of the mucosa.[37,38] Antibiotic coverage is not needed in individuals undergoing GI- or GU-related procedures, specifically vaginal or cesarean section birth and hysterectomy. However, not all authorities agree with these recommendations and call for a more individualized approach until better quality research is available to guide clinical practice.[39]

Management of Cardiovascular Conditions

Because the ongoing management of many cardiovascular conditions is under the purview of a primary care physician or nurse practitioner, the central focus from the perspective of women's health providers should be on primary and secondary prevention, specifically promoting healthy dietary intake and exercise and smoking cessation. Data from the Nurses' Health Study[40] showed an association between daily exercise, healthy dietary intake and weight, and modest alcohol intake and lower rates of CVD. The importance of diet and exercise in the prevention of diabetes, hypertension, and atherosclerotis has been upheld in numerous meta-analyses.[41-43] The type of diet and exercise appears to matter. One meta-analysis of six randomized controlled trials (RCTs), composed of 2650 individuals, found that following a Mediterranean diet was associated with greater reductions in BMI, BP, fasting glucose, and total cholesterol than low-fat diets.[44] Other studies suggest similar findings.[45,46]

Protection against CVD by exercising is dose-dependent, with the greatest benefit seen with higher levels of exercise.[47] Women appear to benefit more than men and have greater reductions in the RR of CVD compared to men no matter how exercise was measured (leisure-type physical activity [LTPA], transport physical activity, or total physical activity) in a meta-analysis of nine studies.[47] Transport physical activity means walking, biking, or other physical activity being used to go someplace, as opposed to driving or taking public transportation. Women meeting the basic recommendations of 150 minutes of moderate-intensity exercise per week had a 20% reduction in their risk of coronary artery disease (RR 0.80; 95% CI, 0.69–0.92) compared to women with no LTPA.[47]

The impact of alcohol intake follows a J-shaped curve. In a meta-analysis of 27 prospective studies reporting data on 1,425,513 individuals, it was found to be protective against stroke at low doses (RR 0.85; 95% CI, 0.75–0.95; P = 0.005), had little or no effect at moderate doses, and increased the risk of stroke at high doses (RR, 1.20; 95% CI, 1.01–1.43; P = 0.034).[48] Encouraging women to become more physically active, to consume a healthier diet, and to moderate their alcohol intake can help prevent CVD.

Decreasing or stopping cigarette smoking can also protect against CVD. Smoking increases the risk of stroke to a greater degree in women than in men. The impact is dose-dependent and rises as the number of cigarettes smoked increases; however, even smoking 1 to 4 cigarettes a day increases the risk by 2–3 times.[4] The risk of MI drops dramatically after cessation, with the risk reduced by 50% at 1 year and essentially the same as never-smokers in 10 years.[4]

The promotion of healthy behaviors forms the foundation of care for women affected by

Table 16-4 Criteria for Optimal Cardiovascular Health in Women

Total cholesterol < 200 mg/dL
Blood pressure < 120/< 80 mmHg
Fasting blood glucose < 100 mg/dL
Body mass index < 25 kg/m^2
Nonsmoker
Physical activity of ≥ 150 min/week moderate intensity, ≥ 75 min/week vigorous intensity, or combination
Healthy diet

Data from Mosca L, Benjamin EJ, Berra K, Bezanson JL, Dolor RJ, Lloyd-Jones DM, et al. Effectiveness-based guidelines for the prevention of cardiovascular disease in women—2011 update: a guideline from the American Heart Association. *J Am Coll Cardiol*. 2011;57(12):1404-1423.

any cardiovascular condition. These healthy behaviors will help promote optimal cardiovascular health in women. The criteria set by the American Heart Association to determine optimal cardiovascular health for women are listed in **Table 16-4**.[49] For women with established CVD, the presentation, workup, and management will vary by specific condition. The following sections address common and severe conditions that present in the context of women's health.

Hypertension

Prevalence rates of hypertension are similar between men and women, affecting approximately 30% of all Americans.[50] Rates are highest among individuals older than 65 years (71.6%) and non-Hispanic black individuals (41.3%).[50] Many individuals with hypertension are uncontrolled; only 36.6% of men and 52.0% of women have BP levels < 140/90 mmHg.[51] Yet, in addition to smoking cessation, BP control is the single most important strategy to prevent future adverse cardiovascular events in women.[52] It is essential that women's health providers monitor BP levels of women in their care and refer as needed to providers skilled in the management of hypertensive disorders.

Physiology

BP is a function of *cardiac output (CO)* and *peripheral vascular resistance (PVR)*. PVR occurs mainly in the small muscular arteries and arterioles. Small changes in arterial diameter have a profound effect on flow. The degree of PVR is determined by the diameter of small arteries and arterioles, which is controlled by the contractile state of their smooth muscle and affected by a complex interplay of local, regional, and systemic neural, humoral, and renal factors. CO is determined by heart rate (regulated by parasympathetic and sympathetic stimulation) and stroke volume (a function of filling pressure and force of contraction of the cardiac muscle).[53] Filling pressure is determined by the amount of blood returning to the heart, which is in turn determined by the intravascular volume and venous capacitance. *Venous capacitance* refers to the degree to which blood can be stored in the venous compartment.[53] Nearly 70% of total blood volume is retained in the venous system due to the thinner walls and larger lumens of veins; constriction of veins increases and dilation decreases venous return.[54] Therefore, stroke volume is dependent on left ventricular pump function, venous return, the contractile state of the ventricular muscle, and aortic input impedance, which is the complex relation between unsteady flow and pressure throughout the cardiac cycle.[55] With ejection, the larger arteries dilate and absorb pressure, which has an end result of reducing the magnitude of pressure changes in the system, damping pressure in the capillaries, and accounts for a large degree of the diastolic

pressure.[55] Over time, changes in CO and PVR result in compensatory changes in the cardiac vasculature and the development of remodeling and hypertrophy.

The regulation of normal BP is due to a dynamic, complex interaction between the arterial and venous compartments of the vascular system, but is also influenced by the renin-angiotensin-aldosterone system. Under normal conditions, a drop in BP or in sodium chloride (NaCl) delivery or stimulation from the sympathetic nervous system increases the release of renin from the kidney. Renin cleaves angiotensinogen (released primarily from the liver) into angiotensin I. Angiotensin-converting enzyme (ACE) is found primarily in the lungs and converts angiotensin I into angiotensin II. Angiotensin II is a potent vasoconstrictor throughout the body. It also helps regulate the glomerular filtration rate, increases the absorption of NaCL from the renal tubules, and stimulates the release of aldosterone from the adrenals. Together, these processes raise BP. Natriuretic peptides found in the brain, heart, and other tissues downregulate the renin-angiotensin-aldosterone system and lower BP by dilating blood vessels and increasing the glomerular filtration rate in the kidney, leading to a loss of sodium and water. Thus, normal BP is a result of a complicated feedback loop involving the sympathetic nervous system, liver, kidneys, vasculature, and the renin-angiotensin-aldosterone sytem.[56]

The exact underlying physiology of hypertension remains unclear, but a number of pathogenic mechanisms have been suggested. Genetics play a large role, accounting for 30% to 60% of the variation in BP readings between individuals.[53] Environmental factors such as dietary intake, exercise, obesity, and cigarette smoking are thought to affect genetic expression and account for another 20% in the variation in BP between individuals.[53] Activation of the sympathetic nervous system, which is associated with primary hypertension, leads to numerous deleterious changes such as peripheral vasoconstriction, an increase in heart rate, high levels of norepinephrine, and an increase in systemic BP. The sympathetic nervous system also has pro-hypertrophic effects on myocardial tissue and contributes to the development of vascular hypertrophy and stiffness and lower arterial distensibility and compliance. In addition, activation of the sympathetic nervous system leads to insulin resistance, renal vasoconstriction, and increased reabsorption of sodium and renin release in the kidney.[53] The role of the renin-angiotensin-aldosterone system in the development of essential hypertension is little understood, because the majority of individuals with essential hypertension have low or normal levels of renin. Some researchers hypothesize that while renin levels overall may be normal, heterogeneity in nephrons can lead some nephrons to under- and others to overproduce renin.[53] Some secondary causes of hypertension such as renin-secreting tumors, renal ischemia, or catecholamine-releasing pheochromocytoma are associated with high levels of renin, whereas others increase levels of aldosterone.[56,57]

Target organ damage associated with hypertension results primarily from events occurring at the microvascular level. Examples include myocardial ischemia, renal damage, retinopathy, and slowly advancing dementia. Another central and early effect of CVD is chronic inflammation.[58] Hypertension has been identified as a risk factor for stroke, MI, renal failure, congestive heart failure, progressive atherosclerosis, retinopathy, and dementia.

Management

The course of hypertension involves insidious damage that can be clinically silent for a decade or more. It typically presents in the fourth decade of life and is often preceded by a period of BP lability. Ninety-five percent of patients with hypertension have primary or essential hypertension, where there is no specific cause for the elevated BP.[11] *Secondary hypertension* occurs rarely and is attributed to illnesses such as Cushing's syndrome, pheochromocytoma, primary aldosteronism, or sleep apnea (Table 16-5).[59] Once hypertension has been diagnosed, appropriate treatment needs to be implemented, usually a combination of medication and lifestyle changes.

Lifestyle modifications such as weight loss, dietary changes, and exercise are critical elements of treatment no matter the stage of essential hypertension. Each strategy is associated with improvements in BP and lipid levels. With a weight reduction of 10 to 12 pounds, women who have an elevated BMI have a demonstrated systolic BP reduction of 5 to 20 mmHg.[60] Following the Dietary Approach to Stop Hypertension (DASH) diet, which includes foods high in potassium such as fruits, vegetables, and low-fat dairy products, can reduce systolic/diastolic BP by 5–6/3 mmHg and low-density lipoprotein (LDL) cholesterol by 11 mg/dL.[61] Further reductions can be seen in individuals who reduce their intake of trans fats. Lowering sodium intake to 1150 mg/day reduces systolic/diastolic BP by 3–4/1–2 mmHg, while aerobic physical activity can decrease BP on average by 2–5/1–4 mmHg and LDL cholesterol by 3–6 mg/dL.[61] These benefits are additive, with the greatest reductions in BP and cholesterol levels seen in those individuals who adopt all of these recommendations.

The JNC guidelines are issued by the National High Blood Pressure Education Program in collaboration with professional organizations and experts in the field. These guidelines set the standard of care in the management of essential hypertension. Each guideline focuses on specific key concepts. The 2014 JNC guideline (JNC 8) focuses exclusively on the pharmacologic treatment of hypertension and evaluates the strength of the evidence that treating individuals with hypertension above a systolic level of 140 and diastolic

Table 16-5 Differential Diagnoses for Secondary Hypertension

Causes of Secondary Hypertension	History or Physical Findings	Diagnostic Studies
Hyperparathyroidism	Kidney stones Osteoporosis Depression Lethargy Muscle weakness Renal dysfunction Abdominal bruits Nocturia Diabetes Hematuria	Protein in urine PTH Elevated creatinine
Renovascular disease and Chronic kidney disease	Edema Elevated BUN and creatinine Proteinuria	Creatinine clearance Renal ultrasound Estimated glomerular filtration rate
Pheochromocytoma	Labile hypertension Family history of endocrine disorders Hypertension after abdominal palpation Headaches Diaphoresis Palpitations	Elevated urine vanillylmandelic acid (VMA)
Hyperaldosteronism	Hypokalemia Hypernatremia Headache Weakness Fatigue Muscle cramps Polyuria Polydipsia Nocturia Paresthesias	Low potassium level
Cushing's syndrome	Weight gain Fatigue Weakness Hirsutism Amenorrhea Moon facies Dorsal hump	Dexamethasone-suppression test
Coarctation of the aorta	Arm blood pressure > leg blood pressure Late systolic murmur Decreased or delayed femoral pulses	Abnormal chest x-ray

(continues)

Table 16-5 Differential Diagnoses for Secondary Hypertension (*continued*)

Causes of Secondary Hypertension	History or Physical Findings	Diagnostic Studies
Hypothyroid	Fatigue Weight loss Hair loss Diastolic hypertension Muscle weakness	Elevated TSH
Hyperthyroid	Heat intolerance Weight loss Palpitations Systolic hypertension, exophthalmos Tremor Tachycardia	TSH levels
Sleep apnea	Snoring Daytime sleepiness	Sleep studies with oxygen saturation
Drugs and substances associated with hypertension	Immunosuppressants including corticosteroids NSAIDs Cox-2 inhibitors Estrogens Weight-loss agents Stimulants—nicotine, amphetamines Bromocriptine Nardil Testosterone Pseudoephedrine Licorice Antidepressants, especially venlafaxine Buspirone Clozapine Ergotamine St. John's wort Anabolic steroids Cocaine Ecstasy	

BUN = blood urea nitrogen, NSAIDs = nonsteroidal anti-inflammatory drugs, PTH = parathyroid hormone, TSH = thyroid-stimulating hormone

Data from Viera A, Neutze D. Diagnosis of secondary hypertension: an age-based approach. *Am Fam Physician.* 2010;82(12):1471-1478.

Box 16-1 Specific JNC 8 Recommendations

1. Individuals ≥ 60 years:
   - Initiate pharmacologic treatment if SPB is ≥ 150 mmHg or DBP is ≥ 90 mmHg.
   - Adjust treatment to achieve SPB < 150 mmHg or DBP < 90 mmHg.
2. Individuals < 60 years:
   - Initiate pharmacologic treatment if DBP is ≥ 90 mmHg.
   - Adjust treatment to reduce DBP to < 90 mmHg.
3. Individuals > 18 years with chronic kidney disease or diabetes:
   - Initiate pharmacologic treatment if SPB is ≥ 140 mmHg or DBP is ≥ 90 mmHg.
   - Adjust treatment to reduce SPB < 140 mmHg and DBP < 90 mmHg.

DBP = diastolic blood pressure, JNC = Joint National Commission, SBP = systolic blood pressure

Data from James P, Oparil S, Carter B, Cushman WC, Dennison-Himmelfarb C, Handler J, et al. 2014 evidence-based guideline for the management of high blood pressure in adults: report from the panel members appointed to the eighth Joint National Committee (JNC 8). *JAMA*. 2014;311(5):507-520.

level of 90 mmHg reduced adverse outcomes.[62] Based on an examination of the evidence, JNC 8 recommends initiating pharmacologic therapy and setting treatment goals based on an individual's age and the presence or absence of underlying chronic conditions, shown in **Box 16-1**.

The classes of medications in use for hypertensive treatment are described in the paragraphs that follow and summarized in **Table 16-6**.

Angiotensin receptor blockers (ARBs) block the action of the renin-angiotensin system and inhibit the action of angiotensin II at the receptor site. They are well tolerated. They do not cause cough and are rarely associated with angioedema. Therefore, they are generally preferable to angiotensin-converting enzyme inhibitors (ACEIs) if they are affordable, although they may be less effective in individuals of African descent compared to Caucasians when used alone in monotherapy. Because they interfere with fetal development by affecting the renin-angiotensin system, their use is contraindicated in pregnancy, particularly in the second and third trimesters.[11] Women of childbearing age who use ARBs or ACEIs should use an effective contraceptive or be transitioned to another medication.

ACEIs block the conversion of angiotensin I to angiotensin II by inhibiting angiotensin-converting enzyme.[11] Cough is common, particularly in women and individuals of Asian and African descent. These medications should not be prescribed to women who have had an episode of angioedema in the past because of the risk of recurrence while on ACEIs. Like the ARBs, these medications appear to be less effective in African Americans when used as monotherapy; however, no racial differences in treatment effects are seen when they are combined with diuretics or calcium channel blockers (CCBs) ACEIs should not be combined with the ARBs, because in combination (but not when prescribed alone) they can worsen kidney disease.[11] This category of medications is contraindicated during pregnancy.

Alpha-blockers (ABs) work by blocking the arterial alpha-adrenergic receptors, thereby reducing vasoconstriction. They are not commonly used, because there is less evidence documenting their clinical benefit in reducing sequelae associated

Table 16-6 Antihypertensive Medications

Antihypertensive Class	Examples—Drug Name (Trade Name)	Pregnancy and Breastfeeding Considerations
Angiotensin-converting enzyme inhibitors (ACEIs)	Benazepril (Lotensin) Captopril (Capoten) Enalapril (Vasotec) Lisinopril (Prinivil, Zestril) Moexipril (Univasc)	Contraindicated in pregnancy for all listed. Probably safe in breastfeeding for all listed.
Angiotensin receptor blockers (ARBs)	Candesartan (Atacand) Eprosartan (Teveten) Irbesartan (Avapro) Losartan (Cozaar) Valsartan (Diovan)	Contraindicated in pregnancy for all listed. Safety in breastfeeding varies by product; check before prescribing.
Alpha-blockers (ABs)	Doxazosin (Cardura) Prazosin (Minipress) Terazosin (Hytrin)	Pregnancy category C for all listed. Safety in breastfeeding unknown for all listed.
Beta-blockers (BBs)	Atenolol (Tenormin)	Contraindicated in pregnancy; probably unsafe with breastfeeding.
	Bisoprolol (Zebeta)	Trimester-specific recommendations; safety in breastfeeding unknown.
	Labetalol (Trandate)	Combined alpha- and beta-blocker. Pregnancy category C; probably safe with breastfeeding.
	Metoprolol (Toprol)	Trimester-specific recommendations; probably safe in breastfeeding.
Calcium channel blockers (CCBs)—non-dihydropyridines	Diltiazem (Cardizem CD, Dilacor XR, Tiazac)	Pregnancy category C; probably safe in breastfeeding.
	Verapamil (Calan, Isoptin)	Pregnancy category C; possibly unsafe in breastfeeding.
Calcium channel blockers (CCB)—dihydropyridines	Amlodipine (Norvasc)	Pregnancy category C; minimal data. Safety in breastfeeding unknown.
	Nifedipine (Procardia)	Pregnancy category C; safe in breastfeeding.
Centrally acting drugs	Clonidine (Catapres) Methyldopa (Aldomet)	Limited safety data; 2nd-line agent Safe in pregnancy (category B); safe in breastfeeding.
Direct vasodilators	Hydralazine (Apresoline)	Pregnancy category C; probably safe in breastfeeding.
Thiazide-type diuretics	Hydrochlorothiazide	Pregnancy category B; safe in breastfeeding but may reduce milk volume.

FDA pregnancy categories are being revised; at this time older drugs continue to be described in this manner. Typically, only categories A, B, and C are prescribed during pregnancy. B = Animal reproduction studies have failed to demonstrate a risk to the fetus and there are no adequate and well-controlled studies in pregnant women. C = Animal reproduction studies have shown an adverse effect on the fetus and there are no adequate and well-controlled studies in humans, but potential benefits may warrant use of the drug in pregnant women despite potential risks.

with hypertension. They are most often prescribed as adjunctive therapy for treatment-resistant hypertension or in men with hypertension who also have benign prostatic hypertrophy, because ABs reduce the size of the prostate gland.[11] They must be used with caution in the elderly, as they increase the likelihood that an older individual might experience postural hypotension causing falls.[63]

Beta-blockers (BBs) have been used for BP reduction for decades. The BBs decrease cardiac output and renin release from the kidney. They are particularly helpful in women with a history of MI, heart failure, or angina, although they are less effective in reducing the risk of stroke than other antihypertensives. They can also worsen glucose metabolism and are not recommended for use in diabetics. Side effects include bronchospasm, decreased libido, and fatigue. The combined alpha- and beta-blocker (labetalol) is safe for the fetus and is commonly used in pregnant and breastfeeding women who require antihypertensive therapy.[11]

Calcium channel blockers (CCBs) block the calcium-dependent contraction of vascular smooth muscle. They are categorized into two groups: 1) dihydropyridines, such as amlodipine and nifedipine, which work by dilating arteries; and 2) nondihydropyridines, such as diltiazem and verapamil, which reduce heart rate and contractility and dilate arteries to some degree. The most common side effect is peripheral edema. They are equally effective in all races and ethnicities, particularly when used in combination with ACEIs or ARBs. They also have the advantage of reducing proteinuria and are helpful in slowing fast heart rates associated with atrial fibrillation. CCBs have also been used in the treatment of conditions other than hypertension. They have been found to reduce the frequency and severity of Raynaud's disease.[64] However, they have several disadvantages. Care must be taken when combining CCBs with other antihypertensive medications. Non-dihydropyridine CCBs

cannot be safely used in combination with BBs.[11] Non-dihydropyridine CCBs also must be used with caution in older women, because, similarly to the ABs, they increase the risk of postural hypotension and subsequent falls compared to other antihypertensive products.

Centrally acting antihypertensive medications, while effective, are less frequently used due to bothersome side effects. Dry mouth and fatigue are common. One of the agents in this class, alpha-methyldopa (Aldomet), is commonly used to treat hypertension in pregnancy.[11]

Direct vasodilators are infrequently used because they often cause fluid retention and tachycardia. Therefore, if they are used, they are prescribed in combination with other products for the treatment of resistant hypertension.[11] In obstetric practice, hydralazine (Apresoline) is commonly used intravenously to manage hypertensive emergencies associated with severe preeclampsia.[65]

Mineralocorticoid receptor antagonists are reserved for use in the treatment of resistant hypertension. These agents block the binding of aldosterone to mineralocorticoid receptors, decrease the reabsorption of sodium, and have a mild diuretic effect. The best-known product in this class is spironolactone. Gynecomastia and sexual dysfunction are commonly reported side effects.[11]

Thiazide diuretics promote vasodilation and block the absorption of sodium.[11] They also block the excretion of calcium in the distal tubule, which has been shown to be somewhat protective against development of osteoporosis in elderly women. The primary side effects include hypokalemia, hypomagnesemia, hyponatremia, and gout.[11] Diuretics are most effective in reducing BP when combined with ARBs or ACEIs.

Deciding which pharmaceutic option is best depends on age, severity of hypertension, and the presence or absence of comorbidities. Usually, one product is started initially and the dose is maximized before adding on a second agent from a different class.[62] However, a two-agent regimen may be needed immediately for individuals with severe hypertension, defined as BP ≥ 160/100 mmHg.[11] Recommendations also differ by race and age. For those with only hypertension, African Americans should be prescribed either a CCB or a thiazide diuretic, white and other non-black individuals younger than age 60 an ARB or ACEI, and white and other non-black individuals 60 years of age or older a CCB or thiazide diuretic. If a second agent is needed to achieve a BP < 140/90 mmHg, then an ARB or ACEI should be added for black individuals, a CCB or thiazide diuretic for white and non-black individuals younger than 60 years, and an ARB or ACEI for white and non-black individuals 60 years of age or older.[11] These recommendations are based on the evidence that the degree of protection afforded by antihypertensives against kidney damage, heart failure, and stroke varies by the class of medication and by characteristics such as race, age, and presence of comorbidities.[11,62]

Women should have an office visit scheduled 2 to 4 weeks after treatment has begun depending on the severity of BP. The initially prescribed dose should be one-half the anticipated maximum dose. Doses can then be titrated upward every 2 to 3 weeks as needed to reach goal BP levels. Ideally, goal BP levels should be reached 6 to 8 weeks after treatment is started.[11] Once goal BP has been reached, office visits can be scheduled every 3 to 6 months. More frequent office visits may be required if BP is difficult to control or if other medical conditions are present. Poor adherence is a common reason for treatment failure and must always be addressed at each visit. Nonadherence can be due to forgetfulness, inability to tolerate side effects, or lack of resources to pay for the medication. Regular visits also provide an opportunity to support women in making healthy lifestyle changes that can lower

BP, which can eliminate or reduce the need for medications.

Midwives and other women's health providers may initiate antihypertensive therapy if that is within their expertise and institutional/jurisdictional scope of practice, and they are able to monitor women who have stable BPs on medications. Women whose BP remains elevated on medications or have abnormal EKG findings or cardiac symptoms should be referred to the cardiologist for an evaluation as soon as possible.

Management Issues Specific to Women

The management of hypertension in women can be challenging. Hypertension limits contraceptive choice, complicates preconception planning, adversely affects fetal and maternal health in pregnancy, and affects the management of menopausal symptoms.

CONTRACEPTION

Reproductive-aged women with hypertension are more limited in their contraceptive choices than normotensive women, particularly if they have end-organ damage. Selecting a contraceptive product that balances the need for safety with ease of use and efficacy can be especially difficult. In order to provide guidance, the World Health Organization (WHO) has established guidelines to provide women with underlying medical conditions the broadest array of options.[66] The Centers for Disease Control and Prevention have adapted these as the United States Medical Eligibility Criteria (US MEC) for contraceptive use.[67] Contraceptive options are rated for their safety in women with different underlying conditions such as migraine headaches, human immunodeficiency virus infection, and diabetes, as well as hypertension. Ratings range from 1 (safest) to

4 (least safe). WHO criteria are defined as follows for each condition:[66]

1. Use is not restricted; any woman can safely use.
2. The benefits generally outweigh associated risks for this contraceptive.
3. Risks outweigh benefits for this method most of the time.
4. The contraceptive method has a level of risk that is too high for safe use.

Of the hormonal options, progestin-only options are deemed safer than estrogen-containing products and can be used in most situations. Progestin-only pills, progestin contraceptive implants, and the Levonorgestrel Intrauterine System (LNG IUS) are rated as Category 1 and medroxyprogesterone (Depo-Provera) as Category 2. However, these ratings drop if the BP rises to ≥ 160/90 mmHg. With severe BP, progestin-only pills, progestin implants, and the LNG IUS drop to Category 2 and Depo-Provera to Category 3. Estrogen-containing products (combined oral contraceptives, vaginal ring, transdermal patch) should not be used if women have hypertension; they are deemed to be Category 3 or Category 4 medications.[66]

CHRONIC HYPERTENSION IN PREGNANCY

None of the first-line agents used in the management of hypertension are recommended for use during pregnancy.[68] ACEIs, ARBs, CCBs, and thiazide diuretics are all associated with theoretical or proven fetal or neonatal morbidities. ACEIs and ARBs have historically been considered unsafe only if used in the second or third trimesters; their use in mid- to late pregnancy has long been known to be associated with intrauterine growth restriction (IUGR), oligohydramnios, anuria, and fetal kidney failure. However, newer evidence suggests that exposure in the first trimester is associated with fetal cardiovascular, kidney, and central nervous system malformations.[69]

Whether diuretics should be used in pregnancy is debated. Diuretics lead to vascular constriction, which may theoretically increase the risk of worsening hypertension in pregnancy and placental hypoperfusion. There is little evidence to support this concern, although the use of thiazide diuretics is very rarely associated with maternal electrolyte disturbances and neonatal thrombocytopenia and hemolytic anemia.[69] Therefore, some authorities conclude that women already on thiazide diuretics may continue their use in pregnancy. Of note, the American College of Obstetricians and Gynecologists (ACOG) did not make any recommendation regarding the use of thiazide diuretics in its most recently released guideline.[68] While not commonly used in the management of hypertension, spironolactone, which has diuretic properties, should be stopped immediately because it is associated with fetal anti-androgen effects.[69]

Because many of the products used in the treatment of hypertension are associated with adverse fetal or neonatal outcomes, many women will need to stop their usual regimen in pregnancy. Whether they should be switched to other safer products or remain off medication is debated. Due to the normal decrease in vascular resistance found in pregnancy, BP levels are typically 10 mmHg lower at the end of the second trimester compared to prepregnancy levels.[65] Therefore, many authorities including ACOG recommend not restarting hypertension medications in women without evidence of end-organ damage unless BP levels exceed 150–160/100–110 mmHg.[65,69]

ACOG recommends the use of three products in pregnancy for the treatment of chronic hypertension: methyldopa, labetalol, or nifedipine.[68] Methyldopa (Aldomet) is a centrally acting antihypertensive medication.[65] While not widely used in the general population, the evidence documenting its safety is robust after more than 30 years of use in pregnancy. However, it may worsen depression and should be avoided or used with caution in women with mood disorders.[65] Another option recommended by ACOG is labetalol (Trandate, a combined AB and BB).[68] However, not all BBs are equally safe in pregnancy; atenolol, for example, is associated with IUGR and should not be used.[69] The other first-line agent recommended by ACOG is nifedipine (Procardia, a CCB). Its major disadvantage is that it complicates the management of superimposed preeclampsia. Women on nifedipine who require magnesium sulfate for the prevention of seizures may develop profound hypotension.[69]

Women who have not been in regular care may enter pregnancy with preexisting but unrecognized hypertension. The diagnosis of chronic hypertension may be masked by the normal decline in BP during the first two trimesters. The diagnosis of chronic hypertension in pregnancy is made on the basis of a prior diagnosis or persistent elevation of BP of at least 140/90 mmHg on 2 occasions more than 24 hours apart, before the 20th week of gestation. Some women may also be suspected of having preexisting chronic hypertension but not meet the definition due to late entry to care. These women can be considered to have developed chronic hypertension if BP elevations persist longer than 6 to 12 weeks postpartum.

Once the diagnosis of chronic hypertension is made, women need to be seen frequently, although the number and spacing of visits are individualized depending on maternal and fetal status. BP and urine protein should be assessed at each visit. Laboratory tests including CBC, platelet count, uric acid, 24-hour urine for protein, and liver enzymes are obtained to establish a baseline and repeated as necessary. Consultation with and/or referral to a physician for management of women with hypertension during pregnancy is essential. Pregnant women with chronic hypertension are at risk for superimposed preeclampsia and fetal growth restriction. Close monitoring for these complications is important. Baseline sonographic evaluation is recommended at 18 to 20 weeks' gestation. A follow-up sonogram can be obtained at 28 to 32 weeks and can be repeated monthly until term to ensure appropriate fetal growth. Nonstress tests and biophysical profiles are not essential in women with mild chronic hypertension as long as there is normal fetal growth and no evidence of preeclampsia. Serial nonstress tests, biophysical profiles, and umbilical artery Doppler velocimetry may be used if there is a suspicion of growth restriction or superimposed preeclampsia. Lifestyle modifications should also be recommended and include moderate exercise, healthy dietary intake, and appropriate weight gain based on a woman's prepregnancy BMI.

PREGNANCY-RELATED HYPERTENSION

Hypertension in pregnancy is classified into four categories:[67]

1. *Chronic hypertension* affects 1% to 5% of all pregnancies and is discussed in detail in the previous section.[65]

2. *Transient hypertension or gestational hypertension* affects 6% to 7% of all pregnancies. It occurs after the 20th week of pregnancy, presents without proteinuria, lacks other features of preeclampsia, and resolves soon after delivery.[65,68] Women who are overweight are at risk for this condition.

3. *Preeclampsia* affects 5% to 7% of all pregnancies.[65] It is defined as the presence of hypertension in conjunction with proteinuria ($\geq$ 300 mg in a 24-hour collection or $\geq$ 1+ in a random urine sample) after 20 weeks' gestation.[68] Edema is no longer one of the diagnostic criteria for preeclampsia because it so common in pregnancy.[65] Also of note is that preeclampsia can occur in the absence

of proteinuria. In the absence of proteinuria, preeclampsia is present if hypertension is associated with thrombocytopenia (platelet count of < 100,000 mcL), impaired liver function (liver transaminases twice normal concentration), renal insufficiency (elevated serum creatinine > 1.1 mg/dL or a doubling of serum creatinine), pulmonary edema, or new-onset cerebral or visual disturbances.[68] Abnormal coagulation studies and liver function tests; symptoms such as headache, visual changes, and epigastric pain; and higher levels of proteinuria make the diagnosis more certain. *Eclampsia* indicates the presence of seizure activity not due to other causes.

4. *Preeclampsia superimposed on chronic hypertension* has the features of both disorders. It is quite common, occurring in up to 25% of women with chronic hypertension.[65] Markers of concern depend on a woman's baseline status. In women who are well controlled, a sudden rise in BP or the development of new-onset proteinuria may indicate the presence of superimposed preeclampsia. The diagnosis in women with preexisting proteinuria or poorer control will be harder to make. In these women, sudden increases in proteinuria, BP levels, or the development of thrombocytopenia or transaminitis suggest superimposed preeclampsia.[65]

As a general rule, midwives and other women's health providers who care for women with hypertensive disorders during pregnancy do so in close consultation with a physician skilled in the management of these problems.[70]

MENOPAUSAL SYMPTOM MANAGEMENT

Women with hypertension are at higher risk for adverse cardiac events, making the management of menopausal symptoms more difficult. Risks can be cumulative—the more risks factors that are present (i.e., obesity, smoking, other comorbidities),

the greater the chance of complications with hormone replacement therapy (HRT). Therefore, the decision to prescribe HRT, the choice of product, and the duration of treatment for women with hypertension are not straightforward.[71] HRT use does not appear to worsen hypertension. In fact, use of HRT products containing drospirenone may slightly decrease BP.[71] However, the Women's Health Initiative trial showed a small, but significant, increased risk of cardiovascular events with HRT use.[72] If after careful consideration of risk a woman decides to use HRT, a transdermal patch may be a safer option.[71]

Alternative Therapies in the Management of Hypertension

The American Heart Association recently convened a panel of experts to review the evidence on the effectiveness of alternative strategies other than diet and medications in lowering BP.[73] They conducted an extensive review of the literature on meditation, acupuncture, exercise, and biofeedback techniques, among other modalities. Overall, the evidence was of insufficient quality to arrive at any conclusion about effectiveness of many alternative therapies. However, enough high-quality data were available to determine that transcendental meditation, some biofeedback techniques, and device-guided slow breathing were associated with modest reductions in BP. Exercise was associated with the greatest reductions in BP.[73]

Very few alternative therapies have been shown to reduce the risk of preeclampsia. Neither vitamin E nor vitamin C reduce the risk of developing preeclampsia in low-risk women.[68] Following a healthy diet was associated with a 33% reduction in risk (RR 0.67, 95% CI 0.53–0.85; $P = 0.001$) of developing preeclampsia in a meta-analysis of 6 studies.[74] Calcium supplementation can reduce the severity of preeclampsia but only in populations with insufficient intakes of calcium. High-risk women with a prior history of preeclampsia and a preterm delivery at < 34 weeks' gestation may benefit from taking daily low-dose aspirin (60 to 80 mg) beginning in the first trimester of pregnancy.[68]

Dyslipidemia

Dyslipidemia affects more than 50% of all women in the United States and increases the risk of subsequent cardiac disease.[75] In one large prospective cohort study (N = 1478), there was a significant dose relationship between length of exposure to dyslipidemia and CVD: After 15 years of follow up, CVD occurred in 4.4% for those with no exposure to elevated cholesterol levels, 8.1% for those with 1 to 10 years of exposure, and 16.5% for those with 11 to 20 years of exposure (P < 0.001).[76] Consequently, lowering cholesterol levels is critically important in preserving the health and wellbeing of women.

Physiology

Cholesterol plays a vital role in the synthesis of cell membranes, bile acids, and hormones. Triglycerides are used as a source of energy for muscles and stored as fat if intake exceeds demand. As important as these substances are for bodily function, neither is easily absorbed from the GI tract or transported in the blood, because they are not water soluble. However, when cholesterol and triglycerides are combined together, they form the lipoproteins, which with the help of the apoproteins are more soluble. The family of lipoproteins include: 1) chylomicrons, 2) very low-density lipoprotein (VLDL), 3) intermediate-density lipoprotein (IDL), 4) LDL, and 5) high-density lipoprotein (HDL). These lipoproteins differ in their composition, with each having various amounts of triglyceride and cholesterol. Each of these lipoproteins plays a role in the absorption, distribution, utilization, or removal of cholesterol from the body.

There are two primary pathways in the formation of lipoproteins: exogenesis and endogenesis. The exogenesis pathway involves the absorption of dietary cholesterol and triglycerides from the GI tract, where after absorption they are assembled together as chylomicrons and enter the lymphatic circulation with the help of apolipoprotein B. Apolipoprotein CII on the chylomicrons activates enzymes that convert triglycerides in the chylomicrons to fatty acids and glycerol that are released and taken up by muscle and fat cells. Thus, the chylomicrons play a role in meeting the energy needs of the body through the release of the triglyceride derivatives, fatty acid, and glycerol. The now triglyceride-depleted remnants of the chylomicrons are returned to and taken up into the liver by the LDL-like receptor cells.[77]

The endogenesis pathway involves the synthesis of lipoproteins within the liver. Excess triglycerides from circulating free fatty acids and chylomicron remnants are released as VLDL from the liver. VLDL is composed of 80% triglycerides and 20% cholesterol.[78] VLDL is hydrolyzed by lipoprotein lipase with help from apolipoprotein CII; this process releases triglycerides to the peripheral tissue and converts VLDL to IDL. IDL is composed of 50% cholesterol and 50% triglycerides. The liver can reabsorb some IDL, but IDL can also be hydrolyzed by hepatic lipase to form LDL. Like with VLDL, this process releases triglycerides for use by the peripheral tissue and lowers the amount of triglycerides within LDL. LDL is composed of 10% triglycerides and 90% cholesterol. Because LDL is composed mostly of cholesterol, it is the primary lipoprotein used in the body for the formation of steroid hormones, cell wall synthesis, and other processes requiring cholesterol.

HDL plays an important role in the reverse cholesterol transport system and by doing so is cardioprotective. HDL is released from the liver and intestine. In its original form, it is composed primarily of phospholipid and apolipoprotein A-1 and has very little cholesterol.[77] "Immature" HDL is then primed to remove unesterified cholesterol from peripheral cells, such as the macrophages, through the ABC1 transporter protein.[77] HDL then returns to the liver where it is processed and its cholesterol is excreted into bile or used to create steroidal hormones. In this process, HDL plays a critical role in lowering the levels of intracellular cholesterol.[78] It also can reduce cardiovascular risk through a number of other pathways: It inhibits LDL and phospholipid oxidation, preserves endothelial function, decreases levels of adhesive proteins, and has antithrombotic and anti-inflammatory properties.[77,79]

Defects in any of these pathways can lead to dyslipidemia. Congenital deficiencies of lipoprotein lipase or apolipoprotein CII can result in severe elevations of triglycerides and chylomicrons. Familial genetic disorders can lead to elevations of LDL cholesterol alone or elevations of LDL and triglycerides. Some individuals may have defects in processes that remove VLDL remnant particles; high levels of VLDL raise cholesterol and triglyceride levels. Other conditions such as diabetes, nephrosis, or medications can result in high levels of triglycerides.[78] Excessive dietary intake of calories and high-fat foods and limited exercise also raise triglycerides. Whatever the process, higher levels of triglycerides are associated with a decrease in the production of HDL, an increase in the production of VLDL and LDL, and insulin resistance.[80]

Excess LDL can lead to plaque formation within the arterial system. Oxidized LDL is deposited under the endothelial cells at arterial branch points, where blood flow is turbulent. In response, the endothelial cells secrete chemical attractants and increase the activity of adhesive proteins. Monocytes are recruited to the site. Once they enter the subendothelial space, they transform to macrophages. The earliest lesion of atherosclerosis is the fatty streak, which is a mass of extracellular lipids, macrophages, and smooth muscle cells. These lesions progress over time to become fibrofatty plaques in the intima of arteries. The accumulation of lipids in the macrophages leads to the formation of foam cells, release of cytokines, and ultimately cell death. This triggers increased migration of macrophages into the region, localized inflammation, and an ever-expanding vicious cycle of LDL deposition, macrophage recruitment, plaque formation, and cell death.[81] Eventually, the deposition becomes large enough to encroach into the lumen of the artery, narrowing and eventually blocking the lumen completely.[78]

Management

The primary treatment modality for dyslipidemia is lifestyle modification with the addition of medications for those with overt CVD or at high risk of progression to overt disease. The National Cholesterol Education Program (NCEP), under the auspices of the National Heart, Lung, and Blood Institute, has released a series of guidelines for the treatment and management of high cholesterol since 1988. Each of the first three guidelines—Adult Treatment Panel I (ATP I), Adult Treatment Panel II (ATP II), and Adult Treatment Panel III (ATP III)—stressed the importance of lowering LDL cholesterol. The National Heart, Lung, and Blood Institute transitioned the responsibility of evaluating the evidence to the American Heart Association and the American College of Cardiology midway through the development of the most current guideline, Adult Treatment Panel IV (ATP IV). In this transition, the ATP IV has been transformed from being a comprehensive guideline, developed from evidence from RCTs supplemented by expert opinion where evidence was lacking, to treatment guidelines focused on medication management. Therefore, clinicians desiring a more comprehensive clinical view of the management of dyslipidemia may still find utility in referencing the ATP III.[82]

Of the previous guidelines, ATP III was the most aggressive, setting cutoffs for total cholesterol, LDL, HDL, and triglyceride levels that were thought to be optimal, acceptable, or elevated based on risk—with those at higher risk having lower goal levels.[83] ATP III also incorporated the presence or absence of risk factors such as smoking, BP, and age into the determination of whether medications were needed. Further, ATP III stressed the importance of lowering LDL levels to goal levels, because elevated LDL levels promote the progression of atherosclerosis. It also recommended treatment of metabolic syndrome.[83] The newest guidelines have abandoned many of these recommendations.

The new guidelines will result in substantive changes in how dyslipidemia is managed in clinical practice.[84] ATP IV has abandoned the "treat to goal" paradigm recommended by ATP III. The treat-to-goal strategy has never been tested in RCTs; rather, the doses of cholesterol-lowering medications in RCTs were based on set doses. Treating to set goals for LDL levels can result in using doses that exceed the doses used in the RCTs, making this strategy more expensive and more likely to be associated with adverse reactions and side effects with no proven benefit. The ATP IV guidelines recommend only two levels of treatment: high intensity for those at highest risk and medium intensity for those at lower risk or who are unable to tolerate high-dose statin therapy. High-intensity therapy usually results in a reduction of LDL cholesterol of more than 50% and medium-intensity therapy a decline in LDL levels of between 30% and 50%.[84] Further, the panel found no high-quality evidence to support the use of other pharmacologic options long used in the management of dyslipidemia—specifically, fibrates, nicotinic acid (niacin), bile acid sequestrants, and omega-3 fatty acids.

ATP IV recommends the use of statin therapy alone. Statins should be *offered* to four high-risk groups:[84]

1. Those 75 years of age or younger with clinical atherosclerotic CVD defined as acute coronary syndromes, history of MI, stable or unstable angina, coronary or other arterial revascularization, stroke, transient ischemic attack, or peripheral arterial disease presumed to be of atherosclerotic origin

2. Those 21 years of age or older with LDL cholesterol ≥ 190 mg/dL

3. Those with diabetes, aged 40 to 75 years, and an LDL cholesterol level between 70 and 189 mg/dL

4. Those with a 10-year risk of atherosclerotic CVD of at least 7.5%, aged 40 to 75 years, no diabetes, and an LDL cholesterol level between 70 and 189 mg/dL

Treatment can also be *considered* in other situations: in individuals between 40 and 75 years of age with a 10-year risk of 5% to 7.5% and in individuals with other risk factors. These include primary LDL cholesterol ≥ 160 mg/dL or other evidence of genetic dyslipidemias, family history of premature atherosclerotic CVD with onset before 55 years of age in a first-degree male relative or before 65 years of age in a first-degree female relative, high-sensitivity CRP ≥ 2 mg/L, a coronary artery score (CAC) ≥ 300 Agatston units, or an ankle-brachial index < 0.9, which is a test used to determine the presence of peripheral artery disease.[84]

The ATP IV no longer recommends "counting" risk factors to determine if statin therapy is needed. Rather, it recommends the use of the new revised 10-year risk calculator (based on Pooled Cohort Equations) to determine whether medication management is warranted.[85] The revised risk calculator adds new cardiovascular endpoints of concern, fatal and nonfatal stroke, to the original ones (nonfatal MI and cardiac death). Consequently, it is expected to identify more individuals at risk and increase the numbers of individuals for whom statins should be considered. Because it has not been tested in prospective trials, some experts believe that the new risk calculator will overestimate the need for statin use in the general population.[86]

Medication Management

Pharmacologic therapy is often required to lower LDL levels to an acceptable level, especially in high-risk individuals. Five classes of medications have historically been prescribed for cholesterol control: nicotinic acid (niacin), bile acid sequestrants, fibric acid derivatives, selective cholesterol absorption inhibitors, and 3-hydroxy-3-methylglutaryl-coenzyme A (HMG CoA) reductase inhibitors (statins). The ATP IV guidelines unequivocally recommend statins as the only first-line option. However, it is possible that medications within the other classes may play a role in the management of dyslipidemia in those individuals who are unable to achieve control on statin regimens or unable to tolerate them.[87] Unfortunately, ATP IV did not address how best to manage these clinical situations. Newer agents such as the peroxisome proliferator-activated receptor (PPAR) dual (alpha/gamma) agonists, also known as the "glitizars," are currently being investigated and may become alternative agents used in statin-intolerant individuals.[88]

NICOTINIC ACID (NIACIN)

Niacin is associated with dramatic improvements in lipid profiles, reducing LDL levels by 20% and triglycerides by 20% to 30% and raising HDL levels by 20% to 25%.[89] It impairs the hepatic synthesis of VLDL, which is essential for the production of LDL. Niacin has been shown to reduce cardiovascular events in numerous studies, but the evidence on the relationship between niacin as monotherapy and reductions in cardiovascular death is weak.[89] Adding niacin to a statin-only regimen has not been shown to improve outcomes and is associated with significantly higher rates of rash, itch, and new-onset diabetes.[89] Even monotherapy at a low dose can cause flushing, which many individuals find intolerable. Therefore, niacin is unlikely to play a significant role in the management of dyslipidemia in the future.

BILE ACID SEQUESTRANTS

Bile acid sequestrants are the oldest available agents and are particularly beneficial in that they lower LDL levels and improve glucose metabolism.[88] They inhibit the return of bile acids from the bowel to the liver, which decreases the production of cholesterol and increases its excretion in the feces. Their chief side effects are GI symptoms, which limit their tolerability. Because their use has not been shown to reduce cardiovascular mortality, they are not recommended as a first-line agent in the treatment for dyslipidemia.[90] However, they could potentially be used as adjunctive therapy, particularly among individuals with both dyslipidemia and diabetes.

FIBRIC ACID DERIVATIVES

Fibric acid derivatives rapidly lower dangerously elevated triglycerides and can also raise HDL levels. They are associated with reductions of 10% to 11% in the incidence of cardiac events such as nonfatal MI and cardiac interventions, but they have not been shown to reduce cardiovascular mortality.[89] In some studies, they are associated with an increase in all-cause mortality.[91] Adding a statin does not seem to improve outcomes. In the future, they are likely to be little used in the management of dyslipidemia, except in the rare instance that an individual also has significantly elevated triglycerides.[90]

SELECTIVE CHOLESTEROL ABSORPTION INHIBITORS

Ezetimibe is the first agent in the class of the selective cholesterol absorption inhibitors. It inhibits the absorption of cholesterol from the GI and biliary tracts. It has been found to be particularly effective in individuals with diabetes or CHD. Compared to statin therapy alone, an ezetimibe-statin combined regimen is associated with a 26% to 28% reduction in LDL cholesterol in these populations. Some studies also suggest that ezetimibe may improve glucose tolerance. However, to date, no improvements in cardiovascular deaths have been reported, although a trial investigating the impact of ezetimibe on cardiovascular death, major coronary events, and stroke is currently underway.[88]

HMG CoA REDUCTASE INHIBITORS (STATINS)

Statins are considered the gold standard of cholesterol management. They are highly effective in lowering LDL and, therefore, the risk for CHD. They inhibit the HMG CoA reductase enzyme, which is essential for the synthesis of cholesterol. They also increase the uptake of LDL by the liver. They have been shown to inhibit adhesion molecules and cytokine production, improve endothelial function, and reduce platelet aggregation and deposition, endothelial vasodilation, and blood viscosity. These processes can prevent thrombin formation, which may be the reason for their effectiveness in stroke prevention.[92]

ATP IV has simplified monitoring of statin monotherapy.[84] Women should be asked about baseline fatigue and muscle aches before initiating therapy. The only recommended baseline laboratory test is a transaminase (alanine transaminase; ALT) level. Further hepatic testing is needed only in individuals who report symptoms suggestive

of hepatotoxicity (i.e., dark urine, fatigue, yellowing of the skin, abdominal pain, or loss of appetite.) ATP IV recommends routine monitoring of glucose metabolism, because statin use raises the risk of developing new-onset diabetes. ATP IV also recommends against routine monitoring with CK in individuals receiving statin therapy; rather, a CK level should be obtained, along with creatinine and urinary myoglobinuria, only if an individual reports muscle pain, tenderness, stiffness, cramping, weakness, or fatigue.[84] These symptoms may indicate rhabdomyolysis. Rhabdomyolysis is a rare but very serious side effect of statin use in which muscle tissue is damaged. Byproducts of skeletal muscle destruction can accumulate in the renal tubules and produce acute renal failure. If rhabdomyolysis is suspected, statin use should be stopped immediately.

One of the most common reasons individuals stop statin use is myalgia. Of the individual statins, simvastatin and pravastatin appear to be better tolerated than others.[93] For those individuals intolerant of statins, a recent systematic review of the literature suggests that combination therapy with a low-dose statin and either a bile acid sequestrant or ezetimibe is likely to be more effective than other approaches. However, the authors point out that these approaches should be used with caution, because there are no clinical data on long-term benefits or harms.[94] Further safety monitoring is more complex in those using dual therapy for dyslipidemia. ATP IV gives specific recommendations about identifying reasonable candidates, baseline testing, and monitoring for each of the classes of commonly used dyslipidemia medications.

Alternative Therapies

The quality of the evidence makes it difficult to determine if vitamins or antioxidants can reduce the risk of CVD. Oxidative stress and the oxidation of LDL have been shown to be important steps in the progression of coronary heart disease. Observational studies on populations with high intakes of omega-3 fatty acids showed a relationship with better cardiovascular health; however, clinical trials on the impact of antioxidant supplementation on the prevention or progression of CVD have had conflicting results.[91] The impact of omega-3 fatty acids on insulin resistance is unclear. Similarly, supplementation with vitamins E, C, and D has not shown consistent improvements in cardiovascular health in the studies conducted to date.[95] Folic acid supplementation has been found to reduce homocysteine levels, but has not consistently been found to reduce cardiovascular events or deaths. Further research is needed to determine if there is a role for supplementation in the promotion of cardiovascular health.

Metabolic Syndrome

The ATP III identified metabolic syndrome as a new secondary target for cardiovascular risk-reduction therapy.[60] *Metabolic syndrome* is a constellation of atherosclerotic risk factors including 1) triglycerides $\geq$ 150 mg/dL, 2) HDL < 50 mg/dL in women, 3) central obesity (waist circumference > 35 inches in women), and 4) hypertension ($\geq$ 130/85 mmHg). The diagnosis is made when three or more of these risk factors are present. Women with this syndrome have an increased risk of developing coronary artery disease and stroke. However, more recently the utility of this designation has been called into question.[96] These risk factors are also risk factors for hypertension and diabetes. Further, the management of these risk factors is no different from current recommendations for the treatment of obesity, dyslipidemia, or hypertension. Given this, ATP IV recommends that individuals be counseled on the reduction of their individual

risks and makes no recommendations specific to the management of metabolic syndrome.[84]

Dyslipidemia and Pregnancy

The identification and management of dyslipidemia in women of reproductive age deserve special attention. While dyslipidemia is a chronic problem, suspension or delaying of treatment due to pregnancy or lactation has not been found to increase maternal mortality. The normal changes that occur during pregnancy cause a significant rise in all the sub-fractions of the total cholesterol profile. These elevations may persist for more than 1 year postpartum. The only recommended treatment for dyslipidemia during pregnancy and lactation is to eat healthy and to stay active. Pharmacologic management during pregnancy and lactation is contraindicated. Cholesterol and other products of cholesterol biosynthesis are essential components for fetal development.

Venous Thromboembolism

VTE occurs when a blood clot forms in a vein. The location can vary and be in the deep veins of the legs or pelvis (DVT), the superficial veins of the legs (superficial venous thromboembolism, SVT), or in the lungs (pulmonary embolism [PE]). DVT is far more prevalent than PE, accounting for 66% of the cases of symptomatic VTE. PE is less common and more deadly with a mortality rate of 12% compared to 6% for DVT. One of the primary sources for a PE is thought to be from a DVT, because 70% of individuals with a PE also have a DVT.[97] Overall, VTE is the third most common vascular disorder; only MI and stroke are more common.[98] It disproportionally affects reproductive-aged women compared to similarly aged men and older populations.[99] Conditions associated with VTE are listed in **Table 16-7**.

Table 16-7 Risk Factors for Thromboembolism

Cancer
Coagulation factor disorders
Infections
Inflammatory disease
Medications: oral contraceptives, hormone
    replacement therapy
Obesity
Pregnancy and postpartum
Prolonged bedrest
Smoking
Surgery
Trauma
Travel

Physiology

The underlying pathophysiology that prompts thromboembolism is the same wherever a clot develops. Any one of the following mechanisms can disrupt normal hemodynamic balance and result in the formation of a clot: 1) stasis and low oxygen tension in the vessel, 2) activation of the endothelium lining the veins, 3) activation of blood platelets, 4) activation of innate and acquired immunity, and 5) change in the concentration and nature of microparticles and pro- and anticoagulant proteins.[98]

Stasis is associated with many conditions such as varicosities, obesity, pregnancy, and travel and contributes to hypoxia within the blood vessels. Areas of hypoxia, particularly behind the deep venous valves, can cause an inflammatory response resulting in activation of the endothelium. Activation of the endothelium results in the release of granules containing von Willebrand factor and P-selectin, the upregulation of other adhesive receptors, and the local recruitment of monocytes, granulocytes, platelets, and microparticles.[98,100] Both von Willebrand factor and P-selectin bind to the endothelial surface and also with other constituents of the blood such as platelets, erythrocytes, and leukocytes. Among the leukocytes, monocytes are the cells that most readily synthesize tissue factor, particularly under hypoxic conditions.[100] In combination with calcium, tissue factor converts Factor VII$_a$ to Factor VII. In turn, Factor VII is converted to Factor X in the presence of calcium and phospholipid.[101] These processes are known as the extrinsic pathway of coagulation.

The intrinsic pathway plays a lesser role in coagulation. Damage to constituents of the blood, such as the granulocytes, from hypoxia and inflammation, releases substances that allow contact between triggers in the blood and Factor XII; these processes then initiate the coagulation cascade within the intrinsic pathway.[101] Substances that can trigger the intrinsic pathway include bacteria; lipoproteins such as chylomicrons, VLDLs, and oxidized LDLs; and inorganic polyphosphates, which are released by activated platelets at the site of the original injury.[98] Processes that trigger the extrinsic pathway, as well as chronic inflammation and acute infection, play a role in activating the intrinsic pathway.[98]

The intrinsic and extrinsic pathways converge into the common pathway at the level of Factor X and Factor Xa. In the common pathway, Factor Xa converts prothrombin to thrombin. In turn, thrombin converts fibrinogen to fibrin.[101] Fibrin is the substance that binds the developing thrombus to the vessel wall. Activated platelets, released at the site of the injury, set in motion a self-renewing process that recruits other platelets to the injury site and results in an ever-enlarging thrombus (**Figure 16-1**).[101]

Conditions that affect these pathways are associated with an increased risk of thromboembolism. Individuals with conditions associated with chronic inflammation such as rheumatoid arthritis, inflammatory bowel disease, and

Figure 16-1 Coagulation cascade/intrinsic and extrinsic pathway.

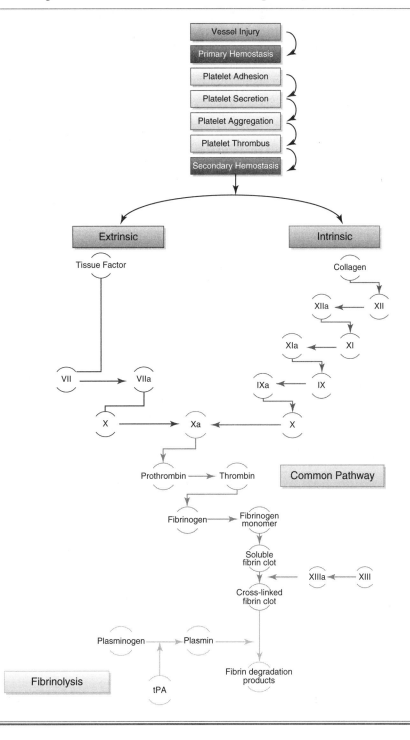

antiphospholipid syndrome are at greater risk of thromboembolism. Microparticles, which are submicron vesicles shed from the surface of intravascular cells (among them platelets, endothelial cells, and leukocytes), are thought to play a role in the increased risk of thromboembolism found in individuals with cancer. Although the exact mechanism is little understood, complexes between tissue factor and microparticles are higher in individuals with cancer than in healthy individuals.[98]

Genetic factors also affect increased risk of thromboembolism. Deficiencies in the natural anticoagulants—antithrombin, protein C, and protein S—are associated with a 10-fold increased risk of thromboembolism.[98] Other genes influence the procoagulant potential of the blood: prothrombin G20201A, Factor V Leiden, and blood group non-O. The risk of thromboembolism is increased two to three times for prothrombin G20210 and three to five times for Factor V Leiden. Blood group non-O doubles the risk of thromboembolism.[98]

Assessment

The symptoms associated with VTE are nonspecific. Fifty percent or more of individuals with DVT report tenderness, pain, and swelling in a lower extremity; about 50% with PE report chest pain, tachypnea, and dyspnea.[101] These symptoms are also present in many other conditions, making it difficult to diagnosis DVT or PE by symptoms alone. Consequently, many advocate the use of pretest probability scoring systems to determine what specific tests are best used in various situations. A number of scoring systems are available. Risk determination is based on a numerical score based on signs and symptoms, the number of risk factors present, and the degree of risk attached to specific risk factors. Weaker risk factors with associated odds ratios of less than 2 for VTE include prolonged bed rest, sitting in a car or airplane for more than 8 hours, age, obesity, pregnancy, and varicose veins. Intermediate risk factors with odds ratios between 2 and 9 include cancer, hormone or oral contraceptive use, pregnancy/postpartum, previous thromboembolism, and thrombophilia. High-risk factors with odds ratios greater than 10 include major general surgery, major trauma, and spinal cord injury.[97]

Deep Vein Thrombosis

The specific test chosen varies not only by the number and quality of risk factors that are present, but also by whether a DVT or PE is the condition of concern. The two test modalities used to evaluate a possible DVT include the D-dimer assay and duplex ultrasonography. *D-dimer assays* measure the presence of fibrin degradation products in the blood. Fibrin degradation products are produced as a result of fibrinolysis, which is the process by which a blood clot is dissolved. A D-dimer assay is fast, reliable, and readily available, making it the first-line choice for evaluating a potential DVT in individuals with low-risk factors. It is a highly sensitive test with a negative predictive value of 94% and therefore can be used to rule out the presence of a DVT in low-risk individuals.[97] However, a positive test in low-risk individuals should be confirmed with additional testing; other conditions such as pregnancy and renal impairment can cause false-positive results. In this situation, duplex ultrasonography is preferred.[21,97,102]

Duplex ultrasonography combines grey-scale imaging using transducer compression maneuvers with color-flow Doppler imaging and Doppler waveform analysis. Transducer compression maneuvers allow for visualization of the intraluminal thrombosis by compression of the veins along their length by the transducer. Color-flow Doppler imaging assesses the blood flow through the thrombosed area and is particularly helpful in areas difficult to reach with compression maneuvers. Normal blood flow can also be assessed via Doppler waveform analysis and should show spontaneous respirophasic flow.[103] A positive test result confirms the presence of DVT.[102]

The investigation of a potential DVT in intermediate- and high-risk women is more complicated because of the greater likelihood that a DVT is present in these women compared to low-risk women. A high-risk profile includes having three or more of the following: active cancer; paralysis, paresis, or cast of lower extremity; immobilization in previous 4 days or major surgery within 4 weeks; localized tenderness along the distribution of deep vein system; entire leg swollen; calf swollen by more than 3 cm; pitting edema; or collateral superficial veins.[102] Low-risk women have none of these conditions, whereas intermediate-risk women have one or two.

Duplex ultrasound is considered to be the first-line test for women at higher risk with a suspected DVT. If it is negative, a D-dimer assay should be obtained. If the D-dimer is negative, DVT can be ruled out. A positive D-dimer assay is highly suggestive, but not diagnostic of, the presence of a DVT. Therefore, a positive D-dimer requires a follow-up duplex ultrasound in 1 week.[97] Sensitivity and specificity of a duplex sonogram are highest in symptomatic individuals. It is less accurate in evaluating potential DVTs if they are located in the calf or upper extremity. It is also difficult to distinguish between an old and new clot.[97,102] Consequently, serial sonograms are sometimes necessary to help determine the diagnosis.

PULMONARY EMBOLISM

A different panel of tests is used to investigate a possible PE; these include an EKG, chest x-ray, blood gases, measurement of oxygen saturation, and other tests. Because of the strain on the right side of the heart, specific EKG changes can be seen with a PE: supraventricular

arrhythmia, P-pulmonale, T-wave inversion on precordial leads, right bundle branch block, and $S_1Q_3T_3$ pattern (although this latter pattern is uncommon).[95,102] Findings on the chest x-ray are nonspecific and may include platelike atelectasis, pleural effusion, and an elevated hemidiaphragm. Hypoxemia is common but may not be present in all cases.[97]

As with DVT, use of a scoring system can aid in the identification of PE. Clinical signs, symptoms, and the presence or absence of risk factors can be used to determine if a woman is at low, intermediate, or high risk.[97,102] The Institute for Clinical Systems Improvement's algorithm suggests that a score of > 4 is highly suggestive of PE. The scoring algorithm is provided in **Table 16-8**.[102]

Which additional tests are ordered is based on the severity of a woman's presentation and her underlying risk profile.[102] D-dimer assays play a limited role in the evaluation of PE and are generally only used as first-line testing in low-risk

Table 16-8 Risk Scoring Algorithm for VTE

Indicator	Score
Clinical signs	3
Alternative diagnosis unlikely	3
Heart rate > 100	1.5
Immobilization previous 4 days	1.5
Previous DVT or PE	1.5
Hemoptysis	1
Cancer treatment for the last 6 months	1

DVT = deep vein thrombosis, PE = pulmonary embolism, VTE = venous thromboembolism

Reproduced from Wells PS, Anderson DR, Bormanis J, et al. Value of assessment of pretest probability of DVT in clinical management. *Lancet*. 1997:350;1795-98. Copyright 1997, with permission from Elsevier.

women. Women who are at low risk of a PE but who have a positive D-dimer assay are recommended to have a follow-up CT pulmonary angiogram.[102] During a CT pulmonary angiogram, an iodine contrast agent is introduced through an IV line and a series of images is obtained of the pulmonary vascular bed.

Urgent evaluation is required if a massive PE is suspected so that treatment can be instituted as soon as possible. A massive PE should be suspected if a woman is hemodynamically unstable (defined as a systolic BP $\leq$ 90 mmHg or a drop of 40 mmHg), reports syncope or respiratory distress, has severe hypoxemia, or whose imaging studies show 50% or more absent perfusion or whose echocardiogram shows right ventricular strain or failure.[102] Individuals who are hemodynamically unstable may only require a bedside echocardiogram to confirm the diagnosis. While not available in all settings, a multidetector CT pulmonary angiogram is the test of choice in less acute situations. It is often the first imaging test performed for high-risk women with a less acute presentation. If it is not available, a ventilation/perfusion (V/Q) scan is an acceptable alternative.[102] The multidetector CT pulmonary angiogram has largely replaced traditional pulmonary angiography and the V/Q scan. It is less invasive than a traditional pulmonary angiography and easier to interpret than a V/Q scan.[97] It also has the advantage of being able to better detect other conditions that can mimic a PE. Because it has high specificity and low sensitivity, it is better at ruling out a PE than it is in diagnosing one. Consequently, a negative multidetector CT pulmonary angiogram requires additional testing to confirm or refute a diagnosis of PE.[102]

SUPERFICIAL VENOUS THROMBOEMBOLISM

SVT is far more common than either DVT or PE. It should be suspected if a tender cord is palpated along a superficial vein on physical exam. Often the area is red and swollen.[104] Historically, it has been thought to be a relatively benign condition, but newer evidence suggests that it is associated with a concomitant DVT in nearly 25% of cases.[104] In addition, 50% of the DVTs accompanying an SVT are not contiguous with the SVT. Therefore, most authorities recommend a duplex ultrasound when evaluating a suspected SVT. D-dimer assays have not been found to be useful in the diagnosis of an isolated SVT.[104]

Treatment

The goals of anticoagulation therapy are to allow natural fibrinolysis to occur and to prevent further growth of the thrombosis, embolism, and future recurrence.[101] While it is beyond the scope of this chapter to discuss treatment of the various thromboembolic conditions in depth, this section highlights several management issues relevant to the treatment of SVT, DVT, and PE.

No consensus has yet been reached on the appropriate treatment of an isolated SVT. If an accompanying DVT is found during the workup, treatment should be the same as for any DVT. However, treatment for an isolated SVT depends on the risk status of the affected individual and the size and location of the SVT. The risk that a DVT is present increases dramatically if the SVT affects the perforating veins or is < 3 cm from the saphenofemoral junction. An SVT located < 3 cm from the saphenofemoral junction or one that is larger than 5 cm has been suggested by some authorities to require treatment, although recommended regimens differ in these two situations. According to Scott, Mahdi, and Alikhan, an SVT close to the saphenofemoral junction requires treatment using a therapeutic anticoagulant regimen, whereas a large clot farther from the saphenofemoral junction requires treatment only with fondaparinux for 45 days.[104] Fondaparinux (Arixtra) is an indirect Factor 10a inhibitor.[105]

A number of treatment options are available for the management of DVT and PE depending on risk profile and suspected condition. For individuals with PE, the American College of Chest Physicians recommends initial treatment with parenteral anticoagulation (i.e., low-molecular-weight heparin, fondaparinux, or intravenous or subcutaneous unfractionated heparin).[106] These same medications, with the addition of oral rivaroxaban, can also be used in the initial management of DVT. The Institute for Clinical Systems Improvement essentially agrees, recommending the use of low-molecular-weight heparin or fondaparinux in the initial management of DVT.[102] These same products (with the addition of unfractionated heparin) are also recommended for the treatment of PE.[102] Low-molecular-weight heparin is a reliable anticoagulant and is given subcutaneously. It has the advantage of requiring no laboratory monitoring except in special circumstances. Unfractionated heparin is given by continuous intravenous infusion. It can provide protection against recurrent thromboembolism within 24 hours after therapeutic levels are reached, which is defined as having an aPTT 1.5 to 2.5 times normal.[102] Fondaparinux is given once daily subcutaneously. The duration of treatment with any of the initial regimens is short, lasting at minimum 5 days from time of diagnosis to the start of maintenance therapy to allow for full anticoagulant effect to be achieved before transitioning to a maintenance regimen.[101]

Warfarin (Coumadin), a vitamin K antagonist, is the most commonly used maintenance product, although newer oral products are becoming available.[105] It can be started immediately—at the time that the initial parenteral regimen begins. While inexpensive, warfarin has a narrow therapeutic window and requires ongoing monitoring throughout treatment. Adequate levels are determined by following the INR; goal INR is 2.5 (range 2.0–3.0). The other newer oral products coming onto the market do not require ongoing monitoring.[105] They appear to be well tolerated. While their use is increasing, what their role will be in the management of PE and DVT is yet to be determined.

Particular care must be used when prescribing warfarin to nonpregnant reproductive-aged women. Women should be counseled that exposure in the first trimester is associated with fetal defects in 25% or more of pregnancies. Therefore, an effective contraceptive plan should be in place for women of reproductive age. Warfarin is classified by the Food and Drug Administration as Category X and should not be prescribed to women during pregnancy. The American Academy of Pediatrics considers warfarin to be compatible with breastfeeding.[107]

Duration of maintenance treatment with warfarin is individualized.[102] One of the factors influencing the duration of treatment is whether the thromboembolic event was thought to be associated with transient, persistent, or unrecognized risk factors. Transient risk factors include recent immobilization, general surgery, use of oral contraceptives, and current or recent pregnancy. Individuals with transient risk factors are generally treated with anticoagulation therapy for 3 to 6 months.[101] Individuals with persistent or unrecognized risk factors receive treatment at minimum for 3 to 6 months of treatment, but may have their treatment regimen extended beyond this time period. No consensus has been reached about what is the best treatment approach for individuals at higher risk of recurrence. Because the recurrence rate for individuals with unprovoked thromboembolism is 10% in the first year and 30% in the 5 years after the index event, some individuals may require indefinite treatment.[105]

Pregnancy and Postpartum

Because pregnancy is a hypercoagulable state, risk of VTE increases 5-fold in pregnancy and 60-fold in the first 3 months postpartum compared to nonpregnant women.[108] During pregnancy, the levels of pro-coagulation factors increase, levels of anticoagulation factors like protein S decrease, and the velocity of blood flow slows in the lower extremities. These changes set the stage for the development of VTE. The risk of VTE is further exaggerated in pregnant women with underlying risk factors. Personal characteristics increase risk of a VTE: age > 35 years (odds ratio [OR] 2.1, 95% CI 2.0, 2.3), smoking 10 to 30 cigarettes a day (OR 2.1, 95% CI1.3, 3.4), and BMI > 30 kg/m^2 (OR 7.7, 95% CI 3.2, 19). Pregnancy-related conditions also increase risk: singleton in vitro fertilization (OR 4.5, 95% CI 2.0, 9.4), preeclampsia (OR 3.1, 95% CI 1.8, 5.3), vaginal delivery with infection (OR 20.2, 95% CI 6.4, 63.5), and postpartum hemorrhage after vaginal delivery of > 1000 mL (OR 4.1, 95% CI 2.3, 7.3).[108]

Diagnosing VTE is more difficult in pregnant than nonpregnant women. Not only are the signs and symptoms of VTE also commonly seen in normal pregnancy, testing is less accurate. The only clinical pearl suggestive of a DVT is if symptoms occur in the left leg, particularly if the calf of the left leg is 2 cm or more larger than the right leg. For unknown reasons, 70% to 80% of DVTs in pregnant women occur in the left leg.[108] Commonly used scoring systems have not been validated in pregnancy, making it more difficult to systematically identify higher risk women. In addition, D-dimer levels normally increase in pregnancy, complicating the interpretation of the assay. Some authorities suggest that a duplex ultrasound should be the first-line test in pregnancy.[108] Both a V/Q scan and multidetector CT pulmonary angiogram, commonly used in nonpregnant women, expose the fetus to low doses of radiation; therefore, magnetic resonance direct thrombus imaging, depending on the suspected location of the VTE, may be preferred over these imaging modalities. However, it should be noted that V/Q scans and multidetector CT pulmonary angiograms are *not* contraindicated in pregnancy, because the risk of death from an undiagnosed VTE is high.[108]

Unfractionated heparin and low-molecular-weight heparin are the two most commonly used medications for the treatment and prophylaxis of VTE in pregnancy. Neither medication crosses the placental barrier, unlike warfarin. Generally, low-molecular-weight heparin is the preferred product, because if given in weight-adjusted doses it does not require laboratory monitoring. Low-molecular-weight heparin is less likely to cause thrombocytopenia or untoward bleeding.[108] Pregnant women require twice-daily dosing due to increased renal clearance in pregnancy.

Adaptations in the regimen need to be made at the end of pregnancy. Because the effects of low-molecular-weight heparin cannot be reversed rapidly, some obstetricians change over to unfractionated heparin as women approach their due date. If this approach is taken, regular monitoring of the aPTT is necessary. Others continue the use of low-molecular-weight heparin throughout pregnancy, stopping at delivery, and resuming 12 to 24 hours after birth if bleeding is normal. Either warfarin or low-molecular-weight heparin should be used at minimum for 6 weeks postpartum with a total treatment time of 6 months. Both warfarin and low-weight-molecular weight heparin are safe to use during lactation.[108] Women should be discharged from the hospital after birth with an effective contraceptive plan, because use of warfarin is associated with a high risk of birth defects in exposed fetuses.

Hypercoagulable States

Acquired and inherited thrombophilias can upset the fine balance between the anticoagulant and pro-coagulant agents in the blood and result in thromboembolism. No consensus has been reached about whether, and if so in whom, testing for these conditions is warranted. This lack of consensus is due to the fact that both thrombophilia and VTE are rare events. Even in the event that VTE occurs, the thrombophilias account for only a very small percentage of these cases. Therefore, screening for these conditions is not recommended for the general public and most high-risk individuals.

While most authoritative bodies recommend against screening, controversy exists. Some experts recommend consideration of screening in specific situations. Screening may be warranted in women who experienced a VTE in pregnancy or after birth, because these women are at high risk of recurrent VTE in a subsequent pregnancy.[108] Other experts recommend testing in families with a high penetration of VTE or in relatives of an individual who has an extremely high-risk thrombophilia profile.[109,110]

Genetic risk factors that are associated with increased risk of thromboembolism include mutations affecting the expression of the pro-coagulants (Factor V Leiden and Factor II mutation, called prothrombin 20210) and the anticoagulants (antithrombin, protein C, and protein S).[101] Factor V Leiden is the most common of the genetic conditions and affects approximately 4% to 5% of the general population, primarily individuals of European, Mediterranean, or Middle Eastern descent. It is rarely seen in individuals of Southeast Asian or $_A$ub-Saharan African ancestry.[109] In Factor V Leiden polymorphism, the clotting factor is inactivated too slowly and results in increased thrombin generation. While this increases the lifetime risk of VTE three- to fivefold, the absolute risk is small: VTE appears to affect only 5% of heterozygous carriers of Factor V Leiden over their lifetime.[109] Homozygous carriers are at greater risk of VTE, but because this expression is very uncommon, it does not increase the overall societal burden of VTE.

Prothrombin G20210A mutations, also called Factor II mutations, are the second most common inherited thrombophilia, affecting 1% to 2% of individuals (primarily of European descent). It is associated with a 30% increase in levels of prothrombin in heterozygous individuals and a 70% increase in prothrombin levels in homozygous individuals.[109] It is associated with a two- to fourfold increased lifetime risk of VTE. However, as with Factor V Leiden, the absolute risk of experiencing a VTE is small for affected individuals.

Other genetic mutations can result in deficiencies in the natural anticoagulants. These conditions are exceedingly rare, affecting at most 0.3% of the general population.[109] Insufficient production of antithrombin from genetic mutations leads to insufficient inhibition of factor Xa and thrombin and increased thrombin activity. Increased thrombin activity also occurs with deficiencies in proteins C and S as a result of insufficient inhibition of Factor Va and Factor VIIIa.[107]

Other risk factors are not genetic in origin, but are acquired over time. The most common of these is antiphospholipid antibody syndrome. Approximately 1% to 5% of individuals carry antiphospholipid antibodies, but only a small minority of these individuals will develop APS. The prevalence of is estimated to be between 40 and 50 cases per 100,000 individuals.[111]

APS is characterized by venous or arterial thrombosis, recurrent pregnancy loss, moderate thrombocytopenia, or other problems in the presence of antiphospholipid antibodies (i.e., lupus anticoagulant, anticardiolipin antibodies, or anti-β_2 glycoprotein-1 antibodies).[111] It can affect multiple organs and is associated with neurologic (migraine, stoke, epilepsy), cardiac (MI, valve dysfunction, myocardiopathy), abdominal (renal conditions, splenic infarction), cutaneous (ulcers, cutaneous necrosis), orthopedic (arthralgia, arthritis), and ophthalmic manifestations. APS may occur in isolation (primary) or may be associated with other conditions (secondary). It is most commonly associated with systemic lupus erythematosus, but it also is seen in association

Table 16-9 Criteria for Antiphospholipid Syndrome

Clinical criteria:

1. Arterial or venous thrombosis

2. Obstetric morbidity:

   a. Unexplained death of a morphologically normal fetus at ≥ 10 weeks' gestation

   b. Preterm birth at ≤ 34 weeks' gestation of a morphologically normal fetus due to severe preeclampsia, severe IUGR, placental insufficiency (indicated by abnormal Doppler flow velocimetry waveform analysis [absent end-diastolic flow in the umbilical artery]), oligohydramnios (an amniotic fluid index ≤ 5 cm), or low birth weight (< 10% for gestational age)

   c. Three or more unexplained consecutive miscarriages at < 10 weeks' gestation

Laboratory criteria:

1. Anticardiolipin IgG and/or IgM present in medium or high titers (> 40 GPL or MPL or > 99%) measured twice at least 12 weeks apart

2. Anti-β_2G1 IgG and/or IgM antibodies at > 99% measured twice at least 12 weeks apart

3. Positive lupus anticoagulant measured twice at least 12 weeks apart (tested following appropriate laboratory guidelines)

anti-β_2G1 = anti-beta$_2$-glycoprotein 1, IgG = immunoglobulin G, IgM = immunoglobulin M, IUGR = intrauterine growth restriction

Data from Miyakis S, Lockshin MD, Atsumi T, Branch DW, Brey RL, Cervera R, et al. International consensus statement on an update of the classification criteria for definite antiphospholipid syndrome (APS). *J Thromb Haemost.* 2006;4(2):295-306.

with other autoimmune disorders, infections, sickle cell disease, certain medications, and diabetes.[112]

According to the Sapporo criteria, the diagnosis of APS can be made if an individual meets at minimum one clinical and one laboratory criterion shown in **Table 16-9**.[113]

While the underlying pathophysiology is unclear, antiphospholipid antibodies are thought to inhibit anticoagulation reactions, affect expression and activation of tissue factor, impair fibrinolysis, and enhance platelet activation and aggregation, among other physiologic effects, which then result in vaso-occlusion.[111] Treatment for APS is based on its presentation—that is, treatment of associated diseases and VTE if present. Some suggest that daily low-dose aspirin may be protective, although the evidence is insufficient to make any

firm recommendation in nonpregnant individuals.[114] While the diagnosis and management of suspected or confirmed coagulopathies should be under the direction of a hematologist, women's health providers should have a high index of suspicion that a woman may have one of these conditions, because they are associated with recurrent miscarriage and adverse pregnancy outcomes.

Pregnancy Considerations

Inherited and acquired thrombophilias are associated with adverse pregnancy outcomes. A workup for APS should be considered if a woman has red flags in her history: recurrent miscarriages, early-onset preeclampsia, IUGR, placental abruption, prolonged coagulation studies, or pregnancy-related thrombosis. See criteria provided in Table 16-9. For women with APS, treatment can markedly improve outcomes. While many treatment modalities have been reported in the literature, the most frequently used appears to be low-dose aspirin and low-dose heparin. The best outcomes also appear to be seen in women using combined aspirin (81 mg) and low-dose heparin. Women with a prior VTE are treated at a higher heparin dose and receive therapeutic anticoagulation. Women should also be advised to take daily calcium to prevent bone loss associated with heparin use. Baseline and serial measurements of aPTT and platelets are needed to monitor coagulation status and to detect heparin-induced thrombocytopenia. Ongoing fetal surveillance is also required beginning at 28 weeks' gestation. Anticoagulation treatment continues postpartum; the duration of postpartum treatment depends on the individual woman's risk profile.[112]

The level of evidence linking Factor V Leiden to adverse pregnancy outcomes is weaker than that for APS. The strongest evidence of risk associated with Factor V Leiden is pregnancy loss, particularly in the last half of pregnancy, and VTE. The presence of Factor V Leiden has been found in 8% to 30% of women with pregnancy loss and 20% to 46% of women with pregnancy-related VTE.[115] The association between Factor V Leiden and preeclampsia, IUGR, and placental abruption is unclear.[115] Given its rarity, routine screening is not recommended in pregnancy but can be considered in those with pregnancy loss or pregnancy-related thromboembolism.

A dearth of studies on the relationship between other thrombophilias and adverse pregnancy outcomes makes it difficult to offer evidence-based recommendations for care. The evidence to date suggests that the risk of preeclampsia or small for gestational age does not appear to be higher in women with prothrombin G20210A, although they may be at higher risk of recurrent pregnancy loss.[116] Deficiencies in protein C and protein S do not appear to be associated with early pregnancy loss, IUGR, or placental abruption, but may be related to increased risk of preeclampsia or stillbirth in the limited number of available studies. Women with antithrombin deficiency are at increased risk of embryonic demise and fetal death, but given the rarity of this disorder, screening is not recommended.[116]

ACOG has published a set of guidelines on how to best manage the inherited thrombophilias in pregnancy.[117] Given the lack of consistent and robust evidence linking the inherited thrombophilias to adverse pregnancy outcomes, their recommendations are directed at preventing VTE in pregnancy and postpartum. The ACOG guidelines categorize the thrombophilias into those considered to be low risk and those considered to be high risk.[117] Low-risk thrombophilias include Factor V Leiden heterozygous, prothrombin G20210A heterozygous, protein C deficiency, and protein S deficiency. Women who fall into this category have two options for care: surveillance only or the receipt of prophylactic heparin. They require postpartum anticoagulation if they have risk factors such as obesity, prolonged immobility, or a family history of thromboembolism in a first-degree relative before the age of 50. Women with low-risk thrombophilia who have had a prior VTE may be managed either with surveillance or prophylactic heparin in pregnancy but require postpartum anticoagulation at an intermediate or therapeutic level.[116]

High-risk thrombophilias include antithrombin deficiency, double heterozygous for prothrombin G20210A mutation and Factor V Leiden, Factor V Leiden homozygous, and prothrombin G20210A mutation homozygous. Women with these thrombophilias require prophylactic heparin in pregnancy and postpartum anticoagulation therapy. If these women have had a prior VTE, they may require a higher dosage of heparin in pregnancy.[116]

Methylenetetrahydrofolate reductase (MTHFR) is an enzyme involved in the metabolism of folic acid. Mutations in this enzyme are associated with elevations in homocysteine levels. It is thought to be a marker, not a cause, of thrombosis. Thus, MTHFR mutations are thought to play a minimal role, if any, in the risk of VTE. They are not associated with pre-eclampsia, IUGR, or placental abruption, but are associated with higher risk of neural tube defects. Therefore, folic acid supplementation is recommended for women with MTHFR mutations.[116]

Consultation with a hematologist and fetal medicine expert should be obtained for women suspected of having any of these conditions in pregnancy.

Varicose Veins

Varicose veins are the most common manifestation of chronic venous disease, affecting 25% to 33% of women.[118] Prevalence increases with age. Varicosities are caused by increased intravenous pressure from prolonged standing, increased intraabdominal pressure from pregnancy or obesity, or familial factors, or they are secondary to a DVT.[118] These factors contribute to the development of failed or incompetent venous valves that do not allow for normal blood flow. Affected individuals may experience heaviness in the legs, aching, burning, swelling, leg cramps, or itching. Symptoms often become progressively worse throughout the day, particularly with standing, and improve with walking and with elevation.

Women seek medical intervention for varicose veins for two reasons: symptom relief and better cosmetic appearance. Without intervention varicosities will worsen over time. Benefit can be derived from simple interventions, including leg elevation and compression stockings. Women should be advised to take frequent breaks during the day to elevate their legs, because this will help to decrease swelling and improve circulation. Compression stockings are graduated stockings

with a higher pressure at the ankle and lower pressure proximally to the knee and the thigh. These specially fitted stockings can be obtained at a medical supply pharmacy. Compression stockings work by decreasing venous pressure, reflux, and residual venous volume of varicosities; however, their benefit only lasts while they are worn. Compression stockings should be put on first thing in the morning, because the veins are at their lowest pressure. They should be removed each evening. Leg elevation following removal is recommended. The use of regular stockings is not recommended, because they do not have any extra compression value. Ace bandages wrapped around the legs do not provide extra support, and the level of compression may actually make the varicosities worse; in rare instances they may cause DVT.

In obese women, weight reduction is a significant aspect of the plan of care and should be incorporated at the beginning. Increasing activity and changing nutritional habits should be encouraged.

Invasive treatments are available, but a full course of conservative treatment should be attempted before seeking surgical intervention. Surgery is indicated in cases when the varicosities are large, symptomatic, and cosmetically troubling. Prior to surgery, veins should also be evaluated by duplex ultrasound of the affected extremity. Imaging can assess the competence and diameter of the vascular bed, determine the degree of reflux at the saphenofemoral and saphenopopliteal junctions, and help determine if superficial thrombophlebitis or a DVT is present.[118]

Several treatment options are available. These include laser treatment, sclerotherapy, endovenous obliteration of the saphenous vein, and surgery. Laser treatments have generally been used in the treatment of telangiectasias and smaller vessels with diameters less than 0.5 mm. Sclerotherapy involves injecting superficial veins with an agent that seals and scars the vein. This technique works best on small- and medium-sized veins (1 to 3 mm). Endovenous obliteration involves inserting a long, thin catheter that emits heat, radio waves, or laser energy. As the catheter is pulled out, the lumen of the vein collapses. Surgery is commonly performed if the saphenous vein is involved. Several techniques can be used. Ligation involves tying off the enlarged veins. Phlebectomy and stripping are techniques that remove the affected veins.[118] Each of these procedures is associated with different rates of efficacy, risk, and recurrence. In order to provide guidance regarding the best option for treatment, the NICE of the United Kingdom conducted a systematic review of the literature on treatment options for varicose views. After balancing the cost, effectiveness, safety, and risks of the various procedures, NICE concluded: 1) endothermal ablation using radiofrequency waves or laser energy was the preferred option; 2) if this approach is unsuitable, then sclerotherapy is another option; and 3) if neither of these options are acceptable, then vein stripping surgery could be considered.[119]

References

1. Centers for Disease Control and Prevention. Women and heart disease fact sheet. 2013. Available at: http://www.cdc.gov/dhdsp/data_statistics/fact_sheets/fs_women_heart.htm. Accessed April 26, 2016.

2. Clarke JL, Ladapo JL, Monane M, Lansky A, Skoufalos A, Nash DB. The diagnosis of CAD in women: addressing the unmet need—A report from the National Expert Roundtable Meeting. *Popul Health Manag.* 2015;18(2):86-92.

3. Canto J, Rogers W, Goldberg R, Peterson ED, Wenger NK, Vaccarino V, et al. Association of age and sex with myocardial infarction symptom presentation and in-hospital mortality. *JAMA.* 2012; 307(8):813-822.

4. Stock EO, Redberg R. Cardiovascular disease in women. *Curr Probl Cardiol.* 2012;37(11):450-526.

5. Weber B, Kapoor W. Evaluation and outcomes of patients with palpitations. *Am J Med.* 1996;100: 138-148.

6. Abramson BL, Melvin RG. Cardiovascular risk in women: focus on hypertension. *Can J Cardiol.* 2014; 30(5):553-559.

7. Flegal K, Carroll M, Kit B, Ogden C. Prevalence of obesity and trends in the distribution of body mass index among us adults, 1999-2010. *JAMA.* 2012; 307(5):491-497.

8. Bates GW, Legro RS. Longterm management of polycystic ovarian syndrome (PCOS). *Mol Cell Endocrinol.* 2013;373(1-2):91-97.

9. US Department of Health and Human Services; National, Heart, Lung, and Blood Institute. *The Seventh Report of the Joint National Committee on Prevention, Detection, Evaluation, and Treatment of High Blood Pressure* (JNC 7). 2004. Available at: http://www.nhlbi.nih.gov/guidelines/hypertension/jnc7full.pdf. Accessed April 26, 2016.

10. McFadden C, Townsend R. Blood pressure measurement: common pitfalls and how to avoid them. *Consultant.* 2003;43:161-165.

11. Weber MA, Schiffrin EL, White WB, Mann S, Lindholm LH, Kenerson JG, et al. Clinical practice guidelines for the management of hypertension in the community: a statement by the American Society of Hypertension and the International Society of Hypertension. *J Hypertens.* 2014;16(1):14-26.

12. Chobanian A, Bakris G, Black HR, Cushman WC, Green LA, Izzo JLJ, et al. The seventh report of the Joint National Committee on Prevention, Detection, Evaluation, and Treatment of High Blood Pressure: The JNC 7 report. *JAMA.* 2003;289(19): 2560-2572.

13. Franklin SS, Thijs L, Hansen TW, O'Brien E, Staessen JA. White-coat hypertension: new insights from recent studies. *Hypertension.* 2013;62(6): 982-987.

14. Staessen J, Asmar R, De Buyzere M, Imai Y, Parati G, Shimada K, et al. Task Force II: blood pressure measurement and cardiovascular outcome. *Blood Press Monit.* 2001;6(6):355-370.

15. National Institute for Health and Care Excellence (NICE). The Clinical Management of Primary Hypertension in Adults. London, United Kingdom: National Institute for Health and Care Excellence (NICE); 2011.

16. Stergiou GS, Bliziotis IA. Home blood pressure monitoring in the diagnosis and treatment of hypertension: a systematic review. *Am J Hypertens.* 2011; 24(2):123-134.

17. Abbott AV. Diagnostic approach to palpitations. *Am Fam Physician.* 2005;71(4):743-750.

18. Wolff A, Cowan C. 10 steps before you refer for palpitations. *Br J Cardiol.* 2009;16(4):182-186.

19. Wallace ML, Ricco JA, Barrett B. Screening strategies for cardiovascular disease in asymptomatic adults. *Prim Care*. 2014;41(2):371-397.

20. Buckley D, Fu R, Freeman M, Rogers K, Helfand M. C-reactive protein as a risk factor for coronary heart disease: a systematic review and meta-analyses for the US Preventive Services Task Force. *Ann Intern Med*. 2009;151(7):483-495.

21. Wilkins JT, Lloyd-Jones DM. Biomarkers for coronary heart disease clinical risk prediction: a critical appraisal. *Prev Cardiol*. 2010;13(4):160-165.

22. Kamal AH, Tefferi A, Pruthi RK. How to interpret and pursue an abnormal prothrombin time, activated partial thromboplastin time, and bleeding time in adults. *Mayo Clin Proc*. 2007;82(7):864-873.

23. Wyant A, Collett D. Identifying and managing chest pain in women. *JAAPA*. 2015;28(1):48-52.

24. Hanson MA, Fareed MT, Argenio SL, Agunwamba AO, Hanson TR. Coronary artery disease. *Prim Care*. 2013;40(1):1-16.

25. Aldous SJ. Cardiac biomarkers in acute myocardial infarction. *Int J Cardiol*. 2012;164(3):282-294.

26. Kumar A, Cannon CP. Acute coronary syndromes: diagnosis and management, part I. *Mayo Clin Proc*. 2009;84(10):917-938.

27. Thygesen K, Alpert JS, White HD, Joint ESC/ACCF/AHA/WHF Task Force for the Redefinition of Myocardial Infarction, Jaffe AS, Apple FS, et al. Universal definition of myocardial infarction. *Circulation*. 2007;116(22):2634-2653.

28. Shah BN. Echocardiography in the era of multimodality cardiovascular imaging. *Biomed Res Int*. 2013;2013:310483.

29. Mieres JH, Gulati M, Bairey Merz N, Berman DS, Gerber TC, Hayes SN, et al. Role of noninvasive testing in the clinical evaluation of women with suspected ischemic heart disease: a consensus statement from the American Heart Association. *Circulation*. 2014;130(4):350-379.

30. Fung E, Järvelin M, Doshi R, Shinbane J, Carlson S, Grazette L, et al. Electrocardiographic patch devices and contemporary wireless cardiac monitoring. *Front Physiol*. 2015;6:149.

31. Patel MR, Bailey SR, Bonow RO, Chambers CE, Chan PS, Dehmer GJ, et al. ACCF/SCAI/AATS/AHA/ASE/ASNC/HFSA/HRS/SCCM/SCCT/SCMR/STS 2012 appropriate use criteria for diagnostic catheterization: a report of the American College of Cardiology Foundation Appropriate Use Criteria Task Force, Society for Cardiovascular Angiography and Interventions, American Association for Thoracic Surgery, American Heart Association, American Society of Echocardiography, American Society of Nuclear Cardiology, Heart Failure Society of America, Heart Rhythm Society, Society of Critical Care Medicine, Society of Cardiovascular Computed Tomography, Society for Cardiovascular Magnetic Resonance, and Society of Thoracic Surgeons. *J Am Coll Cardiol*. 2012;59(22):1995-2027.

32. O'Gara PT, Kushner FG, Ascheim DD, Casey DE, Chung MK, de Lemos JA, et al. 2013 ACCF/AHA guideline for the management of ST-Elevation myocardial infarction: a report of the American College of Cardiology Foundation/American Heart Association Task Force on Practice Guidelines. *Circulation*. 2013;127(4):e362-e425.

33. Wittels K. Aortic emergencies. *Emerg Med Clin North Am*. 2011;29(4):789-800.

34. Raviele A, Giada F, Bergfeldt L, Blanc JJ, Blomstrom-Lundqvist C, Mont L, et al. Management of patients with palpitations: a position paper from the European Heart Rhythm Association. *Europace*. 2011;13(7):920-934.

35. Hayek E, Gring CN, Griffin BP. Mitral valve prolapse. *Lancet*. 2005;365(9458):507-518.

36. Zuppiroli A, Rinaldi M, Kramer-Fox R, Favilli S, Roman MJ, Devereux RB. Natural history of mitral valve prolapse. *Am J Cardiol*. 1995;75(15):1028-1032.

37. Nishimura R, Carabello B, Faxon D, Freed MD, Lytle BW, O'Gara PT, et al. ACC/AHA 2008 guideline update on valvular heart disease: focused update on infective endocarditis: a report of the American College of Cardiology/American Heart Association Task Force on Practice Guidelines endorsed by the Society of Cardiovascular Anesthesiologists, Society for Cardiovascular Angiography and Interventions, and Society of Thoracic Surgeons. *J Am Coll Cardiol*. 2008;52(8):676-685.

38. Wilson W, Taubert KA, Gewitz M, Lockhart PB, Baddour LM, Levison M, et al. Prevention of infective endocarditis: guidelines from the American Heart Association: a guideline from the American Heart Association Rheumatic Fever, Endocarditis, and Kawasaki Disease Committee, Council on Cardiovascular Disease in the Young, and the Council on Clinical Cardiology, Council on Cardiovascular Surgery and Anesthesia, and the Quality of Care and Outcomes Research Interdisciplinary Working Group. *Circulation*. 2007;116(15):1736-1754.

39. Dhoble A, Vedre A, Abdelmoneim SS, Sudini SR, Ghose A, Abela GS, et al. Prophylaxis to prevent infective endocarditis: to use or not to use? *Clin Cardiol*. 2009;32(8):429-433.

40. Forman JP, Stampfer MJ, & Curhan GC. Diet and lifestyle risk factors associated with incident hypertension in women. *JAMA*. 2009;302:401-411.

41. Jhamnani S, Patel D, Heimlich L, King F, Walitt B, Lindsay J. Meta-analysis of the effects of lifestyle modifications on coronary and carotid atherosclerotic burden. *Am J Cardiol.* 2015;115(2): 268-275.

42. Chen L, Pei J-H, Kuang J, Chen H-M, Chen Z, Li Z-W, et al. Effect of lifestyle intervention in patients with type 2 diabetes: a meta-analysis. *Metabolism.* 2015;64(2):338-347.

43. Schellenberg ES, Dryden DM, Vandermeer B, Ha C, Korownyk C. Lifestyle interventions for patients with and at risk for type 2 diabetes: a systematic review and meta-analysis. *Ann Intern Med.* 2013;159(8):841-851.

44. Nordmann AJ, Suter-Zimmermann K, Bucher HC, Shai I, Tuttle KR, Estruch R, et al. Meta-analysis comparing Mediterranean to low-fat diets for modification of cardiovascular risk factors. *Am J Med.* 2011;124(9):841-851.e2.

45. Hooper L, Summerbell CD, Thompson R, Sills D, Roberts FG, Moore H, et al. Reduced or modified dietary fat for preventing cardiovascular disease. *Cochrane Database Syst Rev.* 2011;7:CD002137.

46. Estruch R, Ros E, Salas-Salvadó J, Covas M-I, Corella D, Arós F, et al. Primary prevention of cardiovascular disease with a Mediterranean diet. *N Engl J Med.* 2013;368(14):1279-1290.

47. Sattelmair J, Pertman J, Ding EL, Kohl HW, Haskell W, Lee I-M. Dose response between physical activity and risk of coronary heart disease: a meta-analysis. *Circulation.* 2011;124(7):789-795.

48. Zhang C, Qin Y-Y, Chen Q, Jiang H, Chen X-Z, Xu C-L, et al. Alcohol intake and risk of stroke: a dose–response meta-analysis of prospective studies. *Int J Cardiol.* 2014;174(3):669-677.

49. Mosca L, Benjamin EJ, Berra K, Bezanson JL, Dolor RJ, Lloyd-Jones DM, et al. Effectiveness-based guidelines for the prevention of cardiovascular disease in women—2011 update: a guideline from the American Heart Association. *J Am Coll Cardiol.* 2011;57(12):1404-1423.

50. Gillespie CD, Hurvitz KA. Prevalence of hypertension and controlled hypertension—United States, 2007-2010. *MMWR.* 2013;62(3):144-148.

51. Keenan NL, Rosendorf KA. Prevalence of hypertension and controlled hypertension—United States, 2005-2008. *MMWR.* 2011;60(1):94-97.

52. Engberding N, Wenger NK. Management of hypertension in women. *Hypertens Res.* 2012;35(3):251-260.

53. Singh M, Mensah GA, Bakris G. Pathogenesis and clinical physiology of hypertension. *Cardiol Clin.* 2010;28(4):545-559.

54. Fink G. Sympathetic activity, vascular capacitance and long-term regulation of arterial pressure. *Hypertension.* 2009;53(2):307-312.

55. Mayet J, Hughes A. Cardiac and vascular pathophysiology in hypertension. *Heart.* 2003;89(9): 1104-1109.

56. Atlas SA. The renin-angiotensin aldosterone system: pathophysiological role and pharmacologic inhibition. *J Manage Care Pharm.* 2007;13(8 Suppl B): 9-20.

57. Onusko E. Diagnosing secondary hypertension. *Am Fam Physician.* 2003;67(1):67-74.

58. Ryan M. An update on immune system activation in the pathogenesis of hypertension. *Hypertension.* 2013;62:226-230.

59. Viera A, Neutze D. Diagnosis of secondary hypertension: an age-based approach. *Am Fam Physician.* 2010;82(12):1471-1478.

60. National Cholesterol Education Program (NCEP) Expert Panel on Detection, Evaluation, and Treatment of High Blood Cholesterol in Adults (Adult Treatment Panel III). Third report of the National Cholesterol Education Program Expert Panel On Detection, Evaluation, and Treatment of High Blood Cholesterol in Adults (Adult Treatment Panel III): final report (NIH Publication No. 02-5215). *Circulation.* 2002;106(25):3143-3421.

61. Eckel RH, Jakicic JM, Ard JD, de Jesus JM, Houston Miller N, Hubbard VS, et al. 2013 AHA/ACC Guideline on lifestyle management to reduce cardiovascular risk: a report of the American College of Cardiology/American Heart Association Task Force on Practice Guidelines. *Circulation.* 2014; 129(Suppl 2):S76-99.

62. James P, Oparil S, Carter B, Cushman WC, Dennison-Himmelfarb C, Handler J, et al. 2014 evidence-based guideline for the management of high blood pressure in adults: report from the panel members appointed to the eighth Joint National Committee (JNC 8). *JAMA.* 2014;311(5):507-520.

63. Hajjar I. Postural blood pressure changes and orthostatic hypotension in the elderly patient: impact of antihypertensive medications. *Drugs Aging.* 2005;22(1):55-68.

64. Thompson AE, Pope JE. Calcium channel blockers for primary Raynaud's phenomenon: a meta-analysis. *Rheumatology.* 2005;44(2):145-150.

65. Vest AR, Cho LS. Hypertension in pregnancy. *Cardiol Clin.* 2012;30(3):407-423.

66. World Health Organization. Medical eligibility criteria for contraceptive use, 5th ed. 2015. Available at: http://www.who.int/reproductivehealth/publications/family_planning/MEC-5/en/ Accessed May 3, 2016.

67. Centers for Disease Control and Prevention. United States Medical Eligibility Criteria (US MEC) for Contraceptive Use 2010. Available at: http://www.cdc.gov/reproductivehealth/unintendedpregnancy/usmec.htm. Accessed April 25, 2016.

68. American College of Obstetricians Gynecologists. Hypertension in pregnancy. Report of the American College of Obstetricians and Gynecologists' Task Force on Hypertension in Pregnancy. *Obstet Gynecol.* 2013;122(5):1122-1131.

69. Kattah AG, Garovic VD. The management of hypertension in pregnancy. *Adv Chronic Kidney Dis.* 2013;20(3):229-239.

70. American College of Obstetricians and Gynecologists. *Hypertension in Pregnancy.* Washington, DC: American College of Obstetricians and Gynecologists; 2013. Available at: http://www.acog.org/Resources-And-Publications/Task-Force-and-Work-Group-Reports/Hypertension-in-Pregnancy. Accessed April 25, 2016.

71. MacLennan AH. HRT in difficult circumstances: are there any absolute contraindications? *Climacteric.* 2011;14(4):409-417.

72. Writing Group for the Women's Health Initiative Investigators. Risks and benefits of estrogen plus progestin in healthy postmenopausal women: principal results from the women's health initiative randomized controlled trial. *JAMA.* 2002;288(3):321-333. doi:10.1001/jama.288.3.321.

73. Brook RD, Appel LJ, Rubenfire M, Ogedegbe G, Bisognano JD, Elliott WJ, et al. Beyond medications and diet: alternative approaches to lowering blood pressure: a scientific statement from the American Heart Association. *Hypertension.* 2013; 61(6):1360-1383.

74. Allen R, Rogozinska E, Sivarajasingam P, Khan KS, Thangaratinam S. Effect of diet- and lifestyle-based metabolic risk-modifying interventions on preeclampsia: a meta-analysis. *Acta Obstet Gynecol Scand.* 2014;93(10):973-985.

75. Romero CX, Romero TE, Shlay JC, Ogden LG, Dabelea D. Changing trends in the prevalence and disparities of obesity and other cardiovascular disease risk factors in three racial/ethnic groups of USA adults. *Adv Prev Med.* 2012;2012:8.

76. Navar-Boggan AM, Peterson ED, D'Agostino RB, Neely B, Sniderman AD, Pencina MJ. Hyperlipidemia in early adulthood increases long-term risk of coronary heart disease. *Circulation.* 2015;131(5):451-458.

77. Kwiterovich PO. The metabolic pathways of high-density lipoprotein, low-density lipoprotein, and triglycerides: a current review. *Am J Cardiol.* 2000; 86(12, Suppl 1):5-10.

78. Jain KS, Kathiravan MK, Somani RS, Shishoo CJ. The biology and chemistry of hyperlipidemia. *Bioorg Med Chem.* 2007;15(14):4674-4699.

79. Link JJ, Rohatgi A, de Lemos JA. HDL cholesterol: physiology, pathophysiology, and management. *Curr Probl Cardiol.* 2007;32(5):268-314.

80. AbouRjaili G, Shtaynberg N, Wetz R, Costantino T, Abela GS. Current concepts in triglyceride metabolism, pathophysiology, and treatment. *Metabolism.* 2010;59(8):1210-1220.

81. Yuan Y, Li P, Ye J. Lipid homeostasis and the formation of macrophage-derived foam cells in atherosclerosis. *Protein Cell.* 2012;3(3):173-181.

82. Grundy SM. Then and now: ATP III vs. IV. American College of Cardiology; 2013. Available at: http://www.acc.org/latest-in-cardiology/articles/2014/07/18/16/03/then-and-now-atp-iii-vs-iv?w_nav=LC. Accessed April 26, 2016.

83. Talwalkar P, Sreenivas C, Gulati A, Baxi H. Journey in guidelines for lipid management: from adult treatment panel (ATP)-I to ATP-III and what to expect in ATP-IV. *Indian J Endocrinol Metab.* 2013;17(4):628-635.

84. Stone NJ, Robinson JG, Lichtenstein AH, Bairey Merz CN, Blum CB, Eckel RH, et al. ACC/AHA guideline on the treatment of blood cholesterol to reduce atherosclerotic cardiovascular risk in adults: a report of the American College of Cardiology/American Heart Association Task Force on Practice Guidelines. *J Am Coll Cardiol.* 2014;63(25 Pt B):2889-2934.

85. National Heart, Lung and Blood Institute. Risk assessment tool for estimating your 10-year risk of having a heart attack http://cvdrisk.nhlbi.nih.gov/ Accessed May 2, 2016.

86. Keaney JF, Curfman GD, Jarcho JA. A pragmatic view of the new cholesterol treatment guidelines. *N Engl J Med.* 2014;370(3):275-278.

87. Robinson JG. 2013 ACC/AHA cholesterol guideline for reducing cardiovascular risk: what is so controversial? *Curr Atheroscler Rep.* 2014;16(6):413.

88. Goyal P, Igel L, LaScalea K, Borden WB. Cardiometabolic impact of non-statin lipid lowering therapies. *Curr Atheroscler Rep.* 2014;16(2):1-12.

89. Wierzbicki AS, Viljoen A. Fibrates and niacin: is there a place for them in clinical practice? *Expert Opin Pharmacother.* 2014;15(18):2673-2680.

90. Last A, Ference J, Falleroni J. Pharmacologic treatment of hyperlipidemia. *Am Fam Physician.* 2011; 84(5):551-558.

91. Pisaniello AD, Scherer DJ, Kataoka Y, Nicholls SJ. Ongoing challenges for pharmacotherapy for dyslipidemia. *Expert Opin Pharmacother.* 2015;16(3): 347-356.

92. Gazzerro P, Proto MC, Gangemi G, Malfitano AM, Ciaglia E, Pisanti S, et al. Pharmacological actions of statins: a critical appraisal in the management of cancer. *Pharmacol Rev.* 2012;64(1):102-146.

93. Naci H, Brugts J, Ades T. Comparative tolerability and harms of individual statins: a study-level network meta-analysis of 246,955 participants from 135 randomized, controlled trials. *Circulation.* 2013; 6(4):390-399.

94. Gudzune KA, Monroe AK, Sharma R, Ranasinghe PD, Chelladurai Y, Robinson KA. Effectiveness of combination therapy with statin and another lipid-modifying agent compared with intensified statin monotherapy: a systematic review effectiveness of combination therapy with statin. *Ann Intern Med.* 2014;160(7):468-476.

95. Eilat-Adar S, Sinai T, Yosefy C, Henkin Y. Nutritional recommendations for cardiovascular disease prevention. *Nutrients.* 2013;9:3646-3683.

96. Kahn R, Buse J, Ferrannini E, Stern M, American Diabetes Association, European Association for the Study of Diabetes. The metabolic syndrome: time for a critical appraisal: joint statement from the American Diabetes Association and the European Association for the Study of Diabetes. *Diabetes Care.* 2005;28(9):2289.

97. Wilbur J, Shian B. Diagnosis of deep venous thrombosis and pulmonary embolism. *Am Fam Physician.* 2012;86(10):913-919.

98. Reitsma PH, Versteeg HH, Middeldorp S. Mechanistic view of risk factors for venous thromboembolism. *Arterioscler Thromb Vasc Biol.* 2012;32(3):563-568.

99. Heit JA. Epidemiology of venous thromboembolism. *Nat Rev Cardiol.* 2015;12:464-474.

100. López JA, Chen J. Pathophysiology of venous thrombosis. *Thromb Res.* 2009;123(Suppl 4):S30-S34.

101. Battinelli EM, Murphy DL, Connors JM. Venous thromboembolism overview. *Hematol Oncol Clin North Am.* 2012;26:345-367.

102. Dupras D, Bluhm J, Felty C, Hansen C, Johnson T, Lim K, et al. Institute for Clinical Systems Improvement. Health Care Guideline: Venous Thromboembolism Diagnosis and Treatment. 2013. Available at: https://www.icsi.org/_asset/5ldx9k/VTE0113.pdf. Accessed April 26, 2016.

103. Gornik H, Sharma A. Duplex ultrasound in the diagnosis of lower extremity deep venous thrombosis. *Circulation.* 2014;129:917-921.

104. Scott G, Mahdi AJ, Alikhan R. Superficial vein thrombosis: a current approach to management. *Br J Haematol.* 2015;168(5):639-645.

105. Wells P, Forgie M, Rodger M. Treatment of venous thromboembolism. *JAMA.* 2015;311(7):717-728.

106. Kearon C, Akl EA, Comerota AJ, Prandoni P, Bounameaux H, Goldhaber SZ, et al. Antithrombotic therapy for VTE disease: antithrombotic therapy and prevention of thrombosis, 9th ed: American College of Chest Physicians evidence-based clinical practice guidelines. *Chest.* 2012;141(Suppl 2):e419S-94S.

107. Briggs G, Freeman R. *Drugs in Pregnancy and Lactation.* 10th ed. Philadelphia, PA: Wolters Kluwer; 2015.

108. Marik PE. Venous thromboembolism in pregnancy. *Clin Chest Med.* 2010;31(4):731-740.

109. MacCallum P, Bowles L, Keeling D. Diagnosis and management of heritable thrombophilias. *BMJ.* 2014;349:g4387.

110. Lim MY, Moll S. Thrombophilia. *Vasc Med.* 2015;20(2):193-196.

111. Gómez-Puerta JA, Cervera R. Diagnosis and classification of the antiphospholipid syndrome. *J Autoimmun.* 2014;48-49:20-25.

112. Kutteh WH, Hinote CD. Antiphospholipid antibody syndrome. *Obstet Gynecol Clin North Am.* 2014;41(1):113-132.

113. Miyakis S, Lockshin MD, Atsumi T, Branch DW, Brey RL, Cervera R, et al. International consensus statement on an update of the classification criteria for definite antiphospholipid syndrome (APS). *J Thromb Haemost.* 2006;4(2):295-306.

114. Tripodi A, de Groot PG, Pengo V. Antiphospholipid syndrome: laboratory detection, mechanisms of action and treatment. *J Intern Med.* 2011;270(2): 110-122.

115. Kujovich JL. Factor V Leiden thrombophilia. *Genet Med.* 2011;13:1-16.

116. Davenport WB, Kutteh WH. Inherited thrombophilias and adverse pregnancy outcomes: a review of screening patterns and recommendations. *Obstet Gynecol Clin North Am.* 2014;41(1):133-144.

117. American College of Obstetricians and Gynecologists. Practice Bulletin No. 138: inherited thrombophilias in pregnancy. *Obstet Gynecol.* 122(3):706-716, September 2013.

118. Jones R, Carek P. Management of varicose veins. *Am Fam Physician.* 2008;78(11):1289-1294.

119. Marsden G. Practice guidelines: diagnosis and management of varicose veins in the legs: summary of NICE guidance. *BMJ.* 2013;347:f4279.

CHAPTER 17

GASTROINTESTINAL DISEASES

Barbara K. Hackley | Elaine Leigh

Gastrointestinal (GI)-related problems are among the most common reasons women are seen in the primary care office and/or emergency department. Abdominal pain and functional problems with bowel motility are seen daily in women's health practices. Other symptoms reported by women are less common but still problematic. Complicating the difficulty in arriving at a diagnosis is that abdominal pain and other common GI symptoms may indicate the presence of respiratory, cardiac, or genitourinary conditions. This chapter discusses the evaluation of common GI symptoms and the management of some of the more common GI disorders affecting women in primary care practices.

Clinical Presentation

Common symptoms associated with various GI conditions include nausea and vomiting, diarrhea, dyspepsia and heartburn, dysphagia, abdominal pain, constipation, and rectal bleeding. Understanding the physiologic basis and diagnostic approach to these symptoms can help elucidate the differential diagnoses.

Nausea and Vomiting

Nausea can be defined as an unpleasant sensation of queasiness with the perceived imminent need to vomit. *Vomiting* is defined as the forceful oral expulsion of gastric contents associated with the contraction of the abdominal and chest wall musculature. Nausea and vomiting can be conceptualized as having three components: nausea, *retching* (spasmodic respiratory and abdominal movements, "dry heaves"), and vomiting. However, these three components are neither mutually exclusive nor are all three always present. Vomiting is usually preceded by nausea, although nausea and retching can occur without vomiting. Vomiting includes voluntary and involuntary processes. Vomiting should be distinguished from regurgitation, a passive process where there is retrograde flow of esophageal contents into the mouth, which is common in gastroesophageal reflux disease (GERD).

Vomiting is a reflex that allows the body to rid itself of unwanted contents of the stomach and/or small bowel. The act of vomiting is under control of two medullary centers: the vomiting center in the dorsal portion of the lateral reticular formation including the dorsal vagal complex ("vomiting center") and the chemoreceptor trigger zone (CTZ) in the area of the floor of the fourth ventricle. The vomiting center receives input via the vagus and sympathetic nerves; it is activated directly by signals from the cortex thalamus (anxiety, pain), signals from the GI tract, CTZ, or from the vestibular apparatus of the inner ear (motion sickness, Meniere's disease, benign positional paroxysmal vertigo). Just prior to vomiting, antiperistaltic waves push contents of the small intestine to the duodenum and stomach. Distension within the upper regions of the GI tract trigger the vomiting center and the actual act of vomiting. Individuals vary considerably in the threshold of their vomiting centers to different stimuli.[1]

Toxic substances in the blood (e.g., drugs, chemotherapeutic agents, radiation therapy, uremia) can activate the CTZ. The CTZ can also be affected by signals in the stomach and small intestines via the vagal efferent nerves. Activation of either pathway can lead to emesis. Specific neurotransmitters in the CTZ identify substances as harmful and relay impulses to the vomiting center to initiate the vomiting cycle. The responsible neurotransmitters include serotonin, dopamine, acetylcholine, histamine, and neurokinin-1 neuropeptide. Because stimulation of neurotransmitters induces vomiting, interference with transmission of these neurotransmitters will prevent the vomiting center from being activated. Antiemetics act in this fashion by blocking at least one of the neurotransmitters. Examples include ondansetron (Zofran) as a serotonin antagonist, promethazine (Phenergan) and prochlorperazine (Compazine) as dopamine antagonists, scopolamine as an anticholinergic, and meclizine (Antivert) or dimenhydrinate (Dramamine) as antihistamines.

Nausea and vomiting (NV) may represent a physiologic homeostatic response to an ingested toxin or indicate a disease process of the GI tract, adjacent organs, or the central nervous system (CNS). They are also common symptoms in pregnancy or as a reaction to certain medications. Conditions associated with nausea and vomiting are listed in **Table 17-1**.

Because nausea and vomiting are present in so many different conditions, it is essential to ascertain the evolution and constellation of symptoms a woman may report. Most acute cases of nausea and vomiting, whether caused by infection, toxins, or pregnancy, are self-limited and can be managed with supportive care. If neither dehydration nor electrolyte imbalance is present, symptoms have been present for less than a week, and no alarm symptoms as listed in **Table 17-2** are present, then testing is generally unnecessary.[2] Nausea and vomiting of acute onset are more commonly seen with food poisoning, gastroenteritis, cholecystitis, or pancreatitis. If abdominal pain is present, then organic causes (i.e., cholecystitis, pancreatitis, hepatitis) or obstruction need to be considered. Pain, along with vomiting of bile, feculent material, or undigested or partially digested food, can be present with intestinal obstruction or esophageal strictures. Gastric outlet obstruction tends to be associated with intermittent symptoms, whereas intestinal obstruction tends to present with acute symptoms and severe pain.[3] Vomiting accompanied by diarrhea, myalgia, and headache suggests viral gastroenteritis.[2] CNS conditions also can cause vomiting, which may or may not be accompanied by nausea. Suspect CNS conditions if other focal neurologic signs, projectile vomiting, or headache (particularly if worsened by Valsalva maneuvers or exertion) is present. Conditions affecting the inner ear may present with nausea as well as vertigo. Lastly, migraine and cluster headaches may also be accompanied by nausea and vomiting.[2]

Diarrhea

Diarrhea is defined as passage of unformed or frequent stools ($\geq$ 3 a day).[4] It is characterized by an increase in water content, volume, or frequency

Table 17-1 Differential Diagnosis for Nausea and Vomiting

Drug-enduced Etiologies
Cancer Chemotherapy Agents
Analgesics
Aspirin
Nonsteroidal anti-inflammatory drugs
Anti-gout medications
Cardiovascular Medications
Anti-arrhythmics
Anti-hypertensives
Beta blockers
Calcium channel blockers
Diuretics
Hormonal Medications
Oral contraceptives
Antibiotics
Macrolides
Tetracycline
Sulfonamides
Acyclovir
Nicotine
Narcotics
Radiation Therapy
Alcohol Abuse

Disorders of the Gut and Peritoneum
Mechanical Obstruction
    Small intestinal obstruction
Functional Gastrointestinal (GI) Disorders
    Gastroparesis (Weakness of gastric peristalsis)
    Irritable bowel syndrome
Organic GI Disorders
    Peptic ulcer disease
    Cholecystitis
    Pancreatitis
    Crohn's disease
    Hepatitis

Infectious Etiologies
Viral/bacterial gastroenteritis

Endocrine Etiologies
Pregnancy
Uremia
Diabetic ketoacidosis
Hyperthyroidism

Central Nervous System
Increased intracranial pressure
Emotional/psychiatric
Migraine
Seizure disorder
Labyrinthine disorders
    Motion sickness
    Labyrinthitis
    Meniere's disease

Data from Spieker M. Evaluating dysphagia. *Am Fam Physician*. 2000;61(12):3639-3648; American College of Radiology. ACR appropriateness criteria: Acute (nonlocalized) abdominal pain and fever or suspected abdominal abscess. https://acsearch.acr.org/docs/69467/Narrative/. 2013. Accessed May 5, 2016.

of stools and a decrease in consistency of stools. The underlying cause of diarrhea is an incomplete absorption of water through the intestinal villus from, or an increase in secretion of fluid from the intestinal crypt cells into, the lumen of the intestine. Water is pulled across the intestinal mucosa through the villus by osmotic forces generated by the transport of electrolytes and nutrients from the gut. Secretion into the gut from the intestinal crypt cells occurs simultaneously with absorption. Both mechanisms are in exquisite balance with each other. Diarrhea can result from one or more of the following processes: changes in osmotic forces, where unabsorbed substances draw water from the plasma into the intestinal lumen; secretory processes resulting from disordered electrolyte transport, most often from decreased absorption relative to secretion;

Table 17-2 Alarm Symptoms Associated with Nausea and Vomiting

Abdominal pain
Altered mental state or focal neurologic deficits
Dehydration
- Confusion, lethargy (severe)
- Decreased skin turgor or dry mouth
- Decreased urine output or concentrated urine
- Dizziness, lightheadedness, fatigue, or weakness
- Orthostatic hypotension
- Tachycardia
Feculent vomiting
Gastrointestinal bleeding or melena
Hematochezia
Recent hospitalization or antibiotic use
Persistent vomiting
Progressive dysphagia
Older than 55 years
Unintended weight loss

Data from Anderson WD, Strayer SM. Evaluation of nausea and vomiting in adults: a case-based approach. *Am Fam Physician.* 2013;88(6):371-379.

inflammatory diseases, which damage the endothelium and lead to a mixture of osmotic, exudative, and secretory changes that result in diarrhea; or altered motility of the intestine or colon.[5] Accelerated transit time in the gut can limit absorption, such as can be seen with hyperthyroidism, and lead to diarrhea even if the absorption-secretion processes are otherwise normal.

Diarrhea can be categorized as inflammatory, fatty, or watery (which has two subcategories—secretory or osmotic). Inflammatory diarrhea should be suspected if a woman reports bloody stools, tenesmus, fever, or abdominal pain. Laboratory findings that can confirm inflammatory diarrhea include leukocytes found on examination of the stool, elevated C-reactive protein or sedimentation rates, and low albumin. The intestinal mucosa can be inflamed from conditions such as Crohn's disease and ulcerative colitis or from infections such as *Clostridium difficile,*

cytomegalovirus, or *Entamoeba histolytica.* Follow-up testing with colonoscopy or sigmoidoscopy may be indicated if chronic inflammatory diarrhea is suspected.[5]

Fatty diarrhea should be suspected if a woman reports weight loss and has stools that are bulky, pale, and oily in appearance, are difficult to flush, and leave an oily residue in the toilet. Fatty diarrhea is caused by malabsorption from conditions such as gastric bypass surgery or mucosal diseases such as celiac disease. It can also be due to problems in digestion; for example, from pancreatic exocrine insufficiency seen in chronic pancreatitis or inadequate duodenal bile acid concentration seen in cirrhosis.[5] Special tests can be ordered to detect fecal fat if fatty diarrhea is suspected. Additional tests that may be needed include endoscopy with small bowel biopsies, small bowel aspiration, or hydrogen breath tests.[5]

Watery diarrhea is due to either osmotic problems from the ingestion of poorly absorbed ions or sugars (osmotic diarrhea) or secretory problems that disrupt the epithelial electrolyte transport system and lead to an imbalance between secretion and absorption (secretory diarrhea). In secretory diarrhea, secretion exceeds absorption resulting in diarrhea. One way to distinguish between osmotic and secretory diarrhea is to determine the response to fasting. Diarrhea due to osmotic causes decreases in response to fasting, whereas fasting does not influence the degree of diarrhea in secretory diarrhea. Osmotic diarrhea is often due to either ingesting poorly absorbed ions contained in medications such as laxatives and antacids or difficult-to-absorb sugars such as sorbitol, or malabsorption due to the inability to absorb carbohydrates as in lactose intolerance (LI). The most common cause of acute secretory diarrhea is infection. However, secretory diarrhea can also be chronic and is seen with bile acid malabsorption, inflammatory bowel disease (IBD), some endocrine tumors, cancer (colon, lymphoma), or as a consequence of diabetic neuropathy.[5]

Diarrhea can also be categorized by timing. Acute diarrhea lasts for less than 2 weeks, persistent diarrhea for 2 to 4 weeks, and chronic diarrhea for a month or more.[6] Underlying causes of acute diarrhea include infectious agents such as bacteria, viruses, parasites, and bacterial or chemical toxins, whereas chronic diarrhea is more likely to be due to irritable bowel syndrome (IBS), IBD, nonspecific colitis/microscopic colitis (MC), malabsorption syndrome, and chronic infections (**Table 17-3**).[6]

Antibiotic therapy may also contribute to the development of diarrhea. Antibiotics associated

Table 17-3 Differential Diagnosis of Diarrhea

Timing	Type	Condition	Type	Diagnostic Clues
Acute	Bacterial	*Campylobacter*	Inflammatory	Consumption of undercooked poultry; bloody stools; rectal pain; fever; abdominal pain
		Clostridium difficile	Inflammatory	Consumption of undercooked beef, pork, or poultry; hospital admission or recent antibiotic use; bloody stools; rectal pain
		Listeria	Secretory	Consumption of raw milk, soft cheeses, or undercooked beef, pork, or poultry; pregnancy
		Salmonella	Inflammatory	Consumption of undercooked beef, pork, or poultry; bloody stools; rectal pain; fever; abdominal pain
		Shiga toxin–producing *E. Coli*	Inflammatory	Consumption of bean sprouts or raw ground beef, undercooked pork; bloody stools; abdominal pain
		Shigella	Inflammatory	Bloody stools; rectal pain; fever; abdominal pain; nausea and vomiting
		Vibrio	Secretory	Consumption of raw or undercooked shellfish; rice-water stools
		Yersinia	Inflammatory	Consumption of undercooked beef and pork; bloody stools; fever
	Viral	Norovirus	Secretory	Abdominal pain; nausea and vomiting
	Parasitic	*Cryptosporidium*	Secretory	Watery diarrhea, cramping
		Cyclospora	Secretory	Watery diarrhea, with frequent, sometimes explosive, bowel movements
		Entamoeba histolytica	Inflammatory	Bloody stools; rectal pain
		Giardia	Secretory	Ingestion of contaminated water; rectal pain; abdominal pain

(continues)

Table 17-3 Differential Diagnosis of Diarrhea (*continued*)

Timing	Type	Condition	Type	Diagnostic Clues
Chronic	Cancer	Cancer	Inflammatory	
	GI disorders	Celiac disease	Fatty malabsorption/ osmotic	
		Crohn's disease	Inflammatory/ secretory	
		Irritable bowel syndrome	Functional	
		Lactose intolerance	Fatty malabsorption/ osmotic	
		Obstruction		
		Ulcerative colitis	Inflammatory/ secretory	
	Surgery	Gastric bypass	Fatty malabsorption	
	Other	Hyperthyroidism	Secretory/motility	
		Medications	Secretory	More common medications associated with diarrhea: antacid and nutritional supplements that contain magnesium, antibiotics, proton pump inhibitors, selective serotonin reuptake inhibitors, nonsteroidal anti-inflammatory medications

Data from Guandalini S, Vaziri H, eds. *Diarrhea: Diagnostic and Therapeutic Advances.* New York, NY: Springer; 2011; Juckett G, Trivedi R. Evaluation of chronic diarrhea. *Am Fam Physician.* 2011;84(10):1119-1126; Barr W, Smith A. Acute diarrhea in adults. *Am Fam Physician.* 2014;89(3):180-189; Erickson CD, DuPont HL, Steffen R. *Traveler's Diarrhea.* Hamilton, Ontario: BC Decker, Inc; 2008; Lang F. *Encyclopedia of Molecular Mechanisms of Disease*, Vol. 2. New York, NY: Springer; 2009.

with diarrhea include the cephalosporins, macrolides, amoxicillin, clindamycin, aminoglycosides, and fluoroquinolones.[7] Antibiotics can trigger diarrhea through malabsorption, changes in secretory processes or motility, or alterations in the numbers or function of the normal GI flora (which then encourages an overgrowth of pathogens).[7] Normal GI flora resist overgrowth of pathogens by outcompeting pathogens for microbial nutrients and by secreting potent antimicrobial metabolites that inhibit growth of pathogens.[8] New research indicates that the normal GI flora can directly target and kill specific pathogens such as *C. difficile,* as well as release signals that enhance the innate mucosal immune response of the GI tract.[8] Risk factors for developing antibiotic-associated diarrhea include being older than 50 years of age, recent hospitalization or nursing home stay, immunosuppression, or coexisting GI diseases.[9,10] The most serious antibiotic-associated diarrhea is caused by an overgrowth of *C. difficile,* which can produce a pseudomembranous colitis and other complications such as toxic megacolon.[7] Individuals suspected of having *C. difficile* should be tested using a nucleic acid amplification tests for *C. difficile,* such as polymerase chain reaction, which has greater sensitivity than stool enzyme immunoassays for toxins A + B.[10] Given the seriousness of this condition, women suspected of having diarrhea related to *C. difficile* should be under management of a healthcare provider skilled in the management of GI infections.

Dyspepsia and Heartburn

Dyspepsia is a heterogenous set of symptoms affecting the upper abdomen. The Rome III criteria are used to assist healthcare professionals in assessing and diagnosing functional GI disorders. Dyspepsia can be divided into two categories: organic disease, where an underlying explanation for symptoms can be identified, and functional, where no underlying cause can be identified. Four cardinal symptoms of functional dyspepsia include postprandial fullness, early satiation, epigastric pain, and epigastric burning without evidence of structural disease that is likely to explain the symptoms. Other symptoms include bloating, belching, and, on occasion, nausea and vomiting.[11] If *heartburn,* a burning sensation in the chest caused by stomach acids, is the predominant symptom, then GERD is the most likely cause.[11] GERD is a condition caused by a relaxation of the lower esophageal sphincter allowing a backwash of stomach contents into the esophagus. Heartburn is one symptom of GERD. (See **Table 17-4**.)

Table 17-4 Differential Diagnosis of Dyspepsia

Type	Condition
Organic	Gastroparesis
	Gastroesophageal reflux disease
	Gastric or esophageal cancer
	Infections (*Giardia*)
	Inflammatory disease (Crohn's disease, sarcoidosis)
	Intolerance to foods or drugs
	Pancreatitis or pancreatic cancer
	Peptic ulcer
Functional	Diagnosis of exclusion, no identified pathology

Reproduced from Oustamanolakis P, Tack J. Dyspepsia: organic versus functional. *J Clin Gastroenterol.* 2012;46(3): 175-190.

Dysphagia

Dysphagia is described as difficulty swallowing or an inability to pass solid food or liquid substances from the mouth through the esophagus to the stomach. It is an uncommon symptom in most women seen in obstetric and gynecologic (OB/GYN) practices. It is more common in individuals over the age of 50 years and can be caused by numerous neuromuscular problems, obstructive masses, and medications (i.e., antibiotics, nonsteroidal anti-inflammatory drugs [NSAIDs], theophylline, and others). The underlying causes of symptoms include chronic GERD, tumors, stroke, esophageal strictures or spasms, and degenerative diseases such as multiple sclerosis. Symptoms may initially be intermittent, possibly progressing to more persistent symptoms. With esophageal strictures, solid food products are more likely to get caught than liquid or soft food products. Anyone who has rapidly progressing dysphagia needs an immediate referral and evaluation for esophageal cancer.

Swallowing is assessed as part of the physical examination. Observing the patient and feeling the rise of thyroid cartilage during a swallow can assess the coordination of the swallow processes. Laboratory tests are minimally helpful but could include a complete blood count (CBC) to help rule in inflammatory or infectious processes or a thyroid-stimulating hormone (TSH) test to evaluate the health of the thyroid.

Testing such as barium swallow, upper GI series or endoscopy, or manometry can evaluate the function of the esophageal sphincter and muscles of the esophagus and may be needed to pinpoint the underlying etiology.[12,13]

Abdominal Pain

Abdominal pain is ubiquitous in conditions affecting the GI tract. It can also be present in conditions affecting the respiratory, cardiac, or reproductive systems. Pain can be characterized as acute ($<$ 12 weeks) or chronic ($\geq$ 12 weeks). However, while this categorization may help direct the differential list, it is more useful to determine if the pain is more recent, occurring over the last several days, and worsening, or if the pain has been unchanged for months or years. Some individuals will fall in between these two extremes; in this case, conditions that cause either acute or chronic pain will need to be considered.

Any woman who presents with acute abdominal pain of rapid evolution—particularly if she also has fever, dehydration, and/or unstable vital signs—should be evaluated for cholecystitis, pancreatitis, diverticulitis, obstruction, and peritonitis. Women with obstruction may report anorexia, nausea and vomiting, and bloating. The nature of the vomitus (bilious vs. feculent) varies by location and extent of the obstruction. On examination, distension and high pitched or absent bowel sounds may be noted. *Peritonitis* (inflammation of the peritoneum) may indicate

severe infection, perforation, or intraperitoneal hemorrhage. It can also be seen in women with a ruptured ectopic pregnancy. Women with peritonitis look ill, may be reluctant to move in an attempt to avoid pain, and get little relief from pain medications. (Classic abdominal maneuvers used to evaluate an acute abdomen are described in the section covering the physical examination.) Individuals with severe presentations need to be evaluated thoroughly and rapidly to determine whether emergency surgery is needed.

Location of pain may also help direct the workup and pinpoint the diagnosis. **Table 17-5** lists etiologies commonly presenting with pain in one or more of the four quadrants of the abdomen. One of the difficulties in making a diagnosis based on location is that pain can originate from an organ within a specific quadrant or be referred from another location. For example, pain in the upper abdomen can be a result of problems with the liver or in the biliary tract, but may also be referred from the heart (i.e., myocardial infarction), kidney (i.e., infection or stone), or lung (i.e., pneumonia, pulmonary embolism). Similarly, lower abdominal pain can be related to the intestinal tract but also can be referred down from the upper abdomen or up from pelvic structures. For example, renal colic can be referred downward from the flank through the abdomen to the groin; cystitis, pelvic inflammatory disease, endometriosis, ovarian cysts, or ectopic pregnancy can also present with referred pain to the lower abdomen.

The character of the pain may also provide clues to the underlying cause of abdominal pain. Colicky pain is localized and has a specific pattern (waxes, peaks, and then wanes). It is thought to be due to small muscle contractions resulting from obstruction in the lumen of the intestine (intestinal obstruction), biliary tract (gallbladder stones), or ureter (kidney stones).[14]

If the etiology is not clear after the initial evaluation, imaging may be helpful. The American

Table 17-5 Abdominal Pain by Quadrant

RUQ	LUQ
Acute cholecystitis	Diverticulitis
Biliary colic/stones	Gastric ulcer
Duodenal ulcer	Gastritis
Hepatitis	Herpes zoster
Herpes zoster	Lower lobe pneumonia (left-sided)
Lower lobe pneumonia (right-sided)	Myocardial ischemia
Myocardial ischemia	Nephrolithiasis (left-sided)
Nephrolithiasis (right-sided)	Pancreatitis
Pancreatitis	Pericarditis
Retrocecal appendicitis	Pulmonary embolism
Subphrenic abscess	Splenic rupture
Perforated peptic ulcer	Pyloric obstruction

RLQ	LLQ
Appendicitis	Colon perforation
Cecal perforation	Constipation
Constipation	Early appendicitis
Crohn's disease	Ectopic pregnancy
Diverticulosis	Endometriosis
Ectopic pregnancy	Kidney or ureteral stone
Endometriosis	Ovarian cyst
Intestinal obstruction	Salpingitis
Kidney or ureteral stone	Sigmoid diverticulitis
Ovarian cyst	Sigmoid perforation
Regional enteritis	Strangulated hernia
Salpingitis	Ulcerative colitis
Strangulated hernia	
Perforated duodenal ulcer	
Pelvic inflammatory disease	

Abbreviations: RUQ, right upper quadrant; LUQ, left upper quadrant; RLQ, right lower quadrant; LLQ, left lower quadrant.

Data from Shaw B. Primary care for women: Comprehensive assessment of gastrointestinal disorders. *J Nurse Midwifery.* 1995;40:216–230; Barkauskas VH, Baumann LC, Darling-Fisher CS. *Health and Physical Assessment.* 3rd ed. St. Louis, MO: Mosby; 2002.

College of Radiology (ACR) makes recommendations based on diagnostic yield, safety, and cost.[15] Recommendations vary by presentation:

- *Right upper quadrant pain* suspected to be cholecystitis: initial imaging with an abdominal ultrasound, which can detect gallstones and biliary tract distension. Conditions affecting

the liver or biliary tree are the most common cause of pain in the right upper quadrant (RUQ).[16]

- *Right lower quadrant pain* suspected to be appendicitis: computed tomography (CT) scan with or without intravenous (IV) contrast media in nonpregnant women. To minimize exposure to ionizing radiation, either an abdominal ultrasound or magnetic resonance imaging (MRI) of the abdomen and pelvis without contrast is preferred for pregnant women.[17]

- *Left lower quadrant pain* suspected to be diverticulitis: CT scan of the abdomen and pelvis with contrast. No recommendations are made on the imaging test of preference for pregnant women.[18]
- *Epigastric pain* suspected to be peptic ulcer disease: upper GI (UGI) radiography with barium swallow and fluoroscopy to evaluate for gastric erosions, ulcer, or cancer. Upper GI with small bowel series can be considered if concern exists for Crohn's or other small bowel conditions.[13]
- *Nonlocalized acute abdominal pain with fever* and no recent surgery: CT of the abdomen and pelvis with contrast in nonpregnant women and, to minimize exposure to radiation, use of either an abdominal ultrasound or MRI of the abdomen and pelvis without contrast for pregnant women.[19]

All reproductive-aged women should have a pregnancy test. Other testing may be indicated. For example, an electrocardiogram is ordered if upper abdominal pain is thought to be referred from a myocardial infarction. Pulmonary causes can be evaluated with a chest x-ray (for pneumonia) or D-dimer test (for embolism) depending on associated signs and symptoms. Women with abdominal pain suspected of being referred from the pelvic organs should be evaluated with an abdominal and transvaginal pelvic ultrasound, which can detect ectopic pregnancy, ovarian cysts, or fibroids.[14]

Constipation

Constipation is defined as infrequent or difficult evacuation of feces with bowel movements. When asked to identify symptoms, individuals also include straining or hard stools as part of the definition. The consensus criteria developed by an

Table 17-6 ROME III Criteria for Constipation

Criteria
Duration of symptoms $\geq$ 6 months
Does not meet criteria for irritable bowel syndrome
Rare to no loose stools
Meets at least 2 of the following criteria for $\geq$ 25% of defecations in the last 3 months:
• Straining
• Lumpy, hard stools
• Feeling of incomplete evacuation
• Sensation of anorectal obstruction/blockage
• Manual maneuvers (e.g., digital removal, support of pelvic floor) to effect evacuation
• Fewer than 3 defecations per week

Data from Longstreth GF, Thompson WG, Chey WD, Houghton LA, Mearin F, Spiller RC. Functional bowel disorders. *Gastroenterology.* 2006;130(5):1480-1491.

international expert panel (Rome III) for defining constipation are listed in **Table 17-6**.[20] While most constipation is benign, it can also be a symptom of a number of diseases or a result of structural or neurologic problems.[21] **Table 17-7** lists conditions that should be considered if a woman reports constipation. A history of physical or sexual abuse can also result in increased GI complaints.

The American Gastroenterological Association classifies constipation into three categories: 1) slow transit time, 2) normal transit time, and 3) pelvic floor dysfunction/defecatory disorders.[21] Slow transit times can result from inadequate calorie intake or from colonic motor dysfunction. Healthy individuals have 1 to 15 high-amplitude propagated contractions in the colon daily. Delayed transit is thought to occur from one or more of the following processes: an absence of high-amplitude contractions, retrograde propulsions, reduced spatial overlap of adjacent propagated

Table 17-7 Differential Diagnosis of Constipation

Category	Example
Medical condition	Diabetes
	Hypothyroidism
	Hypokalemia
	Heavy metal poisoning
Medications	Opiates
	Nonsteroidal anti-inflammatory drugs
	Antihistamines
	Antidepressants
	Antihypertensives
Myopathies	Amyloidosis
	Scleroderma
Neuropathies	Cerebrovascular disease
	Multiple sclerosis
	Parkinson's disease
	Spinal cord injury
Obstruction	Anal fissure
	Colon cancer
	Megacolon
	Rectocele
	Strictures

Data from Bharucha A, Pemberton J, Locke G. American Gastroenterological Association technical review on constipation. *Gastroenterology.* 2013;144:218-238.

sequences, or absent responses to ingestion of a meal. Defecatory disorders are thought to be due to poor-quality rectal evacuation forces and/or increased resistance to evacuation. Resistance can be due to high resting pressure, incomplete relaxation, or paradoxical contraction of the anal muscles. Evacuation forces can be affected by excessive straining, which may weaken and damage the pelvic floor, making expulsion difficult.[21] A systematic approach in the primary care setting will help to identify the underlying cause, provide symptomatic relief, exclude serious disease, and minimize unnecessary testing.

Rectal Bleeding

The presentation of GI bleeding depends on the location and volume of bleeding and is categorized by acuity (acute vs. chronic) and by location (upper vs. lower GI tract). Upper GI bleeding originates in the esophagus, stomach, or duodenum. Vomiting of frank blood is most commonly due to disorders affecting the upper GI tract. Lower GI bleeding originates in the mid-gut (small bowel to the terminal ileum) and lower bowel (colon) and most commonly presents as bright red bleeding from the rectum (*hematochezia*).[22] However, hematochezia can also occur if there is rapid, profuse bleeding anywhere in the GI tract. Blood that mixes with stomach acid or acidic intestine secretions can present either as coffee-ground vomitus or as black, "sticky" stool (*melena*). Occult blood loss is unrecognized, but may be detected by a positive fecal occult blood test (FOBT) result and/or iron deficiency anemia.[22]

GI bleeding can also be categorized by underlying causes: mass lesion (cancer, adenoma), inflammation (i.e., ulcers, Crohn's disease, ulcerative colitis, erosive esophagitis, or gastritis), vascular disease (diverticular, vascular ectasia or angiodysplasia, a degenerative structural lesion of previously healthy vasculature of the GI tract; portal hypertensive gastropathy or colopathy), and infection (i.e., parasites).[23,24] (See **Table 17-8.**)

Symptoms associated with GI bleeding reflect the acuity of the bleeding and the underlying etiology. Women with acute and profuse bleeding may become hemodynamically unstable. In chronic bleeding, symptoms of anemia, such as fatigue, dizziness, and angina,

Table 17-8 Common Causes of Rectal Bleeding

Location	Condition	Risk Factors	Presentation
Upper GI tract	Peptic ulcer disease	NSAIDs, aspirin, tobacco	Abdominal pain, heartburn, dyspepsia
	Gastritis/duodenitis		
	Esophageal varices	Alcohol abuse	Jaundice, ascites, palmar erythema, spider angiomata, hepatomegaly, splenomegaly
	Mallory-Weiss tear		Vomiting, retching, or seizures prior to bleeding
	Gastric cancer		Left supraclavicular adenopathy, mass, abdominal pain, weight loss
Small bowel	Angiodysplasia		
	Crohn's disease	Family history	Associated fistulas
Large bowel	Diverticulitis	Age > 60 years	Painless bleeding
	Arteriovenous malformations	Age > 60 years, renal failure	Painless bleeding
	Neoplasms	Inflammatory bowel disease, age > 50 years, adenomatous polyps, family history	Abdominal pain, weight loss, muscle wasting
	Ulcerative colitis	Family history	Abdominal pain, diarrhea with blood and mucus
Anorectal causes	Hemorrhoids	Constipation, pregnancy	
	Anal fissure	Constipation, Crohn's disease, psoriasis, cancer	Sharp pain and sensation of tearing with defecation; commonly starts age 20 to 40 years
	Intestinal worms	Recent foreign travel	

GI = gastrointestinal, NSAIDs = nonsteroidal anti-inflammatory drugs

Data from Bull-Henry K, Al-Kawas F. Evaluation of occult gastrointestinal bleeding. *Am Fam Physician.* 2013;87(6):430-436; Manning-Dimmitt L, Dimmitt S, Wilson G. Diagnosis of gastrointestinal bleeding in adults. *Am Fam Physician.* 2005;71: 1339-1346.

are more common. Individuals with anatomic or vascular causes of bleeding often present with profuse, painless, large-volume blood loss, whereas diarrhea and abdominal pain are more common with inflammatory causes.[22] Black or dark green stools are associated with GI bleeding, but other causes of black stools should be considered and include bismuth (found in antidiarrheal products), licorice, and iron preparations.

The initial evaluation is directed by presentation and suspected location of pathology. Hemodynamically unstable individuals need rapid evaluation to detect the underlying cause and put in place measures to stabilize, and begin treatment for, the affected individual. Appropriate triage can be conducted using standardized assessments to direct the diagnostic approach.[23] The Glasgow-Blatchford Score and other systems use clinical information (i.e., blood pressure, pulse rate, syncope, comorbidities) and laboratory data rapidly obtained after emergency department admission (e.g., CBC, blood urea nitrogen [BUN]) to determine the likelihood that an intervention (endoscopy, transfusion, or surgery) will be needed and the risk of death. The result can be used to help determine timing of testing (e.g., urgent vs. routine endoscopy) and location of care (i.e., inpatient vs. outpatient).[25]

A variety of approaches are recommended to evaluate GI bleeding. An endoscopy is used to evaluate suspected upper GI bleeding, but is limited by the length of the scope. It can best evaluate the esophagus, stomach, and duodenum, but cannot reach down far enough to evaluate the entire small bowel.[23] Bleeding from sources farther down in the GI tract, in the mid to distal small bowel, can be evaluated by push endoscopy, capsule endoscopy, deep enteroscopy, or CT enterography. Push endoscopy, which uses longer scopes than used in endoscopy, can reach the proximal jejunum, but not farther, and has higher complication rates than other procedures; therefore, it is used less frequently. Capsule endoscopy is considered by the American College of Gastroenterology to be a first-line agent in the investigation of small bowel disease,[26] because it is a noninvasive way to evaluate the entire length of the small bowel.[23] The patient is asked to swallow a pill-sized video camera, which will pass out of the body through the stool. The video camera transmits pictures to a device worn around the abdomen by the patient. These pictures are later analyzed and can detect problems located anywhere in the small bowel. With deep enteroscopy, a scope is inserted via an oral or anal route, which can reach deep into the GI tract, as far as the mid and distal small bowel. CT enterography scans can also be used to evaluate the small bowel, but are less accurate in detecting vascular ectasia, which is a common cause of occult bleeding from the small bowel.[23] However, CT and MRI enterography scans have the advantage of being able to evaluate the bowel wall and can detect extra-enteric disease.[22]

All women over the age of 50 should undergo colonoscopy screening for colon cancer. Colonoscopy is also used in the evaluation of lower GI bleeding, suggested by frank rectal bleeding or melena, and in evaluation of occult bleeding, suspected in the presence of iron deficiency anemia or a positive fecal occult blood test. The American Gastroenterological Association recommends colonoscopy in women over age 50 years who have iron deficiency anemia, even if the fecal occult smear is negative, because the risk of colon cancer increases with age.[23,27] Endoscopy is not needed unless upper GI tract bleeding is suspected. However, colonoscopy in combination with endoscopy is recommended in women with a positive fecal occult smear, even if no anemia is present, because occult bleeding can occur from sources anywhere in the bowel.[27] The combination of both tests is useful in detecting disease of both the upper and lower GI tract.[22]

Other tests include CT angiography, catheter angiography, and radionuclide scans. CT angiography is noninvasive and can identify the exact site and cause of bleeding, but it requires a sufficient level of active bleeding to pull contrast into the bowel lumen to identify the site of bleeding. Catheter angiography can detect bleeding sites and can also be used as a therapeutic option, because it allows for infusion of vasoconstrictive medications into the area of active bleeding. Radionuclide imaging can also detect bleeding but cannot identify the underlying cause and is less accurate in localizing the site of bleeding compared to CT.[22]

Essential History, Physical, and Laboratory Evaluation

Because symptoms related to the GI system can represent such diverse conditions, evaluation begins by focusing on the presenting symptoms, their evolution over time, and associated signs and symptoms. What questions are asked, what components of the physical exam are done, and what laboratory or imaging tests, if any, are performed will be driven by the differential diagnosis. Certain constellations of symptoms, physical exam findings, and laboratory results suggest different etiologies. See **Table 17-9** for a description of diagnostic possibilities.

History

The history for GI-related conditions needs to be comprehensive, starting with presenting symptoms and evolution of symptoms over time. Specific questions will vary by primary complaint. Patients presenting with nausea or vomiting should be asked about the presence or absence of nausea, retching and/or vomiting, and symptom onset, duration, and frequency. A diet history should be taken for the 24 hours prior to onset of symptoms and include the patient's ability to eat or drink amidst symptoms. Patients should be asked about associated symptoms such as fever, headache, abdominal pain, constipation, or diarrhea; alleviating or exacerbating factors; and over-the-counter, prescription, or alternative therapies used successfully or unsuccessfully for relief. Many drugs act on the CTZ to cause

nausea and vomiting, including opiates, dopamine agonists, nicotine, digoxin anesthetics, and chemotherapy agents. Other commonly used agents such as aspirin, NSAIDs, and antibiotics cause damage to the gastric mucosa and activate the vomiting center. The clinician should also inquire about possible pregnancy with questions about menstrual history, contraceptive practices, and associated symptoms common to early pregnancy such as breast tenderness, fatigue, or increased urinary frequency. The patient should be assessed for presence of eating disorders, sexual/physical abuse, and substance use or abuse.

Often women have difficulty describing the frequency and characteristics of their stool. The first set of questions when investigating reports of diarrhea or constipation should be directed to determining if indeed a woman truly has constipation or diarrhea or is just having a normal variation of her usual stool pattern. Pictorial descriptions, such as the Bristol Stool Form Scale, can aid with clarity. Once the frequency and consistency of the stool are clear, then additional details gleaned from the clinical history can help to establish the cause of diarrhea or constipation. Many of the questions described earlier in the section on nausea and vomiting should be included (i.e., medical and diet history, symptoms of dehydration, and medication use), as well as symptom duration, pain, fever, weight loss, and travel history.[28] Additional questions include whether diarrhea occurs only during the day or during nighttime sleep, and whether fecal incontinence is occurring due to the frequency and urgency of the stooling. Almost all medications can have diarrhea as a side effect, and some are associated with constipation. Asking about the temporal relationship of medications to the onset of diarrhea or constipation might help establish a link.[5] Determining if others in her household, workplace, or school environment are also ill can help elucidate if diarrhea is

Table 17-9 Abdominal Pain by Main Location with Signs and Symptoms

Diagnosis	Pain Location	Pain Radiates	Symptoms	Signs
Hepatitis	RUQ	Right shoulder	• Fatigue • Malaise • Anorexia	• Hepatic tenderness • Hepatomegaly • Increased bilirubin • Jaundice • Increased liver enzymes
Cholecystitis Cholelithiasis	RUQ Epigastric pain	Back, right scapula, mid-epigastric, sudden onset with associated nausea	• Anorexia • Nausea • Severe pain • Prolonged episodes	• RUQ tenderness • Jaundice • Vomiting • Increased WBC • Peritoneal irritation
Pancreatitis	Mid-epigastric region LUQ	Radiates to back, left shoulder, may have peritonitis, knife-like pain	• Pain radiating to back or chest	• Fever • Rigidity • Rebound tenderness • Nausea • Vomiting • Jaundice • Abdominal distension • Diminished bowel sounds
Gastric Ulcer Duodenal Ulcer	Mid-epigastric LLQ pain	Radiation to back, if posterior ulcer, peritonitis with perforation, may awaken patient from sleep	• Abrupt pain if perforated • Burning pain	• Tenderness in epigastric and/or RUQ
Aortic Aneurysm	Periumbilical – especially into back flanks	Epigastric or back pain, flank, hip pain May be colicky	• Abdominal, back or flank	• Vague to severe GI symptoms

(continues)

Table 17-9 Abdominal Pain by Main Location with Signs and Symptoms *(continued)*

Diagnosis	Pain Location	Pain Radiates	Symptoms	Signs
Appendicitis	Early – periumbilical Late – RLQ at McBurney point	May present with peritoneal signs	• Anorexia • Nausea • Pain	• Vomiting • Localized RLQ guarding and tenderness late • Rovsing sign • Iliopsoas sign • Obturator sign • WBC increased • Left shift • Low grade fever
Crohn's disease or ulcerative colitis	RLQ Central pain	May radiate to back	• Chronic, watery diarrhea with blood, mucus • Anorexia • Weight loss • Fatigue	• Fever • Cachexia • Anemia • Leukocytosis
Diverticulitis	LLQ Rare RLQ	Generalized	• Recurrent LLQ pain	• Fever • Vomiting • Diarrhea • Chills • Tenderness over descending colon
GYN– ovarian cyst, ovarian torsion, ectopic, PID	RLQ, LLQ, suprapubic	Radiation to groin or right shoulder	• Symptoms of pregnancy • Lower abdominal pain • Nausea • Dyspareunia	• Tenderness • Mass • Fever • Cervical motion tenderness • Cervical discharge
Urolithiasis or nephrolithiasis	Flank	Radiates to labia	• Hematuria dysuria	• Flank pain • CVAT
Cystitis	Suprapubic pain		• Urgency • Dysuria • Frequency • Hematuria	• Flank pain

Abbreviations are: RUQ, right upper quadrant; LUQ, left upper quadrant; RLQ, right lower quadrant; LLQ, left lower quadrant; CVAT, costovertebral angle tenderness; PID, pelvic inflammatory disease.

Data from Shaw B. Primary care for women: Comprehensive assessment of gastrointestinal disorders. *J Nurse Midwifery.* 1995;40:216–230; Graber MA. General surgery. In: Graber MA, Toth PP, Herting RL, Eds. University of Iowa. *The Family Practice Handbook.* 3rd ed. St. Louis, MO: Mosby; 1997, pp. 380–411.

due to a viral or food-borne illness. Both diarrhea and constipation can signal the presence of underlying medical problems or cancer. Alarm symptoms include sudden change in bowel habits after age 50 years, unexplained weight loss, anemia, persistent abdominal pain, and family history of colon cancer.[21]

The history for women reporting dyspepsia should include relationship of symptoms to food or medication intake, chronicity, and the presence of alarm symptoms: weight loss, symptoms of bleeding, or dysphagia.[11] Dyspepsia can accompany a wide range of GI infections and conditions. Determining which of the many symptoms are most problematic for a woman with dyspepsia can help narrow the differential diagnosis list. For example, women who primarily experience heartburn or dyspepsia with food intake may have GERD or another upper GI tract disorder.

The history for a woman presenting with abdominal pain is particularly challenging, because abdominal pain can be due to numerous conditions affecting the cardiac, respiratory, GI, musculoskeletal, and reproductive systems. It is particularly important to elicit the timeline of symptoms, their evolution, accompanying symptoms, and the presence or absence of risk factors. For reproductive-aged women, the first set of questions should always focus on the possibility of pregnancy. Whether a woman is pregnant or not affects what diagnoses are under consideration, what additional laboratory or imaging testing is needed, and what components of the physical exam need to be performed. Table 17-9 describes symptoms of common etiologies associated with abdominal pain.

Rectal bleeding encompasses a wide range of presentations ranging from benign (e.g., hemorrhoids, use of NSAIDs) to life threatening (e.g., massive hemorrhage, cancer). Thus, the range of questions is correspondingly broad and should cover medications (e.g., risk of mucosal injury from NSAID use or precipitation of bleeding with anticoagulant use), risk factors for cancer (e.g., family history, IBD), or the presence of other conditions that predispose to bleeding (e.g., gastroenterological conditions, liver disease).[23]

Physical Examination

The physical examination of a patient presenting with GI-related symptoms should be comprehensive and directed by findings elicited by history. It should include at minimum vital signs and examination of the lungs, heart, and abdomen. Based on the history, a complete examination of the head, ears, eyes, nose, and throat; neurologic assessment; and pelvic and rectal examination may also be indicated.

Specific findings can suggest the underlying cause and potential complications. For example, dehydration may be suggested by tachycardia, orthostatic hypotension, and in extreme cases, by poor skin turgor. Dermatitis herpetiformis, an itchy blistering rash, can occur in celiac disease. Erythema nodosum, pyoderma gangrenosum, and psoriasis may accompany IBD. Tremor, goiter, and exophthalmoses can be seen with hyperthyroidism. Lymphadenopathy can be present in acquired immune deficiency syndrome (AIDS) or lymphoma.[6,7] Dyspepsia accompanied by dysphagia might indicate gastric cancer.[11]

A thorough examination of the abdomen is essential. With the patient supine, the abdomen should be inspected for shape, symmetry, gross distension, hernias, pulsations, and visible scars. Next, the abdomen should be auscultated *prior* to palpation or manipulation of the abdomen, because this may disturb intestinal function, thereby affecting bowel sounds. Frequency and character of bowel sounds should be noted in all four quadrants. Generally, the frequency of sounds is increased with diarrhea and early intestinal obstruction and decreased in peritonitis and ileus. Vascular sounds are assessed for bruits, an indication of turbulent flow within the vessel, and the liver and spleen are auscultated for friction rubs if a mass or peritoneal infection is suspected. Percussion may be helpful in distinguishing distension caused by fluid versus air.

Palpation should begin lightly in all quadrants before proceeding to deeper manipulation. Eliciting pain or tenderness can suggest particular entities. Specific maneuvers are described in **Table 17-10**. The presence of hepatomegaly, masses, or ascites on abdominal exam should be noted.

A pelvic exam is mandatory in women reporting abdominal and pelvic pain. A thorough examination is needed to evaluate for gynecologic causes of abdominal pain such as endometriosis, ectopic pregnancy, ovarian masses, fibroids, and pelvic inflammatory disease. The pelvic exam can also detect uterine prolapse, cystocele, and rectocele. Uterine prolapse and reduced pelvic floor strength can impede the ability of a woman to evacuate stool.

A digital rectal exam can assess anal tone.[29] The rectal exam is best performed with the woman lying on her left side with the knees drawn up. The provider should observe the descent of the perineum when asking a woman to simulate stool evacuation and an elevation of the perineum when the woman is asked to squeeze the rectal muscles to simulate retention of stool. The anal verge should be snuggly closed; gaping could indicate a neurogenic cause of constipation. During a digital rectal exam, the resting tone of the sphincter can be evaluated, as can the strength and coordination of the sphincter when the woman is asked to squeeze around the examining finger. The puborectalis

Table 17-10 Maneuvers in Evaluating the Abdomen

Sign	How Elicited	Differential Diagnosis
Rebound	Gentle deep pressure over abdomen with quick release produces severe pain on release	Local or general peritonitis
Guarding	Patient resistance to gentle pressure on abdominal wall	Voluntary or involuntary response to palpation related to perforated viscera (internal organs) or internal bleeding
Murphy sign	Pause in inspiration as examiner palpates under liver	Cholecystitis
Rovsing sign	Palpation of LLQ causes pain in RLQ	Appendicitis
McBurney point	Point at which palpation of RLQ two-thirds distance between umbilicus and right iliac crest causes pain	Appendicitis
Obturator sign	Pain on rotation of flexed thigh, especially with internal rotation	Perforated appendix
Costovertebral angle tenderness (CVAT)	Gentle tap with closed fist bilaterally along the spine in the region of the kidneys	Pain can indicate kidney infection
Psoas sign	Pain on extension of right thigh	Appendicitis

LLQ = left lower quadrant, RLQ = right lower quadrant

muscle should also contract during the squeeze. Acute pain on palpation of the puborectalis muscle could indicate levator ani syndrome. Asking the woman to push the examiner's finger out of the rectum can assess expulsory forces. In addition, the presence of hemorrhoids, rectal bleeding, or an anal fissure may be noted.[21,29]

Laboratory Evaluation

In most cases, the cause of symptoms will be clear from the history and physical examination, but testing may be needed in select cases. Which exact test is needed will vary by presentation and suspected etiology. The following is a list of commonly ordered tests and a description of when, and why, they might be helpful in evaluating potentially GI-related symptoms:[2,3,28]

- *Celiac serologies* (tissue transglutaminase [tTg], endomysial antibodies [EMA]) can be helpful in investigating refractory cases of dyspepsia and diarrhea.[11]
- *Complete blood count* may show hemoconcentration in the presence of dehydration. Elevated white blood cells (WBCs) may indicate the presence of inflammation or infection. Findings suggestive of anemia may indicate the presence of malabsorption or GI bleeding.
- *Electrolyte imbalances* such as acidosis, alkalosis, and hypokalemia can occur with severe vomiting and diarrhea.
- *Erythrocyte sedimentation rate/C-reactive protein* can be elevated with inflammation.
- *Fecal leukocytes, lactoferrin, and calprotectin* are tests that are used to detect the presence of inflammatory diarrhea. Lactoferrin has largely replaced fecal leukocyte testing, because it has higher sensitivity and specificity and results are rapidly available. Lactoferrin is a marker for leukocytes released by damaged or dying cells and increases in bacterial infections.[28] Calprotectin detects the presence of neutrophilic protein in the stool, which is elevated in

inflammatory disease. It is a noninvasive test and particularly useful in distinguishing IBS from inflammatory diarrhea and can also predict disease flares in those with already established inflammatory disease.[30]

- *Fecal occult blood* tests may be performed to detect the presence of blood. Positive results can be present in infection or with damage to the GI tract. In combination with a positive fecal leukocyte or lactoferrin test, a positive result suggests inflammatory diarrhea.[28]
- *Fecal osmotic gap* is useful in the evaluation of chronic diarrhea. An analysis based on fecal electrolytes (i.e., sodium, potassium, anions) can distinguish between osmotic and secretory diarrhea. Fecal electrolytes are high in secretory diarrhea because electrolytes are incompletely absorbed, whereas with osmotic diarrhea electrolyte absorption is unaffected and fecal electrolytes in a stool sample are low.[31] Thus, this test is used to direct the next steps needed to detect the underlying cause of diarrhea.
- *Helicobacter pylori testing* can be obtained through serologic testing, specifically enzyme-linked immunosorbent assay (ELISA), which can detect whether an individual has been exposed to infection, but cannot document cure. Other alternatives include a urea breath test, stool antigen test, and stomach biopsy—all of which are considered adequate for screening and confirming cure after treatment.[32] Of the four test options, serologic testing is the least accurate.[33]
- *Liver enzymes, lipase, and amylase* may be helpful in the evaluation of upper abdominal pain or jaundice to rule out liver or gallbladder disease, infections such as hepatitis, or pancreatitis.
- *Hepatitis panel* should be ordered for initial evaluation of abnormal liver enzymes, signs of jaundice, or exposure to blood products.
- *Pregnancy* tests in reproductive-aged women are commonly performed because early pregnancy is often unrecognized and can cause nausea and vomiting. A positive pregnancy

test can also help differentiate an ectopic pregnancy from appendicitis, which can have similar presentations.

- *Stool for ova and parasites* should be ordered if parasites are suspected to be the underlying cause of persistent diarrhea or chronic anemia. Many tests for ova and parasites do not automatically include tests for *Cryptosporidium* and *Giardia*; therefore, these tests may need to be added to the panel. Shedding may only be sporadic, so collection of samples ideally occurs on 3 consecutive days.[34,35]
- *Stool cultures* are generally unnecessary in the evaluation of acute diarrhea, unless a patient has obviously bloody stools, persistent or severe symptoms, immunosuppression, signs of inflammatory disease, or is elderly. Stool cultures for *C. difficile* should be considered in hospitalized patients with persistent unexplained diarrhea of 3 or more days' duration and in outpatients who have used antibiotics in the previous 3 months.[28]
- *Thyroid-stimulating hormone* can be considered, although thyroid disease is a rare cause of nausea, vomiting, diarrhea, or constipation.
- *Urinalysis* is useful in detecting urinary or kidney infections and in assessing the degree of dehydration if present.
- *Urine culture* is useful if lower or upper urinary infections are suspected, which can cause referred pain to the abdomen.

Imaging/Diagnostic Procedures

Imaging studies are used to evaluate for the presence of lesions, obstruction, or dysfunction of the gallbladder, liver, pancreas, or intestinal tract. These tests include the following:[2,5]

- *Abdominal x-ray is performed* if constipation, bowel obstruction, kidney stones, or a foreign body are suspected. Free air under the diaphragm can be seen with or without GI perforation. Although not always present, calcifications can be seen with gallstones (10%) and kidney stones (90%).[14]
- *Abdominal ultrasonography* is the preferred test to evaluate the possible presence of gallstones. It is also used in the evaluation of palpable abdominal masses, trauma, and suspected abdominal and/or retroperitoneal pathology.[16,36]
- *Chest x-ray* may be considered if aspiration of gastric contents is of concern or pulmonary pathology is suspected.
- *Colonoscopy or flexible sigmoidoscopy* may be ordered if inflammatory diarrhea, such as Crohn's disease or ulcerative colitis, is suspected. Because colonic biopsy and cultures can be obtained via lower endoscopy procedures, these tests can also be helpful in differentiating colitis from *C. difficile*.[28] Sigmoidoscopy may be sufficient as the initial endoscopy test in the evaluation of chronic diarrhea, but colonoscopy should be considered if findings are inconclusive, symptoms persist, or if IBD is suspected. Colonoscopy is the preferred test if colorectal cancer is suspected.[37]
- *Computed tomography scans* are useful in a variety of situations. CT scan with IV contrast media is the initial preferred test in the evaluation of lower right-sided abdominal pain in nonpregnant women, because it has a high detection rate for appendicitis and is more accurate than an abdominal ultrasound in detecting appendicitis. A CT scan (with oral and IV contrast media) is used in the evaluation of lower left-sided pain suggestive of diverticular disease.[14] CT scans can be particularly helpful in evaluating patients with nonspecific pain who need urgent evaluation, because they can provide imaging of the pancreas, spleen, kidneys, intestines, and vasculature.[14] They are also used in the evaluation of possible gallstones or other biliary conditions. However, CT scans

should be used judiciously. An abdominal CT scan exposes a woman to approximately three times the amount of radiation she would receive each year from background radiation.[38] Alternative modalities, particularly ultrasound and MRI, are increasingly being evaluated as potentially safer alternatives to CT scans.[38]

- *Endoscopic retrograde cholangiopancreatography (ERCP)* has a sensitivity of 85% to 87% and specificity of 100% for determining if the biliary tree is healthy and for identifying bile duct obstruction and choledocholithiasis. It can be used for imaging the biliary tree and as a way to remove stones.[39]
- *Esophagogastroduodenoscopy (EGD; also known as an upper endoscopy)* with or without biopsy is used in the management of GERD if the diagnosis is in doubt or if GERD does not resolve with treatment. It may also be helpful in evaluating diarrhea, abdominal pain, upper GI bleeding, or other conditions that affect the upper GI tract. Results can also be used to distinguish causes of chronic diarrhea such as celiac disease, *Giardia* infection, Crohn's disease, Whipple's disease, intestinal amyloid, and pancreatic insufficiency.[37]
- *Hepatobiliary iminodiacetic acid scan (HIDA)* is used to visualize the biliary tree and rule out liver and gallbladder disease. It has a sensitivity of 97% and specificity of 77% for the detection of acute cholecystitis.[39]
- *Magnetic resonance cholangiopancreatography (MRCP)* has a sensitivity of 97% and specificity of 98% for detecting gallstones anywhere in the biliary tract.[39]
- *MRI of the abdomen* is an alternative test to evaluate possible obstruction of the GI tract.
- *MRI or CT of the head* evaluates neurologic causes of nausea and vomiting such as cancer or tumors, only when other signs or symptoms are present that suggest an underlying neurologic cause of nausea and vomiting.

- *Pelvic ultrasound* may be needed if pain related to the uterus or ovaries is suspected. It can help identify the location of a pregnancy (intrauterine or ectopic), fibroids, or ovarian cysts. The transvaginal approach is preferred.
- *Scintigraphy* or gastric emptying study is used to evaluate gastric motility disorders such as gastroparesis. Gastroparesis, or delayed gastric emptying, results in a slowing or cessation of the movement of food from the stomach into the small intestine. The cause of gastroparesis is usually unknown, but it can occur due to damage to the vagus nerve from surgery or as a complication of diabetes. With scintigraphy, the patient is asked to consume a standard meal and then a series of images are obtained to assess gastric emptying time.
- *Upper GI series* is a series of x-rays obtained after swallowing barium, using fluoroscopy, which can evaluate the health of the esophagus, stomach, and upper small intestine. It is used to identify muscle weakness, varices, tumors, strictures, hiatal hernias, or esophageal ulcers and other conditions affecting the upper GI tract that can cause dyspepsia, nausea, vomiting, weight loss, or upper GI bleeding.[13]

Management of Common Gastrointestinal Conditions

The GI conditions covered in this section are organized by their predominant symptom. Although most of these conditions have overlapping symptoms, particularly abdominal pain, this organizational structure will help providers hone in on the differential list for various presentations. The role of midwives and other women's health providers will vary depending on the acuity, severity, and duration of symptoms and whether the condition is a self-limited or chronic condition. Therefore, in some situations the women's health provider will manage and treat the condition independently, and in others the role of the women's health provider will be to provide anticipatory guidance, order baseline tests, and refer to an appropriate specialist.

Conditions Associated with Nausea, Vomiting, and/or Diarrhea

Gastroenteritis

Most cases of acute diarrhea are attributed to viral infections. Viral diarrhea is characterized by the destruction of villous mucosa, which decreases the intestinal surface area available for absorption and ion secretion. Symptoms suggestive of viral gastroenteritis include abdominal pain, fever, anorexia, and myalgia. Noroviruses, which are highly infectious, are the causative agent in 40% to 60% of nonbacterial cases of gastroenteritis.[6]

Bacterial diarrhea causes inflammation of the colon, resulting in red blood cells and WBCs in the stool. Normal feces should have few or no red blood cells or WBCs. In the United States, most bacterial infections are due to ingesting improperly cooked or contaminated food. Common etiologies are *Salmonella, Shigella, Escherichia coli, Yersinia,* and *Campylobacter.*[6] *E. coli* O157:H7, a Shiga toxin–producing *E. coli,* is a frequent cause of severe diarrhea in the United States. Characteristic features of bacterial diarrhea include elevated temperature and multiple stools per day that are bloody and explosive.[28]

Food poisoning occurs when an enterotoxin or protozoa is ingested from contaminated food or water or when infectious agents within the stomach produce enterotoxins. Nausea, vomiting, and abdominal pain may be present along with diarrhea. Ingestion of suspicious food (i.e., raw meats, eggs, or shellfish; unpasteurized milk or juices; improperly stored or refrigerated foods) suggests food poisoning, especially if similar symptoms are present in other persons exposed to the same food. Bacterial or protozoal infections, commonly caused from exposure to contaminated water or food, are the most common cause of traveler's diarrhea found in individuals visiting developing semitropical or tropical countries, particularly Mexico, parts of Africa and the Middle East, and the Indian subcontinent.[6]

Protozoal infections are less common causes of diarrhea in the United States. *Cryptosporidium* and *Giardia lamblia* are the most common causative agents. Both are transmitted via the fecal–oral route.[34,35] They are environmentally hardy, moderately chlorine tolerant, and highly infectious. The primary risk factor for acquiring giardiasis is drinking contaminated water, particularly water from poorly maintained or constructed wells. Other risk factors include exposure through contact with 1) contaminated water during recreational sports in pools, lakes, and ponds; 2) contaminated stool via diaper-changing practices in daycare settings; 3) *Giardia* cysts by engaging in oral-anal sex with an infected individual; and 4) rarely in the United States, food contaminated by infected food service workers.[6,34] Risk factors are similar for *Cryptosporidium*: ingestion of recreational or untreated drinking water, contact with livestock, recent international travel, or contact with infected persons.[6,35]

Because most diarrheal illnesses are viral in origin and self-limited, treatment is usually supportive. Evidence does not support commonly recommended practices such as the avoidance of solid food or dairy or following a BRAT (bananas, rice, applesauce, and toast) or bland diet.[28] The focus is on rehydration. Usually liquids are sufficient, but an oral rehydration solution may be useful in individuals with severe diarrhea, postural lightheadedness, or reduced urination. Oral rehydration solutions can be purchased (e.g., Pedialyte) or made at home.[4] A reduced osmolarity oral rehydration solution approximating World

Health Organization (WHO)–recommended solutions can be created by mixing ½ teaspoon of salt, 6 teaspoons of sugar, and 1 liter of water.[28] If oral rehydration is not sufficient, IV rehydration may be necessary.

Microbiologic investigation (i.e., stool examination for WBCs, ova and parasites, or blood; stool culture) is usually unnecessary. If a woman has significant fever, bloody diarrhea, or suspected traveler's diarrhea, then testing is appropriate for *Salmonella, Shigella, Campylobacter,* or *E. coli* O157:H7, and for *C. difficile* if she reports recent antibiotic use, chemotherapy, or hospitalization and diarrhea of more than 3 days' duration.[28] Testing for parasites (*Giardia, Cryptosporidium, Cyclospora,* or *Isospora belli*) or for inflammatory markers (fecal lactoferrin testing or microscopy for leukocytes) should be considered if diarrhea persists for more than 7 days.[4]

Some medications may provide symptomatic relief. Loperamide, particularly in combination with simethicone, can relieve gas-related symptoms and reduce diarrhea.[28] These products are contraindicated in individuals with bloody diarrhea and can lead to the development of serious complications. Bismuth subsalicylate (Pepto-Bismol) is another safer alternative and can be used with inflammatory diarrhea. The use of probiotics may be helpful in the prevention and treatment of antibiotic-associated diarrhea.[28] Concurrent administration of probiotics along with antibiotics was associated with a 40% reduction in the risk of developing diarrhea in 1 large meta-analysis of 63 randomized controlled trials (RCTs) including 11,811 participants.[40]

Antibiotics are usually avoided in the treatment of acute diarrhea, with the exception of traveler's diarrhea, due to concerns about eradicating normal healthy intestinal flora, encouraging superimposed *C. difficile* infections, and promoting the development of antibiotic resistance.[4] Preventive regimens are generally not given except to immunocompromised individuals.[41] For healthier individuals, antibiotics can be prescribed in advance but only used if diarrhea develops while traveling. Unfortunately, post-treatment colonization with antibiotic-resistant organisms is highly likely.[42] Therefore, some authorities recommend a triage approach to treatment.[43] A clear triage plan should be put in place before a woman travels. This will ensure that unnecessary antibiotic use will be avoided and the woman will understand the parameters of when to seek care if she becomes seriously ill.

Generally, individuals with loose stools, no fever, and only mild constitutional symptoms need only oral rehydration. Individuals with moderate symptoms (defined as having greater than 3 stools in a day with mild constitutional symptoms) can be treated with an antimotility agent such as loperamide for 48 hours. Antibiotics are optional. However, loperamide should not be used for an extended period of time or in the presence of high fever, bloody diarrhea, or other symptoms of inflammatory diarrhea. Misuse is associated with paralytic ileus, severe colitis, and perforation. Those with more severe presentations (defined as six stools a day with or without other symptoms) should be treated with antibiotics and antimotility agents. Symptoms persisting for > 72 hours require evaluation by trained professionals.[43]

If the decision is made that antibiotic treatment for traveler's diarrhea is necessary, the choice of antibiotic will depend on local microbial patterns. *E. coli* and *Campylobacter* have historically been the most commonly identified causative agents, although many other bacterial, viral, and parasitic agents are increasingly being identified in traveler's diarrhea.[41] The drugs of choice where resistant *Campylobacter* is unlikely (i.e., Mexico, Central America, sub-Saharan Africa, and possibly South America) are the fluoroquinolones, whereas azithromycin is recommended for treatment of diarrhea for travelers to South and Southeast Asia where resistant *Campylobacter* is more prevalent.[41,43] Consultation with local travel experts prior to traveling is often helpful in determining what antibiotics, if any, are recommended and if other preventive practices, such as vaccines, are needed.

More intensive care for serious and persistent presentations of gastroenteritis may be needed. Referral to an emergency department is indicated when the individual presents with diarrhea-induced dehydration accompanied by an inability to tolerate oral fluid replacement. Urgent referral is also mandatory if hemolytic uremic syndrome is suspected, which is a rare but potentially fatal complication of diarrhea, primarily associated with diarrhea caused by Shiga toxin–producing *E. coli* or *Shigella dysenteriae*.[44] Most individuals with hemolytic uremic syndrome require blood transfusions. Others are affected by neurologic damage and renal failure, making prompt evaluation and treatment critical in preventing long-term morbidity or death.[44] Some chronic forms of diarrhea (e.g., Crohn's disease, ulcerative colitis, or AIDS) can also present with acute symptoms. If the latter conditions are suspected, referral to a gastroenterologist is warranted.

Conditions Associated with Nausea and Vomiting

GASTROPARESIS

Gastroparesis is a condition of delayed stomach emptying in the absence of mechanical obstruction. A buildup of food and liquid content in the stomach causes bloating, nausea, abdominal distension, vomiting, and early satiety. The etiology of gastroparesis involves several factors and can be characterized in one of three main categories: idiopathic, diabetic, and postsurgical. There is an association between psychologic dysfunction and severity of disease. Patients with gastroparesis often feel socially isolated because of the inability

to eat normally. These feelings of isolation and rejection, food cravings, and stigmatization lead to decreased quality of life.[45]

There are no standardized treatment plans for individuals with gastroparesis. Modification of diet is imperative, avoiding foods with high roughage. Surgical placement of a gastric stimulator has been shown to provide varying improvement of symptoms. Prokinetic medications, such as metoclopramide (Reglan), need to be given cautiously because of the anticholinergic effects, especially in older adults. Individuals with severe presentations may require supplemental feedings, by jejunal feeding tube or parenterally, to maintain nutritional balance.[45]

Conditions Associated with Diarrhea

CELIAC DISEASE/GLUTEN INTOLERANCE

Celiac disease is an immune-mediated disorder triggered by the ingestion of gluten, a protein found in wheat, rye, and barley, in individuals with genetic susceptibility to the disorder. It affects less than 1% of the population but is more common in women than in men.[46] Common symptoms include diarrhea, steatorrhea, weight loss, postprandial abdominal pain, and bloating. Less common manifestations include dermatitis herpetiformis (a blistering rash) and ataxia.[47] Serologic tests are confirmed by obtaining a biopsy of the small intestine during an endoscopy procedure. Treatment consists of avoiding gluten in the diet.[46,47] Most individuals with celiac disease can tolerate eating pure oats uncontaminated by gluten in limited amounts. Adding oats to the diet, if tolerated, can improve dietary quality by adding extra fiber, vitamin B, magnesium, and iron.[47]

Non-celiac gluten sensitivity (NCGS) manifests itself with GI and/or non-GI symptoms. After ingesting foods with gluten, complaints of bloating, diarrhea, and abdominal pain can occur. Symptoms are relieved with a gluten-free diet. NCGS differs from wheat allergy and celiac disease in that it is not the result of allergy or autoimmune disorder. Serologies for celiac disease will be negative, as will biopsies of the small bowel; NCGS is not associated with damage to the small bowel. The diagnosis of NCGS is a diagnosis of exclusion and confirmed if symptoms return after gluten-containing foods are reintroduced to the diet.[48,49]

INFLAMMATORY BOWEL DISEASE

IBD is divided into two types: ulcerative colitis and Crohn's disease. Both conditions can present with abdominal pain and diarrhea. While similar in many aspects, there are distinct differences between the two conditions. *Ulcerative colitis* affects the colon and rectum. The pattern of damage is continuous, usually beginning in the rectum and spreading proximally up the GI tract. Rectal bleeding and bloody diarrhea are common symptoms. In contrast, *Crohn's disease* can affect the entire GI tract. Damage is sporadic and characterized by "skip" lesions of affected tissue alternating with healthy tissue. Lesions are most frequently found in the small intestine and colon, particularly in the terminal ileum and cecum. Perianal disease, fistulas, and strictures are common, but the rectum is usually spared.[50]

Crohn's Disease Crohn's disease is thought to originate with an insult to the GI tract (e.g., alternation in the normal intestinal flora or damage to the mucosal barrier of the GI tract) that triggers an abnormal immune response in genetically susceptible individuals.[50] Affected individuals may report fever, malaise, anorexia, and weight loss, along with abdominal pain and diarrhea.[51] Risk factors for Crohn's disease include a family history of IBD, recent use of NSAIDs, and cigarette smoking. Physical findings indicative of the disease include abdominal fullness or mass or a perianal fissure, mass, or large skin

tags. Other systemic findings that can occur with Crohn's disease include spondylarthritis, arthritis, skin manifestations (erythema nodosum and pyoderma gangrenosum), ocular changes (uveitis, episcleritis, or scleroconjunctivitis), primary sclerosing cholangitis, and hypercoagulability.[52]

Laboratory tests may show anemia, thrombocytosis, or elevated erythrocyte sedimentation rates or C-reactive protein. Testing must be done to exclude other diagnostic possibilities. Commonly ordered tests include markers of intestinal inflammation (fecal calprotectin or lactoferrin), general inflammatory markers (C-reactive protein, elevated segmentation rates), and tests for other causes (ova and parasites, *C. difficile*). Usually a diagnosis is confirmed via colonoscopy and/or imaging of the small bowel and by histopathology findings on biopsy. CT enterography or MRI can be used to determine the extent of damage to the small bowel. Results can help elucidate disease severity, location, and type (penetrating, structuring, or inflammation).[50,52]

The course of the disease fluctuates, with individuals experiencing remissions of variable length of time and eventual relapse. Progression of disease is common, eventually leading to strictures or perforations with subsequent surgery for many individuals. Individuals with Crohn's disease have a two- to threefold increased risk of colon cancer compared to the general population. Surgery is common in severe presentations and is used to treat complications associated with Crohn's disease (i.e., toxic megacolon, intestinal obstruction, strictures, penetrations, uncontrolled bleeding, dysplasia, or cancer).[50]

Treatment options include corticosteroids, thiopurines, methotrexate, anti-tumor necrosis factor (TNF) medications, and combination therapy, as well as surgery.[50] Corticosteroids primarily play a role in inducing remission, but they are ineffective in maintaining remission and are associated with significant adverse effects if used long term. Steroids are weaned off, if possible, as maintenance of remission is accomplished using immunomodulators or biologic agents. The immunomodulators, which include the thiopurines (azathioprine, mercaptopurine) and methotrexate, are used as maintenance therapy in individuals with moderate to severe disease or who are steroid dependent. Adverse effects associated with their use include increased risk of infection, bone marrow suppression, liver toxicity, and increased risk of skin cancers and lymphoma.

Biologic agents include medications that contain monoclonal antibodies directed against TNF. The available anti-TNF agents in the United States include infliximab, adalimumab, and certolizumab pegol. While effective, they increase the risk of infection, psoriasis, and some cancers. Natalizumab, another biologic agent, is a monoclonal antibody directed against alpha-4 integrins that prevents recruitment and transport of leukocytes across the vascular endothelium. It is effective for both induction and maintenance of remission in moderate to severe disease. Because use of natalizumab is associated with progressive multifocal leukoencephalopathy, it is recommended for use only in individuals who have failed treatment with anti-TNF agents.

Controversy exists about which of these treatment options is best in what situations, whether combination therapy with immunomodulators and anti-TNF agents improves outcomes compared to monotherapy, and whether early treatment compared to "watchful waiting" results in improved long-term outcomes.[50,52]

Ulcerative Colitis Like Crohn's disease, ulcerative colitis is hypothesized to be a result of interactions between environmental, genetic, and microbial factors. The exact etiology is unknown. It is characterized by continuous ulcerations starting in the rectum and spreading upward through the colon. Its primary symptom is diarrhea with blood and/or mucus.[53] Affected individuals also commonly report abdominal pain, rectal bleeding,

urgency or tenesmus, fever, and weight loss.[53] Strictures and perforations are uncommon.[50] Many of the other complications associated with Crohn's disease can also occur with ulcerative colitis: toxic megacolon, dysplasia or colorectal cancer, arthritis, skin manifestations (erythema nodosum, pyoderma gangrenosum, oral ulcers), ocular conditions (episcleritis, scleritis, uveitis, iritis), anemia, and coagulation changes.[53]

Several factors may increase the risk of developing or worsening ulcerative colitis. Individuals with a history of inflammatory disease in a first-degree relative or who had an appendectomy at a young age are at greater risk of developing disease. Flares of ulcerative colitis in affected individuals are associated with smoking cessation and use of NSAIDs. Low vitamin D levels appear to increase the risk of developing cancer or *C. difficile* infections in individuals with ulcerative colitis.[54]

Diagnosis is based on results of colonoscopy and biopsy. Findings suggestive of ulcerative colitis on colonoscopy include a uniformly inflamed mucosa starting at the anorectal verge extending proximally with an abrupt or gradual transition to healthy tissue. Erosions and ulcerations can be seen in more severe disease. Often infiltrates, goblet-cell depletion, distorted crypt architecture, and ulcerations are seen on histologic evaluation of biopsy samples.[53] As with Crohn's disease, laboratory tests can help confirm inflammation and exclude other diagnostic possibilities. (See the previous section under Crohn's disease for commonly ordered tests also used in the evaluation of ulcerative colitis.)

Treatment options are similar to those for Crohn's disease with one important exception—sulfasalazine and 5-aminosalicylates are useful in the treatment of ulcerative colitis but not Crohn's disease. These products are considered to be first-line agents in the treatment of ulcerative colitis; remission rates approach 50%. Dosage and route vary depending on the location and severity of the disease. Adjunctive use of probiotics can be helpful in achieving and maintaining remission.[54] Individuals who fail to respond to first-line agents are candidates for corticosteroids and in refractory cases, an immunomodulator or anti-TNF agent.[53-55] (The immunomodulators and anti-TNF agents are described in the previous section on Crohn's disease.) As with Crohn's disease, once remission is achieved, corticosteroids are weaned off and any of the other agents can be used to maintain remission.[53,55] Treatment goals include both clinical remissions but also complete mucosal healing as evidenced by endoscopy findings. Mucosal healing is associated with fewer hospitalizations and lower rates of colectomy.[54]

Surgery may be needed in refractory cases or in those with secondary complications. Up to 20% of individuals may require a colectomy, which can be curative in many cases. Indications for surgery include failure of or inability to tolerate medical therapy, toxic megacolon, perforation, uncontrolled bleeding, persistent strictures, dysplasia, or cancer.[53,55]

Pregnancy and Inflammatory Bowel Disease The course of IBD is unaffected by pregnancy;[56] however, IBD can affect pregnancy outcomes. Women with quiescent disease throughout pregnancy have similar risks to the general population. Active disease is associated with preterm birth, low birth weight, and fetal loss. Women with active Crohn's disease appear to have worse outcomes than women with active ulcerative colitis. Medications used in the treatment of IBD are considered low risk except for thalidomide and methotrexate. While the thiopurines carry a pregnancy category D rating, authorities still recommend their continued use in pregnancy. The D rating is based on the high dosing used to treat leukemia at the time the thiopurines were approved. Lower doses are used to treat autoimmune diseases and may be safer in pregnancy.

However, because active disease poses risk, their use can be continued in pregnancy.[57,58]

Microscopic Colitis There are two types of MC: lymphocytic colitis and collagenous colitis. Symptoms typical of MC include multiple watery stools with or without abdominal pain and weight loss, fecal incontinence, and rectal bleeding.[59] The etiology is unknown; factors attributed include advancing age, female sex, autoimmune disorders affecting the thyroid, and celiac disease. Findings on colonoscopy reveal normal mucosa, but pathology shows abnormality at the cellular level. Treatments vary and will be managed by a GI specialist. In some cases antidiarrheal medications are enough to control symptoms. Other times, medications such as the mesalamines or oral steroids are needed.[59]

Conditions Characterized Primarily by Dyspepsia and Heartburn

FUNCTIONAL DYSPEPSIA

The underlying pathophysiology of functional dyspepsia is complex. Possible mechanisms include delayed gastric emptying, impaired ability for the stomach to accommodate a meal, hypersensitivity to gastric distension, changes in duodenal sensitivity to various nutrients, antral hypomotility, and autonomic nervous system dysfunction.[11] Risk factors for the development of dyspepsia include bacterial gastroenteritis; anxiety, depressive, and somatoform disorders; and the use of NSAIDs.[11]

What testing is needed to exclude organic disease is controversial.[11] Three approaches have been recommended: immediate endoscopy; non-invasive testing for *H. pylori* infection, followed by treatment if testing is positive and endoscopy if symptoms persist after treatment; and empirical treatment and endoscopy in the event of treatment failure. Immediate endoscopy is recommended for those at higher risk of cancer (those who are older than 55 years or younger individuals with a family history of gastric cancer; who have a personal history of partial gastrectomy, previous peptic ulcer, or gastric cancer; who immigrated from a country with a high rate of gastric cancer; or who have alarm symptoms: anemia, weight loss, persistent vomiting, evidence of GI bleeding, lymphadenopathy, abdominal mass, or dysphagia).[11,60,61] Evidence suggests that immediate endoscopy is not a cost-effective strategy in low-risk individuals with dyspepsia, because organic disease is identified in only 30% of endoscopies. Further, the condition of greatest concern, gastric cancer, is rare in younger individuals. The second strategy, testing for *H. pylori,* is unlikely to be useful, because the prevalence of infection has been rapidly declining in the United States, particularly in individuals younger than 30 years. While testing for (and treating) *H. pylori* infections has the advantage of reducing the risk of gastric cancer, it is a cost-effective strategy only in high-prevalence (> 20%) populations.[11] The third approach, empiric treatment, is the recommended approach in the United States in low-risk individuals.[11,61] Treatment with a proton-pump inhibitor (PPI) is more effective than H_2-receptor blockers and provides rapid relief, usually within the first 2 weeks.[11]

Ongoing management depends on severity and persistence of symptoms. Generally, a PPI is continued for 4 to 8 weeks, at which time it can be discontinued and symptoms reassessed. Those with a relapse of symptoms should be tested for *H. pylori* and treated, if needed.[11]

Other medications have been used in a limited way in the treatment of functional dyspepsia. These include the prokinetics, which target gastric motility. The only prokinetic products currently available in the United States are metoclopramide (Reglan), erythromycin, and herbal products containing peppermint. The evidence supporting their use is weak.[60] Women with refractory symptoms are sometimes offered a trial of low-dose tricyclic antidepressants, because these agents have been found to be effective in the treatment of other functional GI disorders.[11]

GASTROESOPHAGEAL REFLUX DISEASE

GERD is one of the most common GI disorders, affecting 10% to 20% of individuals in the Western world.[62] Long-term consequences of untreated GERD include erosive esophagitis, Barrett's esophagitis, and, rarely, the occurrence of esophageal cancer. Barrett's esophagitis is caused by long-term exposure to gastric reflux. In response, the cells of the esophagus become dysplastic, which in turn increases the risk of esophageal cancer. Risk factors for Barrett's esophagitis include age over 50 years, symptoms of GERD for more than 5 to 10 years, obesity, and male sex.[62]

The pathophysiology of GERD is multifactorial. A coordinated closure of the inner and outer sphincter of the lower esophagus effectively prevents gastric reflux. The two sphincters should overlay each other, reinforcing each other, ensuring a strong, effective closure of the esophagogastric junction. Acid reflux can occur if these two sphincters, the lower esophageal sphincter and crural diaphragm, are pushed apart, as happens with hiatal hernia or during transient relaxations of the sphincters. Relaxation of the sphincters occurs normally at the same rate in individuals with and without GERD, but these episodes are twice as likely to be accompanied by gastric reflux in individuals with GERD.[63] Individuals with GERD appear to have a larger gastric acid pocket located closer to the lower esophageal sphincter than do individuals without GERD. Thus, when transient relaxations of the sphincters occur, more acid is available to enter the esophagus. Reflux is also more likely to occur if there are pressure gradient changes between the stomach and esophagus. Conditions that increase the pressure in the stomach and promote retrograde flow include straining and obesity. Even if gastric reflux occurs, damage to the esophagus can be prevented or minimized if gastric contents are rapidly cleared through esophageal peristalsis and gravity or neutralized by salivary bicarbonate.[63] Thus, delays in clearance can also prompt symptoms.

The most common symptoms of GERD include heartburn (retrosternal burning possibly radiating to the neck) and acid regurgitation (the return of gastric contents into the pharynx or esophagus). GERD is also associated with chronic cough, laryngitis, asthma, and, rarely, dental erosions.[64] Heartburn and regurgitation commonly occur after eating, especially after large fatty meals, and are frequently noticed at night. They are exacerbated by recumbency, straining, or bending over and are usually relieved with antacids. When heartburn and regurgitation occur in a typical pattern, the clinician can establish the diagnosis of GERD and begin treatment empirically without further diagnostic testing.[62,64]

Testing can be deferred in straightforward cases, because the diagnostic yield is low in these situations.[64] However, additional testing should be considered in those who are unresponsive to empiric therapy with a PPI, are elderly, or have noncardiac chest pain or other alarm symptoms. Historically, a barium swallow was used in the diagnosis of GERD; however, it has low sensitivity for GERD, although it may be used in those who report dysphagia. The currently recommended test of choice for the evaluation of suspected GERD is endoscopy.[62] Most endoscopies are negative, but GERD is confirmed if erosive esophagitis, strictures, or signs of Barrett's esophagus (columnar-lined esophagus) are seen.[62]

The goals of treatment are to relieve symptoms, promote healing of esophageal erosions, and prevent further complications. Treatment includes weight loss for those who are obese or who have gained weight recently, elevation of head of bed during sleep, and avoidance of meals within 2 to 3 hours of bedtime. Historically, elimination of specific foods was recommended in the treatment

of GERD; however, eliminating foods such as coffee, caffeine, chocolate, spicy foods, citrus, carbonated beverages, fatty foods, or mint from the diet has not been shown to improve clinical symptoms.[62] Therefore, the American College of Gastroenterology concluded that not enough evidence is available to recommend dietary modifications in the management of GERD.[62]

Pharmacologic management, the primary approach to treatment, can help control GERD symptoms by increasing gastric pH (antacids), decreasing acid production (histamine-2 receptor antagonists [H2RAs]), or suppressing acid secretion (PPIs). Table 17-11 lists the commonly used medications for GERD. The American College of Gastroenterology recommends that treatment begin with a PPI, because the PPIs are superior in providing relief of heartburn compared to the H2RAs. All of the PPIs appear to be equally effective.[62] PPIs should be started at a once-daily dose, ideally before the first meal of the day. Many PPIs, depending on the agent chosen, perform best if given 30 to 60 minutes before a meal. For individuals with only a partial response, the provider should confirm that the woman is taking her medications as directed. If compliance is not an issue, then an increase in dose to twice daily or changing to another agent may afford relief. Therapy continues for 8 weeks if symptoms are controlled, and then a downward titration of medication dosage begins.

Referral to a gastroenterologist is helpful in refractory cases, because additional testing, adjunctive therapy, and/or surgery may be needed. In addition, long-term use of PPIs is associated with vitamin and mineral deficiencies, osteoporosis, and infection with *C. difficile* and other pathogens.[62] Therefore, consultation with a gastroenterologist is prudent in patients with long-term symptoms. Commonly, the gastroenterologist will order a 24-hour esophageal pH impedance test. The 24-hour esophageal pH test identifies the amount, duration, and pattern of reflux.

Table 17-11 Medications Used for GERD and Peptic Ulcer Disease

Drug	Mechanism	Comments
Antacids/alginic acids—Treatment of heartburn, reflux		
Bicarbonate—aluminum or magnesium formulations (e.g., Maalox, Mylanta, Rolaids)	• Increases pH • Neutralizes acidic gastric contents	• Frequent dosing needed. • Potential medication interactions. • Bicarbonate can cause sodium retention—avoid in pregnancy.
Histamine H$_2$-receptor antagonists (H$_2$RA)—Treatment of duodenal ulcers, uncomplicated		
Cimetidine (Tagamet) Ranitidine (Zantac) Famotidine (Pepcid) Nizatidine (Axid) All compatible with pregnancy, breastfeeding, and lactation	• Inhibits acid production • Competes with histamine • Binds to H$_2$ receptors of parietal cells	Side effects include diarrhea, headache, drowsiness, fatigue, muscle pain, and constipation. Decrease dose in persons with decreased creatinine clearance.
Proton pump inhibitors (PPIs)—Used in the treatment of gastric and duodenal ulcers and GERD		
Omeprazole (Prilosec) (Low risk in pregnancy, potential toxicity in breastfeeding) Lansoprazole (Prevacid) (Low risk in pregnancy, potential toxicity in breastfeeding) Rabeprazole (Aciphex) (Pregnancy—limited data, suggest low risk Breastfeeding—potential toxicity) Pantoprazole (Protonix) (Suggest low risk in pregnancy; limited data for breastfeeding, but probably compatible)	• Suppresses gastric acid production • Requires acid environment for activation—take dose 30–60 min before meal	• Caution for use in severe hepatic disease and chronic renal failure. • Do not take with H$_2$ antagonists.
Prostaglandin analogs—Prevention of NSAID-induced gastric ulcers		
Misoprostol (Cytotec) (Pregnancy—oral products contraindicated except for cervical ripening) Breastfeeding—potential toxicity (*Pregnancy category X) (*Absolute contraindication in pregnancy)	• Acid suppression • Increases mucosal blood flow—decreased basal and food-stimulated acid secretion	• Care for use in persons < 18 years old and renal failure • Side effects: diarrhea, abdominal pain, cramping, exacerbation of inflammatory bowel disease

Sulfated polysaccharides—Short-term and maintenance treatment of duodenal ulcers	
Sucralfate (Carafate) (Pregnancy—compatible Breastfeeding—probably compatible)	• Viscous gel that adheres to epithelial cells and erosions • Increases mucosal resistance

GERD = gastroesophageal reflux disease, NSAIDs = nonsteroidal inflammatory drugs

Data from Katz PO, Gerson LB, Vela MF. Diagnosis and management of gastroesophageal reflux disease. *Am J Gastroenterol.* 2013;108:308-328; Briggs GG, Freeman RK, Yaffe SJ, eds. *Drugs in Pregnancy and Lactation.* 10th ed. Philadelphia, PA: Wolters Kluwer; 2015; Hart AM. Evidence-based recommendations for GERD treatment. *Nurse Pract.* 2013;38(8):6-34.

If negative, then adjunctive pain management may be helpful. If positive for acid reflux, then a change in PPI dosing may be helpful. Individuals who do not respond to a revised PPI regimen may benefit from the addition of an H₂RA at bedtime or antireflux surgery. Individuals who test weakly positive for reflux on the esophageal impedance pH test may benefit from medications designed to reduce relaxation of the esophageal sphincter, pain management, or antireflux surgery.[65]

HEARTBURN IN PREGNANCY

Heartburn affects the majority of pregnant women. The occurrence of heartburn increases as gestation progresses. Both the physiologic relaxation of the esophageal sphincter under the influence of increased estrogen and the mechanical effects of the gravid uterus increasing intraabdominal pressure play a role. Antacids are considered safe and, along with lifestyle changes, should be first-line treatment. Antacids containing bicarbonate should be avoided in pregnancy due to electrolyte alterations. If additional treatment is needed to control symptoms, H₂RAs and PPIs can safely be utilized. Table 17-11 contains pregnancy safety categories of common medications used for GERD. The major goal of treatment is to relieve symptoms.

LACTOSE INTOLERANCE

Lactose intolerance (LI) is caused by a lactase deficiency. Individuals with LI are unable to digest a sugar found in milk and other dairy products. Approximately 30–50 million Americans, regardless of age, have LI. Lactose intolerance is more commonly found in Africans, African Americans, South Americans, Native Americans, Asians, and those of Mediterranean descent. Not all people with a deficiency in lactase will have symptoms of bloating, diarrhea, and gas. Other associated symptoms include nausea, cramping, or foul-smelling or floating stools. Diagnosis is made on clinical or laboratory grounds. A diagnosis is likely if consuming a diet low in lactose improves symptoms and reintroducing lactose-containing foods triggers a relapse. Alternatively, a diagnosis can be made if a positive result is found on a lactose-hydrogen breath test (obtained after ingesting 50 g of lactose). This test can cause cramping, bloating, gas, and diarrhea, prompting the development of genetic tests based on a venous blood sample. Treatment is directed at prevention of symptoms by avoiding foods known to trigger symptoms and by taking lactase tablets or capsules before eating lactose-containing foods. Lactose intolerance is not a harmful condition, but care should be taken to replace dietary calcium with supplementation to prevent calcium deficiency.[66]

Conditions Characterized Primarily by Dysphagia

ESOPHAGEAL STRICTURE

Strictures cause a delay in esophageal clearing and present with symptoms of dysphagia, regurgitation, and heartburn. Esophageal stricture is a long-term complication of GERD. PPIs are considered an important first step in treating GERD, but, if symptoms persist, evaluation with EGD (upper endoscopy) may be indicated. If a stricture is found to be present on EGD, it is most often treated with esophageal dilation. Strictures may need only a single stretching or dilations may be required periodically.[67]

ESOPHAGEAL CANCER

Several types of cancer affect the esophagus, primarily squamous cell carcinoma and adenocarcinoma. Risk factors vary by type: 1) squamous cell carcinoma—tobacco and alcohol use, caustic injury, poor oral hygiene, and being from certain parts of the world (Turkey, Kazakhstan, northern and central China, or southern or eastern Africa); 2) adenocarcinoma—symptomatic GERD, Barrett's esophagus, obesity, tobacco use, diet low in fruits and vegetables, male sex, and living in the United States or western Europe. Rates are increasing, particularly for adenocarcinomas.[68]

Esophageal cancer can be insidious in its presentation, aggressive, and can rapidly metastasize. Therefore, healthcare providers should be vigilant and refer women with suspicious symptoms quickly, particularly if a woman reports rapidly progressing and worsening dysphagia. Unexplained weight loss is another warning sign. Individuals may or may not have a history of long-term reflux symptoms. The preferred test is a barium swallow, although an upper endoscopy with biopsy is needed to confirm the diagnosis.

Mortality rates are dependent on the rapidness of diagnosis and intervention.[68]

Conditions Characterized Primarily by Abdominal Pain

IRRITABLE BOWEL SYNDROME

IBS is a functional disorder of the GI tract in which no identifiable cause of symptoms can be identified. It is characterized by persistent changes in bowel habits and abdominal pain or discomfort. The criteria for the diagnosis of IBS, Rome III, were revised in 2006;[20] these criteria are listed in **Table 17-12**.[69] IBS is classified into 4 types: IBS-C (constipation in > 25% of stools); IBS-D (diarrhea > 25% of stools); IBS-mixed (alternating rapidly between constipation and diarrhea); and unclassified (neither loose nor hard stools > 25% of the time).[70] Women with primarily constipation may report bloating, incomplete stool evacuation, and straining, while women with primarily diarrhea experience loose stools, gas, urgency, and in a minority of cases, loss of bowel control.[70]

Table 17-12 Criteria for Irritable Bowel Syndrome

Rome III Criteria

Symptoms have been occurring for ≥ 6 months.

Recurrent abdominal pain or discomfort for at least 3 days per month for the past 3 months associated with 2 or more of the following criteria:
- Change in stool frequency since onset of symptoms
- Change in stool form since onset of symptoms
- Improvement with defecation

Modified from Longstreth GF, Thompson WG, Chey WD, Houghton LA, Mearin F, Spiller RC. Functional bowel disorders. *Gastroenterology.* 2006;130(5):1480-1491. Copyright 2006, with permission from Elsevier.

Several factors increase the risk of developing IBS. It is more common in women than men, in individuals younger than 50 years of age, and in less socioeconomically advantaged individuals.[71] IBS is also more common post-gastroenteritis.[70]

Individuals with IBS have intermittent symptoms, which are often worsened by stress. The underlying etiology is unclear. It has been thought to be due to changes in gut motility and visceral hypersensitivity, exacerbated by psychosocial factors.[70] Delays in gastric emptying and increases in small bowel and colon motility have been found in individuals with IBS.[70] Visceral sensitivity plays a major role in the development of chronic pain and is likely due to localized tissue injury and inflammation, sensitivity, and hyperalgesia at the site of the injury. This peripheral sensitization can spread to the surrounding tissue. Stress reactivity magnifies these responses.[70] The importance of stress in IBS is supported by evidence that shows that IBS is more common in those exposed to childhood abuse and current life stressors and improves with exercise.[70] Newer evidence suggests that other mechanisms, in addition to those already described, may play a role in the development of symptoms; these include subtle IBD, changes in the mucosal immune activation and permeability of the small bowel and colon, serotonin and/or central dysregulation, malabsorption or maldigestion, bacterial overgrowth, and genetic factors.[70,72]

Many of the symptoms associated with IBD also occur with other GI conditions, making the diagnosis challenging. Diagnosis is made on clinical criteria. Generally, testing is not recommended unless alarm symptoms are present (i.e., older than 50 years of age, GI bleeding, weight loss, fever, anemia, or an abdominal mass) or the presentation suggests another possible etiology. Some authorities recommend routinely testing for celiac disease in individuals with suspected IBS-D or IBS-M, because the presentations of IBS and celiac disease are similar but risk is

higher with celiac disease.[73] In some studies, risk of celiac disease in individuals with IBS is up to three times higher compared to individuals without IBS.[71] Tests that should be considered in the presence of alarm symptoms include CBC, comprehensive metabolic profile, inflammatory markers (C-reactive protein or segmentation rate), and TSH. Stool cultures, fecal leukocytes, and/or fecal calprotectin or lactoferrin should be considered if IBD is suspected in individuals with risk factors for more serious disease.[71,74] Endoscopy is not needed in individuals younger than 50 years of age without alarm symptoms. Individuals over 50 years may need routine colon cancer screening or diagnostic evaluation with colonoscopy depending on whether organic disease is suspected.[73,74]

Treatment modalities include use of stress management techniques, probiotics, and medications. Most individuals with IBS make dietary changes in an attempt to control symptoms. Unfortunately, few high-quality data are available to determine if following certain dietary practices can significantly improve symptoms.[75] Food triggers for some individuals include wheat and dairy products and foods containing hard-to-absorb food components such as fructose, lactose, fructo- and galacto-oligosaccharides, sorbitol, mannitol, and other ingredients.[70] However, not enough evidence exists yet to recommend that individuals follow gluten-free or low-FODMAP (fermentable oligosaccharides, disaccharides, monosaccharides, and polyols) diets. Psyllium and soluble (but not insoluble) fibers appear to afford relief for some individuals.[75] Probiotics have been found to relieve symptoms, particularly bloating and flatulence, but the quality of the evidence is low.[70,75] Studies have used various probiotics (*Bifidobacteria*, *Saccharomyces boulardii*, *Lactobacilli*, and combinations of probiotics), making it difficult to recommend a specific probiotic or combination of probiotics.[74,75] A number of psychologic interventions (cognitive behavioral therapy, psychoeducation, mind–body therapy, hypnotherapy, and psychodynamic interpersonal therapy) have been shown to reduce abdominal pain and symptom severity and improve quality of life for individuals with IBS in two meta-analyses.[76,77]

Medications recommended for the treatment of IBS by the American Gastroenterological Association include antispasmodic medications, tricyclic antidepressants, and various products for the symptomatic management of diarrhea or constipation, depending on the predominant symptom.[78] However, many of these recommendations are conditional. Antispasmodic medications (conditional recommendation) are suggested for use in the treatment of abdominal pain and cramping.[78] Tricyclic antidepressants can alter pain perception independently of their impact on depression or anxiety.[70] They are associated with a modest improvement in global symptoms and abdominal pain when used in the treatment of IBS and are given a conditional recommendation for use by the American Gastroenterological Association.[78] Some have advised the use of the selective serotonin reuptake inhibitors as an alternative. However, several RCTs have not demonstrated improvement in symptoms with use of the selective serotonin reuptake inhibitors. Consequently, the American Gastroenterological Association recommends against their use in the management of IBS.[78]

Based on a systematic review of the literature, the American Gastroenterological Association recommends for the treatment of IBS-C:[78]

- Linaclotide, a guanylate cyclase C agonist (strong recommendation, high-quality evidence)
- Lubiprostone (conditional recommendation, moderate-quality evidence)
- Polyethylene glycol (PEG) laxatives (conditional recommendation, low-quality evidence)

For IBS-D, the American Gastroenterological Association suggests using:[78]

- Rifaximin (conditional recommendation, moderate-quality evidence)
- Alosetron (conditional recommendation, moderate-quality evidence)
- Loperamide (conditional recommendation, low-quality evidence)

Alosetron, a 5HT3 receptor antagonist, is reserved for use only in individuals with IBS-D who have failed other treatment modalities, because it is associated with an increased risk of ischemic colitis.[70] To be able to prescribe alosetron, providers must be enrolled in the Alosetron Risk Evaluation and Mitigation Strategy (REMS) program and attest that they have the skills to recognize and manage/refer complications associated with use of alosetron and agree to follow certain prescribing practices.

The impact of IBS on pregnancy has not been reported in the literature, nor is it known if pregnancy relieves or exacerbates symptoms. Treatment should be supportive with an emphasis on stress management techniques, healthy eating, and exercise.

GALLBLADDER DISEASE

The gallbladder is a pear-shaped organ lying beneath the liver on the right side of the abdomen. It functions as a storage reservoir for bile produced by the liver to aid in digestion. There is a high concentration of bile salts, pigments, and cholesterol within the bile storage pool. When foods high in fat content are eaten, the gallbladder contracts and bile salts are ejected into the intestine. Bile acids aid in the biliary excretion of cholesterol and are important in the intestinal absorption of fat, particularly cholesterol, and fat-soluble vitamins.

Gallstones are formed from three primary mechanisms: 1) abnormal bile composition, due mainly from excessive biliary excretion of cholesterol; 2) accelerated nucleation of solid monohydrate crystals, a precursor to gallstones; and 3) hypomotility within the gallbladder. Gallstones are composed of a mixture of cholesterol, calcium bilirubinate, proteins, and mucin. They can be classified by presence or absence of cholesterol and whether their color is black or brown. Most stones are thought to have a mixed composition. In industrialized countries, cholesterol-based stones account for the majority of gallstones. Black-pigmented stones are formed in the gallbladder and result from hemolysis.[79] They are associated with sickle cell disease and liver cirrhosis. Brown-pigmented stones are associated with bacterial or parasitic infections of the biliary tract and are more commonly seen in Asians. Brown stones usually form in the intrahepatic bile duct.[79]

The incidence of *cholelithiasis* (i.e., symptomatic gallstones) is greater in women than men and increases with age. Risk factors include genetic predisposition, diabetes, sedentary lifestyle, diet rich in animal and refined sugars, cirrhosis, and certain medications.[39,80] Obese women and those who have undergone gastric bypass surgery have a high incidence of developing gallstones.[80] A contributing factor in the latter situation is rapid weight loss, which appears to increase levels of bile mucin, a glycoprotein that promotes nucleation, a critical step in the formation of gallstones. Ursodeoxycholic acid may be recommended in patients going through rapid weight loss to decrease this effect.[80]

Pregnant women and those using oral contraceptives and other hormone-replacement therapies are also at higher risk of gallstones.[39] Estrogen contributes to super saturation of the bile with cholesterol, while progesterone reduces gallbladder contractions and increases stasis; both processes increase the risk of developing gallstones.[80] Gallbladder stasis contributes to gallstone formation, because it allows sludge (muddy sediment, which is a precursor to stones) and crystals to build up in the gallbladder longer than necessary and adds to delay in normal emptying times.[79] Sludge can be detected by ultrasound and is composed of cholesterol and calcium bilirubinate in a thick mucin gel. Although sludge can lead to

gallstones, it can also disappear spontaneously. Sludge is primarily seen in pregnancy.

Most gallstones do not cause symptoms. However, when they do, women often report biliary colic—colicky, stabbing, spasmodic pain in the epigastric area or the RUQ of the abdomen, often radiating to the right scapular area, and lasting from 2 to 4 hours per episode. This colicky pain is caused primarily from the impaction of gallstones in the cystic duct leading to gallbladder distension. Often the impacted stone will float free and symptoms subside.[39] See **Figure 17-1**.

Gallstones are associated with complications such as cholecystitis, cholangitis, and pancreatitis depending on the duration and site of blockage. *Cholecystitis* is an inflammation of the gallbladder caused by prolonged occlusion of the bile ducts. With cholecystitis, women may experience anorexia, dyspepsia, and low-grade fever. Some, but not all women, report nausea and vomiting. Patients may have localized tenderness or guarding in the RUQ area, often following a fatty or heavy meal. A positive Murphy's sign may be seen in acute cholecystitis, which is determined by whether tenderness is elicited on deep palpation under the right costal margin upon inspiration; this maneuver brings the inflamed gallbladder into contact with the examiner's hand.

Gallstones can also cause complications such as cholangitis, choledocholithiasis, and pancreatitis. *Cholangitis* is an infection of the bile duct that occurs when the obstructed bile duct becomes contaminated with bacteria ascending from the intestine. *Choledocholithiasis* is a condition in which stones have migrated from the gallbladder down the cystic duct and become lodged in the common bile duct, causing obstruction; it too is associated with the development of cholangitis. Cholangitis should be suspected if a woman develops fever, jaundice, and severe RUQ pain. Pancreatitis can also develop if a stone descends even

Figure 17-1 The biliary tract.

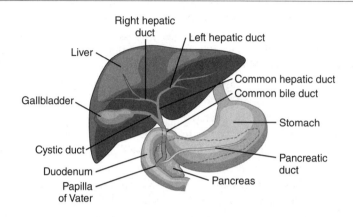

farther down the biliary tract and becomes lodged at the sphincter of Oddi, where the common bile duct from the liver and gallbladder merge with the pancreatic duct before draining into the small intestine. Women with gallbladder-related pancreatitis will present with epigastric pain and have elevated serum levels of lipase and amylase.[39]

Laboratory testing includes a CBC, liver function tests, and liver enzymes. Results of the CBC may show leukocytosis with a left shift. Elevations of serum bilirubin and alkaline phosphatase, in particular, can signal potential gallbladder disease and are often noted during biliary obstruction. Serum amylase and lipase should also be ordered and may be elevated in pancreatitis.[39]

Ultrasound detects gallstones with a specificity and sensitivity of more than 95%.[39] Confirmation of gallbladder disease on ultrasound includes gallbladder wall thickening or edema and a sonographic Murphy's sign, where a positive Murphy's sign is seen during palpation with the ultrasound transducer. If the diagnosis is unclear or if complications are suspected, other imaging tests may be needed. If choledocholithiasis develops from a stone blocking the common bile duct

or pancreatitis is suspected, an ERCP test may be used. Ultrasounds cannot visualize the bile ducts. However, during an ERCP a camera is advanced down the endoscope and allows visualization, and in some cases, removal of gallstones lodged deeper in the biliary tree. Other imaging options can also evaluate the biliary tree; these include MRCP, which is becoming increasingly popular, and CT scans. On occasion a plain abdominal x-ray may be ordered to rule out other causes of an acute abdomen.[39]

A careful evaluation of clues elicited on the history, physical examination, laboratory, and imaging tests should make the diagnosis clear. Other conditions causing similar symptoms such as biliary colic, peptic ulcer disease, GERD, esophageal spasm, acute pancreatitis-related gallstone disease, myocardial infarction, and pneumonia need to be ruled out. Once the diagnosis is made, the treatment of choice is usually surgery. The exact procedure will depend on the location of the gallstones and if complications are present, but often the procedure of choice is laparoscopic cholecystectomy for individuals with acute cholecystitis or complications related to bile stones.

Other treatment options are still used in selected populations. Individuals who are not surgical candidates or who have small stones can be considered for treatment with oral dissolution therapy. Treatment is long, lasting 6 to 12 months, and has a recurrence rate of 50%. Similarly, extracorporeal shock wave lithotripsy also has a high rate of recurrence and may not completely clear the bile duct. Sometimes, this procedure is done to make the stones fragment into smaller pieces and easier to remove by ERCP, thereby avoiding surgery.

Gallbladder disease is the second most common cause of surgery in pregnancy. Gallstones occur in 12% to 15% of women. Ultrasound is the preferred imaging technique.[56] Symptomatology is unchanged in pregnancy. Treatment choices include conservative management with IV hydration, analgesia, and possibly antibiotics, ERCP, and surgical management. Surgery is associated with preterm labor. The risks and benefits of the various approaches must be balanced and take into consideration severity of disease, general health status, and gestational age at time of symptom onset.[81-83]

PEPTIC ULCER DISEASE

Peptic ulcer disease is a result of ulcerations occurring in the stomach or duodenum. The etiology of ulcer formation remains unclear. Disruptions in the normal protective mechanisms allow acid to reach and damage the mucosa and result in ulcerations.[84] The two primary risk factors in the United States for peptic ulcer disease are use of NSAIDs or aspirin and infection with *H. pylori*. Other factors (smoking, stress, excessive alcohol use) have been implicated, but none have been found to independently contribute to the development of the disease.[84]

Presenting symptoms include varying degrees of mild to severe symptoms. Upper abdominal pain or discomfort is the most common presenting complaint in peptic ulcer disease. Dyspepsia and heartburn are also common. With duodenal ulcers, pain often occurs at night or with fasting and is relieved by eating. However, many peptic ulcers are asymptomatic until the affected individual presents with complications such as bleeding or penetration. Other complications such as gastric outlet obstruction or fistulas are less common and suggest other etiologies.[84] For example, while gastric outlet obstructions can occur with peptic ulcer disease, they are more commonly seen in gastric cancer.[32]

The preferred diagnostic test in the evaluation of suspected peptic ulcer disease is endoscopy. Findings on endoscopy suggestive of peptic ulcer disease include ulcerations with smooth, regular, rounded edges with a base often filled with exudate. The ulcerations extend through the muscularis submucosa into the deeper layers of the wall.[84] Biopsies are obtained during endoscopy for *H. pylori* infection, and if the appearance of the lesions is suspicious, for cancer. The workup may need to be extended if other causes are suspected. Conditions such as celiac disease, cancer, IBS, GERD, and drug-induced dyspepsia may have similar symptoms to peptic ulcer disease.[85]

Whether endoscopy is always needed is debated. High-risk individuals and those with severe symptoms would likely benefit from endoscopy. However, some advocate following a protocol similar to that discussed earlier for dyspepsia: treating presumptively with a trial of a PPI for 4 weeks and testing with endoscopy only for those with alarm symptoms or who fail the initial trial of a PPI.[33] The American College of Gastroenterology recommends that all individuals with peptic ulcer disease be tested and treated for *H. pylori*.[86]

Treatment includes lifestyle modifications and medication management. Individuals with peptic ulcer disease should be counseled to quit smoking, avoid alcohol, and stop the intake of NSAIDs.[32] Diet has not been shown to relate to ulcer development or healing, but avoiding foods that aggravate dyspeptic symptoms is recommended. Empiric pharmacologic therapy consists of a PPI for 4 to 8 weeks to decrease acid secretion (see Table 17-11). Other agents are used to strengthen the mucosal barrier, including the prostaglandin analogues (misoprostol), which promote mucosal resistance, and the bismuth salts (subcitrate, subsalicylate), which promote ulcer healing by enhancing mucosal repair.[84]

Treatment of *H. pylori* infection is also needed in those who test positive. A number of regimens have been approved. The first-line treatment for *H. pylori* has long been triple therapy (PPI, amoxicillin, clarithromycin twice daily) for 7 to 10 days. However, increasing resistance to clarithromycin is undermining the effectiveness of this regimen. Therefore, the exact regimen used will depend on local antibiotic resistance patterns. Adjunctive use of probiotics also appears to increase cure rates.[85] Table 17-13 lists regimens recommended by the American College of Gastroenterology.[86]

Peptic ulcer disease is rare in pregnancy. Women with active disease often go into remission in pregnancy.[82]

Table 17-13 Treatment Regimens for *H. Pylori*

First-Line Recommendations
Proton pump inhibitor, clarithromycin, and amoxicillin or metronidazole for 14 days
Proton pump inhibitor or H$_2$-receptor antagonist, bismuth, metronidazole, and tetracycline for 14 days

Data from Chey WD, Wong BC, the Practice Parameters Committee of the American College of Gastroenterology. American College of Gastroenterology guideline on the management of *Helicobacter pylori* infection. *Am J Gastroenterol*. 2007;102:1808-1825.

APPENDICITIS

Appendicitis poses a lifetime risk of 7% and is more common in adolescents and young adults; males are more affected than females. It is the most common acute abdominal emergency in the United States.[87]

The appendix is an approximately 9-cm long diverticulum originating from the cecum, located near the ileocecal valve. Because the end is free, the tip of the appendix can be oriented toward different locations in the lower abdomen—most frequently, in the paracolic gutter lateral to the cecum (35%), posterior to the cecum (30%), or in or close to the pelvis (30%).[88]

The appendix's orientation toward the pelvis, which occurs in a significant minority of cases, makes the diagnosis of appendicitis particularly challenging in women. Many of the signs and symptoms of appendicitis are nonspecific; right lower quadrant pain and other common symptoms seen in appendicitis can also be present in ectopic pregnancy, simple and complex right ovarian masses, right ovarian torsion, endometriosis, urinary tract disease, and pelvic inflammatory disease. Other nongynecologic conditions that can mimic appendicitis are Crohn's disease, diverticulosis, intestinal obstruction, Meckel diverticulum, pyelonephritis, gastroenteritis, right lower lobe pneumonia, and strangulated hernia, among other conditions.[88]

The first symptoms of appendicitis may be mild, with minor cramping and gradual onset of pain or slight nausea, feelings of indigestion, and anorexia. Symptoms worsen and progress to periumbilical pain, vomiting, and low-grade fever. The most predictive symptom is migration of pain from the periumbilical region to the right lower quadrant and pain before vomiting.[88] The most predictive findings on physical exam include rebound tenderness and a positive psoas sign, described in Table 17-10.[89] Other findings can also suggest appendicitis (i.e., positive obturator,

McBurney and/or Rovsing signs, flank tenderness in lower right side, patient preference for being in a position with the knees drawn up).[90]

Laboratory findings are often nonspecific. Mild leukocytosis, elevated neutrophils, and a shift to the left are commonly seen in appendicitis. Markers of inflammation (e.g., C-reactive protein) can also be present. Often a urinalysis is performed to rule out renal calculi and pyelonephritis. In addition, all reproductive-aged women, regardless of whether they have had a sterilization procedure or not, should be queried about their last menstrual period, sexual history, and use of contraceptives or condoms, and they should take a pregnancy test. Ectopic pregnancy can occur even after a sterilization procedure. Although this is rare, ectopic pregnancy is a life-threatening condition requiring early recognition and treatment.

Given that so many conditions have a similar presentation to appendicitis, several strategies have been proposed to narrow the diagnoses under consideration. The use of the Alvarado scoring system is one such strategy; it scores prognostic clinical and laboratory findings on a scale from 1 to 10 (see **Table 17-14**). The higher the score, the more likely an individual has appendicitis. Individuals with scores less than 5 are unlikely to have appendicitis. Intermediate scores of 5 and 6 warrant admission to the hospital for observation, whereas scores of 7 or more suggest the need for surgery.[91,92] A meta-analysis of 42 studies evaluating the sensitivity and specificity of the Alvarado Scoring System concluded that the scoring system was much better at ruling out appendicitis (99% sensitivity in women), but was much less accurate at "ruling in" appendicitis. Using a cutoff score of 7 or above as an indicator of the need for surgery, the specificity of the Alvarado Scoring System in women was only 57%. The authors concluded that the Alvarado score at intermediate- and high-risk cutoffs overpredicted appendicitis in women.[91]

Table 17-14 Alvarado Scoring System for Appendicitis

Component	Possible Points
Symptoms	
Migration of pain to right lower quadrant	1
Anorexia	1
Nausea or vomiting	1
Signs	
Tenderness right lower quadrant	2
Rebound pain	1
Elevated temperature	1
Laboratory	
Leukocytosis	2
Left shift	1
Total Score	*10*

Reproduced Reprinted from Alvarado A. A practical score for the early diagnosis of acute appendicitis. *Ann Emerg Med.* 1986;15:557-564. Copyright 1986, with permission from Elsevier.

Another strategy to narrow the differential list is to use a combination of laboratory tests.[93] WBCs are typically higher than 10,000 mm³ in appendicitis. Neutrophilia of > 75% and a C-reactive protein level of > 25/liter are almost always present. An abnormal result on any one of these tests is predictive of appendicitis. If all three tests are examined as a set and each is abnormal, the sensitivity rises to 97% to 100%.[88]

Imaging is useful when the diagnosis is in doubt. The preferred test according to the American College of Radiology is a CT scan of the abdomen and pelvis with or without contrast.[17] A normal appendix has thin walls and a less than 6-mm wall-to-wall diameter on CT scan.[87] An ultrasound is often used in women, because it is safer in pregnant women than a CT scan and is better at detecting other common gynecologic conditions that can mimic appendicitis. MRI is occasionally ordered.

The pathophysiology of appendicitis is multifactorial. Historically, it has been thought to be due to obstruction, most commonly from fecaliths—hard stony lumps of feces—within the appendix or from other sources of obstruction such as seeds, cancer, worms, or hypertrophy of lymphoid tissue.[87] Obstruction leads to inflammation, distension, bacterial overgrowth, necrosis, and over time perforation.[89] Recent studies have shown that neither increased intraluminal pressures nor fecaliths were identified in the majority of patients with appendicitis. Nor does perforation seem to be inevitable in all cases. Therefore, some propose that there are two distinct entities—nonperforated appendicitis and perforated appendicitis, with perforated appendicitis occurring in those with inflammation or an altered colonic microbiome.[89]

This new understanding of the disease is changing the management of appendicitis in select situations. Historically, the treatment was surgical, which is still the recommended approach for most individuals with uncomplicated appendicitis.[89] However, accumulating evidence from small RCTs suggests an "antibiotic-first" strategy (with surgery for those without improvement) may safely be considered in those without suspected perforation, abscess, sepsis, or peritonitis.[89,93] Studies comparing an antibiotic-first strategy to immediate surgery have found similar reported rates of complications, including perforations, between the two approaches, although between 0% and 53% of individuals randomized to the antibiotic-first strategy in various trials had an appendectomy within 48 hours. In addition, relapse may be high in those successfully treated with antibiotics. Clinical trials have reported rates of appendectomy of 10% to 37% within 4 to 7 months after successful antibiotic treatment of appendicitis.[89] Therefore, larger clinical trials comparing surgical and antibiotic-based strategies

are needed to determine the utility and safety of the antibiotic-first strategy and to develop consensus on which strategy is best in which circumstance.[93] However, the evidence is strong enough that an antibiotic-first strategy could be considered in those who are not surgical candidates or in those who are strongly opposed to surgery.[89,93] The recommended surgical approach is either an open or laparoscopic appendectomy.[88]

Appendicitis occurs in 1 out of 1500 pregnancies and is the most common cause of nonobstetric-related surgery in pregnancy.[94] It occurs most commonly in the second trimester of pregnancy.[94] It is challenging to diagnose due to its variable presentation. The appendix is often displaced superiorly from its normal position. Therefore, pain can occur anywhere in the abdomen, not just in the right lower quadrant. Further, leukocytosis normally occurs in pregnancy and can mask the mild leukocytosis commonly seen in appendicitis. However, C-reactive protein and neutrophilia, commonly seen in appendicitis, do not appear to be changed by pregnancy and if elevated may help pinpoint the diagnosis. The imaging modality of choice is ultrasound. MRI is another alternative, although CT scans are avoided if possible.[56] If there is a delay in diagnosis and perforation occurs, maternal and perinatal morbidity and mortality can be high. Consequently, appendectomy may be performed when suspicion is high even if the diagnosis is not confirmed.[82]

Diverticular Disease

Risk factors for diverticular disease include advancing age, obesity, and genetic susceptibility.[95] The formation of *diverticula* (small "out-pouches" in the digestive tract, which occur most commonly in the sigmoid colon in the US population) is poorly understood. They are thought to occur as a result of several factors—age-related changes in the mucosal wall, neurologic degeneration of the nerves that affect gastric motility, and increases in colon pressure—that result in bulging at sites of weakness and mucosal herniation in the colon. Stasis can result in altered colonic microbiota, production of abnormal metabolites, and subsequent inflammation. Further inflammation occurs from damage caused by trapped fecaliths within the diverticulum and results in acute diverticulitis.[96] More extensive inflammation of the surrounding tissue can result in abscess, fistula, or peritonitis. Repeated episodes of recurrent inflammation can lead to fibrosis and strictures.[96]

Diverticular disease encompasses a range of entities depending on the extensiveness of the disease, whether it is a single or recurrent episode, and the presence or absence of inflammation; these entities include asymptomatic diverticulosis, symptomatic uncomplicated diverticular disease, and diverticulitis. Almost all older adults have asymptomatic diverticula (*diverticulosis*). Up to 5% of individuals with diverticulosis will experience rectal bleeding. Rectal bleeding can be profuse, accounting for 30% to 50% of cases of massive rectal bleeding. Low-dose aspirin and NSAIDs increase the risk. Some individuals develop symptomatic uncomplicated disease that presents with symptoms similar to IBS (i.e., pain, change in bowel habits) but no inflammation is present. *Diverticulitis* results from inflammation of the diverticulum and can be acute or chronic and uncomplicated or complicated.[96]

The most common symptoms of diverticulitis include left lower quadrant pain or tenderness, fever, and elevated WBC count with possible left shift. Diarrhea is more common, but constipation can occur. Women may report dysuria from bladder irritation secondary to an inflamed colon. Other signs include a tender, palpable mass and distension. Complications occur in a subset of women and include pericolonic abscess with localized peritonitis, perforation and generalized peritonitis and sepsis, obstruction, and fistula.[96]

Other conditions present with similar symptoms, including appendicitis, bowel obstruction, cancer, ectopic pregnancy, gastroenteritis, IBD, IBS, pancreatitis, ovarian torsion, and tubo-ovarian abscess.[95] CT scan is recommended, which can help exclude other diagnostic possibilities and document the location and severity of disease. A colonoscopy is also used to rule out colon cancer, but it is commonly avoided during an episode of acute diverticulitis to prevent perforation. It is usually done 6 to 8 weeks later, after resolution of the episode.[96] Newer evidence suggests that colonoscopy may be needed only in those with complicated disease, other risk factors for colon cancer, or for age-appropriate screening.[95]

Management is directed toward resolution of symptoms. Acute diverticulitis can be managed on an outpatient basis with bowel rest, analgesia, and antibiotics, reserving inpatient management for severe presentations. Smaller abscesses can be managed with IV antibiotics, but some may require percutaneous drainage done with the aid of a CT scan or ultrasound. Surgery will be required to manage larger abscesses and fistulas. Rectal bleeding usually resolves spontaneously but may require use of endoscopic procedures or surgery to achieve hemostasis. Obstruction usually resolves with conservative management but may require surgery or an endoscopic procedure if the underlying cause is due to strictures.[96]

To prevent recurrence of disease, the American Gastroenterological Association recommends extra dietary fiber, vigorous exercise, and the avoidance of NSAIDs.[97] The American Gastroenterological Association concludes that there is not enough evidence to support recommending any of the following to prevent recurrence of disease in individuals with acute uncomplicated diverticulitis: probiotics, mesalamine (an anti-inflammatory medication), rifaximin (a poorly absorbed oral antibiotic), or the avoidance of seeds, nuts, or popcorn in the diet.[97] However, this recommendation is made with the caveat that these recommendations apply only to acute uncomplicated disease. Other authorities concluded that mesalamine and rifaximin can be useful in preventing recurrence.[96]

PANCREATITIS

The pancreas is an elongated organ lying in the back of the mid-abdomen and sits outside the posterior curve of the stomach, behind the duodenum and the spleen. It has three entities: the head, body, and tail. Functions include production of digestive enzymes and certain hormones, including insulin responsible for regulating blood glucose. The pancreas has an endocrine pathway: the islets of Langerhans produce insulin, glucagon, and somatostatin, which are secreted into the systemic circulation. It also has an exocrine pathway: the acinar cells, which produce and secrete digestive enzymes outwardly through excretory ducts emptying into the GI tract. Digestive enzymes flow down the main pancreatic duct, which joins the common bile duct at the ampulla of Vater, and then on into the duodenum (Figure 17-1). These digestive enzymes are activated in the duodenum and are essential for digestion.

Acute pancreatitis is defined as an acute inflammation. While the underlying pathophysiology is not completely clear, an insult to the acinar cells leads to early activation of the digestive enzymes found inside the acinar cells and damages the surrounding gland and nearby tissue. The underlying trigger can be a toxic substance (e.g., alcohol), metabolic derangements (i.e., hyperlipidemia, hypercalcemia, drugs), mechanical obstruction (i.e., gallstones, congenital malformations, ampullary dysfunction, and stenosis), and genetic disorders, among other causes (**Table 17-15**).[98] Alcohol abuse and gallstones account for 70% to 75% of all cases in the United States.[98] Because the gallbladder and pancreas share a common drainage duct, gallstones blocking this duct will back up pancreatic enzymes. Serum triglyceride levels above 1000 mg/dL can also initiate attacks of acute pancreatitis, but the etiology of this action is unclear. Hypertriglyceridemia-induced pancreatitis is more likely to occur in individuals with abnormal lipids who also have a second

Table 17-15 Primary Causes of Acute Pancreatitis

- Gallstones
- Alcohol-induced
- Drug-related
- Hereditary conditions
- Post ERCP-induced
- Infections (viral, mumps, mononucleosis)
- Hyperlipidemia
- Hypercalcemia
- Pregnancy
- Idiopathic
- Trauma
- Venom (spider, scorpion, reptile bites)
- Hypertriglyceridemia

Abbreviation: ERCP, endoscopic retrograde cholangiopancreatography

Data from Nam J, Murthy S. Acute pancreatitis—the current status in management. *Expert Opin Pharmacother.* 2003;4:235–241; Riela A, Zinsmeister A, Melton L, DiMagno E. Etiology, incidence and survival of acute pancreatitis in Olmsted County, Minnesota [abstract]. *Gastroenterology.* 1991;100:A296; Gullo L, Migliori M, Pezzilli R, Olah A, Farkas G, Levy P, et al. An update on recurrent acute pancreatitis: Data from five European countries. *Am J Gastroenterol.* 2002;97:1959–1962; Cole L. Unraveling the mystery of acute pancreatitis. *Nursing.* 2001;31:58–63; Toskes P. Hyperlipidemic pancreatitis. *Gastroenterol Clin North Am.* 1990:9:783–791; Choudari CP, Yu A, Imperiale T, Fogel E, Sherman S, Lehman G. Significance of heterozygous cystic fibrosis gene in idiopathic pancreatitis [abstract]. *Gastroenterology.* 1998;114 G1818, Part 2, Suppl S:A447; Hozumi Y, Kawang M, Saito T, Miyata M. Effect of tamoxifen on serum lipid metabolism. *J Clin Endocrinol Metab.* 1998; 83:1633–1635.

risk factor for hypertriglyceridemia (i.e., obesity, alcohol, diabetes mellitus, or medication).[99]

The presentations associated with acute pancreatitis range from mild and self-limiting to severe disease with significant risk of mortality. Commonly, a woman with pancreatitis presents with severe epigastric or left upper quadrant pain. The pain is constant and radiates to the back, chest, or flanks.[100] In those with gallstone-related pancreatitis, RUQ pain may occur initially. Women may also report nausea, vomiting, indigestion, abdominal fullness, clay-colored stools, and decreased urine output. Bowel sounds are often decreased. Distension and jaundice may be present. Some individuals may present with Cullen's sign (ecchymosis and edema in the subcutaneous tissue around the umbilicus) and Grey Turner's sign (ecchymosis of the flank). Both are signs of severe disease and result from intraabdominal or retroperitoneal bleeding.[101]

Most individuals respond rapidly to care and are substantially better within 48 hours of disease onset.[100] Up to 15% of individuals with acute pancreatitis develop severe disease. Some develop a systematic inflammatory response that affects distant organs, leading to respiratory distress, renal failure, upper GI bleeding, myocardial depression, and/or shock.[98] Others develop focal or diffuse necrosis of the pancreas. If infected necrosis occurs, mortality is high.[98] To identify those at risk for severe disease as early as possible, several scales have been developed to predict the risk of developing complications; these include the Glasgow, Ranson, and APACHE scales. One of the simplest to use is a bedside scale composed of only five variables. High-risk findings on this scale include: 1) BUN > 25 mg/dL, 2) impaired mental status, 3) age > 60 years, 4) presence of pleural effusion on x-ray, and 5) signs of systemic inflammation (i.e., tachycardia, temperature < 36°C or > 38°C, leukopenia or leukocytosis, or hyperventilation).[98]

A comprehensive set of laboratory tests is often ordered to gauge severity of the presentation, identify the underlying cause, and predict disease course. Commonly ordered tests are listed in **Table 17-16**. Two of the most helpful are levels of amylase and lipase. Serum amylase rises within a few hours after onset of symptoms for most individuals with acute pancreatitis and normalizes within 3 to 5 days. Lipase remains elevated longer.[100] Of the two tests, lipase is more sensitive and specific than amylase. Values of either test greater than three times normal are generally considered strongly indicative of acute pancreatitis.[100,101] Other conditions that cause elevations of lipase and amylase levels may need to be considered: renal disease, diseases of salivary glands (amylase), appendicitis, cholecystitis, peptic ulcer, intestinal obstruction, and gynecologic diseases. Because of its variable presentation, the American College of Gastroenterology states that two of the following criteria must be met to diagnose acute pancreatitis: 1) abdominal pain consistent with the disease, 2) serum amylase and/or lipase levels at minimum three times the upper limit of normal, and 3) characteristic findings seen on imaging.[100]

An abdominal ultrasound is done to confirm the presence or absence of gallstones, which are the underlying cause of acute pancreatitis in 40% to 70% of cases.[100] If the etiology is in doubt or if the patient is still acutely ill at 48 to 72 hours,

Table 17-16 Laboratory Tests Used in the Evaluation of Acute Pancreatitis

Amylase

Complete blood count

Comprehensive metabolic panel

C-reactive protein

Lactate dehydrogenase

Lipase

Liver function tests

Renal function tests

Triglyceride level

Urinalysis

Data from Cruz-Santamaría D, Taxonera C, Giner M. Update on pathogenesis and clinical management of acute pancreatitis. *World J Gastrointest Pathophysiol.* 2012;3(3):60-70; Quilan J. Acute pancreatitis. *Am Fam Physician.* 2014;90(9):632-639.

other tests may be employed. The recommended test in these situations is either a contrast-enhanced computed tomographic (CE-CT) scan and/or an MRI of the pancreas.[98]

Treatment options are determined by the underlying etiology. Supportive care is provided to manage nausea, vomiting, and pain; correct fluid and electrolyte imbalances; and treat infection, if present. One of the immediate goals of care is to reduce BUN levels through aggressive IV hydration. Individuals able to tolerate foods can continue to eat. If cholangitis is suspected, ERCP may need to be done within 24 hours of admission to remove an impacted stone. Cholecystectomy is recommended once the patient is stable to prevent recurrent attacks.[98,100]

Pancreatitis is extremely rare in pregnancy, occurring in 1 in 1000–10,000 women. More than 70% of cases are due to gallstones. Ultrasound is the first initial test done in pregnancy. It can identify biliary dilation and gallstones, but has low diagnostic yield for pancreatitis. If the diagnosis is in doubt, MRCP should be ordered because it can examine pancreatic parenchyma and the common bile duct with more accuracy than an ultrasound. Generally, pancreatitis in pregnancy is a self-limiting disease, but it can be associated with poor maternal and perinatal outcomes. Management is supportive with IV fluids, bowel rest, and correction of electrolyte and calcium imbalances.[56,82]

Bowel Obstruction

Bowel obstruction can occur anywhere in the intestinal tract, but more commonly affects the small bowel. It occurs when a blockage exists in either the large or small intestine. Failure of intestinal contents to pass beyond the obstruction leads to a buildup of accumulated air and secretions and delays or stops the passage of flatus and feces. While passage of feces is impeded, some feces and secretions may still escape, depending on the degree of obstruction, but are more likely to be liquefied and have an abnormal appearance. (See **Table 17-17** for a description of the types of intestinal obstruction.) Subsequent vomiting and loss of absorptive capacity in the bowel lead to dehydration and electrolyte imbalances. Stasis promotes bacterial overgrowth. Edema of the bowel wall can lead to ischemia, necrosis, and perforation.[102]

The most common cause is adhesions from prior surgeries such as appendectomies, gynecologic procedures, hernia repairs, and colorectal

Table 17-17 Types of Intestinal Obstruction

Term	Definition
Simple obstruction	Bowel obstruction with an intact blood supply
Strangulating obstruction	Bowel obstruction with resultant ischemia
Closed-loop obstruction	A segment of bowel occluded at two points along its course with the sites of obstruction adjacent to each other
Partial obstruction	Luminal narrowing, permitting the passage of some gas and intestinal contents
Complete obstruction	Total luminal occlusion
Obturation obstruction	Bowel obstruction caused by an intraluminal mass
Functional obstruction	Symptoms of mechanical obstruction in the absence of luminal occlusion or compression

surgeries. Other causes include cancer, herniation, and IBD.[102] Very rarely, intussusception or volvulus can result in a bowel obstruction. With *intussusception*, one portion of the bowel "telescopes" over the next, resulting in edema and obstruction and eventually to bowel ischemia. *Volvulus* refers to torsion of a segment of the intestinal tract.

The most common symptoms are abdominal distension, cramping abdominal pain, nausea, vomiting, difficulty in passing flatus, and obstipation (extreme constipation). The symptoms vary depending on the location of the obstruction. If it is more proximal in the intestine, vomiting is more common. Distension and pain are common if the obstruction is more distal. Other physical findings include fever, tachycardia, hypotension, oliguria, and dehydration. Abdominal inspection may reveal surgical scars or distension. Tympany may be elicited on percussion. Bowel sounds may be exaggerated. Laboratory tests including a CBC, electrolytes, renal studies, and urinalysis are commonly ordered to assess degree of dehydration, the presence of sepsis, and electrolyte imbalance.[102]

Imaging is necessary in the evaluation of bowel obstruction. While a CT scan is the preferred approach, an upright abdominal x-ray is often ordered, because results can be obtained quickly. The x-ray can accurately diagnose obstruction in 60% of cases.[102] Whenever possible, the American College of Radiology recommends a CT scan of the abdomen and pelvis with contrast, although contrast should be withheld if a high-grade small intestinal obstruction is suspected because the contrast will not reach the site of concern and will add to the patient's discomfort.[103] A CT scan has the added advantage of being able to better locate the site of obstruction, its extensiveness, and the presence of other complications such as strangulation, necrosis, and perforation.[102] Other imaging modalities sometimes used include ultrasonography, contrast fluoroscopy, and MRI.

The primary goal of treatment is to relieve the obstruction. Supportive measures include correction of metabolic abnormalities, bowel rest, rehydration, and treatment with antibiotics if superimposed infection from bacterial overgrowth is suspected. Conservative management with nasogastric suction and IV fluid is successful in 40% to 70% of clinically stable patients. If obstruction persists for more than 24 to 48 hours despite conservative management, surgery is most often indicated.[102] Surgery is required if strangulation is suspected to prevent necrosis and bowel death.

Bowel obstruction is rare in pregnancy, occurring in 1 out of every 1500–3000 pregnancies. It most often occurs in the third trimester. Adhesions are the primary cause, accounting for 60% to 70% of small bowel obstructions in pregnancy. Often an abdominal x-ray is the first test ordered, although an MRI may be needed if the diagnosis is not clear.[94] Bowel obstruction is associated with increased risk of perinatal and maternal mortality.[56]

ACUTE ABDOMINAL PAIN IN PREGNANCY

Pregnancy can complicate the evaluation of acute abdominal pain. The differential list will need to include OB/GYN-related causes (i.e., ectopic pregnancy, ovarian cyst or torsion of the ovary, degenerating fibroid), conditions that can be exacerbated by pregnancy (i.e., GERD, gallbladder disease, kidney stones, urinary tract infections), and those that can also occur in the nonpregnant patient (i.e., appendicitis, gastroenteritis). Evaluation is further complicated by the normal physiologic changes that accompany pregnancy. For example, the expanding uterus can change the position of the gallbladder and appendix and therefore change the location of pain of these conditions in pregnancy. The interpretation of various tests can be more difficult, because normal laboratory values can change in pregnancy. Lastly, the availability of imaging tests may be more limited due to concerns about fetal safety.

Each of the sections in this chapter on specific conditions associated with abdominal pain briefly addresses the impact of pregnancy on the presentation, evaluation, and management of nonobstetric causes of abdominal pain in pregnancy. The details of obstetric management in cases of acute abdominal pain are beyond the scope of this chapter. This section discusses how pregnancy impacts the choice of imaging modalities frequently used in the evaluation of abdominal pain.

CT scans expose the mother and fetus to ionizing radiation and are generally avoided if possible.[94] The impact of radiation in pregnancy depends on gestational age, dosage, and outcome of concern. Some outcomes occur only if radiation exposure exceeds a threshold level; these include pregnancy loss, congenital malformations, neurobehavioral abnormalities, and fetal growth retardation.[94] Exposures of less than 5 rad are not thought to be associated with an increase in fetal anomalies or pregnancy loss. The most vulnerable period of exposure for these outcomes is between 8 and 15 weeks' gestation.[94] Other adverse outcomes related to radiation exposure, such as cancer and mutagenic defects, can occur at any level of exposure and at any gestational age. For example, exposure to 1 to 2 rads of radiation is thought to increase the risk of childhood leukemia by a factor of 1.5 to 2 over background incidence and result in 1 case of leukemia in 2000 children exposed to ionizing radiation in utero.[94] Commonly used diagnostic tests have various exposure levels: chest x-ray, 2 view, 0.02–0.07 mrad; single-view abdominal film 100 mrad; CT scan of abdomen and lumbar spine 3.5 rad; and CT pelvimetry 250 mrad. Some of these tests are below background levels of radiation, which is estimated to be 0.1 rad (or 100 mrad) over the course of pregnancy.[94]

Ultrasound and MRI and are the imaging modalities of choice in pregnancy. Ultrasound is used whenever possible. The American College of Radiology advises against unnecessary use of MRI in pregnancy. MRI uses magnetic fields and pulsed radiofrequency gradients. No known deleterious effects have been identified; theoretical risks include miscarriage and "heating effects" on the fetus.[94] MRI without contrast should be used only if the information cannot be gained by ultrasound and the information provided by MRI will guide management of care in the current pregnancy.[104]

The use of contrast agents should be avoided if possible.[94] Contrast agents are known to cross the placental barrier and go into the fetal bloodstream. After entering the fetal bloodstream, they are excreted through the urine and swallowed by the fetus. The impact of fetal exposures is unknown.[105]

Conditions Characterized by Constipation

FUNCTIONAL CONSTIPATION

The majority of individuals diagnosed with constipation complain of mild symptoms that are not associated with structural abnormalities, intestinal motility disorders, or systemic disease. A detailed history should include a description of symptoms from the individual's own point of view, as well as a description of the characteristics of the stool and timing, frequency, and completeness of evacuation. Completion of a symptom diary can assist this process. Follow-up questions should include a description of current prescription and nonprescription medications, regimens used to relieve symptoms, presence or absence of alarm symptoms (e.g., rectal bleeding, weight loss, anemia), and whether metabolic or neurologic diseases that can cause constipation are suspected.

A CBC may be the only test needed. Historically, a fasting glucose, TSH, and calcium level have commonly been ordered, but the cost-effectiveness these laboratory tests has been recently called into question.[21] A colonoscopy is needed if a woman meets age-based recommendations, has an abrupt onset of symptoms, or if alarm symptoms are present. Healthy individuals younger than 50 years old with mild symptoms and no evidence of other disease processes can be started with a trial of fiber supplements and/or laxatives. Only if these therapies fail to provide relief are other tests needed.[29]

Treatment measures consist of dietary alterations, additional fiber and laxatives, and exercise. Response is not immediate and adjustments may need to be made in treatment regimens. Side effects include increased gaseousness and distension that diminishes after several days. The initial approach focuses on adding fiber through dietary changes or by using a fiber supplement. A twice-daily dose of fiber should be given with meals or water and adjusted after 7 to 10 days. If fiber alone is not satisfactory, then an osmotic agent (i.e., PEG-based solutions, magnesium citrate–based products, sodium phosphate–based products, and nonabsorbable carbohydrates) can be added to the regimen.[21] Of all the available products, psyllium (fiber) and PEG osmotic laxatives (e.g., MiraLax) have been the most extensively studied.[21,106] Stimulant laxatives, used as rescue medications, appear to be safe for long-term use. These include bisacodyl and glycerine suppositories. Other newer products (secretagogues, serotonin 5-HT4 receptor agonists) are reserved for use in refractory cases. **Table 17-18** lists common medications used for constipation.

Referral to a gastroenterologist or colorectal surgeon is needed for persistent symptoms. Testing for constipation may include sigmoidoscopy, colonoscopy, or a barium enema to evaluate the structure of the colon. Colonic transit time can be evaluated using timed passage of radiopaque

Table 17-18 Commonly Used Medications for Constipation

Type	Generic (Trade) Name	Side Effects and Comments
Fiber	Bran	Bloating, flatulence
	Psyllium (Metamucil)	Bloating, flatulence
	Methylcellulose (Citrucel)	Minimal bloating
	Calcium polycarbophil (Fibercom)	Bloating, less gas
Stool surfactant	Docusate sodium (Colace)	May cause pneumonia, if aspirated
	Mineral oil	
Stimulants	Bisacodyl (Dulcolax)	Abdominal cramps
	Docusate and senna (Peri-Colace)	
	Senna (Senokot, Exlax)	Possible cramping, avoid daily use
Osmotic laxative	Magnesium (Milk of Magnesia, Epsom salt)	Abdominal cramps
Enemas	Tap water	Mechanical lavage
	Phosphate enema (Fleet)	For acute constipation
	Soap suds enema	Impaction
Hyperosmolar	Sorbitol	Cramps, bloating, flatulence
	Polyethylene glycol (GoLYTELY, MiraLax)	Used before colonoscopy
	Magnesium citrate	Lemon flavored

Data from Locke GR 3rd, Pemberton JH, Phillips SF. AGA technical review on constipation. *Gastroenterology*. 2000; 119: 1761–1766; McQuaid KR. Alimentary tract. In: Tierney LM, McPhee SJ, Papadakis MA, Eds. *Current Medical Diagnosis and Treatment*. 42nd ed. New York: McGraw-Hill; 2003; Wolf JL. Bowel function. In: Carlson KJ, Eisenstat SA, Frigoletto FD, Schiff I, Eds. *Primary Care of Women*. 2nd ed. St. Louis: Mosby; 2002. pp. 133–141.

markers or scintigraphy. Treatment is based on identified cause. Higher doses of laxatives or the use of newer products are recommended for those with slow transit time. Generally, if conservative management is ineffective, an anorectal manometry and a rectal balloon expulsion test are recommended.[29] During this procedure, a small catheter with a balloon on the end is gently inserted into the rectum. The patient is asked to perform a series of maneuvers (relaxing, squeezing in, pushing out), and pressures are recorded. With the balloon expulsion test, a small amount of water is inserted into the balloon and then the patient is asked to evacuate the balloon as she would for a bowel movement. Prolonged time to expulsion can indicate rectal dysfunction. Occasionally, a defecography is ordered to evaluate the defecatory processes. Individuals with defecatory disorders can benefit from biofeedback and pelvic floor muscle retraining.[21,29]

Conditions Characterized Primarily by Rectal Bleeding

HEMORRHOIDS

Hemorrhoids are a common cause of minor rectal bleeding. They are the result of enlargement and displacement of the normal anal cushions, which are specialized vascular structures in the upper anal canal. The anal cushions are held in place by strong muscular fibers. They are thought to play a role in anal continence by maintaining closure of the anal canal. As a consequence of aging or aggravating conditions such as pregnancy, obesity, constipation, or diarrhea, the muscle fibers that attach the anal cushions to the anal sphincter become stretched and deteriorate, allowing the anal cushions to prolapse into the anal canal. Congestion, edema, and bleeding then ensue.[107]

Hemorrhoids are classified by their location as being internal or external. The dentate line is the demarcation line that distinguishes between

Table 17-19 Internal Hemorrhoid Classification

Grade	Description
Grade I	Visible with anoscope; may extend into anal canal
Grade I	Prolapses outside anal canal; may reduce spontaneously
Grade III	Same degree of prolapse; requires manual reduction
Grade IV	Unable to be reduced; may strangulate

Data from Wald A, Bharucha AE, Cosman BC, Whitehead WE. Management of benign anorectal disorders. *Am J Gastroenterol.* 2014:1-17; Rivadeneira DE, Steele SR, Ternent C, Chalasani S, Buie WD, Rafferty J, et al. Practice parameters for the management of hemorrhoids (revised 2010). *Dis Colon Rectum.* 2011;54(6):1059-1064.

external and internal hemorrhoids. Internal hemorrhoids arise above, and external hemorrhoids below, this line. Internal hemorrhoids are graded by severity. This classification system is used to guide management (**Table 17-19**).[108]

The symptoms of hemorrhoids are caused by the edema and displacement of the submucosal lining of the anal canal. The painless bleeding seen with this disease is usually from internal hemorrhoids. Women will often describe minimal bright red bleeding noted on the toilet tissue or around stools. Other symptoms of internal hemorrhoids include prolapse, itching, and a mucus discharge. The itching of the perianal skin is caused by exposure to leakage of rectal contents around the hemorrhoid. If harsh cleaning or scratching occurs, the skin may become more inflamed and a recurrent cycle develops. Severe pain may occur if the prolapsed internal hemorrhoid becomes strangulated.

External hemorrhoids are dilations of the inferior (external) hemorrhoidal plexus, below the dentate line, and are covered with squamous epithelium that contains many pain receptors.[107] External hemorrhoids may become thrombosed, and extreme pain usually is seen in the acute phase of this condition. A thrombosed external hemorrhoid can be recognized as a painful blue mass located at the anal verge. Eventually, symptoms improve when the overlying anoderm sloughs; at this time bleeding may occur. Anal skin tags are the result of healing redundant skin. Their only significance is the potential impact on hygiene after defecation.

The diagnosis of hemorrhoids is made on clinical grounds. No testing is needed unless red flags are present that suggest inflammatory disease, cancer, or other serious anorectal disorders. If any of these conditions are suspected, a colonoscopy should be ordered and referral made to a gastroenterologist.[109]

Nonsurgical therapy for hemorrhoids consists of increased dietary fiber, lubricant rectal suppositories with or without steroids, and warm sitz baths. Local anesthetics can be used for symptomatic relief from the discomfort of painful external hemorrhoids. Choices include 5% Lidocaine ointment, dibucaine ointment or cream (0.5–1.0%), benzocaine, dyclonine, and pramoxine. Witch hazel acts as an astringent and may be more soothing if kept cold in the refrigerator prior to applying. Use of a topical steroid may reduce inflammation. Topical steroids and analgesic creams or ointments should not be used for more than 1 week because of the potential for tissue inflammation or thinning of the skin.

Anoscopic therapy may be needed for acutely thrombosed external hemorrhoids or for hemorrhoids that are persistent and painful. Individuals who present urgently within 3 days of onset of symptoms of an acutely thrombosed external hemorrhoid benefit from excision, which gives rapid relief of symptoms and reduces the chance of recurrence. The procedure can be done under local anesthesia in the office or emergency department.[109] However, if the patient is seen later— 3 or more days after symptom onset, excision is not recommended. No treatment is needed

other than sitz baths if symptoms are resolving.[109] Individuals with internal hemorrhoids grades 1 to 3 can be treated with banding, sclerotherapy, or infrared coagulation.[110] Of these choices, ligation appears to be the most effective option. Surgical procedures (i.e., hemorrhoidectomy) are more appropriate for hemorrhoids that are accompanied by large symptomatic external tags or are severe (defined as a large 3rd-degree hemorrhoid or a 4th-degree hemorrhoid of any size).[109,110]

ANAL FISSURES

Anal fissures are tears or rents in the distal anal canal. They may be caused by trauma from the passage of firm stool and are seen in patients with constipation, Crohn's disease, tuberculosis, and cancer. Fissures can be either acute or chronic in nature. Examination of the anal tissue is difficult to perform in many patients because of the severe discomfort at the site of the fissure.[109] On inspection, a new fissure has the appearance of a recent laceration. If the fissure has become chronic, its appearance will include a slightly raised area around the defect, and white horizontal fibers of the internal anal sphincter are seen at the base of the defect. The location where the fissures are most often seen is at the midline, primarily in the posterior aspect and secondarily in the anterior aspect of the anal canal. Spasm occurs at the site of the exposed internal sphincter muscle. The spasm is painful and also causes the fissure to pull further apart, thus aggravating the condition and preventing healing from occurring.[109]

Medical therapy of anal fissures is designed to promote healing and disrupt the cycle of spasm and resultant inadequate or failed healing of the defect. Relaxation of the anal sphincter, atraumatic passage of stool, and analgesia are the main goals of medical therapy. Sitz baths help to promote relaxation of the sphincter, stool softeners and bulking agents prevent firm stools, and topical anesthetic creams provide pain relief.[108,109]

Various modalities have been employed in the treatment of chronic anal fissures. Topical nitrates (0.2% nitroglycerin ointment) twice daily for 6 to 8 weeks appear to promote healing of chronic anal fissures.[109] Botulinum toxin is an alternative, but it is associated with temporary fecal or flatus incontinence in some individuals.[108] Topical application of a calcium channel blocker also affords relief for some. If healing does not occur with medical approaches, surgical therapy is recommended. The goal of surgery is to achieve relaxation of the internal anal sphincter. The most commonly recommended procedure is lateral internal sphincterotomy, which involves the division, and then repair, of the internal anal sphincter from its distal-most end for a distance equal to the length of the fissure.[108] The aim is to reduce anal sphincter pressures, not close the fissure. Once the sphincter relaxes, healing of the fissure will occur.

Colon Cancer

Colon cancer is the third most common cancer found in women after lung and breast cancer, yet only 65% of women between 50 and 75 years of age have been screened with a sigmoidoscopy or colonoscopy in the past 10 years or with a fecal occult blood test within the last year.[111] Early detection of colorectal cancer and removal of adenomatous polyps save lives; therefore, women should be offered and encouraged to get appropriate screening. The selection of a particular screening modality and the time that screening starts depend on patient preferences, age, availability, and the presence or absence of risk factors and/or clinical disease. Factors that increase the risk of developing colon cancer include IBD, personal or family history of colorectal cancer or polyps, genetic syndromes, and lifestyle factors, such as tobacco and alcohol use, insufficient exercise, overweight and obesity, and unhealthy dietary practices (low-fiber, high-fat, and low fruit and vegetable intake).[111]

The American College of Gastroenterology makes a distinction between screenings for the prevention, as opposed to the detection, of cancer. It recommends using modalities that do both; colonoscopy, flexible sigmoidoscopy, and CT colonography can detect precancerous lesions (polyps, adenomas) and cancer. If polyps are identified, they may be able to be removed at the time of the procedure (colonoscopy) or referred later for removal (if a flexible sigmoidoscopy or CT colonography was done). Only if an individual declines one of these "cancer prevention" tests should she be offered cancer detection tests. Cancer detection tests cannot identify precursor lesions to cancer. The preferred cancer detection test is an annual fecal immunochemical test (FIT). It has a markedly higher sensitivity than older guaiac-based hemoccult cards, which are no longer recommended for colorectal cancer screening. Other tests have limited data on their effectiveness (Hemoccult II SENSA, a highly sensitive fecal occult blood test) or are expensive (fecal DNA test) and are not recommended by the American College of Gastroenterology.[112] See **Table 17-20** for a description of available tests.

Not all authorities recommend the same screening tests or schedules. Screening recommendations also vary by risk profile and screening results. **Table 17-21** lists recommendations of selected authorities, but the reader is strongly advised to refer to newer guidelines as they change periodically as new evidence becomes available. Of note, the recommendations listed here from the US Preventive Services Task Force are the 2015 draft statement, the most current available at the time of publication.[113] Referral for a consultation with a gastroenterologist, and possibly a genetic counselor, is recommended in complex cases.

Colon cancer is typically silent in the earliest stages. It is diagnosed either as a result of the clinical workup for suspicious symptoms or as a consequence of indicated routine screening. Presenting signs and symptoms of colorectal cancer

Table 17-20 Tests Used in Colon Cancer Screening

Test	Use	Advantages	Disadvantages
Colonoscopy	Cancer prevention and detection	Examines the entire colon and can detect right-sided lesions that can be missed on sigmoidoscopy Single-session diagnosis and treatment (can remove identified polyps at time of colonoscopy) Long interval between screenings	Requires sedation Requires adequate colon cleansing or detection of polyps will be compromised Rare risk of colonic perforation and bleeding Variability in skill of examiner
CT colonography	Cancer prevention and detection	Lower risk of perforation than colonoscopy Recommended by ACG only for individuals who decline colonoscopy	Evidence stronger for use of colonoscopy Can't detect small polyps (polyps $\geq$ 5 mm account for 80% of colorectal cancers) Less likely to be covered by insurance plans Requires bowel preparation Increases radiation exposures
Double contrast barium enema	Not recommended		No longer recommended as it is less effective at detecting polyps than other modalities
Fecal DNA testing	Cancer detection	Not recommended	Expensive Requires collection of entire stool FIT tests have better sensitivity and specificity No well-established evidence-based recommendation on appropriate timing of screening using DNA tests Positive results require follow-up colonoscopy
Fecal immuno-chemical test (FIT)	Cancer detection	Replaces older fecal occult blood testing guaiac-based tests, which have lower sensitivity and specificity in colorectal cancer screening Results not affected by diet or medications	Detects bleeding from the lower GI tract, may not detect bleeding from upper GI sources Requires ongoing annual assessments Requires 1 sample obtained at home, cannot be acquired during an office examination

(continues)

Table 17-20   Tests Used in Colon Cancer Screening (*continued*)

Test	Use	Advantages	Disadvantages
Flexible sigmoidoscopy	Cancer prevention and detection	No sedation necessary	Detects only 60% to 70% of the cancers detected by colonoscopy Cannot detect lesions beyond the distal colon Need partial or complete bowel preparation Positive findings require further investigation by colonoscopy Small risk of perforation Requires repetition in 5 to 10 years depending on the skill of the examiner
Hemoccult II SENSA	Cancer detection	New improved more sensitive guaiac-based test	Less evidence supporting its use than FIT

ACG = American College of Gastroenterology, CT = computed tomography, DNA = deoxyribonucleic acid, FIT = fecal immunochemical test, GI = gastrointestinal

Data from American College of Obstetricians and Gynecologists. Committee opinion no 609: colorectal cancer screening strategies. *Obstet Gynecol.* 2014;124(4):849-855; Rex DK, Johnson DA, Anderson JC, Schoenfeld PS, Burke CA, Inadomi JM. Colorectal cancer screening. *Am J Gastroenterol.* 2009;104:739-750; Turgeon DK, Ruffin MT. Screening strategies for colorectal cancer in asymptomatic adults. *Prim Care.* 2014;41(2):331-353.

in the majority of patients are nonspecific and include abdominal pain and distension, change in bowel habits, hematochezia or melena, weakness, and weight loss. Abdominal pain can be caused by partial obstruction, peritoneal dissemination, or intestinal perforation. Laboratory findings include iron deficiency anemia and a positive fecal occult blood stool sample. Because the recognition of colorectal cancer is challenging and, unfortunately, often delayed, a high index of suspicion is required of an astute clinician and prompt referral for consultation and/or colposcopy is suggested.

Colonoscopy, which is recommended to start at the age of 50, allows removal of polyps and adenomas and histologic evaluation of risk. Most polyps in the sigmoid and rectum are small

hyperplastic polyps that have a low potential of developing into dysplasia or cancer. Adenomas have malignant potential. They are categorized as tubular adenomas (with a low conversion rate to cancer of 4.8%), tubulovillous (less common but with a conversion rate of 19%), and villous (also less common but with a high conversion rate of 38.4%).[114] Findings on colposcopy that suggest the presence of cancer include: 1) adenomas that are large ($\geq$ 10 mm), have villous elements, or have high-grade dysplasia; 2) findings of $\geq$ 3 adenomas on a single examination; or 3) serrated polyps that are large or have dysplasia. These findings dictate at minimum earlier surveillance, if not treatment.[114] Interested readers are referred to a medical/surgical textbook for further details on the management of colorectal cancer.

Table 17-21 Colon Cancer Screening Recommendations by Various Authorities

Organization	Low-Risk Individuals	High-Risk Individuals: Risk Profile with Recommended Action

ACG	Start age 50 for general population and age 45 for African Americans.
	Cancer prevention:
	• Preferred test: Colonoscopy every 10 years
	• Alternative tests:
	  ▪ CT colonography every 5 years
	  ▪ Flexible sigmoidoscopy every 5 to 10 years
	Cancer detection:
	• Preferred test: FIT
	• Alternative: Annual fecal occult blood testing with highly sensitive test
		Single first-degree relative with CRC or advanced adenoma* ≥ 60 years:
		• Screen as low-risk individual.
		Single first-degree relative with CRC or advanced adenoma < 60 years or 2 first-degree relatives with CRC or advanced adenoma:*
		• Begin age 40 years or 10 years earlier than age at diagnosis of youngest relative with colonoscopy every 5 years.
		Familial adenomatous polyposis:
		• Refer for genetic counseling and possible testing.
		• Refer to gastroenterologist for consultation; may require annual flexible sigmoidoscopy or colonoscopy.
		Family history of hereditary nonpolyposis colorectal cancer:
		• Refer for genetic counseling and possible testing.
		• Refer to gastroenterologist for consultation; may require colonoscopy biannually between ages 20 and 40 years, and annually thereafter.

ACOG	Start at age 50 for low-risk individuals and age 45 for African Americans until age 75 years. • Preferred test: colonoscopy every 10 years • Alternative testing: Describes options. Preferred testing strategy is to use a modality that can prevent and detect cancer, does not indicate preference for 1 test over another in this category.	Does not address
ACP	Start at age 50 and end at age 75. Screening should not be done in individuals not in good health with a life expectancy of less than 10 years. No preference among following options: • Annual high-sensitivity fecal occult blood test or FIT • Flexible sigmoidoscopy every 5 years • Colonoscopy every 10 years	Does not address

(continues)

Table 17-21 Colon Cancer Screening Recommendations by Various Authorities *(continued)*

Organization	Low-Risk Individuals	High-Risk Individuals: Risk Profile with Recommended Action
USPSTF	Start at age 50 and end at 75 years. Recommends screening for adults between 76 and 85 years be individualized after consideration of screening history and health status. Individuals who have never been screened or are healthy are likely to benefit most. Discusses options but does not indicate preference among the following modalities: • FIT or highly sensitive fecal occult blood test every year • Flexible sigmoidoscopy every 10 years with FIT every year • Colonoscopy every 10 years	Does not address

ACG = American College of Gastroenterology, ACP = American College of Physicians, ACOG = American College of Obstetricians and Gynecologists, CRC = colorectal cancer, CT = computed tomography, FIT = fecal immunochemical test, USPSTF = US Preventive Services Task Force

*Advanced adenoma is defined as adenoma ≥ 1 cm in size or high-grade dysplasia or villous elements.

Data from American College of Obstetricians and Gynecologists. Committee opinion no 609: colorectal cancer screening strategies. *Obstet Gynecol.* 2014;124(4):849-855; Rex DK, Johnson DA, Anderson JC, Schoenfeld PS, Burke CA, Inadomi JM. Colorectal cancer screening. *Am J Gastroenterol.* 2009;104:739-750; US Preventive Services Task Force. Draft Recommendation Statement: Colorectal cancer screening. Available at: http://www.uspreventiveservicestaskforce.org/Page/Document/draft-recommendation-statement38/colorectal-cancer-screening2. 2015. Accessed May 5, 2016; Wilt T, Harris R, Qaseem A. High Value Care Task Force of the American College of Physicians. Screening for cancer: advice for high-value care from the American College of Physicians. *Ann Intern Med.* 2015;162(10):718-725.

INTESTINAL PARASITES

Intestinal parasites are uncommon but not unknown in the United States. They may cause GI symptoms and anemia from chronic blood loss. This section describes three infections: roundworm, hookworm, and pinworms.

Roundworm Roundworm (*Ascaris lumbricoides*) disease occurs mostly in developing countries. Transmission is via the fecal-oral route. Adult worms inhabit the small intestine and, once fertilized, pass their eggs through feces to contaminate soil. The eggs mature into larvae that are

the infectious stage. In poor sanitary conditions, larvae are spread from a human via soil (fertilizer or poor hygiene) to another human host. Once ingested, the larvae migrate through the lungs during their maturation process, are coughed up and swallowed, and settle in the small intestine where they develop into adults.

Clinical manifestations of infection are generally asymptomatic, but some individuals report cough or abdominal discomfort. Many individuals do not have evidence of clinical disease unless there is a heavy worm infestation. A heavy worm load can be associated with bowel obstruction and with hepatobiliary and pancreatic ascariasis. Diagnosis is based on identifying ova or mature worms in stool specimens. Treatment includes mebendazole and albendazole.

Hookworm Human hookworm disease (*Ancylostoma duodenale* and *Necator americanus*) is widely distributed in underdeveloped tropical and subtropical parts of the world and was historically epidemic in the Southeastern United States. Infections in developed countries are more common in immigrants and travelers returning from areas where infections are endemic.

Hookworms are small (1 cm), long, creamy white nematodes that live in the upper small intestine attached to the mucosa. Adult worms lay eggs that pass in feces to hatch in warm, moist topsoil. In this larval stage, they become infective to humans. Contact with contaminated soil can allow the skin to be penetrated by the larvae. These larvae are carried through venous circulation to the lungs, where they can make their way up to the pharynx and esophagus to be swallowed. They enter the small intestine where they mature into adults. Worms remain in the gut for up to 2 years.

The spread of infection is most prevalent in areas with poor sanitary practices—that is, cultures where infected individuals defecate in areas frequented by others and those that use human excrement as fertilizer for crops. The incidence decreases once adequate sanitation procedures are utilized.

Most infections are asymptomatic until the worm burden is large. The major clinical findings attributed to hookworm disease are iron deficiency anemia, eosinophilia, and chronic protein malnutrition. Diagnosis is based upon fecal smear examination for hookworm ova. The drugs of choice for treatment are mebendazole and albendazole. Iron replacement is recommended for the anemia.

Pinworms Pinworms, also known as *Enterobiasis vermicularis*, are the most common nematode in the United States. Infestation occurs mostly commonly in children and household members of infected children. The infection is spread via the fecal–oral route. The worms live in the cecum of the large intestine. At night the females migrate to lay eggs on the perineum, which can cause perianal pruritus. An easy way to determine if an infestation is present is to touch cellophane tape to the perianal area right after awakening. The tape is then placed on a slide and examined under the microscope for eggs. This should be repeated for 3 consecutive days. Infections are easily treated with mebendazole, pyrantel pamoate, and albendazole.

Miscellaneous

Nonalcoholic Fatty Liver Disease

Nonalcoholic fatty liver disease is thought to affect 20% to 30% of adults in developed countries. Risk factors include male gender, visceral obesity, high body mass index, Hispanic ethnicity, and diabetes.[115] It is an asymptomatic disease. A subset of individuals with nonalcoholic fatty liver disease will develop steatohepatitis, which increases the risk of progressive liver disease. Fat accumulates in the liver and over time results in hepatocellular injury, ballooning, and inflammation that can lead to cirrhosis, hepatocellular carcinoma, and liver transplantation.[116]

Nonalcoholic fatty liver disease is most often detected as an incidental finding on laboratory tests or ultrasounds done for another reason. Common laboratory changes seen with nonalcoholic fatty liver disease include elevated fasting blood glucose, low high-density lipoprotein (HDL) cholesterol, and high levels of triglycerides. Hepatic steatosis is seen on ultrasound in fatty liver disease, although it is an unreliable indicator of fatty liver disease unless 30% or more of the liver is affected.[115] Neither CT scans nor MRIs reliably assess steatohepatitis and fibrosis. Liver biopsy can confirm the diagnosis, but is expensive, invasive, and associated with procedural-related complications. Therefore, controversy exists about when, whether, and how to confirm the diagnosis of nonalcoholic fatty liver disease. Currently, alternative biomarkers are being investigated because of the limitations of current testing modalities.[116,117]

Other causes of fatty liver disease need to be ruled out. In addition to alcohol abuse, medications, hepatitis C, Wilson's disease, Reye's syndrome, HELLP (hemolysis, elevated liver enzymes, low platelet count) syndrome, and pregnancy can lead to fatty liver disease.[117] Nonalcoholic fatty liver disease can be distinguished from that caused by excessive intake of alcohol by laboratory findings; with excessive alcohol use, the aspartate transaminase/alanine transaminase ratio is > 1 and high HDL cholesterol is seen together with hypertriglyceridemia.[118]

No treatment specifically for nonalcoholic fatty liver disease is currently available. Rather, treatment is supportive and directed as needed against comorbidities. Affected women are advised to increase exercise, lose weight, and improve the quality of their diet.[116] Weight loss of 3% to 5% is needed to improve steatosis, but weight loss of 10% is needed to reduce liver inflammation.[117]

Other options are helpful if progressive liver disease is present. The American Gastroenterological Association recommends the use of vitamin E and pioglitazone in individuals with biopsy-confirmed steatohepatitis.[117] Studies have shown that use of vitamin E in nondiabetic patients with nonalcoholic fatty liver disease is associated with lower levels of aminotransferases; improvements in steatosis, inflammation, and ballooning; and resolution of steatohepatitis, but does not affect hepatic fibrosis. Similar findings are seen with pioglitazone.[117] Metformin is not recommended, because it has not been shown to be associated with improvements in markers of liver health. Preliminary evidence suggests that bariatric surgery is associated with improvements in histologic markers of hepatic steatosis, but the American Gastroenterological Association concluded that it is premature to recommend bariatric surgery (unless an individual meets already established criteria) as a management approach for nonalcoholic fatty liver disease until better quality evidence is available.[116,117]

References

1. Becker D. Nausea, vomiting, and hiccups: a review of mechanisms and treatment. *Anesth Prog.* 2010;57(4):150-157.

2. Anderson WD, Strayer SM. Evaluation of nausea and vomiting in adults: a case-based approach. *Am Fam Physician.* 2013;88(6):371-379.

3. Scoriza K, Williams A, Phillips J, Shaw J. Evaluation of nausea and vomiting. *Am Fam Physician.* 2007;76:76-84.

4. Guerrant RL, Van Gilder T, Steiner TS, Thielman NM, Slutsker L, Tauxe RV, et al. Practice guidelines for the management of infectious diarrhea. *Clin Infect Dis.* 2001;32(3):331-351.

5. Sweetser S. Evaluating the patient with diarrhea: a case-based approach. *Mayo Clin Proc.* 2012;87(6):596-602.

6. Guandalini S, Vaziri H, eds. *Diarrhea: Diagnostic and Therapeutic Advances.* New York, NY: Springer; 2011.

7. Juckett G, Trivedi R. Evaluation of chronic diarrhea. *Am Fam Physician.* 2011;84(10):1119-1126.

8. Buffie C, Pamer E. Microbiota-mediated colonization resistance against intestinal pathogens. *Nat Rev Immunol.* 2013;13(11):790-781.

9. McFarland L. Epidemiology, risk factors and treatments for antibiotic-associated diarrhea. *Dig Dis.* 1998;16:292-307.

10. Surawicz CM, Brandt LJ, Binion DG, Ananthakrishnan AN, Curry SR, Gilligan PH, et al. Guidelines for diagnosis, treatment, and prevention of *Clostridium difficile* infections. *Am J Gastroenterol.* 2013; 108:478-498.

11. Oustamanolakis P, Tack J. Dyspepsia: organic versus functional. *J Clin Gastroenterol.* 2012;46(3): 175-190.

12. Spieker M. Evaluating dysphagia. *Am Fam Physician.* 2000;61(12):3639-3648.

13. American College of Radiology. ACR practice parameter for the performance of esophagrams and upper gastrointestinal examination of the upper gastrointestinal examination in adults. 2014. Available

at: http://www.acr.org/~/media/ACR/Documents/PGTS/guidelines/Esophagrams_Upper_GI.pdf. Accessed May 5, 2016.

14. Cartwright S, Knudson M. Evaluation of acute abdominal pain in adults. *Am Fam Physician.* 2008;77(7):971-978.

15. American College of Radiology. Appropriateness Criteria. Available at: https://acsearch.acr.org/list. Accessed May 5, 2016.

16. American College of Radiology. ACR Appropriateness Criteria Right Upper Quadrant Pain. 2013. Available at: https://acsearch.acr.org/docs/69474/Narrative/. Accessed May 5, 2016.

17. American College of Radiology. ACR Appropriatens Criteria: Right Lower Quadrant Pain—Suspected Appendicitis. 2013. Available at: https://acsearch.acr.org/docs/69357/Narrative/. Accessed May 5, 2016.

18. American College of Radiology. ACR Appropriateness Criteria: Left Lower Quadrant Pain—Suspected Diverticulitis. 2013. Available at: https://acsearch.acr.org/docs/69356/Narrative/. Accessed May 5, 2016.

19. American College of Radiology. ACR Appropriateness Criteria: Acute (Nonlocalized) Abdominal Pain and Fever or Suspected Abdominal Abscess. 2013. Available at: https://acsearch.acr.org/docs/69467/Narrative/. Accessed May 5, 2016.

20. Longstreth GF, Thompson WG, Chey WD, Houghton LA, Mearin F, Spiller RC. Functional bowel disorders. *Gastroenterology.* 2006;130(5):1480-1491.

21. Bharucha A, Pemberton J, Locke G. American Gastroenterological Association technical review on constipation. *Gastroenterology.* 2013;144:218-238.

22. Kim BSM, Li BT, Engel A, Samra JS, Clarke S, Norton ID, et al. Diagnosis of gastrointestinal bleeding: a practical guide for clinicians. *World J Gastrointest Pathophysiol.* 2014;5(4):467-478.

23. Bull-Henry K, Al-Kawas F. Evaluation of occult gastrointestinal bleeding. *Am Fam Physician.* 2013;87(6):430-436.

24. Manning-Dimmitt L, Dimmitt S, Wilson G. Diagnosis of gastrointestinal bleeding in adults. *Am Fam Physician.* 2005;71:1339-1346.

25. Laine L, Jensen DM. Management of patients with ulcer bleeding. *Am J Gastroenterol.* 2012;107:345-360.

26. Gerson LB, Fidler JL, Cave DR, Leighton JA. ACG clinical guideline: diagnosis and management of small bowel bleeding. *Am J Gastroenterol.* 2015;110(9):1265-1287.

27. Raju G, Gerson L, Das A, Lewis B. American Gastroenterological Association (AGA) Institute medical position statement on obscure gastrointestinal bleeding. *Gastroenterology.* 2007;133:1694-1698.

28. Barr W, Smith A. Acute diarrhea in adults. *Am Fam Physician.* 2014;89(3):180-189.

29. The AGA Institute Medical Position Panel, Bharucha AE, Dorn SD, Lembo A, Pressman A. American Gastroenterological Association medical position statement on constipation. *Gastroenerology.* 2013;144:211-217.

30. Konikoff M, Denson L. Role of fecal calprotectin as a biomarker of intestinal inflammation in inflammatory bowel disease. *Inflamm Bowel Dis.* 2006;12(6):524-534.

31. Schiller LR. Definitions, pathophysiology, and evaluation of chronic diarrhoea. *Best Pract Res Clin Gastroenterol.* 2012;26(5):551-562.

32. Najm WI. Peptic ulcer disease. *Prim Care Clin Office Pract.* 2011;38:383-394.

33. Ramakrishnan K, Salinas R. Peptic ulcer disease. *Am Fam Physician.* 2007;76(7):1005-1012.

34. Painter JE, Gargano JW, Collier SA, Yoder JS. Giardiasis surveillance—United States, 2011–2012. *MMWR.* 2015;64(SS03):15-25.

35. Painter JE, Hlavsa MC, Collier SA, Xiao L, Yoder JS. Cryptosporidiosis surveillance—United States, 2011–2012. *MMWR.* 2015;64(SS03):1-14.

36. American College of Radiology. ACR–AIUM–SPR–SRU Practice Parameter for the performance of an ultrasound examination of the abdomen and/or retroperitoneum. 2014. Available at: http://www.acr.org/~/media/ACR/Documents/PGTS/guidelines/US_Abdomen_Retro.pdf. Accessed May 5, 2016.

37. American Society for Gastrointestinal Endoscopy. The role of endoscopy in the management of patients with diarrhea. *Gastrointest Endosc.* 2010;71(6):887-889.

38. Cartwright S, Knudson M. Diagnostic imaging of acute abdominal pain in adults. *Am Fam Physician.* 2015;91(7):452-459.

39. Abraham S, Rivero HG, Erlikh IV, Griffith L, Kondamudi VK. Surgical and nonsurgical management of gallstones. *Am Fam Physician.* 2014;89(10):795-802.

40. Hempel S, Newberry S, Maher A, Wang Z, Miles JN, Shanman R, et al. Probiotics for the prevention and treatment of antibiotic-associated diarrhea: a systematic review and meta-analysis. *JAMA.* 2012;307(18):1959-1969.

41. Hill D, Beeching NJ. Travelers' diarrhea. *Curr Opin Infect Dis.* 2010;23(5):481-487.

42. Kantele A, Lääveri T, Mero S, Vilkman K, Pakkenan SH, Ollgren J, et al. Antimicrobials increase the risk of ESBL-PE colonization in travelers. *Clin Infect Dis.* 2015;60:837-846.

43. Kollaritsch H, Paulke-Korinek M, Wiedermann U. Traveler's diarrhea. *Infect Dis Clin North Am.* 2012;26(3):691-706.

44. Walker C, Applegate J, Black R. Haemolytic-uraemic syndrome as a sequela of diarrhoeal disease. *J Health Popul Nutr.* 2012;30(3):257-261.
45. Bennell J, Taylor C. A loss of social eating: the experience of individuals with gastroparesis. *J Clin Nurs.* 2013;22:2812-2821.
46. Fasano A, Catassi C. Celiac Disease. *N Engl J Med.* 2012;367:2419-2426.
47. Rubio-Tapia A, Hill ID, Kelly CP, Calderwood AH, Murray JA. Diagnosis and management of celiac disease. *Am J Gastroenterol.* 2013;108:656-676.
48. Sapone A, Bai J, Ciacci C, Dolinsek J, Green P, Hadjivassiliou M, et al. Spectrum of gluten-related disorders: consensus on new nomenclature and classification. *BMC Med.* 2012;10:13.
49. Capili B, Chang M, Anastasi J. A clinical update: nonceliac gluten sensitivity—is it really the gluten. *J Nurse Prac.* 2014;10(9):666-673.
50. Cheifetz A. Management of active Crohn disease. *JAMA.* 2013;309(20):2150-2158.
51. Mowat C, Cole A, Windsor A, Ahmad T, Arnott I, Driscoll R, et al. Guidelines for the management of inflammatory bowel disease in adults. *Gut.* 2011;60(5):571-607.
52. Lichtenstein GR, Hanauer SB, Sandborn WJ. The Practice Parameters Committee of the American College of Gastroenterology. Management of Crohn's disease in adults. *Am J Gastroenterol.* 2009;104(2):465-483.
53. Danese S, Fiocchi C. Ulcerative colitis. *N Engl J Med.* 2011;365(18):1713-1725.
54. Iskandar H, Dhere T, Farraye F. Ulcerative colitis: update on medical management. *Curr Gastroenterol Rep.* 2015;17(11):1-11.
55. Kornbluth A, Sachar DB. Ulcerative colitis practice guidelines in adults: American College of Gastroenterology, Practice Parameters Committee. *Am J Gastroenterol.* 2010;105(3):501-523.
56. Masselli G, Derme M, Laghi F, Framarino-dei-Malatesta M, Gualdi G. Evaluating the acute abdomen in the pregnant patient. *Radiol Clin North Am.* 2015;53(6):1309-1325.
57. Beaulieu DB, Kane S. Inflammatory bowel disease in pregnancy. *Gastroenterol Clin North Am.* 2011;40(2):399-413.
58. Chaudrey K, Kane S. Safety of immunomodulators and anti-TNF therapy in pregnancy. *Curr Treat Options Gastro.* 2015;13(1):77-89.
59. Farrukh A, Mayberry J. Microscopic colitis: a review. *Colorectal Dis.* 2014;16:957-964.
60. Loyd R, McClellan D. Update on the evaluation and management of functional dyspepsia. *Am Fam Physician.* 2011;83(5):547-552.
61. Talley NJ, Vakil N, the Practice Parameters Committee of the American College of Gastroenterology.

62. Katz PO, Gerson LB, Vela MF. Diagnosis and management of gastroesophageal reflux disease. *Am J Gastroenterol.* 2013;108:308-328.
63. Boeckxstaens GE, Rohof WO. Pathophysiology of gastroesophageal reflux disease. *Gastroenterol Clin North Am.* 2014;43(1):15-25.
64. Vakil N. The initial diagnosis of GERD. *Best Pract Res Clin Gastroenterol.* 2013;27(3):365-371.
65. Hershcovici T, Fass R. Step-by-step management of refractory gastroesophageal reflux disease. *Dis Esophagus.* 2013;26(1):27-36.
66. Mattar R, de Campos Mazo D, Carrilho F. Lactose intolerance: diagnosis, genetic, and clinical factors. *Clin Exp Gastroenterol.* 2012;5:113-121.
67. Patrick L. Gastroesophageal reflux disease (GERD): a review of conventional and alternative treatments. *Altern Med Rev.* 2012;16(2):116-134.
68. Pennathur A, Gibson MK, Jobe BA, Luketich JD. Oesophageal carcinoma. *Lancet.* 2013;381:400-412.
69. Rome III Diagnostic Criteria for Functional Gastrointestinal Disorders. Available at: http://www.rome criteria.org/assets/pdf/19_RomeIII_apA_885-898.pdf. Accessed May 5, 2016.
70. Laskaratos F-M, Goodkin O, Thoua NM, Murray CD. Irritable bowel syndrome. *Medicine.* 2015;43(5):266-270.
71. Burbige E. Irritable bowel syndrome: diagnostic approaches in clinical practice. *Clin Exp Gastroenterol.* 2010;3:127-137.
72. Camilleri M. Peripheral mechanisms in irritable bowel syndrome. *N Engl J Med.* 2012;367(17):1626-1635.
73. El-Salhy M. Irritable bowel syndrome: diagnosis and pathogenesis. *World J Gastroenterol.* 2012;18(37):5151-5163.
74. Saha L. Irritable bowel syndrome: pathogenesis, diagnosis, treatment, and evidence-based medicine. *World J Gastroenterol.* 2014;20(22):6759-6773.
75. Ford AC, Moayyedi P, Lacy BE, Lembo AJ, Saito YA, Schiller LR, et al. American College of Gastroenterology monograph on the management of irritable bowel syndrome and chronic idiopathic constipation. *Am J Gastroenterol.* 2014;109(S1):S2-S26.
76. Altayar O, Sharma V, Prokop LJ, Sood A, Hassan Murad M. Psychological therapies in patients with irritable bowel syndrome: a systematic review and meta-analysis of randomized controlled trials. *Gastroenterol Res Pract.* 2015;10(2):1-19.
77. Ford AC, Quigley EMM, Lacy BE, Lembo AJ, Saito YA, Schiller LR, et al. Effect of antidepressants and psychological therapies, including hypnotherapy, in irritable bowel syndrome: systematic review and

Guidelines for the management of dyspepsia. *Am J Gastroenterol.* 2005;100:2324-2337.

meta-analysis. *Am J Gastroenterol.* 2014;109(9): 1350-1365.

78. Weinberg DS, Smalley W, Heidelbaugh JJ, Sultan S. American Gastroenterological Association Institute guideline on the pharmacological management of irritable bowel syndrome. *Gastroenterology.* 2014; 147(5):1146-1148.

79. Van Erpecum KJ. Pathogenesis of cholesterol and pigment gallstones: an update. *Clin Res Hepatol Gastroenterol.* 2011;35(4):281-287.

80. Wittenburg H. Hereditary liver disease: gallstones. *Best Pract Res Clin Gastroenterol.* 2010;24(5):747-756.

81. Kilpatrick CC, Orejuela F. Management of the acute abdomen in pregnancy: a review. *Curr Opin Obstet Gynecol.* 2008;20(6):534-539.

82. Devarajan S, Chandraharan E. Abdominal pain in pregnancy: a rational approach to management. *Obstet Gynaecol Reprod Med.* 2011;21(7):198-206.

83. Augustin G, Majerovic M. Non-obstetrical acute abdomen during pregnancy. *Eur J Obstet Gynecol Reprod Biol.* 2007;131(1):4-12.

84. Malfertheiner P, Chan FKL, McColl KEL. Peptic ulcer disease. *Lancet.* 2009;374(9699):1449-1461.

85. Fashner J, Gitu J. Diagnosis and treatment of peptic ulcer disease and *H. pylori* infection. *Am Fam Physician.* 2015;91(4):236-242.

86. Chey WD, Wong BC, the Practice Parameters Committee of the American College of Gastroenterology. American College of Gastroenterology guideline on the management of *Helicobacter pylori* infection. *Am J Gastroenterol.* 2007;102:1808-1825.

87. Deshmukh S, Verde F, Johnson PT, Fishman EK, Macura KJ. Anatomical variants and pathologies of the vermix. *Emerg Radiol.* 2014;21:543-552.

88. William R. *Digestive Diseases—Research and Clinical Developments: Appendicitis: Symptoms, Diagnosis, and Treatments.* New York, NY: Nova; 2011.

89. Flum DR. Acute appendicitis—appendectomy or the "antibiotics first" strategy. *N Engl J Med.* 2015; 372(20):1937-1943.

90. Hardin D. Acute appendicitis: review and update. *Am Fam Physician.* 1999;60(7):2027-2034.

91. Ohle R, O'Reilly F, O'Brien K, Fahey T, Dimitrov E. The Alvarado score for predicting acute appendicitis: a systematic review. *BMC Med.* 2011;9:139.

92. Alvarado A. A practical score for the early diagnosis of acute appendicitis. *Ann Emerg Med.* 1986;15: 557-564.

93. Grönroos J. Clinical suspicion of acute appendicitis— is the time ripe for more conservative treatment? *Minim Invasive Ther Allied Technol.* 2011;20:42-45.

94. Khandelwal A, Fasih N, Kielar A. Imaging of acute abdomen in pregnancy. *Radiol Clin North Am.* 2013;51(6):1005-1022.

95. Wilkins T, Embry K, George R. Diagnosis and management of acute diverticulitis. *Am Fam Physician.* 2013;87(9):612-620.

96. Gaglia A, Probert CS. Diverticular disease. *Medicine.* 2015;43(6):320-323.

97. Stollman N, Smalley W, Hirano I, Adams MA, Dorn SD, Dudley-Brown SL, et al. American Gastroenterological Association Institute guideline on the management of acute diverticulitis. *Gastroenterology.* 2015;149(7):1944-1949.

98. Cruz-Santamaría D, Taxonera C, Giner M. Update on pathogenesis and clinical management of acute pancreatitis. *World J Gastrointest Pathophysiol.* 2012;3(3):60-70.

99. Kota S, Kota S, Jammula S, Krishna S, Modi K. Hypertriglyceridemia-induced recurrent acute pancreatitis: a case-based review. *Indian J Endocrinol Metab.* 2012;16(1):141-143.

100. Tenner S, Baillie J, DeWitt J, Swaroop S. American College of Gastroenterology Guideline: management of acute pancreatitis. *Am J Gastroenterol.* 2013;108:1400-1415.

101. Quilan J. Acute pancreatitis. *Am Fam Physician.* 2014;90(9):632-639.

102. Jackson PG, Raiji M. Evaluation and management of intestinal obstruction. *Am Fam Physician.* 2011;82(2):159-165.

103. American College of Radiology. ACR Appropriateness Criteria: Suspected Small-Bowel Obstruction. 2013. Available at: http://www.acr.org/~/media /832f100277004bc69a8c818c7c9bff33.pdf. Accessed May 5, 2016.

104. Expert Panel on MR Safety, Kanal E, Barkovich J, Bell C, Borgstede JP, Bradley WG, et al. ACR guidance document on MR safe practices: 2013. *J Magn Reson Imaging.* 2013;37:501-530.

105. American College of Radiology. *ACR Manual on Contrast Material, Version 10.1.* Available at: http:// www.acr.org/~/media/ACR/Documents/PDF /QualitySafety/Resources/Contrast Manual/2015 _Contrast_Media.pdf/. Accessed May 5, 2016.

106. Tack J, Müller-Lissner S, Stanghellini V, Boeckxstaens G, Kamm MA, Simren M, et al. Diagnosis and treatment of chronic constipation—a European perspective. *Neurogastroenterol Motil.* 2011;23(8):697-710.

107. Lohsiriwat V. Hemorrhoids: from basic pathophysiology to clinical management. *World J Gastroenterol.* 2012;18(17):2009-2017.

108. Fargo M, Latimer K. Evaluation and management of common anorectal conditions. *Am Fam Physician.* 2012;85(6):624-630.

109. Wald A, Bharucha AE, Cosman BC, Whitehead WE. Management of benign anorectal disorders. *Am J Gastroenterol.* 2014:1-17.

110. Rivadeneira DE, Steele SR, Ternent C, Chalasani S, Buie WD, Rafferty J, et al. Practice parameters for the management of hemorrhoids (Revised 2010). *Dis Colon Rectum.* 2011;54(6):1059-1064.

111. American College of Obstetricians and Gynecologists. Committee opinion no 609: colorectal cancer screening strategies. *Obstet Gynecol.* 2014;124(4): 849-855.

112. Rex DK, Johnson DA, Anderson JC, Schoenfeld PS, Burke CA, Inadomi JM. American College of Gastroenterology guideline for colorectal cancer screening 2009. *Am J Gastroenterol.* 2009;104:739-750.

113. US Preventive Services Task Force. Draft Recommendation Statement: Colorectal cancer screening. 2015. Available at: http://www.uspreventiveservices taskforce.org/Page/Document/draft-recommendation -statement38/colorectal-cancer-screening2. Accessed May 5, 2016.

114. Short M, Layton M, Teer B, Domagalski J. Colorectal cancer screening and surveillance. *Am Fam Physician.* 2015;91(2):93-100.

115. Lonardo A, Bellentani S, Argo CK, Ballestri S, Byrne CD, Caldwell SH, et al. Epidemiological modifiers of non-alcoholic fatty liver disease: focus on high-risk groups. *Dig Liver Dis.* 2015;47(12):997-1006.

116. Ahmed A, Wong RJ, Harrison SA. Nonalcoholic fatty liver disease review: diagnosis, treatment, and outcomes. *Clin Gastroenterol Hepatol.* 2015;13(12): 2062-2070.

117. Chalasani N, Younossi Z, Lavine JE, Diehl AM, Brunt EM, Cusi K, et al. Diagnosis and management of non-alcoholic fatty liver disease: practice guideline by the American Association for the Study of Liver Diseases, American College of Gastroenterology, and the American Gastroenterological Association. *Am J Gastroenterol.* 2012;107:811-826.

118. Preiss D, Sattar N. Non-alcoholic fatty liver disease: an overview of prevalence, diagnosis, pathogenesis, and treatment considerations. *Clin Sci.* 2008; 115:5.

CHAPTER 18

OBESITY AND WEIGHT MANAGEMENT

Diane Berry

Overweight/obesity is a serious public health concern. Proper weight management requires a balance between nutrition and regular exercise. Midwives and other women's health providers are in a unique position to evaluate and manage obesity in the primary care setting. Intervention in overweight and obesity includes accurate diagnosis and an intervention that teaches the woman to find her personal balance of nutrition and exercise. This chapter focuses primarily on the management of overweight and obesity in women who are not pregnant; pregnancy-related concerns are also addressed.

Overweight and obesity in the United States have reached epidemic proportions, with the number of overweight children, adolescents, and adults increasing continuously and dramatically since the 1970s. Overweight is defined as a body mass index (BMI) $\geq$ 25 to 29.9 kg/m^2, and obesity is defined as a BMI $\geq$ 30.0 kg/m^2 (see **Table 18-1**).[1] Obesity is further divided into risk categories: Class 1 (BMI 30.0–34.9), Class 2 (BMI 35.0–39.9), and Class 3 (BMI $\geq$ 40). Overweight and obesity affect more than 68.8% of the US population over the age of 20 years.[2]

Obesity is prevalent in both sexes, affects all ages, crosses all ethnic groups, and has increased dramatically since the mid-1990s. Currently, 80% of African American and 78% of Hispanic women are overweight or obese, compared with 60.3% of non-Hispanic White women.[2] Obesity is a risk factor for hypertension, lipid abnormalities, type 2 diabetes mellitus, coronary heart disease, stroke, cholecystitis, osteoarthritis, sleep apnea

---

Table 18-1 Nonpregnant Women: Body Mass Index and Weight Status

Body Mass Index	Weight Status
Below 18.5	Underweight
18.5–24.9	Normal
25.0–29.9	Overweight
30.0 and above	Obese

Data from US Department of Health and Human Services, Public Health Service, National Center for Health Statistics. *Vital and Health Statistics: Anthropometric Reference Data and Prevalence of Overweight United States, 1976–80.* Hyattsville, MD: US Department of Health and Human Services; 1987.

and respiratory problems, and some cancers.[3,4] Obese individuals tend to suffer increased psychologic effects such as depression and low self-esteem when compared with normal weight individuals.[5]

Healthy People 2020 reports that overweight and obesity are major contributors to preventable causes of death and recommends reducing the proportion of children, adolescents, and adults who are overweight or obese through healthy diet and regular exercise.[6] The National Task Force on Prevention and Treatment of Obesity recommends weight loss and lasting lifestyle change through improved nutrition and increased activity.[7]

Obesity is a complex problem with etiologic factors that include the interaction of predisposing genetic and metabolic factors with a changing environment. Heredity, environmental and socioeconomic factors, energy intake, and energy expenditure all influence the continued increase in overweight and obese individuals in the United States.

Heredity plays a major role in the development of obesity, with genes, gender, and population being influential. Genes passed from parents to children provide a basis for genetic inheritance, but diet and exercise provide additional variation. There is direct evidence to demonstrate a strong genetic contribution to the metabolic profile at birth.[8] The relationship between parental and childhood adiposity at birth is moderate, weakens during the first 2 years, and then strengthens at ages 3–4 years.[9] Identical twins are more highly correlated in body composition than fraternal twins or other siblings.[10] Overweight or obese children with overweight or obese parents have an increased risk of developing adult obesity.[9] When both parents are of normal weight, their child has the lowest risk of developing obesity as an adult. Overweight and obesity in adolescence increases the risk for the development of obesity in adulthood regardless of parental weight status.[11] In addition, women have higher body fat

percentages than men,[12] which may be related to an autosomal obesity gene that interacts with sex hormones to increase fat accumulation in women.[13]

The increased availability of processed food, fat, and calories coupled with the decrease in physical activity and an increase of sedentary activity since the 1980s have fueled the obesity epidemic. The importance of environment and cultural change is evidenced by Pima Indians living in Arizona who, due to increased food intake and decreased physical activity, weigh 25 kg more than Pima Indians living in their traditional culture in Mexico.[14] The environmental influence of proper maternal nutrition during pregnancy may minimize the risk of obesity for the developing child.[15,16] Low birth weight is associated with the development of increased abdominal fat later in life.[17]

There is also a strong association between gender, ethnicity, socioeconomic factors, and obesity. In developed societies, women of lower socioeconomic status tend to be more obese than men or children of the same socioeconomic group.[18] The degree of socioeconomic inequality in obesity varies across gender, age, and ethnic groups. Women have an inverse association between socioeconomic status and obesity.[19] There is a higher prevalence of obesity in ethnic minority youth, with females being more obese than males.[20] Young African American females tend to gain weight at a faster rate than either African American males or Caucasian females or males.[21]

Energy intake includes food choices, total dietary consumption, feeding style, and the environment. Since the 1980s, energy intake has increased as the consumption of fast food has increased and fewer meals are eaten at home.[17,22] Fast food restaurants are open at all hours. Advertisements promote excessive intake. However, caloric and fat content of meals are now available to consumers so they can make more informed choices regarding their food intake.

Energy expenditure results from any physical activity; the greatest expenditures occur with strenuous activities. Most studies have found that obese individuals are less physically active than those of normal weight.[23] Physical activity has decreased and sedentary activities such as television viewing and computer games have increased since the 1990s. Reduction of sedentary activities and an increase in physical activity have been found to reduce BMI.[24]

Pathophysiology of Obesity

Body weight regulation is complex and relates to energy intake and energy expenditure. Obesity is classified as either an exogenous condition resulting from an excessive intake of calories or an endogenous condition due to metabolism.[25] Structure and distribution of adipose tissue can be defined as either *hyperplastic*, having a greater than normal number of fat cells, or *hypertrophic*, having a larger than normal size of fat cells. There are multiple theories to explain the pathophysiology of obesity:

- The *fat-cell theory* suggests that overweight and obese individuals have an excessive number of fat cells, which increase whenever a positive energy balance occurs.[26]
- The *lipoprotein-lipase theory* proposes that enzymes regulate the size of fat cells to maintain a constant cell size, thereby thwarting weight-loss attempts by obese individuals. Lipoprotein-lipase is an enzyme that is synthesized by fat cells and hydrolyzes triglycerides into free fatty acids and glycerol, which then enter fat cells and are re-esterified into triglycerides, promoting fat storage.[27] When obese individuals lose weight, lipoprotein-lipase levels rise in the cells, which stimulate the fat cells to return to their normal size, thereby preventing weight-loss maintenance.
- The *lipostatic theory* suggests that everyone has a biologic set point controlled by the ventromedial hypothalamus that regulates appetite and maintains body weight.[28] Obese individuals have a higher set point and have more difficulty maintaining weight loss.
- The *thermogenesis of brown adipose tissue theory* postulates that individuals with a larger number of subcutaneous brown fat cells release excess energy through heat production instead of converting energy to fat stores, and that obese individuals have fewer brown fat cells when compared with lean individuals.[29,30] Therefore, individuals with more subcutaneous fat cells expend more energy, produce fewer fat stores, and are leaner.
- The *sodium-potassium-adenosine triphosphatase pump theory* states that sodium is pumped out of the cell and potassium is pumped into the cell, which splits adenosine triphosphate and releases energy.[31] Obese individuals have fewer sodium-potassium-adenosine triphosphatase pumps and a decreased energy release.
- Psychologic theories propose that obese individuals may be more directed by external cues, such as sight, smell, and taste of food, than by internal cues such as hunger or satiety and that eating may create a desire to eat more.[17]

Since the early 2000s, there has been landmark research on the genetic and metabolic control systems that regulate body weight. The central nervous system is responsible for appetite regulation through three categories of neurotransmitters, which include gamma-aminobutyric acid, monoamines, and neuropeptides.[32] Gamma-aminobutyric acid functions throughout the central nervous system as an on/off switch for neural circuits and maintains a state of arousal. Monoamines include norepinephrine, dopamine, and serotonin, which function as a form of "volume control" on a variety of systems and behaviors. Dopamine has been found to be important in relation to the reward characteristics of feeding. Both norepinephrine and serotonin are present in the hypothalamus and are involved in body weight regulation. These two transmitters have a complex physiology with multiple receptor subtypes and reuptake sites. Neuropeptides have effects on specific behaviors and body functions through receptor subtypes and interactions with other neural circuits.[32]

Other research focuses on the other substances active in regulating dietary intake. Leptin, which is produced in fat cells, alters liver glucose production and fat metabolism in skeletal muscle, liver, and pancreatic beta cells.[33,34] Neuropeptide Y is a hypothalamic neurotransmitter and a potent orexigenic peptide that alters appetite, peripheral metabolism, and fat storage through alteration in adipose tissue lipoprotein lipase, thereby decreasing energy expenditure.[35] Neuropeptide Y responds to leptin stimulation by altering neuropeptide Y production. Insulin production increases in response to food intake and produces satiety as part of a coordinated response to food ingestion. Insulin acts in the brain primarily to reduce food intake, which is important in body weight regulation.[32] Excessive intake of foods rich in fat and carbohydrates stimulates hyperinsulinemia. Through a negative-feedback mechanism, excessive insulin levels decrease the number of insulin receptor sites on adipose tissue cells, thereby decreasing the amount of glucose that can enter the cell. As glucose levels rise, excess glucose is either stored as glycogen in the liver or as triglycerides in adipose cells, which enhances hypertrophy and hyperplasia of fat cells.[32,36]

Office-Based Obesity Care

Measurement of Obesity

Opportunities to work with women who are overweight and obese present themselves to health providers daily. A team approach with a comfortable environment and proper equipment coupled with sensitive, professional behavior provide the most effective therapeutic environments. Evaluation of obesity must start with some form of measurement that quantifies the extent of the problem. The following sections describe currently available measurements.

Body Mass Index (BMI)

BMI is a simple calculation that determines height-to-weight ratio. The index correlates physical stature with mortality ratios based on actuarial studies. BMI has now become the fifth vital sign. BMI is calculated as follows:

$$BMI = weight\ (kg)/height\ squared\ (m^2)$$

To estimate BMI from pounds and inches use:

$$[weight\ (pounds)/height\ squared\ (inches^2)] \times 703$$

(See **Table 18-2**.) BMI calculators are also available online at the Centers for Disease Control and Prevention (CDC) website.[37] When explaining BMI, important information includes the normal weight range, how the woman's weight and BMI compare, and how this affects her risk of morbidities. BMI provides a general idea of obesity or excess fat. However, it may be overestimated in individuals who are very muscular or have edema, and underestimated in older individuals who have lost lean body mass and fat mass.

Waist Circumference

Recent evidence suggests that the single best predictor of adverse health effects from excess body fat is visceral adiposity through a waist circumference measurement.[38] A high waist circumference is associated with an increased risk for type 2 diabetes, dyslipidemia, hypertension, and coronary heart disease. Abdominal fat has three compartments, which include visceral, retroperitoneal, and subcutaneous fat.[39] Approximately 47% of the variance in insulin resistance among healthy subjects without diabetes can be

Table 18-2 Body Mass Index

Weight (lbs)

	120	130	140	150	160	170	180	190	200	210	220	230	240	250	260	270	280	290	300	310	320	330
4'5"	30	33	35	38	40	43	45	48	50	53	55	58	60	63	65	68	70	73	75	78	80	83
4'6"	29	31	34	36	39	41	43	46	48	51	53	56	58	60	63	65	68	70	42	75	77	80
4'7"	28	30	33	35	37	40	42	44	47	49	51	54	56	58	61	63	65	68	70	72	75	77
4'8"	27	29	31	34	36	38	40	43	45	47	49	52	54	56	58	61	63	65	67	70	72	74
4'9"	26	28	30	33	35	37	39	41	43	46	48	50	52	54	56	59	61	63	65	67	69	72
4'10"	25	27	29	31	34	36	38	40	42	44	46	48	50	52	54	57	59	61	63	65	67	69
4'11"	24	26	28	30	32	34	36	38	40	43	45	47	49	51	53	55	57	59	61	63	65	67
5'0"	23	25	27	29	31	33	35	37	39	41	43	45	47	49	51	53	55	57	59	61	63	65
5'1"	23	25	27	28	30	32	24	36	38	40	42	44	45	47	49	51	53	55	57	59	61	62
5'2"	22	24	26	27	29	31	33	35	37	38	40	42	44	46	48	49	51	53	55	57	59	60
5'3"	21	23	25	27	28	30	32	34	36	37	39	41	43	44	46	48	50	51	53	55	57	59
5'4"	21	22	24	26	28	29	31	33	34	36	38	40	41	43	45	46	48	50	52	53	55	57
5'5"	20	22	23	25	27	28	30	32	33	35	37	38	40	42	43	45	47	48	50	52	53	55
5'6"	19	21	23	24	26	27	29	31	32	34	36	37	39	40	42	44	45	47	49	50	52	53
5'7"	19	20	22	24	25	27	28	30	31	33	35	36	38	39	41	42	44	46	47	49	50	52
5'8"	18	20	21	23	24	26	27	29	30	32	34	35	37	38	40	41	43	44	46	47	49	50
5'9"	18	19	21	22	24	25	27	28	30	31	33	34	36	37	39	40	41	43	44	46	47	49
5'10"	17	19	20	22	23	24	26	27	29	30	32	33	35	36	38	39	40	42	43	45	46	47
5'11"	17	18	20	21	22	24	25	27	28	29	31	32	34	35	36	38	39	41	42	43	45	46
6'0"	16	18	19	20	22	23	24	26	27	29	30	31	33	34	35	37	38	39	41	42	43	45

(continues)

Table 18-2 Body Mass Index Weight (lbs) *(continued)*

	120	130	140	150	160	170	180	190	200	210	220	230	240	250	260	270	280	290	300	310	320	330
6'1"	16	17	19	20	21	22	24	25	26	28	29	30	32	33	34	36	37	38	40	41	42	44
6'2"	15	17	18	19	21	22	23	24	26	27	28	30	31	32	33	35	36	37	39	40	41	42
6'3"	15	16	18	19	20	21	23	24	25	26	28	29	30	31	33	34	35	36	38	39	40	41
6'4"	15	16	17	18	20	21	22	23	24	26	27	28	29	30	32	33	34	35	37	38	39	40
6'5"	14	15	17	18	19	20	21	23	24	25	26	27	29	30	31	32	33	34	36	37	38	39
6'6"	14	15	16	17	19	20	21	22	23	24	25	27	28	29	30	31	32	34	35	36	37	38
6'7"	14	15	16	17	18	19	20	21	23	24	25	26	27	28	29	30	32	33	34	35	36	37
6'8"	13	14	15	17	18	19	20	21	22	23	24	25	26	28	29	30	31	32	33	34	35	36
6'9"	13	14	15	16	17	18	19	20	21	23	24	25	26	27	28	29	30	31	32	33	34	35
6'10"	13	14	15	16	17	18	19	20	21	22	23	24	25	26	27	28	29	30	31	32	34	35

Data from US Department of Health and Human Services, Public Health Service, National Center for Health Statistics. *Vital and Health Statistics: Anthropometric Reference Data and Prevalence of Overweight United States, 1976–80.* Hyattsville, MD: US Department of Health and Human Services; 1987.

explained by intra-abdominal fat.[40] As subcutaneous fat increases, leptin levels also increase leading to increased insulin resistance. See **Figure 18-1** for an explanation of correct measurement technique to assess waist circumferences. A high-risk waist circumference for women is greater than 35 inches (88 cm) and for men is greater than 40 inches (102 cm). Waist circumference loses its predictive power in determining comorbid conditions once the BMI reaches 35 or greater.[2] If the woman is pregnant, her prepregnant weight is used for assessment.

ANTHROPOMETRY

The caliper method is based on the assumption that the thickness of the subcutaneous fat reflects a constant proportion of the total body fat.[41] Using handheld calipers that exert a standard pressure, the skinfold thickness is measured in the triceps, biceps, subscapula, axilla, iliac crest, supraspinale, abdominal, front thigh, medial calf, or chest (see **Figure 18-2**). The technique is described in **Box 18-1**. Body fat percentage based on the sum of three measurements is then calculated (**Table 18-3**).

Skinfold measurements are easy to do and inexpensive, but may not be a valid predictor of body fat percentage. Unfortunately, reliability may be subjective depending on the experience of the individual doing the testing and the quality of the calipers. However, these measurements can be used to provide information about change in body composition over time.

NEAR-INFRARED INTERACTANCE

Near-infrared interactance uses a fiber-optic probe connected to a digital analyzer that indirectly measures fat and water tissue composition.[41] The bicep is the most often used site. The near-infrared interactance light penetrates the skin and is reflected off the bone to the detector. The data are entered into a computer using a prediction equation that includes the woman's height, weight, frame size, and level of activity, and an estimate of body fat percentage is provided. The amount of pressure applied, skin color, and hydration may affect results.

Figure 18-1 Waist circumference.

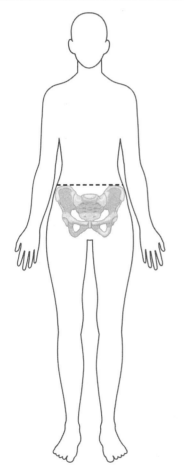

Palpate the upper hipbone to locate the right illiac crest. At the lateral border of the right illiac crest and the midaxillary line, the tape is placed horizontally around the waist approximately 1 inch above the umbilicus at normal minimal respiration.

Figure 18-2 Skinfold measurement sites.

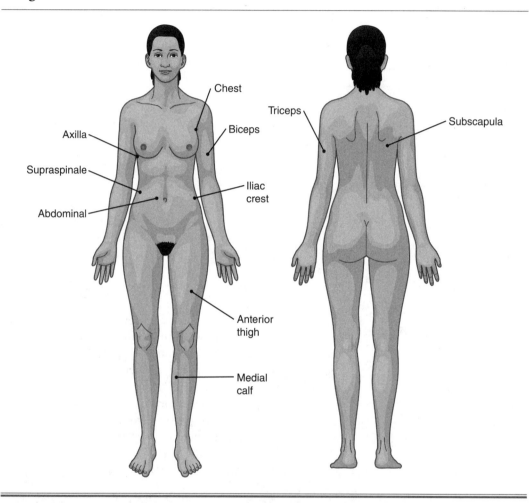

Box 18-1 Technique for Skinfold Measurement

- Choose the site you will use for skinfold measurement.
- Firmly pinch the skinfold between your thumb and forefinger and place the calipers over the skinfold, while continuing to hold the skinfold with your other hand.
- Press with your thumb until you feel a click. The caliper slide will automatically stop at the correct measurement.
- After reading the measurement, return the caliper slide to the far-right starting position.
- Repeat three times and use the average of your measurements.

Refer to **Table 18-3** to determine body fat percentage for women.

Table 18-3 Calculation of Female Body Fat Percentage Skinfold in Millimeters

Age ⇩	2–3	4–5	8–9	10–11	12–13	14–15	16–17	18–19	20–21	22–23	24–25	26–27	28–29	30–31	32–33	34–35
Up to 20	11.3	13.5	15.7	19.7	21.5	23.2	24.8	26.3	27.7	29.0	30.2	31.3	32.3	33.1	33.9	34.6
21–25	11.9	14.2	16.32	20.3	22.1	23.8	25.5	27.0	28.4	29.6	30.8	31.9	32.9	33.8	34.5	35.2
26–30	12.5	14.8	16.9	20.9	22.7	24.5	26.1	27.6	29.0	30.3	31.5	32.5	33.5	34.4	35.2	35.8
31–35	13.2	15.4	17.6	21.5	23.4	25.1	26.7	28.2	29.6	30.9	32.1	33.2	34.1	35.0	35.8	36.4
36–40	13.8	16.0	18.2	22.2	24.0	25.7	27.3	28.8	30.2	31.5	32.7	33.8	34.8	35.6	36.4	37.0
41–45	14.4	16.7	18.8	22.8	24.6	26.3	27.9	29.4	30.8	32.1	33.3	34.4	35.4	36.3	37.0	37.7
46–50	15.0	17.3	19.4	23.4	25.2	26.9	28.6	30.1	31.5	32.7	34.0	35.0	36.0	36.9	37.6	38.3
51–55	15.6	17.9	20.0	24.0	25.9	27.6	29.2	30.7	32.1	33.3	34.6	35.6	36.6	37.5	38.3	38.9
56 and Up	16.3	18.5	20.7	24.6	26.5	28.2	29.8	31.3	32.7	34.0	35.2	36.3	37.2	38.1	38.9	39.5
⇐	Lean		⇒ ⇐	Ideal		⇒ ⇐	Average		⇒ ⇐	Overweight		⇒				

Data from US Department of Health and Human Services, Public Health Service, National Center for Health Statistics. *Vital and Health Statistics: Anthropometric Reference Data and Prevalence of Overweight United States, 1976–80.* Hyattsville, MD: US Department of Health and Human Services; 1987.

HYDRODENSITOMETRY

Hydrodensitometry is based on the assumption that densities of fat mass and fat-free mass are constant. The method measures whole body density by determining body volume. The densities of bone and muscles are higher than that of water, while fat is less dense. A woman who has more bone and muscle will have a higher body density and a lower fat percentage. She will weigh more when submerged in water than a woman of the same weight who has less bone and muscle and more fat. The woman is weighed outside the tank in a bathing suit, and is weighed again in a chair or sling in the tank using underwater scales. A body fat percentage is calculated from the body density using either Siri or Brozek standard equations.[41,42] It is important to take into consideration the amount of air that is left in the lungs after exhaling during underwater weighing. Hydrodensitometry has been considered the most accurate technique for body fat measurement. However, athletes typically have denser bones and muscles, which may lead to an underestimation of body fat. In contrast, women with osteoporosis (i.e., less bone density) may have their body fat overestimated.

AIR DISPLACEMENT

Air displacement uses the same principles as underwater weighing and is quite costly.[42] The BOD POD® is a fiberglass plethysmograph that measures body volume by changes in pressure in a closed chamber. Computerized sensors are used to measure how much air is displaced; then body density and body fat are calculated.

DUAL ENERGY X-RAY ABSORPTIOMETRY (DEXA)

DEXA is based on a three-compartment model that divides the body into total body mineral mass, fat-free lean mass, and fat tissue mass.[42]

DEXA is based on the assumption that bone mineral content is directly proportional to the amount of photon energy absorbed by the bone being studied. DEXA uses a whole body scanner, which has 2 low-dose x-rays that read bone and soft tissue mass simultaneously, and takes between 10 and 20 minutes. DEXA is the new gold standard in body composition analysis, because it provides a higher degree of precision in one measurement and provides information about where fat is distributed throughout the body. DEXA scanning is expensive and involves limited exposure to radiation.

BIOELECTRICAL IMPEDANCE ANALYSIS

Bioelectrical impedance analysis (BIA) is a quick, simple, and accurate way to determine body composition. The individual removes shoes and socks, gel electrodes are placed on the hands and feet, and a mild, safe electrical current (50 kHz) is sent through the body. Impedance is greatest in fat tissue, which contains only 10–20% water. Fat-free mass contains 70–75% water, which allows the current to pass easily. The differences in conduction between the two tissues provide a measure of electrical impedance, which is then applied to a formula with height, weight, gender, age, and fitness level to calculate the percentage of body fat, fat-free mass, and hydration level.[43] The Tanita leg-to-leg bioimpedance analysis uses two footpad electrodes that are on an electronic scale.[44] The woman stands with bare feet on the electrodes and the scale automatically measures weight and impedance. The woman's height, weight, fitness level, gender, and age are entered, and the scale determines body fat percentage based on equation formulas. The Tanita BIA is quick, portable, and inexpensive. Dehydration may cause overestimation of body fat percentage. Women with pacemakers or internal cardiac defibrillators should not use BIA.

In summary, the primary care provider has several measurements of obesity available. Lean body mass, high levels of athleticism, osteoporosis, and other factors can affect results, requiring the practitioner to carefully assess each patient's degree of physical activity when interpreting results. Waist circumference measurement is an inexpensive technique to estimate risk. Anthropometry is another cost-effective way to measure body fat percentage. Near-infrared interactance, hydrodensitometry, air displacement, and DEXA scanning are not routinely used for obesity screening due to cost and inconvenience. BIA is a cost-effective way to measure body fat percentage in the office but is not commonly used in primary care.

Associated Disease Risks

Every woman who presents with obesity needs a thorough history. A physical examination to rule out associated disease risks should also be completed. Associated disease risks of obesity include prediabetes, type 2 diabetes, hypertension, and hyperlipidemia. Hypothyroidism and Cushing's syndrome should also be ruled out. These conditions are not sequelae of obesity, but effective treatment may improve weight status and thus, overall health.

PREDIABETES AND TYPE 2 DIABETES MELLITUS

Prediabetes is the impairment of the response of insulin on glucose, lipids, protein metabolism, and vascular endothelial function.[3] Genetics and the environment interact in ways that lead to the development of prediabetes. Individuals with a genetic predisposition to obesity who overconsume carbohydrates, fats, and calories and who have decreased physical activity and increased sedentary activity are at an increased risk. Prediabetes starts with hyperinsulinemia

and normal glucose tolerance. As the disease progresses, β-cell function is impaired; insulin levels start to decline as impaired glucose tolerance increases.[3]

Type 2 diabetes mellitus is increasing proportionally to the increase in obesity in the United States, with African Americans, Hispanics, and Native Americans at higher risk than Whites. Further risk factors for the development of type 2 diabetes include a family history of type 2 diabetes, ethnic minority group, prediabetes, central adiposity, and obesity.[3]

Diagnosis of type 2 diabetes may be made by a fasting plasma glucose (FPG) level of ≥ 126 mg/dL or a glycosylated hemoglobin level ≥ 6.5% on 2 separate days or a 2-hour oral glucose tolerance test (OGTT) with glucose ≥ 200 mg/dL at 2 hours.[3] A random glucose ≥ 200 mg/dL accompanied by classic diabetes symptoms of weight loss, polydipsia, and/or polyuria are diagnostic of type 2 diabetes.[3]

Nutrition education, exercise prescription, and referrals to a certified diabetes educator (CDE) and endocrinologist for management are warranted.

HYPERTENSION

Overweight and obesity are risk factors for the development of hypertension. Weight loss decreases the incidence of hypertension.[4] Hypertension is an independent risk factor for the development of coronary heart disease; as blood pressure increases, so does the risk of myocardial infarction, heart failure, stroke, and kidney disease.[45] As with diabetes, hypertension increases as BMI and age increase.[45] African American and Hispanic populations have higher prevalence. Elevated blood pressure is also an important factor in the early appearance of atherosclerotic lesions in the coronary arteries.[4]

Hypertension is confirmed by two or more properly measured blood pressure readings on each of two or more office visits. Before instituting medication therapy for hypertension, the woman should have an electrocardiogram, urinalysis, blood glucose, hematocrit, serum potassium, serum creatinine, serum calcium, and a fasting lipid profile that includes total cholesterol, high-density lipoprotein (HDL) cholesterol, low-density lipoprotein (LDL) cholesterol, and triglycerides. Recently, blood pressure management has been revised in the 2014 Evidence-Based Guideline for the Management of High Blood Pressure in Adults, based on randomized controlled trials.[46]

HYPERLIPIDEMIA

The development of hyperlipidemia is an independent risk factor for the development of coronary artery disease and premature mortality.[47] Overweight or obese women should have a lipid level drawn at least annually, more often if elevated. Lipid levels should include total cholesterol, LDL, HDL, and triglycerides. The Third Report of the National Cholesterol Education Program (NCEP) Expert Panel on the Detection, Evaluation, and Treatment of High Blood Cholesterol in Adults (Adult Treatment Panel III) should be used as a guide for diagnosis and management of hyperlipidemia.[48] Based on the LDL level (**Table 18**-4) and the presence of clinical coronary heart disease, symptomatic coronary heart disease, peripheral arterial disease, or abdominal aortic aneurysm and major risk factors such as cigarette smoking, hypertension (blood pressure > 140/90 mmHg or on antihypertensive medication), low HDL (< 40 mg/dL), family history of premature coronary heart disease, diabetes, or age with men above 45 and women above 55, individuals are targeted for intensive therapeutic lifestyle changes.[48] The American College of Cardiology and American Heart Association have published Guidelines for Lifestyle Management to address cardiovascular risks.[49] Medical management is discussed elsewhere in this text.

HYPOTHYROIDISM

The prevalence of hypothyroidism is higher in women than men and increases with age.[25] Primary hypothyroidism is caused by an impairment to thyroid function such as Hashimoto's thyroiditis, postpartum thyroiditis, radiation-induced hypothyroidism, subacute thyroiditis, or a subtotal thyroidectomy. Secondary hypothyroidism, caused by an interruption to the hypothalamic

Table 18-4 Lipid Levels

Test	Optimal	Near Optimal	Borderline High	High	Very High
Total cholesterol	< 200		200–239	≥ 240	
Low-density lipoprotein (LDL)	< 100	100–129	130–159	160–189	≥ 190
High-density lipoprotein (HDL)	≥ 60*				
Triglycerides	< 150		150–199	200–249	≥ 500

* Higher is better (low is ≤ 40)

Data from National Cholesterol Education Program, National Heart, Lung, and Blood Institute, National Institutes of Health. *Third Report of the National Cholesterol Education Program Expert Panel on the Detection, Evaluation, and Treatment of High Blood Cholesterol in Adults (Adult Treatment Panel III).* Washington, DC: US Department of Health and Human Services; 2002.

pituitary axis, is often the result of an injury to thyrotrophic cells by either a nonfunctioning or functioning pituitary adenoma. A thorough history will include asking about signs and symptoms such as cold intolerance, fatigue, constipation, hair loss, dry skin, joint swelling, hyperlipidemia, congestive heart failure, or hypertension. The diagnosis of primary hypothyroidism is demonstrated by increased thyroid-stimulating hormone (TSH) and low T_4 levels. If the TSH is abnormal, then thyroid peroxidase antibodies (TPO) should be drawn, which will provide evidence of an autoimmune process. The diagnosis of secondary hypothyroidism is suspected when the TSH level is low and the woman exhibits signs and symptoms of hypothyroidism or has amenorrhea, galactorrhea, postural hypotension, or a change in visual fields. Subclinical hypothyroidism can be diagnosed with an elevated TSH level and otherwise normal free thyroid hormone concentration. Women with hypothyroidism should be referred to an endocrinologist for further workup.

Cushing's Syndrome

Cushing's syndrome is caused by the overproduction of cortisol by the adrenal glands resulting from a pituitary tumor-secreting adrenocorticotropic hormone (ACTH), ectopic production of ACTH, or a tumor in one of the adrenal glands. It is difficult to evaluate women for Cushing's syndrome, because overweight and obesity can produce hypercortisolism. In addition, overweight and obesity and Cushing's syndrome can have similar symptoms such as central obesity, moon facies, supraclavicular fat pads, buffalo hump, central obesity, diabetes, and depression. Cushing's syndrome includes several specific symptoms, which include proximal muscle weakness and wide violaceous striae. Screening tests include the overnight dexamethasone suppression test and the 24-hour urinary free cortisol. The dexamethasone

suppression test is conducted by giving the woman a 1-mg dose of dexamethasone at 2300 hours, and drawing serum cortisol at 0800. A normal value is less than 5 ng/dL.[50] The 24-hour urinary free cortisol test is collected over a 24-hour period; a value less than 100 is considered normal.[50] False-positive tests can result from obesity, alcohol, or depression. If either test is positive, an immediate referral to an endocrinologist is warranted.

Management of Obesity

Treatment goals for obesity include decreasing weight, improving nutrition, increasing physical activity, and decreasing sedentary activity to decrease the incidence of type 2 diabetes, hypertension, and hyperlipidemia. Management of obesity includes dietary changes, behavioral modification, and exercise interventions to assist women to balance their energy, lose weight, increase physical activity, and decrease sedentary activity.

The office environment must be comfortable for overweight and obese women. Modifications include a stable scale with a large floor plate capable of weighing heavier individuals in a private room, large gowns, large blood pressure cuffs, and armless chairs in the waiting room. Health care should be delivered using a team approach in a nonjudgmental manner.

Providers need to be empathetic with patients and assume that they know they are overweight or obese. At the same time, women should hear from their provider about weight control. They can be asked the following question: What do you think about your weight? Open-ended questions provide an opportunity to assess the woman's interest and motivation for weight control in a nonjudgmental manner. The client's perspective is important to hear first, before making recommendations or describing the complications of overweight and obesity. Commonly, the presenting complaint is not weight management, but a health condition affected by weight. The focus should be on factors that affect both the presenting problem and the weight issue. Identification of barriers to success provides insight into the client's personal struggle and provides opportunities to institute healthy behavior change. Working closely with the woman to develop a diet and exercise plan acceptable to her may improve adherence. A journal of dietary intake and exercise should be brought to each visit for review. Providers can use the detailed data in these diaries to provide specific support and encouragement. Providers need to clearly describe what weight loss can accomplish, how much weight loss a patient can reasonably expect to achieve, and focus on nonweight outcomes such as improved lipids, blood sugar control, and blood pressure. Providers need to be empathetic about dissatisfaction with weight and shape and encourage weight-independent self-esteem, which reinforces that a patient's worth is not measured on a scale.

The role of the provider with obese women is as a consultant and coach. A good consultant recognizes that he or she is not the decision maker, not in control, and not ultimately responsible for the outcome. A good consultant is an expert and a good listener who believes that the woman has good reason for doing whatever she is currently doing, although the decisions may also have adverse consequences. The first step in consulting is to understand the motives for the client's actions. The next step is working with the woman to appreciate the implications of behaviors on health, and moving that behavior in a direction that would promote health. When a clinician is counseling about behavior change, the woman needs to be in control, with the provider as the facilitator providing education, support, and encouragement. Behavior change takes time and is constantly evolving and changing. Overweight and obesity are lifelong problems that require a strong commitment by the provider to

the woman and by the woman to a balance of proper dietary intake, exercise, and behavioral modification.

Dietary Interventions

Dietary interventions are based on the evidence that overweight and obesity result when energy intake exceeds energy expenditure. A negative energy balance is needed for weight loss. General caloric restriction, decreased fat intake, healthier eating habits, and non-diet approaches have all been used to foster weight loss. Women have to make lifestyle changes they can incorporate into their daily lives. One exception is that women who are pregnant should never diet to lose weight, although healthier food choices and exercise can be encouraged to improve maternal and fetal health. Referral to a registered dietitian provides the woman with in-depth counseling on dietary principles. The US Department of Agriculture Dietary Guidelines for Americans 2010 contain in-depth information on nutrition and dietary guidelines.[22]

General dietary principles include eating a healthy diet that includes 5–7 servings of fruits and vegetables each day. Whole grains should take precedence over refined, processed carbohydrates. Fiber intake is important to improve bowel regularity and should be increased to 25–30 grams daily. Fluid intake should be increased to at least 64 ounces daily of water. Three servings of low-fat dairy per day provide a good source of calcium. Animal protein should include low-fat chicken and turkey, and fish at least twice a week. Sodium should be limited to no more than 2400 mg per day.[22] There is no single food choice that is essential. Individuals who avoid animal protein, dairy, wheat, or other foods can still have a balanced and healthy weight-loss diet.

Weight-loss diets use moderate calorie reduction. A deficit of 500–1000 kcal per day will achieve 1–2 pounds of weight loss per week. That is a realistic and reasonable weight loss.

In the absence of exercise, a diet that contains 1400–1500 calories per day results in weight loss. The calorie deficit is produced through altering food choices and shrinking food portions.

Altering patterns and behaviors such as nighttime eating, binge eating, trigger foods, large portions, emotional eating, too many snacks, meal skipping, too many liquid calories, activities while eating, and dining out often are all areas in which the clinician can provide support. If an eating disorder is suspected, the provider should talk with the patient and make the appropriate referral to an eating disorder specialist or psychologist.

Making small, continuous, incremental improvements in behaviors is an effective way to produce a calorie deficit, improve the overall quality of the diet, and assist the woman in developing a healthy dietary plan that works for her. Weight loss is hard work and may require long-term counseling. Referral to a weight-loss program sometimes works very well. The clinician needs to be prepared to be flexible and provide support as the woman embarks on a journey toward improved health.

COMMERCIAL DIETS

Commercial diet programs can be useful adjuncts for individuals who need nutrition education, weight monitoring, and social support (see Table 18-5). A survey of individuals who would consider a commercial diet found that safety, cost, and the prescribed diet were considered most important to know about, as well as any behavioral modification program and anticipated weight loss.[51] Some programs meet weekly and others make contact by telephone or electronic media. Take Off Pounds Sensibly, or TOPS (www.tops.org), founded in 1948, uses dietary education and a weekly weigh-in during a group meeting. Weight Watchers (www.weightwatchers.com), founded in 1963, uses a point system to deliver 1200–2200 calories per day that are tracked in a daily food journal daily and brought to a weekly weigh-in and group meeting. They also offer an activity program and online program. Jenny Craig (www.jennycraig.com) offers a program in centers or via telephone that includes 20 minutes of weekly individual counseling; uses pre-prepared foods comprising 60% carbohydrates, 20% fat, and 20% protein; and includes an activity program. Nutrisystem (www.nutrisystem.com) is a predominately online weight-loss program, which provides Internet-based counselors, personalized exercise programs, and food journals. Pre-prepared food is mailed to the woman's home. This program follows the same dietary guidelines as Jenny Craig. Overeaters Anonymous (www.oa.org) is patterned after the 12-step program of Alcoholics Anonymous. Overeaters Anonymous is a weekly group recovery program that tries

Table 18-5 Comparison of Commercial Weight-Loss Programs

Program	Meeting	Nutrition Education	Exercise Program	Pre-Prepared Foods
Take Off Pounds Sensibly	Weekly	Yes	No	No
Weight Watchers	Weekly/online	Yes	Yes	No
Jenny Craig	Weekly	Yes	Yes	Yes
Nutrisystem	Online	No	Yes	Yes
Overeaters Anonymous	Weekly	No	No	No

to address the emotional, spiritual, and physical aspects of overeating and has no official diet. In making recommendations for commercial diet resources, the provider should evaluate the level of support that each woman needs to be successful in weight loss. Suggestions should be made that would move them toward their goals in a manner that they feel comfortable with and can afford.

MEAL REPLACEMENTS

Meal replacements are an effective adjunct to diet programs because they address inaccurate calorie counting and oversized portions, which lead to weight-loss failure. Meal replacements include shakes, bars, soups, or frozen portion-controlled meals and provide an established caloric count. For weight loss, a 1200–1500 calorie meal plan is recommended. Fat calories should provide no more than 20% of total calories. Meal replacements with fewer than 300 calories allow fresh fruits and vegetables to be included in a meal.

SPECIFIC DIETS

Currently, many popular diet books and websites are available to the public. Many women will seek advice on the Atkins or South Beach diets. There is little or no long-term research to back up the claims of these diets other than the Ornish diet. Most popular diets are similar in structure, with an introduction from the author, an idea, and a diet plan.[52] It is important to listen to the woman's concerns and be knowledgeable about current trends, while advocating for balanced nutrition, better food choices, portion control, calorie counting, and exercise as research-based ways in which to lose and maintain weight loss.

The Atkins diet is based on eating a high-protein and high-fat diet and decreasing carbohydrates.[53] In contrast, the South Beach diet is based on eating high protein—primarily lean chicken, turkey, and fish—and encouraging a balanced diet that includes fruits, vegetables,

whole grains, nuts, and healthy oils.[54] The Ornish diet,[55] which grew out of the Pritikin diet,[56] follows a very low-fat (10%) vegetarian diet. The Glucose Revolution diet is centered around the glycemic index.[57] The glycemic index ranks carbohydrates based on their immediate effect on blood glucose levels. Carbohydrates that break down rapidly during digestion have a higher glycemic index than carbohydrates that break down slowly and release glucose gradually. The Sugar Busters diet uses the glycemic index coupled with an increased consumption of fruits, vegetables, and whole-grain foods.[58] The Zone diet advocates a diet balanced to include 30% protein, 30% fat, and 40% carbohydrates.[59] The Eat Right for Your [blood] Type diet is based on food recommended by blood type and genetic makeup.[60] The Volumetrics weight-control plan includes foods that are high in fiber and water.[61]

The Mediterranean diet focuses on a diet rich in fresh fruit and vegetables, grains, nuts, seeds, low-fat dairy, poultry, and fish.[62] In addition to being publicized as a popular diet method, research has demonstrated significant benefits from making the food choices that are consistent with this diet plan. These benefits include decreased cardiac risk, cancer risk, and overall mortality.[63,64]

Very low-calorie diets (VLCDs) can be used for severely obese (BMI > 30 kg/m^2) women who require rapid weight loss for medical or behavioral reasons. Individuals on VLCDs are referred to a weight-loss center and are evaluated at the clinic at least weekly. Each woman requires a comprehensive history and physical exam with laboratory testing, which may include a complete blood count, chemistry profile, urinalysis, and an electrocardiogram. VLCDs usually last between 12 and 16 weeks and include 800 calories or less per day, high protein content (0.8–1.5 g/kg of ideal body weight per day), vitamins, minerals, electrolytes, and fatty acids, and replace usual food intake with 5 drinks a day plus an additional 64 ounces of noncaloric fluids. Adverse effects include fatigue, weakness, dizziness, constipation, hair loss, dry skin, nausea, diarrhea, change in menses, and cold intolerance. Complications may include gout, gallstones, and cardiac disturbances.[65]

Behavioral Modification Interventions

Behavioral principles for the treatment of overweight and obesity grew out of Learning Theory.[66,67] Eating and exercise have a learned component, which can be relearned by altering environmental cues and reinforcements that control these behaviors.[68] Initially, behavioral programs lasted 10 weeks with weight loss averaging 4.5 kg.[69] Since the mid-1990s, the length of behavioral programs has increased to 6 months, with weekly meetings that focus on energy balance. Behavioral strategies include planning, self-monitoring, stimulus control, problem solving, prevention of relapse in relation to diet and physical activity behavior, and motivational strategies.[68]

DIETARY BEHAVIOR

Calorie reduction, structured meal plans, and meal replacements with behavioral programs have all been used to modify dietary intake with varying success. Most behavioral weight-loss programs encourage caloric reduction through the consumption of 1000–1500 kcal/day.[68] VLCDs providing between 400 and 800 kcal/day in a liquid formula have been found to be effective for an initial weight loss of 20 kg over 12 weeks.[70] These diets are expensive and require continuous medical monitoring. A structured meal plan provides the client with information on how to follow a low-calorie and low-fat diet. Clients learn to eat regularly and balance portions, calories, protein, carbohydrates, and fat. Meal replacements use prepared meals or liquid replacement meals and provide approximately 900 kcal/day, decreasing the need for medical monitoring. Providing food

simplifies dietary adherence. Many individuals regain weight rapidly after discontinuation of the program. In two studies there were no differences found in weight loss when comparing caloric-reduction diets and VLCDs.[71,72]

PHYSICAL ACTIVITY

Increasing physical activity has been the best predictor of long-term maintenance of weight loss. The combination of changes in diet and physical activity improves weight loss and long-term maintenance. Encouraging exercise adherence by the use of a personal trainer and prescribing short-bout activity also improve weight-loss outcomes.[73] Setting and meeting higher physical activity goals support better weight loss and long-term weight-loss maintenance.

MOTIVATIONAL STRATEGIES

Motivational strategies used for weight loss and maintenance include social support and weight-loss satisfaction. Social support has been found to improve long-term weight loss maintenance.[74,75] Social support from other overweight or obese individuals can be instrumental in both weight loss and long-term weight-loss maintenance. Satisfaction with weight loss increases when women are able to set reasonable goals to improve their health.[74]

Exercise Interventions

Exercise maintains cardiovascular health, increases flexibility and muscle strength, and improves sense of wellbeing. Exercise in the absence of dietary change does not have a significant impact on weight loss. However, when exercise is combined with dietary changes, weight loss is enhanced. Diet and exercise interventions have been found to be effective in controlling blood glucose in 15% of women for a few months or longer if they lost at least 7–10% of their body weight.[76] Less structured exercise and reducing sedentary activity appear to be more effective than higher-intensity aerobic exercise.[77]

Exercise increases flexibility and muscle strength, and improves a sense of wellbeing. The benefits of exercise include weight management, improved cardiovascular and respiratory fitness, and reduction of morbidity and mortality. Exercise has been found to reduce resting blood pressure, blood glucose levels, insulin sensitivity, and triglycerides, as well as increase HDL cholesterol.[77]

DEVELOPING AN EXERCISE PROGRAM

An effective exercise program takes into consideration the woman's physical activity history, level of fitness, and current weight status. The current fitness level serves as a baseline. Clinical information such as height, weight, BMI, heart rate, and blood pressure are measured. In addition, posture, flexibility, strength, past injuries, and any concerns about exercise should be assessed and goals established. Barriers to physical activity also need to be identified. A short self-reported questionnaire to use in primary care should include questions regarding leisure and exercise history. Minimum recommendations for exercise include 30 minutes of moderate-intensity physical activity on most or all days of the week.[77]

The most common barriers reported are lack of time, convenience, or need for equipment. Many women work full-time and have multiple family or community responsibilities and limited uncommitted time. Recommendations for an initial exercise program might include starting with a 10-minute walk before breakfast, a second 10-minute walk during lunch, and a third 10-minute walk after dinner, totaling 30 minutes of exercise a day. Lack of convenience is another problem mentioned. With every spare moment in the day spoken for, many women do not feel they can join a gym. A treadmill, stationary bicycle, or a stair climber for home use increases access. Lack of enjoyment is another common concern. Each individual should try various activities to find those she can envision herself doing on a daily basis. Pedometers are an inexpensive way to track and challenge oneself to consistently increase activity.

Previous Level of Exercise Leading questions can help establish a framework. What type of exercise did the woman engage in before? For how many days a week and how many minutes per day did she engage in exercise? How vigorous was the activity? Activity levels can be categorized as sedentary, low activity, moderate activity, or athlete level. A sedentary level includes activities of daily living and minimal physical activity. A low-activity level includes one to two 30-minute sessions of yoga, stretching, or gentle walking per week. A moderate-activity level includes 3 or more 30-minute sessions of running, aerobics, step aerobics, or power walking. An athlete level includes daily 30-minute moderate- to high-intensity workouts.[78]

Clearance Health clearance must precede starting an exercise program for any obese individual. In addition to a comprehensive history and physical examination, risks associated with increasing exercise level should be assessed. Low-risk women are those under the age of 55 who do not experience cardiovascular symptoms and have no more than one coronary artery disease risk factors such as obesity, sedentary lifestyle, impaired glucose tolerance, hypertension, hyperlipidemia, smoking, or a family history of coronary artery disease. Moderate-risk women are those over 55 years old and those with more than one coronary artery disease risk factor. High-risk women have a history or signs of cardiovascular, pulmonary, or metabolic disease.[77] The risk assessment may include a questionnaire similar to the one shown in **Table 18-6** that provides information on her potential risk in participating in exercise.

Table 18-6 Medical Clearance Questionnaire

Age and Exercise

1. Are you age 46 or older? Yes __ No __
2. How many days are you currently exercising each week? _____
3. How intense is the exercise you do each week on a scale from 1 to 5? _____
   (1 = very low, 2 = low, 3 = medium, 4 = high, 5 = very high)

Disease

1. Do you have diabetes? Yes __ No __
2. Do you have heart trouble? Yes __ No __
3. Have you had a stroke? Yes __ No __
4. Do you have asthma or exercise-induced asthma? Yes __ No __
5. Do you have chronic bronchitis or emphysema? Yes __ No __
6. Do you have a pacemaker or cardiac defibrillator? Yes __ No __

Symptoms

1. Do you ever have pain in your chest or heart? Yes __ No __
2. In the last year, how many times have you had shortness of breath,
   which happened when you were resting? Yes __ No __
3. Do you faint or have dizzy spells? Yes __ No __
4. In the last year, have you had shortness of breath at night? Yes __ No __
5. Have you ever had back or joint pain? Yes __ No __
6. Have you ever had a heart murmur? Yes __ No __
7. Has your heart ever "raced" or "skipped" beats? Yes __ No __

Risk Factors

1. Have you ever smoked? Yes __ No __
2. Have you ever had high blood pressure? Yes __ No __
3. Have you ever had high cholesterol? Yes __ No __
4. Have you ever had high triglycerides? Yes __ No __
5. Has anyone is your family had heart disease or had a heart attack
   before the age of 55? Yes __ No __

Medications

1. Have you ever taken medication for high blood pressure? Yes __ No __
2. Have you ever taken medication for high cholesterol? Yes __ No __
3. Have you ever taken medication for high blood sugar? Yes __ No __
4. Have you ever taken medication for a heart condition? Yes __ No __
5. Have you ever taken medication for asthma? Yes __ No __

How would you rate your overall health?

Excellent __ Good __ Fair __ Poor __

Medical clearance is required before beginning an exercise program if you answered YES to any of the previous questions.

A graded exercise test (GET) provides information on specific responses to physical activity. A GET should be conducted before starting an exercise program if the woman has a medical history of coronary heart disease or a metabolic disorder.[77] The test consists of walking on a treadmill or riding a stationary bike while on a cardiac monitor to determine if a heart condition exists. The level of work increases gradually until symptoms such as chest pain or shortness of breath occur or the patient reaches a predetermined heart rate. A morbidly obese woman may reach the target heart rate simply by walking. She should thus start an exercise program with gentle walking and stretching or exercising in a pool to decrease stress on joints and muscles. Physical activity is increased as health improves.

Goals   Exercise programs with goals that are designed by the individual provide a firm foundation upon which to build a program that motivates her and maintains interest. In addition, self-generated goals provide the woman with an opportunity to adjust and change as her program progresses. Goals should include both short-term, highly achievable targets and longer term endpoints. She can evaluate her own progress with the expertise and support of a personal trainer or exercise physiologist.

Posture   Maintaining good posture is important for all women. One of the more obvious changes in women who are overweight or obese is a change in posture: Posture changes as the weight of the abdomen and breast increase the curvature of the lower back (lumbar lordosis) and the forward rounding of the upper spine and shoulders (kyphosis) become more pronounced. Posture can be assessed by asking the woman to stand against a wall as the healthcare provider reviews her body shape and angle from the side.[77] See **Table 18-7** and **Figure 18-3** for a comparison of poor and

Table 18-7 Assessment of Posture

Poor Posture	Good Posture
Head tilted forward, chin toward chest	Head aligned with body
Shoulders rounded forward	Shoulders pulled back and erect
Chest concave	Chest straight
Pelvis tilts forward	Pelvis tucks directly under the torso
Lordosis of the back	Natural spinal curve—not exaggerated

Figure 18-3 Good and bad posture.

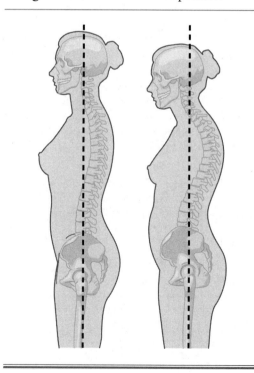

good posture. Abdominal and back muscle weakness is a contributing factor in the development of poor posture.

Flexibility Evaluation of flexibility includes two important stretches that provide baseline information. Increased joint laxity, whether it is benign hyperlaxity, Ehlers-Danlos syndrome, or another condition, can lead to an increased risk of injury; a history of joint hyperflexion should be determined before evaluating stretches.[77] Ask the woman to sit on the floor with her legs together and straight out in front of her. With her arms stretched straight out in front of her, ask her to bend at the waist. She is very flexible if she can extend her hands past her toes. Second, ask her to sit on the floor with her legs spread out in front of her in a "V." With a straight back, ask her to bend at the waist and see how far her chest can go toward the floor. If her chest can touch the floor, then she is very flexible. The woman should be sure not to overstretch, always be aware of her movements, and keep control to prevent injury due to increased joint laxity. If the woman is inflexible, then it is important to design a program that gently increases flexibility over time. An inflexible person would not be able to touch her toes when sitting in a "V" position. If she is inflexible, careful attention should be paid to ensure an adequate warm-up period and performing the exercises in a slow and controlled manner.

Strength An evaluation of the woman's strength includes questioning whether she has lifted weights before. If she has never lifted weights, or has not done so recently, she may begin by lifting either 1- or 2-pound free weights, with 10 to 12 repetitions for 2 to 3 sets, resting between sets. She may increase if she is comfortable and does not feel challenged. However, if she can only manage part of the exercise sets before tiring, then she should decrease the amount of weight or resistance and decrease the number of repetitions; she may then increase the number of sets. Working with a trainer is advised to make sure the exercises are being performed correctly—increasing or decreasing the amount of weight as needed. A trainer will ensure that body mechanics, breathing, and intensity are maintained at proper levels throughout the workout.

Frequency, Intensity, Duration, and Type of Activity The frequency, intensity, duration, and type of activity are all considered in establishing an exercise program.[77] Most women, regardless of BMI, should engage in an exercise program on most days of the week. Body weight stabilizes as energy expenditure increases. Exercise intensity should be prescribed on the percentage of maximal heart rate.[23] An individual's target heart rate is the ideal range of heart beats per minute during exercise based on age (**Table 18-8**). Current thinking indicates that the traditional maximum and target heart rates based on age may not reflect accurately women's responses, and that maximum heart rate may be slightly lower in younger women than generally indicated in unified scales. Gulati and colleagues recommend the following formula:[79]

$$\text{maximum heart rate} = 206 - (0.88 \times \text{age})$$

Moderate-intensity exercise leads to heart rates ranging between 55% and 69% of maximum and vigorous intensity between 70% and 89%. Women can manually check their pulses or wear a heart rate monitor and learn how to calculate the percentage of maximal heart rate to ensure that they are challenging themselves during exercise sessions. Both aging and deconditioning lead to loss of cardiac reserve (cardiac functional capacity above that required for activities of daily living), and thus to decreased tolerance. The Borg 15-point category scale is an alternative to gauge exercise intensity.[77,80]

Table 18-8 Target Heart Rate

Age	Target 50–85%	Average Maximum Heart Rate, 100%
20 years	100–170 beats per minute	200 beats per minute
30 years	95–162 beats per minute	190 beats per minute
35 years	93–157 beats per minute	185 beats per minute
40 years	90–153 beats per minute	180 beats per minute
45 years	88–149 beats per minute	175 beats per minute
50 years	85–145 beats per minute	170 beats per minute
55 years	83–140 beats per minute	165 beats per minute
60 years	80–136 beats per minute	160 beats per minute
65 years	78–132 beats per minute	155 beats per minute
70 years	75–128 beats per minute	150 beats per minute

Duration of activity is inversely related to the intensity of the activity in energy expenditure. Women unable to tolerate 30 minutes of moderate-intensity activity can begin by engaging in activity for at least 10 minutes and increase as tolerance increases. Research demonstrates that cardiac and respiratory fitness can be improved by accumulating exercise in 10-minute bouts.[81,82]

The type of activity suggested should provide both physiologic benefits and be enjoyable. Walking is a good initial activity. It requires little equipment or skill and can be performed anywhere and at any intensity. Resistance training, yoga, or flexibility training may improve strength and endurance when added to walking or another form of aerobic activity. Lifestyle activities to decrease sedentary activity, such as taking the stairs instead of the elevator or parking on the other side of the parking lot when shopping, provide additional physical activity. Pedometers provide visual feedback on daily activity levels and are relatively inexpensive. A reasonable target is 10,000 steps per day. Sedentary individuals take between 3000 and 6000 steps, moderately active individuals 7000–10,000, and very active individuals take between 11,000 and 15,000 steps per day.[83] Pedometer step goals should be increased weekly.

TYPES OF EXERCISE

A successful exercise program includes cardiovascular endurance, strength, muscular endurance, and flexibility through a cross-training program of aerobic, anaerobic, resistance, and flexibility exercises.[77] Cardiovascular endurance depends on the system's ability to pump blood and deliver oxygen to the body. A well-conditioned heart beats 40 to 70 times per minute. Strength training uses a muscle or group of muscles to exert an amount of force in a one-time burst of effort. Weight training and resistance training, which are types of strength training, increase muscle and bone strength and muscle mass. Skeletal muscle contains fast- and slow-twitch fibers, which play different roles in exercise capacity and endurance. Fast-twitch fibers provide the explosive force used in weight lifting. Slow-twitch fibers are for endurance. When weights are lifted, muscle fibers are stretched and slightly injured and heal stronger secondary to microscopic scarring. Muscular endurance is achieved with exercise and increases the ability of the body to resist fatigue while holding a position, carrying something for a long period of time, or repeating a movement without getting tired. Flexibility is the ability of joints and muscles to achieve full range of motion.

Aerobic exercise is any exercise that uses large muscles and is sustained for 2 minutes or longer. The heart and lungs work to supply oxygen to the body. As the heart and lungs work harder, they are conditioned and strengthened. Aerobic activities include walking, hiking, jogging, running, bicycling, or swimming. A session of aerobic activity should last from 20 to 60 minutes. At least 3 or more hours of aerobic activity per week will strengthen the heart. The benefits of aerobic activity include lowering the risk of heart attack by improving the cholesterol profile, and increasing bone strength.

Anaerobic exercise is any exercise that requires short bursts of power, such as weight training or sprinting, and does not require a significant increase in oxygen delivery to the muscle. Because energy supplies in the muscles are limited, anaerobic exercises can be sustained for only a short period of time. Obese women may not be efficient at taking in oxygen and thus reach their anaerobic threshold while exercising at very low levels of intensity. As these women increase their level of fitness, they will be able to supply more oxygen to muscles and use less stored energy. Although anaerobic training improves performance, it does not provide the same health benefits as aerobic exercise.

Resistance training or strength training increases muscle strength and mass, bone strength, and metabolism. It is useful in improving weight loss, body image, and self-esteem. Resistance training increases muscle strength by putting strain on the muscle, which increases to load and stimulates the growth of protein in the muscle cells, in turn increasing the ability of the muscle to generate force.

Resistance training uses free weights, weight machines, and calisthenics. When lifting free weights, the individual controls the bar, weights, and the body positioning through the range of motion. Weight machines control the motion performed during lifting. Calisthenics use the person's own body weight as the resistance force through the motion of performing chin-ups, sit-ups, or push-ups. Resistance tubing uses an elastic band that provides resistance to active muscles. Two to three 30-minute resistance workouts per week, incorporating 3 sets of 8 to 15 repetitions and increasing weight with each set, will increase muscle endurance and tone. Regular weight training increases HDL and metabolic rate, burns calories, reduces fat tissue, and increases bone mineral content.

Isometric, isotonic, and isokinetic exercises are also used in strength training. In *isometric* exercises the muscles contract, but the joints do not move and muscle fibers maintain a constant length. Isometric exercises are performed against an immovable surface (e.g., a wall) and have been found effective in developing total strength of a particular muscle or muscle group. In *isotonic* exercises, the body part is moved and the muscle shortens or lengthens. Lifting free weights, sit-ups, push-ups, and pull-ups are isotonic exercises. Isokinetic exercises require a machine that controls the speed of contraction within the range of motion and are not readily available to the public.

Flexibility exercises use stretching movements to increase the length of the muscles and are effective in increasing joint range of motion. The goal of stretching is to lengthen the connective tissue surrounding muscle tissues and should be done only after the muscles have been warmed up by 5–10 minutes of gentle, low-impact aerobic activity. Stretching should not be done when the muscles are cold or injuries may occur. Each stretching exercise should take between 1 and 2 minutes. Stretching at least three times a week may improve mobility, movement, and posture, and prevent injury. Yoga and dance classes provide an excellent source of stretching exercises.

HYDRATION AND FOOD INTAKE

Current recommendations on hydration and food intake before exercise include individualizing hydration; drinking an appropriate amount of fluids before, during, and after exercise; and recognizing the signs and symptoms of dehydration. Adequate hydration in daily exercise optimizes performance and minimizes the incidence of heat illness. Fluids are lost through perspiration and urine and should be replaced on an individual basis. The sweat rate allows calculation for a range of environmental conditions and practices:[78]

$$\text{sweat rate} = (\text{pre-exercise body weight} - \text{post-exercise body weight} + \text{fluid intake} - \text{urine volume}) \div \text{exercise time in hours}$$

Individuals can use the sweat rate to prevent dehydration when engaging in high-intensity physical exercise or running in hot, humid climates.

Drinking the appropriate amount before, during, and after exercise is important in maintaining hydration and improving recovery. A woman should consume 17 to 20 ounces at least 2 to 3 hours before exercising and another 7 to 10 ounces after warming up. During exercise, she needs 28 to 40 ounces for every hour of exercise or 7 to 10 ounces for every 10 to 15 minutes of exercise. After exercise, fluids lost through sweat and urine can be replaced within 2 hours by drinking 20 to 24 ounces for every pound lost through sweat. The optimal oral hydration solution should include water, carbohydrates, and electrolytes (70 to 1266 mg sodium and 14 to 17 g of carbohydrates) before, during, and after exercise.[84]

The signs and symptoms of dehydration include thirst, irritability, headache, weakness, dizziness, cramps, chills, vomiting, nausea, head or neck sensations, decreased performance, or general discomfort. Interventions include stopping exercise immediately, lying down, increasing fluid intake, and notifying medical personnel when appropriate.

Food intake before exercise needs proper timing to prevent nausea, cramps in the side, and general discomfort.[84] After eating a meal, blood is directed to the stomach to facilitate digestion. If an individual exercises too soon after eating, the blood is redirected to the working muscles, which may cause nausea and cramps. It is best to have nothing in the stomach or intestines for 2 to 3 hours before high-intensity exercise. This allows the body time to digest and avoid feeling hungry. However, exercising on an empty stomach may leave an individual feeling energy depleted. Eating a small snack with carbohydrates, such as fruits, vegetables, and grains, 2 to 3 hours before exercise will provide the energy needed to complete an exercise session.

Nonprescription Weight-Loss Products

Over-the-counter (OTC) nonprescription herbal and alternative medicine weight-loss products have developed into a multimillion dollar industry in the United States.[85] Providers may not be aware that their patients are using these products; asking specifically about OTC medications is part of the medication history. There is limited research supporting claims of effectiveness in achieving weight loss using OTC products. Among the OTC products recommended for weight loss are caffeine, catechins, garcinia, and chromium picolinate.

Many weight-loss products use caffeine. Scientific evidence suggests that caffeine increases oxygen consumption and fat oxidation and stimulates the nervous system at the cortex, medulla, and spinal cord. Using caffeine and ephedra, although possibly effective for weight loss, can lead to small, possibly clinically significant, changes in blood pressure and pulse rate.[86]

Green tea catechins are widely consumed throughout Asia and now in the United States. Green tea leaves of *Camellia sinensis* belong to the family of compounds of epigallocatechin gallate and are considered a powerful antioxidant. Catechins increase energy expenditure by enhancing the sympathetic nervous system at the level of the fat-cell adrenoreceptor. Caffeine plus green tea catechins have a demonstrated modest effect on weight loss; the evidence is less clear for green tea without the addition of caffeine.[87]

Garcinia cambogia contains hydroxycitric acid, which is an extract from the rind of the brindall berry. Hydroxycitric acid has been found to inhibit lyase, which is the enzyme involved in the synthesis of fatty acid outside the mitochondrion. For weight loss, studies provide conflicting evidence on the utility of garcinia; pregnancy data are inadequate to recommend it.[88]

Chromium picolinate has been found to enhance the effectiveness of the insulin response to glucose in diabetic women. Although it is considered safe for short-term use, including during pregnancy and lactation, chromium picolinate has not been found to be effective in the treatment of obesity.[89]

Beta-hydroxy-beta-methylbutyrate (HMB) is a metabolite of leucine, which burns fat, builds strength and muscle tissue, and has been found to reduce muscle catabolism and increase fat-free mass during weight lifting.[85] This effect appears to be most marked in those who are beginning exercise as opposed to those who are already fit. This product should be avoided in pregnancy and lactation.[90]

Chitosan has been advertised as a fat blocker. Acetylated chitin is harvested from shrimp exoskeletons and should be avoided by those with shellfish allergies. Chitosan binds lipids such as cholesterol and triglycerides in the intestines. To date, the data are not sufficient to recommend for use in weight-loss programs; no pregnancy safety data are available.[91]

Pharmacologic Therapy

Pharmacologic therapy should be guided by the principles of beneficence (benefits) and nonmalfeasance (risks). Benefits may include the reduction in health risks, such as hyperlipidemia, hypertension, and coronary artery disease, and improvement in psychosocial benefits, such as an improved quality of life or decrease in depression. (Table 18-9 summarizes available medications.) Centrally acting anorexiants increase satiety and decrease hunger, thereby reducing calorie intake and providing a greater sense of control. The ventromedial and lateral hypothalamic regions in the central nervous system are targeted by centrally acting anorexiants and augment the neurotransmission of norepinephrine, serotonin, and dopamine, thereby decreasing food intake. Adrenergic drugs either stimulate norepinephrine release or block its reuptake, which results in improved appetite control.

Orlistat (Xenical, Alli) is the first nonsystemic drug that acts directly in the gastrointestinal tract for weight loss.[92] It has been found to decrease total cholesterol, LDL, blood pressure, glucose, and insulin. As a pentanoic acid ester, orlistat forms a covalent bond with the active serine residue site of gastric and pancreatic lipases, inhibiting their activity and preventing reabsorption of about 30% of dietary fat (22 g fat or 200 calories in a 2000-calorie, 30% fat diet). Orlistat also negatively reinforces women when they eat a high-fat meal, due to the side effects of anal leakage and diarrhea. Malabsorption of vitamins A, D, E, and K and beta-carotene occurs with Orlistat; vitamin supplementation at bedtime is recommended. Orlistat should be started with lifestyle modifications when a woman has a BMI of 30 or above, or 27 or above in the presence of other risk factors. Lifestyle modifications, including a low-fat, low-cholesterol diet and exercise to increase weight loss, minimize the side effects of Orlistat. The drug should be discontinued for any side effects

Table 18-9 Pharmacologic Agents for Weight Loss

Generic (Trade)	Dosage (DEA Schedule)	Class/Action
Phenylpropanolamine (Acutrim)	75 mg SR daily (OTC)	Centrally acting adrenergic
Phenylpropanolamine (Dexatrim)	75 mg SR daily or 25 mg tid (OTC)	Alpha-1 agonist
Phenylpropanolamine (Prolamine)	37.5 mg daily (OTC)	
Phentermine (Adipex-P)	37.5 mg daily (IV)	Centrally acting adrenergic
Phendimetrazine (Bontril)	105 mg SR daily (III)	Stimulates norepinephrine release
Benzphetamine (Didrex)	25–50 mg daily–tid (III)	
Phentermine (Fastin)	30 mg daily (IV)	
Phentermine (Ionamin)	15–30 mg daily (IV)	
Phendimetrazine (Plegine)	105 mg SR daily (III)	
Phendimetrazine (Prelu-2)	105 mg SR daily (III)	
Diethylpropion (Tenuate)	75 mg SR daily or 25 mg tid (IV)	
Phentermine/Topiramate (Qsymia)	3.75 mg/23 mg	
	7.5 mg/46 mg	
	11.25 mg/69 mg	
	15.0 mg/92 mg	
Mazindol (Mazanor)	1 mg tid (IV)	Centrally acting adrenergic
Mazindol (Sanorex)	1 mg daily (IV)	Blocks norepinephrine reuptake
Orlistat (Xenical)	120 mg tid (not scheduled)	Lipase inhibitor
		Gastric and pancreatic lipase inhibitor

DEA = Drug Enforcement Administration, OTC = over the counter, SR = slow release, tid = 3 times per day

Data from Staff Physician's Desk Reference. *Physician's Desk Reference.* Montvale, NJ: Medical Economics Company; 2013.

and when the woman's BMI is within normal limits or within 2 years.

Qsymia is a new drug that combines phentermine to decrease appetite and extended-release topiramate to reduce food cravings.[93] Phentermine is an appetite suppressant similar to an amphetamine. Topiramate is an anticonvulsant. The medication has extensive contraindications and side effects and requires careful patient counseling. Qsymia should not be prescribed if the patient has used a monoamine oxidase inhibitor such as furazolidone (Furoxone), isocarboxazid (Marplan), phenelzine (Nardil), rasagiline (Azilect), selegiline (Eldepryl, EMSAM, Zelapar), or tranylcypromine (Parnate) in the last 14 days. Before prescribing Qsymia (Food and Drug Administration pregnancy category X), a pregnancy test should be negative and effective birth control should be used while taking this medication. Qsymia can cause irregular vaginal bleeding when used simultaneously with hormonal contraception. Qsymia should not be prescribed if a woman has a history of glaucoma, overactive thyroid, high blood pressure, heart disease (coronary artery disease, heart rhythm problems, congestive heart failure, pulmonary hypertension), diabetes, liver or kidney disease, hypokalemia, a stroke in the past 6 months, or is pregnant or breastfeeding. Individuals taking Qsymia have reported experiencing sensations of a pounding heart rate or fluttering in the chest, depressed mood, thoughts of suicide, trouble concentrating, problems with thinking or speech, dizziness, blurred vision, eye pain, seeing halos around light, symptoms of low blood sugar (headache, hunger, weakness, sweating, confusion, irritability, dizziness, fast heart rate, or feeling jittery), severe lower back pain, red or pink urine, feeling very hot, being unable to urinate, heavy sweating or hot and dry skin, low potassium, confusion, uneven heart rate, extreme thirst, increased urination, leg discomfort, muscle weakness or limp feeling, dangerously high blood pressure, severe headache, blurred vision, buzzing in ears, anxiety, confusion, chest pain, shortness of breath, or seizures.[93]

Surgical Treatment

Bariatric surgery should be considered only for individuals with a BMI > 30 kg/m² and severe comorbidities.[3] In the absence of comorbidities, surgery is recommended only for a BMI > 40 kg/m². It has been demonstrated to have favorable outcomes relative to conservative treatment in terms of absolute weight loss and remission of metabolic disease.[94,95] A multidisciplinary team that incorporates medical, nutritional, and psychologic providers should thoroughly examine the woman before a decision is reached. Bariatric surgery patients require long-term follow up to maintain success and treat any complications; the ability to manage dietary changes and adhere to care recommendations is essential to selecting appropriate candidates. The surgery reduces stomach storage capacity and narrows the stomach exit diameter, with the goal of decreasing volume and rate of food intake. All of the surgeries are effective in producing an average loss of approximately 50% of excess body weight that is maintained in 60% of clients for at least 5 years.[96] Impressive

weight losses over the first 3 years following surgery have been demonstrated: Roux-en-Y gastric bypass (RYGB) patients have an average loss of 41 kg (90 lbs), and those with vertical banded gastroplasty (VBG) have an average loss of 32 kg (71 lbs).[94] Up to 25% of bariatric surgeries fail due to overconsumption of food, which effectively stretches the stomach and allows an increased intake of calories and volume.

Currently, there are three common surgical approaches: RYGB, VBG, and vertical sleeve gastrectomy (VSG).[96] RYGB surgery creates a small stomach pouch connected to the distal small intestine and the upper part of the small intestine, which creates a Y-shaped configuration. It is a malabsorptive procedure; by altering the anatomy of the digestive tract, nutritional absorption is decreased. Malabsorptive procedures tend to lead to more weight loss than restrictive procedures. Dumping syndrome (rapid stomach emptying causing cramping and diarrhea) occurs when high-sugar foods are eaten after RYGB. There are more vitamin deficiencies in RYGB than VGB and VSG surgeries, including fat-soluble vitamins, thiamine, folate, iron, and vitamin B_{12}. For these reasons, among others, the frequency with which RYGB is performed is decreasing.[97]

Restrictive procedures reduce oral intake by limiting gastric volume, produce early satiety, and leave the alimentary canal in continuity, minimizing the risks of metabolic complications. The VBG surgery includes stapling the stomach to permanently create a smaller pre-stomach pouch. The lap band procedure (gastric band) is a laparoscopic variation in which a silicone band is inserted that restricts the amount of food that can enter the stomach. The band can be tightened or loosened through the injection or removal of saline through a port just under the skin. The VSG surgery reduces the stomach to about 15% of its original size by permanently removing a large portion of the stomach. This procedure is permanent and not reversible and is performed laparoscopically.[96]

Immediately after bariatric surgery, the patient consumes a clear-liquid diet for several days and then progresses to a pureed diet for approximately 2 weeks. After the 2-week period, the diet progresses to a high-protein, low-fat diet. Alcohol consumption is discouraged. Overeating may cause nausea and vomiting. In the first month, many patients struggle with dehydration as they adapt to decreased gastric volume. Patients are encouraged to drink a minimum of 48–64 ounces of fluid throughout the day.[96]

Complications from bariatric surgery include gastric dumping syndrome (20%), leaks at the surgical site (12%), incisional hernia (7%), infection (6%), pneumonia (4%); osteopenia and hyperparathyroidism secondary to reduced absorption of calcium have been reported in RYGB.[96] Surgically related mortality is less than 1%.[94]

Weight-Loss Maintenance

The National Weight Control Registry (NWCR) was founded in 1994 by Doctors Wing and Hill to follow clients who succeeded at long-term weight loss.[98] The NWCR now includes more than 10,000 subjects who have maintained a minimum weight loss of 30 pounds for at least 1 year. Successful weight loss was accomplished by eating a low-fat, high-carbohydrate diet, monitoring weight and food intake, and regularly engaging in high levels of exercise.

Currently, many online obesity resources are available for both women and providers to assist in weight loss and maintenance. These provide general information including nutrition, exercise, and surgery, and some are organizations dedicated to the treatment of obesity (see **Table 18-10**).

Table 18-10 Obesity Websites

Name of Organization	Website
Academy of Nutrition and Dietetics	http://www.eatright.org
American College of Sports Medicine	http://www.acsm.org/
American Council on Exercise	http://www.acefitness.org/
American Society for Metabolic and Bariatric Surgery	https://asmbs.org/
Centers for Disease Control and Prevention Division of Nutrition, Physical Activity, and Obesity	http://www.cdc.gov/nccdphp/dnpa/
Food and Nutrition Information Center	https://fnic.nal.usda.gov/
Health.gov, Office of Disease Prevention and Health Promotion	http://www.health.gov/dietaryguidelines/
National Institute of Diabetes and Digestive and Kidney Diseases	http://www.niddk.nih.gov/health/nutrit/pubs/presmeds.htm
Obesity Medicine Association	http://obesitymedicine.org
The Obesity Society	http://www.obesity.org/
Nutrition.gov	http://nutrition.gov
Partnership for Healthy Weight Management	http://www.consumer.gov/weightloss/
World Obesity Federation	http://www.worldobesity.org/

Management of Obesity in Pregnancy

Overweight and obesity in pregnancy are increasing at an alarming rate. More than half of pregnant women are overweight or obese.[3] Young women who are either overweight or obese have been found to have higher rates of prediabetes, type 2 diabetes, hypertension, hypercholesterolemia, and polycystic ovarian syndrome.[99] The Institute of Medicine (IOM) recommends that BMI before pregnancy be used as a guide to calculate the amount of weight to be gained during pregnancy.[100] The IOM suggests that underweight (BMI < 18.5 kg/m^2) women should gain 28–40 pounds total at a rate of 1–1.3 pounds per week in the 2nd and 3rd trimesters, normal weight (BMI 18.5–24.9 kg/m^2) women should gain 25–35 pounds total at a rate of 0.8–1.0 pounds per week in the 2nd and 3rd trimesters, overweight (BMI 25.0–29.9 kg/m^2) women should gain 15–25 pounds total at a rate of 0.5–0.7 pounds per week in her 2nd and 3rd trimesters, and obese (BMI > 30.0 kg/m^2) women should gain 11–20 pounds total at a rate of 0.4–0.6 pounds per week in her 2nd and 3rd trimesters.[101] Some authors have suggested that even 20 pounds is excessive weight gain for obese gravidas.[102]

Obese women are more likely to develop preeclampsia and to require a cesarean section, their pregnancies are more likely to end in miscarriage or fetal death, and their babies are more likely to be macrosomic and to develop obesity later in childhood.[99,103] Excessive gestational weight gain increases the likelihood that women will retain weight postpartum, with minority women who have lower incomes retaining the most weight.[100]

Treatment goals for overweight and obese pregnant women include stabilizing weight gain, improving nutrition, increasing physical activity, and decreasing sedentary activity. It is important for women who are pregnant not to diet, but to follow a nutritious dietary plan that provides healthy whole foods that encourage weight stabilization.

Dietary Interventions

Pregnant women who are overweight or obese should follow the same basic guidelines of proper nutrition as nonpregnant overweight or obese women with the following differences. Women who are pregnant should consume sufficient calories to gain the proper amount of weight and sustain the growing child. Approximately 300 additional calories per day are suggested to meet this goal.[22] Nutrients are best in their natural form, and enriching the diet with whole grains, fruits, and vegetables will increase fiber intake and help prevent constipation. Women require about 64 to 80 ounces of fluid per day and more in hot weather and when exercising.[22]

Behavioral Modification Interventions

Behavioral modification interventions during pregnancy include dietary and exercise behaviors and motivational strategies to encourage proper weight gain during pregnancy. Dieting during pregnancy is not recommended. Assisting women in learning portion control; adding an additional 300 calories per day; eating whole grains, fruits, and vegetables; and drinking an adequate amount of fluid are all important ways to positively modify dietary behavior. Foods that should be avoided during pregnancy include soft unpasteurized cheese, processed food, and raw or undercooked meat or fish.[22] If the pregnant woman is healthy, she should be encouraged to partake in exercise daily.

Exercise Interventions

As stated earlier in the chapter, exercise alone does not have a significant impact on weight stabilization. However, when regular exercise is combined with healthy dietary changes, weight stabilization is enhanced. Exercise during pregnancy can assist in achieving a healthy weight gain, determined by the pregnant woman's prepregnancy BMI.

Exercise should never be used for weight loss during pregnancy.

The American College of Obstetricians and Gynecologists has provided guidelines for exercise during pregnancy and the postpartum period,[104] recommending that healthy pregnant women may continue an already-established exercise routine including an average of 150 minutes of exercise spread over several days of the week. Each woman enters pregnancy with an individual medical and exercise history, and each pregnancy progresses differently. Most healthy women can continue their prepregnancy routine with some adaptations throughout their entire pregnancy as long as there are no medical complications.[104-106]

Some activities that a woman may engage in prepregnancy that are unsafe during pregnancy include scuba diving and skydiving (due to changes in oxygen pressure) and any activity that puts pregnant women at risk for falling or receiving a blow to the abdomen. A thorough evaluation and careful program design can provide a safe exercise regimen that will support a woman's desire to remain physically active throughout her entire pregnancy.

Absolute contraindications to exercise during pregnancy include hemodynamically significant heart disease, restrictive lung disease, incompetent cervix or cerclage, multiple gestation at risk for premature labor, persistent second or third semester bleeding, placenta previa after 26 weeks' gestation, premature labor during current pregnancy, ruptured membranes, pregnancy-induced preeclampsia, and hypertension.[104,106] Relative contraindications during pregnancy include severe anemia, unevaluated maternal cardiac arrhythmias, chronic bronchitis, poorly controlled type 1 diabetes, extreme morbid obesity, extreme underweight (BMI $\leq$ 12), history of an extremely sedentary lifestyle, intrauterine growth restriction in current pregnancy, poorly controlled hypertension, poorly controlled seizure disorder, poorly controlled hyperthyroidism, and heavy smoking.[104,106] These women should begin with a gentle program of stretching and ambulation at their comfort level.

Exercise does not need to be continuous to be beneficial. Short (10-minute) periods of moderate activity will produce health benefits and may burn more than 150 calories. Moderate activities include pushing a stroller for 1 mile in 30 minutes, swimming laps for 20 minutes, stair climbing for 15 minutes, or walking briskly for 30 minutes. If the woman regularly engaged in weight training before pregnancy, then she may continue to do so during pregnancy, provided she is comfortable and doing it correctly.[73]

EDUCATION FOR PREGNANT WOMEN EXERCISING

Women who are pregnant should be taught about adaptations needed in order to exercise safely in pregnancy. These adaptations include avoiding the use of the Valsalva maneuver, sitting, and back-lying positions while exercising; using appropriate measures to determine a safe level of exertion; and using correct body mechanics, proper posture, and exercise techniques in order to prevent worsening of backache and diastasis recti, which commonly occurs in pregnant women.

The Valsalva maneuver is performed when an individual exhales forcibly against a closed glottis while no air enters through the nose or mouth. Individuals can perform the Valsalva maneuver while lifting heavy weights, straining during a bowel movement, or strenuous coughing. During the Valsalva maneuver, return of venous blood to the heart is decreased and the woman may feel lightheaded; in pregnancy, oxygen to the fetus may be decreased. The woman needs to breathe without holding her breath. Counting aloud while exercising can prevent forcible exhalation.

Heart Rate Versus Perceived Exertion   It is no longer an accepted standard that a heart rate of 140 beats per minute is appropriate for pregnant women. Borg's scale of the rate of perceived exertion (see Table 18-9) is recommended to help women to judge their exercise intensity.[77] Individuals should be taught to rate their own perception of exertion and how heavy and strenuous the exercise feels for them, including feelings of physical stress, effort, and fatigue.

Sitting Versus Standing   During pregnancy, extended periods of motionless standing are not recommended. Motionless standing decreases venous return and causes edema in the lower extremities. The tailor sit position is a much better position in which to exercise. The tailor sit places the woman in a seated position, with her weight on her buttocks, legs crossed in front of her, and her back extended and relaxed. Most exercises can be modified to a seated position.

Back Lying   The back-lying position can cause a decrease in cardiac return by putting pressure on the inferior vena cava. Pressure from the weight of the uterus and fetus also decreases blood flow to the uterus, placenta, and fetus. If any signs or symptoms of dizziness occur, then the woman can roll into a side-lying position. Exercising in the back-lying position is acceptable throughout pregnancy provided the woman stays attuned to the possible warning signs of the vena cava syndrome.

Body Mechanics and Posture   One of the more obvious changes during pregnancy is a change in posture and adjustment in center of gravity. During pregnancy, a woman's center of gravity shifts upward and forward. She should always be aware of her posture and should try to stand with her feet hip-width apart and her weight evenly distributed over the pelvis, with her knees held softly and not locked. Her head should be centered over her shoulders, the shoulders in a relaxed position, and her chest should be pointed upward. Her umbilicus should be pulled back toward the spine.

Diastasis Recti   A separation of the rectus abdominis muscle is known as diastasis recti. When the abdominal muscles are weaker than the back muscles, poor posture may ensue. Abdominal muscles that are stronger during pregnancy assist the women during labor and the birthing process.

The main abdominal muscles involved in diastasis recti are the rectus abdominis and the transverse muscle. The rectus abdominis is a longitudinal muscle, divided in two halves, and connected by a soft, fibrous band called the linea alba. The transverse muscle wraps around the body at the level of the umbilicus. **Figure 18**-4 illustrates the assessment of diastasis recti. If there is more than a 2½ finger

Figure 18-4 Assessment of diastasis recti.

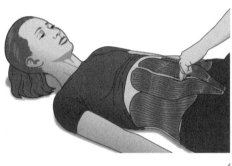

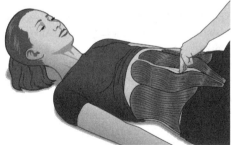

Have the woman rest at ease, arms to her sides, knees bent, and feet flat. Facing the woman's head, palpate the mid abdomen at the level of the umbilicus. Ask her to raise her head about four inches and assess the width of separation.

separation of the rectus muscle, the woman would benefit from seeing a prenatal fitness trainer before doing abdominal exercises to ensure she is performing the exercises correctly. Common actions such as coughing, sneezing, getting up from an examination table, or any movement that pushes the transverse muscle against the recti can cause further separation.[25]

Several activities can be modified to reduce the development of diastasis recti. When a woman is getting up from an exam table, she should roll into a side-lying position and push up with both arms rather than using the abdominal muscles. When moving sitting on the floor to a standing position, the woman should roll onto her hands and knees and bring one foot forward to the floor with hands on the knee. Then, push up with the arms to a standing position. When exercising, each stretch and exercise should begin with diaphragmatic breathing, which will bring the transverse muscle back toward the spine during exhalation.

Specific Exercises in Pregnancy

Aerobic Exercises   There are many low-risk aerobic exercises such as dancing, cycling, swimming, and walking. Aerobic dancing and low-impact aerobics provide a complete workout when they include a warm-up, aerobic exercise, and cool down. Cycling is an excellent exercise, but stationary or recumbent bikes are suggested toward the latter part of pregnancy, because increased joint laxity and changes in the center of gravity may place the woman at risk of falling. Swimming uses many different muscles; the water provides support as the pregnant woman gets a full-body workout. Walking is another exercise that can be gentle or more vigorous depending on how the woman is feeling and her level of fitness.

Weight Training   Free weights are an excellent way in which to strengthen muscles. Women should start out with 1- to 2-pound weights and increase the weight over time. Free weights are usually 0.5, 1, 2, 3, 5, or 10 pounds. Adding weight should be done according to what feels comfortable. However, the exercises should be challenging, slow, and controlled. If the prescribed number of repetitions and sets is comfortable, additional weight may be added. If additional weight makes the exercises painful or uncontrolled, then the weights should be decreased to the previous level. If free weights are not available, the woman may try items found in her own home, such as soup cans or bottles of water.

Resistance   Resistance training is a specialized method of conditioning designed to increase muscle strength, muscle endurance, and muscle power. Resistance training can be performed using resistance bands, resistance machines, or the woman's own body weight. Resistance bands are easy to use, inexpensive, and can be easily adjusted to increase or decrease the amount of resistance desired. It is important to remind the woman that her wrists should remain straight without applying pressure on the wrist. The increase in relaxin can cause increased laxity and may injure the wrists. During exercise with resistance bands, the wrist should remain in a neutral position with thumbs pointing out straight and in line with the hand.

Hydration and Food Intake

Woman who are pregnant need to keep well hydrated during exercise. In addition to the daily eight 8-ounce glasses of water, pregnant women should drink 14 to 22 ounces of fluid 2 hours before exercise, 6 to 12 ounces every 15 to 20 minutes during exercise, and 16 to 24 ounces for every pound lost after exercise.[107,108] In addition, women who are pregnant need to eat before exercising so the body does not burn fat, because weight loss is not a goal. Eating approximately 2 hours to 3 hours before exercise will ensure adequate availability of calories for a workout. Light, high-water-content fruits (peaches or watermelon); fruit yogurt; cottage cheese; raisins; a bagel with low-fat cheese; a bowl of cereal with low-fat milk; yogurt with graham crackers; a fruit smoothie with nonfat yogurt; and whole-wheat toast are examples of good choices.

Warning Signs

If at any time during exercise a woman experiences chest pain or tightness; dizziness; headache; increased shortness of breath; muscle weakness or tingling pain; or redness, warmth, or swelling of the calf, she should stop exercising immediately and seek medical attention. If the woman is pregnant and feels decreased fetal movement, fluid leakage from the vagina, one-sided headache, blurred vision, uterine contractions (not Braxton Hicks), or vaginal bleeding, she should stop exercising immediately and seek medical attention. After the woman is examined by her midwife and medically cleared, she may resume her exercise regimen. She may need to alter, decrease, or discontinue certain activities.

Sciatica   Pain from sciatica is caused at the location where the sciatic nerve passes through and emerges from the lumbar vertebrae. The pain travels below the knee and may involve the foot. In addition, there may be numbness or weakness of the lower leg muscles. A prolapsed intervertebral disc or a herniated nucleus pulposus may cause sciatica. During pregnancy, the enlarging uterus coupled with a change in posture and center of gravity may cause women to experience these symptoms. It is important to rule out any disc involvement before exercising. Comfort measures for women with nonpathologic presentations include stretching and bending the affected leg at the knee while keeping the opposite leg extended and pulling the affected leg across the body.[25] Another stretch includes getting onto all fours or stretching the lower back by getting in the knee–chest position to change the pressure of the uterus and baby.

Program Evaluation

Program evaluations should occur at regular intervals when an exercise regimen has been developed. The first reason is to evaluate whether the woman's goals are being met and she is satisfied with her current exercise regimen. Second, it provides an opportunity to determine how she should proceed with her exercise regimen and make adjustments if she is pregnant. Third, it is important to determine if the number of repetitions and the amount of weight or resistance are appropriate. Lastly, a pregnant woman will need to monitor her diastasis as she progresses through her pregnancy and exercise program.

References

1. National Heart, Lung, and Blood Institute. *Clinical Guidelines on the Identification, Evaluation and Treatment of Overweight and Obesity in Adults—The Evidence Report*. Bethesda, MD: National Institutes of Health; 1998. http://www.nhlbi.nih.gov/guidelines/obesity/ob_gdlns.pdf. Accessed May 8, 2016.
2. Flegal KM, Carroll MD, Kit BK, Ogden CL. Prevalence of obesity and trends in the distribution of body mass index among US adults, 1999–2010. *JAMA*. 2012;307(5):491-497.
3. American Diabetes Association. Standards of medical care in diabetes 2013. *Diabetes Care*. 2013;36: S11-S66.
4. Jensen MD, Ryan DH, Apovian CM, Ard JD, Comuzzie AG, Donato KA. 2013 AHA/ACC/TOS guideline for the management of overweight and obesity in adults: a report of the American College of Cardiology/American Heart Association Task Force on Practice Guidelines and The Obesity Society. *Circulation*. 2014;129(25 Suppl 2):S102-S138.

5. US Department of Health and Human Services Office of Disease Prevention and Health Promotion. *Healthy People 2020: Nutrition and Weight Status*. https://www.healthypeople.gov/2020/topics-objectives/topic/nutrition-and-weight-status. Accessed May 8, 2016.

6. Adamus-Leach HJ, Wilson PL, O'Connor DP, Rhode PC, Mama SK, Lee RE. Depression, stress and body fat are associated with binge eating in a community sample of African American and Hispanic women. *Eat Weight Disord*. 2013;18(2):221-227.

7. National Institute of Diabetes and Digestive and Kidney Diseases. Overweight, obesity, and health risk: national task force on prevention and treatment of obesity. *Arch Intern Med*. 2000;160:898-904.

8. Alul FY, Cook DE, Shchelochkov OA, Fleener LG, Berberich SL, Murray JC, et al. The heritability of metabolic profiles in newborn twins. *Heredity*. 2013;110(3):253-258.

9. Whitaker RC, Wright JA, Pepe MS, Seidel KD, Dietz WH. Predicting obesity in young adulthood from childhood and parental obesity. *N Engl J Med*. 1997;337(13):869-873.

10. Stunkard AJ, Harris JR, Pederson NL, McClearn GE. The body-mass index of twins who have been reared apart. *N Engl J Med*. 1990;322: 1483-1487.

11. Berkowitz RI, Stunkard AJ. Development of childhood obesity. In: Wadden TA, Stunkard AJ, eds. *Handbook of Obesity Treatment*. New York, NY: The Guilford Press; 2002.

12. Bray GA. Obesity. *Curr Ther Endocrinol Metab*. 1994;5:465-474.

13. Chehab FF. Leptin as a regulator of adipose mass and reproduction. *Trends Pharmacol Sci*. 2000;21(8): 309-314.

14. Esparza J, Fox C, Harper IT, Bennett PH, Schulz LO, Valencia ME, et al. Daily energy expenditure in Mexican and USA Pima Indians: low physical activity as a possible cause of obesity. *Int J Obes Relat Metab Disord*. 2000;24:55-59.

15. Ravelli AC, van der Meulen JH, Osmond C, Barker DJ, Bleker OP. Obesity at the age of 50 in men and women exposed to famine prenatally. *Am J Clin Nutr*. 1999;70:811-816.

16. Ravelli GP, Stein ZA, Susser MW. Obesity in young men after famine exposure. *N Engl J Med*. 1976; 295:349-353.

17. Akabas SR, Lederman SA, Moore BJ. *Textbook of Obesity*. Ames, IA: Wiley-Blackwell; 2012.

18. Sobal J, Stunkard AJ. Socioeconomic status and obesity: a review of the literature. *Psychol Bull*. 1989; 105:260-275.

19. Zhang Q, Wang Y. Socioeconomic inequality of obesity in the United States: do gender, age and ethnicity matter? *Soc Sci Med*. 2004;58:1171-1180.

20. Gordon-Larsen P, Adair LS, Popkin BM. The relationship of ethnicity, socioeconomic factors, and overweight in US adolescents. *Obes Res*. 2003; 11:121-129.

21. Ambrosius WT, Newmans SA, Pratt JH. Rates of change in measures of body size vary by ethnicity and gender. *Ethn Dis*. 2001;11:303-310.

22. US Department of Agriculture, US Department of Health and Human Services. *Dietary Guidelines for Americans 2010*. Washington, DC: US Government Printing Office; 2010.

23. Jakicic JM, Gallagher KI. Physical activity considerations for management of body weight. In: Bessesen DH, Kushner R, eds. *Evaluation and Management of Obesity*. Philadelphia, PA: Hanley & Belfus; 2002:73-87.

24. Jakicic JM, Clark K, Coleman E, Donnelly JE, Foreyt JP, Melanson E, et al. American College of Sports Medicine position stand: appropriate intervention strategies for weight loss and prevention of weight gain for adults. *Med Sci Sports Exerc*. 2001;33:2145-2156.

25. Esherick JS, Clark DS, Slater ED. *Current Practice Guidelines in Primary Care 2013*. New York, NY: McGraw-Hill; 2013.

26. Faust IM, Johnson PR, Stern JS, Hirsch J. Diet-induced adipocyte number increases in adult rats: a new model for obesity. *Am J Physiol*. 1978;235: E279-E286.

27. Schwartz RB, Brunzell JD. Increase of adipose tissue in lipoprotein lipase activity with weight loss. *J Clin Invest*. 1981;67:1425.

28. Keesey RE. A set-point theory of obesity. In: Brownell KD, Foreyt JP, eds. *Handbook of Eating Disorders*. New York, NY: Basic Books; 1986: 63-87.

29. Himms-Hagen J. Brown adipose tissue metabolism and thermogenesis. *Annu Rev Nutr*. 1985;5:69-84.

30. Miller DS. Thermogenesis and obesity. *Bibl Nutr Dieta*. 1979;27:25-32.

31. De Luise M, Blackburn GL, Flier JS. Reduced activity of the red cell sodium-potassium pump in human obesity. *N Engl J Med*. 1980;303:1017.

32. Bessesen DH. Regulation of appetite by the central nervous system. In: Bessesen DH, Kushner R, eds. *Evaluation and Management of Obesity*. Philadelphia, PA: Hanley and Belfus; 2002:155-166.

33. Elmquist JK, Elias CF, Saper CB. From lesions to leptin: hypothalamic control of food intake and body weight. *Neuron*. 1999;22:221-232.

34. Ahima RS, Flier JS. Leptin. *Annu Rev Physiol.* 2000;62:413-437.

35. Schwartz MW, Woods SC, Porte D, Deely RJ, Baskin DG. Central nervous system control of food intake. *Nature.* 2000;404(6778):661-671.

36. Kushner R. Defining the scope of the problem of obesity. In: Bessesen DH, Kushner R, eds. *Evaluation and Management of Obesity.* Philadelphia, PA: Hanley and Belfus; 2002:1-8.

37. Centers for Disease Control and Prevention. Healthy weight—It's not a diet, it's a lifestyle! Available at: http://www.cdc.gov/media/subtopic/matte/pdf/031210-Healthy-Weight.pdf. Accessed May 8, 2016.

38. Snijder MB, Zimmet PZ, Visser D, Dekker JM, Seidell JC, Shaw JE. Independent and opposite associations of waist and hip circumferences with diabetes, hypertension and dyslipidemia: the AusDiab Study. *Int J Obes Relat Metab Disord.* 2004;28(3):402-409.

39. Lean ME, Han TS, Morrison CE. Waist circumference as a measure for indicating need for weight management. *BMJ.* 1995;311:158-161.

40. Cnop M, Landchild MJ, Vidal J, Havel PJ, Knowles NG, Carr DR, et al. The concurrent accumulation of intra-abdominal and subcutaneous fat explains the association between insulin resistance and plasma leptin concentrations: distinct metabolic effects of two fat compartments. *Diabetes.* 2002;51(4):1005-1015.

41. Davies PSW, Cole TJ. *Body Composition Techniques in Health and Disease.* New York, NY: Cambridge University Press; 1995.

42. US Department Health Human Services, Public Health Services, NHANES III. *Anthropometric Procedures Video* (Stock Number 017-022-01335-5). Washington, DC: Government Printing Office; 1996.

43. Burke L, Deakin V. *Clinical Sports Nutrition.* 2nd ed. Rosehill, Australia: McGraw-Hill Publishers; 2000.

44. Nunez C, Rubiano M, Horlick J, Thornton J, Heymsfield SB. Leg-to-leg bioimpedance system validity in children. In: *Experimental Biology.* New York, NY: Experimental Biology; 1999.

45. National High Blood Pressure Education Program. *JNC 7 Express: The Seventh Report of the Joint National Committee on Prevention, Detection, Evaluation, and Treatment of High Blood Pressure.* Washington, DC: US Department of Health and Human Services, National Institutes of Health, National Heart, Lung, and Blood Institute; 2003.

46. James PA, Oparil S, Carter BL, Cushman WC, Dennison-Himmelfarb C, Handler J, et al. 2014 evidence-based guideline for the management of high blood pressure in adults: report from the panel members appointed to the Eighth Joint National Committee (JNC 8). *JAMA.* 2014;311(5):507-520.

47. Go AS, Mozaffarian D, Roger VL, Benjamin EJ, Berry JD, Blaha MJ, et al. Heart disease and stroke statistics—2014 update. *Circulation.* 2014;129:e28-292.

48. US Department of Health and Human Services, Public Health Service, National Institutes of Health, National Heart, Lung, and Blood Institute. *Third Report of the National Cholesterol Education Program Expert Panel on the Detection, Evaluation, and Treatment of High Blood Cholesterol in Adults (Adult Treatment Panel III).* Washington, DC: US Department of Health and Human Services; 2002.

49. Eckel RH, Jakicic JM, Ard JD, Hubbard VS, de Jesus JM, Lee IM, et al. 2013 AHA/ACC guideline on lifestyle management to reduce cardiovascular risk: a report of the American College of Cardiology, American Heart Association Task Force on Practice Guidelines. *Circulation.* 2013;129(25 Suppl 2):S76-99.

50. Pagana KD, Pagana TJ. *Mosby's Diagnostic and Laboratory Test Reference.* 11th ed. St. Louis, MO: Elsevier-Mosby; 2013.

51. Wang SS, Wadden TA, Womble LG, Nonas CA. What consumers want to know about commercial weight-loss programs: a pilot investigation. *Obes Res.* 2003;11:48-53.

52. Bessesen DH. Talking to patients about popular diet books. In: Bessesen DH, Kushner R, eds. *Evaluation and Management of Obesity.* Philadelphia, PA: Hanley & Belfus; 2003:59-69.

53. Atkins RC. *Dr. Atkins' New Diet Revolution.* New York, NY: M. Evans and Company; 2002.

54. Agatston A. *The South Beach Diet.* Emmaus, PA: Rodale Press; 2003.

55. Ornish D. *Dr. Dean Ornish's Program for Reversing Heart Disease: The Only System Scientifically Proven to Reverse Heart Disease Without Drugs or Surgery.* 2nd ed. New York, NY: Ballantine Books; 1996.

56. Monte T, Pritikin I. *Pritikin: The Man Who Healed America's Heart.* Emmaus, PA: Rodale Press; 1988.

57. Brand-Miller J, Wolever TMS, Foster-Powell K, Colagiuri S. *The New Glucose Revolution: The Authoritative Guide to the Glycemic Index—The Dietary Solution for Lifelong Health.* New York, NY: Marlowe & Company; 2003.

58. Steward HL, Bethea MC, Andrews SS, Balart LA. *The New Sugar Busters: Cut Sugar to Trim Fat.* New York, NY: The Ballantine Publishing Group; 2003.

59. Sears B. *A Week in the Zone.* New York, NY: Harper-Collins; 2000.

60. D'Adamo PJ, Whitney C. *Eat Right for Your Type.* New York, NY: G.B. Putnam's Sons; 2003.

61. Rolls BJ, Barnett RA. *Volumetrics Weight Control Plan.* New York, NY: HarperCollins; 2000.

62. Cloutier M, Adamson E. *The Mediterranean Diet.* New York, NY: HarperCollins; 2004.

63. Yang J, Farioli A, Korre M, Kales SN. Modified Mediterranean diet score and cardiovascular risk in a North American working population. *PLoS ONE.* 2014;9(2):e87539.

64. Mitrou PN, Kipnis V, Thiébaut AC, Reedy J, Subar AF, Wirfält E, et al. Mediterranean dietary pattern and prediction of all-cause mortality in a US population: results from the NIH-AARP Diet and Health Study. *Arch Intern Med.* 2007;167:2461-2468.

65. Bessesen DH, Kushner R. *Evaluation and Management of Obesity.* Philadelphia, PA: Hanley & Belfus; 2003.

66. Ferster CB, Nurnberger JI, Levitt EB. The control of eating. *J Math.* 1962;1:87-109.

67. Stuart RB. Behavioural control of overeating. *Behav Res Ther.* 1967;5:357-365.

68. Wing RA. Behavioral weight control. In: Wadden TA, Stunkard AJ, eds. *Handbook of Obesity Treatment.* New York, NY: The Guilford Press; 2002:301-316.

69. Wing RR, Jefferey RW. Outpatient treatments of obesity: a comparison of methodological and clinical results. *Int J Obes.* 1979;3:261-279.

70. Wadden TA, Stunkard AJ, Brownell KD. Very low calorie diets: their efficacy, safety, and future. *Ann Intern Med.* 1983;99:675-684.

71. Wadden TA, Foster GD, Letizia KA. One-year behavioral treatment of obesity: comparison of moderate and severe caloric restriction and the effects of weight maintenance therapy. *J Consult Clin Psychol.* 1994;62:165-171.

72. Wing RR, Blair E, Marcus MD, Epstein LH, Harvey J. Year-long weight loss treatment for obese patients with type II diabetes: does inclusion of an intermittent very low calorie diet improve outcome? *Am J Med.* 1994;97(4):354-362.

73. Centers for Disease Control and Prevention. *Physical Activity Guidelines for Americans: Adults.* Washington, DC: Centers for Disease Control and Prevention; 2008.

74. Berry D. An emerging model of behavior change in women maintaining weight loss. *Nurs Sci Q.* 2004;17(3):242-252.

75. Wing RR, Jeffery RW. Benefits of recruiting participants with friends and increasing social support for weight loss maintenance. *J Consult Clin Psychol.* 1999;67:132-138.

76. Rosenbloom AL, Silverstein JH. *Type 2 Diabetes in Children and Adolescents: A Guide to Diagnosis, Epidemiology, Pathogenesis, Prevention, and Treatment.* Alexandria, VA: American Diabetes Association; 2003.

77. American College of Sports Medicine. *Guidelines for Exercise Testing and Prescription.* 7th ed. New York, NY: Lippincott Williams and Wilkins; 2006.

78. Cowlin A. Women and exercise. In: Varney H, Kriebs JM, Gregor CL, eds. *Varney's Midwifery.* 4th ed. Sudbury, MA: Jones and Bartlett Publishers; 2004:187-247.

79. Gulati M, Shaw LJ, Thisted RA, Black HR, Merz CN, Arnsdorf MF. Heart rate response to exercise stress testing in asymptomatic women: the St. James Women Take Heart Project. *Circulation.* 2010;122:130-137.

80. Borg GV. Borg's perceived exertion chart. *Med Sci Sports Exerc.* 1982;14:377-387.

81. Jakicic JM, Winters C, Lang W, Wing RR. Effects of intermittent exercise and use of home exercise equipment on adherence, weight loss, and fitness in overweight women: a randomized trial. *JAMA.* 1999;266:1535-1542.

82. Jakicic JM, Wing RR, Butler BA, Robertson RJ. Prescribing exercise in multiple short bouts versus one continuous bout: effects on adherence, cardiorespiratory fitness, and weight loss in overweight women. *Int J Obes Relat Metab Disord.* 1995;19(12):893-901.

83. Schneider PL, Crouter SE, Bassett DR. Pedometer measures of free-living physical activity: comparison of 13 models. *Med Sci Sports Exerc.* 2004;36:331-335.

84. Eston R, Reilly T. *Kinanthropometry and Exercise Physiology Laboratory Manual: Tests, Procedures, and Data.* London, UK: Chapman & Hall; 1996.

85. Physicians Desk Reference Staff. *Nonprescription Drugs, Dietary Supplements and Herbs.* Montvale, NJ: Medical Economics Company; 2011.

86. Natural Medicines Comprehensive Database. Caffeine. Available at: http://naturaldatabase.therapeuticresearch.com/nd/Search.aspx?cs=SCHOOLNOPL%7EUMD&s=ND&pt=9&Product=caffeine. Accessed May 8, 2016.

87. Natural Medicines Comprehensive Database. Catechins. Available at: http://naturaldatabase.therapeuticresearch.com/nd/Search.aspx?cs=SCHOOLNOPL-UMD&s=ND&pt=100&id=960&ds=&name=Epigallo+Catechin+Gallate+(GREEN+TEA)&searchid=45847224. Accessed May 8, 2016.

88. Natural Medicines Comprehensive Database. Garcinia. Available at: http://naturaldatabase.therapeuticresearch.com/nd/Search.aspx?cs=SCHOOLNOPL-UMD&s=nd&pt=100&id=818. Accessed May 8, 2016.

89. Natural Medicines Comprehensive Database. Chromium. Available at: http://naturaldatabase.thera peuticresearch.com/nd/Search.aspx?cs=SCHOOL NOPL-UMD&s=nd&pt=100&id=932. Accessed May 8, 2016.

90. Natural Medicines Comprehensive Database. HMB (Hydroxymethylbutyrate). Available at: http://natural database.therapeuticresearch.com/nd/Search.aspx? cs=SCHOOLNOPL-UMD&s=ND&pt=9& Product=hmb&btnSearch.x=0&btnSearch.y=0. Accessed May 8, 2016.

91. Natural Medicnes Comprehensive Database. Chitosan. Available at: http://naturaldatabase.therapeuti-cresearch.com/nd/Search.aspx?cs=SCHOOLNO PL-UMD&s=nd&pt=100&id=625. Accessed May 8, 2016.

92. US Food and Drug Administration. Xenical: Full Prescribing Information. Available at: http://www.accessdata.fda.gov/drugsatfda_docs/label /2013/020766s033lbl.pdf. Accessed May 8, 2016.

93. Vivus. Qysmia: Full Prescribing Information. Available at: https://www.qsymia.com/pdf/prescribing-information.pdf. Accessed May 8, 2016.

94. Maggard MA, Shugarman LR, Suttorp M, Maglione M, Sugerman HJ, Livingston EH, et al. Meta-analysis: surgical treatment of obesity. *Ann Intern Med.* 2005;142(7):547-559.

95. Gloy VL, Briel M, Bhatt DL, Kashyap SR, Schauer PR, Mingrone G, et al. Bariatric surgery versus non-surgical treatment for obesity: a systematic review and meta-analysis of randomised controlled trials. *BMJ.* 2013;347:f5934.

96. Lavazzo CR, ed. *Bariatric Surgery: From Indications to Postoperative Care (Surgery Procedures, Complications and Results).* Hauppauge, NY: Nova Science Publishers; 2013.

97. Buchwald H, Oien DM. Metabolic/bariatric surgery worldwide 2008. *Obes Surg.* 2009;19(12): 1605-1611.

98. Thomas JG, Wing RR. Maintenance of long-term weight loss. *Med Health R I.* 2009;92(2):56-57.

99. Kriebs J. Obesity in pregnancy: addressing risks to improve outcomes. *J Perinat Neonat Nurs.* 2014;28: 32-4082.

100. Institute of Medicine. *Weight Gain During Pregnancy: Reexamining the Guidelines.* Washington, DC: National Academies Press; 2009.

101. National Academy of Sciences. *Nutrition During Pregnancy: Weight Gain and Nutrient Supplements.* Washington, DC: National Academy Press; 1990.

102. Kominiarek MA, Seligman NS, Dolin C, Gao W, Berghella V, Hoffman M, et al. Gestational weight gain and obesity: is 20 pounds too much? *Am J Obstet Gynecol.* 2013;209:214.e1-e11.

103. Oken E, Rifas-Shiman SL, Field AE, Frazier AL, Gillman MW. Maternal gestational weight gain and offspring weight in adolescence. *Obstet Gynecol.* 2008;112(5):1-8.

104. American College of Obstetricians and Gynecologists. Committee Opinion No. 650: Physical Activity and Exercise During Pregnancy and the Postpartum Period. *Obstet Gynecol.* 2015 Dec;126(6):e135-e142. doi:10.1097/AOG.0000000000001214.

105. Artal R, Clapp JF, Vigil DV. Exercise during pregnancy: ACSM current comment. Indianapolis, IN: American College of Sports Medicine; 2013. Available at: https://www.acsm.org/docs/current-comments/exerciseduringpregnancy.pdf. Accessed May 8, 2016.

106. American College of Obstetricians and Gynecologists. Committee Opinion No. 549. Obesity in pregnancy. *Obstet Gynecol.* 2013;121:213-217.

107. Coleman E. *Exercise and Fitness.* Ashland, OR: Nutrition Dimension; 1990.

108. Convertino VA, Armstrong LE, Coyle EF, Mack GW, Sawka MN, Senay LC, Jr, et al. American College of Sports Medicine position stand. Exercise and fluid replacement. *Med Sci Sports Exerc.* 1996;28(1):i-vii.

CHAPTER 19

BREAST HEALTH AND DISEASE

Jan M. Kriebs

Women often present with breast concerns in the ambulatory setting, and these often relate to perceived risk of cancer. In fact, women are more likely to die of complications related to obesity, diabetes, and hypertension than of breast cancer. Many times, women are experiencing symptoms caused by normal hormone fluctuations or other benign changes. These range from normal adolescent development to cyclic mastalgia and fibrocystic changes (FCCs) to adenomas. However, some presentations are serious and may indicate breast cancer.

In primary care, conversations regarding breast awareness and normal changes are part of health promotion. Helping women understand their specific risks, the role of genetic risk, the effectiveness of screening and diagnostic techniques, benefits of treating confirmed disease, and lifetime cancer prevalence are important components of providing exemplary care to women of all ages. Primary care providers are called upon to screen, evaluate, and manage benign breast symptoms, and to manage general breast health including recommendations for breast examination, mammography, genetic counseling, and

other diagnostic tools as appropriate. They are responsible for ordering tests, explaining their results, and for coordinating care between women and breast specialists for invasive procedures such as fine-needle aspiration (FNA), biopsy, and surgery. This chapter presents the background needed by women's health providers to provide care for women with breast-related concerns.

Breast Development and Anatomy

Breast development begins in utero, with the formation of the mammary ridge, external nipples, and milk ducts. Until puberty, the breast tissue remains basically unchanged. The stages of breast development are described by Tanner staging, named for the pediatric endocrinologist who first consolidated descriptions of male and female sexual maturation (**Table 19-1**). Thelarche (breast development) begins at age 8.8 years on average in African American girls, 9.3 years in Hispanic ethnic girls, and 9.7 years in whites and Asians.[1] Body mass index (BMI) also influences onset of breast

Table 19-1 Tanner Staging of the Female Breast

Stage 1 Nipple tip is raised above skin (prepubescent).

Stage 2 Breast bud appears, raising the breast and nipple above the chest wall; the areola darkens and becomes more prominent.

Stage 3 Glandular tissue develops, increasing breast size.

Stage 4 Nipple and areola form a separate mound above the breast.

Stage 5 Mature breast shape emerges with prominent nipple above areola, which forms part of the rounded breast.

development, with higher BMI (> 85 percentile) associated with earlier development. The average age at thelarche is decreasing among white, non-Hispanic girls and appears to be associated with increasing BMI.[1] Endocrine-disrupting chemicals have been associated with disruption of pubertal development and timing.[2,3] The complex interactions of variation in exposures and timing make this a difficult area to study.

Under the influence of estrogen from the maturing ovaries, breast connective tissue begins to accumulate fat tissue- at the same time that the milk glands are maturing. Adolescent breasts tend to be dense, with predominant glandular tissue and minimal fat deposits. Often, breast development is associated with complaints of breast tenderness and with asymmetric changes as the breasts mature. Girls can be reassured that in most cases, when they are fully developed, their breasts will be similar in size and shape. Fibroadenomas (FAs) commonly develop in late adolescence and may cause anxiety, but breast cancers are rare in this age group.[4]

The mature breast is supported within two layers of fascia—one subcutaneous and one next to the chest wall. *Cooper's ligaments* weave between the lobes connecting the two layers of fascia to provide breast support. Lymphatic drainage is primarily to the axillary lymph nodes. The functional glandular tissue is clustered behind

the nipple, with multiple small lobules ending in alveoli. The milk ducts reach into the glandular tissue, drawing milk to the nipple during lactation. Most women have 5–9 ductules opening into each nipple (**Figure 19-1**). The majority of women have nipples that rise above the surrounding areola and become firm and erect with arousal or during nursing. Some women have nipples that lie flat against the areola and display minimal erection, or that are inverted (**Figure 19-2**). The areola contains the *Montgomery's tubercles*, sebaceous glands that provide lubrication for the nipple and have been reported to produce olfactory cues for the nursing infant.[5]

During pregnancy the breast enlarges with the development of the milk supply and may become tender. The breasts may begin to leak colostrum prior to birth. After childbirth and weaning, many mothers will note that their breasts are smaller and softer, as well as having less structural support than before breastfeeding. This can be an effect of increased relaxin secretion and increased breast weight during pregnancy. Other factors associated with breast sagging include advancing age, significant weight loss, higher BMI, larger breast size, number of pregnancies, and smoking. Breastfeeding, prenatal weight gain, and lack of exercise were not associated with breast sagging in these studies.[6,7]

Figure 19-1 Anatomy of the female breast.

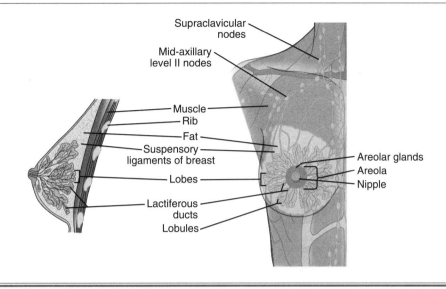

Figure 19-2 Appearance of the female nipple.

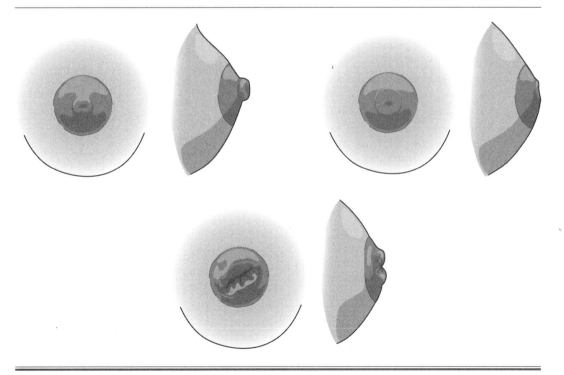

As women age, the relative proportion of fat in the breast tissue increases as the glandular component shrinks. With menopause, skin thinning and loss of elasticity may lead to visible changes in the texture of the skin.

Epidemiology of Common Breast Conditions

As women move through the reproductive years and into their elder years, breast symptomatology changes and with it the risk of various conditions. Benign breast disease can be sorted into four categories: nonproliferative, proliferative without atypia, atypical proliferative disease, and a group of miscellaneous problems. As women age, the risk of breast cancer increases.

Benign Breast Conditions

Among benign conditions, FCC is the most common. It was historically called fibrocystic disease, until researchers identified a prevalence of greater than 50% in reproductive-aged women on examination and greater than 90% on histology. It is most common among women 20–50 years of age.[8] Given the frequency of occurrence, it is easier to cite protective factors, which include combined hormonal contraceptives and menopause, than risk factors. The use of hormone replacement therapy (HRT) post-menopause may cause a recurrence of clinical symptoms in affected women. Similarly, the prevalence of discrete breast cysts is highest in adult women ages 20–50 years. During the peak age range of 35–50 years, as many as one-third of all women will have at least 1 cyst. FA is the most common breast tumor in women under the age of 30. FA, a form of proliferative breast disease, peaks at a slightly younger age, between 15 and 35 years, with a 25% prevalence.[8] Complex or multiple FAs are linked to a slightly higher risk of breast cancer.

Breast Cancer

Ninety-nine percent of breast cancer diagnoses occur in women. In 2015, the estimate for new diagnoses of any breast cancer in the United States was 231,840, based on prior data and population age.[9] Risk factors for cancer are shown in Table 19-2. As our understanding of the interactions of genetics, lifestyle, and the environment increases, this list becomes longer. In contrast, an active lifestyle and healthy weight as well as prolonged breastfeeding may decrease risk. Table 19-3 shows the relative incidence of breast cancer by age.[9] Figure 19-3 shows the distribution of these

Table 19-2 Risk Factors for Breast Cancer

Female sex

Increasing age

White and black race, as compared to Asian, Native American, or Hispanic

Obesity

Alcohol use

Tobacco exposure

Lack of regular exercise

Radiation therapy of the chest for Hodgkin's lymphoma

Early menarche

Late menopause

Delayed or absent childbearing

Limited or absent breastfeeding

Use of hormone replacement therapy

Dense breasts

Proliferative breast disease

First-degree family history of breast cancer

BRCA1 or BRCA2 gene mutations

Personal history of breast cancer

Personal history of ovarian or colon cancer

Table 19-3 Rate of Invasive Breast Cancer Diagnoses by Age, Among US Women 2009–2011

Birth–49 years	1.9%	(1 in 53)
50–59 years	2.3%	(1 in 44)
60–69 years	3.5%	(1 in 29)
70+ years	6.7%	(1 in 15)
Lifetime risk	12.3%	(1 in 8)

Data from Siegel RL, Miller KD, Jemal A. Cancer statistics, 2015. *CA Cancer J Clin.* 2015;65:5-29. doi:10.3322/caac.21254.

diagnoses for black and white women by age.[10] The National Cancer Institute's (NCI's) Surveillance, Epidemiology, and End Results (SEER) Program website provides additional information on cancer epidemiology.[11]

The estimate of deaths from breast cancer for 2015 was 40,290, about 29% of all cancer deaths in women.[10] It is only between the ages of 20 and 60 years, a group for whom the frequency of disease is relatively lower, that breast cancer is the most common cause of cancer death in women. At both younger and older ages, diseases of the lung are more common. **Figure 19-4** shows relative mortality rates by race and age. Note that although rates of breast cancer are higher among white women, African Americans have higher mortality both overall and at younger ages.

Five-year breast cancer survival rates among white women are 92%; among black women, the rate is significantly lower at 80%.[9] Increased cancer mortality among black women has been associated with delay in diagnosis to a later disease stage and inadequate or delayed treatment; in other words, the mortality rate is associated with healthcare access barriers.[12] However, studies have found that even when controlling for social and economic risk factors, black women have higher rates of more aggressive tumors.[12-14] The

counseling and decisions that are part of a screening program are discussed in the section on breast cancer screening, later in this chapter.

Essential History, Physical, and Laboratory Evaluation

Breast examination is a key part of a woman's health examination. Beyond that, women themselves are commonly the first to notice a breast abnormality. In a study of women under the age of 40 years, 80% of masses were self-identified, while the other 20% were first discovered during an office visit.[15] Women also commonly seek care for other changes such as nipple discharge and breast pain. A thorough evaluation of these problems is dependent on understanding the normal physiologic changes that occur over time, characteristics of various breast-related problems, and particular patient profiles that raise concern.

A note of caution is warranted when interpreting clinical and test results: Many of the benign conditions have a spectrum of disease that ranges from no additional cancer risk to a multiple-fold risk or have symptoms that suggest systemic disease. Age, family history, and other factors also play a role in interpreting these results. For example, FCCs may mask a developing mass; galactorrhea may be a result of prolonged breastfeeding or a symptom of pituitary tumor. When in doubt, a breast specialist should be involved in care at an early stage.

History

Breast evaluation is an excellent example of the importance of genetic and reproductive screening during the health history. The personal history related to breast disease includes age at menarche (and menopause when relevant), use of hormonal contraception, parity and age at first birth, breastfeeding duration, mammography or breast sonography or magnetic resonance

Figure 19-3 Incidence of breast cancer by age.

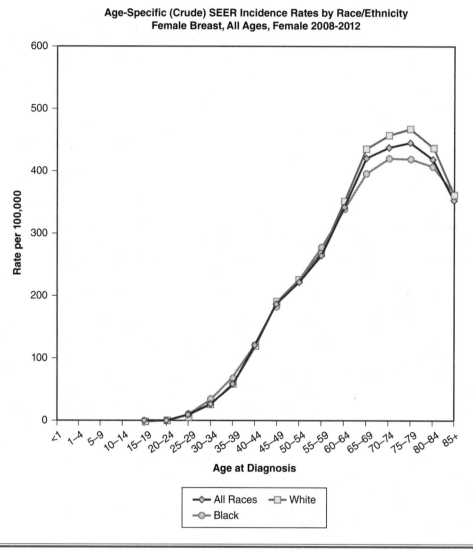

Age-Specific (Crude) SEER Incidence Rates by Race/Ethnicity
Female Breast, All Ages, Female 2008-2012

imaging (MRI), and any breast injuries, infections, nipple discharge, or masses. Prior diagnoses of breast diseases and conditions must be obtained. The surgical history for women includes asking specifically about breast biopsy or aspiration, any surgery to augment or reduce breast size, and removal of any mass. The family history of cancer should be detailed for both

Figure 19-4 Age- and race-specific mortality for breast cancer in women 2008–2012.

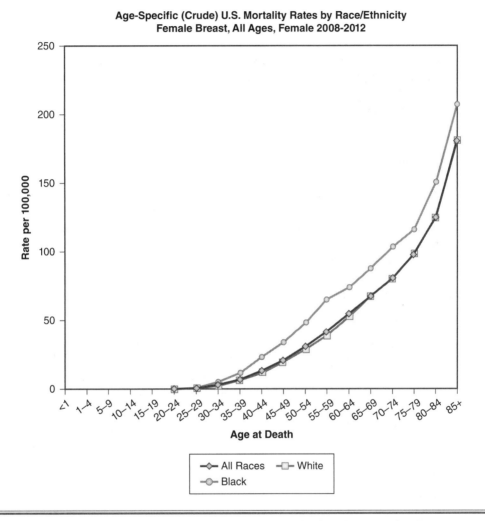

Reproduced from National Cancer Institute. Surveillance, Epidemiology, and End Results Program. http://seer
.cancer.gov/faststats/selections.php?series=cancer. n.d. Accessed May 8, 2016.

maternal and paternal relatives. Familial breast and ovarian cancer links through inherited genetic mutations have been well studied.[16] Early-onset prostate and colon cancer have also been proposed as sharing genetic risks, although the association is not well demonstrated, particularly for colon cancer.[16-18]

When a chief complaint is related to the breast or when the review of symptoms elicits a current breast complaint, detailed questions should be asked. Even if the woman has not expressed concerns, a clinical finding on examination elicits the same queries. For a breast mass, these include the onset, duration, whether cyclic or constant, any related pain or tenderness, and any change in size or in the appearance of the breast.

If a woman reports breast tenderness, inquiries should be made regarding onset, frequency, and area of concern. Whether there is an association to the menstrual cycle is important. Some women experience physiologic tenderness during the luteal phase as a result of gonadotropin effects on the mammary lobules, stroma, and ducts. While pregnancy and lactation also can cause physiologic breast tenderness, childbearing women should be screened for signs of mastitis when complaining of breast tenderness, nipple pain, or inflammation.

Nipple discharge can be physiologic or pathologic. History and symptoms specific to breast discharge include onset, color, and characteristics; the amount of discharge; whether the discharge is continuous or intermittent; whether both breasts are affected; and whether a mass is present. The provider should also determine if the discharge is spontaneous or if it must be expressed and if only one or many ducts are affected. To be significant, a discharge should be true, spontaneous, persistent, and not associated with lactation. It can be milky, multicolored and sticky, purulent, clear (watery), yellow (serous), pink (serosanguineous), or bloody (sanguineous). Purulent, bloody, or serosanguineous discharge is always pathologic and requires further evaluation. **Table 19-4** provides some differential diagnoses associated with common signs and symptoms.

Physical Examination

Clinical breast examination (CBE) is detailed in the appendix to this chapter. Examination includes observation of the woman sitting erect and with arms at her waist. The breasts are then observed while the patient is still sitting and leaning forward to see if there is any area that is attached to the wall of the chest. Upon inspection, whether sitting or supine, the following should be noted: size and symmetry of the breasts, contour (masses, dimpling, or retraction), edema, venous pattern, and the shape and size of the nipples as well as any lesions or discharge on the nipples.

Next, examination requires flattening the breast tissue against the woman's chest while she is in a supine position. This is of particular importance for the woman with larger breasts. To palpate the lateral portion of the large-breasted woman, having her roll onto her contralateral hip and rotate her shoulder back while placing her hand on her forehead allows for the best flattening of the tissue. To examine the medial portion of the breast, the woman should rest flat on her back so that the breast falls laterally in the larger breasted woman.

Upon finding an area that is clearly suspicious or even mildly suspicious, careful documentation is necessary; it should describe the characteristics of the area of concern and whether similar findings are present in the opposite breast. It is often helpful to draw the lesion on a schematic of the breast, including descriptors such as size, shape, and other qualities (i.e., cystic or solid, solitary, discrete, firm, hard, sensitive or not).

Breast masses are more difficult to discern during pregnancy and lactation because of the normal physiologic changes. There is increased glandular and areolar development, an overall increase in the parenchymal-to-adipose tissue ratio, and an increase in vascular flow. A lactating woman presenting with a mass is more likely to have a benign problem such as mastitis or a galactocele than cancer.

Laboratory and Imaging

The clinical evaluation of breast abnormalities is more likely to require imaging, an aspiration, or biopsy than laboratory testing. However, specific

Table 19-4 Breast Symptoms as Diagnostic Features

Symptom	Associated Findings	Possible Diagnoses
Swelling	Cyclic premenstrual	Normal hormonal change
	Lactation	Fullness before nursing, engorgement
Breast pain	Lactation	Engorgement, clogged duct, mastitis
	Nonlactating	Mastalgia (may be cyclic), Mondor's disease
Nipple pain	Lactation	Early lactation, normal finding
		After lactation established: fungal infection of nipple, improper latch, irritation or cracking, Raynaud's
	Nonlactating	Eczema, dermatitis, Paget disease
Nipple scaling		Eczema, Paget disease
Nipple discharge	Milky	Galactorrhea
	Dark green or black	Draining cyst, inflamed duct or ductal ectasia
	Bloody	Ductal carcinoma in situ, nipple injury
Skin texture changes	Generalized erythema, shiny	Engorgement (lactation only)
	Focal edema or redness	Mastitis, inflammatory breast cancer
	Peau d'orange	Mondor's disease, inflammatory breast cancer
Increased vascularity	Lactation	Normal increased blood supply for milk production
	Nonlactating	Breast cancer
Mass or lump	Cyclic	Fibrocystic changes, cyst
	Noncyclic	Cyst, fibroadenoma, lymph node, breast cancer
	Subcutaneous cord	Mondor's disease
	Lactation	Infectious mastitis, clogged ducts, galactocele
Nodularity		Fibrocystic changes, multiple cysts or fibroadenomas
Inflammation	Localized	Mastitis, breast abscess, inflammatory breast cancer
	Generalized	Engorgement

findings may require laboratory confirmation. These include prolactin and thyroid levels when galactorrhea is present outside of the cycle of pregnancy and breastfeeding, and culture of breast discharge with mastitis. The practice of collecting a cytology specimen for breast discharge has been shown to have a high false-positive rate and poor sensitivity, and should not be used as a sole method of diagnosing abnormal discharge.[19]

Mammography is the current standard screening mechanism for breast cancer. Regulations under the Mammography Quality Standards Act (MQSA) define minimum quality standards and required training of the professionals who perform and interpret mammograms. The use of digital, rather than film, images has increased diagnostic accuracy for pre- and perimenopausal women who have denser breasts.[20] Although women may express concerns regarding radiation exposure, the total dose in a standard screening test is quite low in modern equipment. Mammography is also used, in conjunction with ultrasound, for the evaluation of benign breast masses and localization for aspiration or biopsy. Screening recommendations are discussed in the section of this chapter on breast cancer.

In a screening mammogram, each breast is compressed for two digital views: craniocaudal and lateral. Adequate compression is required for high-quality imaging, often leading to complaints from women about discomfort associated with the test. Calcifications, masses, and breast density are reported. Macrocalcifications are associated with age-related changes, inflammation, or breast injury. More than half of women over age 50 years have macrocalcifications, as do 10% of younger women. Microcalcifications are a greater concern; the number, shape, and location provide evidence to suggest cancer. Masses may be either cystic or solid. Density is described based on the proportions of fatty tissue to fibroglandular tissue.

About 10% of women having a mammogram will require further evaluation.[21] A diagnostic mammogram is ordered either to follow a suspicious screening test or to evaluate clinical findings. More views are taken and at different angles as well as magnification of a suspicious area. The diagnostic mammogram answers the question, "does this mass require a biopsy or is a follow-up diagnostic study sufficient?" A repeat study may be recommended in a certain period of time to show resolution, stability, or heightened concern that may require a biopsy. Mammogram reports are presented in terms of Breast Imaging Reporting and Data System (BI-RADS) categories. In addition to the categories shown in **Table 19-5**, they comment on breast density, masses, calcifications, and the appropriate interval for reevaluation.[22]

Breast ultrasound is used in conjunction with a mammogram for women with denser breasts and when it is necessary to evaluate whether a mass is solid or cystic. Simple cysts are diagnosed if four criteria are met: round or oval in shape, sharply defined margins, lack of internal echoes, and posterior acoustic enhancement. This technique can also be used to guide FNA or biopsy and to assess lymph nodes in the axilla. Although not as sensitive as MRI, it is relatively inexpensive, safe, and noninvasive. Ultrasound results are coded using the same BI-RADS terminology as mammograms.

MRI provides exquisitely detailed images of the breast tissue. It can be used to assess breast tumors identified on mammogram, may be used to support a needle biopsy, and can also be used

Table 19-5 BI-RADS Scoring

0   Incomplete exam; additional images or comparison to other prior studies are needed

1   Negative

2   Benign changes: a negative exam but with changes not associated with an increased risk of cancer such as simple cysts or macrocalcifications

3   Probably benign: < 2% chance that the findings indicate cancer, but need short-interval follow up (usually every 6 months for 2 years, to be sure the changes are stable)

4   Suspicious abnormality: sometimes further subdivided into a, b, c categories; indicates need for further evaluation, usually including biopsy

5   Highly suggestive of malignancy: > 95% chance of breast cancer, requires tissue diagnosis

6   Known biopsy-proven malignancy

Data from Sickles EA, D'Orsi CJ, Bassett LW, et al. ACR BI-RADS® Mammography. In: *ACR BI-RADS® Atlas, Breast Imaging Reporting and Data System.* Reston, VA: American College of Radiology; 2013; National Cancer Institute. Mammograms. Bethesda, MD: US Department of Health and Human Services. http://www.cancer.gov/types/breast/mammograms-fact-sheet#q6. 2014. Accessed July 14, 2016.

with mammography in high-risk women (> 20% lifetime risk) as part of their regularly scheduled testing. The false-positive rate (findings that suggest cancer turn out to be benign) is high enough that, coupled with cost, it is not in use as a screening methodology.

Other less common types of imaging may be ordered by breast specialists, such as thermal imaging or direct imaging of the ducts (galactogram, ductogram). Positron emission tomography (PET) and computerized axial tomography (CAT) may be used after breast cancer diagnosis to help identify metastasis.

Biopsies are performed for diagnosis of a palpable or sonographically localized mass. Of the 10% of women requiring further imaging after a screening mammogram, 8–10% will require biopsy to further assess a mass.[21] FNA and *core biopsy* (CB) can both be performed in a physician's office, if the provider has appropriate training and experience. FNA uses a narrow-gauge hollow needle to aspirate fluid or take a small tissue sample. CB collects a larger (up to 1/16-inch diameter) solid sample. A vacuum-assisted CB allows the provider to acquire a larger sample. FNA is most appropriately used when there is low suspicion of cancer in a symptomatic lesion; the advantages are less pain associated with the procedure and the possibility of same-day diagnosis if a cytopathologist is available. Further, if the ultrasound appearance is of a simple cyst, the fluid is nonbloody (either clear or greenish black), and the cyst resolves, then no further workup is necessary.[23,24] CB provides a sample large enough for both histology and receptor testing and should be used when there is a higher suspicion of cancer or FNA findings are inconclusive.[23]

An open or *excisional biopsy* is undertaken when complete removal of a mass is desired. Excisional biopsy provides a complete pathologic assessment. When the mass is not palpable on examination, stereotactic or ultrasound-guided biopsy or mammographic localization is used.

Historically, the recommendation has been to consider surgical excision for any lesion with a greater than 2% risk of breast cancer.[25] Lesions suspicious for malignancy are removed with at least a 1-cm margin, while lesions such as an FA need only minimal margins. The whole lesion is removed intact. Stereotactic biopsy uses *x*, *y*, and *z* coordinates on the mammogram to find a nonpalpable mass. After a benign breast biopsy report, women should have follow-up mammography. Some authors recommend increased surveillance at 6 months, but the most current evidence suggests that annual follow up is appropriate.[26,27]

The term *triple testing* is used to describe the combination of clinical evaluation, imaging, and biopsy (either FNA or CB). During biopsy, samples may have histologic and biochemical analyses, which may determine receptor status or markers for increased cancer risk.

Evaluation of Breast Masses in Pregnancy

The most common breast masses found during pregnancy are FA, lactating adenoma, cysts, infarctions, or galactocele.[28] Ultrasound is used as the initial imaging mode, and mammography for further evaluation, with appropriate shielding.[28,29] Mammograms are generally considered less sensitive because of increased breast density and other physiologic changes,[30] although a small study by Swinford and colleagues showed no increased mammographic density in half the pregnant women studied.[31] Regardless of whether a woman is pregnant or lactating, an ultrasound can tell the difference between a solid or cystic mass.[30] If strict BI-RADS scoring is used, ultrasound should be adequate with a BI-RADS score of 1 or 2; a BI-RADS score of 4 warrants biopsy to identify malignancies.[28] If the results are indeterminate or suspicious, a biopsy is performed to rule out malignancy. Contrast-enhanced MRI is not routinely used during pregnancy. The gadolinium contrast material crosses the placenta, although there is no evidence for teratogenicity.[32]

Classification and Management of Benign Breast Conditions

Breast conditions are typically divided into categories based on their characteristics and risk of subsequent development of breast cancer. The main classifications for benign disorders include: 1) nonproliferative, 2) proliferative without atypia, 3) and proliferative with atypia. These classifications are listed in **Table 19-6**. It should be noted that some authors assign specific conditions to different categories. For example, simple FAs may be placed in the nonproliferative category rather than all of these tumors being identified as proliferative, and some authors will not distinguish between mild ductal hyperplasia and moderate or florid hyperplasia. Some experts now include carcinoma in situ with malignancies. In addition, a group of other symptoms and infectious diseases is not covered by these categories but is of concern both to women and their practitioners. These include FCCs, mastalgia, breast asymmetry, breast discharge, mastitis, and unconfirmed masses.

Women's health clinicians need to arrange for consultation and referral for women with many of these findings. Counseling women with breast findings on examination is discussed later in this chapter.

Fibrocystic Breasts

As stated earlier, more than half of all women of reproductive age experience clinically apparent changes often described as nodularity, or "glandular" changes. These FCCs increase prior to the menstrual cycle and may be affected by hormonal

Table 19-6 Categories of Benign Breast Disease

Nonproliferative
  Apocrine metaplasia
  Cyst
  Fat necrosis
  Mammary duct ectasia
  Mild hyperplasia of the usual type
  Non-sclerosing adenosis
  Phylloides tumor, benign
  Solitary central papilloma
Proliferative lesions without atypia
  Fibroadenoma
  Lactating adenoma
  Moderate or florid ductal hyperplasia of the usual type
  Multiple papillomas
  Radial scars
  Sclerosing adenosis
Proliferative disease with atypia
  Atypical ductal hyperplasia (ADH)
  Atypical lobular hyperplasia (ALH)
  Lobular carcinoma in situ (LCIS)

contraception. The symptoms are typically bilateral. Women may complain of discrete cysts or of thickened, "lumpy" tissue; of increased pain or breast tenderness prior to menses; and occasionally of a dark nipple discharge. Tissue changes associated with FCC include cysts, fibrosis (flat, firm mats of scar-like fibrous tissue), ductal or lobular hyperplasia, calcifications, and adenosis (enlargement) of the breast lobules. FCCs are not associated with increased risk of breast cancer unless there are atypical changes associated with ductal or lobular hyperplasia. Guray and Sahin consider that because FCC incorporates many individual types of lesions, it ought to be assessed based on the specific characteristics of each woman as to whether it is nonproliferative, proliferative without atypia, or proliferative with atypia.[8] When symptoms such as discolored or bloody nipple discharge, cysts, or distortion of breast tissue are present in FCC, referral for further evaluation is prudent.

There is no specific treatment that is effective for management of FCC. The use of hormonal contraception may decrease symptoms, although there is not good evidence for their use. Decreased caffeine and dietary fat intake and smoking cessation have also been recommended. Vitamin E and evening primrose oil have been studied for relief of the associated cyclic mastalgia;[33] their use can be recommended, although, again, there is no definitive evidence. Over-the-counter nonsteroidal anti-inflammatory drugs (NSAIDs), acetaminophen, a supportive bra, and the application of mild heat may offer the best comfort.

Nonproliferative Changes

Nonproliferative lesions can occur anywhere in the breast, including the ducts, lobes, and stroma. They include cysts, papillary apocrine changes, apocrine metaplasia, ductal ectasia, and calcifications. Another benign inflammatory condition, fat necrosis, is sometimes included in this category, as are tumors such as hemangiomas and lipomas. Nonproliferative changes are not considered to greatly increase risk of subsequent breast cancer, although women with a first-degree relative with breast cancer are at higher risk, even if their current findings are nonproliferative.[34] In an evaluation that combined nonproliferative and proliferative lesions without atypia, Wang and colleagues reported a relative risk (RR) of developing breast cancer for all women of 1.60 (95% confidence interval [CI] 1.17–2.19), increasing to an RR of 1.95 (95% CI 1.29–2.93) for women over 50 years.[35] Similarly, the meta-analysis by

Dyrstad and colleagues reported an RR for women with nonproliferative disease of 1.76 (95% CI 1.58–1.95).[36]

Cysts

Breast cysts are round or ovoid, fluid-filled epithelial structures that form in the terminal duct of breast lobules following an obstruction. The incidence has been reported to be between 25% and 47% in different series, and the nonclinical incidence (cysts too small or asymptomatic to attract attention) may be much higher.[37,38] They respond to the hormonal changes of the menstrual cycle; women may notice both increasing size and tenderness prior to the menses. They may be singular or multiple and are frequently bilateral. Palpable macrocysts may be ≥ 2.5 mm and can be identified on ultrasound with 98% accuracy.[39] Although peak incidence is among women 35–50 years of age, postmenopausal women, particularly those using hormone replacement, may also have palpable cysts.[37] On examination, cysts palpate as smooth, movable, clearly defined lesions, which may or may not be painful. Normal cyst fluid is clear, cloudy, and yellow or green in color.

If cysts are large, painful, or concerning to the woman, they can be managed by sonographic confirmation and FNA to remove the fluid. For simple cysts, this is the only required treatment unless the cyst recurs. Cysts that persist and grow in size require further evaluation, as do cysts treated with FNA if bloody fluid is obtained or if the mass has solid portions. Thick walls, septations, partially solid masses, and internal nodules are atypical findings and classified as BI-RADS 4 (suspicious).[37,40] Cysts that have thick walls and are hyperechoic on ultrasound have a 10-fold increase in risk of breast cancer.[41] These cysts and those with atypical cells on aspiration should not be followed with short-interval imaging, but have excisional biopsy.[38,42]

PHYLLODES TUMOR (BENIGN)

Phyllodes tumors (also called phylloides tumors) are a mixture of stroma and glandular tissue, sometimes mistaken for FA on clinical examination. They make up less than 1% of all breast masses. The most common timing of occurrence is in women between 30 and 50 years of age; in one series, average age at diagnosis was 39.7, with a range from 14–71 years.[43] Phyllodes tumors are more common among Hispanic women.[44] Although benign phyllodes tumors are considered a nonproliferative finding, rates of malignancy associated with phyllodes tumors range up to 16% in different populations.[44-46] Diagnosis with a sampling biopsy may not adequately describe the mass. Excisional biopsy is necessary to eliminate the risk of a malignant tumor and to prevent recurrence.

FAT NECROSIS

Fat necrosis is a benign inflammatory response in fatty breast tissue. It is most common in midlife and in older women, with an overall incidence of 2.75% of breast masses.[47] It is commonly seen in the subareolar region or in superficial tissue. The presentation can range from firm, smooth nodules to irregular, fixed masses. Skin or nipple retraction may be present. On imaging, its appearance can be confused with malignancies; CB or excision is required to confirm the diagnosis.[48]

MAMMARY DUCT ECTASIA

Duct ectasia occurs most commonly in perimenopausal women, when the ductal opening is widened and the walls thicken. The ductules of the breast fill with desquamated ductal epithelium and secretory proteinaceous contents, which may produce a black or green nipple discharge. Skin bacteria collecting in the duct may cause mastitis, leading to swelling, pain, and malaise. The most common bacteria found are *Staphylococcus aureus* and *Staphylococcus epidermidis*.[49] Nipple or skin changes may be noted if the underlying inflammation causes retraction. Often, duct ectasia is an incidental finding on a mammogram. Biopsy may be needed to distinguish mammary duct ectasia from cancer if tissue scarring creates a hard, irregular lump. Peripheral placement, irregular margin of the duct, and a focal thickening increase the likelihood of malignancy.[50] Women can be counseled to wear a supportive bra and use heat, positioning, and mild pain relievers as needed for discomfort. Smoking cessation should be recommended, because there is a positive association between current smoking and symptoms of ductal ectasia.[51]

OTHER NONPROLIFERATIVE CONDITIONS

Mild hyperplasia of the usual type refers to an overgrowth of the cells that line either the milk ducts or lobules. Typically, ducts have 2 layers of epithelial cells; in mild hyperplasia 1–2 additional layers are present.[39] It may be seen on mammogram. On microscopic examination, the cells appear normal. Mild hyperplasia of the usual type is not associated with breast cancer.

Non-sclerosing adenosis refers to an increase in the glandular tissue within breast lobules, without tissue scarring. When seen on mammography, the calcifications may make it difficult to distinguish from breast cancer. It is found on biopsies of fibrocystic breast changes.

Apocrine metaplasia is the overgrowth of columnar secretory apocrine cells in the lining of microcysts or acini. These cell types are normally found in the axillary sweat glands and the periareolar glands. It is a common finding in fibrocystic breasts, particularly in women over 25 years—so much so that some authors consider this a normal finding. As an isolated finding, it is not associated with breast cancer.[52] *Papillary apocrine change* refers to further development of the metaplasia (three or more cell thickness) without associated cellular atypia. [52]

A *solitary central papilloma* is a wart-like tumor of the terminal milk duct containing both glandular and fibrovascular features. It may be associated with a unilateral clear or bloody discharge. If palpable, it is felt as a small lesion behind the nipple. Diagnosis by biopsy or ductogram is followed by excision of the mass.

Calcifications are small calcium deposits within the breast. Although microcalcifications may appear as an indicator of increased cancer risk, they are also seen in a number of benign conditions. In addition, the majority of women over 50 will have macrocalcifications. The appearance, number, and distribution are used to stratify risk on imaging.[53] On mammography, calcifications are described both by appearance and distribution. The appearance of benign calcifications may be as a thin, shell-like rim around a cyst; popcorn-shaped deposits in a degenerating FA; or linear or rod-shaped or "milk of calcium" teacup-shaped deposits inside a cyst. Fine linear or amorphous calcifications are more likely to suggest malignancy.[54]

Proliferative Lesions Without Atypia

Proliferative lesions are those that have grown beyond what is considered normal and are characterized by a tendency to bridge and distend the involved tissue. As a group, proliferative disease without atypia is thought to indicate a 1.5–2-fold greater risk of breast cancer than that of a woman without breast changes.[55,56] Dyrstad and colleagues' recent meta-analysis gave an RR for the class of 1.76 (95% CI 1.58–1.95). This type of lesion includes FA, moderate or florid usual ductal hyperplasia, intraductal papilloma, sclerosing adenosis, radial scars, and lactating adenoma.[36]

Fibroadenoma (FA)

FAs develop within the breast lobules and contain both epithelial and stromal cells; they present as hyperplastic breast lobules and are considered to be an aberration of normal development and involution. The prevalence, including asymptomatic lesions, is 25%.[57] Clinical FAs are more common among African American women. The peak incidence is in women 20–30 years of age, and they often develop during adolescence. Adolescent women with FA can be reassured that they resolve in up to 40% of cases. Given the very low incidence of breast cancer in this population, they can be followed clinically unless the mass is large or rapidly progressing.[58]

Clinically, FAs are firm, soft mobile lesions found either as a result of breast self-awareness that brings a woman in for evaluation or as an examination finding. Most are 2–3 cm when found on examination. Giant FAs are 10 cm in diameter, more likely to appear in late adolescence, and more likely to continue rapid expansion.[8] Approximately 20% of women will have multiple or bilateral lesions.[8] *Juvenile FA* is a term given to rapidly expanding lesions seen in adolescents.

Evaluation of FA includes observation through an entire menstrual cycle, to confirm persistence (as opposed to cyclic FCC); in young women ultrasound is the preferred imaging. On ultrasound, FAs appear as round or oval, circumscribed, homogenous, solid masses with low-level internal echoes in a uniform distribution and intermediate acoustic attenuation.[59] Particularly for adolescents, MRI and mammography have limited utility secondary to breast density in this population.[58] Stable masses that do not demonstrate other abnormalities on imaging can be followed conservatively, with or without confirmatory biopsy.

Simple single FA is unlikely to substantially increase cancer risk. CB can confirm the nature of the lesion, and it can rule out atypia and other diagnoses such as phylloides that can be confused on examination. Even enlarging lesions with no atypia on biopsy can be followed conservatively if the woman prefers.[60] However, approximately 50% of FAs contain other proliferative tissue, such as sclerosing adenosis or ductal hyperplasia.[8] Kabat and colleagues found a relative increase of 1.74 (CI: 0.94–3.22) in breast cancer risk with complex FA without atypia.[55] Dupont and colleagues found a relative breast cancer risk of 3.10 (95% CI, 1.9–5.1) among patients with complex FAs that remained elevated over time; those at highest risk had additional proliferative breast changes or a family history of breast cancer.[61] Reports by Nassar and colleagues[62] and by Collins and colleagues[63] also showed that a family history and additional atypical findings associated with complex FA increased long-term risk of cancer.

Criteria for excisional biopsy include age over 35 years, poorly circumscribed or immobile masses on examination, inconclusive biopsy, and size > 2.5 cm, because these characteristics may indicate more aggressive disease.[42,64] Cryoablation is a newer technique available for triple-testing negative FA that conserves the appearance of the breast.[65] Women nearing menopause with stable FA that is triple-testing confirmed may be counseled that menopause will likely lead to involution of the mass as her hormonal status changes.[64]

OTHER PROLIFERATIVE CONDITIONS WITHOUT ATYPIA

Moderate and florid *ductal epithelial hyperplasia of the usual type* (without atypia) are variants of proliferative lesions in which there is an increased number of cells relative to what is normally seen above the basement membrane. They have an increased risk of invasive breast cancer of between 0.5 and 2 times normal. Moderate hyperplasia is

present when there are 3 more than the expected layers of cells above the basement membrane; with florid hyperplasia, 70% of the duct lumen is involved.

Multiple *intraductal papillomas* may appear as multiple formations in the smaller peripheral ducts or as diffuse areas of papillomatosis. When they are multiple, they are more peripheral, more bilateral, and appear to be more susceptible to malignant transformation. Diagnosis is by ductogram or biopsy. Treatment involves removal of the associated duct structures.

Lactating adenoma is a rare presentation demonstrated as a small, firm, mobile mass noted during pregnancy or the postpartum period. These are well-differentiated benign tumors of secretory mammary epithelium. They are thought to occur either as a new pregnancy stimulated change or when a preexisting tubular adenoma or FA develops morphologic changes resulting from the physiologic state of pregnancy. Sonogram evaluation as soon as possible after identification followed by FNA is a preferred method for evaluation. In most cases, the mass will resolve spontaneously. Large or rapidly growing tumors will require excision.[66,67]

Radial scars, also called complex sclerosing lesions, are rare lesions diagnosed on mammogram or biopsy specimens. The name *radial scar* derives from the appearance of the cells when stained. Their imaging appearance is not distinct from the appearance of breast cancer. Work by King and colleagues had suggested that if a radial scar was an incidental finding on biopsy (i.e., not seen mammographically), then the risk of cancer was low.[68] However, other reports have suggested that relying on biopsy to exclude cancer underestimates the actual incidence of coexisting breast cancer, and all such lesions should have complete excisional biopsy.[69,70] A Mayo Clinic study found an RR of 1.99 (95% CI 1.49–2.61) for breast cancer associated with a radial scar found with a biopsy and recommended against excision, given that this risk is similar to the risk with other proliferative types. This decision should be made between the woman and the breast specialist to whom she is referred.[71]

Sclerosing adenosis is a proliferation of glandular and stromal elements that enlarges and distorts the lobular units and is associated with diffuse calcifications. It may be palpable or a finding on mammography. The scarring of fibrous tissue is the distinguishing factor that makes this a proliferative condition. The risk of cancer is commonly reported to be 1.5–2 times that of unaffected women. Biopsy is generally required to differentiate sclerosing adenosis from cancer; even then, histologic changes may make the diagnosis difficult.[8,21]

Proliferative Lesions with Atypia—Hyperplasia and Carcinoma In Situ

Atypical hyperplasia (AH) can occur either in the ducts (atypical ductal hyperplasia, ADH) or in the lobules (atypical lobular hyperplasia, ALH) of the breast. In this type of hyperplastic cellular growth, cell structure becomes distorted. Both ADH and ALH are typically diagnosed on biopsy after CBE or mammography; the lesion is identified in about 8–10% of post-mammography samples.[72] When biopsy results show AH, women have an RR risk of breast cancer 4–5 times that of other women.[56] Dyrstad and colleagues give an RR for AH, not otherwise specified, as 3.93 (95% CI 3.24–4.76).[36] Kabat and colleagues placed the risk in premenopausal women under 50 even higher, with an RR greater than 7.[55] Risk factors for progression to cancer include younger age, those with multiple foci of atypia, and those with less age-related lobular involution.[72] Women with AH, multiple foci of atypia, and the presence of

histologic calcifications may be at very high risk (> 50% risk at 20 years), regardless of family history.[73]

The current recommendation of the National Comprehensive Cancer Network for ADH is complete surgical excision with a wide margin.[74] This recommendation is based on rates of upgrading the diagnosis to ductal carcinoma in situ (DCIS) or invasive cancer at the time of surgery, ranging from 15–30%.[75]

ALH and *lobular carcinoma in situ* (LCIS) together are described as lobular neoplasia (LN). In contrast to ADH, there has not been consensus on the best way to manage these lesions. Despite their status as potential precursor lesions for breast cancer, there has not been a consistent recommendation for excision. One recent study places the likelihood of upgrading an LN to breast cancer at about 3% (95% CI, 0–9%) if the histology on biopsy agreed with mammographic findings, but 38% (95% CI, 9–76%) if they did not agree.[76] Lewis and colleagues reported on findings after excision of LN that included upgrading previously identified lesions in 8% of ALH and 19% of LCIS cases.[77] Hartmann and colleagues point out that the risk among women with ALH is highest within the first 5 years and includes risk of both DCIS and more advanced cancers.[75] Data show that LCIS progresses to breast cancer at rates similar to those for ductal disease.[78,79] Taken together these data suggest that women with LN should be counseled carefully about both the risks and benefits of complete excisional biopsy (lumpectomy).[75] Although excision is currently the standard for all women, there are trials of close follow up for the women with lowest risk of progression.[75,80] The use of prophylactic medications to prevent breast cancer—selective estrogen receptor modulators (SERM) and aromatase inhibitors (AI)—is an option. When data for women with a history of AH were analyzed separately in trials, use of hormonal therapy showed risk reduction of 41–79%.[6]

DUCTAL CARCINOMA IN SITU (DCIS)

DCIS in situ is either a cancer precursor lesion or an early malignancy occurring inside of the milk ducts and confined to that space. If DCIS and LCIS were considered as cancers rather than precursors, as some experts now suggest, DCIS would comprise 15–20% of that larger number of malignancies. Although it may present with a small nodular lump or bloody unilateral nipple discharge, it is most commonly found on screening mammogram. A cluster of irregular microcalcifications is an indication for further evaluation for DCIS.

The current age-adjusted incidence rate of DCIS is 32.5 per 100,000 women. Incidence rates are highest among women 50–64 years of age. The prevalence is highest among white women. Long-term outcomes are worse when DCIS is diagnosed based on symptoms and when the woman is younger at diagnosis.[81] Li and colleagues reported that women diagnosed before age 40 and women who are African American or Hispanic are more likely to be diagnosed with subsequent cancer at an advanced stage.[78]

When DCIS is present, the risk of progression to breast cancer is poorly understood; the natural history is difficult to study, because most women receive definitive treatment. One study found a 40% incidence of cancer among a group of women with clinical symptoms, whose biopsies were originally read as benign, but on review were found to have shown DCIS.[82] Women whose DCIS is found only on mammogram have a lower risk of progression.

When DCIS is a possibility based on symptoms or imaging, prompt referral to a breast specialist is indicated. Management will include biopsy to verify the diagnosis; sometimes an excisional biopsy with a wide tissue margin is done, rather than sampling. Therapy for confirmed DCIS includes lumpectomy, with or without radiation or tamoxifen treatment, or mastectomy. Counseling for therapeutic decisions includes the woman's age, spread of disease, and her preference regarding the available options. Tamoxifen has been demonstrated to lower subsequent cancer risk among women with estrogen receptor–positive DCIS, with or without radiation therapy.[83]

Other Symptoms and Conditions

MASTALGIA

Mastalgia is the term used to describe pain within the breast tissue, regardless of the underlying cause. More than 50% of all women will experience breast pain at least once.[84] One study reported a prevalence of cyclic mastalgia of 79%.[85] Women reporting breast pain tend to have larger breasts and be less physically active.[84] Ader and Shriver reported that among the 30% of women who experienced significant mastalgia, 33% noted interference with sexual activity and 29% with physical activity.[85]

Evaluation of breast pain begins with history and should include the type of pain, relationship to menses, duration, location, and relationship to other medical problems. The provider should establish whether the woman wants specific treatment or if reassurance that the pain does not represent a more serious problem is acceptable. While the patient is sitting and again while lying supine, the physical exam starts with a general exam of the breast and then proceeds to the affected area. If the woman is then turned half on her side so that the breast tissue can fall away from the chest wall, it is possible to discern whether the pain is located in the breast tissue, chest wall, or rib area. Some women have nodularity at the site of the pain.

Cyclic mastalgia is caused by hormonal stimulation and may be a presenting symptom with FCC; discomfort begins late during the luteal phase of the menstrual cycle and resolves after the menses. The breast may feel full, tender, or achy, particularly in the outer aspects and axilla. Increased nodularity may be present during the clinical examination. Alternatively, fluid retention at this time of the menstrual cycle may be the cause of pain without associated clinical findings.

Noncyclic mastalgia occurs primarily in women between 30 and 50 years of age, and may also occur in postmenopausal women.[86] It is more likely to be reported as localized and sharp. Multiple associations have been proposed, including parity, prior surgeries, medications, and ductal ectasia. Isolated breast pain is not associated with increased cancer risk.

Extramammary mastalgia describes pain that is not in the breast tissue but is referred from an underlying structure or organ. Examples include costochondritis, cardiac pain, and pleuritic pain. It may also be used to refer to pain from conditions such as *Mondor's disease*, a subcutaneous sclerosing thrombophlebitis of the anterior chest wall. The diagnosis of Mondor's disease is based on palpation of a tender, subcutaneous cord or linear skin dimpling. It is a benign finding that will resolve in several weeks with NSAIDs and heat.[87]

Women with sharp, persistent, focal pain and women who have a family history of breast cancer, are over 35, or have other risk factors for breast cancer should have imaging to exclude underlying disease. When appropriate, a pain diary along with a pain analogue chart and a menstrual diary should be recommended for a few months, so that the woman can note any association of the pain with the menstrual cycle or other precipitating factors.

Treatment for mastalgia—after excluding disease, encouraging the use of a supportive bra, and offering reassurance—can include the use of NSAIDs, which has been shown to reduce breast pain.[88] Adjustments in the estrogen dose or overall hormone exposure in contraception can be considered for women with cyclic pain. Evening primrose oil and vitamin E show some promise as an alternative therapy.[89] Fat restriction and caffeine avoidance have been recommended, although the evidence for their benefit is not strong.[86]

Danazol, tamoxifen, goserelin, bromocriptine, and other hormonally active drugs have been studied for use with severe mastalgia, and danazol has been approved by the US Food and Drug Administration for that use. When prescribed off-label, short-term tamoxifen is usually the first choice; side effects include hot flashes, menstrual irregularity or amenorrhea, weight gain, nausea, vaginal dryness, bloating, and (rare) thromboembolic events. Side effects of danazol include weight gain, menstrual irregularity/amenorrhea or menorrhagia, vocal changes, and hot flashes.[90] Consultation is recommended before prescribing these medications for mastalgia.

GALACTORRHEA

Galactorrhea is a milky or clear discharge, usually bilateral, that is normally associated with pregnancy and lactation. Outside of these time periods, galactorrhea can persist after breastfeeding for months or years as an ability to express milky fluid. Frequent nipple stimulation with sexual activity can also cause either a recurrence or new onset. Beyond these associations, the clinical evaluation will require assessment of a variety of causes. Numerous medications are associated with this condition. A list of commonly associated drugs is given in **Table 19-7**.[91,92] Some common herbs, including blessed thistle, fennel, fenugreek seed, marshmallow, nettle, red clover, and red raspberry may also induce galactorrhea;[92] several of them are in use as galactogogues by women trying to increase milk supply.

Hypothyroidism and occasionally thyrotoxicosis are associated with milk secretion. Pituitary adenoma and renal insufficiency are other medical causes included in the initial evaluation. If the prolactin level is normal and no medication cause is

Table 19-7 Medications Associated with Galactorrhea

Antidepressants and anxiolytics	Contraceptives
Alprazolam	Medroxyprogesterone
Buspirone	Combined hormonal contraceptives
Selective serotonin reuptake inhibitors (citalopram, fluoxetine, others)	Hormone replacement therapy
Tricyclic antidepressants	Conjugated equine estrogen and medroxyprogesterone
Antihypertensives	Opiates
Atenolol	Codeine
Methyldopa	Heroin
Reserpine	Morphine
Verapamil	Amphetamines
Antipsychotics	Anesthetics
Butyrophenones (e.g., haloperidol)	Cannabis
Phenothiazines (e.g., chlorpromazine)	Cyclobenzaprine
Risperidone	Danazol
Histamine H2-receptor blockers	Isoniazid (INH)
Cimetidine	Metoclopramide
Famotidine	Rimantadine
Ranitidine	Sumatriptan
	Valproic acid

Data from Peña KS, Rosenfeld JA. Evaluation and treatment of galactorrhea. *Am Fam Physician*. 2001;63(9):1763-1770; Huang W, Molitch ME. Evaluation and management of galactorrhea. *Am Fam Physician*. 2012;85(11):1073-1080.

found, no further evaluation is indicated. Elevated prolactin level is followed with thyroid hormone levels and creatinine level. If neither of these indicate a cause, the woman should be referred for MRI of the pituitary.[93] The timing of consultation and referral to an endocrinologist is based on clinical and laboratory findings and scope of care of the practitioner; in no case should it occur later in timing than the ordering of pituitary imaging.

ABNORMAL NIPPLE DISCHARGE

Discolored nipple discharge is associated with several of the conditions discussed earlier in this chapter, including intraductal papilloma, ductal ectasia, and FCCs. Any associated symptoms, whether systemic or related to the breast, may suggest alternative diagnoses to be considered, such as neurologic and visual changes from a pituitary tumor. Bloody, serous, or serosanguineous discharge can be associated with DCIS, breast cancer, and papilloma, and warrants referral to a breast specialist. Concern is highest in postmenopausal women, and when the discharge is spontaneous and occurs only in one breast. Ductography and ductoscopy are methods that have high positive predictive value but may still miss cancers.[42] The usual management is with ductal excision for histologic evaluation.[93,94] Amin and colleagues recommend discussion with younger women who may plan to breastfeed in the future before the extent of surgery is finalized, so that they may balance risk of recurrence against ability to nurse a child.[42] Dupont and colleagues identified a small subset of women with abnormal discharge for whom conservative observation may be warranted. This included women with a serous discharge whose imaging and CB results gave a cancer risk of < 2% and who had no prior cancer history and no BRCA mutation.[95]

GALACTOCELE

Galactocele is an uncommon milk-filled retention cyst caused by a duct clogged by protein, containing thickened milk and chronic inflammatory infiltrate in the ductal wall. It is formed by an overdistension of a lactiferous duct and presents as a firm, nontender lesion. It usually occurs during late pregnancy or lactation and is diagnosed during weaning. Galactostasis is milk retention, while galactocele represents a further stage of retention. The lesions are known to occur singly or in multiples, generally in only one breast. Diagnostic aspiration is often curative. Needle aspiration followed by excision should the cyst recur is the standard method of diagnosing and treating galactocele.

MASTITIS

According to the Academy of Breastfeeding Medicine, the true definition of *mastitis* is inflammation of the breast—a spectrum of conditions that ranges from engorgement to abscess.[96] In clinical practice, the term commonly refers to an infection of the breast. The true incidence of infectious mastitis as opposed to clogged, painful milk ducts; yeast infections of the nipple and milk ducts; or other conditions is unclear, because there is little high-quality research and because many women are diagnosed and treated without examination or breast milk culture. This facilitates treatment and promotes breastfeeding but increases the risk of misdiagnosis.

Infectious mastitis occurs most commonly during lactation or weaning; it is caused by bacterial contamination of the milk ducts. Mastitis typically involves the interlobular connective tissue of the breast parenchyma along a peripheral wedge of the breast, although multiple lobules and ducts may be affected. A prospective 12-week study found the incidence of bacterial mastitis in lactating women to be 9.6%.[97] Other studies have reported much higher rates; a prospective study in Australia found a 20% rate of mastitis.[98] Historically 33% has been given as a rate; however, this is based on retrospective surveys of lactation specialists.[99]

Bacteria associated with the condition are most likely to be *S. aureus*, other *Staphylococcus* species, and *Streptococcus*. *Enterobacter* species, *Escherichia coli*, and *Mycobacterium tuberculosis* have also been identified as possible pathogens. The diagnosis is typically made empirically based on symptoms or clinical evaluation, with culture reserved for cases where supportive measures and antibiotics prove ineffective. As many as 50% of lactating women are colonized by *S. aureus*.[100]

In the history, prior mastitis (with either the current or a previous child) and family history of mastitis may be associated with increased risk. Factors related to the current situation that may be associated with mastitis are shown in **Table 19-8.**

Common symptoms include breast tenderness, fever, malaise, chills, redness, and a localized "hot spot" of inflamed, swollen, tender tissue, most commonly on the outer quadrant of the breast.[97,98,101] A purulent nipple discharge or lymphadenopathy may also be present. Mastitis is not diagnosed solely on the basis of breast tenderness. The woman should be evaluated for additional risk factors. When possible, the woman should be seen prior to beginning therapy to

Table 19-8 Risk Factors for Mastitis

Delayed lactation

Separation from the infant for more than 24 hours

Maternal or infant illness

Maternal stress and fatigue

Poor latch, or weak or uncoordinated suckling

Infrequent or scheduled feeding

Limited use of different nursing positions

Use of breast creams or antifungals

Blocked nipple pore or duct, milk blister

Damaged or cracked nipple, especially if colonized with *S. aureus*

Milk oversupply leading to engorgement

Rapid weaning

Constant pressure on the breast

Excess milk supply

Data from Amir LH, Academy of Breastfeeding Medicine Protocol Committee. ABM Clinical protocol #4: mastitis, revised March 2014. *Breastfeed Med.* 2014;9(5):239-243. doi:10.1089/bfm.2014.9984; Foxman B, D'Arcy H, Gillespie B, Bobo JK, Schwartz K. Lactation mastitis: occurrence and medical management among 946 breastfeeding women in the United States. *Am J Epidemiol.* 2002;155(2):103-114; Kinlay JR, O'Connell DL, Kinlay S. Risk factors for mastitis in breastfeeding women: results of a prospective cohort study. *Aust N Z J Public Health.* 2001;25(2):115-120.

verify the diagnosis, but treatment should not be delayed if an office visit is impractical. A recent Cochrane Review notes that there is minimal research supporting the benefits of antibiotic therapy or validating preferred regimens.[102] This is not a reason to defer treatment, but it is a reason to be sure there is an indication to treat.

Treatment for mastitis is both supportive and medical. All women with symptoms suggestive of plugged ducts or mastitis are counseled to apply moist heat compresses before feeding, massage the tender or firm area regularly to encourage milk expression, and breastfeed freely.[96] Breastfeeding is safe so long as pus is not observed at the nipple. Cracked or bleeding nipples are not a contraindication. If the woman finds nursing too painful, milk can be pumped or hand expressed to empty the milk ducts. If the milk is not removed, the milk stasis will promote bacterial growth. The most common antibiotic used is dicloxacillin 500 mg orally 4 times daily for 10–14 days. Antibiotic choices are listed in **Table 19-9**. Pain and fever relief with NSAIDs or acetaminophen is appropriate. There is a brief but significant increase in risk of aggressive breast cancer immediately following pregnancy, an effect of the hormonal changes involved.[103] If presumed mastitis does not rapidly resolve after treatment is initiated, both antibiotic-resistant organisms and the possibility of a malignancy must be considered. Mammography may be recommended to exclude

Table 19-9 Outpatient Antibiotics for Mastitis

First-line therapy:

  Dicloxacillin 500 mg PO qid for 10–14 days

  Cephalexin 500 mg PO qid for 10–14 days

  Amoxicillin-clavulanate 875 mg PO bid for 10–14 days

If beta-lactam allergy is present:

  Clarithromycin 500 mg PO bid for 10–14 days

If MRSA is suspected:

  Clindamycin 300 mg PO tid for 10–14 days

  Trimethoprim-sulfamethoxazole 1 DS tablet PO bid for 10–14 days

bid = twice daily, DS = double-strength, MRSA = methicillin-resistant *Staphylococcus aureus*, PO = per os (by mouth), qid = 4 times per day, tid = 3 times per day

malignancy in women over 30 or otherwise at increased risk.[104]

Untreated, mastitis may progress to abscess. In a combined randomized controlled trial (RCT) and survey of a cohort of women, Amir and colleagues reported an incidence of 0.4% in all breastfeeding women and 2.9% among women treated for mastitis, which is lower than historical estimates of 11% risk of abscess following mastitis.[105] Primiparity, maternal age > 30 years, gestation > 41 weeks, African American race, and tobacco use are all associated with increased risk.[105-107] The suspicion of a breast abscess is an indication for referral to a specialist able to manage the treatment. Management includes identification on ultrasound, aspiration of small collections, and possibly surgical incision and drainage of larger (> 5 cm) pockets. Antibiotic therapy is continued and intravenous antibiotics may be needed for persistent or severe abscess.[104,108]

Nonlactational mastitis may present as subareolar abscess with tenderness, redness, and swelling; a palpable mass usually is not accompanied by fever or malaise. Subareolar abscess is often associated with nipple inversion or retraction. A peripheral abscess may occur anywhere in the breast tissue with pain, tenderness, and swelling. Non-lactational mastitis can occur as a result of nipple stimulation, piercing, or other manipulation of the nipple. Smoking, African American race, and obesity have been associated with this form of mastitis and progression to abscess.[107,109] Women with a mass other than in the periareolar area should be assessed for systemic diseases that predispose them to abscess development, such as diabetes and immunosuppression. Although less common than lactational mastitis, the risk of recurrence and progression may be higher. It must be distinguished from ductal ectasia, inflammatory breast cancer (IBC), and granulomatous mastitis. Mammography may be recommended to exclude malignancy.[104] Infection with anaerobes, *Proteus* species, and mixed colonies of bacteria are associated with abscess in this population.[107] The woman should have imaging to follow resolution of the abscess as clinically indicated.[104]

Idiopathic granulomatous mastitis (IGM) is a rare, chronic breast condition. Other granulomatous processes in the breast may be associated with infection or implants.[8] Women with IGM are more likely to be younger than those with periductal mastitis or ductal ectasia and less likely to smoke.[110] The condition may be triggered by inflammation, infection, or hormonal factors. Corticosteroids and methotrexate are used in its treatment, with or without surgery to remove affected tissue.[111]

CANDIDA INFECTIONS OF THE NIPPLE AND BREAST

Candida infections of the nipple and ducts are a cause of sharp, stabbing, or burning pain associated with breastfeeding.[100] Risk factors include early mixed feeding methods and prolonged pregnancy.[112] Because *Candida albicans* and other *Candida* species are commensals, and because they are difficult to identify in breast milk except by polymerase chain reaction, empiric diagnosis based on reported symptoms is common. Francis-Morrill and colleagues reported a high positive predictive value when a constellation of three or more of the following symptoms was present: burning, stabbing, pain, or soreness, especially if they were associated with flaky or shiny skin of the nipple/areola.[113] Betzold's review and meta-analysis found that severe, deep pain on breastfeeding was associated with detection of *Candida* and with *S. aureus*.[114] Treatment for yeast infections during lactation can begin with topical nystatin (often prescribed for infants with thrush), with all-purpose "triple-nipple" cream (compounded of mupirocin 2% ointment, betamethasone 0.1% ointment, and miconazole *or* fluconazole powder to a final concentration of 2%), or with oral fluconazole.

RAYNAUD'S PHENOMENON OF THE NIPPLE

Raynaud's phenomenon is an exaggerated vasoconstriction in response to a trigger, causing temporary tissue ischemia. Primary Raynaud's is more common in women than men and onset usually occurs between ages 15 and 25 years. Secondary Raynaud's is typically seen in men and women over 35, and is associated with a variety of causes including several autoimmune diseases. The response is triggered by cold or stress.

As a cause of breastfeeding pain, it must be differentiated from *Candida* infection and other causes of breast pain by verification of correct breastfeeding technique, presence of Raynaud's symptoms other than during lactation, occurrence in response to cold stimulus, and the typical blanching followed by cyanosis and/or erythema during an exacerbation.[115] When diagnosis is confirmed, nifedipine has been reported to offer relief.[115,116] Counseling includes avoidance of cold and smoking cessation.

THE UNCONFIRMED MASS

Unconfirmed mass is a problem of clinical significance. It can be anything from a local lymph node to a small cancerous mass that the woman recognizes because she is familiar with her own breast. In this case, the patient presents with a breast mass that is not palpable on CBE. Should the provider convince the patient that the findings of the CBE are correct? What should be done if she has breast pain? The provider should always take this concern seriously, documenting a careful history with regard to onset, duration, and exacerbating circumstances. If the woman feels a lump and it is not discernible on palpation, the location of the mass should be documented with a diagram or descriptive narrative. A standard examination should be conducted with particular emphasis on the area the woman best feels the lump. This area should be compared to the same area in the other breast. If the patient is still concerned, then a follow-up appointment should be made. If she is of reproductive age, then the examination should be repeated in the follicular phase of her cycle. In every such case, the woman should be reassured that her concern is appropriate and respected. A consult with a collaborating physician and referral to a breast evaluation program are appropriate if the concern persists. If the woman is over 40 years of age, then a screening mammogram is appropriate prior to consultation.

Breast Cancer Screening

Breast cancer screening is an evolving process. The epidemiology of breast cancer was briefly discussed earlier in this chapter. Although breast cancer is not the leading cause of death among women, it may be the one most women are aware of or are concerned about. After steady, decades-long increases in the breast cancer rate, attributable not only to more effective screening programs, but changes in childbearing patterns, perimenopausal HRT use, and obesity rates, the rate stabilized in 2003, when there was a sharp decrease in the use of HRT.[117,118]

The first step in screening for breast cancer is to collect a complete history and review of symptoms as discussed in the section on the essential evaluation. (Refer back to Table 19-2 for a list of risk factors to consider.) The second step is completion of a CBE. (See the **Appendix** at the end of this chapter.) CBE has not been standardized and techniques can differ widely. Furthermore, the sensitivity of CBE is far from perfect, and providers vary considerably in the prevalence of abnormalities they find on CBE. Barton and colleagues reported that the sensitivity of CBE is approximately 54% and the specificity of the exam is about 94%. Duration of the exam may correlate with accuracy of lump detection.[119] Clinical examination poses potential risks for either missed findings or unnecessary testing. When the choice is there, it is always best to err on the side of careful examination and testing, while advising the woman that the test may not reveal any abnormality. It is also beneficial to remind women that no screening test can 1) find every abnormality or 2) always identify a benign finding. The contribution of the CBE to breast cancer diagnosis is not clear; the impact of the teaching opportunity is.

The final step in the clinical examination is to teach breast awareness to the woman. All women should be counseled about breast awareness, including self-examination if she wishes to perform breast self-examination (BSE), and be encouraged to pay attention to any changes she notices. BSE is no longer part of the routine preventive recommendations for prevention of breast cancer, based on evidence that the performance of BSE does not affect cancer mortality and that it increases the number of biopsies for benign disease.[120]

Although BSE is no longer recommended, women who are attentive to the appearance and shape of their breasts are more likely to notice changes that occur between clinical visits. Particularly among young, low-risk women, this may benefit the individual who finds a suspicious change or mass. A study from 2001 of recently diagnosed breast cancer patients found that the majority had first identified symptoms at home.[121] Women need to feel confident that if or when they notice a change they can call for an immediate appointment. Self-identification is followed by clinical examination and a discussion of options for imaging.

Risk Factors for Breast Cancer

Increased understanding of the complex interweaving of demographic, lifestyle, and genetic factors has shown that breast cancer is not monolithic, and that screening programs should reflect individual risk rather than population norms. All women need to receive age- and risk-appropriate screening. Several models for risk evaluation are currently in use, based on demographic, genetic, and lifestyle factors. Some of the breast cancer risk factors, such as obesity, sedentary lifestyle, or excessive alcohol use, are modifiable ones for which counseling can facilitate risk reduction.[122] Obesity and weight gain during midlife are associated with postmenopausal breast cancer, presumably through the role of fat tissue in storing estrogens.[123,124] Hyperinsulinemia, with or without overt type 2 diabetes, has been identified as increasing risks among older women.[45,125] Alcohol consumption, even at moderate ($<$ 1 drink/day) levels is associated with lifetime cancer risk.[126] Early onset of tobacco use and exposure to secondhand smoke have been associated with increased risk of breast cancer.[122,127,128] These should be addressed with all women, because they affect not only breast cancer risk but many other health conditions. Other lifestyle factors believed to affect breast cancer risk include nightshift or rotating day/nightshift work;[129]

the increased risk is believed to be associated with melatonin disruption.[130]

The risk factors for which there is most evidence are not as amenable to risk reduction. As shown in the epidemiology section, breast cancer risk rises steadily with age. Two-thirds of invasive breast cancers occur in women over 55 years of age and only 1 in 8 among women under 45. Some experts find that the incidence decreases with advanced age > 85, while others find that this may be an effect of decreased screening in elderly women.

Race and ethnicity are related to breast cancer risk, both generally and with regard to onset and prognosis. White women have the highest lifetime breast cancer risk in the United States. African American women have slightly lower risks overall, but have higher rates of aggressive premenopausal cancer and poorer overall survival. Poorer survival is attributed to later diagnosis, less access to high-quality care, genetic differences in the disease, and lifestyle factors such as obesity and diet that can impact survival.[13,131,132] The incidence of BRCA1 and BRCA2 genes in the African American community appears to be higher than among non-Hispanic whites. Among African American women with early-onset breast cancer, family history, or triple-negative cancer, 25% had mutations in BRCA1 and BRCA2 or another breast cancer gene.[132] Pal and colleagues found a 12% incidence of these genes among premenopausal black women in Florida with a breast cancer diagnosis.[133] Cancer risks among Hispanic women are more difficult to quantify; women of Hispanic ethnicity are multicultural and multi-ethnic, and traditional risk factors do not appear to completely explain risks in this population.[134] It is possible that the burden of poverty and difficulty affording or accessing care affect populations of color in ways not fully appreciated.

Increased breast density has been identified as an independent risk factor for breast cancer.[135,136] It masks underlying lesions, but more importantly has been identified as having a positive association with familial breast cancer risk.[137] Using percentage density, a meta-analysis found that RR for

those whose breast density was greater than the 75th percentile was 4.64 (95% CI 3.64–5.91) compared to those with the least dense breasts.[138] Another study found similar risk stratification and noted that the risk persisted regardless of age or menopausal status over a 10-year period. The increased risk related to high density of the breast parenchyma was independent of family history, age at first birth, alcohol consumption, and benign breast disease.[139] Estimating the volume of dense fibroglandular tissue is a newer and more accurate technique that increases accuracy in predicting risk. An increasing number of states have mandated that providers explain breast density as a risk factor to women. In a survey published in 2015, differences existed by education, race/ethnicity, and income related to women's knowledge.[140]

As previously discussed, several of the benign breast diseases are associated with increased risk of breast cancer. Hartmann and colleagues reported categorical associations as follows: The RR of breast cancer in a cohort of 9000+ women with benign disease was 1.56 (95% CI, 1.45–1.68), persisting for > 25 years after first diagnosis. The RR associated with atypia was 4.24 (3.26–5.41), as compared with an RR of 1.88 (1.66–2.12) for proliferative changes without atypia and of 1.27 (1.15–1.41) for nonproliferative lesions. Among women with nonproliferative lesions, increased risk was associated with family history.[34] These numbers are consistent with other reports.

Genetic risks represent a more complex area than initially understood. Any family history of a first-degree relative with breast cancer gives an increased RR of 1.7.[141] BRCA1 and BRCA2 together explain 5–10% of breast cancer risk.[141] Both are highly complex genes with multiple possible mutations. In a pooled analysis of 22 studies, lifetime cancer risk with BRCA1 has been estimated at ~65%, with higher rates in early onset; BRCA2 carries a ~45% lifetime risk. RR declines with age in BRCA1 carriers, but not with BRCA2.[142] RR is higher in families with multiple affected members and a pattern of early onset.

Based on the specific mutations and lifestyle factors, estimates of personal risk may be as low as 26% or as high as 80–90%.[143] Work by Friebel and colleagues suggests that for women who carry the BRCA1 gene and wish to bear children, delaying first birth may decrease risk. The same meta-analysis found that for BRCA2 carriers, smoking increased risk.[144] Multiple other genetic mutations have been identified, although none with the penetrance of BRCA1 and BRCA2. Li-Fraumeni and Cowden syndromes are rare autosomal dominant mutations that confer high risk of breast cancer.

When the history or examination suggests increased genetic risk, referral to a breast genetics counselor or specialist team for counseling regarding the benefits and risks of testing is appropriate. Genetic counseling has been found to decrease distress, improve risk perception, and reduce intention to be tested.[145] Women should have the opportunity to discuss their risks, understand the possible stresses involved in learning about familial cancers, and make an informed personal choice. The US Preventive Services Task Force (USPSTF) review regarding BRCA testing found that intensive screening had some negative effects, including increased false positives, unnecessary imaging, and unneeded surgery.[145]

The NCI's Breast Cancer Risk Assessment Tool (BCRAT) is based on the *Gail Model*, and has been validated in white and Asian Pacific populations.[146] It may underestimate cancer risk in African American women who have had breast biopsies already. It is not yet completely validated for Hispanic women and for certain other subpopulations.[147] Because this model relies on demographic information, such as age, race, age at menarche, and age at first live birth plus one generation of familial history, and does not evaluate genetic risks, it has limitations, but is still an effective first-line tool for clinicians to use in a general population.[148] It can be accessed online at http://www.cancer.gov/bcrisktool/.

Barlow and colleagues demonstrated that in a population having screening mammograms, breast density and knowledge of combination HRT use improved accuracy of breast cancer risk assessment.[149] The *Tyrer-Cuzick* model, also called the *International Breast Cancer Intervention Study (IBIS)*, includes extended family history and BRCA1/BRCA2 genetic status plus factors such as age, age at menarche, parity, age at first live birth, age at menopause, history of HRT use, history of hyperplasia/AH, history of LCIS, height, and BMI.[150] It has been shown to be more accurate in predicting risk across stratified risk groups, including among average-risk women who are normally given risk predictions based on BCRAT, particularly if the score is adjusted to reflect breast density.[148,151] It is not, however, as adaptable to primary care use.

Other models focus specifically on the genetic risks and are more appropriate for use in high-risk women. For example, the *Claus model* looked at genetic susceptibility based on pattern of cancer among first- and second-degree relatives,[152] and the *BRCAPRO* (a statistical model) includes history of breast and ovarian cancer and details about the diagnoses.[153] The NCI currently advises use of the Breast and Ovarian Analysis of Disease Incidence and Carrier Estimation Algorithm (BOADICEA) developed by the Centre for Cancer Genetic Epidemiology at the University of Cambridge. It combines BRCA1 and BRCA2 mutation carrier probabilities and age-specific risks of breast and ovarian cancer.[154,155] The tool is further explained and can be accessed at http://ccge.medschl.cam.ac.uk/boadicea/.

Imaging in Breast Cancer Screening

Which women should have breast imaging, when, and how often are questions whose answers are not fixed. Women are not well served by a one-size-fits-all approach. Standard recommendations for breast screening timing and intervals are shown in **Table 19-10**.[156-159] The American

Table 19-10 Mammography Screening Guidelines for Breast Cancer in Average-Risk Women

	ACS	USPSTF	ACOG	WHO*
CBE	Not recommended for average-risk women at any age (qualified)**	Insufficient evidence to recommend for or against	20–39: every 1–3 years 40+: annually	
Mammogram	Age 40: offer option (qualified) Age 45: begin screening (strong) Age 45–54: annual screening (qualified) Age 55+: Biennial screening or annual if desired, continuing as long as the woman is healthy and has a life expectancy of 10 years (qualified)	Ages 40–49: individual decision Ages 50–74: biennial Age 76+: insufficient evidence	Age 40: annually	Ages 40–49: with shared decision making Ages 50–69: biennial screening Age 70+: with shared decision making
MRI	Lifetime risk > 20%: annually beginning at age 30 Risk < 15%: not indicated	No recommendation	Not advised	

ACS = American Cancer Society; ACOG = American College of Obstetricians and Gynecologists, CBE = clinical breast examination, MRI = magnetic resonance imaging, USPSTF = US Preventive Services Task Force, WHO = World Health Organization.

*WHO guidelines are for resource-rich countries that have implemented a program of research, monitoring, and evaluation to determine the relative balance of risks versus benefits in women ages 40–49 and 70+ years.

**Recommendations in ACS Guidelines are strong (consensus that benefits outweigh any risks) or qualified (consensus that there is a benefit, but not on balance of benefits and harms).

Data from American College of Obstetricians and Gynecologists. Breast cancer screening. Practice Bulletin No. 122. *Obstet Gynecol.* 2011;118:372-382; Oeffinger KC, Fontham EH, Etzioni R, Herzig A, Michaelson JS, Shih Y-CT, et al. Breast Cancer Screening for Women at Average Risk: 2015 Guideline Update From the American Cancer Society. JAMA. 2015;314(15):1599-1614; Smith RA, Manassaram-Baptiste D, Brooks D, Doroshenk M, Fedewa S, Saslow D, et al. Cancer screening in the United States, 2015: a review of current American Cancer Society guidelines and current issues in cancer screening. *CA Cancer J Clin.* 2015;65:30-54; US Preventive Services Task Force. Breast Cancer: Screening. http://www.uspreventiveservicestaskforce.org/Page/Document/RecommendationStatementFinal/breast-cancer-screening1. February 2016. Accessed May 10, 2016; World Health Organization. WHO position paper on mammography screening. Geneva, Switzerland: WHO. http://www.guideline.gov/content.aspx?f=rss&id=49209&osrc=12. 2014. Accessed May 10, 2016.

College of Obstetricians and Gynecologists guideline is the most commonly recognized in women's health settings. Both the USPSTF Guidelines[158] and the American Cancer Society guidelines were updated in 2015.

Uptake of screening with mammography is influenced by several factors, including provider recommendation, age, socioeconomic status, and insurance status. The Patient Protection and Affordable Care Act has placed routine mammography within the reach of many women who were formerly prevented by cost. However, providers should not assume that women of limited means or education will automatically avail themselves of resources they are not familiar with, or that there are no other financial and transportation barriers. In 2010, only 72.4% of eligible women were screened for breast cancer; that rate was based on women between 50 and 74 years of age having at least 1 mammogram within 2 years.[160]

Interventions that have been shown to increase participation in breast cancer screening are summarized in the Guide to Community Preventive Services.[161] Evidence-based interventions that can be undertaken in a provider's office include one-on-one and group education, provision of brochures or videos in the office, having the provider remind women of the need for mammography, and re-calling women who have missed screening appointments to reschedule.[161]

Routine imaging, when there is not a clinical finding, is recommended to begin either at 40 or 50 years among low-risk women and occur either at 1- or 2-year intervals. When discussing screening, it is important to provide an accurate description of the procedure and review both risks and benefits. Electing not to begin screening until age 50 increases the risk of missing an early, aggressive cancer, although absolute rates are low. Having more mammograms increases the risk of unnecessary follow-up testing or surgeries for a false positive. Women need to be aware that increased frequency of testing with mammography

increases overall radiation exposure that may carry a personal health risk. The USPSTF argues for reduced frequency and years of screening, based on a strict evaluation of cost-benefit that considers only mortality. In contrast, other groups place greater weight on early intervention and morbidity. In no case should the interval between screenings exceed 2 years.

In women with a lifetime risk greater than 20%, enhanced screening should begin between ages 25 and 30 (or 10 years prior to the earliest family diagnosis) and may include sonogram, mammography, and MRI as well as short-interval (6 month) monitoring with CBE and possible imaging. For women at intermediate risk (15–20%), the discussion becomes more complex, because the risk of false positives increases as breast cancer risk declines. Short-interval CBE and annual mammography at age 40 should be a minimum standard in this group.

Prevention of Breast Cancer

Preventive measures against breast cancer fall into three categories: lifestyle changes, preventive medication, and prophylactic surgery.

The lifestyle changes any woman may reasonably undertake to protect her health and decrease breast cancer risk are recommendations that hold true for many diseases. These include counseling to lose weight in midlife and decrease alcohol and tobacco exposure.

Physical activity has been studied as a protective mechanism. A review of 76 studies found that the majority supported ongoing physical activity for risk reduction.[162] Multiple pathways for benefit have been proposed including positive effects on sex hormone levels, immune function, inflammation, obesity, and insulin-related hormones.[162,163]

The evidence for various dietary changes, whether decreasing fats and red meat, increasing soy and antioxidant intake, or other recommendations, is mixed. The publication of data from the PREDIMED RCT in Spain provides support for recommendation of a Mediterranean diet high in olive oil.[164] The data are not definitive, but such a diet—high in plant-based foods including nuts and legumes, low in salt intake, and replacing other fats with olive oil—is healthy for many reasons.

Unlike other hormonal factors that may be protective during the childbearing years, such as age at menarche or early age at first birth, breastfeeding is an intervention that most women who bear children can undertake. Duration of breastfeeding greater than 6 months confers a measurable benefit that increases with duration.[165,166]

Limiting the use of HRT during menopause may reduce risk, because persistence of higher estrogen levels in combined HRT has been associated with risk of postmenopausal breast cancer.[167,168] A recent review of the NCI's SEER data by Wachtel and colleagues suggests that current rates of lobular and ductal breast cancer do not support this link.[169] Further confounding the issue is the short-term reduction in breast cancer risk among women who take estrogen following hysterectomy.[170] The same review of long-term follow up from the Women's Health Initiative found that long-term risk remained elevated for both combined and estrogen-only HRT.[170]

Another way to affect cancer risk for women with high-risk findings based on history or nonmalignant changes is chemoprevention. Chemoprevention of breast cancer has been studied, with both SERM (including raloxifene, lasofoxifene, and arzoxifene) and aromatase inhibitors AIs (such as exemestane or anastrozole) showing benefit.[171-173] For women carrying the BRCA mutations, invasive breast cancer incidence is reduced by 30–68% using SERM.[145] Women should be counseled on the known risks and side effects before choosing these medications. These include increased incidence of thromboembolism for all SERM medications, increased risk for endometrial cancer and cataracts with tamoxifen, possible increased fracture risk with AIs, and increased vasomotor symptoms with all drugs.

Prophylactic surgery may be recommended to reduce risk of breast and ovarian cancers among women at highest risk. Counseling around this issue needs to take into consideration women's childbearing plans, because the surgeries will prevent breastfeeding and/or childbearing. A study by Schwartz and colleagues found that 80% of women given positive results on BRCA testing had had risk-reduction surgery within 5 years.[174] The USPSTF found that risk-reducing mastectomy reduced breast cancer by 85–100% and breast cancer mortality by 81–100%; risk-reducing salpingo-oophorectomy reduced breast cancer by 37–100% and all-cause mortality by 55–100%.[145]

Invasive Breast Cancer

As discussed earlier, there is, if not a clear progression, then an increased risk of invasive cancer with certain benign lesions. The types of invasive cancer are outlined here, although the management of cancer is outside the realm of primary care. Women with breast cancer will often have multidisciplinary teams that include surgeons, radiation oncologists, and medical oncologists and pharmacists to manage the various aspects of their care. The teams often include genetic counselors, nurse practitioners, and therapists to address the woman's needs during recovery.

Cancer is definitively diagnosed with a tissue sample following an examination or imaging study that has raised concern. Most breast cancers are adenocarcinomas, indicating their origin in glandular tissue. Invasive (or infiltrating) ductal carcinoma (IDC) comprises 80% of breast cancers in women. It arises within the milk duct before breaking into the fatty breast tissue from which it can metastasize. Invasive lobular carcinoma (ILC) arises deeper in the breast within the milk lobules; it makes up about 10% of invasive cancers. The most common second cancer in women with a new breast cancer is cancer of the contralateral breast. At 10 years, the risk is considered to be 3–10%; use of adjuvant therapy in estrogen-receptor-positive tumors has decreased that rate in recent years.[175]

Categorization of cancers is by stages. Staging of invasive cancer is a way to communicate systematically through measurements and clinical evaluation. The tumor itself is sized; spread to axillary lymph nodes is assessed; and distant organs such as liver, brain, lung, or spine may be evaluated with PET, computed tomography, or MRI. **Table 19-11** and **Table 19-12** describe

Table 19-11 Breast Cancer Staging

Stage	Primary Tumor	Nodes	Metastases
Noninvasive			
Stage 0 (DCIS and LCIS)	In situ (T_{is})	No regional node metastasis (N_0)	No distant metastases
Early Invasive			
Stage IA	Tumor $\leq$ 20 mm in greatest dimension (T_1)	No regional node metastasis (N_0)	No distant metastases
Stage IB	No primary tumor (T_0) or T_1	Micrometastasis (none greater than 2.0 mm) (N_1 mi)	
Stage IIA	T_0 or T_1 or tumor > 20 mm but $\leq$ 50 mm (T_2)	Metastasis in up to 1–3 axillary or internal mammary lymph nodes (N_1)	
Stage IIB	T_2 or tumor > 50 mm (T_3)	N_0 or N_1	
Locally Advanced Invasive			
Stage IIIA	T_0–T_3 (tumor of any size)	N_0, N_1, or metastasis in 4–9 axillary or internal mammary lymph nodes (N_2)	No distant metastases
Stage IIIB	Tumor of any size with direct extension to chest wall and/or to skin (T_4)	N_0–N_2	
Metastatic stage IV	Any size tumor	Any configuration of local node metastasis	Distant metastasis present

Abbreviations: T describes the original primary tumor, and N describes whether the cancer has reached nearby lymph nodes.

Reproduced from Edge SB, Byrd DR, Compton CC, eds. *AJCC Cancer Staging Manual.* 7th ed. New York, NY: Springer; 2010. Reproduced with permission of Springer.

the terminology used.[176] Stage 0, I, and II cancers generally have better prognoses. At the time of biopsy or surgery, tissue typing for histology and hormone receptor status further categorizes the nature of the malignancy.

Hormone Receptor Status and Prognosis

Estrogen and progesterone receptors (ER, PR) may be present in the tumor, as may overexpression or amplification of human epidermal growth factor type 2 receptor (HER2/neu). After typing, tumors are classified as hormone-receptor positive, HER2 positive, or triple negative (ER, PR, and HER2/neu negative).[177] Because the receptors permit the use of targeted HER2 or hormonal adjuvant treatment, triple-negative cancers are more difficult to treat. Approximately 15–20% of all breast cancers are triple negative. Women

most at risk are younger, African American or Hispanic, or carry one of the BRCA genes.

The size of tumors, spread to surrounding or distant tissue or lymph nodes, and hormone receptor status all inform decisions that a woman will need to make with her cancer team regarding treatment. They also provide information to guide discussions around an individual prognosis.

Most breast cancers are treated with a combination of surgery, radiation, and adjuvant therapy, whether chemotherapy, hormonal, or targeted immunotherapy. Early identification of a cancer can permit breast-conserving surgery. Current evidence is that nonclinical factors such as access to an academic center, private insurance, and socioeconomic status play a role in the uptake of this option.[178] After breast-conserving surgery, use of radiation decreases risk for recurrence by 50%.[11] Women who choose mastectomy do not commonly receive radiation except for late-stage

Table 19-12 Breast Cancer Staging: Tumor/Nodes/Metastasis (TMN)

T_x	No primary tumor found
T_{is}	Cancer in situ (ductal, lobular, or Paget's)
T_1	≤ 2 cm (T_{1a} < 0.5 cm, T_{1b} > 0.5–1.0 cm, T_{1c} > 1.0–2 cm)
T_2	> 2–5 cm
T_3	> 5 cm
T_4	Direct extension of tumor (T_{4a} = chest wall; T_{4b} = skin including ulcer, peau d'orange, infiltration, nodules; T_{4c} = both chest wall and skin; T_{4d} = inflammatory disease)
N_0	No metastasis to regional nodes
N_1	Palpable and mobile ipsilateral axillary nodes
N_2	Fixed ipsilateral axillary nodes
N_3	Ipsilateral infraclavicular, mammary, or supraclavicular nodes
M_o	No evidence of distant metastasis
M_1	Evidence of distant metastasis by clinical, radiological, or histologic determination

tumors. Radiation can produce skin burns or rashes and fatigue, and has potential long-term risks including heart damage, lymphedema, and rib fractures.

The choice of pharmacologic treatment is based on tumor type, staging, and receptor status. Chemotherapeutic drugs are cytotoxic, so they may be used before surgery to shrink tumors or following surgery to remove any remaining tumor cells. Depending on the specific drug, side effects may include nausea, hair loss, fatigue, mouth sores, premature menopause, thrombocytopenia, or leukopenia. Targeted drugs for HER2 receptors, such as trastuzumab (Herceptin), pertuzumab (Perjeta), and ado-trastuzumab emtansine (Kadcyla) are monoclonal antibodies. Risks associated with these drugs include heart damage leading to congestive heart failure. Lapatinib (Tykerb), another drug in this group, carries a risk of liver failure and dehydration from intense diarrhea.

Less Common Cancers

Inflammatory breast cancer (IBC) is the diagnosis in 1–6% of breast cancers.[179] IBC is diagnosed at a slightly younger age than more common cancers (average age 57 years).[180] African Americans are at higher risk than other racial groups.[179] IBC presents as an edematous, thickened, inflamed breast tissue, not unlike the appearance of mastitis. The term *peau d'orange* (orange peel) is used to describe this skin appearance. It is less likely to be noted on mammogram. The breast may feel firm or warm to the touch. The nipple may retract from tension as the breast distends. The cancer is aggressive and has a relatively poorer prognosis than more common types; 5-year survival is only 34%, because the cancer is almost always at stage III or IV when diagnosed.[180] In young women who are suspected of having mastitis, IBC must be a consideration if antibiotics do not promptly resolve the infection.

Paget disease is a skin cancer of the nipple and areola, accounting for 1–3% of all breast cancers.[181] It is most often seen in women who also have DCIS or IDC. Chen and colleagues, in 2006, reported the incidence of Paget disease without associated malignancies in the United States at about 13%, which is higher than previously estimated.[182] One hypothesis is that although Paget disease most commonly arises from an underlying ductal malignancy, earlier identification and treatment of DCIS and small IDC have decreased secondary development of nipple disease as a cause. The prognosis is tied to the presence and staging of an underlying tumor. Paget disease of the nipple presents as unilateral erythema and scaling. Although usually not painful, it can be pruritic, exudative, or ulcerative. Induration and infiltration may be present, and an underlying nodule may be palpated in later stages.

Psychosocial Aspects of Breast Cancer

Although modern therapies are less disfiguring than the original radical mastectomy, and chemotherapeutic agents are less toxic, there are still physical effects of treatment, which may be challenging both for women and their partners. In addition, disruption of work and family life increases stress. Younger age at diagnosis, prior mental health issues, comorbid illnesses, and limited social support have been shown to impact coping.[183] Ganz summarizes the common psychosocial issues as treatment-related concerns, fear of recurrence, persistent anxiety about the illness and thoughts of mortality, disruption of body image and feelings of vulnerability, sexual dysfunction, and communication difficulties.[183] Other authors have also noted that the woman and her partner need to be considered as a dyad in terms of coping with cancer.[184,185]

It is in the primary care setting that women most commonly present with their concern about a mass or change that may be breast cancer, and primary care providers are frequently involved in women's lives throughout and after treatment. It is part of the primary care provider's role, even as care is handed off to specialists, to maintain awareness during future visits of the need to assess coping and the potential need for additional mental health, counseling, or community resources.

Missed Diagnoses and Liability

Breast cancer receives significant media attention. On the positive side, this has led to increased surveillance and detection, but it also has increased anxiety on the part of women regarding the disease and providers who may be fearful of missing significant breast disease. First, every practitioner needs to know the standard of practice in the clinical setting and in the community in which she or he works. Second, every provider of women's health care should be aware of the resources locally or regionally for breast evaluation and management of breast cancer. Third, every provider should always assume that the medical record will be read by another. Interdisciplinary teams are frequently available, with advanced practice nurses and genetic counselors seeing many of the women who come for care.[42]

Screening for breast cancer is not synonymous with mammographic screening. Documentation of a personal and family history with attention to reproductive and breast conditions in addition to a CBE is essential. Because most specialty boards recommend regular mammographic screening for women who are between the ages of 40 and 69, women's health providers should discuss it with all women in that age range. Although there is no consensus for women younger than 50 and older than 69 years, breast imaging can still be part of an individualized plan. A woman's risk factors

and personal preference should be taken into consideration, and the discussion documented. Recommendations for additional counseling and additional testing should be followed up to confirm either that the woman chose to go, or that her refusal is documented.

The acronym FACT (factual, accurate, complete, and timely) should be used when recording breast findings. Each entry should include the time and date and be signed. The women's health provider should record all efforts to contact the patient and any follow up that is done. Entries should include significant changes in condition for the better or worse. The patient's emotional response should be recorded if it is significant. Any contact made with other professionals about the breast condition should be recorded; this includes supervisory or consultative conversations. The woman should be informed of diagnostic and treatment risks and alternative therapies when appropriate. Limiting factors (e.g., "patient declines mammogram, biopsy"; "interview terminated prior to obtaining complete history"; "patient distracted due to children in exam room with her—plan finish interview/exam in 1 hour/2 days") should be documented. Charting the characteristics of a breast mass may include modifiers such as "cystic or solid, solitary, discrete, firm/hard."

Medical malpractice cases are governed by civil law, specifically tort law, the primary claim of which is negligence.[186] Reasons for lawsuits include dissatisfaction with rapport (the hurried provider), lack of ability to administer care and treatment consistent with expectations, suspicion of cover-up, need for information, desire to protect others, and inability to effectively communicate with the provider.[187,188] A lawsuit may be the result of an adverse outcome, but the litigation is concerned not with outcome but with conduct of providers.[186] Gynecologic liability cases against midwives are infrequent, representing fewer than 5% of reported claims in a national survey.[189]

Most relate to in-office procedures. The probable causes for low rates of these claims include high rates of referral to physicians for identified abnormalities and not performing surgery.[190] As more midwives and women's health practitioners provide care to midlife and older women, the risks of failing to correctly identify and refer increase with exposure.

Delay in diagnosis is the leading cause of malpractice litigation.[186] In a closed claims review by Gandhi and colleagues, most legal claims were found to be the results of multiple process failures and system errors.[191] Process failures, or breakdowns, refer to the acts required for patient care to flow smoothly. Contributing factors are not the acts themselves but characteristics of the provider, the patient, or the system. The frequency of diagnostic process breakdowns included: failure to order an appropriate diagnostic test (55%), failure to create a proper follow-up plan (45%), failure to obtain an adequate history or perform an adequate physical examination (42%), and failure to correctly understand and act on diagnostic tests (37%). The leading factors that contributed to the errors were failures in judgment (79%), vigilance or memory (59%), knowledge (48%), patient-related factors (46%), and handoffs (20%). Multiple events (median three of both process errors and contributing factors) contributed to each claim.[191]

Another important aspect of litigation is standard of care, which means care that is reasonable and prudent and that another provider would exercise under similar circumstances. The benchmark for conduct is reasonableness. It is the duty of the clinician to obtain a reasonable history, perform a reasonable exam, and arrive at a reasonable management plan. The management plan should be developed with the patient, ensuring that she understands the goals and rationale. A patient should never be advised to "return as needed," because the healthcare provider is considered to have "superior knowledge" that a patient might not comprehend.

Abandonment may be found if a clinical condition exists and appropriate transfer of care is not successfully completed. This means that the primary provider is responsible for providing an appropriate referral for screening or care and following up to be sure the appointment was kept, or sending a reminder if the woman does not go for testing.

The main reasons for failure to diagnose or correctly manage a breast pathology include the following: no pathology identified when pathology is present, misidentified pathology, severity of problem not recognized, failure to advise patients of findings, improper reporting, failure to advise of limited scope of assessment, failure to advise of follow-up care needed, failure to advise of alternatives or appropriateness of requested care or evaluation, and failure to communicate assessments or recommendations in a timely fashion.

The primary care provider will be judged on the written record. Midwives and other women's health providers carry major responsibility for recording the problem, getting the woman to the proper care, and providing appropriate communication with all of the team members—including the woman—throughout the entire process. Specific plans for follow up should always be documented—whether it involves a return appointment in a certain time period, a consultation, or a referral.

Conclusion

Part of providing women's health care is attention to those aspects that are unique to women, or less frequently addressed by other professionals. This includes education about normal physiologic changes associated with maturation, pregnancy, and aging; information about the available modalities for breast and genetic evaluation; discussion of the risks of both benign and malignant breast conditions; and support for informed decision making.

Midwives and nurse practitioners, as primary care providers, are responsible for breast health, screening, and referral. The evaluation of benign lesions and management of problems such as mastitis are well within the scope of practice.

All at-risk women benefit from early detection and treatment of cancer, and midwives are ideally positioned to help women to access the best care. This requires being knowledgeable about the signs of disease, the best risk-reduction strategies, the latest referral guidelines, and the best

resources available in the community to maximize the best prognosis possible.

One aspect of the primary care role is coordination of care. Ensuring that communication between providers is maintained and that referrals are completed (and appointments kept) is part of that coordination. Communicating with women about clinical assessment, test results, associated risks, and management options is essential to the role and will serve to optimize the flow of care and follow-up evaluation and to minimize error, confusion, and delay in the quality of care.

References

1. Biro FM, Greenspan LC, Galvez MP, Pinney SM, Teitelbaum S, Windham GC, et al. Onset of breast development in a longitudinal cohort. *Pediatrics*. 2013;132(6):1019-1027. doi:10.1542/peds.2012-3773.

2. Fisher MM, Eugster EA. What is in our environment that effects puberty? *Reprod Toxicol*. 2014;44:7-14.

3. Fenton SE, Reed C, Newbold RR. Perinatal environmental exposures affect mammary development, function, and cancer risk in adulthood. *Annu Rev Pharmacol Toxicol*. 2012;52:455-479. doi:10.1146/annurev-pharmtox-010611-134659.

4. Duflos C, Plu-Bureau G, Thibaud E, Kuttenn F. Breast diseases in adolescents. *Endocr Dev*. 2012;22:208-221. doi:10.1159/000326690.

5. Doucet S, Soussignan R, Sagot P, Schaal B. The secretion of areolar (Montgomery's) glands from lactating women elicits selective, unconditional responses in neonates. In: Hausberger M, ed. *PLoS ONE*. 2009;4(10):e7579. doi:10.1371/journal.pone.0007579.

6. Rinker B, Veneracion M, Walsh CP. Breast ptosis: causes and cure. *Ann Plast Surg*. 201;64(5):579-584. doi:10.1097/SAP.0b013e3181c39377.

7. Rinker B, Veneracion M, Walsh CP. The effect of breastfeeding on breast aesthetics. *Aesthet Surg J*. 2008;28(5):534-537. doi:10.1016/j.asj.2008.07.004.

8. Guray M, Sahin AA. Benign breast diseases: classification, diagnosis, and management. *Oncologist*. 2006;11:435-449; doi:10.1634/theoncologist.11-5-435

9. Siegel RL, Miller KD, Jemal A. Cancer statistics, 2015. *CA Cancer J Clin*. 2015;65:5-29. doi:10.3322/caac.21254.

10. Howlader N, Noone AM, Krapcho M, Garshell J, Miller D, Altekruse SF, et al., eds. *SEER Cancer Statistics Review, 1975–2012*. Bethesda, MD: National Cancer Institute. Available at: http://seer.cancer.gov/csr/1975_2012/. Accessed May 8, 2016.

11. National Cancer Institute. Surveillance, Epidemiology, and End Results Program. Available at: http://seer.cancer.gov/faststats/selections.php?series=cancer. Accessed May 8, 2016.

12. Daly B, Olopade OI. A perfect storm: how tumor biology, genomics, and health care delivery patterns collide to create a racial survival disparity in breast cancer and proposed interventions for change. *CA Cancer J Clin*. 2015;65(3):221-238. doi:10.3322/caac.21271.

13. Dunn BK, Agurs-Collins T, Browne D, Lubet R, Johnson KA. Health disparities in breast cancer: biology meets socioeconomic status. *Breast Cancer Res Treat*. 2010;121(2):281-292. doi:10.1007/s10549-010-0827-x.

14. Chlebowski RT, Chen Z, Anderson GL, Rohan T, Aragaki A, Lane D, et al. Ethnicity and breast cancer: factors influencing differences in incidence and outcome. *J Natl Cancer Inst*. 2005;97:439-448. doi:10.1093/jnci/dji064.

15. Marrow M, Wong S, Venta L. The evaluation of breast masses in women younger than forty years of age. *Surgery*. 1998;124:634.

16. Valeri A, Fournier G, Morin V, Morin JF, Drelon E, Mangin P, et al. Early onset and familial predisposition to prostate cancer significantly enhance the probability for breast cancer in first degree relatives. *Int J Cancer*. 2000;86(6):883-887.

17. Scott RJ, Ashton KA. Familial breast and bowel cancer: does it exist? *Hered Cancer Clin Pract.* 2004;2(1):25-9. doi:10.1186/1897-4287-2-1-25.

18. Beebe-Dimmer JL, Yee C, Cote ML, Petrucelli N, Palmer N, Bock C, et al. Familial clustering of breast and prostate cancer and risk of postmenopausal breast cancer in the Women's Health Initiative Study. *Cancer.* 2015;121(8):1265-1272. doi:10.1002 /cncr.29075.

19. Moriarty AT, Schwartz MR, Laucirica R, Booth CN, Auger M, Thomas N, et al. Cytology of spontaneous nipple discharge—Is it worth it? *Arch Pathol Lab Med.* 2013;137:1039-1042. doi:10.5858 /arpa.2012-0231-CP.

20. Pisano ED, Hendrick RE, Yaffe MJ, Baum JK, Acharyya S, Cormack JB, et al. Diagnostic accuracy of digital versus film mammography: exploratory analysis of selected population subgroups in DMIST. *Radiology.* 2008;246(2):376-383. doi:10.1148/radiol. 2461070200.

21. Neal L, Tortorelli CL, Nassar A. Clinician's guide to imaging and pathologic findings in benign breast disease. *Mayo Clin Proc.* 2010;85(3):274-9. doi:10.4065/mcp.2009.0656.

22. Sickles EA, D'Orsi CJ, Bassett LW, et al. ACR BI-RADS® Mammography. In: *ACR BI-RADS® Atlas, Breast Imaging Reporting and Data System.* Reston, VA: American College of Radiology; 2013.

23. Kocjan G, Bourgain C, Fassina A, Hagmar B, Herbert A, Kapila K, et al. The role of breast FNAC in diagnosis and clinical management: a survey of current practice. *Cytopathology.* 2008;19(5):271-8. doi: 10.1111/j.1365-2303.2008.00610.x.

24. Heisey RE, McCready DR. Office management of a palpable breast lump with aspiration. *CMAJ.* 2010;182(7):693-696. doi:10.1503/cmaj.090416.

25. Sickles EA. Periodic mammographic follow-up of probably benign lesions: results in 3,184 consecutive cases. *Radiology.* 1991;179:463-8.

26. Shin S, Schneider HB, Cole FJ, Laronga C. Follow-up recommendations for benign breast biopsies. *Breast J.* 2006;12:413-7. doi:org/10.1111/j.1075-122X.2006. 00302.x.

27. Johnson JM, Johnson AK, O'Meara ES, Miglioretti DL, Geller BM, Hotaling EN, et al. Breast cancer detection with short-interval follow-up compared with return to annual screening in patients with benign stereotactic or US-guided breast biopsy results. *Radiology.* 2015;275:54-60.

28. Langer A, Mohallem M, Berment H, Ferreira F, Gog A, Khalifa D, et al. Breast lumps in pregnant women. *Diagn Interv Imaging.* 2015;96(10): 1077-1087. doi:10.1016/j.diii.2015.07.005.

29. Litton JK, Theriault RL, Gonzalez-Angulo AM. Breast cancer diagnosis during pregnancy. *Womens Health (Lond Engl).* 2009;5(3):243-249. doi:10.2217 /whe.09.2.

30. Joshi S, Dialani V, Marotti J, Mehta TS, Slanetz PJ. Breast disease in the pregnant and lactating patient: radiological-pathological correlation. *Insights Imaging.* 2013;4(5):527-538. doi:10.1007 /s13244-012-0211-y.

31. Swinford AE, Adler DD, Garver KA. Mammographic appearance of the breasts during pregnancy and lactation: false assumptions. *Acad Radiol.* 1998; 5(7):467-472.

32. Vashi R, Hooley R, Butler R, Geisel J, Philpotts L. Breast imaging of the pregnant and lactating patient: imaging modalities and pregnancy-associated breast cancer. *Am J Roentgenol.* 2013;2:321-328.

33. Pruthi S, Wahner-Roedler DL, Torkelson CJ, Cha SS, Thicke LS, Hazelton JH, et al. Vitamin E and evening primrose oil for management of cyclical mastalgia: a randomized pilot study. *Altern Med Rev.* 2010;15(1):59-67.

34. Hartmann LC, Sellers TA, Frost MH, Lingle WL, Degnim AC, Ghosh K, et al. Benign breast disease and the risk of breast cancer. *N Engl J Med.* 2005;353(3):229-237.

35. Wang J, Costantino JP, Tan-Chiu E, Wickerham DL, Paik S, Wolmark N. Lower-category benign breast disease and the risk of invasive breast cancer. *J Natl Cancer Inst.* 2004;96:616.

36. Dyrstad SW, Yan Y, Fowler AM, Colditz GA. Breast cancer risk associated with benign breast disease: systematic review and meta-analysis. *Breast Cancer Res Treat.* 2015;149(3):569-575. doi:10.1007/ s10549-014-3254-6.

37. Berg WA, Sechtin AG, Marques H, Zhang Z. Cystic breast masses and the ACRIN 6666 experience. *Radiol Clin North Am.* 2010;48(5):931-987. doi:10.1016/j.rcl.2010.06.007.

38. Rinaldi P, Ierardi C, Costantini M, Magno S, Giuliani MM, Belli P, et al. Cystic breast lesions: sonographic findings and clinical management. *J Ultrasound Med.* 2010;29:1617-1626.

39. Ferara A. Benign breast disease. *Radiol Technol.* 2011;82(5):447M-62M.

40. Houssami N, Irwig L, Ung O. Review of complex breast cysts: implications for cancer detection and clinical practice. *ANZ J Surg.* 2005;75:1080-5. doi: 10.1111/j.1445-2197.2005.03608.x.

41. Tea MK, Grimm C, Heinz-Peer G, Delancey J, Singer C. The predictive value of suspicious sonographic characteristics in atypical cyst-like breast lesions. *Breast.* 2011;20(2):165-9.

42. Amin AL, Purdy AC, Mattingly JD, Kong AL, Termuhlen PM. Benign breast disease. *Surg Clin North Am.* 2013;93:299-308.

43. Ben Hassouna J, Damak T, Gamoudi A, Chargui R, Khomsi F, Mahjoub S, et al. Phyllodes tumors of the breast: a case series of 106 patients. *Am J Surg.* 2006;192:141-147.

44. Pimiento JM, Gadgil PV, Santillan AA, Lee MC, Esposito NN, Kiluk JV, et al. Phyllodes tumors: race-related differences. *J Am Coll Surg.* 2011;213(4): 537-542.

45. Guillot E, Couturaud B, Reyal F, Curnier A, Ravinet J, Laé M, et al. Management of phyllodes breast tumors. *Breast J.* 2011;17(2):129-137. doi:10.1111/j .1524-4741.2010.01045.x.

46. Ferroni P, Riondino S, Buonomo O, Palmirotta R, Guadagni F, Roselli M. Type 2 diabetes and breast cancer: the interplay between impaired glucose metabolism and oxidant stress. *Oxid Med Cell Longev.* 2015;2015:183928. doi:10.1155/2015/ 183928.

47. Tan PH, Lai LM, Carrington EV, Opaluwa AS, Ravikumar KH, Chetty N, et al. Fat necrosis of the breast—a review. *Breast.* 2006;15(3):313-8. doi:10.1016/j.breast.2005.07.003.

48. Kerridge WD, Kryvenko ON, Thompson A, Shah BA. Fat necrosis of the breast: a pictorial review of the mammographic, ultrasound, CT, and MRI findings with histopathologic correlation. *Radiol Res Pract.* 2015;2015:613139. doi:10.1155/2015/ 613139.

49. Rahal RM, Júnior RF, Reis C, Pimenta FC, Netto JC, Paulinelli RR. Prevalence of bacteria in the nipple discharge of patients with duct ectasia. *Int J Clin Pract.* 2005;59(9):1045-1050.

50. Ferris-James DM, Iuanow E, Mehta TS, Shaheen RM, Slanetz PJ. Imaging approaches to diagnosis and management of common ductal abnormalities. *Radiographics.* 2012;32(4):1009-1030.

51. Rahal RM, de Freitas-Júnior R, Paulinelli RR. Risk factors for duct ectasia. *Breast J.* 2005;11(4):262-265.

52. Wells CA, El-Ayat GA. Non-operative breast pathology: apocrine lesions. *J Clin Pathol.* 2007; 60(12):1313-20. doi:10.1136/jcp.2006.040626.

53. Tse GM, Tan PH, Pang AL, Tang AP, Cheung HS. Calcification in breast lesions: pathologists' perspective. *J Clin Pathol.* 2008;61(2):145-151.

54. Nalawade YV. Evaluation of breast calcifications. *Indian J Radiol Imaging.* 2009;19(4):282-286. doi:10.4103/0971-3026.57208.

55. Kabat GC, Jones JG, Olson N, Negassa A, Duggan C, Ginsberg M, et al. A multi-center prospective cohort study of benign breast disease and risk of subsequent breast cancer. *Cancer Causes Control.* 2010;21(6): 821-828. doi:10.1007/s10552-010-9508-7.

56. Schnitt SJ. Benign breast disease and breast cancer risk: morphology and beyond. *Am J Surg Pathol.* 2003;27(6):836.

57. El-Wakeel H, Umpleby HC. Systematic review of fibroadenoma as a risk factor for breast cancer. *Breast.* 2003;12:302-307.

58. Cerrato F, Labow BI. Diagnosis and management of fibroadenomas in the adolescent breast. *Semin Plast Surg.* 2013;27(1):23-5. doi:10.1055/ s-0033-1343992.

59. Cole-Beugler C, Soriano RZ, Kurtz AB, Goldberg BB. Fibroadenoma of the breast: sonomammography correlated with pathology in 122 patients. *Am J Roentgenol.* 1983;140:369-375.

60. Sanders LM, Sara R. The growing fibroadenoma. *Acta Radiol Open.* 2015;4(4):2047981615572273. doi:10.1177/2047981615572273.

61. Dupont WD, Page DL, Parl FF, Vnencak-Jones CL, Plummer WD, Rados MS, et al. Long-term risk of breast cancer in women with fibroadenoma. *N Engl J Med.* 1994;331:10-15. doi:10.1056/NEJM 199407073310103.

62. Nassar A, Visscher DW, Degnim AC, Frank RD, Vierkant RA, Frost M, et al. Complex fibroadenoma and breast cancer risk: a Mayo Clinic benign breast disease cohort study. *Breast Cancer Res Treat.* 2015;153:397-405.

63. Collins LC, Baer HJ, Tamimi RM, Connolly JL, Colditz GA, Schnitt SJ. The influence of family history on breast cancer risk in women with biopsy-confirmed benign breast disease. *Cancer.* 2006;107: 1240-7. doi:10.1002/cncr.22136.

64. Hubbard JL, Cagle K, Davis JW, Kaups KL, Kodama M. Criteria for excision of suspected fibroadenomas of the breast. *Am J Surg.* 2015;209(2):297-301. doi: 10.1016/j.amjsurg.2013.12.037.

65. Kaufman CS, Littrup PJ, Freeman-Gibb LA, Smith J S, Francescatti D, Simmons R, et al. Office-based cryoablation of breast fibroadenomas with long-term follow-up. *Breast J.* 2005;11(5):344-350. doi:10.1111/j.1075-122X.2005.21700.x.

66. Manipadam MT, Jacob A, Rajnikanth J. Giant lactating adenoma of the breast. *J Surg Case Rep.* 2010;9:8. doi:10.1093/jscr/2010.9.8.

67. Baker TP, Lenert JT, Parker J, Kemp B, Kushwaha A, Evans G, et al. Lactating adenoma: a diagnosis of exclusion. *Breast J.* 2001;7:354-7. doi:10.1046/j. 1524-4741.2001.20075.x.

68. King TA, Scharfenberg JC, Smetherman DH, Farkas EA, Bolton JS, Fuhrman GM. A better understanding of the term radial scar. *Am J Surg.* 2000;180(6):428-432; discussion 432-3.

69. Nassar A, Conners AL, Celik B, Jenkins SM, Smith CY, Hieken TJ. Radial scar/complex sclerosing lesions: a clinicopathologic correlation study from a single institution. *Ann Diagn Pathol.* 2015;19(1): 24-8. doi:10.1016/j.anndiagpath.2014.12.003.

70. Linda A, Zuiani C, Furlan A, Londero V, Girometti R, Maching P, et al. Radial scars without atypia diagnosed at imaging-guided needle biopsy: how often is associated malignancy found at subsequent surgical excision, and do mammography and sonography predict which lesions are malignant? *Am J Roentgenol.* 2010;194:1146-1151.

71. Berg JC, Visscher DW, Vierkant RA, Pankratz VS, Maloney SD, Lewis JT, et al. Breast cancer risk in women with radial scars in benign breast biopsies. *Breast Cancer Res Treat.* 2008;108(2):167-174.

72. Hartmann LC, Radisky DC, Frost MH, Santen RJ, Vierkant RA, Benetti LL, et al. Understanding the premalignant potential of atypical hyperplasia through its natural history: a longitudinal cohort study. *Cancer Prev Res (Phila).* 2014;7(2):211-7. doi: 10.1158/1940-6207.CAPR-13-0222.

73. Degnim AC, Visscher DW, Berman HK, Frost MH, Sellers TA, et al. Stratification of breast cancer risk in women with atypia: a mayo cohort study. *J Clin Oncol.* 2007;25(19):2671-2677.

74. Bevers TB, Anderson BO, Bonaccio E, Buys S, Daly MB, Dempsey PJ, et al. NCCN clinical practice guidelines: breast cancer screening and diagnosis. *J Natl Compr Canc Netw.* 2009 Nov;7(10):1060-1096.

75. Hartmann LC, Degnim AC, Santen RJ, Dupont WD, Ghosh K. Atypical hyperplasia of the breast—risk assessment and management options. *N Engl J Med.* 2015;372(1):78-89. doi:10.1056/NEJMsr 1407164.

76. Murray MP, Luedtke C, Liberman L, Nehhozina T, Akram M, Brogi E. Classic lobular carcinoma in situ and atypical lobular hyperplasia at percutaneous breast core biopsy. *Cancer.* 2013;119:1073-9. doi:10.1002/cncr.27841.

77. Lewis JL, Lee DY, Tartter PI. The significance of lobular carcinoma in situ and atypical lobular hyperplasia of the breast. *Ann Surg Oncol.* 2012;19(13): 4124-4128. doi:10.1245/s10434-012-2538-5.

78. Li CI, Malone KE, Saltzman BS, Daling JR. Risk of invasive breast carcinoma among women diagnosed with ductal carcinoma in situ and lobular carcinoma in situ, 1988–2001. *Cancer.* 2006;106:2104-2112. doi:10.1002/cncr.21864.

79. Cutuli B, De Lafontan B, Kirova Y, Auvray H, Tallet A, Avigdor S, et al. Lobular carcinoma in situ (LCIS) of the breast: is long-term outcome similar to ductal carcinoma in situ (DCIS)? Analysis of 200 cases. *Radiat Oncol.* 2015;10:1.

80. Shah-Khan MG, Geiger XJ, Reynolds C, Jakub JW, Deperi ER, Glazebrook KN. Long-term follow-up of lobular neoplasia (atypical lobular hyperplasia/lobular carcinoma in situ) diagnosed on core needle biopsy. *Ann Surg Oncol.* 2012;19:3131-3138.

81. Allegra CJ, Aberle DR, Ganschow P, Hahn SM, Lee CN, Millon-Underwood S, et al. National Institutes of Health State-of-the-Science conference statement: diagnosis and management of ductal carcinoma in situ September 22–24, 2009. *J Natl Cancer Inst.* 2010;102(3):161-9. doi:10.1093/jnci/djp485.

82. Sanders ME, Schuyler PA, Dupont WD, Page DL. The natural history of low-grade ductal carcinoma in situ of the breast in women treated by biopsy only revealed over 30 years of long-term follow-up. *Cancer.* 2005;103(12):2481-2484.

83. Allred DC, Anderson SJ, Paik S, Wickerham DL, Nagtegaal ID, Swain SM, et al. Adjuvant tamoxifen reduces subsequent breast cancer in women with estrogen receptor—positive ductal carcinoma in situ: a study based on NSABP Protocol B-24. *J Clin Oncol.* 2012;30(12):1268-1273. doi:10.1200 /JCO.2010.34.0141.

84. Scurr J, Hedger W, Morris P, Brown N. The prevalence, severity, and impact of breast pain in the general population. *Breast J.* 2014;20(5):508-513. doi: 10.1111/tbj.12305.

85. Ader DN, Shriver CD. Cyclical mastalgia: prevalence and impact in an outpatient breast clinic sample. *J Am Coll Surg.* 1997;185(5):466-470.

86. Smith RL, Pruthi S, Fitzpatrick LA. Evaluation and management of breast pain. *Mayo Clin Proc.* 2004; 79:353-372.

87. Santen RJ, Mansel R. Benign breast disorders. *N Engl J Med.* 2005;353(3):275-285.

88. Colak T, Turgut I, Kanik A, Ogetman Z, Aydin S. Efficacy of topical nonsteroidal antiinflammatory drugs in mastalgia treatment. *J Am Coll Surg.* 2003; 196(4):525-530.

89. Pruthi S, Wahner-Roedler DL, Torkelson CJ, Cha SS, Thicke LS, Hazelton JH, et al. Vitamin E and evening primrose oil for management of cyclical mastalgia: a randomized pilot study. *Altern Med Rev.* 2010;15(1):59-67.

90. Rosolowich V, Saettler E, Szuck B, Lea RH, Levesque P, Weisberg F. Mastalgia. *J Obstet Gynaecol Can.* 2006;28(1):49-71.

91. Leung AKC, Pacaud D. Diagnosis and management of galactorrhea. *Am Fam Physician.* 2004;70: 543-550.

92. Peña KS, Rosenfeld JA. Evaluation and treatment of galactorrhea. *Am Fam Physician.* 2001;63(9): 1763-1770.

93. Huang W, Molitch ME. Evaluation and management of galactorrhea. *Am Fam Physician.* 2012; 85(11):1073-1080.

94. Foulkes RE, Heard G, Boyce T, Skyrme R, Holland PA, Gateley CA. Duct excision is still necessary to rule out breast cancer in patients presenting with spontaneous bloodstained nipple discharge. *Int J Breast Cancer.* 2011;2011:495315.

95. Dupont SC, Boughey JC, Jimenez RE, Hoskin TL, Hieken TJ. Frequency of diagnosis of cancer or high-risk lesion at operation for pathologic nipple discharge. *Surgery.* 2015;158(4):988-994. doi:10.1016/j.surg.2015.05.020.

96. Amir LH. ABM Clinical protocol #4: mastitis, revised March 2014. *Breastfeed Med.* 2014;9(5):239-243. doi:10.1089/bfm.2014.9984.

97. Foxman B, D'Arcy H, Gillespie B, Bobo JK, Schwartz K. Lactation mastitis: occurrence and medical management among 946 breastfeeding women in the United States. *Am J Epidemiol.* 2002; 155(2):103-114.

98. Kinlay JR, O'Connell DL, Kinlay S. Risk factors for mastitis in breastfeeding women: results of a prospective cohort study. *Aust N Z J Public Health.* 2001;25(2):115-120.

99. Kvist LJ. Re-examination of old truths: replication of a study to measure the incidence of lactational mastitis in breastfeeding women. *Int Breastfeed J.* 2013;8:2. doi:10.1186/1746-4358-8-2.

100. Amir LH, Donath SM, Garland SM, Tabrizi SN, Bennett CM, Cullinane M, et al. Does *Candida* and/or *Staphylococcus* play a role in nipple and breast pain in lactation? A cohort study in Melbourne, Australia. *BMJ Open.* 2013;3(3):e002351. doi:10.1136/bmjopen-2012-002351.

101. Mediano P, Fernández L, Rodríguez JM, Marín M. Case–control study of risk factors for infectious mastitis in Spanish breastfeeding women. *BMC Pregnancy Childbirth.* 2014;14:195. doi:10.1186/1471-2393-14-195.

102. Jahanfar S, Ng CJ, Teng CL. Antibiotics for mastitis in breastfeeding women. *Cochrane Database Syst Rev.* 2013;2:CD005458.

103. Polyak K. Pregnancy and breast cancer: the other side of the coin. *Cancer Cell.* 2006;9:151-153.

104. Trop I, Dugas A, David J, El Khoury M, Boileau JF, Larouche N, et al. Breast abscesses: evidence-based algorithms for diagnosis, management, and follow-up. *Radiographics.* 2011;31(6):1683-1699. doi: 10.1148/rg.316115521.

105. Amir LH, Forster D, McLachlan H, Lumley J. Incidence of breast abscess in lactating women: report from an Australian cohort. *BJOG.* 2004; 111(12):1378.

106. Kvist LJ, Rydhstroem H. Factors related to breast abscess after delivery: a population-based study. *BJOG.* 2005;112(8):1070-1074.

107. Bharat A, Gao F, Aft RL, Gillanders WE, Eberlein TJ, Margenthaler JA. Predictors of primary breast abscesses and recurrence. *World J Surg.* 2009;33(12):2582-2586. doi:10.1007/s00268-009-0170-8.

108. Lam E1, Chan T, Wiseman SM. Breast abscess: evidence based management recommendations. *Expert Rev Anti Infect Ther.* 2014;12(7):753-762. doi:10.1586/14787210.2014.913982.

109. Gollapalli V, Liao J, Dudakovic A, Sugg SL, Scott-Conner CE, Weigel RJ. Risk factors for development and recurrence of primary breast abscesses. *J Am Coll Surg.* 2010;211(1):41-48. doi:10.1016/j.jamcollsurg.2010.04.007.

110. Al-Khaffaf B, Knox F, Bundred MJ. Idiopathic granulomatous mastitis: a 25-year experience. *J Am Coll Surg.* 2008;206:269-273.

111. Sheybani F, Sarvghad M, Naderi HR, Gharib M. Treatment for and clinical characteristics of granulomatous mastitis. *Obstet Gynecol.* 2015;125(4): 801-807.

112. Morrill JF, Heinig MJ, Pappagianis D, Dewey KG. Risk factors for mammary candidosis among lactating women. *J Obstet Gynecol Neonatal Nurs.* 2005; 34(1):37-45.

113. Francis-Morrill J, Heinig MJ, Pappagianis D, Dewey K. Diagnostic value of signs and symptoms of mammary candidosis among lactating women. *J Hum Lact.* 2004;20:288-295.

114. Betzold CM. Results of microbial testing exploring the etiology of deep breast pain during lactation: a systematic review and meta-analysis of non-randomized trials. *J Midwifery Womens Health.* 2012;57:353-64. doi:10.1111/j.1542-2011.2011.00136.x.

115. Anderson JE, Held N, Wright K. Raynaud's phenomenon of the nipple: a treatable cause of painful breastfeeding. *Pediatrics.* 2004;113:360-364.

116. Page SM, McKenna DS. Vasospasm of the nipple presenting as painful lactation. *Obstet Gynecol.* 2006; 108(3 Pt 2):806-808.

117. Kohler BA, Sherman RL, Howlader N, Jemal A, Ryerson AB, Henry KA, et al. Annual report to the nation on the status of cancer, 1975–2011, featuring incidence of breast cancer subtypes by race/ethnicity, poverty, and state. *J Natl Cancer Inst.* 2015;107:djv048. doi:10.1093/jnci/djv048.

118. Ravdin PM, Cronin KA, Howlader N, Berg CD, Chlebowski RT, Feuer EJ, et al. The decrease in breast-cancer incidence in 2003 in the United States. *N Engl J Med.* 2007;356(16):1670-1674.

119. Barton MB, Harris R, Fletcher SW. The rational clinical examination. Does this patient have breast cancer? The screening clinical breast examination: Should it be done? How? *JAMA.* 1999;282(13): 1270-1280.

120. US Preventive Services Task Force. Screening for breast cancer: U.S. Preventive Services Task Force Recommendation Statement. *Ann Intern Med.* 2009;151:716-726.

121. Coates RJ, Uhler RJ, Brogan DJ, Gammon MD, Malone KE, Swanson CA, et al. Patterns and predictors of the breast cancer detection methods in women under 45 years of age (United States). *Cancer Causes Control.* 2001;12(5):431-442.

122. Luo J, Margolis KL, Wactawski-Wende J, Horn K, Messina C, Stefanick ML, et al. Association of active and passive smoking with risk of breast cancer among postmenopausal women: a prospective cohort study. *BMJ.* 2011;342:d1016. doi:10.1136/bmj.d1016.

123. Ahn J, Schatzkin A, Lacey JV Jr, Albanes D, Ballard-Barbash R, Adams KF, et al. Adiposity, adult weight change, and postmenopausal breast cancer risk. *Arch Intern Med.* 2007;167(19):2091.

124. Emaus MJ, van Gils CH, Bakker MF, Bisschop CN, Monninkhof EM, Bueno-de-Mesquita HB, et al. Weight change in middle adulthood and breast cancer risk in the EPIC-PANACEA study. *Int J Cancer.* 2014;135(12):2887-2899. doi:10.1002/ijc.28926.

125. Lawlor DA, Smith GD, Ebrahim S. Hyperinsulinaemia and increased risk of breast cancer: findings from the British Women's Heart and Health Study. *Cancer Causes Control.* 2004;15(3):267-275.

126. Chen WY, Rosner B, Hankinson SE, Colditz GA, Willett WC. Moderate alcohol consumption during adult life, drinking patterns, and breast cancer risk. *JAMA.* 2011;306(17):1884.

127. Gaudet MM, Gapstur SM, Sun J, Diver WR, Hannan LM, Thun MJ. Active smoking and breast cancer risk: original cohort data and meta-analysis. *J Natl Cancer Inst.* 2013;105(8):515-525.

128. Johnson KC, Miller AB, Collishaw NE, Palmer JR, Hammond SK, Salmon AG, et al. Active smoking and secondhand smoke increase breast cancer risk: the report of the Canadian Expert Panel on Tobacco Smoke and Breast Cancer Risk (2009). *Tob Control.* 2011;20(1):e2.

129. Hansen J, Stevens RG. Case-control study of shift-work and breast cancer risk in Danish nurses: impact of shift systems. *Eur J Cancer.* 2012;48(11): 1722-1729.

130. Schernhammer ES, Hankinson SE. Urinary melatonin levels and breast cancer risk. *J Natl Cancer Inst.* 2005;97(14):1084.

131. Menashe I, Anderson WF, Jatoi I, Rosenberg PS. Underlying causes of the black–white racial disparity in breast cancer mortality: a population-based analysis. *J Natl Cancer Inst.* 2009;101(14):993-1000. doi:10.1093/jnci/djp176.

132. Churpek JE, Walsh T, Zheng Y, Moton Z, Thornton AM, Lee MK, et al. Inherited predisposition to breast cancer among African American women. *Breast Cancer Res Treat.* 2015;149:31-9. doi:10.1007/s10549-014-3195-0.

133. Pal T, Bonner D, Cragun D, Monteiro AN, Phelan C, Servais L, et al. A high frequency of BRCA mutations in young black women with breast cancer residing in Florida. *Cancer.* 2015;121(23):4173-4180. doi:10.1002/cncr.29645.

134. Haile RA, John EM, Levine AJ, Cortessis VK, Unger JB, Gonzales M, et al. A review of cancer in U.S. Hispanic populations. *Cancer Prev Res.* 2012; 5(2):150-163; doi:10.1158/1940-6207.

135. Vacek PM, Geller BM. A prospective study of breast cancer risk using routine mammographic breast density measurements. *Cancer Epidemiol Biomarkers Prev.* 2004;13:715-722.

136. Tice JA, Cummings SR, Ziv E, Kerlikowske K. Mammographic breast density and the Gail model for breast cancer risk prediction in a screening population. *Breast Cancer Res Treat.* 2005;94: 115-122.

137. Martin LJ, Melnichouk O, Guo H, Chiarelli AM, Hislop G, Yaffe MJ, et al. Family history, mammographic density, and risk of breast cancer. *Cancer Epidemiol Biomarkers Prev.* 2010;19:456-463; doi:10.1158/1055-9965.EPI-09-0881.

138. McCormack VA, dos Santos Silva I. Breast density and parenchymal patterns as markers of breast cancer risk: a meta-analysis. *Cancer Epidemiol Biomarkers Prev.* 2006;15:1159-69. doi:10.1158/1055-9965. EPI-06-0034.

139. Byrne C, Schairer C, Wolfe J, Parekh N, Salane M, Brinton LA, et al. Mammographic features and breast cancer risk: effects with time, age, and menopause status. *J Natl Cancer Inst.* 1995;87(21):1622-1629. doi:10.1093/jnci/87.21.1622.

140. Rhodes DJ, Breitkopf CR, Ziegenfuss JY, Jenkins SM, Vachon CM. Awareness of breast density and its impact on breast cancer detection and risk. *J Clin Oncol.* 2015;33(10):1143-1150.

141. Jardines L, Goyal S, Fisher P, Weitzel J, Royce M, Goldfarb SB. Breast Cancer Overview: Risk Factors, Screening, Genetic Testing, and Prevention. Cancer Network; June 1, 2015. Available at: http://www.cancernetwork.com/cancer-management/breast-cancer-overview-risk-factors-screening-genetic-testing-and-prevention. Accessed May 10, 2016.

142. Antoniou A, Pharoah PDP, Narod S, Risch HA, Eyfjord JE, Hopper JL, et al. Average risks of breast and ovarian cancer associated with BRCA1 or BRCA2 mutations detected in case series unselected for family history: a combined analysis of 22 studies. *Am J Hum Genet.* 2003;72(5):1117-1130.

143. Eccles DM. Identification of personal risk of breast cancer: genetics. *Breast Cancer Res.* 2008;10(Suppl 4): S12. doi:10.1186/bcr2172.

144. Friebel TM, Domchek SM, Rebbeck TR. Modifiers of cancer risk in BRCA1 and BRCA2 mutation carriers: a systematic review and meta-analysis. *J Natl Cancer Inst.* 2014;106:dju091. doi:10.1093 /jnci/dju091.

145. Nelson HD, Fu R, Goddard K, et al. *Risk Assessment, Genetic Counseling, and Genetic Testing for BRCA-Related Cancer: Systematic Review to Update the U.S. Preventive Services Task Force Recommendation* [Internet]. Rockville, MD: Agency for Healthcare Research and Quality; 2013.

146. National Cancer Institute. Breast Cancer Risk Assessment Tool. Available at: http://www.cancer.gov /bcrisktool/Default.aspx. Accessed May 10, 2016.

147. National Cancer Institute. Breast Cancer Risk Assessment Tool. About the Tool. Available at: http://www.cancer.gov/bcrisktool/about-tool.aspx. Accessed May 10, 2016.

148. Evans DG, Howell A. Can the breast screening appointment be used to provide risk assessment and prevention advice? *Breast Cancer Res.* 2015;17(1):84. doi:10.1186/s13058-015-0595-y.

149. Barlow WE, White E, Ballard-Barbash R, Vacek PM, Titus-Ernstoff L, Carney PA, et al. Prospective breast cancer risk prediction model for women undergoing screening mammography. *J Natl Cancer Inst.* 2006;98(17):1204-1214. doi:10.1093/jnci/djj331.

150. Tyrer J, Duffy SW, Cuzick J. A breast cancer prediction model incorporating familial and personal risk factors. *Stat Med.* 2004;14:1111-1130. doi:10.1002/sim.1668.

151. Quante AS, Whittemore AS, Shriver T, Strauch K, Terry MB. Breast cancer risk assessment across the risk continuum: genetic and nongenetic risk factors contributing to differential model performance. *Breast Cancer Res.* 2012;14(6):R144. doi:10.1186 /bcr3352.

152. Claus EB, Risch N, Thompson WD. The calculation of breast cancer risk for women with a first degree family history of ovarian cancer. *Breast Cancer Res Treat.* 1993;28:115-120. doi:10.1007 /BF00666424.

153. Parmigiani G, Berry D, Aguilar O. Determining carrier probabilities for breast cancer-susceptibility genes BRCA1 and BRCA2. *Am J Hum Genet.* 1998;62(1):145-158.

154. Antoniou AC, Pharoah PP, Smith P, Easton DF. The BOADICEA model of genetic susceptibility to breast and ovarian cancer. *Br J Cancer.* 2004;91: 1580-1590.

155. Lee AJ, Cunningham AP, Kuchenbaecker KB, Mavaddat N, Easton DF, Antoniou AC, et al. BOADICEA breast cancer risk prediction model: updates to cancer incidences, tumour pathology and web interface. *Br J Cancer.* 2014;110(2):535-545. doi:10.1038/bjc.2013.730.

156. American College of Obstetricians and Gynecologists. Breast cancer screening. Practice Bulletin No. 122. *Obstet Gynecol.* 2011;118:372-382.

157. Smith RA, Manassaram-Baptiste D, Brooks D, Doroshenk M, Fedewa S, Saslow D, et al. Cancer screening in the United States, 2015: a review of current American Cancer Society guidelines and current issues in cancer screening. *CA Cancer J Clin.* 2015;65:30-54. doi:10.3322/caac.21261.

158. US Preventive Services Task Force. Breast Cancer: Screening. Available at: http://www .uspreventiveservicestaskforce.org/Page/Document /UpdateSummaryFinal/breast-cancer-screening. Accessed May 10, 2016.

159. Agency for Healthcare Research and Quality. WHO position paper on mammography screening. Available at: http://www.guideline.gov/content.aspx?f=r ss&id=49209&osrc=12. Accessed May 10, 2016.

160. Centers for Disease Control and Prevention (CDC). Cancer screening—United States, 2010. *MMWR.* 2012;61(3):41-45.

161. The Guide to Community Preventive Services. Cancer Prevention and Control. Available at: http:// www.thecommunityguide.org/cancer/index.html. Accessed May 10, 2016.

162. Loprinzi PD, Cardinal BJ, Smit E, Winters-Stone T. Physical activity and breast cancer risk. *J Exerc Sci Fitness.* 2012;10:1-7.

163. Lynch BM, Neilson HK, Friedenreich CM. Physical activity and breast cancer prevention. *Recent Results Cancer Res.* 2011;186:13-42. doi:10.1007 /978-3-642-04231-7_2.

164. Toledo E, Salas-Salvadó J, Donat-Vargas C, Buil-Cosiales P, Estruch R, Ros E, et al. Mediterranean diet and invasive breast cancer risk among women at high cardiovascular risk in the PREDIMED trial: a randomized clinical trial. *JAMA*

Intern Med. 2015;175(11):1752-1760. doi:10.1001/jamainternmed.2015.4838.

165. Collaborative Group on Hormonal Factors in Breast Cancer. Breast cancer and breastfeeding: collaborative reanalysis of individual data from 47 epidemiological studies in 30 countries, including 50302 women with breast cancer and 96973 women without the disease. *Lancet.* 2002;360:187-195.

166. Scoccianti C, Key TJ, Anderson AS, Armaroli P, Berrino F, Cecchini M, et al. European Code against Cancer 4th Edition: Breastfeeding and cancer. *Cancer Epidemiol.* 2015;39(Suppl 1):S101-6. doi:10.1016/j.canep.2014.12.007.

167. Beral V for the Million Women Study Collaborators. Breast cancer and hormone-replacement therapy in the Million Women Study. *Lancet.* 2003;362:419-427.

168. Chlebowski RT, Hendrix SL, Langer RD, Stefanick ML, Gass M, Lane D, et al. Influence of estrogen plus progestin on breast cancer and mammography in healthy postmenopausal women: the women's health initiative randomized trial. *JAMA.* 2003;289:3243-3253.

169. Wachtel MS, Yang S, Dissanaike S, Margenthaler JA. Hormone replacement therapy, likely neither angel nor demon. *PLoS ONE.* 2015;10(9):e0138556. doi:10.1371/journal.pone.0138556.

170. Chlebowski RT, Rohan TE, Manson JE, Aragaki AK, Kaunitz A, Stefanick ML, et al. Breast cancer after use of estrogen plus progestin and estrogen alone: analyses of data from 2 Women's Health Initiative randomized clinical trials. *JAMA Oncol.* 2015;1(3):296-305. doi:10.1001/jamaoncol.2015.0494.

171. Fisher B, Costantino JP, Wickerham DL, Cecchini RS, Cronin WM, Robidoux A, et al. Tamoxifen for the prevention of breast cancer: current status of the National Surgical Adjuvant Breast and Bowel Project P-1 study. *J Natl Cancer Inst.* 2005;97:1652-1662.

172. Martino S, Cauley JA, Barrett-Connor E, Powles TJ, Mershon J, Disch D, et al. Continuing outcomes relevant to Evista: breast cancer incidence in postmenopausal osteoporotic women in a randomized trial of raloxifene. *J Natl Cancer Inst.* 2004;96:1751-1761.

173. Goss PE, Ingle JN, Ales-Martinez JE, Cheung AM, Chlebowski RT, Wactawski-Wende J, et al. Exemestane for breast-cancer prevention in postmenopausal women. *N Engl J Med.* 2011;364: 2381-2391.

174. Schwartz MD, Isaacs C, Graves KD, Poggi E, Peshkin BN, Gell C, et al. Long term outcomes of BRCA1/BRCA2 testing: risk reduction and surveillance. *Cancer.* 2012;118(2):510-517. doi:10.1002/cncr.26294.

175. Nichols HB, de González AB, Lacey JV, Rosenberg PS, Anderson WF. Declining incidence of contralateral breast cancer in the United States from 1975 to 2006. *J Clin Oncol.* 2011;29(12):1564-1569. doi:10.1200/JCO.2010.32.7395.

176. American Joint Committee on Cancer. *Breast Cancer Staging.* 7th ed. 2009. Available at: https://cancerstaging.org/references-tools/quickreferences/Documents/BreastMedium.pdf. Accessed May 10, 2016.

177. National Cancer Institute. Breast Cancer Treatment—for health professionals (PDQ®). Available at: http://www.cancer.gov/types/breast/hp/breast-treatment-pdq#cit/section_1.84. Accessed May 10, 2016.

178. Lautner M, Lin H, Shen Y, et al. Disparities in the use of breast-conserving therapy among patients with early-stage breast cancer. *JAMA Surg.* 2015;150(8):778-786. doi:10.1001/jamasurg.2015.1102.

179. Wingo PA, Jamison PM, Young JL, Gargiullo P. Population-based statistics for women diagnosed with inflammatory breast cancer (United States). *Cancer Causes Control.* 2004;15(3):321-328.

180. National Cancer Institute. Inflammatory Breast Cancer. Available at: http://www.cancer.gov/types/breast/ibc-fact-sheet. Accessed May 10, 2016.

181. National Cancer Institute. Paget Disease of the Breast. Available at: http://www.cancer.gov/types/breast/paget-breast-fact-sheet#r2. Accessed May 10, 2016.

182. Chen CY, Sun LM, Anderson BO. Paget disease of the breast: changing patterns of incidence, clinical presentation, and treatment in the U.S. *Cancer.* 2006;107:1448-1458. doi:10.1002/cncr.22137.

183. Ganz PA. Psychological and social aspects of breast cancer. *Oncology (Williston Park).* 2008;22(6):642-6, 650; discussion 650, 653.

184. Fergus KD, Gray RE. Relationship vulnerabilities during breast cancer: patient and partner perspectives. *Psychooncology.* 2009;18(12):1311-1322. doi:10.1002/pon.1555.

185. Belcher AJ, Laurenceau JP, Graber EC, Cohen LH, Dasch KB, Siegel SD. Daily support in couples coping with early stage breast cancer: maintaining intimacy during adversity. *Health Psychol.* 2011;30(6):665-673. doi:10.1037/a0024705.

186. Brenner RJ. Breast cancer evaluation: medical legal issues. *Breast J.* 2004;10(1):6-9.

187. Hickson GB, Clayton EW, Githens PB, Sloan FA. Factors that prompted families to file medical malpractice claims following perinatal injuries. *JAMA*. 1992;267(10):1359-1363.

188. Hickson GB, Federspiel CF, Pichert JW, Miller CS, Gauld-Jaeger J, Bost P. Patient complaints and malpractice risk. *JAMA*. 2002;287(22):2951-7.

189. Guidera M, McCool W, Hanlon A, Schuiling K, Smith A. (2012). Midwives and liability: results from the 2009 Nationwide Survey of Certified Nurse-Midwives and Certified Midwives in the United States. *J Midwifery Womens Health*. 2012;57: 345-352. doi:10.1111/j.1542-2011.2012. 00201.x.

190. McCool WF, Guidera M, Griffinger E, Sacan D. Closed claims analysis of medical malpractice lawsuits involving midwives: lessons learned regarding safe practices and the avoidance of litigation. *J Midwifery Womens Health*. 2015;60:437-444. doi:10.1111/jmwh.12310.

191. Gandhi TK, Kachalia A, Thomas EJ, Puopolo AL, Yoon C, Brennan TA, et al. Missed and delayed diagnoses in the ambulatory setting: a study of closed malpractice claims. *Ann Intern Med*. 2006;145(7):488.

APPENDIX 19-A

BREAST EXAMINATION

Clinical examination of the breasts takes place while taking into consideration any concerns expressed by the woman, any relevant personal or family history, and review of any prior records or reports. Routine formal breast self-examination is no longer recommended, but rather has been replaced by "breast awareness" as a way to recognize abnormal changes between clinical evaluations. There is no consensus about the frequency and effectiveness of clinical breast examinations[1-3]; for more information on breast evaluation and diagnosis, see the *Breast Conditions* chapter.

Procedure for Breast Examination

1. Wash hands prior to beginning the examination.
2. The woman should be seated on the examining table so that she is facing the examiner. Her chest area should be entirely exposed. Throughout the examination, use the drape or gown to cover any parts of the woman's body not being examined.
3. Have the woman sit erect, facing the examiner. Look at the breasts with her arms loose at her sides, raised overhead, and then with her hands on her hips so that her elbows are extended 90 degrees from the plane of her abdomen. Ask her to lean forward to check that the breasts hang freely.
   - With her arms raised, the pectoral fascia is elevated. If there is a carcinoma that has attached to the fascia, the breast may show an indentation in the contour or skin retraction. When her hands are pressed against her hips, the pectoral muscles contract and if there is a carcinoma that is fixed to the

underlying fascia, the breast may elevate more than expected or skin dimpling or nipple deviation may occur. Similarly, when leaning over, the breasts will normally fall freely away from the chest but may exhibit asymmetry or retraction if the fibrosis of a breast lesion is present.
   - Note any visible scars.
4. Palpate the lymph nodes above and below the clavicle on both sides.
5. Ask the woman to lie supine on the table, and have her raise one arm and fold it behind her head or across her forehead.
   - If she has expressed concern about a possible mass or lesion, the opposite breast should be examined first.
6. Gently palpate the axillary lymph nodes. Move your palpating hand within the axilla to press anteriorly for the pectoral nodes, posteriorly for the subscapular nodes, along the upper arm for the lateral brachial nodes, and deep in the middle for the central axillary nodes (**Figure 19A-1**).
   - Small isolated lymph nodes that are palpable may reflect irritation from shaving or a localized infection. They should be reevaluated within 1 month.
7. Inspect the appearance of the nipples and areolae.
   - Nipples may be erect, flat, or inverted. The appearance changes with reproductive maturity, pregnancy, breastfeeding, and aging.
   - Spontaneous discharge, cracking, lesions, and bleeding are abnormal.
   - Do not squeeze the nipple in an attempt to elicit discharge.

Figure 19A-1

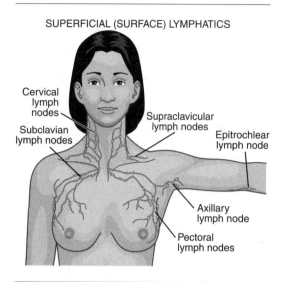

SUPERFICIAL (SURFACE) LYMPHATICS

Cervical lymph nodes

Subclavian lymph nodes

Supraclavicular lymph nodes

Epitrochlear lymph node

Axillary lymph node

Pectoral lymph nodes

Figure 19A-2

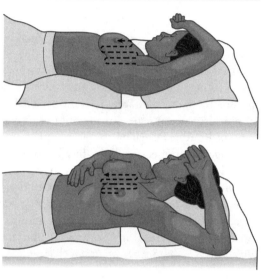

8. Inspect the appearance of the breasts.
   - Skin texture and appearance change over time.
   - Edema, redness, retracted or collapsed areas, visible sores, and masses are all abnormal observations.
9. The most effective pattern for clinical breast examination works up and down the breast, beginning under the axilla and working to- ward the sternum, and from the clavicle to below the inframammary ridge (**Figure 19A-2**).
10. Palpate each breast for texture and masses. Using the flat surface of the fingers, gently palpate each area being assessed with a circular motion (**Figure 19A-3**).
11. The full depth of the breast to the underlying rib cage is examined (**Figure 19A-4**).
    - Breast tissue has texture. Some young women will have very smooth tissue, while an older woman who has breastfed-may have an all-over nodular texture. The texture of the breast should be consistent.

Figure 19A-3

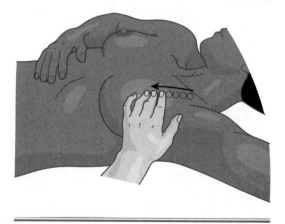

- Prior to the menses, coarse nodularity or firmness may be more noticeable.
- Palpable masses of any kind need to be evaluated further (**Figure 19A-5**).

Figure 19A-4 Palpating breast tissue to three different levels of pressure.

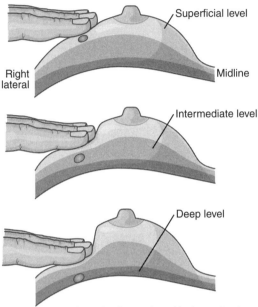

Apply pressure in a circular motion with the pads of your fingers to increasing levels, making three circles: superficial, intermediate, and deep pressure.

Figure 19A-5 "Lumpy" breast texture versus a mass.

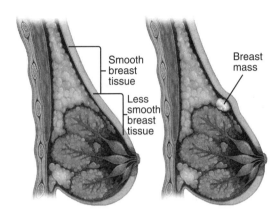

12. While performing the breast evaluation, the examiner describes what is being felt and explains how a woman can recognize breast changes. If the woman wishes to learn self-examination, this is the appropriate time to illustrate the procedure.

References

1. American College of Obstetricians and Gynecologists Practice Bulletin No. 122. Breast cancer screening. *Obstet Gynecol.* 2011;118(2P1):372-382.
2. U.S. Preventive Services Task Force. Screening for breast cancer: US Preventive Services Task Force recommendation statement. *Ann Intern Med.* 2009;151(10):716-726, W-236.
3. Barton MD, Harris R, Fletcher SW. Does this patient have breast cancer? The screening clinical breast examination: should it be done? how? *JAMA.* 1999;282:1270-1280.

CHAPTER 20

URINARY SYSTEM

Megan Sapp Madsen | Jan M. Kriebs

The urinary or renal system includes the kidneys, ureters, bladder, and urethra. Common problems include infections of the bladder and kidney, renal stones, and interstitial cystitis (IC). Women experience urinary symptoms more often than men; the overall burden among adults accounts for about 8 million adult outpatient office visits each year.[1] Half of all women self-report having had at least one infection.[2] Women also experience urinary incontinence (UI) more commonly than men, partly as a result of pregnancy and childbirth. Chronic or acute kidney failure, glomerular nephritis (an inflammatory process originating with an immune response), and kidney neoplasms are beyond the scope of this chapter and are not addressed.

Basics of Anatomy and Physiology

The renal system can be thought of as having two main divisions: the kidneys and the urinary tract. The kidneys function to filter urea, other wastes, and fluid; regulate blood pressure and blood volume; and maintain electrolyte and acid-base balance, while the ureters, bladder, and urethra form the urinary tract, responsible for collecting and excreting urine.

The kidneys are retroperitoneal abdominal organs. Structurally, the kidney is contained within a fibrous capsule, within which the renal cortex surrounds the medulla, divided in turn into several pyramids. Urine drains from the kidney through the renal pelvis into the ureters. See **Figure 20-1**.

Each renal cortex is filled with more than one million nephrons, consisting of a cluster of blood capillaries called a glomerulus and a small, curved tube called a renal tubule. The glomerulus acts as a nonspecific filter, while the various segments of the tubules rebalance and concentrate urine. This includes nearly complete reabsorption of organic nutrients and the hormonally controlled reabsorption of water and ions. Most nephrons lie deep within the cortex and cross into the medulla at the point of collection tubes; the juxtamedullary nephrons have larger glomeruli and greater medullary exposure of the tubules, and do proportionally more to concentrate urine.

Figure 20-1 The kidney and nephron.

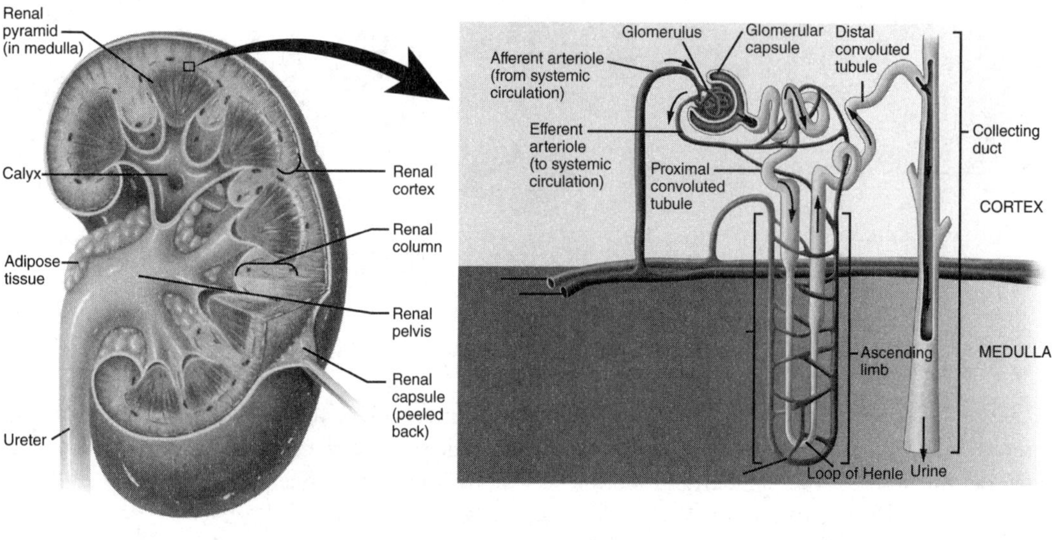

The renal pelvis and its calyces, along with the ureters, contract muscular fibers to move urine along to the bladder.

When voided, urine contains water, urea, sodium, and potassium, along with other chemical compounds. Urine has traditionally been considered to be sterile unless bacteria are cultured using standard technique. Recently, evidence of a urinary microbiome has emerged. Using deoxyribonucleic acid (DNA) sequencing and extended culture techniques, multiple species of bacteria have been reliably identified. These findings hold true for women who have no symptoms and for those with symptomatic complaints such as overactive bladder (OAB).[3-5]

The kidneys produce calcitriol, the active form of vitamin D, and erythropoietin, which stimulates red blood cell (RBC) production; the kidneys also secrete the enzyme renin in response to abnormally low blood pressure. The kidneys are acted on in their turn by antidiuretic hormone, aldosterone, angiotensin II, and the cardiac hormone atrial natriuretic peptide (ANP).

Essential History, Physical Examination, and Laboratory

Symptoms related to many of the conditions discussed in this chapter, such as renal stones or acute urinary infections, are a presenting complaint for women. However, UI may be a difficult topic for a woman to introduce, even when it is affecting her quality of life. Just as with other sensitive topics, working through the history from general questions to specifics, and from less to more potentially embarrassing is key. The woman's health provider is probably best placed to elicit information; the intimate nature of much of the gynecologic history and examination can break down barriers to discussing problems that are uncomfortable to address.

History

In addition to collecting information that will assist in the diagnosis and treatment of presenting symptoms, primary care providers can identify risks for chronic disease and facilitate referral to appropriate specialists. History specific to the renal system includes prior infections or renal stones and any family history of kidney disease such as polycystic kidneys. Conditions that can predispose to kidney disease include diabetes, hypertension, sickle cell trait or disease, systemic lupus erythematosus, and heart disease. A reproductive history that includes both sexual and birth information informs the provider about risk factors for lower urinary tract infections (LUTIs) and incontinence.

Overuse of acetaminophen and nonsteroidal anti-inflammatory drugs (NSAIDs) can damage kidneys. A large number of other medications also increase risk of kidney damage. A complete medication list should be reviewed whenever acute or chronic kidney disease is suspected. Lifestyle factors that may predispose to renal disease include smoking and obesity. Substance abuse is also a contributor, particularly opioids, inhalants, ecstasy (3,4-methylenedioxymethamphetamine, or MDMA), and phencyclidine (PCP).[6]

The review of systems includes questions about voiding patterns; pain with urination, in the lower back, or above the symphysis; and odor or discoloration of the urine. Additionally, questions about vaginal discharge and symptoms may help to clarify the source of an infection.

Physical Examination

The physical examination includes assessment for suprapubic or abdominal pain, and for costovertebral angle pain (pain over the kidneys). See **Figure 20-2** for the performance of this technique. Inguinal lymph nodes are evaluated when infection is suspected. A speculum examination is required if there is a suspicion that genital infections may be present. For example, a genital herpes outbreak near the urethra may cause pain during voiding; *Trichomonas* may infect the bladder as well as the vagina. In menopausal women, inspection of the external genitalia and vagina for evidence of atrophic changes is appropriate.

Laboratory and Imaging Studies

Laboratory studies that may be required include urine and blood samples. Blood tests are ordered for specific diagnoses and are discussed in the section on specific conditions. Frequently ordered urine tests include urinalysis, urine culture, and 24-hour urine.

A *urinalysis* is collected using the midstream clean-catch method. The method of cleaning the perineal area should be carefully described. If a woman is on her menses or has significant vaginal discharge, then a sterile tampon can be placed into the vagina prior to cleaning the perineum. If this is not possible, or the woman is otherwise unable to clean herself, a catheterized specimen can be considered. When available, a first morning urine specimen is desirable, because it will be more concentrated. Dilute urine from frequent voiding or large-volume fluid intake can produce false-negative results.

Urinalysis provides visual, chemical, and microscopic information. **Table 20-1** describes the contents of the urinalysis report. Causes of discolored urine include foods such as fava beans (brown); beets, blackberries, and rhubarb (red); and carrots (bright yellow). Certain medications also alter the color of urine. In addition to the well-known effect of Pyridium, phenothiazines may also cause orange urine. Other examples include metronidazole, nitrofurantoin, methyldopa, and senna (brown); amitriptyline and intravenous (IV) cimetidine or promethazine

Figure 20-2 Assessing for costovertebral tenderness.

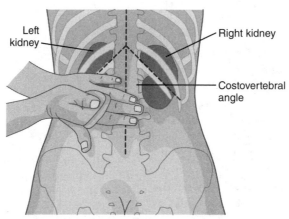

Left kidney

Right kidney

Costovertebral angle

Choose the technique that is most comfortable for both examiner and patient.
1. With the woman seated on the exam table, place the palm of one hand over her costovertebral angle on one side. Make a fist out of your other hand. Use the ulnar surface of your fist for striking. Strike the back of the hand that is over the costovertebral angle with the fist of your other hand.
OR
2. Put your hands around the woman's waist and locate, by palpation, the costovertebral angles with the flat part of your index and middle fingers on each hand. Alternately strike each costovertebral angle with your fingers by a sudden, upward motion of your hand.

(blue/green); and rifampin (red).[7] **Table 20-2** describes the findings associated with common conditions affecting the urinary tract.

Urine culture provides evidence of infection. The specimen needs to be collected as a clean catch to prevent overgrowth of perineal bacteria, yeast, or parasites. A report of low levels of multiple bacteria, or showing normal flora, needs to be repeated. Susceptibility testing is performed when an organism predominates at high levels. Bacterial counts of 10^5 are considered the gold standard for urinary tract infections (UTIs) when the specimen is voided, or 10^2 if the specimen is catheterized. Lower counts in midstream specimens may still be associated with symptomatic infection that requires treatment. Dilute urine, current antibiotic use, and high vitamin C intake may cause falsely negative or low bacterial counts. If an initial urine sample is contaminated, the subsequent urine should be collected after a sufficient amount of time has elapsed for bacterial levels in the urinary tract to rise to detectable levels.

A 24-hour urine collection can be used for evaluation of kidney damage. Protein, creatinine, cortisol, signs of predisposition to kidney stones, and other findings can guide diagnostic protocols.

Several imaging studies can be used in diagnosis of renal disease. Ultrasound can identify hydronephrosis, abnormal placement or size of the kidneys, and polycystic kidneys. Although the

Table 20-1 Report from a Urinalysis

Component	Item Measured	Interpretation Corresponding to Microscopy
Visual inspection	Color	Changes in color may be related to foods, fluid intake, medication, blood in urine, urinary concentration. Lack of any color suggests kidney damage or uncontrolled diabetes.
	Clarity	Cloudiness suggests pus, mucus, crystals, infection, or blood.
	Odor	Off odors may be caused by food, infection.
Dipstick	pH	Normal range is 4.6–8.0, tending to be slightly more acid in morning hours.
	Specific gravity	Normal: 1.005–1.03 Concentration suggests dehydration.
	Protein	Normal: absent Presence can suggest infection, cancer, glomerulonephritis, hypertension, or other diseases, including preeclampsia during pregnancy.
	Glucose	Normal: negative, trace Presence associated with diabetes, adrenal, kidney, or liver disease; may be trace positive in pregnancy.
	Ketones	Normal: negative Presence associated with eating disorders, starvation, uncontrolled diabetes; may be trace normal during pregnancy. Reflects oxidative stress, not a direct indicator of dehydration.
	Bilirubin	Normal: negative Presence suggests liver disease.
	Nitrites	Normal: negative Positive suggests cystitis, pyelonephritis, contamination with vaginal secretions.
	Leukocyte esterase	Normal: negative Presence demonstrates presence of WBCs.
	Blood	Normal: negative Positive may be cystitis, pyelonephritis, kidney stones, exercise induced, hemolytic disease, malignancy or other bladder lesions, polycystic kidneys, sickle cell disease.
Microscopy	Presence or absence of cells, crystals, other components	Normal: no findings; minimal numbers of crystals, RBCs or WBCs, or casts are considered normal. Abnormal: > 3–5 RBCs, > 5 WBCs, mucus, casts, crystals, bacteria, yeasts, trichomonads Squamous cells indicate inadequate cleaning.

RBCs = red blood cells, WBCs = white blood cells.

Note: The list of interpretations is not comprehensive.

Table 20-2 Risk Factors for Asymptomatic Bacteriuria and Cystitis

Female sex

Sexual activity

Use of condoms and nonoxynol-9 spermicide

Older age

Urinary retention

Diabetes mellitus

Neurogenic bladder

Hemodialysis

Urinary catheter use:

    Indwelling

    Intermittent

kidney, ureter, and bladder (KUB) x-ray is named for the renal system, its primary use in renal disease is the identification of stones. An *intravenous pyelogram (IVP)* uses contrast medium to diagnose kidney and bladder stones, cysts, and tumors. Computerized tomography (CT) and magnetic resonance imaging (MRI) are used to diagnose a variety of renal issues including renal vein thrombosis, masses and cysts, and stones.

Tests for UI include post-void residual (PVR), Q-Tip test, and urodynamic testing. They are discussed in the section on UI.

Infections of the Urinary Tract

Definitions

Urinary tract infection is actually a global term, but is commonly used to describe infections in the bladder. Conditions affecting the lower urinary tract include uncomplicated and complicated cystitis, asymptomatic bacteriuria (ASB),

and urethritis. Infection of the upper tract, specifically the kidney, is termed *pyelonephritis*.

Acute cystitis, or LUTI, is a symptomatic infection of the bladder. It is considered uncomplicated in nonpregnant, premenopausal, immune-competent women who do not have comorbid conditions that would increase risk. Further criteria include normal renal anatomy without obstruction or a history of instrumentation. A UTI is complicated if structural or functional abnormalities exist. Examples of these abnormalities include polycystic kidney disease, neurogenic bladder, diabetes, pregnancy, nephrolithiasis, immunosuppression, or indwelling urinary catheter.[8,9]

An upper UTI, or *pyelonephritis*, is infection of one or both kidneys. It is further described as acute or chronic, where chronic implies multiple recurrences of disease.

Asymptomatic bacteriuria (ASB) in women is defined by the Infectious Diseases Society of America (IDSA) as 2 consecutive voided urine specimens with isolation of the same bacterial strain in quantitative counts of 10^5 colony-forming units (cfu) per mL, or in a single catheterized specimen with a count of 10^2 cfu/mL.[10] The diagnosis requires that no urinary symptoms be present. The presence or absence of pyuria on microscopy does not affect the diagnosis.

Urethritis is inflammation and infection of the urethra, diagnosed by isolation of the causative agent.

Risk Factors

Symptoms of UTIs are common complaints both in emergency care facilities and primary care settings. Half of all women will experience at least 1 UTI in their lifetime, and 1 in 3 women will experience her first UTI by age 24.[11]

Female anatomy predisposes to a greater incidence of LUTI than in men, because the shorter length of the urethra increases the possibility of bacteria penetrating to the bladder. Anatomic and hormonal changes associated with pregnancy increase the risk that bacteria in the urine will progress to a more serious infection, in part due to increased stasis and *vesicouretereal reflux* (movement of urine back from the bladder toward the kidney). Sexual activity increases risk in several ways. Bacterial contamination of the periurethral area is increased during sexual acts, which also increases risk for sexually transmitted infections that involve the bladder or urethra. Multiple sexual partners, a new partner, and practicing anal intercourse add risk. Use of the female diaphragm, condoms, and nonoxynol-9 spermicides are also associated with increased incidence.[12,13] Advancing age increases risk of UTI in women, as decreased estrogen promotes atrophy of the walls of the urinary tract. Older women with UI, prolapse, or incomplete voiding (increased post-void residual urine) have further increased risk.[14,15] Table 20-2 summarizes the risks for urinary infections and ASB.[16,17]

Some medical conditions may predispose to infection if bladder innervation is affected and/or chronic catheter use is required; examples include multiple sclerosis, Parkinson's, and spinal cord injury. Suppression of the immune system, whether from uncontrolled diabetes, human immunodeficiency virus (HIV), or therapeutic immunosuppression are additional medical factors.[11] Specific to the renal history, kidney stones, procedures involving the bladder, and abnormal renal or bladder anatomy also increase UTI risk. Examples of childhood conditions increasing adult risk of infection include anatomical and/or functional abnormalities such as vesicoureteral reflux and unilateral kidney agenesis. Less important factors include blood group secretor status (a determinant of immunologic susceptibility to various diseases), genetic predisposition, and anatomic factors such as distance from urethra to anus.

Etiology

Bacteria commonly reach the urethra as a result of contamination from the rectum. Bacterial colonization of the lower urinary tract is through adhesion to the uroepithelium, mediated by the papillae on the bacterial cell wall.[17] The formation of a biofilm, production of proteases, and toxins that damage tissue to release nutrients and offer a foothold for bacterial invasion and dissemination, allow for persistence and colonization in an otherwise unfriendly environment.[18] A normally functioning urinary system works to prevent infection through several mechanisms. Fluid intake dilutes any bacteria that are present, and frequent voiding flushes the system. Bacterial growth is inhibited by the high urea content and osmolality of urine. Organic acids from mucosal cells and local antibody responses along with polymorphonuclear leukocytes in the bladder wall also destroy bacteria.[16] Urothelial mucosal cells secrete the tissue factors responsible for prohibiting or actively preventing attachment of bacteria to the mucosal surface. These cells have been found to be deficient in women who experience UTIs, especially recurrent infections.[17] A failure of some or all of these protective mechanisms, in addition to bacterial load and virulence, allows UTIs to develop.

Escherichia coli, by far the most common pathogen, is seen in 80% of uncomplicated infections, followed by *Staphylococcus saprophyticus*, which has an incidence of 10% to 15%.[19] Other Enterobacteriaceae, such as *Proteus mirabilis* and *Klebsiella pneumoniae*, are less common; other genera of Gram-negative and Gram-positive species are rarely isolated in uncomplicated UTIs.[19]

Complicated UTIs have a more diverse etiology; bacteria and fungi that are unlikely causes of UTI in healthy women can readily infect individuals with anatomic abnormalities, metabolic conditions such as diabetes, or immunologic disease. For example, among adults with diabetes mellitus, *E. coli* is still the single most common organism, but an increased percentage of infections is caused by *Klebsiella* species, *Enterobacter* species, *Proteus* species, Group B Streptococci, and *Enterococcus faecalis*.[20] Among older women, polymicrobial UTIs are common, with *E. coli* remaining the primary causative organism. Fungal UTIs are responsible for up to 7% of total complicated UTIs.[21] *Staphylococcus epidermidis*, diphtheroids, lactobacilli, and anaerobes are organisms commonly found on the skin and in the distal portion of the urethra and, therefore, represent probable contamination when seen in culture. The presence of *Trichomonas* and yeast may indicate vaginal contamination and can also cause urethritis.

Cystitis

SIGNS AND SYMPTOMS

The most common presenting symptom of LUTI is dysuria, pain, or difficulty when urinating. Women may also report frequency and urgency secondary to irritation of the urinary tract, as well as suprapubic pain or pressure. Women rarely experience gross hematuria. Fever rarely occurs with LUTI and should increase the suspicion for pyelonephritis.

ESSENTIAL HISTORY AND REVIEW OF SYSTEMS

Information obtained from the history dictates the physical examination and the laboratory and imaging tests to be performed. In addition to evaluating current symptoms, the history determines whether any factors are present that increase the risk of infection as discussed earlier.

Current symptoms, including the onset, severity, and duration of dysuria, and urgency should be investigated. Less common complaints include nocturia, low back pain, and loss of appetite. Systemic symptoms such as fever, malaise, chills, flank pain, or vomiting point to an upper tract infection. Details of any attempt at self-treatment should be elicited, especially the use of herbal or homeopathic substances.

The time since a previous infection should be determined, as well as whether a culture was performed and all medication prescribed was taken. UTIs are recurrent if there are $\geq$ 2 infections in 3 months or $\geq$ 3 infections in 1 year. Other renal conditions that can have symptoms similar to UTIs include acute pyelonephritis, urethritis, and IC. Dysuria has a broad differential diagnosis that includes chemotherapy for pelvic or bladder cancer, endometriosis, atrophic vaginitis, genital herpes, and infectious vaginitis.[22,23] A history of frequent or recurrent UTIs should be corroborated by information from the culture prior to treatment.

PHYSICAL EXAMINATION

Specific to LUTI, the lower abdomen is palpated, particularly in the suprapubic area. Assessment for costovertebral angle tenderness (CVAT) is indicated to rule out upper tract infection. A pelvic examination including inspection for lesions, bimanual exam for pelvic tenderness, and screening for vaginitis and for sexually transmitted diseases are appropriate in all sexually active women. In menopausal women, inspection of the external genitalia and vagina for evidence of atrophic changes is appropriate.

LABORATORY EXAMINATION

Urinalysis is the first step in assessment. Presence of both leukocyte esterase (LE) and nitrites on urine dipstick is a cost-effective screen, because LE is a sensitive but not particularly specific finding, whereas the presence of nitrites is more specific.[7] Positive results identify a subset of samples that need to be examined microscopically for the presence of white blood cells (WBCs), epithelial cells, RBCs, casts, crystals, and bacteria. On a microscopic exam, five or more WBCs per high-power field (HPF) from a centrifuged, uncontaminated sample reflect true pyuria.[24] **Table 20-3** relates

Table 20-3 Dipstick and Microscopic Findings Seen in Common Urinary Tract Conditions

Conditions	Laboratory Findings on Dipstick					Laboratory Findings on Microscopy				Comments
	Blood	Protein	Leukocytes	Esterace	Nitrates	WBC	RBC	Bacteria	Epithelial	
Vaginal contamination	+/-	+/-	+/-	+/-	+/-	+/-	+/-	+/-	+++	Need to repeat the sample.
Urinary tract infection	+/-	+/-	++	++	++/-	++	++/-	+/-	0 to few	Pyuria is common in both cystitis and urethritis; however, hematuria differs according to what site is infected. Hematuria is common in cystitis but not urethritis.[24]
Acute pyleonephritis	+/-	+/-	++	++	++/-	+++/-	++/-	++	0 to few	Pyuria is common. WBC casts may be present.
Kidney disease	++	++	-	-	-	+/-	++/-	-/-	0 to few	RBC casts are indicative of upper tract disease.

the findings on urinalysis to various conditions of the urinary tract.

Reproductive-aged women, particularly those who are pregnant, are more likely to obtain samples that are contaminated by vaginal fluids, making the laboratory results less accurate and more difficult to interpret. Contamination cannot be determined by dipstick evaluation of a urine sample; however, microscopic findings of moderate to large numbers of epithelial cells indicate contamination. In this case, repeating the sample using better clean-catch technique or catheterization may result in more accurate findings. A high ratio of WBCs to epithelial cells in a contaminated sample suggests infection. In this case, the sample should be repeated and treatment individualized.

The decision to proceed with culture and sensitivity identification depends on risk status. Pregnant women, those with recurrent UTIs or failure of short-course therapies, women unable to accurately identify their symptoms as being bladder related, women with suspected renal involvement, and patients with recent urologic instrumentation require a urine culture. Culture is also indicated if the patient will be undergoing urologic surgery.

Diagnosis

Bent and colleagues reviewed nine studies to evaluate diagnosis based on symptoms alone. In their analysis, women with at least one symptom of a UTI—frequency, dysuria, hematuria, or back pain—had a probability of a confirmed UTI of at least 50%. Combinations of symptoms, specifically dysuria plus frequency, raised the probability of culture-proven LUTI to more than 90%.[25]

Although often diagnosed in a physician's office based on typical symptoms, culture-proven diagnosis has traditionally required the presence of 10^5 cfu/mL in a midstream-voided specimen.[26] The criterion for treatment can be lowered to 10^2 to 10^4 organisms/mL of urine in women who are

symptomatic.[27,28] Dysuria, frequency, hematuria, nocturia, and urgency increase the probability of LUTI. The presence of vaginal discharge makes LUTI less likely.[28]

In general, those with uncomplicated UTIs can be treated based on history and urinalysis findings and do not require a culture, whereas those suspected of having a complicated UTI or underlying conditions that make eradication of infection more difficult should have a culture performed. The danger of relying on symptoms alone in diagnosing UTIs is the risk of overuse of antibiotics in a time when resistance is increasing. Culture should also be performed for symptomatic women whose urinalyses are negative.

Treatment of Uncomplicated Cystitis

If clinical suspicion is high based on symptoms, history, and office evaluation, it is reasonable to initiate empiric treatment. As discussed earlier, the incidence of infection in this circumstance is as high as 90%. Women who meet the criteria for having a complicated UTI are at higher risk of being infected with less common or antibiotic-resistant bacteria and require culture, even when empiric treatment is begun.

Common treatment regimens recommended by the IDSA for uncomplicated cystitis are shown in **Table 20-4**.[19] Notably, adherence to evidence-based treatment is limited; a 2015 study found that only 33% of clinicians were prescribing based on the IDSA guidelines.[29] Three- to 5-day regimens are adequate for uncomplicated cystitis in nonpregnant women; fosfomycin is the only recommended 1-day regimen and has decreased efficacy compared to 3- to 5-day treatments. Beta-lactam agents, such as amoxicillin-clavulanate, cefaclor, and cefpodoxime-proxetil, in 3- to 7-day regimens are appropriate choices for therapy when other recommended agents cannot be used. The fluoroquinolones are no longer considered first-line

Table 20-4 IDSA First-Line Recommendations for Treatment
of Uncomplicated LUTI

- Nitrofurantoin macrocrystals (Macrobid) 1 tablet bid for 5 days
- Trimethoprim-sulfamethoxazole 160/800 (Bactrim DS) 1 tablet bid for 3 days, *if* local resistance is < 20% *or* culture-proven susceptibility
- Fosfomycin trometamol or fosfomycin tromethazine 3 g in a single dose—may have decreased efficacy compared to 3-day therapy

bid = 2 times per day, DS = double strength

Data from Gupta K, Hooton TM, Naber KG, et al. International clinical practice guidelines for the treatment of acute uncomplicated cystitis and pyelonephritis in women: a 2010 update by the Infectious Diseases Society of America and the European Society for Microbiology and Infectious Diseases. *Clin Infect Dis.* 2011;52(5):e103-e120.

regimens and should be used only when no other option is available. Neither ampicillin nor amoxicillin are recommended.[19] Longer courses do not seem to be more effective in eradicating infection or preventing recurrences and are associated with higher rates of adverse effects.[30] Pregnant women and women over 60 years of age generally require longer therapy, as do those with complicated UTIs.

Empiric therapy is based on knowledge of common urinary pathogens and local susceptibility patterns. As many as 33% of bacterial strains associated with uncomplicated cystitis and pyelonephritis in the United States exhibit resistance to amoxicillin and sulfonamides.[31] Resistance to trimethoprim-sulfamethoxazole (TMP-SMX) in outpatient settings has been estimated to be about 24% nationally[32] and continues to rise. A recent Canadian study found rates of resistance for *E. coli* isolates in British Columbia as high as 27% to ciprofloxacin, 26% to TMP-SMX, and 46% to ampicillin.[33] Ceftriaxone resistance is also increasing and was reported in one study of acute pyelonephritis to be 5% overall, but 18.8% among those with risk factors.[34] Among the risks for having a drug-resistant UTI are older age, prior UTI, exposure to antimicrobials, comorbidities such as diabetes or immune suppression, recent hospitalization, and long-term care residence.[35]

Supportive therapy in the treatment of UTIs includes intake of adequate amounts of fluids to help flush the bacteria out of the urinary tract and also during administration of sulfonamides. Phenazopyridine, a urinary tract analgesic that is available over the counter, may be used for a short (less than 2-day) course in patients who have normal renal function. Two hundred milligrams may be administered by mouth three times per day as needed. The woman should be warned that this medication will turn her urine a deep, reddish-orange color.

Recurrent Infections

Once a woman has had one UTI, the risk of recurrent infection is at least 25%.[36] The risk is higher when the first infection is caused by *E. coli* than by other organisms.[37] Most recurrent infections occur within 2–3 months.[38] *Relapse* is defined as a second infection within 2 weeks with the same microorganism. It is distinguished from *reinfection*, in which a different bacterium causes the infection or the same organism causes infection after treatment and several weeks without symptoms.

Risk factors for recurrent UTI are dependent on age and menopausal status. Behavioral risks factors such as recent sexual intercourse, a new sexual partner, and use of spermicide place young women at greater risk of recurrent infection.[37,39] Decreased estrogen in tissue and incomplete bladder emptying result in greater risk for postmenopausal women.[40] A shorter than average anatomic distance from the urethra to the anus also increases the risk of recurrent UTIs.[38] Lifestyle changes, such as voiding after sexual activity, more frequent voiding, and avoiding chemical products such as bubble baths or douching, have not been shown to be effective in reducing risk but will not be harmful.[41]

Prophylaxis for Recurrent UTI

Management strategies for recurrent UTIs start with attempts at prevention. Whenever possible, non-antimicrobial methods should be tried before prescribing, because resistance is an increasing concern. Decreasing or avoiding the use of spermicidal cream or jelly either alone or with diaphragms may help. The use of vaginal estrogens is beneficial in postmenopausal women; estrogen supports the urothelial defense against bacterial adherence.[42,43] All currently available products have been shown to reduce nocturia and recurrent UTI.[44]

Cranberry juice or supplements containing cranberries have been suggested to decrease the risk of developing UTIs by decreasing bacterial adherence to the bladder wall.[45] A recent Cochrane review found no clear evidence of effectiveness. However, poor adherence or inadequate amounts of the active ingredient may have affected results. Also, many of the studies are small and short term, limiting the power of the study.[46] A review by Wang and colleagues, during the same time period, found that cranberry products appeared more effective among women with recurrent UTI, cranberry juice drinkers, and individuals who used cranberry-containing products more than twice daily.[47] Both dried cranberries and juice have been studied, as well as supplements of cranberry extract. The evidence suggests utility, but there is

not sufficient evidence to recommend a specific product.[48-51]

Acupuncture has been evaluated and found to be efficacious.[52] Other nonantibiotic recommendations include the use of *Lactobacillus crispatus* intravaginal suppositories in premenopausal women, or oral *L. rhamnosus* GR-1 and *L. reuteri* RC-14A.[53]

Antimicrobial treatment for recurrent infections can be provided in a variety of ways. Prophylaxis is appropriate for those women who have had either 2 infections in the prior 6 months or 3 infections in the prior 12 months. There are three options for prophylactic regimens: continuous, postcoital, and acute self-treatment.[54]

A Cochrane review showed little difference between the efficacy of antibiotic types.[55] The woman's preference, medication tolerance, side effects, and pregnancy plans should be considered when selecting a regimen. Continuous prophylaxis is usually administered for 6 to 12 months; longer durations have been safely used.[55] **Table 20-5** provides recommended regimens. Adherence is key. Long-term use can promote the development of bacterial resistance.

Table 20-5 Continuous Antimicrobial Prophylaxis Regimens

Trimethoprim-sulfamethoxazole 40 mg/200 mg daily *or* 3 times per week

Trimethoprim 100 mg daily

Nitrofurantoin 50 mg *or* 100 mg daily

Cefaclor 250 mg once daily

Cephalexin 125 mg once daily

Cephalexin 250 mg once daily

Only if no other effective drug is available:

Norfloxacin 200 mg once daily

Ciprofloxacin 125 mg once daily

Eells and colleagues provided a cost-effectiveness analysis of preventive strategies for women who had three or more LUTIs per year. Their data showed daily antibiotic use to be the most effective strategy for recurrent UTI prevention compared to daily cranberry pills, estrogen therapy, or acupuncture.[48]

Postcoital antibiotics are taken as a single dose following each act of intercourse, but not more often than daily. Because they are taken only intermittently, there may be fewer medication-related side effects. See **Table 20-6**.

Self-administered treatment for acute infection is a reasonable option for women who are comfortable recognizing their symptoms and initiating short-course medications.[56] The patient is instructed to begin treatment when symptoms present. If symptoms do not resolve within 48 hours, the woman should notify her provider and be evaluated.

Other concerns with long-term use of antimicrobial prophylaxis exist. TMP-SMX has the potential to reduce the effectiveness of estrogens by interrupting the enterohepatic recycling of estrogen.[57] It is possible that broad-spectrum antibiotics may reduce the bioavailability of estrogen, but probably only in the first 2 weeks of use. At the present, the World Health Organization considers that the use of most broad-spectrum antibiotics does not significantly affect the efficacy of combined hormonal contraceptives.[58] Extended use of nitrofurantoin is associated with adverse events including hepatitis, respiratory symptoms, and neuropathy. Any long-term antibiotic may increase risk of *Clostridium difficile* infection. Among the significant risks associated with fluoroquinolone use are tendonitis, tendon rupture, central nervous system reactions, peripheral neuropathy, myasthenia gravis exacerbation, liver damage, and prolonged QT interval. Fluoroquinolones should not be prescribed for LUTI when another choice can be made.

Women who experience 3 or more infections in 1 year with the same organism may be candidates for further urologic evaluation including an IVP or renal ultrasound and cystoscopy. While young women rarely have anatomic defects that require further evaluation, older women may need referral to a practitioner specializing in urology or urogynecology.

Complicated Urinary Tract Infections

Complicated urinary tract infections (cUTIs) are characterized by pyuria and a documented microbial pathogen and are accompanied by fever, chills, malaise, flank pain, and/or CVAT that occur in the presence of a functional or anatomic abnormality of the urinary tract or in the presence of catheterization. Examples of complicated UTIs are infections that occur in pregnant women, diabetics, and elderly women; in those who have structural or neurologic abnormalities, obstruction, or stones; or in persons with other immune or metabolic complications.[38] Patients with pyelonephritis, regardless of underlying abnormalities of the urinary tract, are considered a subset of patients with cUTIs, according to the US Food and Drug Administration (FDA).[59]

Risks for the development of cUTIs are a history of polycystic renal disease, nephrolithiasis,

Table 20-6 Postcoital Antimicrobial Prophylaxis Regimens

Trimethoprim-sulfamethoxazole 40 mg/200 mg *or* 80 mg/400 mg

Nitrofurantoin 50 mg or 100 mg

Cephalexin 250 mg

Ciprofloxacin 125 mg

Norfloxacin 200 mg

Ofloxacin 100 mg

neurogenic bladder, and recent urinary instrumentation or indwelling catheter. Infection in these individuals is more challenging to manage because of the higher rate of treatment failure.[60] A greater variety of organisms cause cUTIs, and an increased rate of antimicrobial resistance can be seen in these infections.[61,62] Some of the organisms involved are *E. coli, Klebsiella, Proteus, Serratia, Pseudomonas*, enterococci, and staphylococci.[21]

Both urinalysis and culture and sensitivity should be obtained when evaluating women at risk for cUTI.[60] Empiric therapy can be started while waiting for culture results. Although recommendations for fluoroquinolone use may be changing, at this time, they are considered appropriate for use in cUTI. If symptoms are mild, an oral fluoroquinolone for a minimum of 5 to 14 days is an appropriate first-line therapy. Fluoroquinolones should not be used if they have recently been prescribed. While there is no definitive evidence to support the exact length of therapy, a 7-day regimen is generally appropriate for women with complicated LUTI, while a 14-day regimen is preferable for those with symptoms of upper UTI.[60] Women given fluoroquinolones should be counseled about the risks associated with their use prior to the prescription being provided. Other appropriate medications include third-generation cephalosporins and piperacillin plus a penem bicyclic β-lactamase inhibitor.[63] A culture should be repeated 2 to 4 weeks after finishing the medication to confirm a cure.

Hospitalization is indicated in more severe infections, because progression to urosepsis is associated with 30–40% fatality rate.[64] Women receiving outpatient treatment for cUTI should be instructed to call immediately with worsening symptoms or if no relief is obtained from treatment.

Asymptomatic Bacteriuria

Asymptomatic bacteriuria is associated with being female, pregnancy, aging, and diabetes. By definition it does not present as a chief complaint or on review of systems, but is an incidental finding. Table 20-2 lists risk factors for ASB and cystitis. The presence of a dominant organism in quantities $\geq 10^5$ cfu/mL is sufficient for diagnosis; sterile pyuria is not.

The incidence of ASB in reproductive-aged women is approximately 5%.[13] Among type 2 diabetics, a recent review reported a range of 8–26%.[65] In the elderly, ASB is often transient.[14] The incidence is increased 5 times in women over 70 years. Studies put the long-term likelihood of an older woman having ASB at 30–50%; in this population, treatment has not been shown to affect outcomes.[14]

According to the IDSA and the US Preventive Services Task Force, the only specific indication for screening is early pregnancy.[10,66]

With very limited exceptions, treatment of ASB offers no benefits. In one study, treatment increased risk of recurrent symptomatic UTI over a 12-month period.[67] Use of antibiotics eradicates the bacteria, but in a Cochrane review treatment was associated with increased adverse events compared to nontreatment; not treating did not increase risk of progression to symptomatic UTI, complications, or death.[68] In contrast, evidence does exist for treating pregnant women and those preparing for a urologic procedure that may damage or irritate the bladder mucosa; in these limited circumstances, treatment limits disease progression.[69]

Urethritis

Risk factors for urethritis include inadequate personal hygiene, irritation of the urethra (such as from medication or personal products), and sexual activity. Symptoms include external irritation, pain or irritation on initiation of voiding, urgency, and possibly a discharge from the urethra. Women often describe vaginal infections, cystitis, and urethritis similarly.

The history includes whether the woman is sexually active, has any history of sexually transmitted infections, has a new partner or multiple partners, and whether a male condom is used during intercourse. Additional questions call attention to hygiene and any use of personal hygiene, spermicidal, or laundry products that may cause irritation.

Examination includes visual assessment of the urethral meatus for signs of inflammation. Inspection of the perineum for lesions, with attention to evaluation of the urethra and Bartholin's and Skene's glands for discharge, is essential. Vaginal speculum examination to collect samples for wet mount and bimanual examination are indicated. Because the symptoms overlap with other urinary conditions, samples for *Neisseria gonorrhoeae* and *Chlamydia trachomatis*, urinalysis, and urine culture should be collected.

The diagnosis may be as simple as bacterial contamination with the same agents that produce LUTI. Gonorrhea, chlamydia, *Trichomonas*, and herpes are other common infections associated with urethritis.

Pyelonephritis

Acute pyelonephritis is an upper tract infection that may or may not be associated with ASB or cystitis. Commonly, it is an ascending infection arising from the urethra, moving to the bladder, and then to the kidneys. The causative uropathogen in up to 80% of cases of pyelonephritis is *E. coli*. Other uncommon routes of infection are hematogenous—for example, in debilitated or immunocompromised patients or as a result of bacteremia or fungemia—or lymphatic in origin.[70]

Not all cases of pyelonephritis are accurately diagnosed. Estimates of annual incidence in one study were 15–17 cases per 10,000 women.[71] Signs and symptoms of pyelonephritis include complaints of cystitis and back pain or more significant findings such as nausea and vomiting,

flank pain, fever greater than 38°C (100.4°F), and CVAT. A study of women presenting to an emergency department for symptoms of pyelonephritis found that the presence of fever was strongly correlated with the diagnosis.[72] Symptoms of pyelonephritis can develop rapidly. The duration of symptoms prior to presentation for care is frequently less than 4 days. Symptoms of cystitis may or may not be present in patients with pyelonephritis. They may precede, be coincident with, or follow the development of pyelonephritis. Acute disease may be accompanied by systemic symptoms such as malaise, chills and shaking, flank pain, or vomiting associated with a high fever.

Certain laboratory findings are more suggestive of pyelonephritis. The standard criterion of 100,000 cfu/mL of pathogen is seen in 80–90% of cases.[73] Results suggestive of pyelonephritis on urine dipstick include protein, blood, nitrates, and LE. Microscopic results from the urinalysis usually show significant levels of leukocytes and bacteria. White cell casts can be seen in association with pyelonephritis and are generally considered pathognomonic; however, their absence does not rule out the diagnosis.[60]

All women in whom the diagnosis of pyelonephritis is suspected should have urine cultures obtained prior to the initiation of antibiotic therapy. Blood cultures should be considered in women who have a high fever and/or require hospitalization.

Management of uncomplicated pyelonephritis is straightforward. A urine culture is sent, and a 10- to 14-day course of antibiotic treatment is started immediately; treatment is not delayed pending results. Knowledge of local resistance patterns is essential in making appropriate treatment choices. Healthy, nonpregnant women who have mild symptoms without high fever, nausea, or vomiting may be treated on an outpatient basis after initial rehydration. This may be administered in an urgent care setting.[60] Treatment can be started with a single IV dose of a long-acting drug such as IV ciprofloxacin, ceftriaxone, or an aminoglycoside; where the local resistance to fluoroquinolones exceeds 10%, one of the alternative agents should always be used.[19] Whether or not that dose is given, a 7-day course of ciprofloxacin 500 mg twice daily is appropriate if fluoroquinolone resistance is low. Alternatives include TMP-SMX if the pathogen is susceptible or possibly a beta-lactam agent; these therapies are given for 14 days and preceded by an IV antibiotic dose.[19]

Follow-up cultures are only necessary for those whose symptoms do not resolve after the antimicrobial course. If symptoms re-present within a few weeks of treatment, a different antibiotic should be prescribed to avoid resistant infection.[60]

COMPLICATED PYELONEPHRITIS

Women should be admitted for inpatient therapy of acute uncomplicated pyelonephritis if they are pregnant, have a cUTI, are unable to maintain oral hydration, are debilitated, are not likely to be adherent to outpatient therapy, or do not have appropriate resources for home care and transportation for return visits.

Chronic pyelonephritis is defined by inflammation and fibrosis. Urinary tract obstruction, vesicoureteral reflux, and recurrent or persistent kidney infection may contribute to the development. Most commonly it occurs in those who have anatomic abnormalities. It may have the same symptoms as acute pyelonephritis, but also include nonspecific symptoms such as malaise, fatigue, or abdominal pain. One type of complicated pyelonephritis, xanthogranulomatous pyelonephritis, is caused by an obstructing stone that on radiologic exam may appear to be a mass-like lesion. The advantage of treatment with ciprofloxacin in the case of complicated or chronic pyelonephritis is its ability to provide broad-spectrum coverage of many Gram-negative and Gram-positive organisms.[74] Subsequent antibiotic suppression may be considered. Patients who experience recurrent pyelonephritis are candidates for further urologic evaluation.

Renal Stones

Etiology

Urolithiasis (urinary tract stones) can form either in the upper or lower urinary tract. In the developed world, most stones develop in the kidney and are referred to as *nephrolithiasis* or kidney stones. Kidney stones are formed by the crystals of salt precipitates that aggregate into large masses that have difficulty in clearing the lower tract. **Table 20-7** lists the common types of kidney stones.[75,76] About 80% of the kidney stones in the United States are composed of calcium, either as calcium oxalate or less commonly calcium phosphate.[76] The method by which calcium stones form is not well understood. One theory of stone formation is that calcium stones evolve from a crystallization process that begins in the loop of Henle or in the distal part of the distal tubule. At this point, the urine is usually supersaturated with calcium salts. As these large crystals develop, they move slowly down the nephron and can adhere to the collecting duct walls. An injury to the tissue provides a site for attachment and development. An alternative theory is that calcium phosphate crystals form in the medulla and attach to the renal papillae, creating a film known as Randall's plaque, where further aggregation occurs.[77,78]

Epidemiology

The most recently reported National Health and Nutrition Examination Survey data put the incidence of kidney stones at 7.1% in American women and 10.6% in men.[79] Rates are highest among non-Hispanic Caucasians, although the incidence is increasing among other groups. Obesity

Table 20-7 Common Kidney Stones

Type	Incidence	Comments
Calcium oxalate	80%	60% increased incidence of urinary calcium; serum level can be normal. Seen in hypercalcemia, hyperparathyroidism, hyperthyroidism sarcoidosis, increased bone demineralization.
Struvite	2%–20%	Responsible for the majority of staghorn calculi. Caused by urease producing bacteria in UTIs.
Uric acid	6% (seen in 20% of patients with gout)	Formed by supersaturation of excess uric acid, low urine volume
Cystine	1%	Autosomal recessive inherited disorder
Miscellaneous: Xanthine Silicate Indinavir	Less than 1%	

Data from Manthey D, Teichman J. Nephrolithiasis. *Emerg Med Clin North Am.* 2001;19(3):633-654; Coe F, Parks J, Asplin J. The pathogenesis and treatment of kidney stones. *N Engl J Med.* 1992;327(16):1141-1152.

and diabetes are consistently associated with urolithiasis.[79] Other risk factors include family history; chronic dehydration associated with inadequate fluid intake; and diet high in protein, sodium, or sugar or low in calcium.[80] Type of beverage intake appears to be a factor, with grapefruit juice increasing risk by 44%.[81] A more extensive list of associated risks is provided in **Table 20-8**. Genetic factors are thought to play a major role in risk of developing stones.[82] Recurrence rates are 35–50%.[83]

Characteristics of Disease

The primary symptom of urinary stones is acute flank pain radiating to the groin area. The pain may localize to the lower abdominal area in the vicinity of the stone or radiate to the pelvis. As the stone travels down the tubule, it may cause lower quadrant pain that radiates to the urethra or labia. Nausea/vomiting, urinary frequency, urgency, dysuria, and CVAT are often present.

Stones as small as 1 mm in diameter can cause pain.[80,84] The differential diagnosis for renal stones is shown in **Table 20-9**.

Stone size and location in the renal system influence the natural progression of the disease. Stones that are less than 6 mm in diameter and located in the distal ureter have the highest rate of spontaneous passage.[85] Stones that are less than 5 mm pass spontaneously 75–90% of the time.[85] By comparison, approximately 50% of stones 5 to 10 mm in diameter require intervention to aid expulsion.[85] Sixty-six percent of stones that pass spontaneously do so within the first 4 weeks after onset of symptoms.[86] Complications such as renal function deterioration, sepsis, and ureteral stricture are seen at a cumulative rate of 20%.[87]

Diagnosis

Diagnosis is suggested by history and examination and confirmed by laboratory findings and

Table 20-8 Risk Factors for Kidney Stones

Family history

High protein intake

High sodium intake

High oxalate intake (dark green vegetables)

Obesity

Diabetes, insulin resistance

Osteoporosis

Sarcoid

Sjögren's syndrome

Hyperthyroidism

Hyperparathyroidism

Hypertension

Cushing's disease

Medications (e.g., lithium, acetazolamide, long-term steroids, anticonvulsants)

Malignancy

Malabsorption (gastric bypass, inflammatory bowel disease)

Anorexia, bulimia

Kidney abnormalities (horseshoe kidney, medullary sponge)

Gout (uric acid stones)

Cystinuria (cysteine stones, familial)

Urinary tract infections (struvite stones)

Immobility

Table 20-9 A Partial Differential Diagnosis for Kidney Stones

Pyelonephritis

Ectopic pregnancy

Ovarian torsion

Intra-kidney bleeding

Appendicitis

Diverticulitis

Bowel obstruction

Cholecystitis

imaging. The history asks about risk factors including prior stones, family history of renal disease, and diet, as well as those listed in Table 20-8. A complete examination of the abdomen includes assessment of CVAT, as shown in Figure 20-2 earlier in the chapter. A pelvic examination is done to rule out other causes of groin or pelvic pain such as pelvic inflammatory disease. Laboratory evaluation for nephrolithiasis includes blood for electrolytes (sodium, potassium, chloride, bicarbonate), calcium, creatinine, and uric acid; urinalysis; urine culture when indicated; and 24-hour collection of urine.[88] Findings on urinalysis include hematuria in 90% of cases, but the absence of blood in the urine does not exclude the diagnosis.[86] In all women of childbearing age (menarche through menopause), a pregnancy test is performed before imaging studies are ordered.

Radiologic examination of the kidneys and collecting system is used to evaluate the function and presence of anatomic abnormality. It also serves to confirm the diagnosis, helps to rule out other diagnoses with similar symptoms, has the potential to determine obstruction or infarction, and can identify the location of the stone. The preferred imaging study for confirmation of the diagnosis of kidney stone is a noncontrast helical CT of the abdomen and pelvis.[89,90] The sensitivity and specificity for noncontrast CT in detection of renal calculi are 97% and 98%, respectively.[88] A low-dose CT is recommended for women with a body mass index (BMI) less than 30 kg/m^2, while standard CT yields higher sensitivity and specificity in those with BMI greater than 30 kg/m^2.[88] Follow up with a plain x-ray of KUB will determine if the stone is radiopaque and aids in the diagnosis of the type of stone.

Stones composed of calcium, magnesium salts, and uric acid are radiolucent.

Pregnant women should have an ultrasound as the initial evaluation to avoid radiation exposure of the pelvis. It is considered a first-line test and can also be used if other abdominal processes, such as gallstones or a torsed or ruptured ovary, are suspected.[91]

Other studies, including a KUB x-ray or IVP, are no longer considered first-line tests. The KUB provides less information than CT, and IVP has both the risk of reaction to a contrast medium and higher levels of radiation. They are used as adjunctive tests, or, in the case of KUB, when CT is not available.

Management

Acute management at the time of passing a renal stone includes pain management, usually with an NSAID or an opioid, or with a combination of the two. NSAIDs have the advantages of discouraging individuals who are drug seeking, fewer side effects, and relaxing smooth muscles (spasm of the ureter is a direct cause of stone pain).[92] Other nonopioids are not recommended.[93]

Individuals may be asked to strain their urine for a period of time to determine that the stone has passed. Medical therapy with alpha-blockers or calcium channel blockers has been studied and remains the standard recommendation during expectant management of stones < 10 mm in diameter.[90] These drugs are thought to shorten the time to stone passage. A recent large trial found that neither was superior to placebo in promoting stone passage during a 4-week interval.[94]

When renal colic (the acute pain of nephrolithiasis) or other symptoms suggest kidney stones in nonpregnant women, referral is made to an emergency department for acute pain or to a urologist for milder symptoms. The role of women's health practitioners is limited to providing information about expected care and following up with future screening and dietary counseling. Pregnant women suspected of having a kidney stone should be sent to a labor and delivery unit for assessment and management or to an emergency department if pain is acute, depending on the local standards.

Observation is often all that is required after the passage of a first stone. The medical management of a first kidney stone in nonpregnant women consists of increasing fluid intake combined with dietary modifications. The goal of increasing fluid is increased urine output of at least 2–2.5 liters/day.[95,96]

When women are prone to stone formation, dietary counseling may help to reduce recurrences. Dietary changes are thought to affect the excretion of calcium, oxalate, and uric acid, all of which are substances thought to promote stone development.[97] Dietary restrictions vary with stone type and urinary analysis, so initial plans should be made by a clinician familiar with the composition of stones and test results.

Diets that contain large amounts of refined carbohydrates, animal proteins, and salt and a low intake of vegetables and fruit increase the risk of *hypercalciuria* and the development of calcium oxalate stones.[97] Calcium intake should equal 1000–1200 mg daily.[96] Low-calcium diets are believed to provoke *hyperoxaluria*, which can promote the development of stones and also may lead to a negative calcium balance and subsequent bone loss.[76] Examples of high oxalate-containing foods to limit include walnuts, hazelnuts, peanuts, almonds, nut butters, soy products, strawberries, beets, spinach and other dark leafy greens, rhubarb, parsley, chives, chocolate, cocoa, wheat germ, brown rice, and both green and black tea. Hyperoxaluria is treated with avoidance of these foods, a reduction in the intake of carbohydrates and animal protein, and encouragement of normal intake of calcium.[97] An observational study was able to show an association between the dietary intake of at least 40 mg pyridoxine (vitamin B_6)

per day and the reduction of oxalate.[98] Uric acid stone disease is treated with limitation of meats and other foods high in purine.[97] A potassium-enriched diet derived from fruit, fruit juices, and vegetables can improve hypocitraturia.[97] Higher levels of citrate are thought to protect against calcium stones. Cystinuria treatment includes reduction of the intake of cystine and methionine amino acids and common salt.[97] The National Institute of Diabetes and Digestive and Kidney Diseases (NIDDK) recommends that individuals prone to stone formation follow the Dietary Approaches to Stop Hypertension (DASH) diet.[99]

Medications are used when nephrolithiasis is accompanied by urinary abnormalities that diets have failed to ameliorate. Thiazides and indapamide have been shown to be effective in the reduction of stone recurrence.[97] Side effects of these medications include hypotension, muscular cramps, asthenia, hypokalemia, hyponatremia, hypomagnesemia, hyperuricemia, hyperglycemia, and hypercholesterolemia.[97]

Uric acid stones can be treated by alkalinizing the urine, because an alkaline state dissolves pure uric acid stones. Alkali, in the form of sodium bicarbonate or acetazolamide, can be used to elevate the urinary pH. If the daily uric acid level is greater than 1000 mg despite dietary reduction of purine and increased fluid intake, allopurinol may be administered to reduce uric acid production.[97] Side effects seen with the use of this drug include pruritus, urticaria, maculopapular and exfoliative skin eruptions, dyspepsia, and abdominal pain. If this treatment fails, the approach to therapy should be the same as for radiopaque stones.[86]

Surgical Management of Stones

Obstruction is an indication for hospitalization. Open renal and ureteral surgery is the gold standard for definitive treatment of large stones. Three modalities are available for the treatment of stones that are too large to pass through the renal system: percutaneous nephrostolithotomy, rigid and flexible ureteroscopy, and shockwave lithotripsy. Percutaneous nephrostolithotomy is a technique in which an incision is made in the flank, a nephroscope is inserted into the kidney, and the stone is broken up and removed using a laser, ultrasound probe, or pneumatic device. Ureteroscopy is a procedure used to access middle and distal ureteral stones.[85] Shockwave lithotripsy uses high-energy shockwaves, delivered through a water medium, with the guidance of biplanar fluoroscopy. The stones are fragmented by the energy delivered to the surface of the stone. Open surgery is used for the management of complicated renal and ureteral calculi that cannot be resolved with the use of the prior techniques.[100] Morbidly obese patients may need open surgery, because their body habitus may preclude localization by fluoroscopy or ultrasonography. Shockwave lithotripsy may fail because of wave attenuation by the excess tissue.[96]

Interstitial Cystitis/Painful Bladder Syndrome

Etiology and Epidemiology

The definition of *interstitial cystitis/painful bladder syndrome* (IC/PBS) from the American Urological Association (AUA) is: "An unpleasant sensation (pain, pressure, discomfort) perceived to be related to the urinary bladder, associated with lower urinary tract symptoms of more than 6 weeks duration, in the absence of infection or other identifiable causes."[101] The terminology is changing to reflect the unclear etiology and primary symptoms of the condition. Suprapubic pain or pressure, frequency > 10 times daily, urgency, and nocturia are consistent symptoms; dyspareunia may also occur. IC/PBS should be suspected if the woman reports multiple treatment failures for cystitis and her urine culture fails to demonstrate infection. The term *interstitial cystitis* is used when specific additional criteria are met, including ulcerative lesions (Hunner's ulcers) and glomerulations (pinpoint hemorrhages) of the urothelium.[102] IC/PBS is a diagnosis of exclusion in most cases, when no other findings explain the signs and symptoms.

The etiology of IC is unclear but may include an autoimmune reaction against bladder antigens and a deficiency in the glycosaminoglycan layer of the bladder surface that allows toxins to penetrate the mucosa. Subsequent mast cell infiltration and activation lead to histamine release and local bladder wall damage from bacteria.[103,104] Pelvic floor dysfunction and neural hypersensitivity may also play a role.[105] The NIDDK states that IC/PBS may be a bladder manifestation of generalized inflammatory conditions such as irritable bowel or fibromyalgia.[102] Submucosal hemorrhages or ulcers are commonly seen on cystoscopy. Histopathology from biopsy confirms the diagnosis.

More than 3 million American women have symptoms that would support the diagnosis of IC/PBS.[106] About 9 out of 10 individuals diagnosed with the disorder are female.[103] Peak incidence is generally considered to occur in adults 30–60 years of age, although recent evidence shows that IC occurs across adulthood. Better identification of characteristics of IC/PBS contributes to earlier recognition and to reassignment of diagnosis among older women.[107] Painful intercourse, external genitalia pain, pain on voiding, urgency, and increased voiding frequency are more common in younger patients; nocturia, incontinence, and bladder wall ulceration are more common in the older population.[107] Symptoms can remit and relapse irregularly and may worsen with menstruation. A study designed to investigate the natural history of IC reported that in a group of 374 women, the symptoms of IC progressed rapidly and then seemed to plateau within 5 years of onset of disease.[108] The differential diagnosis for IC/PBS includes sexually transmitted disease, endometriosis, bladder cancer, and recurrent UTIs.

Evaluation

A detailed history of the symptoms experienced by the woman and information about any prior attempts at diagnosis should be obtained. It is important to gently ask about the possibility of prior abuse, because sexual abuse has been linked to symptoms typical of IC/PBS.[109,110] Data about foods that may be bladder irritants should be collected. A urogenital examination is done to rule out gynecologic or neurologic pathology. A voiding diary is completed to provide quantitative information about the frequency, amount of voided urine, and pattern of pain symptoms.

Bladder irritants include caffeine, chocolate, citrus fruits, alcoholic beverages (especially red wine), spicy foods, tomatoes, aspartame, saccharine, monosodium glutamate, nuts, vinegar, onions, and soy sauce. Smoking is also commonly reported to aggravate symptoms.[102] By eliminating potential irritants from the diet and then gradually reintroducing them one at a time, it may be possible to identify dietary changes that will reduce symptoms.

A urinalysis and culture are obtained to evaluate for infection or hematuria. If hematuria is present in IC, urine cytology should be done to look for cancerous or precancerous cells, because hematuria can be a symptom of bladder cancer. Infection is not consistent with a diagnosis of IC/PBS, although UTI and IC/PBS can coexist. Cystoscopy to rule out bladder cancer can be performed. Bladder wall biopsy confirms the absence of cancer.[102] A voiding cystogram may be ordered to evaluate for the presence of urethral defects. Urodynamic testing may screen for a neurogenic bladder, bladder instability, outlet obstruction, and the presence of sensory instability. Women suspected of having IC require a complete workup and should be referred to a specialist practice.

The NIDDK recommends diagnosis based on inclusion and exclusion of particular symptoms, cystoscopic findings of bladder wall inflammation, biopsy, and the absence of other diseases that can cause similar symptoms.[102] The AUA states that cystoscopy and urodynamics are not required in straightforward cases.[101] The most complete information is obtained if biopsies are performed at the time of the cystoscopy and if the cystoscopy is done using hydrodistension.[104] Because chronic inflammation may cause a contracted bladder with reduced capacity, evaluating the bladder capacity may help in the diagnosis.

Management

Management is planned to proceed in stages, and an essential component of early management is counseling women that this is a chronic condition, no one treatment is universally effective, and multiple techniques may need to be tried. The associated psychosocial effects have major negative impacts on quality of life; pain management is an ongoing component of care.[111]

The AUA provides treatment guidelines that describe a stepwise approach. The first steps include lifestyle and behavioral changes that may offer relief of symptoms. Irritant foods that can be excluded were listed earlier; smoking cessation can be recommended. Stress management techniques should be discussed.[101] Measures that reduce the acidity of the urine may make voiding more comfortable. Increasing fluid intake can dilute urine, making it less acidic.

Physical therapy to release muscle contractures and trigger points is part of the "second-line" therapies recommended by the AUA.[101] Kegel exercises should not be recommended, because increased muscle tone may increase symptoms.

Women can use their voiding diary and autodilation to increase the timespan between voidings. Autodilation refers to the process by which the patient gradually increases the time interval between voiding. In this way, the bladder is very gradually distended in small increments over a prolonged period of time. Patients should be seen frequently in order to monitor whether they are adhering to the voiding schedule and to receive support and encouragement.

Initial attempts at medication therapy take an empiric approach, with the use of anti-inflammatory medications, narcotic pain relievers, and antidepressants and antihistamines. The latter are believed to reduce pain, increase bladder capacity, and generally reduce symptoms.[102] Use of transcutaneous electrical nerve stimulation (TENS) is an effective nonpharmacologic option.[102] Hydrodistension ameliorated the symptoms in a subset of patients in the short term.[112] Dimethyl sulfoxide has been approved by the FDA for instillation into the bladder. While the mechanism of action is unclear, its ability to permeate the bladder wall may make it reduce pain and inflammation more effectively. Initial instillations are performed in the urologist's office. Some women learn to perform the procedure at home. Pentosan polysulfate sodium (Elmiron) is an oral medication that provides relief from pain and frequency for some patients. Relief may take several months to develop, so long-term trials are necessary for the woman wishing to use this medication. The mechanism of action is unknown.[102]

In rare instances, a surgical approach is utilized. Fulguration of the bladder and excision of lesions are typical procedures.[102]

Urinary Incontinence

UI is a relatively common problem among mature women. As many as 25% of all young women experience some degree of incontinence, with athletes at greatest risk. Prevalence increases to approximately 50% in middle-aged women and more than three-quarters of elderly women.[113-115] Both UI and OAB negatively affect quality of life across psychological, professional, and personal parameters.[116,117]

Definitions and Etiology

Stress urinary incontinence is defined by the AUA as "leakage of urine during events that result in increased abdominal pressure such as sneezing, coughing, physical exercise, lifting, bending and even changing positions."[118] *Urge urinary incontinence* is "involuntary leakage accompanied by or immediately preceded by urgency"[118] where urgency is a difficult-to-delay, overwhelming desire to void or the need to void for fear of leaking urine. Mixed incontinence is a combination of the symptoms of each.[118] *Overactive bladder* is the term used for a sense of urgency, with or without actual incontinence. It can be accompanied by frequency and/or nocturia.[119]

Stress incontinence is the result of inadequate pelvic floor support for the urethra and bladder neck (urethral hypermobility) or of intrinsic weak tone of the sphincter between the bladder and urethra. Loss of muscle tone and connective tissue strength can be caused by persistent, increased pressure downward. Sphincter damage is usually related to damage to the nerves and muscle of the urethra. Urge incontinence is related to overactivity of the detrusor muscle, causing inappropriate contraction during bladder filling.

Risk factors for UI and OAB in women include advancing age, childbearing (with vaginal birth increasing risk more than cesarean), hysterectomy, pelvic organ prolapse, obesity, frequent UTI, chronic cough, straining from constipation, cognitive impairment, neurologic disability, stroke, and diabetes.[120,121] Because many women do not seek help for mild or even moderate symptoms, questioning women about this issue becomes an important service.

Evaluation for UI/OAB

HISTORY

The history for UI/OAB includes general and lifestyle factors that might play a role in risk. Further questions include the symptoms noted, such as urgency, loss of urine with urge, fear of leaking, loss of urine when bearing down (e.g., coughing, squatting, running), frequency, amount, hesitancy, precipitating triggers, nocturia, intermittent or slow stream, incomplete emptying, continuous urine leakage, and straining to void;[122] the frequency of the symptoms; and how they affect her life. The target group for questioning is middle-aged and older women, although asking young women is an appropriate way to provide education about preventive measures and their reproductive health. Women should be asked specifically about current and previous symptoms, keeping in mind that mild UI is an intermittent issue.

PHYSICAL AND LABORATORY EXAMINATION

The physical examination includes a complete pelvic, evaluating for factors such as prolapse, atrophy, and masses. If there is a suspicion of neurologic involvement, then a neurologic examination is warranted. Simple office evaluations that can be performed by an experienced clinician include the bladder stress test. Laboratory testing includes blood for chemistries and kidney function, a urinalysis, and culture to rule out infection as a cause.

The bladder stress test is performed by asking the woman to drink enough fluid for her bladder to feel full, and then directly observing her perineum as she performs Valsalva maneuvers multiple times. The presence of leaked urine is a positive test. This test is useful for confirming stress incontinence but is usually negative in pure urge incontinence.[123]

Additional tests may be performed as part of a comprehensive workup by a urogynecology team if the diagnosis is unclear or surgery may be required. These include a Q-Tip test, postvoid residual, renal imaging, and urodynamics. The *Q-Tip test* evaluates anatomic strength of the musculature at the junction of bladder and urethra; the urethrovesical angle widens with stress when the muscle tone is poor (urethral hypermobility). To perform the test, the urethral meatus is cleaned, and a sterile, lubricated cotton swab is inserted gently until resistance is met. The woman is asked to bear down; if the swab changes direction by more than 30°, the test is positive (**Figure 20-3**). *Postvoid residual* is a catheterized collection immediately postvoid to determine whether the bladder is emptying completely. An alternative is a bladder ultrasound. When available, ultrasound assessment is preferable, because it is noninvasive; however, no sterile specimen is obtained with this technique. If one is needed for other tests, a sterile catheterization should be performed.

Urodynamics are a series of tests to evaluate bladder pressure, urine flow, and urethral function.[124] Cystometry measures the bladder's ability to serve as a reservoir. The test assesses detrusor activity, bladder capacity, and compliance. Uroflowmetry measures the rate of flow of urine throughout a single voiding episode to evaluate muscle tone, outlet obstruction, and sphincter spasm. The bladder pressure test combines cystometry and uroflowmetry.

Figure 20-3 Q-Tip test.

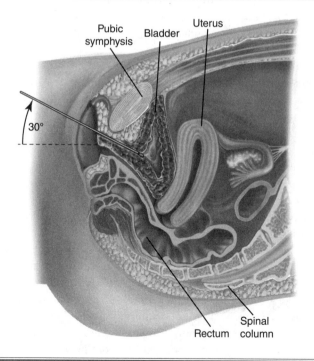

Management

While stress incontinence is diagnosed based on patient history and examination as well as a stress test, the report of urgency-related urine loss is the most sensitive screen for urge incontinence. If incontinence is suspected based on history, physical examination, and performance of a bedside bladder stress test, then initial discussion of management is within the scope of women's health practitioners or may appropriately be referred to a specialist physician or nurse practitioner. Some women must be referred for further evaluation, including those with fistula, pelvic prolapse, neurologic dysfunction, pain, or hematuria. In every case, unless the practitioner is skilled in this area, consultation and referral are advisable.

Initial management includes lifestyle counseling, pelvic floor exercises, maintenance of a voiding diary and bladder training (urge UI), and topical estrogen for postmenopausal women. Modifiable risk factors such as constipation or urinary infections are treated. Lifestyle counseling includes weight loss, smoking cessation, decreased fluid intake, and avoidance of dietary irritants such as caffeine, carbonated beverages, or artificial sweeteners.[124,125] There is little evidence that these methods, other than weight loss, are beneficial.[126] Pelvic floor exercises have been shown to be beneficial for both stress and mixed incontinence. Electrical stimulation, biofeedback, and use of vaginal cones may help women who are unable to complete the exercises successfully.[127,128] Depending on the level of incontinence, dual therapy can improve outcomes and may need to be instituted early in the course of retraining.[128] Bladder training is a behavioral therapy. It requires the woman to void immediately on rising, and at specified intervals, gradually increasing the time between voids as she is able to hold her urine when she feels urgency. Relaxation techniques can be taught as a tool for delaying urination.

Medical therapy for stress UI includes the use of alpha-blockers such as pseudoephedrine, pessary fitting, and tampon use to apply physical pressure to the bladder neck. When these are ineffective, referral for injection of a bulking agent or surgical repair is indicated.[124]

Medical therapy for urge UI begins with the use of an antimuscarinic or anticholinergic medication. Antimuscarinics include solifenacin, tolterodine, fesoterodine, oxybutynin, and trospium. All of these drugs have significant side effects of dry mouth, constipation, stomach pain or upset, headache, and somnolence. Anticholinergic hyoscyamine is an alternative. Side effects are similar and also include flushing and visual changes. Both categories also have significant contraindications that should be reviewed with patients before prescribing.[124]

Pregnancy Considerations Related to the Renal System

Anatomic and physiologic changes of pregnancy influence the frequency of infections. Pregnancy causes an increase in the volume, weight, and size of the kidney. The ureters, calyces, and renal pelvises undergo dilation. Because of the slight dextrorotation of the uterus during pregnancy and the more acute angle of the right ureter as it passes over the pelvic brim, dilation is usually seen more on the right. The dilated collecting system is responsible for up to an additional 200-mL volume of urine in the bladder. Both the glomerular filtration rate and blood flow are increased, but, simultaneously, higher progesterone levels seen in pregnancy contribute to decreased ureteral peristalsis and prolonged transit time of urine from the kidneys to the bladder. Incomplete bladder emptying and subsequent stasis of urine increase the risk for UTIs. The higher renal threshold for glucosuria seen in pregnancy somewhat mimics a diabetic state with its concomitant increase in UTIs. Late in pregnancy, the distended uterus may contribute to a syndrome in which the patient experiences abdominal discomfort, hydronephrosis, and possibly hypertension and an increase in serum creatinine levels.

ASB occurs in 2–10% of pregnant women.[129] Pregnancy is the only indication for screening and treatment of ASB.[10,66] When a woman has been treated during pregnancy, periodic rescreening is appropriate. Treatment is associated with decreases in the rates of preterm birth and low birth weight.[130,131]

Women who have sickle cell trait or disease have an increased incidence of UTIs and should be screened each trimester in pregnancy.

Current estimates of the incidence of *cystitis* in pregnancy range from 1–4 %.[132] Treatment of UTIs in pregnancy is unchanged from nonpregnant women, with the exception that pharmacologic choices are limited by safety for the fetus.[133] When sensitivities are not available or empirical treatment is indicated, regional antibiotic resistance patterns should be considered. Repeat urine cultures should be obtained 1 to 2 weeks after completion of the drug therapy. Culture is then repeated at least once in each subsequent trimester of the pregnancy. Two culture-confirmed LUTIs during pregnancy are an indication for suppression until the birth; nitrofurantoin macrocrystals are the preferred regimen unless there is evidence of resistance in the previous infections. Women on suppression should have a dipstick urinalysis each visit that includes nitrates and LE, or at least one culture in the third trimester, to prevent bacterial breakthrough.

Pregnant women with ASB have an increased incidence of pyelonephritis compared to nonpregnant women. Untreated ASB in pregnancy has a rate of progression to pyelonephritis that can be as high as 40%; treatment reduces this rate to 3–4%.[132,134]

The incidence of *pyelonephritis* in pregnancy is estimated to be between 0.5% and 2%; more than 80% occur in the second and third trimesters.[129,132,135] Risk factors include maternal age, first birth, sickle cell anemia, diabetes, nephrolithiasis, illicit drug use, history of pyelonephritis, and maternal urinary tract defects.[132] The signs and symptoms of pyelonephritis in pregnant women are similar to those found in nonpregnant women. CVAT may be more pronounced on the right than the left. Symptoms of cystitis may be present. Most patients will have improvement of symptoms and become afebrile within 48 hours, at which point discharge to home with a 7- to 10-day course of oral antibiotic therapy is reasonable. Urine culture should be obtained before discontinuing oral therapy. After one episode of pyelonephritis in pregnancy or any recurrent infection, patients should receive antibiotic suppression for the remainder of the pregnancy with nitrofurantoin monohydrate 100 mg nightly or TMP-SMX double strength 160/800 mg nightly. An acceptable alternative to antibiotic suppression is culturing the urine every 2 weeks and screening for symptoms at every prenatal visit. These interventions have demonstrated significant reduction in recurrence of pyelonephritis.

Pregnant women with *urolithiasis* usually present with abdominal and flank pain. The symptoms of urolithiasis can be mistaken for appendicitis, diverticulitis, or placental abruption. Also included in the differential diagnosis of urolithiasis are UTI, pyelonephritis, pelvic inflammatory disease, abdominal aortic aneurysm, and bladder cancer. Ultrasound of the kidneys and pelvis is the preferred method of imaging in pregnancy, because it provides adequate imaging of the calculi and avoids radiation exposure from abdominal x-rays. Internal ureteral stents or a nephrostomy tube can be placed if the patient is unable to pass a ureteral calculus, although most pass spontaneously.[136,137] Because of the associated risk of asymptomatic UTI, patients should be screened for infection at appropriate intervals during the pregnancy. Adequate pain relief and hydration are necessary for the treatment of urolithiasis in pregnancy. When necessary, ureteroscopy can be safely used during the intrapartum period.[137]

Role of the Women's Health Provider in Management of Renal Conditions

The role of the women's health provider in the management of various urinary conditions depends on the condition in question and the system in which he or she practices. Certainly, independent management of UTIs is within the scope of practice in all practice settings. ASB and recurrent lower tract infections occurring in the nonpregnant population can be managed independently, as can uncomplicated pyelonephritis that responds appropriately to outpatient treatment. Complicated lower UTIs in the nonpregnant or pregnant women that do not respond to appropriate treatment may warrant further consultation or referral. Complicated cases of pyelonephritis in the nonpregnant woman and all cases of pyelonephritis in pregnancy should involve consultation, comanagement, or referral to a specialist. Knowledge of the risk factors for each type of UTI supports the delivery of health care to affected women in a safe, efficient, and cost-effective manner.

Renal stones require evaluation and management beyond the scope of women's health. These women should be referred upon diagnosis. There is a role in follow-up support and advice regarding nutritional and lifestyle activities to prevent recurrence.

Given the chronicity and disability associated with IC for many women, those suspected of having this condition should have a thorough evaluation by a urogynecologist. Follow-up care should be individualized and may be best managed using a team approach. Comprehensive care of patients with IC should include psychosocial assessments and multidisciplinary interventions, including behavioral and chronic pain counseling.

References

1. Schappert SM, Rechtsteiner EA. *Ambulatory medical care utilization estimates for 2007. Vital Health Statistics 2011.* Atlanta, GA: National Center for Health Statistics.
2. Foxman B, Brown P. Epidemiology of urinary tract infections: transmission and risk factors, incidence, and costs. *Infect Dis Clin North Am.* 2003;17:227-241.
3. Hilt EE, McKinley K, Pearce MM, Rosenfeld AB, Zillox MJ, Mueller ER, et al. Urine is not sterile: use of enhanced urine culture techniques to detect resident bacterial flora in the adult female bladder. Munson E, ed. *J Clin Microbiol.* 2014;52(3):871-876.
4. Khasriya R, Sathiananthamoorthy S, Ismail S, Kelsey M, Wilson M, Rohn JL, et al. Spectrum of bacterial colonization associated with urothelial cells from patients with chronic lower urinary tract symptoms. *J Clin Microbiol.* 2013;51:2054-2062.
5. Lewis DA, Brown R, Williams J, White P, Jacobson SK, Marchesi JR, et al. The human urinary microbiome; bacterial DNA in voided urine of asymptomatic adults. *Front Cell Infect Microbiol.* 2014;3:41.
6. National Institute on Drug Abuse. Medical Consequences of Drug Abuse. Available at: http://www.drugabuse.gov/publications/medical-consequences-drug-abuse/kidney-damage. Accessed May 23, 2016.
7. Simerville J, Maxted W, Pahira J. Urinalysis: a comprehensive review. *Am Fam Physician.* 2005;71(6):1153-1162.

8. Colgan R, Williams M. Diagnosis and treatment of acute uncomplicated cystitis. *Am Fam Physician.* 2011;84(7):771-776.

9. Johansen TE, Botto H, Cek M, Grabe M, Tenke P, Wagenlehner FM, et al. Critical review of current definitions of urinary tract infections and proposal of an EAU/ESIU classification system. *Int J Antimicrob Agents.* 2011;38(Suppl):64-70.

10. Nicolle LE, Bradley S, Colgan R, Rice JC, Schaeffer A, Hooton TM. Infectious Diseases Society of America guidelines for the diagnosis and treatment of asymptomatic bacteriuria in adults. *Clin Infect Dis.* 2005;40(5):643-654. doi:10.1086/427507.

11. Foxman B. Epidemiology of urinary tract infections: incidence, morbidity, and economic costs. *Am J Med.* 2002;113(Suppl 1A):5S-13S.

12. Handley MA, Reingold AL, Shiboski S, Padian NS. Incidence of acute urinary tract infection in young women and use of male condoms with and without nonoxynol-9 spermicides. *Epidemiology.* 2002;13(4):431-436.

13. Hooton TM, Scholes D, Stapleton AE, Roberts PL, Winter C, Gupta K, et al. A prospective study of asymptomatic bacteriuria in sexually active young women. *N Engl J Med.* 2000;343:992-997.

14. Mody L, Juthani-Mehta M. Urinary tract infections in older women: a clinical review. *JAMA.* 2014;311(8):844-854. doi:10.1001/jama.2014.303.

15. Cove-Smith A, Almond M. Management of urinary infections in the elderly. *Trends Urol Gynaecol Sex Health.* 2007;12:4:31-34.

16. Colgan R, Nicolle LE, McGlone A, Hooton TM. Asymptomatic bacteriuria in adults. *Am Fam Physician.* 2006;74:985-990.

17. Schaeffer A. Infection and inflammation of the genitourinary tract. *J Urol.* 2001;165(4):1374-1381.

18. Flores-Mireles AL, Walker JN, Caparon M, Hultgren SJ. Urinary tract infections: epidemiology, mechanisms of infection and treatment options. *Nat Rev Microbiol.* 2015;13:269-284. doi:10.1038/nrmicro3432.

19. Gupta K, Hooton TM, Naber KG, et al. International clinical practice guidelines for the treatment of acute uncomplicated cystitis and pyelonephritis in women: a 2010 update by the Infectious Diseases Society of America and the European Society for Microbiology and Infectious Diseases. *Clin Infect Dis.* 2011;52(5):e103-120. doi:10.1093/cid/ciq257.

20. Hoepelman AIM, Meiland R, Geerings SE. Pathogenesis and management of bacterial urinary tract infections in adult patients with diabetes mellitus. *Int J Antimicrob Agents.* 2003;22:35-43.

21. Imam TH. Bacterial Urinary Tract Infections. Merck Manual. Available at: http://www.merckmanuals.com/professional/genitourinary-disorders/urinary-tract-infections-uti/bacterial-urinary-tract-infections. Accessed May 23, 2016.

22. Butrick C. Patients with chronic pelvic pain: endometriosis or interstitial cystitis/painful bladder syndrome? *JSLS.* 2007;11(2):182-189.

23. Kodner CM, Thomas Gupton EK. Recurrent urinary tract infections in women: diagnosis and management. *Am Fam Physician.* 2010;82(6):638-643.

24. Kass E, Finland M. Asymptomatic infections of the urinary tract. *J Urol.* 2002;168(2):420-424.

25. Bent S, Nallamothu BK, Simel DL, Fihn SD, Saint S. Does this woman have an acute uncomplicated urinary tract infection? *JAMA.* 2002;287(20):2701-2710.

26. Hooton TM, Roberts PL, Cox ME, Stapleton AE. Voided midstream urine culture and acute cystitis in premenopausal women. *N Engl J Med.* 2013;369(20):1883-1891.

27. Wilson ML, Gaido L. Laboratory diagnosis of urinary tract infections in adult patients. *Clin Infect Dis.* 2004;38(8):1150-1158. doi:10.1086/383029.

28. Giesen LG, Cousins G, Dimitrov BD, van de Laar FA, Fahey T. Predicting acute uncomplicated urinary tract infection in women: a systematic review of the diagnostic accuracy of symptoms and signs. *BMC Fam Pract.* 2010;11:78. doi:10.1186/1471-2296-11-78.

29. Kim M, Lloyd A, Condren M, Miller MJ. Beyond antibiotic selection: concordance with the IDSA guidelines for uncomplicated urinary tract infections. *Infection.* 2015;43(1):89-94. doi:10.1007/s15010-014-0659-4. Epub 2014 Jul 18.

30. Fihn S. Acute uncomplicated urinary tract infection in women. *N Engl J Med.* 2003;349:259-266.

31. Gupta K, Hooton T, Roberts P, Stamm W. Patient initiated treatment of uncomplicated recurrent urinary tract infections in young women. *Ann Intern Med.* 2001;135(1):9-16.

32. Sanchez GV, Master RN, Karlowsky JA, Bordon JM. In vitro antimicrobial resistance of urinary escherichia coli isolates among U.S. outpatients from 2000 to 2010. *Antimicrob Agents Chemother.* 2012;56:2181-2183.

33. British Columbia Centre for Disease Control. *Antimicrobial Resistance Trends in the Province of British Columbia, 2011.* Vancouver, Canada: Communicable Disease Prevention and Control Services, British Columbia Centre for Disease Control; 2012.

34. Moran G, Krishnadasan A, Mower M, Abrahamian F, Takhar S, Talan D. Prevalence of fluoroquinolone- and ceftriaxone-resistant *E. coli* among U.S. Emergency Department Patients with Acute Pyelonephritis.

Poster Abstract Session, October 10, 2014, Philadelphia, PA. Available at: https://idsa.confex.com/idsa/2014/webprogram/Paper46971.html. Accessed May 23, 2016.

35. Patrick DM, Chambers C, Purych D, Chong M, George D, Marra F. Value of an aggregate index in describing the impact of trends in antimicrobial resistance for *Escherichia coli*. *Can J Infect Dis Med Microbiol*. 2015;26(1):33-38.

36. Foxman B. Recurring urinary tract infection: incidence and risk factors. *Am J Public Health*. 1990;80:331.

37. Foxman B, Gillespie B, Koopman J, Zhang L, Palin K, Tallman P, et al. Risk factors for second urinary tract infection among college women. *Am J Epidemiol*. 2000;151:1194.

38. Nosseir SB, Lind LR, Winkler HA. Recurrent uncomplicated urinary tract infections in women: a review. *J Womens Health*. 2012;21(3):347-354. doi:10.1089/jwh.2011.3056.

39. Scholes D, Hooton T, Roberts P, Stapleton A, Gupta K, Stamm W. Risk factors for recurrent urinary tract infection in young women. *J Infect Dis*. 2000;182(4):1177-1182.

40. Raz R, Gennesin Y, Wasser J, Stoler Z, Rosenfeld S, Rottensterich E, et al. Recurrent urinary tract infections in post menopausal women. *Clin Infect Dis*. 2000;30:152-156.

41. Society of Obstetricians and Gynaecologists of Canada. Recurrent urinary tract infection. Clinical Practice Guideline No. 250. *JOGC*. 2010;1082-1090.

42. Raz R, Stamm WE. A controlled trial of intravaginal estriol in postmenopausal women with recurrent urinary tract infections. *N Engl J Med*. 1993;329(11):753-756.

43. Lüthje P, Brauner H, Ramos NL, Ovregaard A, Gläser R, Hirschberg AL, et al. Estrogen supports urothelial defense mechanisms. *Sci Transl Med*. 2013;5(190):190ra80. doi:10.1126/scitranslmed.3005574.

44. Rahn DD, Carberry C, Sanses TV, Mamik MM, Ward RM, Meriwether KV, et al. Vaginal estrogen for genitourinary syndrome of menopause: a systematic review. *Obstet Gynecol*. 2014;124(6):1147-1156. doi:10.1097/AOG.0000000000000526.

45. National Center for Complementary and Integrative Health. Cranberry. Available at: https://nccih.nih.gov/health/cranberry. Accessed May 23, 2016.

46. Jepson RG, Williams G, Craig JC. Cranberries for preventing urinary tract infections. *Cochrane Database Syst Rev*. 2012;10:CD001321. doi:10.1002/14651858.CD001321.pub5.

47. Wang CH, Fang CC, Chen NC, Liu SS, Yu PH, Wu TY, et al. Cranberry-containing products for prevention of urinary tract infections in susceptible populations: a systematic review and meta-analysis of randomized controlled trials. *Arch Intern Med*. 2012;172(13):988-996. doi:10.1001/archinternmed.2012.3004.

48. Eells SJ, Bharadwa K, McKinnell JA, Miller LG. Recurrent urinary tract infections among women: comparative effectiveness of 5 prevention and management strategies using a Markov Chain Monte Carlo Model. *Clin Infect Dis*. 2014;58(2):147-160. doi:10.1093/cid/cit646.

49. Foxman B, Cronenwett AE, Spino C, Berger MB, Morgan DM. Cranberry juice capsules and urinary tract infection after surgery: results of a randomized trial. *Am J Obstet Gynecol*. 2015;213(2):194.e1-8. doi:10.1016/j.ajog.2015.04.003.

50. Ledda A, Bottari A, Luzzi R, Belcaro G, Hu S, Dugall M, et al. Cranberry supplementation in the prevention of non-severe lower urinary tract infections: a pilot study. *Eur Rev Med Pharmacol Sci*. 2015;19(1):77-80.

51. Burleigh AE, Benck SM, McAchran SE, Reed JD, Krueger CG, Hopkins WJ. Consumption of sweetened, dried cranberries may reduce urinary tract infection incidence in susceptible women—a modified observational study. *Nutr J*. 2013;12(1):139. doi:10.1186/1475-2891-12-139.

52. Alraek T, Soedal LIF, Fagerheim SU, Digranes A, Baerheim A. Acupuncture treatment in the prevention of uncomplicated recurrent lower urinary tract infections in adult women. *Am J Public Health*. 2002;92(10):1609-1611.

53. Geerlings SE, Beerepoot MA, Prins JM. Prevention of recurrent urinary tract infections in women: antimicrobial and nonantimicrobial strategies. *Infect Dis Clin North Am*. 2014;28(1):135-147.

54. Lichtenberger P, Hooton TM. Antimicrobial prophylaxis in women with recurrent urinary tract infections. *Int J Antimicrob Agents*. 2011;38(Suppl):36-41.

55. Albert X, Huertas I, Pereiró II, Sanfélix J, Gosalbes V, Perrota C. Antibiotics for preventing recurrent urinary tract infection in non-pregnant women. *Cochrane Database Syst Rev*. 2004;3:CD001209.

56. Gupta K, Hooton TM, Roberts PL, Stamm WE. Patient-initiated treatment of uncomplicated recurrent urinary tract infections in young women. *Ann Intern Med*. 2001;135:9-16. doi:10.7326/0003-4819-135-1-200107030-00004.

57. The Medical Letter. *Handbook of Adverse Drug Interaction*. Marlborough, MA: Skyscape; 2000:196.

58. World Health Organization Department of Reproductive Health and Research. *Medical Eligibility Criteria for Contraceptive Use*. 5th ed. Available at: http://

www.who.int/reproductivehealth/publications/family_planning/MEC-5/en/. Accessed May 23, 2016.

59. US Department of Health and Human Services, Food and Drug Administration, Center for Drug Evaluation and Research. *Complicated Urinary Tract Infections: Developing Drugs for Treatment: Guidance for Industry*. Silver Spring, MD: US Food and Drug Administration; 2015. Available at: http://www.fda.gov/downloads/Drugs/.../Guidances/ucm070981.pdf. Accessed May 23, 2016.

60. Wang A, Nizran P, Malone M, Riley T. Urinary tract infections. *Prim Care*. 2013;40(3):687-706.

61. Stamm W, McKevitt M, Roberts P, White N. Natural history of recurrent urinary tract infections in women. *Rev Infect Dis*. 1991;13:77-84.

62. Nicolle L. A practical guide to antimicrobial management of complicated urinary tract infection. *Drugs Aging*. 2001;18(4):243-254.

63. Wagenlehner FM, Umeh O, Steenbergen J, Yuan G, Darouiche RO. Ceftolozane-tazobactam compared with levofloxacin in the treatment of complicated urinary-tract infections, including pyelonephritis: a randomised, double-blind, phase 3 trial (ASPECT-cUTI). *Lancet*. 2015;385 (9981):1949-1956.

64. Wagenlehner FM, Lichtenstern C, Rolfes C, Mayer K, Uhle F, Weidner W, et al. Diagnosis and management for urosepsis. *Int J Urol*. 2013;20:963-970. doi:10.1111/iju.12200.

65. Nitzan O, Elias M, Chazan B, Saliba W. Urinary tract infections in patients with type 2 diabetes mellitus: review of prevalence, diagnosis, and management. *Diabetes Metab Syndr Obes*. 2015;8:129-136.

66. US Preventive Services Task Force. Screening for asymptomatic bacteriuria in adults: US Preventive Services Task Force Reaffirmation Recommendation Statement. *Ann Intern Med*. 2008;149:43-47.

67. Cai T, Mazzoli S, Mondaini N, Meacci F, Nesi G, D'Elia C, et al. The role of asymptomatic bacteriuria in young women with recurrent urinary tract infections: to treat or not to treat? *Clin Infect Dis*. 2012;55(6):771-7. doi:10.1093/cid/cis534.

68. Zalmanovici Trestioreanu A, Lador A, Sauerbrun-Cutler MT, Leibovici L. Antibiotics for asymptomatic bacteriuria. *Cochrane Database Syst Rev*. 2015;4:CD009534.

69. Trautner BW, Grigoryan L. Approach to a positive urine culture in a patient without urinary symptoms. *Infect Dis Clin North Am*. 2014;28(1):15-31. doi:10.1016/j.idc.2013.09.005.

70. Nicolle L, AMMI Canada Guidelines Committee. Complicated urinary tract infection in adults. *Can J Infect Dis Med Microbiol*. 2005;16(6):349-360.

71. Czaja CJ, Scholes D, Hooton TM, Stamm WE. Population-based epidemiologic analysis of acute pyelonephritis. *Clin Infect Dis*. 2007;45:273-280.

72. Pinson A, Philbreak J, Lindbeck G, Schorling J. Fever in the clinical diagnosis of acute pyelonephritis. *Am J Emerg Med*. 1997;1(2):148-151.

73. Levi M, Redington J, Reller L. The patient with urinary tract infection. In: Schrier R, ed. *Manual of Nephrology*. Philadelphia, PA: Lippincott Williams & Wilkins; 2005:91-114.

74. McLaughlin S. Urinary tract infections in women. *Med Clin North Am*. 2004;88(2):417-429.

75. Manthey D, Teichman J. Nephrolithiasis. *Emerg Med Clin North Am*. 2001;19(3):633-654.

76. Coe F, Parks J, Asplin J. The pathogenesis and treatment of kidney stones. *N Engl J Med*. 1992;327(16):1141-1152.

77. Coe FL, Evan AP, Worcester EM, Lingeman JE. Three pathways for human kidney stone formation. *Urol Res*. 2010;38(3):147-160. doi:10.1007/s00240-010-0271-8.

78. Strakosha R, Monga M, Wong MYC. The relevance of Randall's plaques. *Indian J Urol*. 2014;30(1):49-54. doi:10.4103/0970-1591.124207.

79. Scales CD, Smith AC, Hanley JM, Saigal CS. Urologic diseases in America Project. Prevalence of kidney stones in the United States. *Eur Urol*. 2012;62(1):160-165. doi:10.1016/j.eururo.2012.03.052.

80. Fink HA, Wilt TJ, Eidman KE, et al. Recurrent nephrolithiasis in adults: comparative effectiveness of preventive medical strategies. *Comparative Effectiveness Reviews, No. 61*. Rockville, MD: Agency for Healthcare Research and Quality; 2012. Available at: http://www.ncbi.nlm.nih.gov/pubmedhealth/PMH0048744/. Accessed May 23, 2016.

81. Curhan GC, Willett WC, Speizer FE, Stampfer MJ. Beverage use and risk for kidney stones in women. *Ann Intern Med*. 1998;128:534-540. doi:10.7326/0003-4819-128-7-199804010-00003.

82. Attanasio M. The genetic components of idiopathic nephrolithiasis. *Pediatr Nephrol*. 2011;26(3):337-346. PMID: 20563734.

83. Uribarri J, Oh MS, Carroll HJ. The first kidney stone. *Ann Intern Med*. 1989;111(12):1006-1009.

84. Coll DM, Varanelli MJ, Smith RC. Relationship of spontaneous passage of ureteral calculi to stone size and location as revealed by unenhanced helical CT. *AJR Am J Roentgenol*. 2002;178(1):101-103.

85. Segura J, Preminger G, Assimos D, Dretler SP, Kahn RI, Lingeman JE, et al. Ureteral Stones Clinical Guidelines Panel summary report on the management of ureteral calculi. *J Urol*. 1997;158(5):1915-1921.

86. Teichman J. Clinical practice. Acute renal colic from ureteral calculus. *N Engl J Med*. 2004;350(7):684-693.

87. Ueno A, Kawasmura T, Ogawa A, Takayasu H. Relation of spontaneous passage of ureteral calculi to size. *Urology*. 1977;10(6):544-546.

88. Fulgham PF, Assimos DG, Pearle MS, Preminger GM. Clinical effectiveness protocols for imaging in the management of ureteral calculous disease: AUA technology assessment. *J Urol*. 2013;189:1203-1213.

89. Vieweg J, Teh C, Freed K, Leder R, Smith R, Nelson R, et al. Unenhanced helical computerized tomography for the evaluation of patients with acute flank pain. *J Urol*. 1998;160(3 Pt 1):679-684.

90. Preminger GM, Tiselius HG, Assimos DG, Alken P, Buck C, Gallucci M, et al. 2007 Guideline for the management of ureteral calculi. *J Urol*. 2007;178(6):2418-2434.

91. Curhan G. Imaging in the emergency department for suspected nephrolithiasis. *N Engl J Med*. 2014;371(12):1154-1155.

92. Holdgate A, Pollock T. Systematic review of the relative efficacy of non-steroidal anti-inflammatory drugs and opioids in the treatment of acute renal colic. *BMJ*. 2004;328(7453):1401. doi:10.1136/bmj.38119.581991.55.

93. Afshar K, Jafari S, Marks AJ, Eftekhari A, MacNeily AE. Nonsteroidal anti-inflammatory drugs (NSAIDs) and non-opioids for acute renal colic. *Cochrane Database Syst Rev*. 2015;6:CD006027. doi:10.1002/14651858.CD006027.pub2.

94. Pickard R, Starr K, MacLennan G, Lam T, Thomas R, Burr J, et al. Medical expulsive therapy in adults with ureteric colic: a multicentre, randomised, placebo-controlled trial. *Lancet*. 2015;386(9991):341-9. doi:10.1016/S0140-6736(15)60933-3.

95. Borghi L, Meschi T, Amato F, Briganti A, Novarini A, Giannini A. Urinary volume, water and recurrences in idiopathic calcium nephrolithiasis: a 5-year randomized prospective study. *J Urol*. 1996;155(3):839-843. PMID: 8583588.

96. Pearle MS, Goldfarb DS, Assimos DG, Curhan G, Denu-Ciocca CJ, Matlaga BR, et al.; American Urological Association. Medical management of kidney stones: AUA Guideline. *J Urol*. 2014;192(2):316-324.

97. Borghi L, Meschi T, Schianchi T, Allegri F, Guerra A, Maggiore U, et al. Medical treatment of nephrolithiasis. *Endocrinol Metab Clin North Am*. 2002;31(4):1051-1064.

98. Goldenberg R, Girone J. Oral pyridoxine in the prevention of oxalate kidney stones. *Am J Nephrol*. 1996;16(6):552-553.

99. National Institute of Diabetes and Digestive and Kidney Diseases. Diet for Kidney Stone Prevention. Available at: http://www.niddk.nih.gov/health-information/health-topics/urologic-disease/diet-for-kidney-stone-prevention/Pages/facts.aspx. Accessed May 23, 2016.

100. Metlaga B, Assimos D. Changing indications of open stone surgery. *Urology*. 2002;59(4):490-493.

101. Hanno PM, Burks DA, Clemens JQ, Dmochowski RR, Erickson D, FitzGerald MP, et al. Diagnosis and treatment of interstitial cystitis/bladder pain syndrome. Available at: https://www.auanet.org/education/guidelines/ic-bladder-pain-syndrome.cfm. Accessed June 1, 2016.

102. Moore K. *Urogynecology: Evidence Based Clinical Practice*. London, UK: Springer; 2013:200-204.

103. Bouchelouche K, Nordling J. Recent developments in the management of interstitial cystitis. *Curr Opin Urol*. 2003;13(4):309-313.

104. Dyer AJ, Twiss CO. Painful bladder syndrome: an update and review of current management strategies. *Curr Urol Rep*. 2014;15(2):384.

105. Berry SH, Elliott MN, Suttorp M, Bogart LM, Stoto MA, Eggers P, et al. Prevalence of symptoms of bladder pain syndrome/interstitial cystitis among adult females in the United States. *J Urol*. 2011;186:540-544.

106. Rais-Bahrami S, Friedlander JI, Herati AS, Sadek MA, Ruzimovsky M, Moldwin RM. Symptom profile variability of interstitial cystitis/painful bladder syndrome by age. *BJU International*, 2012;109:1356-1359.

107. Koziol J, Clark D, Gittes R, Tan E. The natural history of interstitial cystitis: a survey of 374 patients. *J Urol*. 1993;149(3):465-469.

108. Peters KM, Kalinowski SE, Carrico DJ, Ibrahim IA, Diokno AC. Fact or fiction—is abuse prevalent in patients with interstitial cystitis? Results from a community survey and clinic population. *J Urol*. 2007;178(3 Pt1):891-895.

109. Mayson BE, Teichman JM. The relationship between sexual abuse and interstitial cystitis/painful bladder syndrome. *Curr Urol Rep*. 2009;10:441-447.

110. Clemens JQ, Link CL, Eggers PW, Kusek JW, Nyberg LM Jr, McKinlay JB. Prevalence of painful bladder symptoms and effect on quality of life in black, Hispanic and white men and women. *J Urol*. 2007;177:1390-1394.

111. Ottem DP1, Teichman JM. What is the value of cystoscopy with hydrodistension for interstitial cystitis? *Urology*. 2005 Sep;66(3):494-499.

112. Carls C. The prevalence of stress urinary incontinence in high school and college-age female athletes in the Midwest: implications for education and prevention. *Urol Nurs*. 2007;27(1):21-4, 39.

113. Kinchen KS, Lee J, Fireman B, Hunkeler E, Nehemiah JL, Curtice TG. The prevalence, burden, and treatment of urinary incontinence among

women in a managed care plan. *J Womens Health (Larchmt)*. 2007;16(3):415-422. PMID: 17439386.

114. Boyington JE, Howard DL, Carter-Edwards L, Gooden KM, Erdem N, Jallah Y, et al. Differences in resident characteristics and prevalence of urinary incontinence in nursing homes in the southeastern United States. *Nurs Res*. 2007;56(2):97-107.

115. Coyne KS, Wein AJ, Tubaro A, Sexton CC, Thompson CL, Kopp ZS, et al. The burden of lower urinary tract symptoms: evaluating the effect of LUTS on health-related quality of life, anxiety and depression: EpiLUTS. *BJU Int*. 2009;103:4-11.

116. Coyne KS, Sexton CC, Irwin DE, Kopp ZS, Kelleher CJ, Milsom I. The impact of overactive bladder, incontinence and other lower urinary tract symptoms on quality of life, work productivity, sexuality and emotional well-being in men and women: results from the EPIC study. *BJU Int*. 2008;101:1388-1395. doi:10.1111/j.1464-410X.2008.07601.x.

117. Appell RA, Dmochowski RR, Blaivas JM, Gromley EA, Karram MM, Juma S, et al. Guideline for the Surgical Management of Female Stress Urinary Incontinence: Update (2009). American Urological Association. Available at: https://www.auanet.org/education/guidelines/incontinence.cfm. Accessed May 23, 2016.

118. Abrams P, Andersson KE, Birder L, Brubaker L, Cardozo L, Chapple C, et al. Fourth International Consultation on Incontinence Recommendations of the International Scientific Committee: Evaluation and treatment of urinary incontinence, pelvic organ prolapse, and fecal incontinence. *Neurourol Urodyn*. 2010;29(1):213-240.

119. Shamliyan T, Wyman J, Bliss DZ, Kane RL, Wilt TJ. *Prevention of Urinary and Fecal Incontinence in Adults* (Evidence Reports/Technology Assessments, No. 161.). Rockville, MD: Agency for Healthcare Research and Quality; 2007. Available at: http://www.ncbi.nlm.nih.gov/books/NBK38514/. Accessed May 23, 2016.

120. Coyne KS, Kaplan SA, Chapple CR, Sexton CC, Kopp ZS, Bush EN, et al. Risk factors and comorbid conditions associated with lower urinary tract symptoms: EpiLUTS. *BJU Int*. 2009;103(Suppl 3): 24-32. doi:10.1111/j.1464-410X.2009.08438.x.

121. Nygaard I. Clinical practice. Idiopathic urgency urinary incontinence. *N Engl J Med*. 2010;363(12):1156.

122. Holroyd-Leduc JM, Tannenbaum C, Thorpe KE, Straus SE. What type of urinary incontinence does this woman have? *JAMA*. 2008;299(12):1446-1456. doi:10.1001/jama.299.12.1446.

123. Gormley EA, Lightner DJ, Burgio KL, Chai TC, Clemens JQ, Culkin DJ, et al. Diagnosis and Treatment of Overactive Bladder (Non-Neurogenic) in Adults: AUA/SUFU GUIDELINE. Available at: http://www.auanet.org/education/guidelines/overactive-bladder.cfm. Accessed May 23, 2016.

124. American Urogynecologic Society. Urinary Incontinence in Women. Available at: http://eguideline.guidelinecentral.com/i/76622-augs-urinary-incontinence. Accessed May 23, 2016.

125. Imamura M, Williams K, Wells M, McGrother C. Lifestyle interventions for the treatment of urinary incontinence in adults. *Cochrane Database Syst Rev*. 2015;12:CD003505.

126. Singh N, Rashid M, Bayliss L, Graham P. Pelvic floor muscle training for female urinary incontinence: Does it work? *Arch Gynecol Obstet*. 2015;293(6):1263-1269.

127. Di Benedetto P. Female urinary incontinence rehabilitation. *Minerva Ginecol*. 2004;56(4):353-369.

128. Schnarr J, Smaill F. Asymptomatic bacteriuria and symptomatic urinary tract infections in pregnancy. *Eur J Clin Invest*. 2008;38(Suppl 2):50-7. doi: 10.1111/j.1365-2362.2008.02009.x.

129. Smaill F. Asymptomatic bacteriuria in pregnancy. *Best Pract Res Clin Obstet Gynaecol*. 2007;21(3):439-450.

130. Sheiner E, Mazor-Dreyb, Levy A. Asymptomatic bacteriuria during pregnancy. *J Matern Fetal Neonatal Med*. 2009;22(5):423-427.

131. Matuszkiewicz-Rowińska J, Małyszko J, Wieliczko M. Urinary tract infections in pregnancy: old and new unresolved diagnostic and therapeutic problems. *Arch Med Sci*. 2015;11(1):67-77. doi:10.5114/aoms.2013.39202.

132. Widmer M, Gülmezoglu AM, Mignini L, Roganti A. Duration of treatment for asymptomatic bacteriuria during pregnancy. *Cochrane Database Syst Rev*. 2011;(12):CD000491.doi:10.1002/14651858.CD000491.pub2.

133. Smaill F, Vazquez JC. Antibiotics for asymptomatic bacteriuria in pregnancy. *Cochrane Database Syst Rev*. 2007;2:CD000490.

134. Hill JB, Sheffield JS, McIntire DD, Wendel GD Jr. Acute pyelonephritis in pregnancy. *Obstet Gynecol*. 2005;105(1):18-23.

135. N'gamba M, Lebdai S, Hasting C, Panayotopoulos P, Ammi M, Sentilhes L, et al. Acute renal colic during pregnancy: management and predictive factors. *Can J Urol*. 2015;22: 7732-7738.

136. Lewis DE, Robichaux AG, Jaekle RK, Marcum NG, Steadman CM. Urolithiasis in pregnancy: diagnosis, management and pregnancy outcome. *J Reprod Med*. 2003;48(1):28-32.

137. McAleer S, Loughlin K. Nephrolithiasis and pregnancy. *Curr Opin Urol*. 2004;14(2):123-127.

CHAPTER 21

INFECTIOUS DISEASES IN WOMEN

Jan M. Kriebs

This text has addressed a variety of infectious complaints, ranging from colds and flu to *Helicobacter pylori*. In this chapter, infections of the female genital tract and some other serious chronic infections are discussed. Every woman's healthcare provider is—or should be—familiar with these topics. A comprehensive survey of infectious diseases would fill its own text; here, those most likely to be addressed in a women's healthcare setting are reviewed.

Vaginal Microbiome

The female lower genital tract is a complex environment. A balanced mix of vaginal flora helps maintain the normal pH, prevent adherence of infectious organisms to the epithelial cells, prevent overgrowth of bacteria and yeasts, and contribute to the normal vaginal discharge. The dominant organisms in the healthy vagina, especially among white and Asian women, are *Lactobacillus* species (spp.), including *L. crispatus*, *L. jensenii*, *L. gasseri*, and *L. iners*.[1] These hydrogen peroxide (H_2O_2)–producing strains of lactobacilli play an active role

in supporting normal flora; the release of H_2O_2 acts to decrease bacterial adherence to epithelial cells. Glycogen stores in the mucosal tissue are metabolized into lactic acid by these bacteria, helping to maintain an acidic environment. The prevalence of more diverse vaginal microbiota is significantly higher in black and Hispanic women. A wide variety of bacterial species, including others that produce lactic acid, are found in healthy, asymptomatic women with fewer lactobacilli species.[2] Additionally, *Prevotella* sp., *Gardnerella vaginalis*, *Atopobium vaginae*, *Bacteroides ureolyticus*, and *Mobiluncus curtisii* are present in the healthy vaginal biota, as are *Candida* species. It has been pointed out by Ravel and others that it is necessary to rethink what is normal in terms of the vaginal microbiome and not assume that lack of lactobacilli or increased numbers of diverse bacteria are in themselves a marker for disease.[2-4] Increased diversity and the associated decrease in lactobacilli increase the opportunity for dysregulation of the vaginal microbiome and thus contribute to an increased risk for infection and possibly for preterm birth.[1,4-7] The relative quantity of various microorganisms and their efficiency in producing

Figure 21-1 Normal vaginal wet mount.

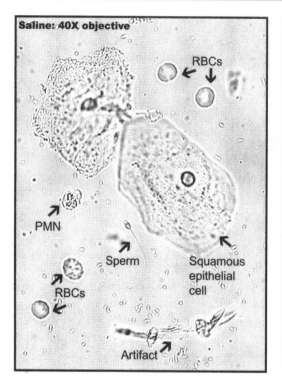
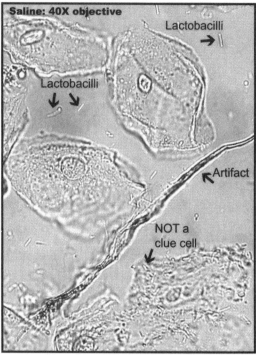

antibacterial substances or utilizing their environment act to control the constituents of the microflora.[8,9] On examination, a wet mount of the vaginal discharge can provide information about the health of the biome. A normal vaginal wet mount is shown in **Figure 21-1**.

Vaginal pH changes with age. During the reproductive years, vaginal pH hovers between 3.8 and 4.2. After menopause, declining serum estradiol is associated with a shift in the vaginal pH to between 5.0 and 6.5,[10] as well as thinning of the vaginal tissue and decreased viscosity of cervical-vaginal secretions. Decreased lactobacilli and increased *Escherichia coli* are present.[11,12]

The vaginal microbiota also change with age. Young girls have a mix of skin and vaginal flora on the vulva, with lactic acid producing bacteria in the vagina, and by the age of menarche display a pattern similar to that of reproductive-aged women.[13] After menopause, the use of topical or systemic hormone therapy plays a role in bacterial composition. Research differs as to the risk of bacterial vaginosis (BV) in the absence of hormone replacement.[14,15]

Events that affect the hormonal balance of the vagina or disrupt the growth of normal flora are associated with increased risk of infection. During pregnancy, the presence of H_2O_2-producing lactobacilli has been demonstrated to decrease the likelihood of BV and *Chlamydia* infections.[2,16]

Other aspects of vaginal anatomy and physiology also play a role in disease transmission risk. These include the exposed columnar epithelium found in adolescent women, increased ectropion with combined hormonal contraception and in pregnancy, and the thin epithelium of postmenopausal women and anyone with decreased estrogen status (e.g., breastfeeding women).

Counseling and Testing for Infectious Diseases

When women present to the clinical setting with complaints such as vaginal irritation or odor, pelvic pain, or an abnormal discharge, the physical examination and laboratory testing frequently can be driven by symptomatology and the woman's history. Other women present requesting testing for "everything" based on suspicion of partner infidelity or fear of a prior exposure. In the absence of specific patient concerns, counseling to address risks of serious infection is frequently omitted, based on provider assumptions about which women are at risk for infection and for which infections the woman is at risk. No group of sexually active women can be presumed to be risk free. The US Preventive Services Task Force (USPSTF) recommends intensive behavioral counseling for at-risk adults and for all sexually active adolescents.[17] *At risk* is defined as women who have more than one sexual partner and/or have had a sexually transmitted infection (STI) diagnosis within 1 year. This author would add any woman whose partner has had more than one partner—a fact she may not know. However, in one study, both obstetrician-gynecologists and general medical practitioners frequently omitted questions about sexual history that would lead them to offer STI prevention messages.[18]

Further, many women may not recognize their own risks or seek out information. Whiteside and

colleagues surveyed 103 women at several urban clinic sites.[19] Although this population was known to be at risk for STIs, one-third had not heard of pelvic inflammatory disease (PID) and almost 80% were unaware of any adverse sequelae to STIs. More than half could not identify any method to prevent infection; only 18% mentioned use of a barrier contraceptive for this purpose.

Many clinicians associate the phrase "counseling and testing" with human immunodeficiency virus (HIV), but the general population's risk of HIV is statistically small. Concerns regarding possible sexual transmission of infections should be addressed by counseling prior to the examination and laboratory testing as well as in the management phase of the visit. The functions of such counseling are to educate the woman about her own health, help her understand why certain tests are performed or recommended, and reduce the risk of future STIs. Introducing these topics before the examination allows the woman to participate in the decision-making process regarding testing. It also offers the opportunity to explain which tests are performed. For example, herpes simplex virus (HSV) culture testing is not routine in an asymptomatic woman, although type-specific glycoprotein G (gG) serology can be offered as part of a comprehensive screen. Doing so requires the explanation that this will test for exposure but not determine the timing of infection. Human papillomavirus (HPV) testing is part of a Papanicolaou (Pap) smear, but those are usually performed at multi-year intervals. A list of tests that should be discussed with women when ordering STI testing is provided in **Table 21-1**.

When considering the importance of effective counseling and testing for infections, it is important to remember that of the five steps to prevent and control the spread of STIs, the first is risk assessment, education, and counseling. See **Table 21-2**.[20]

Table 21-1 Components of a Comprehensive STI Screen

Gonorrhea

Chlamydia

Trichomoniasis

Syphilis

Human immunodeficiency virus (HIV)

Hepatitis B & C

Herpes simplex antibody (gGT) testing

Human papillomavirus (HPV) (under specific circumstances)

Table 21-2 Strategies to Prevent and Control the Spread of Sexually Transmitted Infections (STIs)

- Accurate risk assessment, education, and counseling of persons at risk on ways to avoid STDs through changes in sexual behaviors and use of recommended prevention services
- Pre-exposure vaccination of persons at risk for vaccine-preventable STDs
- Identification of asymptomatically infected persons and persons with symptoms associated with STDs
- Effective diagnosis, treatment, counseling, and follow up of infected persons
- Evaluation, treatment, and counseling of sex partners of persons who are infected with an STD

Reproduced from Centers for Disease Control and Prevention. Sexually transmitted diseases treatment guidelines, 2015. *MMWR Recomm Rep*. 2015;64(No. RR-3):1-137. http://www.cdc.gov/std/tg2015/clinical.htm. 2015. Accessed May 19, 2016.

Evaluation for Reproductive Tract Infections

History

When screening for infections is done as part of an annual examination, a complete health history is taken or reviewed, and additional questions are incorporated as needed to obtain a complete picture. Often, visits relating to genital infections occur as isolated problem visits. At that time, focusing on aspects of health history that affect the gastrointestinal and genitourinary systems is appropriate. This medical history should emphasize prior urinary infections, hepatitis or jaundice, and a history of unexplained pelvic or lower abdominal pain. When recurrent candidal infections are the complaint, additional questions might include diabetes, chronic antibiotic use, immunosuppressive drugs, and HIV status. The social history should include questions about substance use that provides direct risks (e.g., risk of HIV or hepatitis C (HCV) transmission with intravenous [IV] drug use) as well as indirect risks associated with decreased inhibitions when using substances that reduce self-control (e.g., alcohol).

It is important to assess prior obstetric and gynecologic history whenever infection is a consideration; equally, one should anticipate the possibility of prior genital infections in any history taken in the gynecologic setting. Many of the questions asked to completely assess risk of STIs are quite personal. These questions need to be asked after other aspects of the history have been explored, when the woman is aware of her provider's interest in her general health. They can be introduced with a comment about asking all women questions that can help identify risks. The woman should be reassured that asking these questions is not a reflection on her as an individual. As with any sensitive topic, the clinician works from the most general question to the most specific, and from the least invasive to those that are more intimate. The woman's behaviors should be observed for signs of distress or withdrawal, and her emotional concerns addressed before further questions are asked.

The obstetric history is useful to identify whether infection may have played a role in any adverse reproductive outcome. Gynecologic history questions include any history of vaginal infections, STI, PID, or abnormal Pap smears. The sexual history links to these questions and includes age at onset of sexual activity, number and sex of partners, number of current partners, and use of a protective barrier for sexual activity. Women should be reassured that these questions are always asked as part of a comprehensive history. Asking about partner behaviors assesses risk associated with sexual activity. At least among adolescents, underreporting of STIs and pregnancies has been documented.[21]

Table 21-3 lists questions that are asked to assess sexual risk factors.[22,23] Note that the last question is a direct offer to be tested. This offer should be made explicitly at every visit with a woman who is or may be sexually active, regardless of her age. It may be easier for her to consent to testing that is offered, even if she would not ask for herself. The Centers for Disease Control and Prevention (CDC) offers an excellent *Guide to Taking a Sexual History*, which can be accessed online. The link is listed in the online resources section. It provides examples of dialogue to help make these questions more acceptable to women.

Women who self-identify as lesbian or report having a female partner (sexual minority women) also need to be asked these questions. Many of these women have had previous experience in heterosexual relationships;[24] some are bisexual throughout their sexual lives. Many have limited understanding of sexual risk in the context of a same-sex relationship; they may also lack information about healthy sexual practices.[25] Bisexual women have increased risks of STIs and depression relative to lesbian women, and are less likely to seek health care than other women, possibly for cost reasons.[26] Adolescent sexual minority women are at particular risk, because they may still be exploring gender identity and have been found to be at greater risk for substance use, sexual risk taking or victimization, and depressive disorders.[27,28] Transmission of infections between partners of the same sex is well documented, regardless of whether heterosexual

Table 21-3 Sexual Risk Assessment

When were you and your partner last tested for an STI and/or for HIV?

Are you sexually active at this time?

How long ago were you last sexually active?

Are your sex partners male, female, or both?

Do you have vaginal sex? Oral sex? Anal sex?

Do you have sex with people you don't know well, or with someone you just met?

Do you and your partner talk about preventing infections?

What do you use to protect yourself during sex?

Do you use condoms? Always? How often?

When was the last time you had unprotected sex?

Do you or your partner have any symptoms you don't recognize?

Would you like to be tested today?

HIV = human immunodeficiency virus, STI = sexually transmitted infection

Data from University of Washington STD Prevention Training Center. *STD/HIV Risk Assessment: A Quick Reference Guide.* Seattle, WA: University of Washington Center for Health Education and Research; Anderson JR. *A Guide to the Clinical Care of Women with HIV.* Rockville, MD: US Department of Health and Human Services, Health Resources and Services Administration; 2001.

behavior is present. Cervicovaginal and oral secretions can transmit infections either directly or on sexual toys.[25,29]

Review of Systems

The review of systems serves as a bridge between prior history and the physical examination. Gastrointestinal or genitourinary complaints need to be elicited and explored for the following: onset, duration, quality, factors that improve or worsen the symptom, recurrence, and related symptoms or activities. With regard to STIs, this offers an additional time to incorporate questions about symptoms the current partner may be experiencing. For example, if the woman complains of an open sore, it is prudent to ask whether she has noticed similar lesions on her partner, regardless of her partner's gender identity or sexual orientation.

Physical Examination

Physical examination for possible STIs goes well beyond an examination of the genitalia, because symptoms of various diseases appear in a variety of organ systems. Thus, the skin is inspected for jaundice, rashes, open sores, vesicles, solid lesions, or scarring from prior lesions. The presence or absence of lymphadenopathy is noted. Abdominal examination specifically includes assessment of hepatomegaly, any tenderness to shallow or deep palpation, and the location of any palpable masses.

During the genital examination, the first step in assessing for disease is to inspect the appearance of the external genitalia. Excoriation, lesions, visible discharge, changes in skin color, and any alteration in anatomy need to be noted. Edematous or swollen areas should be palpated; the Bartholin and Skene glands and the urethra should be checked for discharge.

As the speculum is inserted, attention should be paid to the tone and appearance of the vaginal walls. During the speculum examination, the speculum can be gently rotated to view all aspects of the vaginal wall and search for lesions or masses. Abnormalities of the cervix are noted, as is the presence or absence of any discharge. Characteristics of the discharge such as appearance, color, texture, quantity, adherence to tissue, and odor are noted. The amount of ectropion present should be observed. Friability, erosion, and lesions are all recorded.

Samples for microscopic analysis or laboratory testing are collected from the appropriate location within the vagina and cervix. Wet mount specimens for yeast, BV, and *Trichomonas* are collected from the lateral vaginal wall or pooled discharge in the posterior fornix. Rapid testing of vaginal samples for *Trichomonas* provides a highly specific methodology, if relatively expensive for the clinical site; it improves sensitivity relative to microscopy and should be considered.[30] Nucleic acid amplification tests (NAAT) for gonorrhea, *Chlamydia*, and *Trichomonas* are collected from the vagina or endocervix. Unless a full pelvic examination is being performed, either self- or clinician-performed vaginal specimens are acceptable and have been shown to have similar sensitivity and specificity.[30,31] First-catch urine samples are acceptable but are reported to have approximately 10% lower sensitivity for *Chlamydia*.[32] Cultures for HSV are taken from visible lesions; when checking for asymptomatic shedding, both the vulva and cervix are swabbed. When testing for group B *Streptococcus*, the sample is taken from the outer third of the vagina and the rectum.

Vaginal pH can be evaluated at the same time. Samples for pH are taken in the posterior fornix or along the vaginal wall. The pH of the cervix is approximately 7.0, while the normal vaginal pH of reproductive-aged women is 3.8 to 4.2. The material obtained is applied directly to the nitrazine paper or swab.

The bimanual examination that follows allows the examiner to assess for cervical motion tenderness, uterine size and shape, and adnexal pain or masses.

In-Office Laboratory Testing

Use of light microscopy to identify vaginal pathogens (and for fern tests) is considered a moderately complex test by the Centers for Medicare and Medicaid Services under the Clinical Laboratory Improvement Amendments (CLIA) regulations. There are specific requirements for maintaining an on-site microscope that can be reviewed on the CDC's website.[33] Most gynecologic offices will need to maintain CLIA approval to expedite treatment of common infections.

The saline wet mount is used to identify the presence or absence of normal epithelial cells, lactobacilli, red or white blood cells (WBCs), clue cells, and *Trichomonas vaginalis*. *Candida* species may also be seen on wet mount, although use of a potassium hydroxide (KOH) preparation is preferred for accuracy. The slide is prepared by placing the vaginal sample into a test tube with a small amount of saline and plating that specimen within 15 minutes. Delay in proceeding to visualization of the slide can cause a loss of cellular integrity. A slide can be plated at the same time with a drop of KOH solution added to the specimen. The slide should be allowed to stand while the saline specimen is examined to allow for lysis of cells. Both slides are examined under 10× and 40× power.

This specimen can also be used to perform the "*whiff*" test for BV. A positive whiff test is recognized by the release of amines from the lysed anaerobic bacteria when an alkaline solution is added, causing a potent fishy odor.

Laboratory tests used to diagnose specific diseases are discussed further in the sections that follow. **Table 21-4** compares symptoms of the common vaginal infections with those of atrophic vaginitis.

Infections Characterized by Discharge

Changes in vaginal discharge are among the first symptoms noticed by women concerned that they may have acquired an infection. Odor; irritation; and changes in texture, color, or amount of fluid may be introduced as the reason for a visit. The

Table 21-4 Signs and Symptoms of Common Vaginal Infections

	Candidiasis	**Bacterial Vaginosis**	**Atrophic Vaginitis**
Primary complaint	Itching, pain	Odor, burning	Irritation, burning, bleeding
Discharge	Internal only	Visible at introitus	with intercourse
Mucosal irritation	Significant erythema common	Absent	Internal only
Color	White or cream	Gray	
Viscosity	Thick	Thin	Thin
Consistency	Clumps	Homogenous	Decreased rugae
pH	~4.0	> 4.5	> 6.0+/−
"Whiff" test	Absent	Present	Decreased
Wet mount	Pseudohyphae, spores, best seen with KOH	Clue cells, *Mobiluncus*,	Thin, watery
	C. glabrata—spores only	decreased white cells	Decreased superficial cells
Other diagnostic techniques	Culture for severe, resistant infection	Gram stain Culture less useful than PCR	Pap testing, serum estrogen level

KOH = potassium hydroxide, PCR = polymerase chain reaction

Data from Brotman RM, Klebanoff MA, Nansel TR, Yu FK, Andrews WW, Zhang J, et al. Bacterial vaginosis assessed by gram stain and diminished colonization resistance to incident gonococcal, chlamydial, and trichomonal genital infection. *J Infect Dis.* 2010;202:1907-1915; Clark LR, Brasseux C, Richmond D, Getson P, D'Angelo LJ. Are adolescents accurate in self-report of frequencies of sexually transmitted diseases and pregnancies? *J Adolesc Health.* 1997;21:91-96.

woman's description of vaginal discharge can contribute to the plan of evaluation and be a foundation of the differential diagnosis. The astute clinician will remember that menarche, hormonal contraception, topical irritation by chemicals or latex, foreign objects left in the vagina, pregnancy, and menopause all produce changes in vaginal discharge that must be distinguished from infection. Some of these changes may precipitate infection; others are benign variations.

Candida albicans *and Other Yeasts*

The majority of women will experience one or more infections with vulvovaginal candidiasis (VVC) during their lifetime. *Candida* spp. are considered normal in small amounts in the vagina, although colonization is heavier in women prone to recurrent infection. Giraldo and colleagues found that polymerase chain reaction (PCR) testing identified *Candida* in about 30% of women, regardless of prior history.[34] Beigi and colleagues identified a 70% colonization rate in young women over the course of a year, although less than 5% were colonized at every study visit.[35]

More than three-quarters of vaginal yeast infections are the result of *C. albicans* overgrowth when lactobacilli are reduced. *C. glabrata* and *C. tropicalis* are other species known to cause vaginal infections. The incidence of non-albicans infections has been increasing, possibly as a result of selective resistance to antifungal medications and immune suppression with HIV.[36-38]

While *Candida* infections (VVC) are commonly reported to be about 40% of all benign vaginal infections, this cannot be easily confirmed, because many cases are self-diagnosed or diagnosed by clinicians without laboratory confirmation.[36-39] Self-diagnosis and inadequate triage leading to misdiagnosis contribute to unclear data regarding frequency and treatment effectiveness.[40,41]

A clear etiology for uncomplicated VVC is often not seen. Onset of sexual activity, hormonal contraception, diaphragm use, and antibiotic use all have been associated with infection; the roles of douching, tight clothing, feminine hygiene products, and diet have not been confirmed as contributors.[37,42,43] At least one study found an association with current or recent infection with gonorrhea and current BV.[44]

EVALUATION

Presenting symptoms among women with VVC include painful itching and a thick, clumpy (sometimes called curdy or cottage cheesy), white vaginal discharge. Other symptoms include dyspareunia, dysuria, and swelling. Women presenting with VVC often have symptoms they may be embarrassed to reveal; they also may have concerns regarding the etiology of their infection. The history may not provide specific clues to the diagnosis; however, uncontrolled diabetes and immune suppression are both associated with increased risk and with persistent recurrences.

On examination, localized edema, fissures, and excoriation of the vulva may be noted. Inflammatory changes may be present in the vagina and surrounding the introitus. The characteristic discharge is thickened, clumped, and white or cream colored. It is frequently adherent to the vaginal walls or cervix. Wet mount findings include yeast hyphae and spores. These are best seen on KOH preparation, when other structures have been dissolved. Vaginal pH is in the normal range. Microscopy is the most accurate diagnostic technique in the clinical setting (**Figure 21-2**). Culture is useful when frequent recurrences or failure to heal with first-line therapy indicate a more complicated infection.

TREATMENT

For treatment purposes, uncomplicated VVC should be distinguished from complicated. Uncomplicated VVC is defined as being sporadic in nature, mild to moderate in severity, and caused

Figure 21-2 Vulvovaginal candidiasis (VVC).

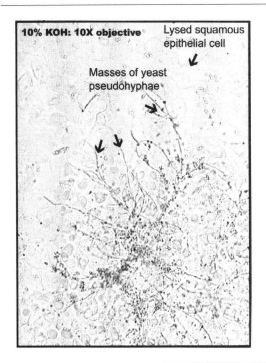

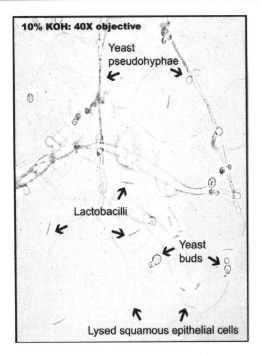

by *C. albicans*. In contrast, complicated VVC recurs frequently, is more severe, is frequently caused by a non-albicans species, and is associated with uncontrolled diabetes, immune suppression, physical debilitation, or corticosteroid use. Although pregnancy is not listed as a complicating factor, the frequency of VVC in pregnancy affects treatment recommendations.[20]

The use of over-the-counter (OTC) antifungals has been widely promoted by the pharmaceutical industry and by clinicians for the treatment of uncomplicated yeast infections. There is evidence that women are frequently mistaken in their self-diagnosis, even when they read the package information and have had prior infections.[38] For this reason, initial prescriptions for new patients should never be provided without office examination, and multiple recurrent infections or inadequate response should be reevaluated clinically, not by symptoms alone.

The topical azoles, whether prescribed or OTC, have similar effectiveness rates. Short-course therapies should be reserved for uncomplicated infections in healthy nonpregnant women. Oral single-dose fluconazole is popular with women who can then avoid "messy" creams or suppositories. A review of oral and intravaginal methods found similar effectiveness rates in the treatment of uncomplicated VVC. Oral and intravaginal products cure about 80% of infections in the short term.[45] However, neither short-course, narrow-spectrum topical products, or oral fluconazole treat non-albicans infections as effectively. Additionally, there is evidence of developing resistance to fluconazole among women treated for long periods with maintenance dosing.[46] The lack of alternatives suggests that lifestyle changes and management of comorbidities to decrease the frequency and severity of recurrences are worth pursuing when counseling women with complicated VVC.

Any factor associated with increased risk of infection or persistent recurrences should be treated initially with a 7-day course of therapy; some experts now recommend extending treatment to 14 days. Sequential doses of fluconazole (one 100-, 150-, or 200-mg tablet orally on days 1, 4, and 7) have improved outcomes relative to a single oral dose.[20] Terconazole is preferable for use with recurrent infections, because it has a broader antifungal spectrum. During pregnancy,

7-day vaginal therapy for VVC can be used safely. Table 21-5 lists the currently available therapies for vaginal yeast infections.[20]

ALTERNATIVE THERAPIES

Boric acid has been used as a remedy for women with persistent VVC and has good efficacy against *Torulopsis glabrata* (also known as *C. glabrata*).[47] It requires access to a compounding pharmacy to obtain the vaginal preparation, which is a gelatin capsule with 600 mg of boric acid. These are inserted vaginally at bedtime for 14 days. Vaginal irritation is an uncommon side effect. Boric acid is poisonous if taken by mouth. A clear explanation of how to use the capsules is mandatory prior to prescribing.

Ingestion and vaginal application of plain yogurt and probiotics have been studied with inconsistent results. Oral ingestion of yogurt is

Table 21-5 Medications for Treatment of Uncomplicated Vulvovaginal Candidiasis

Choose any one from among the following:

Over-the-counter intravaginal agents:

- Clotrimazole 1% cream 5 g intravaginally daily for 7–14 days
- Clotrimazole 2% cream 5 g intravaginally daily for 3 days
- Miconazole 2% cream 5 g intravaginally daily for 7 days
- Miconazole 4% cream 5 g intravaginally daily for 3 days
- Miconazole 100 mg vaginal suppository, 1 suppository daily for 7 days
- Miconazole 200 mg vaginal suppository, 1 suppository for 3 days
- Miconazole 1,200 mg vaginal suppository, 1 suppository for 1 day
- Tioconazole 6.5% ointment 5 g intravaginally in a single application

Prescription intravaginal agents:

- Butoconazole 2% cream (single-dose bioadhesive product), 5 g intravaginally in a single application
- Terconazole 0.4% cream 5 g intravaginally daily for 7 days
- Terconazole 0.8% cream 5 g intravaginally daily for 3 days
- Terconazole 80 mg vaginal suppository, 1 suppository daily for 3 days

Oral agent:

- Fluconazole 150 mg orally in a single dose

Reproduced from Centers for Disease Control and Prevention. Sexually transmitted diseases treatment guidelines, 2015. *MMWR Recomm Rep.* 2015;64(No. RR-3):1-137.

benign, with the exception of gastric distress in some women with lactose intolerance. Early studies have shown some benefit to the use of specific probiotics in treating recurrent VVC.[48,49]

PATIENT COUNSELING

While yeast can be transmitted between partners, it is in no way an STI. Patient counseling includes hygiene measures appropriate for all women, self-care during the infection, prevention of recurrent infection, consideration of changing contraceptive measures, testing for diabetes and HIV when appropriate, and reassurance that this is a common and essentially benign complaint.

Bacterial Vaginosis

BV is a noninflammatory vaginal condition characterized by overgrowth of any of several anaerobic and facultative bacteria and decreased presence of lactobacilli. Commonly identified associations with BV include sexual activity, especially without a condom; early onset of sexual activity; menses; multiple sexual partners; prior STIs and positive HSV2 serology; female sexual partner; practicing cunnilingus; douching; smoking; and African American ethnicity.[50-52] BV is found in virginal women, indicating that the infection is not a strictly sexually transmitted condition.[53] Recolonization after treatment is not uncommon; conversely, BV will resolve spontaneously without recurrence in many women.

The development of our understanding of diversity within the healthy vaginal microbiome has clarified our understanding of normal and healthy, while at the same time revealing reasons for relative risk of symptomatic BV. Koumans and colleagues placed the overall incidence of BV by Gram stain (Nugent's criteria) at 29.2%, with 85% of those infections being asymptomatic.[53] If, however, asymptomatic "infections" are actually a reflection of the biome types found more commonly among African American and Hispanic women, then the incidence of true disease may be much lower than reported.[3] Nugent criteria use the presence or absence of lactobacilli as a scoring point. Amsel's criteria, still the most readily available method of clinical diagnosis, can be positive without gynecologic symptoms or odor. In a letter to the editor, Forney and colleagues state, "Although numerous studies have shown that women with high numbers of *Lactobacillus* species do not have BV, it is a logical fallacy to conclude that women whose vaginal communities have few or no *Lactobacillus* species have BV."[4] They further note that the incidence of healthy vaginal microbiota lacking significant lactobacilli is approximately 30%. At the same time, lactobacilli-deficient biomes are more prone to conditions permitting overgrowth of the bacteria associated with BV (**Table 21-6**). **Figure 21-3** illustrates the transition effect of differing microbiomes on the risk of infection.[1]

Table 21-6 Bacteria Associated with Bacterial Vaginosis

Gardnerella vaginalis

Prevotella spp.

Mobiluncus spp.

Ureaplasma urealyticum

Mycoplasma hominis

Streptococcus spp.

Atopobium vaginae

Eggerthella

Megasphaera

Leptotrichia

Dialister

Bifidobacterium

Slackia

Clostridia (BVAB1, BVAB2, BVAB 3)

Figure 21-3 Effect of microbiota on vaginal health.

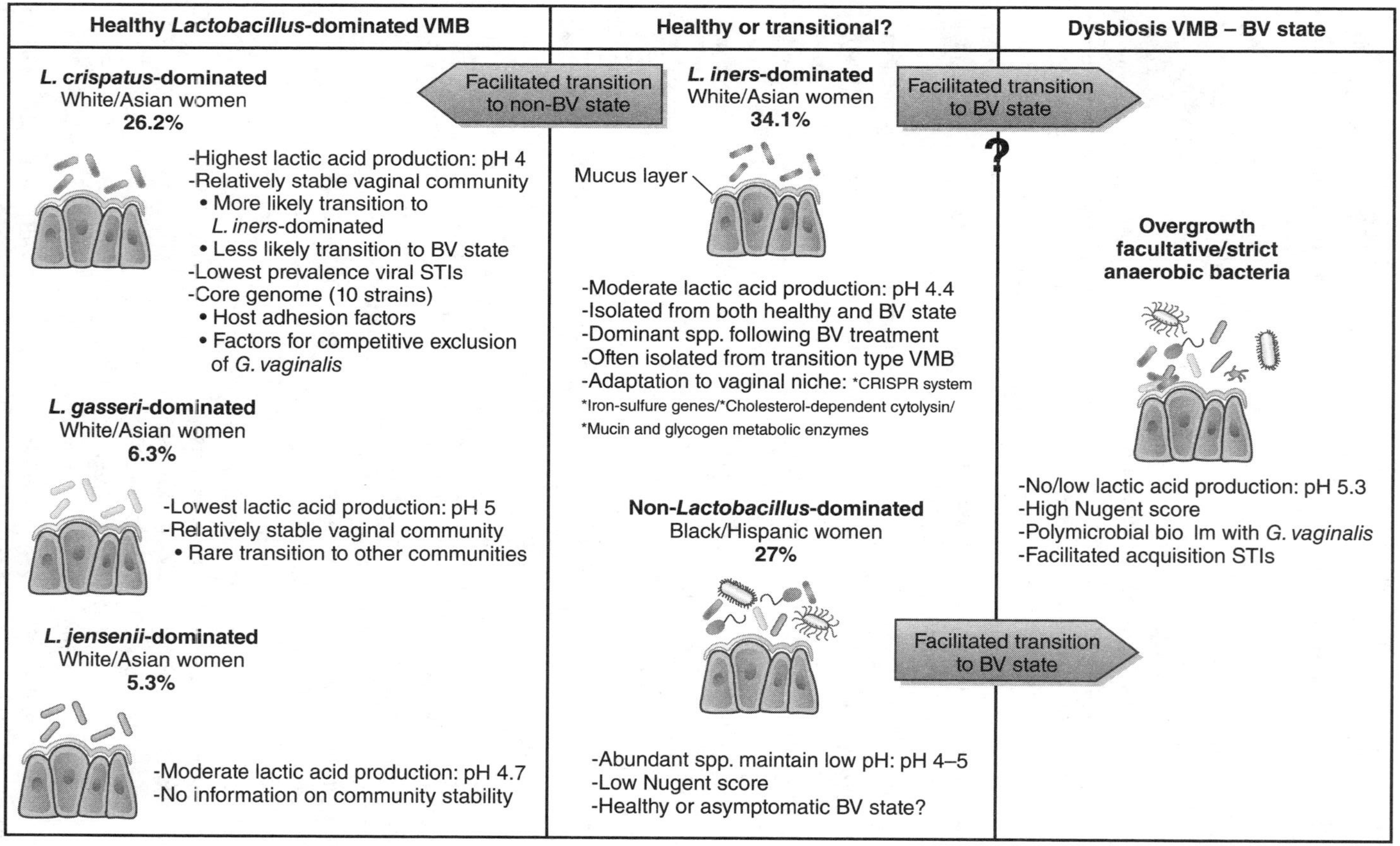

Healthy *Lactobacillus*-dominated VMB	Healthy or transitional?	Dysbiosis VMB – BV state

Facilitated transition to non-BV state

Facilitated transition to BV state

Facilitated transition to BV state

***L. crispatus*-dominated**
White/Asian women
26.2%

-Highest lactic acid production: pH 4
-Relatively stable vaginal community
 • More likely transition to
   L. iners-dominated
 • Less likely transition to BV state
 • Lowest prevalence viral STIs
-Core genome (10 strains)
 • Host adhesion factors
 • Factors for competitive exclusion
   of *G. vaginalis*

***L. gasseri*-dominated**
White/Asian women
6.3%

-Lowest lactic acid production: pH 5
-Relatively stable vaginal community
 • Rare transition to other communities

***L. jensenii*-dominated**
White/Asian women
5.3%

-Moderate lactic acid production: pH 4.7
-No information on community stability

***L. iners*-dominated**
White/Asian women
34.1%

Mucus layer

-Moderate lactic acid production: pH 4.4
-Isolated from both healthy and BV state
-Dominant spp. following BV treatment
-Often isolated from transition type VMB
-Adaptation to vaginal niche: *CRISPR system
*Iron-sulfure genes/*Cholesterol-dependent cytolysin/
*Mucin and glycogen metabolic enzymes

Non-*Lactobacillus*-dominated
Black/Hispanic women
27%

-Abundant spp. maintain low pH: pH 4–5
-Low Nugent score
-Healthy or asymptomatic BV state?

**Overgrowth
facultative/strict
anaerobic bacteria**

-No/low lactic acid production: pH 5.3
-High Nugent score
-Polymicrobial bio lm with *G. vaginalis*
-Facilitated acquisition STIs

Reproduced from Petrova M, Lievens E, Malik S, Imholz N, Lebeer S. *Lactobacillus* species as biomarkers and agents that can promote various aspects of vaginal health. *Front Physiol.* 2015;6:81. http://www.ncbi.nlm.nih.gov/pmc/articles/PMC4373506/figure/F1/. Accessed May 20, 2016. Creative Commons Attribution License available at https://creativecommons.org/licenses/by/3.0/us/

Beigi and colleagues have suggested that the presence or absence of H_2O_2-producing lactobacilli is a factor in coinfection with or increased risk of transmission of HIV and other STIs.[54] The presence of symptomatic BV is considered to indicate an increased risk for the acquisition of STIs including gonorrhea, chlamydia, trichomoniasis, and HIV.[6,55] Disruption of the mucosal barrier and cytokine responses are postulated as reasons for this association with HIV.[55] BV is a strong predictor of infections with *N. gonorrhoeae* and *Chlamydia* when the partner has symptoms of urethritis.[56] Conversely, women whose vaginal biome is characterized by high *Lactobacillus* counts have been found to have lower prevalence of HIV/STI acquisition.[57] In addition, BV is associated with a variety of gynecologic and obstetric complications, including PID, post-abortion infections, post-surgical infections, endometritis, abnormal vaginal bleeding, spontaneous abortion, preterm birth, preterm premature rupture of membranes, and chorioamnionitis.[5-7,58]

Evaluation

Women with BV often complain of a foul, "fishy" odor and associate it with sexual activity or onset of the menses. Burning or irritation is also noted. Some women may complain of feeling "wet." Just as with yeast, the symptoms are not pathognomonic. As indicated by the epidemiology, sexual activity is an essential piece of the history to collect.

On examination, a thin, white discharge may be evident at the introitus. Inflammation or erythema of the vaginal tissue is absent. The release of amines associated with a higher vaginal pH is often noticeable as the examiner approaches the perineum, and will be readily identified on preparation of a KOH specimen.

Clinically, BV is diagnosed by a combination of findings known as *Amsel's criteria* (**Table 21-7**) or in the laboratory with the use of Gram staining using *Nugent criteria*. Culture is relatively

Table 21-7 Amsel's Criteria to Diagnose Bacterial Vaginosis

Thin, white vaginal discharge
Amine release (positive "whiff" test)
Vaginal pH > 4.5
Clue cells on wet mount

Three out of four indicators are required to diagnose BV.

less useful, because many of the species found in BV are also found in normal flora. Collection of material for diagnosis with Amsel's criteria is described in the section on examination of the patient; both a saline wet prep and KOH evaluation are performed. No additional procedures are necessary. Gram staining detects BV by comparing the frequency of *Lactobacillus* morphotypes to those of *Gardnerella* and *Bacteroides*, and to curved Gram-variable rods.[59] Use of Gram staining eliminates the possibility of subjectivity in applying clinical criteria.[60] PCR-based methods are used in the laboratory and have greatly expanded the number of organisms understood to be associated with the development of BV, but are not available for clinical use. Neither Pap smears nor the cards for in-office testing are reliable for use in diagnosis.[20]

Gutman and colleagues have suggested that if vaginal pH is obtained first, then a pH greater than 4.5 plus any other criterion (discharge, amines, clue cells) gives equivalent results to assessment of all four of Amsel's criteria.[61] Others have reported that a positive whiff test plus the presence of clue cells offer an effective tool for rapid diagnosis.[62] In this study, the use of Gram staining to identify bacterial morphology to quantify relative numbers of lactobacilli versus others, or to identify clue cells, did not improve outcomes. Both of these studies described vaginal discharge as being the least useful criterion in making a diagnosis.

Wet mount findings associated with a diagnosis of BV include clue cells, decreased lactobacilli, possible *Mobiluncus*, and no increase in WBCs. When WBCs are seen on a slide that meet the criteria for BV, other vaginal or cervical infections should be suspected, including trichomoniasis, yeast, chlamydia, and gonorrhea.[63] In identifying clue cells, the clinician must recognize most visible cells as covered with adherent bacteria, causing loss of a regular cell outline and obscuring the nucleus. **Figure 21-4** illustrates clue cells.

Figure 21-4 Clue cells.

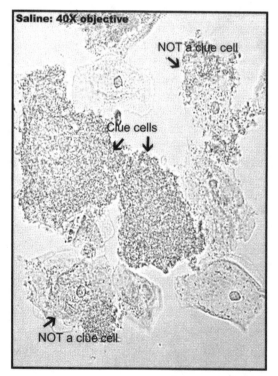

TREATMENT

Treatment of BV can be accomplished with any of several regimens, of which the traditional standard therapy has been a 7-day course of oral metronidazole. The single-dose regimen is less effective in treating BV. For women with infrequent and uncomplicated infections, the use of a vaginal preparation is a reasonable option. Oral metronidazole and vaginal metronidazole gel have similar efficacy, while vaginal clindamycin cream is less effective and increases the risk of resistance.[20,64] **Table 21-8** contains the CDC recommendations for the treatment of BV.[20] Women taking oral metronidazole need to be reminded not to ingest any alcohol during and 24 hours after completing their treatment. Women using vaginal clindamycin cream need to be aware that it is oil based, and that there is increased risk of breakage with use of a latex condom within 72 hours. Treatment of male partners does not affect resolution or recurrence of symptoms and is not recommended.

The question of whether to treat asymptomatic colonization has been a matter of some debate. The clinician must decide whether the risks associated with asymptomatic, and possibly transient, colonization outweigh the value of treatment on an individual basis. Routine screening of women, either during gynecologic examinations or pregnancy, is not recommended.

The use of oral *Lactobacillus* cultures in yogurt and vaginal *Lactobacillus* capsules or suppositories has been shown to have some efficacy against BV and reduce recurrence.[65,66]

PREGNANCY-RELATED CONCERNS

During pregnancy, a prior adverse pregnancy outcome associated with infection should increase watchfulness. Any woman who presents with BV symptoms should be evaluated and treated at the first prenatal visit if possible. Treatment early in pregnancy may be more effective than

Table 21-8 Treatment for Bacterial Vaginosis

Recommended regimens—any one of the following:

- Metronidazole 500 mg orally twice a day for 7 days
- Metronidazole gel 0.75%, 1 full applicator (5 g) intravaginally, once a day for 5 days
- Clindamycin cream 2%, 1 full applicator (5 g) intravaginally at bedtime for 7 days

Alternative regimens—any one of the following:

- Tinidazole 2 g orally once daily for 2 days
- Tinidazole 1 g orally once daily for 5 days
- Clindamycin 300 mg orally twice daily for 7 days
- Clindamycin ovules 100 mg intravaginally once at bedtime for 3 days*

* Clindamycin ovules use an oleaginous base that might weaken latex or rubber products (e.g., condoms and vaginal contraceptive diaphragms). Use of such products within 72 hours following treatment with clindamycin ovules is not recommended.

Reproduced from Centers for Disease Control and Prevention. Sexually transmitted diseases treatment guidelines, 2015. *MMWR Recomm Rep.* 2015;64(No. RR-3):1-137.

in the mid-trimester, when bacteria may already have colonized the cervix and lower uterine segment. Brocklehurst and colleagues reported in a systematic review that early use of clindamycin decreased the risk of late preterm, but not early preterm, birth.[67] The CDC does not consider the evidence to be conclusive, although more studies favor early treatment. The CDC recommendation is to treat with oral metronidazole or clindamycin for symptomatic infections during pregnancy.[20] The 2013 Cochrane review found little benefit to global screening and treatment of BV during pregnancy.[67] Many clinicians prefer to defer metronidazole until organogenesis is complete, although there is no evidence that first-trimester use of metronidazole has risks for the fetus; tinidazole should not be used during pregnancy. Women treated in the first trimester should be evaluated for recolonization 1 month after treatment is complete.

Patient Counseling

Patient counseling includes information about sexual transmission of infections, use of condoms to decrease risks of infection, the fact that BV is not an STI, and that partner treatment is not required. Women should be counseled about the avoidance of douching. Specific information about precautions for metronidazole use is essential, as is information about common side effects such as stomach upset and metallic taste. Recent information suggests that there may be an increase in preterm deliveries with metronidazole use.[68,69] At this time, the recommendations have not changed; however, clinicians need to be aware of the potential risk and counsel women accordingly.

Trichomonas vaginalis

T. vaginalis is a flagellate protozoan that inhabits the vagina, urethra, and Bartholin and Skene glands. It is the most common nonviral STI. The prevalence is estimated at 2.3 million (3.1%) among reproductive-aged US women. Up to 85% of infections are asymptomatic.[70] Associations with *Trichomonas* infections include older age, African American ethnicity, current or previous STI, and substance abuse. Sexual transmission from male to female is more effective (67%–100%) than the reverse (14%–60%).[71] Although it is considered an STI (as opposed to VVC and BV), there is some evidence that it can live in moist conditions for varying lengths of time. Untreated *Trichomonas* can persist in the genitourinary tract. Same-sex couples can transmit *Trichomonas* during sexual activities.

A variety of sequelae are reported for trichomoniasis, including PID, preterm birth, preterm premature rupture of membranes, low-birthweight babies, and increased likelihood of HIV transmission.[72-74]

EVALUATION

Presenting symptoms may include odor, irritation, dysuria, and a discolored vaginal discharge. This is a disease for which assessment of sexual relations is essential to eradicate the infection; without partner treatment, the woman will soon be reinfected.

On examination, the clinician may notice a malodorous, profuse, often frothy discharge that ranges in color from gray to yellow or green and vulvar irritation. The vaginal pH will usually be > 5.0. However, findings on speculum examination are often the first suggestion of the presence of *Trichomonas*. These findings can include friable vaginal and cervical tissue, and, occasionally, the presence of a "strawberry" cervix, the punctate surface of which is so damaged as to have visible petechiae. These are most commonly seen with colposcopy.

When microscopy is performed immediately after the specimen is collected, the clinician will see moving teardrop-shaped bodies, with four anterior flagella in motion (**Figure 21-5**). If the specimen has been left to sit for long, the death of the trichomonads will make diagnosis more difficult. The CDC puts the diagnostic sensitivity of wet mount at 51–65%.[20] NAATs are preferable whenever available. The Aptima Combo 2 assay provides greater than 98% sensitivity and

Figure 21-5 *Trichomonas.*

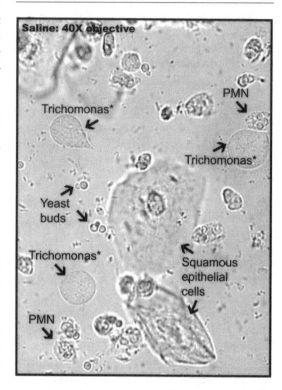

specificity from vaginal secretions; the OSOM rapid test can be performed in a physician's office, takes 10 minutes, and offers similar sensitivity and specificity. Even when cost issues make office-based microscopy the first-line test, consideration should be given to performing a confirmatory NAAT test for high-risk individuals or women whose symptoms suggest an STI when the met mount is negative.[20]

Pap test reports of trichomonads are not generally sensitive enough to be useful in making a diagnosis.[75] In high-prevalence areas (> 20%), treatment based on Pap testing can be recommended.[76]

When a Pap smear result suggests the presence of *T. vaginalis*, the woman can be contacted and offered a screening visit; both false negatives and false positives occur in Pap readings for *Trichomonas*. This should be distinguished from combined Pap/STI testing that includes *Trichomonas* performed by NAAT.

Treatment of trichomoniasis involves the woman and her partner(s). If the midwife does not prescribe for male partners, a referral for the woman's partner to another provider or the local STI clinic is necessary. Because asymptomatic disease is common and the sensitivity of microscopy low, a note stating the reason for recommended treatment should be provided. Recurrence rates are high, running 36% in one study of HIV-infected women.[77] Because most reinfection involves an untreated partner, the issue of partner treatment cannot be overstated.

The oral imidazoles are the only effective treatment available for *T. vaginalis*. **Table 21-9** identifies the current CDC-recommended treatments for trichomoniasis. Resistance occurs in 4–10% of cases treated with metronidazole, and 1% of those treated with tinidazole.[20] In cases where persistent infection rather than reinfection

is suspected, the CDC recommends a 7-day regimen of metronidazole 500 mg twice daily, and, if a third course is needed, metronidazole or tinidazole at 2 grams daily for 7 days. Tinidazole has fewer gastrointestinal side effects than metronidazole. Alcohol should be avoided, and possible drug interactions should always be reviewed. Long-term use of imidazoles has been associated with neuropathy; warning signs should be stressed when repeat courses are prescribed. Liver function testing and a complete blood count should be performed if multiple courses of imidazoles are given. Metronidazole gel is not an effective treatment for *T. vaginalis* infection.

PREGNANCY CONSIDERATIONS

Vaginal trichomoniasis is associated with adverse pregnancy outcomes similar to those found in BV, particularly preterm premature rupture of the membranes, preterm birth, and low-birth-weight babies. Women who are symptomatic should be treated according to the CDC guidelines.[20] The use of metronidazole in the absence of symptoms is debatable. The incidence of adverse outcomes, at least among asymptomatic women, is not lessened by treatment. It has been suggested that an inflammatory response or release of toxins from dying organisms is responsible for the failure to reduce preterm birth.[78]

Mucopurulent Cervicitis

The presence of purulent discharge from the cervix is a clear indicator of cervical infection. *N. gonorrhoeae*, *C. trachomatis*, and BV species are all associated with the presence of cervicitis. *Mycoplasma* was identified by one study of archived cervical specimens as being a factor associated with mucopurulent cervicitis in the absence of other identified causes.[79] Regardless of the cause, diagnosis and treatment are essential to prevent the ascending infections that can lead to

Table 21-9 Treatment for *T. vaginalis*

Recommended regimens—any one of the following:

- Metronidazole 2 g orally in a single dose
- Tinidazole 2 g orally in a single dose

Alternative regimen:

- Metronidazole 500 mg orally twice a day for 7 days

All require abstinence until treatment is complete, partners are treated, and symptoms are resolved. After that time, use of condoms or another effective barrier is advisable.

Reproduced from Centers for Disease Control and Prevention. Sexually transmitted diseases treatment guidelines, 2015. *MMWR Recomm Rep.* 2015;64(No. RR-3):1-137.

chronic pain, infertility, and ectopic pregnancy. If BV species are identified along with any STI, treatment of BV will improve resolution of the cervicitis.[80]

Gonorrhea

Neisseria gonorrhoeae is the cause of about 330,000 new STIs per year in the United States.[81] It is most commonly diagnosed in young adults 15 to 24 years old. In addition to youth, non-white ethnicity and concurrent infection with other STIs are risk factors. Male-to-female transmission is more common than female-to-male, with estimates of transmission as high as 50% per contact.[82] Gonorrhea is associated with increased risk of PID, coinfection with other STIs and HIV, preterm labor and birth, chronic pelvic pain, infertility, and ectopic pregnancy.

Infected men are frequently symptomatic and complain of dysuria or a discharge from the penis. Gonorrhea infections in women are found most commonly on routine screening, or because the woman has nonspecific complaints or a history suggesting STI exposure, or because she has been told by her partner that he is infected.

EVALUATION

On speculum examination, a mucopurulent cervical discharge is frequently seen and indicates the presence of either gonorrhea or another cervicitis, most commonly chlamydia. The presence of BV with increased leukorrhea or increased WBCs on wet mount is also associated strongly with the presence of either gonorrhea or chlamydia.[56,83] The bimanual examination may identify mild cervical, uterine, or adnexal tenderness that does not meet the criteria for cervical motion tenderness. Women with these findings can and should be treated empirically for both gonorrhea and chlamydia.

Diagnosis with culture or NAAT probe is standard. Both can produce false-negative findings with inadequate sampling or improper technique. NAAT testing is available for cervical, vaginal, and urinary specimens, but is not US Food and Drug Administration (FDA)-approved for rectal or oropharyngeal testing at this time. Culture specimens are collected at the endocervix. If other body sites (i.e., rectum, throat) have been exposed, these sites should also be tested. In the symptomatic woman, treatment is not delayed while waiting for culture results. While testing for *C. trachomatis* is not routine, treatment for both infections is accomplished simultaneously on the presumption that the two are frequently associated. Although a test of cure is not routine, if necessary, it should be performed 14 or more days following treatment. Suspected treatment failures are retested using both culture (with sensitivities) and NAAT. A culture with sensitivities for gonorrhea should be performed when a woman diagnosed with gonorrhea and treated appropriately returns a positive test of cure more than 7 days post treatment, and she denies sexual activity since treatment.[81]

TREATMENT

Treatment regimens for *N. gonorrhoeae* are outlined in **Table 21-10**. The rise in rates of resistance to previously recommended regimens means that only a two-drug regimen, consisting of ceftriaxone and azithromycin is standard. The recommendation to use two drugs with different methods of action is intended to slow the rise of further resistance. According to the CDC, only individuals with an immunoglobulin E (IgE) mediated allergy to penicillins or another cephalosporin need to avoid the recommended therapy; the recommendation is to consult an infectious disease specialist for treatment.[20] IgE-mediated allergies include anaphylaxis, Stevens-Johnson syndrome, and toxic epidermal necrolysis.

Table 21-10 Treatment for *Neisseria gonorrhoeae*

Recommended regimen:

- Ceftriaxone 250 mg intramuscularly in a single dose, *plus*:
- Azithromycin 1g orally in a single dose

Alternative regimen if ceftriaxone is not available:

- Cefixime 400 mg orally in a single dose, *plus*:
- Azithromycin 1 g orally in a single dose

Notes:

1. In the case of azithromycin allergy, doxycycline (100 mg orally twice a day for 7 days) can be substituted as a second drug.
2. Spectinomycin is not produced in the United States and is not generally available. When obtainable, it can be used in individuals with an IgE-mediated allergy to penicillin or cephalosporin to treat urogenital/anorectal infections.

Reproduced from Centers for Disease Control and Prevention. Sexually transmitted diseases treatment guidelines, 2015. *MMWR Recomm Rep.* 2015;64(No. RR-3):1-137.

Pregnancy-Related Concerns

In pregnancy, women are treated with the standard regimen; a test of cure is warranted to prevent neonatal exposure. Exposure at birth to infectious cervical secretions can cause ophthalmia neonatorum, which manifests within a few days after birth. The associated risk is infant blindness. When an infant is positive for gonococcal conjunctivitis, the risk of disseminated disease, including sepsis, meningitis, and joint inflammation, should be considered.[20]

Patient Teaching

Patient teaching for gonococcal infections includes safe sex practices, avoidance of all sexual activity until treatment is complete and all current partners have been treated, risks of untreated infection, and side effects of the medication prescribed. All partners within the last 60 days should be seen and evaluated. The importance of having a single, stable, faithful partner is also an essential message. Many young women define single partner and long-term relationship very differently than a clinician will.

Chlamydia

C. trachomatis is an obligate intracellular parasitic bacterium. It is the single most commonly diagnosed STI in women, with 1,401,906 new cases in the United States in 2013.[84] The primary associations are with young age and concurrent or prior STI, and the sequelae are essentially the same as those for gonorrhea. Because of the high incidence of chlamydia in the United States, it is believed to be a major factor in the development of infertility, ectopic pregnancy, and pelvic pain, although high-quality data are limited.

Chlamydia is rarely symptomatic until ascending infection has damaged the upper genital tract. The prevalence of the infection in adolescents and women under 25 means that clinicians must be sensitive to any history suggesting unprotected sexual activity and to any partner complaints of penile discharge or burning.[85]

On examination, yellowish mucopurulent cervicitis may be seen (**Figure 21-6**). The cervix is particularly friable. One study suggested that opacity of the discharge is also a valid clinical indicator and can be used to assist in evaluation for empiric therapy.[86]

Annual testing for chlamydia is recommended for all women under age 25,[87] and for others with risk factors such as new sexual partners, multiple partners, or risky sexual and lifestyle behaviors. NAAT testing of cervical, vaginal, or first-void urine is standard for chlamydia. A test

Figure 21-6 Chlamydia cervicitis.

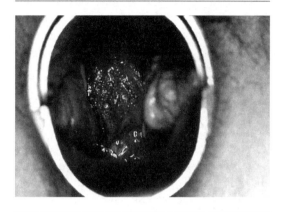

Courtesy of CDC/Dr. Lourdes Fraw, Jim Pledger

Table 21-11 Treatment for *Chlamydia trachomatis*

Recommended regimens—any one of the following:

- Azithromycin 1 g orally in a single dose
- Doxycycline 100 mg orally twice a day for 7 days

Alternative regimens—any one of the following:

- Erythromycin base 500 mg orally 4 times a day for 7 days
- Erythromycin ethylsuccinate 800 mg orally 4 times a day for 7 days
- Levofloxacin 500 mg orally once daily for 7 days
- Ofloxacin 300 mg orally twice a day for 7 days

Treatment during pregnancy:

- Recommended regimen:
  - Azithromycin 1 g orally in a single dose
- Alternative regimens—any one of the following:
  - Amoxicillin 500 mg orally 3 times a day for 7 days
  - Erythromycin base 500 mg orally 4 times a day for 7 days
  - Erythromycin base 250 mg orally 4 times a day for 14 days
  - Erythromycin ethylsuccinate 800 mg orally 4 times a day for 7 days
  - Erythromycin ethylsuccinate 400 mg orally 4 times a day for 14 days

Reproduced from Centers for Disease Control and Prevention. Sexually transmitted diseases treatment guidelines, 2015. *MMWR Recomm Rep.* 2015;64(No. RR-3):1-137.

of cure is not required unless noncompliance or reinfection is suspected; however, any such retesting should be delayed 3–4 weeks following initial therapy to avoid false-positive results from nonviable bacteria remaining in the urogenital tract.[88] The high incidence of reinfection in adolescents and young adults has led to recommendations for rescreening 3 months after an initial treatment or at the next medical visit if that is not possible.[20]

Treatment for chlamydial infection is shown in **Table 21-11**. The opportunity for directly observed therapy, particularly in an adolescent population, reinforces the real utility of using azithromycin.

PREGNANCY-RELATED CONCERNS

During pregnancy, the tetracycline antibiotics are contraindicated. Pregnancy considerations include the very real risk of preterm birth, premature preterm rupture of membranes, low birth weight, and decreased infant survival.[89] In addition, infants exposed to *C. trachomatis* at birth have a risk of ophthalmia neonatorum that approaches 50% and of neonatal pneumonia.

PATIENT COUNSELING

In addition to the patient counseling discussed for gonorrhea, women and girls with chlamydia need to be clear that partners may have no symptoms and deny any problems. Avoidance of intercourse or other sexual activity for a full 7 days post treatment if given a single dose of azithromycin or for the full 7 days of tetracycline treatment is essential. Partner treatment, a mutually monogamous relationship, and condom use cannot be overemphasized in this situation.

Infections Characterized by Lesions

Just as some infections are most commonly described by the characteristics of the associated discharge, others are identified, at least in part, by the lesions produced. Visual inspection and laboratory evaluation combine to make the diagnosis. Women's healthcare providers should be prepared to diagnose, initiate treatment, and appreciate complications requiring referral for each of these diseases.

Syphilis

The bacterium *Treponema pallidum*, a spirochete, is responsible for syphilis. Rates of syphilis in the United States are increasing, primarily among the population of men at least one of whose sexual partners is a man (MSM); approximately 75% of the 17,375 newly reported cases of primary and secondary (P&S) syphilis in 2013 were in this category. Overall, 56,471 cases were reported. Latent-phase syphilis can go undetected unless the infected person is tested in a screening program, so analyses of rates of infection are based on the two symptomatic stages indicative of newly acquired infection. The rate of infection in women has remained unchanged at 0.9/100,000. Black women and women ages 20–24 are at highest risk.[90]

Syphilis is a moderately infectious disease, and the chance of infection from an infected partner who has an open lesion has been reported to be as high as 60%.[91] Syphilis transmission occurs when mucous membranes are exposed to the bacterium or when abraded skin is exposed to infectious lesions. Mother-to-child transmission is possible during pregnancy and birth. Because the disease passes through stages of greater and less infectivity

and is frequently asymptomatic, diagnosis is often delayed, increasing risks of further transmission. While syphilis is curable, undiagnosed cases will persist and cause progressive damage.

After inoculation with *T. pallidum*, the time until the chancre of primary syphilis appears can be up to 90 days, but averages 3 weeks. The chancre is a flat, erythematous, circular open lesion with slightly raised edges. More than one may be present. It is not painful, and women often do not notice an extragenital or vaginal chancre. Spontaneous resolution occurs within a few weeks. Lymphadenopathy, with small rubbery nodes, is common during primary syphilis. Primary syphilis is the period of highest infectivity.

Secondary syphilis is the term given to the next symptomatic phase, which can occur weeks or months after the primary lesion resolves. At this point, syphilis has ceased being a localized disease and become systemic. During this second period of heightened infectivity, a reddish, painless, peeling rash appears, extending from the trunk to head, neck, and limbs, including the palms of the hands and soles of the feet (see **Color Plate 10**). Other signs of secondary syphilis include condyloma lata (round, smooth surfaced, moist lesions arising in the genital area) (see **Color Plate 3**), patchy alopecia, and mucous lesions of the mouth, throat, and cervix (**Figure 21-7**).

The term used to describe the less infectious resting periods of syphilis is *latent phase*. Early latent phase is an asymptomatic period of less than 1 year following exposure to syphilis. Late latent phase must be presumed when there is not a known time of exposure and occurs at any time after the first year of untreated disease. Recurrent signs of secondary syphilis may appear during latency. Although it is rare to see today, tertiary syphilis involves injury to liver, bones, heart, brain, and skin; gummous tumors; and chronic central nervous system damage. The damage occurring during tertiary syphilis can be treated but not reversed.

Figure 21-7 Signs of syphilis.

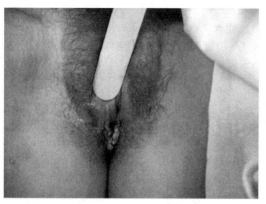

Primary syphilis: chancre (also note condyloma accuminata at posterior of introitus [dual infection])

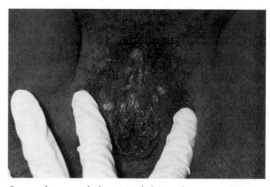

Secondary syphilis: condyloma lata

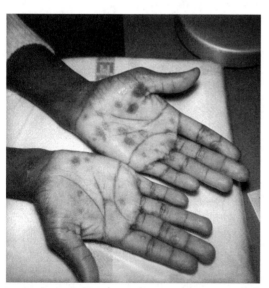

Secondary syphilis: disseminated rash

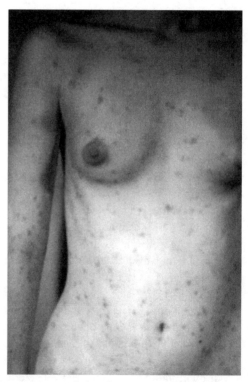

Secondary syphilis: disseminated rash

Top left: Courtesy of CDC/Susan Lindsley. Top right: Courtesy of University of Washington STD Prevention Training Center. Bottom left: Courtesy of CDC/Susan Lindsley. Bottom right: Courtesy of CDC/Susan Lindsley.

EVALUATION

Diagnosis of syphilis most commonly occurs for women during screening or as part of an STI evaluation. Because the primary lesion is painless, it is not always significant enough to bring women in for testing. In parts of the country where syphilis is more prevalent, screening during pregnancy is routine. Women presenting for STI screening or with a presumptive or diagnosed STI should also be tested as part of a complete evaluation. Both syphilis and HIV testing are often omitted from these evaluations because of their relatively low rates. Unfortunately, these are among the most damaging of all STIs. Women diagnosed with pityriasis rosea, which is a benign and self-limiting rash with an appearance similar to that of secondary syphilis, should always be tested for syphilis. See **Figure 21-8**.

Laboratory evaluation is a two-step process. A nonspecific treponemal antibody test (known as non-treponemal tests) is followed by an antigen-specific fluorescent antibody test or particle agglutination test.

Figure 21-8 Pityriasis rosea, showing "herald patch."

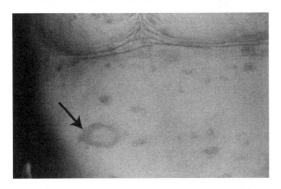

Courtesy of CDC

The most commonly used non-treponemal antibody tests are venereal disease research laboratory (VDRL) and rapid plasma reagin (RPR) tests. Positive results on these tests must be confirmed by a positive result on a treponemal-specific test, of which several are currently approved. False-positive treponemal tests can result from infections such as Lyme disease and Epstein-Barr virus, autoimmune diseases, immunizations, pregnancy, injection drug use, and older age.[92,93]

In addition to serving as the initial test, the non-treponemal tests can be used to follow infectivity. Quantitative reporting should be done by the same lab whenever possible to reduce variation. A rise or fall of two dilutions (fourfold change) indicates a true change in disease progress. A rise from 1:32 to 1:128 would be significant, as would a fall from 1:16 to 1:4. Non-treponemal tests usually become negative over time, although some women will have persistent low titers for life, even after a cure has been effected. Treponemal tests usually remain positive for life.

TREATMENT

Treatment with IM penicillin G is always the preferred technique, so much so that the CDC recommends desensitizing allergic persons to the drug. Treatment guidelines are provided in **Table 21-12**. Alternative therapies exist; these include 14 days of doxycycline or tetracycline or cephalosporins. Unless complete adherence can be ensured, a penicillin allergy desensitization regimen is recommended.

Partner identification and treatment should extend back for the presumed period of symptoms plus 90 days. Thus, if primary syphilis is diagnosed, partners for the prior 90 days plus the current duration of symptoms should be identified. For secondary cases, the reach back period is 6 months plus symptom duration, and for early latent syphilis it is 1 year. Effectiveness of

Table 21-12 Treatment for Syphilis

Recommended regimen for adults
Primary and secondary syphilis:
• Benzathine penicillin G 2.4 million units IM in a single dose
Early latent syphilis:
• Benzathine penicillin G 2.4 million units IM in a single dose
Late latent syphilis or latent syphilis of unknown duration:
• Benzathine penicillin G 7.2 million units total, administered as 3 doses of 2.4 million units IM each at 1-week intervals

IM = intramuscular

Reproduced from Centers for Disease Control and Prevention. Sexually transmitted diseases treatment guidelines, 2015. *MMWR Recomm Rep.* 2015;64(No. RR-3): 1-137.

treatment is tracked with repeat testing at 6, 12, and 24 months.[20] The rate of decrease in titers is dependent on stage of disease and initial titers. A sustained reduction at that point indicates a true cure; for the small proportion of individuals with persistent elevations, further testing, including HIV testing and evaluation for neurosyphilis, is indicated. Retreatment may be required; an infectious disease expert should be consulted.

PREGNANCY-RELATED CONCERNS

During pregnancy, penicillin therapy is necessary, because it is the only agent proven to affect the fetus.[20] Treatment is the same as for nonpregnant women. Untreated or inadequately treated syphilis can cause fetal syphilis (seen on ultrasound as hepatomegaly, ascites, and hydrops), preterm labor or stillbirth, and congenital syphilis. Signs of congenital syphilis include nonimmune hydrops, rhinitis (snuffles), rash, liver or splenic enlargement, and jaundice. The initial infant tests can be positive from maternal antibodies, so

testing of the asymptomatic infant continues every 3 months until a negative result is obtained. In 2013, there were 348 cases of congenital syphilis in the United States, reflecting the decline in rates among women.[90]

An uncommon but significant febrile reaction to therapy is the Jarisch-Herxheimer reaction. Muscle aches and headache may accompany the fever. It may trigger preterm labor or fetal distress when it occurs during the second half of pregnancy.[20]

PATIENT COUNSELING

Women diagnosed with syphilis may need assistance in locating and arranging treatment for their partners; available resources in the city or state should be reviewed. The importance of completing treatment and coming for follow-up monitoring should be stressed. All patients who test positive for syphilis should also be tested for HIV.

Chancroid

Chancroid is a rare disease in the United States, with only 10 diagnoses in 2013, the most recent reporting year; however, it is likely to be underdiagnosed.[94] Most cases are found in discrete outbreaks; cases occurred in four states or jurisdictions in 2013. Minority ethnicity, multiple sexual partners, prostitution, and drug use (primarily cocaine) are risk factors associated with chancroid. The disease is more common in the developing world, particularly in Africa and the Caribbean. It is included here to remind the reader that when evaluating a patient with open vulvovaginal lesions, herpes and syphilis are not the only possible diagnoses. Because the diagnosis of chancroid is made by exclusion, testing for *T. pallidum*, herpes, and HIV should be automatic.

Haemophilus ducreyi is difficult to culture, and no other approved tests are available. The

Table 21-13 Treatment for Chancroid

Recommended regimens—any one of the
following:

- Azithromycin 1 g orally in a single dose
- Ceftriaxone 250 mg intramuscularly in a single
  dose
- Ciprofloxacin 500 mg orally twice a day for
  3 days
- Erythromycin base 500 mg orally 3 times a day
  for 7 days

Reproduced from Centers for Disease Control and Prevention. Sexually transmitted diseases treatment guidelines, 2015. *MMWR Recomm Rep.* 2015;64(No. RR-3):1-137.

diagnosis is made by the presence of a painful genital ulcer, negative tests for syphilis and herpes, and bilateral inguinal lymphadenopathy. The ulcer is usually deeper, softer at the edges, and more irregular than a syphilitic chancre. It is always painful. One or more lesions may be present. If the adenopathy is suppurative (i.e., open and draining purulent discharge), the clinical presentation is classic.[20,95]

Table 21-13 lists the approved regimens for treatment of chancroid. Following treatment, the woman should be reexamined within 1 week. If treatment is successful, marked improvement will already be apparent. Complete resolution, however, may take several weeks. All sex partners during a period of time extending back 10 days prior to the appearance of symptoms should be treated.[20]

Genital Herpes Simplex

Although HSV type 2 is thought of as "genital herpes," both serotypes can be responsible for HSV infections on any part of the body. More than 775,000 individuals acquire HSV annually; the reported rate of HSV-2 in the United States is 15.5%, a decrease from previous estimates,

although this number is believed to be an underrepresentation of the rate of disease.[96,97] More than 85% of those with serologically confirmed herpes do not have identifiable symptoms.[98] An increasing percentage of infections is caused by HSV-1, particularly among adolescents; many of the HSV-1 infections initially occur during childhood.[99,100] A recent study reported that among seronegative women enrolled in a vaccine trial, clinically recognized HSV-1 was three times more likely to present as a genital infection than orally; rates of acquisition of HSV-2 were higher in non-Hispanic blacks, but HSV-1 was more common among non-Hispanic whites.[101] Most infections were not identified clinically, but on serology.

Among risk factors for HSV-2 are African American ethnicity, female sex, older age, multiple lifetime sexual partners, young age at onset of sexual activity, less education, history of STIs, an uncircumcised male partner, smoking, douching, abnormal vaginal flora (e.g., group B streptococcus or BV), and lack of HSV-1 antibody.[102,103] Rates among African Americans remain higher even when controlling for other factors affecting rates.[104] The incidence is doubled in women relative to men as a result of anatomic susceptibility and increased efficiency of transmission.[98]

TRANSMISSION

Transmission of HSV occurs through viral contact with mucous membranes or nonintact skin. Oral–genital transmission occurs, as can occupational transmission if abraded skin is inoculated with the virus. Subclinical shedding of HSV can also be responsible for transmission. Wald and colleagues found that, overall, women with HSV experienced subclinical shedding as much as 2% of the time, or one-third of all days that the virus was reactivated.[105] The duration of episodes of viral shedding was similar (1.5 vs. 1.8 days), whether or not symptoms were present. More recent infection and more frequent clinical recurrences were both associated with increased risk of shedding. In another study, the same team identified similar risks of viral shedding in seropositive persons without a history of clinical HSV.[106]

Prevention of all HSV transmission is not possible when couples are discordant. Prior HSV-1 infection may reduce a woman's chance of acquiring HSV-2 from a partner.[107] Condom use reduces but does not eliminate risk.[108] Subclinical shedding exposes partners who are relying on condoms to prevent infection. Suppression with valacyclovir has been demonstrated to reduce heterosexual transmission.[109] For this reason, the American College of Obstetricians and Gynecologists recommends that serodiscordant couples use suppressive therapy for the infected partner as an additional protective mechanism.[110]

The presentation of HSV is diverse, both at the time of infection and during recurrences of shedding. Approximately one-third of those with an initial HSV-2 infection experience a primary outbreak with multiple lesions, severe pain, and systemic effects such as myalgia, lymphadenopathy, and malaise. Many others who have clinical symptoms present with the classic blisters but do not experience more severe symptoms. Still others have no recognizable symptoms.[101]

Many women with clinical outbreaks notice a prodrome of burning, pain, paresthesias, or irritation along the nerve line where the virus lies dormant, lasting 12 to 24 hours prior to the onset of clinically apparent lesions. HSV lesions are typically multiple round vesicles that erode to form exquisitely tender ulcers (see **Color Plate 12**). As the infection progresses, these develop a golden crust before resolving. In recurrent infection, the number of vesicles is fewer, and some women have only prodromal symptoms—stinging or irritation—along the nerve line, or reddened, irritated tissue. Single isolated, deep ulcers may also represent herpetic infection. Extragenital lesions are common.[111] An illustration of herpes is provided in **Figure 21-9**.

EVALUATION

Diagnosis of HSV should not be limited to observation of the lesions, because this will miss many infected persons.[111] Culture is most sensitive during the vesicular stage and decreases in sensitivity as the infection progresses. NAAT and PCR testing are increasingly available and are more accurate in confirming a clinical diagnosis than culture.[20] Type-specific gG-based serologic assays should also be performed at this time. Knowing the viral type influences counseling and the anticipated lifetime course of the infection. Over time, the incidence of recurrence will be much lower if HSV-1 is the causative agent.

TREATMENT

Pharmacotherapy for management of HSV is shown in **Table 21-14**. Antiviral therapy is always indicated for initial outbreaks and can be prescribed empirically for women with a classic presentation. Severe disease (usually seen in primary infection and with immune suppression) requires IV therapy and physician management in a hospital.

Management of recurrent episodes can decrease the healing time. Suppressive therapy for those with frequent recurrences reduces the frequency and severity of outbreaks, and 70% to 80% of recurrences can be eliminated with suppression therapy. However, neither intermittent nor suppressive therapy will protect against recurrences when medication is stopped.

PREGNANCY-RELATED CONCERNS

During pregnancy, the greatest risk of transmission of HSV to the newborn is at the time of birth. Transmission is most common among women who do not have a history of clinical outbreaks. Transmission risk is highest—up to 50%—when new infection occurs in the third trimester. Women with a history of recurrent herpes, or

Figure 21-9 Herpes lesions of vulva and cervix.

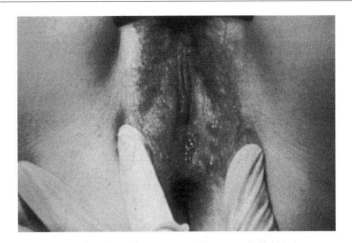

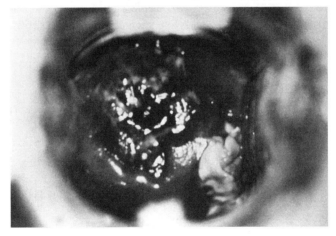

Top: Courtesy of CDC. Bottom: Courtesy of CDC/Dr. Paul Wiesner.

new infections in early pregnancy, rarely transmit. Suppressive therapy for women with frequent recurrences can be used in the late third trimester to decrease the risk of perinatal transmission. On admission in labor, all women should be evaluated for lesions or prodrome as part of the admission examination. Cesarean birth is recommended for those women who have evidence of active HSV.

PATIENT COUNSELING

Patient counseling and education for HSV include the natural history and incurable nature of the infection, modes of transmission, and ways to decrease risks. The CDC summary of counseling following HSV diagnosis is shown in **Table 21-15**.[20] The extensive nature of this list

Table 21-14 Treatment for Genital Herpes Simplex

First clinical episode

Recommended regimens—any one of the following:*

- Acyclovir 400 mg orally 3 times a day for 7–10 days
- Acyclovir 200 mg orally 5 times a day for 7–10 days
- Valacyclovir 1 g orally twice a day for 7–10 days
- Famciclovir 250 mg orally 3 times a day for 7–10 days

Episodic therapy for recurrent outbreaks

Recommended regimens—any one of the following:

- Acyclovir 400 mg orally 3 times a day for 5 days
- Acyclovir 800 mg orally twice a day for 5 days
- Acyclovir 800 mg orally 3 times a day for 2 days
- Valacyclovir 500 mg orally twice a day for 3 days
- Valacyclovir 1 g orally once a day for 5 days
- Famciclovir 125 mg orally twice daily for 5 days
- Famciclovir 1 g orally twice daily for 1 day
- Famciclovir 500 mg once, followed by 250 mg twice daily for 2 days

Suppressive therapy

Recommended regimens—any 1 of the following:

- Acyclovir 400 mg orally twice a day
- Valacyclovir 500 mg orally once a day†
- Valacyclovir 1 g orally once a day
- Famciclovir 250 mg orally twice a day

---

* Treatment can be extended if healing is incomplete after 10 days of therapy.

† Valacyclovir 500 mg once a day might be less effective than other valacyclovir or acyclovir dosing regimens in persons who have very frequent recurrences (i.e., ≥ 10 episodes per year).

Reproduced from Centers for Disease Control and Prevention. Sexually transmitted diseases treatment guidelines, 2015. *MMWR Recomm Rep.* 2015;64(No. RR-3):1-137.

demonstrates the need to allow time for effective counseling, which should be planned with *any* STI diagnosis. Although the evidence does not support concerns about lasting harm from the diagnosis,[112] the emotional impact of the diagnosis for many women dictates that community resources be offered and supportive counseling provided. Online resources, such as the American Sexual Health Association website (www.ashasexualhealth.org), can be offered. Many women have concerns about the safety of childbearing and about transmission to future sexual partners. An international study of patient satisfaction with care found that having educational materials easily available, taking the time for counseling at the initial visit, and effective diagnosis and treatment methods all improved patient perception of quality of care.[113]

Molluscum Contagiosum

Molluscum contagiosum is found most commonly in tropical areas, although the distribution is worldwide. A member of the poxviruses, it is frequently seen in children as a skin infection. Among adults, sexual transmission is more common. Overcrowding, poverty, and inadequate resources for good hygiene are all associated with higher rates of infection.[114]

The virus causes a benign infection of the skin. Firm, raised, flesh-colored nodules with a softly indented (umbilicated) center form from small papules. The average size is less than 0.5 cm. The central area is filled with a soft, curd-like material that can be expressed. The nodules can appear on the genitals, buttocks and thighs, or chest. In immunosuppressed patients, large lesions may be seen on the face. See **Figure 21-10** for an image of molluscum contagiosum.

Transmission occurs through contact with infected skin. In addition to sexual transmission, it can be transferred from personal objects that have been in contact with lesions, and by skin-to-skin contact. The infection can be spread on the body by touching infected areas and then touching other body parts before washing. The incubation period averages 2 to 3 months after the initial exposure.[115]

Table 21-15 Counseling for HSV Diagnosis

The following topics should be discussed when counseling persons with genital HSV infection:

- The natural history of the disease, with emphasis on the potential for recurrent episodes, asymptomatic viral shedding, and the attendant risks of sexual transmission
- The effectiveness of suppressive therapy for persons experiencing a first episode of genital herpes in preventing symptomatic recurrent episodes
- Use of episodic therapy to shorten the duration of recurrent episodes
- Importance of informing current sex partners about genital herpes and informing future partners before initiating a sexual relationship
- Potential for sexual transmission of HSV to occur during asymptomatic periods (asymptomatic viral shedding is more frequent in genital HSV-2 infection than genital HSV-1 infection and is most frequent during the first 12 months after acquiring HSV-2)
- Importance of abstaining from sexual activity with uninfected partners when lesions or prodromal symptoms are present
- Effectiveness of daily use of valacyclovir in reducing risk for transmission of HSV-2 and the lack of effectiveness of episodic or suppressive therapy in persons with HIV and HSV infection in reducing risk for transmission to partners who might be at risk for HSV-2 acquisition
- Effectiveness of male latex condoms, which when used consistently and correctly can reduce (but not eliminate) the risk for genital herpes transmission
- HSV infection in the absence of symptoms (type-specific serologic testing of the asymptomatic partners of persons with genital herpes is recommended to determine whether such partners are already HSV seropositive or whether risk for acquiring HSV exists)
- Risk for neonatal HSV infection
- Increased risk for HIV acquisition among HSV-2 seropositive persons who are exposed to HIV (suppressive antiviral therapy does not reduce the increased risk for HIV acquisition associated with HSV-2 infection)

HIV = human immunodeficiency virus, HSV = herpes simplex virus.

Reproduced from Centers for Disease Control and Prevention. Sexually transmitted diseases treatment guidelines, 2015. *MMWR Recomm Rep.* 2015;64(No. RR-3):1-137.

A presumptive diagnosis can be made on clinical presentation. Staining of the material expressed from the nodules can identify typical "molluscum" bodies in the cytoplasm. The most accurate diagnosis is by biopsy and histopathology.[115]

Because molluscum is a benign disease with a limited course, it will resolve spontaneously after weeks or months. The potential for auto-inoculation and ease of spread through intact skin, and the appearance of the lesions, are reasons for treatment. In particular, genital lesions should be treated to prevent transmission to a sexual partner. Cryotherapy, laser, curetting the lesions, podophyllotoxin cream (0.5%) at home, imiquimod cream, and other methods are equally successful.[115] Individuals who are immunosuppressed may have lesions that are both larger and more persistent.

Lymphogranuloma Venereum

Lymphogranuloma venereum (LGV) is caused by some subgroups of *C. trachomatis* and is rarely seen in the United States. A genital ulcer may appear at the site of initial infection, but it quickly resolves. The more recognizable presentation

Figure 21-10 Molluscum contagiosum.

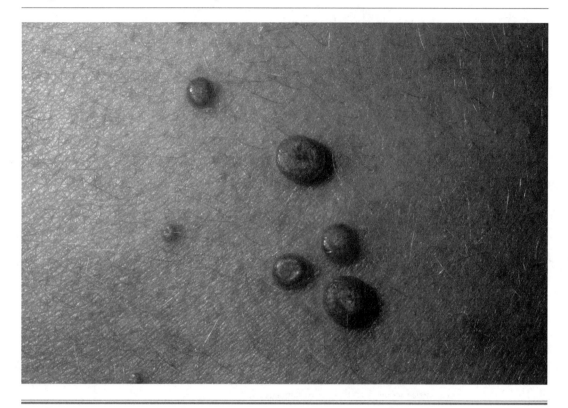

© Dr. P. Marazzi/Science Source

is tender lymphadenopathy, typically unilaterally, in the inguinal/femoral area but also perianally. Diagnosis is by exclusion of other causes of lymphadenopathy and genital ulcers or by culture, direct immunofluorescence, or NAAT.[20]

LGV is treated with doxycycline 100 mg orally twice a day for 21 days or erythromycin base 500 mg orally 4 times a day for 21 days. The patient is seen regularly until all symptoms resolve. All partners counting back 60 days from onset of symptoms should be tested for chlamydia and other STIs and treated as above. During pregnancy, the azithromycin regimen for chlamydia is given.[20]

External Genital Warts (Human Papillomavirus Infection)

Most sexually active adults in the United States have been infected with at least one HPV strain. More than 100 strains are known to exist; at least 40 of these strains are found predominantly in the anogenital area.[116] Their effects range from visible warts to cervical dysplasia. Oncogenic strains are the cause of most female genital cancers and oropharyngeal cancers. The association of HPV with cervical cancer is not addressed here. Non-oncogenic strains such as 6 and 11 are responsible for the visible warts found on the external genitalia and perianal region, vaginally, and at the cervix. Many more women have subclinical infections without any obvious lesions.

The appearance of visible warts is of a fleshy, exophytic mass that is easily friable and nontender unless injured or secondarily infected (see **Color Plate 11**). Warts found on mucous tissue are moister in appearance, but have a similar pattern of growth. Other HPV types produce flat lesions best seen with application of acetic acid or during colposcopy. These can occur both externally and inside the vagina. Internal HPV frequently has an associated dirty-appearing vaginal discharge; this discharge is exaggerated by the presence of coinfections with vaginitis or STIs. Over time, HPV may improve spontaneously or may form progressively larger masses.

EVALUATION

Diagnosis of HPV lesions is most commonly accomplished by visual inspection. HPV must be distinguished from condyloma lata of secondary syphilis and from neoplastic lesions. Biopsy and viral typing are not necessary to make an initial diagnosis, but they can be useful when lesions do not resolve with treatment, or when the appearance of the lesions is not clearly that of HPV. An illustration of visible genital warts is provided in **Figure 21-11**.

PREVENTION AND TREATMENT

HPV infection with the most common viral types can be prevented with vaccination. The Advisory Committee on Immunization Practices (ACIP) recommendation is to provide the 3-dose series of vaccine to both young men and young women between the ages of 11 and 12 prior to the onset of sexual activity, or beginning as early as 9 years of age, and to vaccinate anyone not previously vaccinated up to the age of 26.[117] Vaccines are available that prevent infection with 2 (16, 18), 4 (6, 11, 16, 18), and 9 (6, 11, 16, and 18, 31, 33,

Figure 21-11 HPV Genital warts.

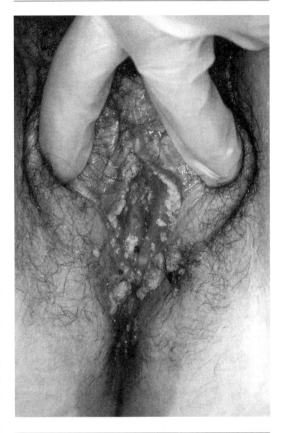

Courtesy of CDC/Joe Millar

45, 52, and 58) strains. Use of the most comprehensive vaccine protects against 81% of cervical cancers and 90% of genital warts.[20] The quadrivalent and 9-valent versions are approved for both sexes.

Treatment plans for HPV focus on resolving symptomatic warts. Often treatment is followed by a period without new lesions. Most recurrences happen within the first 90 days after treatment. It is not clear whether treating warts will reduce infectivity.[20] Individuals with perianal warts should be referred for a digital or anoscopic evaluation for internal warts.

Many women may prefer to use a home-based method such as imiquimod (Aldara) cream, rather than return to the office for repeated treatments. In that case, careful instructions as to use and the period of time after which the woman should return for reevaluation should be documented. Imiquimod cream is an immune modulator that may work by stimulating alpha-interferon production. The most common side effect of imiquimod use is an erythematous "sunburn" rash over the area of application. Cure rates with this method are equivalent to office-applied therapies, and recurrence rates may be lower.[118]

Table 21-16 lists the standard treatment regimens for external warts. Use of cryotherapy, excision, or laser ablation can remove intravaginal lesions or large masses of external warts. Treatment of partners does not appear to change the natural history of infection.

Table 21-16 Treatment for External Genital Warts

Recommended regimens—any one of the following:

Patient-applied:

- Imiquimod 3.75% or 5% cream*
- Podofilox 0.5% solution or gel
- Sinecatechins 15% ointment*

Provider-administered:

- Cryotherapy with liquid nitrogen or cryoprobe
- Surgical removal either by tangential scissor excision, tangential shave excision, curettage, laser, or electrosurgery
- Trichloroacetic acid (TCA) or bichloroacetic acid (BCA) 80–90% solution

* Might weaken condoms and vaginal diaphragms.

Reproduced from Centers for Disease Control and Prevention. Sexually transmitted diseases treatment guidelines, 2015. *MMWR Recomm Rep* 2015;64(No. RR-3): 1-137.

During pregnancy, office-applied treatment is limited to trichloroacetic acid. There is inadequate safety evidence for imiquimod, and podofilox and sinecatechins are contraindicated. Use of cryotherapy, laser, or excision is not contraindicated. Cesarean section is not recommended unless the mass of warts blocks the birth canal or produces excessive bleeding. Transmission to the fetus or newborn is rare.

PATIENT COUNSELING

Patient counseling includes the information that although HPV is sexually transmitted, genital warts are not always visible, and that it is not possible to state when or from which partner an exposure occurred. Women need to be informed that visible lesions may recur, because treatment does not eradicate the virus.

Pelvic Inflammatory Disease (PID)

PID includes any infection of the upper genital tract that has ascended from the vagina and cervix, whether of the endometrium, fallopian, tubes or peritoneum, and tubo-ovarian abscesses. PID is most common among women ages 15 to 24. Table 21-17 lists organisms associated with the development of PID. The diversity of these organisms combined with the often vague symptoms can make acute PID difficult to diagnose when laboratory screening tests are negative or are omitted. In addition, subclinical PID can persist and cause damage. The etiologies of acute and subclinical PID are similar.[119]

While STIs are associated with most cases of PID, the risk factors for acquiring upper genital tract infection vary with the organisms involved. Studies have identified race, young age, early onset of sexual activity, multiple sexual partners, sex during the menses, short duration of symptoms, and history of *N. gonorrhoeae* infection with prior PID as risk factors for a sexually transmitted bacterial infection causing PID.[120-122] Intrauterine

Table 21-17 Organisms Associated with the Development of Pelvic Inflammatory Disease (PID)

Neisseria gonorrhoeae
Chlamydia trachomatis
Gardnerella vaginalis
Prevotella species
Haemophilus influenzae
Escherichia coli
Streptococcus agalactiae
S. pyogenes
S. pneumoniae
Cytomegalovirus
Mycoplasma hominis
Ureaplasma urealyticum
Other vaginal anaerobes associated with BV and enteric Gram-negative rods

The most current information on the CDC STD treatment guidelines can be accessed at http://www.cdc.gov/std.

device (IUD) use and recent pelvic surgery have been implicated in non-STI-related PID.[122] The risk associated with IUD use appears restricted to the period immediately following insertion and is related to the introduction of vaginal flora into the uterine cavity. Antibiotic prophylaxis does not appear to alter this risk.[123] Consistent use of a barrier contraceptive reduces risk of PID. However, no single characteristic, whether it be historical, physical, or laboratory based, is adequate to make the diagnosis of PID or to exclude it.[20]

Evaluation

The presentation of acute PID can be vague enough that the diagnosis will be missed when clinicians are not alert to the possibility of upper genital tract disease. Vague lower abdominal pain

or pain with intercourse may be the presenting symptom, as can an abnormal vaginal discharge (particularly when BV organisms are involved) or unexplained vaginal bleeding. In some women, acute lower abdominal pain, especially in the adnexa, may signal tubal disease.

On examination, vaginal discharge or mucopurulent cervicitis suggests the need for appropriate testing. Uterine or adnexal tenderness or cervical motion tenderness on bimanual examination in sexually active women prompts empiric treatment for acute PID while laboratory results are pending. A pregnancy test must also be performed to exclude ectopic pregnancy from the differential diagnosis. Whenever the question of PID arises, cultures or DNA screens should be collected from the cervix, and a wet mount should be performed.

The CDC recommends the use of additional criteria to improve diagnostic accuracy.[20] These include:

- Oral temperature > 101°F
- Mucopurulent discharge
- Increased WBCs on wet mount
- Elevated erythrocyte sedimentation rate
- Elevated C-reactive protein
- Positive test for gonorrhea or chlamydial infections

Laparoscopy, endometrial biopsy, or imaging can be used to obtain definitive diagnosis when indicated.

Alternative diagnoses need to be considered as explanations for pelvic pain, bleeding, and/or abnormal discharge. These include ectopic pregnancy, appendicitis, endometriosis, bladder infections or interstitial cystitis, and pelvic masses.

Beckmann and colleagues reported on data from the National Hospital Ambulatory Medical Care Survey related to emergency department care for adolescents with STIs.[124] Among their findings was incomplete or incorrect treatment for PID in as many as 65% of all adolescent females with that diagnosis. In addition, less than half of these sexually active teens had a pregnancy test, and only 1% had HIV testing. These findings underscore the need for careful, thorough assessment of women presenting with symptoms suggestive of PID as well as the importance of considering other possible diagnoses (e.g., ectopic pregnancy) and complete STI screening.

TREATMENT

Treatment for PID incorporates broad-spectrum antibiotics, with verification of efficacy not later than 72 hours after beginning medication. Patients should be asked to return for follow up in that timeframe. **Table 21-18** lists regimens recommended for acute uncomplicated PID. Unless anaerobic bacteria have been excluded as a cause, metronidazole is included as a third medication to ensure appropriate coverage.[125] If *N. gonorrhoeae* is implicated, the regimen must include two medications suitable for treatment.[20]

Midwives and other women's health practitioners should consult regarding PID management and refer women who need hospitalization or those for whom invasive procedures such as laparoscopy are required. Partner therapy is necessary, including all partners for two months prior to the diagnosis. IUDs do not need to be removed initially in order to adequately treat PID; however, if there is no improvement in symptoms, then removal can be considered.[126,127]

At times, hospitalization is required to effectively manage upper genital tract disease. During pregnancy, an initial period of hospital-based IV therapy is appropriate because of the risks of chorioamnionitis and preterm birth from intrauterine infection. Women unable to accurately take medications at home or who are too unwell to do so need hospitalization. Tubo-ovarian abscess diagnosed with sonography or other imaging modalities and an acute (surgical) abdomen also warrant hospitalization.

Table 21-18 Regimens for the Treatment of Mild to Moderate Pelvic Inflammatory Disease

Recommended Intramuscular/Oral Regimens

Any one of the following:

- Ceftriaxone 250 mg IM in a single dose
- Cefoxitin 2 g IM in a single dose and probenecid 1 g orally administered concurrently in a single dose
- Other parenteral third-generation cephalosporin (e.g., ceftizoxime or cefotaxime)

Plus:

- Doxycycline 100 mg orally twice a day for 14 days

*With** or *without:*

- Metronidazole 500 mg orally twice a day for 14 days

IM = intramuscular

* Note: All of these regimens include two or three medications to provide an adequate spectrum of coverage.

Reproduced from Centers for Disease Control and Prevention. Sexually Transmitted Diseases Treatment Guidelines, 2015. *MMWR Recomm Rep.* 2015;64(No. RR-3): 1-137.

Sequelae of PID include tubal factor infertility, ectopic pregnancy, and chronic pelvic pain. Because this diagnosis represents an ascending infection that has already affected the uterus and fallopian tubes, even prompt treatment may not prevent these future problems. Prevention of STI transmission greatly reduces the incidence of PID and is thus the best preventive for its sequelae.

Hepatitis and HIV as Sexually Transmitted Diseases

HIV and several forms of hepatitis are transmitted sexually. For convenience, hepatitis A, which is transmitted through the oral–fecal route, has been grouped in this section with other forms of liver infections that are transmitted through blood and body fluids. The severity and chronic nature of these and many other conditions means that midwives, nurse practitioners, or physician assistants are unlikely to be the sole care provider over time. Many women have both a specialist for their chronic disease and a primary provider for their general health needs. Any clinician providing care for women needs to be familiar with the diagnosis, natural course, and general principles of management for hepatitis and HIV in order to facilitate appropriate coordination of care.

Hepatitis

The term *hepatitis* refers to viral infections of the liver and to other inflammatory conditions. Hepatitis can result from generalized infection by viruses, including cytomegalovirus, Epstein-Barr virus, HSV, and measles virus. Nonviral causes of liver infection include bacterial sepsis and syphilis. Hepatitis can also be chemically induced by chronic alcohol ingestion or by medications, such as aspirin (acetylsalicylic acid), acetaminophen (Tylenol), phenytoin (Dilantin), isoniazid (INH), and rifampin, or occur as an autoimmune response. Viral hepatitis is actually a group of pathogenic viruses, identified by the letters A through G. Hepatitis A and E are spread by the fecal–oral route; B, C, and D are spread by contact with blood and body fluids and can be contracted sexually.

The discussion here is limited to the three most common viral hepatic infections: hepatitis A, B, and C. Taken together, these three strains are responsible for 95% of new viral hepatitis diagnoses in the United States.[128] Fewer cases of hepatitis C are reported each year, but it becomes chronic about 75–85% of the time, in contrast to hepatitis B, which develops as a chronic state in 2–6% of adult cases.[128] While all healthcare providers should know the basics of hepatitis diagnosis and

treatment, the responsibility for managing these diseases lies outside the scope of midwifery and most other women's healthcare providers. Hepatitis D occurs as a coinfection with hepatitis B or as a secondary infection, and requires the presence of hepatitis B for transmission. It is uncommon in the general population of North America, although it may occur in intravenous drug users (IVDUs) and persons with frequent exposure to blood products (e.g., hemophiliacs) as well as their sexual contacts.[129] Immigrants from areas with higher prevalence—the Mediterranean basin, eastern Europe, or Central America—are more likely to present with hepatitis.[130]

Hepatitis E is an enterically transmitted virus, often associated with contaminated water sources. It is most common in Asia, the Middle East, South America, and Latin America and has been diagnosed in the United States primarily in individuals traveling from developing countries.[131] Data from the third National Health and Nutrition Examination Survey showed antibodies in more than 20% of those tested,[132] suggesting that there is a greater incidence of food-based transmission in the United States than is recognized. Hepatitis E is frequently associated with only mild symptoms and does not result in a carrier state.

HEPATITIS A

Hepatitis A virus (HAV) is a ribonucleic acid (RNA) virus transmitted via the fecal–oral route, and most cases are part of community-wide outbreaks. In 2014, there were an estimated 2500 infections in the United States.[133] Contaminated water and food (especially shellfish) are common sources of infection. Most cases are the result of close personal contact with an infected person, although bloodborne transmission has been documented in infants and adults.[134] One study found that the single most common risk factor was international travel, followed by case contact, daycare center exposure, food- or waterborne community outbreak, and MSM.[135]

Clinical Illness   HAV has an incubation period of 28 days (range of 15–50 days) with virus shed through the feces approximately 2 weeks prior to clinical symptoms. HAV has a short acute phase of 10 to 15 days, with symptoms resolving within 2 months, although 10–15% of symptomatic persons have persistent or recurrent disease lasting up to 6 months.[133] Viremia persists for at least 1 week following onset of symptoms, and may persist for several months if an individual relapses.[136] There is no chronic state. The symptoms of acute viral hepatitis, shown in **Table 21-19**, are similar for other viral hepatitis forms as well.

Diagnosis   Serologic testing with a positive immunoglobulin M (IgM) antibody is required to confirm acute HAV infection. IgM anti-HAV usually becomes detectable 5 to 10 days before the onset of symptoms and can persist for up to 6 months after infection. Immunoglobulin G (IgG) anti-HAV appears early in the course of the

---

Table 21-19 Clinical Signs and Symptoms Associated with Viral Hepatitis

Initial	As Liver Involvement Increases
Low-grade fever	Jaundice
Weakness/fatigue	Upper right quadrant abdominal pain
Muscle aches	Dark urine
Joint pain	Clay-colored bowel movements
Nausea/vomiting	
Loss of appetite	
Urticaria	

---

disease and indicates lifelong protection against the disease.[137]

Prevention and Treatment   Since 1995, two licensed inactivated HAV vaccines have been available in the United States. In 1996 ACIP recommended HAV vaccination for specific groups at high risk for exposure such as international travelers and individuals working in countries where HAV is endemic. ACIP now recommends routine vaccination of children and vaccination of individuals at increased risk of disease.[137] When given within 2 weeks of exposure, immune globulins provide passive immunity and decrease the risk of HAV transmission by 85%.[138]

There is no medication available for HAV. Because HAV is an acute and not a chronic disease, care includes symptomatic treatment and monitoring for worsening liver disease. The course is worse in those who become infected in the developing world, those with underlying liver damage, and in older adults. The elderly have an increased risk of hospitalization during the acute infection, severe complications (e.g., pancreatitis, ascites, and cholecystitis), and death.[139,140]

Pregnancy does not affect the course of HAV, nor does HAV affect the fetus. Vertical transmission has not been documented. Breastfeeding is not contraindicated.[141,142]

Patient instructions include avoidance of exposure and the importance of vaccination for high-risk persons. Unfortunately, neither good general hygiene nor condom use will prevent transmission during sexual activity.

HEPATITIS B

Hepatitis B virus (HBV) has a reported incidence of about 1.0/100,000, for an incidence in 2014 of 2953 cases reported to CDC; the overall incidence is believed to be much higher—approximately 19,200 cases.[143] Transmission occurs through exposure to blood, blood by-products, contaminated needles, saliva, vaginal secretions, and semen. Those at highest risk include persons with exposure to blood, semen, saliva, or vaginal secretions from an infected person (e.g., unprotected sex, multiple sexual partners, IVDUs, MSM, women who are intimate with MSM, infants born to infected mothers, hemodialysis patients, and residents in an endemic area [including immigrants from those areas]). Currently, prevalence among adults is highest among 30–39 year olds, reflecting the increasing effect of childhood immunization.[144] Prevalence in immigrant groups from areas of endemic disease may run as high as 10–15%, and is almost certainly underidentified in estimates of overall disease burden.[145] Almost 80% of newly diagnosed individuals report high-risk sexual behaviors or drug use.[137]

Infection with HBV may result in a chronic or carrier state with an increased risk for chronic active hepatitis, chronic liver disease, cirrhosis of the liver, and hepatocellular carcinoma. Chronic hepatitis B presently affects between 700,000 and 1.4 million persons in the United States.[146,147] Risk factors for progression to chronic infection include perinatal transmission, older age at infection, coinfection with HCV or hepatitis D, HIV, alcohol consumption, and high HBV viral load.[148]

Clinical Illness Hepatitis B has an incubation period of 90 days (range 60–150 days). About half of those with acute HBV will be asymptomatic.[137] The clinical symptoms and jaundice generally disappear in 1 to 3 months. Most individuals with chronic disease remain asymptomatic, unless they develop progressive liver damage.

Diagnosis Hepatitis B surface antigen (HbsAg) and hepatitis B e-antigen (HbeAg) usually appear in the infected person's blood from 1 to 10 weeks after an acute exposure to HBV, before the onset of clinical symptoms or elevation of the liver enzyme serum alanine aminotransferase (ALT). Persistence of HbsAg for more than 6 months implies progression to chronic HBV infection. HbeAg is a marker for viral replication and infectivity. Hepatitis B core antibody (IgM class) appears during the midphase of the clinical course, with hepatitis B core antibody (IgG class) becoming predominant late in normal recovery. IgM core antibody may remain detectable for 2 years following acute infection; IgG will persist and will also be present in chronic infection. Reports of seroconversion from acute to chronic hepatitis B vary from 5–10%. HbsAg will usually disappear by 4 to 6 months and be followed by the presence of hepatitis B surface antibody (anti-HBs), which will confer lifelong immunity. Hepatitis B core antibody and anti-HBs may persist in noncarriers for many years.[148] **Table 21-20** illustrates the interpretation of these values.

Prevention and Treatment In 2005, the ACIP proposed a comprehensive strategy to eliminate HBV disease, recognizing that prior to the availability of vaccines, perinatal and childhood acquisition of the infection led to much higher rates of chronic disease than adult infection.[149] In 1991, childhood vaccination had become the standard recommendation. Current recommendations include prevention of perinatal transmission by prenatal screening and immunoprophylaxis for all newborns of mothers whose status is positive or unknown, infant vaccination, childhood/adolescent vaccination of those not vaccinated as infants, and adult vaccination of those at risk.[149] Adult vaccination is recommended for those at high risk, such as STI/HIV testing and treatment facilities, drug-abuse treatment and prevention settings, healthcare settings targeting services at IVDUs, healthcare settings targeting services at MSM, and correctional facilities.[150]

Table 21-20 Interpretation of Hepatitis B Serologic Test Results

Test	Results	Interpretation
HBsAg	Negative	Susceptible
Anti-HBc	Negative	
Anti-HBs	Negative	
HBsAg	Negative	Immune due to
Anti-HBc	Positive	natural infection
Anti-HBs	Positive	
HBsAg	Negative	Immune due to
Anti-HBc	Negative	hepatitis B
Anti-HBs	Positive	vaccination
HBsAg	Positive	Acutely infected
Anti-HBc	Positive	
IgM anti-HBc	Positive	
Anti-HBs	Negative	
HBsAg	Positive	Chronically infected
Anti-HBc	Positive	
IgM anti-HBc	Negative	
Anti-HBs	Negative	
HBsAg	Negative	Interpretation
Anti-HBc	Positive	unclear;
Anti-HBs	Negative	4 possibilities:
		1. Resolved infection (most common)
		2. False-positive anti-HBc, thus susceptible
		3. "Low-level" chronic infection
		4. Resolving acute infection

anti-HBc = hepatitis B core antibody, anti-HBs = hepatitis B surface antibody, HBsAg = hepatitis B surface antigen, IgG = immunoglobulin G, IgM = immunoglobulin M

Reproduced from Centers for Disease Control and Prevention. Interpretation of Hepatitis B serologic test results. http://www.cdc.gov/hepatitis/hbv/profresourcesb.htm. 2015. Accessed May 24, 2016.

Hepatitis B immune globulin (HBIG) is recommended for post-exposure prophylaxis in unvaccinated individuals.

During the acute phase of the disease, palliative care is often all that is required. Fulminant liver disease is rare. Most chronic HBV carriers are asymptomatic or have only vague complaints. Chronic HBV can be treated with nucleoside analogues or interferon-α to reduce the risk of disease progression to cirrhosis, liver failure, or carcinoma. Because these medications are suppressive, not curative, they are used when risk of disease progression is high and the individual's ability to adhere to medication is clear.[151] The World Health Organization has recently released guidelines for the medical management of chronic hepatitis B, which requires an experienced infectious diseases team.[152]

Pregnancy-Related Concerns The course of pregnancy is unchanged by HBV, unless liver damage already exists. The vaccine is safe for administration during pregnancy.[149] The primary concern during pregnancy is transmission to the newborn, because 40% of exposed infants will develop chronic disease.[143] This risk can be reduced by 85–95% with the administration of immune globulins immediately after the birth and initiation of a vaccination series. HBV-infected mothers can safely breastfeed.[149]

Hepatitis C

HCV is rarely identified at the time of exposure, because only 20–30% of individuals manifest acute symptoms.[153] In 2014, 2,194 new cases were reported; after adjusting for underreporting and asymptomatic infection, the CDC estimates approximately 30,500 cases actually occurred. Of the 2.7 million Americans with chronic HCV, the majority were probably exposed during the 1970s and 1980s when rates were highest.[153,154] Risk factors include IV drug use, sexual contact with a person having HCV, and healthcare workers who are exposed to blood. Hemodialysis patients and those living with HIV are also at risk.[153,155] Sexual transmission is lower among monogamous sero-discordant couples than among those with multiple partners or other risk factors.[156] There is an association of tattooing and HCV transmission, although the degree of causality is unclear at this time.[157] Needlestick risk to a healthcare worker is 1.8%.[153]

Clinical Illness The period of incubation for HCV ranges from 2 weeks to 6 months. Chronic disease occurs in 70–85% of those infected, develops slowly, and is more likely to progress in men and those infected after the age of 40. Excessive alcohol use, smoking (either tobacco or marijuana), insulin resistance, hepatic steatosis, coinfection with hepatitis B or HIV, and obesity are modifiable factors that affect disease progression.[158] Other diseases may occur more commonly in those with HCV of which diabetes mellitus, occurring three times more frequently, is the most common.[153] According to the CDC, the risk of cirrhosis is 5–20%, and the risk of hepatocellular carcinoma is 1–5%.[153]

Diagnosis Screening is usually targeted to groups at risk (**Table 21-21**). Diagnosis is made by enzyme immunoassay (EIA) or enhanced chemiluminescence immunoassay (CIA) and verified with qualitative/quantitative HCV-RNA PCR. If this confirms the antibody to HCV, then because of the high incidence of chronic disease, serum ALT and quantification of HCV-RNA (viral load) should be performed. Anti-HCV will be positive within 4–10 weeks after exposure in most cases. Chronic disease is defined by persistent HCV-RNA presence for 6 months after diagnosis.[153] Liver function tests will fluctuate and may remain normal for up to a year post-diagnosis.

Prevention and Treatment At this time, there is no vaccine for HCV. Prevention counseling, including use of barriers with sexual activity and avoiding sharing IV drug paraphernalia, is key.

Table 21-21 Testing for Hepatitis C

Indications for HCV testing:

- Adults born during 1945 through 1965—one time
- Current or historic IVDU, even if rare or in distant past
- History of long-term hemodialysis
- Receipt of clotting factor concentrates produced before 1987
- Persistent elevation of alanine aminotransferase (ALT) levels
- HIV
- Recipient of organ transplant
- Blood transfusion prior to 1992 or from an HCV-positive donor
- Exposure to needlesticks or sharps, or mucosal exposures to HCV-positive blood
- Children born to HCV-positive women

Potential indications:

- Receipt of transplanted tissue (e.g., corneal, musculoskeletal, skin, ova, sperm)
- Use of intranasal cocaine and other non-injecting illegal drug
- History of tattooing or body piercing
- History of multiple sex partners or sexually transmitted diseases
- Long-term steady sex partners of HCV-positive persons

HCV = hepatitis C virus, IVDU = intravenous drug users

Modified from Centers for Disease Control and Prevention. Testing recommendations for Hepatitis C Virus Infection. http://www.cdc.gov/hepatitis/hcv/guidelinesc .htm. 2015. Accessed July 14, 2016.

When HCV is identified in the acute stage, the same therapies can be used as during chronic disease. For this reason, any individual testing positive should be referred to an expert in hepatitis for management. Regimens that include nucleoside analogues, pegylated interferon, ribavirin, and protease inhibitors have demonstrated sustained virologic response. Effectiveness depends on the HCV genotype, stage of disease, and adherence.

As with other infections managed with chronic medication, the individual's willingness to adhere to treatment is essential. The recent expansion of therapeutic options has led to increased costs for the healthcare system, but also to the potential for curative treatment.

Pregnancy   During pregnancy, new-onset infection in the last trimester, with the accompanying high viral loads of acute disease, may carry a risk of mother-to-child transmission as high as 33%, although 6% transmission is cited as a background rate in antibody-positive women.[153,159] Infants are not tested for antibodies until 18 months of age, in order for maternal antibodies to have cleared; PCR testing can be performed at 1–2 months and repeated serially if positive. Infected mothers can safely breastfeed.

Patient Counseling for Viral Hepatitis   Patient education for both HBV and HCV deals with transmission risks to sexual partners, prevention of coinfections, signs of disease progression, and long-term sequelae. The importance of lifetime care when chronic disease is present should be emphasized, and promoting access to specialist care should be prioritized.

Human Immunodeficiency Virus/ Acquired Immune Deficiency Syndrome (HIV/AIDS)

In the United States, HIV is a disease that has disproportionately affected women who are poor, urban, and of color. These are all markers for social conditions that leave individuals at greater risk within our society. Data from the CDC show that more than 80% of women living with HIV in the United States were exposed through heterosexual behavior. Of the approximately 48,000 diagnoses of HIV in the United States in 2014, 20% were among women. Black women were about 19 times more likely to be affected than white women, and more than five times more at risk than Hispanics.[160] Other risk factors for HIV infection include young age, IV drug abuse, and sexual activity including having multiple partners or partners who are MSM. Infections with STIs and BV and loss of lactobacilli have been demonstrated to be associated with increased risk of HIV acquisition and viral shedding.[161-163] Among the societal factors that increase risk of transmission are lack of understanding regarding risks and sexual inequity. In addition, the CDC recommends offering testing universally in any setting where the prevalence of HIV exceeds 1%.[164]

Of those women living with HIV, fewer than half are in care, and even fewer are virally suppressed.[165] When a women's health provider is participating in the care of HIV-positive women, whether during pregnancy or for family planning and well-woman care, it is essential that the woman also has access to a primary care provider experienced in HIV management on whom the clinician can call for therapeutic concerns.

Natural History

HIV is an RNA retrovirus that preferentially attacks T helper lymphocytes (CD4 cells) and other cell types. The natural history of HIV begins as an initial viral syndrome within the first month after exposure, including fever, muscle aches, sore throat, lymphadenopathy, and other nonspecific symptoms. During this time, the virus is rapidly reproducing, causing a drop in the CD4 count and a high viral load.[166] Except in cases where the risk of transmission is appreciated, these early symptoms are generally interpreted as a simple viral infection and treated symptomatically. As the body mounts an immune response, the viral load subsides and the CD4 cell number increases.

For a period of time that may exceed 10 years, the disease remains hidden. Although the virus

Figure 21-12 Natural history of HIV infection.

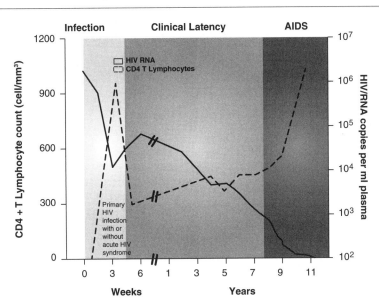

continues to replicate and destroy CD4 cells, these are rapidly replaced until the immune system is too worn down to maintain its protective effect. Over time, as the immune system begins to decline, viral replication again becomes dominant and the CD4 count decreases. A normal CD4 count is above 500 cells/mm[3]. In the later stages of the disease, falling CD4 levels reach a point at which the body can no longer defend itself from common ailments or from diseases that do not commonly attack humans (opportunistic infections). A diagnosis of Stage 3 HIV disease (AIDS) is made based on the occurrence of conditions unlikely to occur in healthy adults or by a CD4 cell count less than 200.[167] In the 21st century, it is far more common for the CD4 count to be the only indicator for this diagnosis.

Figure 21-12 depicts the natural history of HIV infection in the human body.[168] Many factors play a role in determining the length of time spent in an asymptomatic state. Age, sex, race, and strain of HIV all play a role; in general, women with equivalent viral loads progress more rapidly toward AIDS than men.[169] Primary care for women living with HIV includes regular assessment of disease progression, referral for early treatment, monitoring for adverse events related to medication use, and observation for complications. Among the most common HIV complications in women are persistent, difficult-to-treat yeast infections; rapid progress of HPV infections and associated Pap smear abnormalities; and pneumonia.[163] Many women are still asymptomatic when their CD4 count has dropped low enough to become an AIDS-defining condition.

Heterosexual Transmission

Transmission of HIV occurs sexually, through exposure to blood or other body fluids, and perinatally. For women, sexual transmission is the dominant mode. On diagnosis, many women report no known risk, which is to say that they are not involved in drug use, nor are they involved in sex work, nor do they recall any cutaneous exposure. Younger age is associated with increased sexual risk, as are multiple partners, partners with known risk factors, history of STIs, and failure to use a protective barrier during intercourse. It has been estimated that the approximately 25% of HIV-positive individuals who do not know their diagnosis are 3.5 times more likely to transit HIV to an infected partner.[170]

Rates of transmission between heterosexual partners are affected by level of infectivity in the affected partner, use of a protective latex barrier such as a condom, and concurrent infections with other STIs.[171,172] STIs all share a common risk—exposure to more than one sexual partner, either individually or through one's own partner—and all STIs can be cofactors for HIV transmission, particularly those that produce vaginal or cervical lesions.

Irrespective of cofactors, a transmission risk of 5.64 per 100 person-years (95% confidence interval [CI] 3.28–9.70) was reported in one meta-analysis of studies. The risk was directly related to overall viral load, and couples in which the infected partner had a viral load less than 400 had a transmission risk of 0.16 (95% CI 0.02–1.13) per 100 person/years.[173] The recent advent of pre-exposure prophylaxis (PrEP) for use in serodiscordant couples should offer further reductions. PrEP is intended for use in high-transmission-risk settings, such as in a couple who desire to conceive. Women offered PrEP should be tested for HIV and pregnancy prior to beginning therapy and every 3 months thereafter, tested for hepatitis B status and have normal renal function, and counseled about condom use and the risks of drug resistance if they become HIV positive during therapy. The current PrEP recommendation is for tenofovir disoproxil fumarate/emtricitabine (Truvada) daily as a single dose.[174]

HIV Testing Recommendations

The CDC strongly recommends universal screening for all adults ages 13–65 based on an opt-out methodology (**Figure 21-13**). In other words, testing should be regularly offered and performed as part of the general consent for care rather than requiring written evidence of agreement or specific pretest counseling. Women with specific risk factors such as a diagnosis of STIs, substance abuse, or multiple sexual partners should be tested at least yearly.[164] Clinicians should not make value judgments about individual risk. Unless a heterosexual transmission rate of less than 0.1% can be documented for a jurisdiction, routine screening is an important public health activity.[164]

The CDC recommends use of an HIV-1 antigen/antibody combined immunoassay. This format permits more accurate diagnosis of acute infection, fewer indeterminate and false-positive results, and faster turnaround. Follow-up testing with DC4 cell count, viral load, and resistance testing confirm the diagnosis and permit treatment. Rapid HIV testing offers an opportunity to extend testing to settings where immediate post-test counseling is beneficial, and to times when intervention can be facilitated—such as on labor and delivery units; these offer a preliminary result that must be confirmed with the combination immunoassay.[164]

After the test is complete, women who test negative should have counseling that reinforces risk reduction. When a woman tests positive, she presents greater challenges in post-test counseling. For many women, the emotional impact of being told that an HIV test is positive

Figure 21-13 Testing algorithm for HIV.

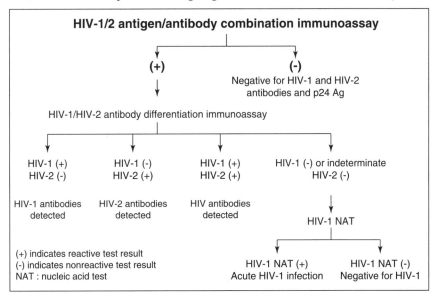

Recommended Laboratory HIV Testing Algorithm for Serum or Plasma Specimens

1. Laboratories should conduct initial testing for HIV with an FDA-approved antigen/antibody combination immunoassay* that detects HIV-1 and HIV-2 antibodies and HIV-1 p24 antigen to screen for established infection with HIV-1 or HIV-2 and for acute HIV-1 infection. No further testing is required for specimens that are nonreactive on the initial immunoassay.

2. Specimens with a reactive antigen/antibody combination immunoassay result (or repeatedly reactive, if repeat testing is recommended by the manufacturer or required by regulatory authorities) should be tested with an FDA-approved antibody immunoassay that differentiates HIV-1 antibodies from HIV-2 antibodies. Reactive results on the initial antigen/antibody combination immunoassay and the HIV-1/HIV-2 antibody differentiation immunoassay should be interpreted as positive for HIV-1 antibodies, HIV-2 antibodies, or HIV antibodies, undifferentiated.

3. Specimens that are reactive on the initial antigen/antibody combination immunoassay and nonreactive or indeterminate on the HIV-1/HIV-2 antibody differentiation immunoassay should be tested with an FDA-approved HIV-1 nucleic acid test (NAT).

   • A reactive HIV-1 NAT result and nonreactive HIV-1/HIV-2 antibody differentiation immunoassay result indicates laboratory evidence for acute HIV-1 infection.

   • A reactive HIV-1 NAT result and indeterminate HIV-1/HIV-2 antibody differentiation immunoassay result indicates the presence of HIV-1 infection confirmed by HIV-1 NAT.

   • A negative HIV-1 NAT result and nonreactive or indeterminate HIV-1/HIV-2 antibody differentiation immunoassay result indicates a false-positive result on the initial immunoassay.

4. Laboratories should use this same testing algorithm, beginning with an antigen/antibody combination immunoassay, with serum or plasma specimens submitted for testing after a reactive (preliminary positive) result from any rapid HIV test.

Exception: As of April 2014, data are insufficient to recommend use of the FDA-approved single-use rapid HIV-1/HIV-2 antigen/antibody combination immunoassay as the initial assay in the algorithm.

Reproduced from Centers for Disease Control and Prevention. Quick reference guide—Laboratory testing for the diagnosis of HIV infection: updated recommendations. http://stacks.cdc.gov/view/cdc/23446. June 27, 2014. Accessed July 14, 2016.

overshadows any other information they are given. A second encounter may be necessary to present basic information and make referrals for care. Among the topics to discuss are interpretation of test results, monitoring health and disease progression, what treatment is available, where to find competent care, disclosure, partner notification, discrimination, and behavior changes to protect her health and prevent transmission. Observation for emotional distress or depression is essential.

DISCLOSURE

Issues of disclosure are frequently difficult for newly diagnosed women. Indeed, some women will go for months or years without revealing their status to anyone. O'Brien and colleagues found that advancing disease was an incentive for disclosure and that young age was linked with nondisclosure. In this study, immediate family members and primary sexual partners were most likely to be told, but less than one-quarter of the patients told casual sexual partners.[175] Risky sex without disclosure has also been found to be the case for nonexclusive partners, with nondisclosure rates of 13% in serodiscordant couples.[176] Many women decrease sexual activity or increase their use of barriers after diagnosis, whether or not they have disclosed their status. Fear of violence or disruption of a stable relationship may influence some women's decisions not to share their diagnosis. Clinicians need to be aware of resources for supportive counseling and partner notification programs that women can use to inform partners of HIV exposure.

MONITORING HIV PROGRESSION

The CD4 cells are one group of the T lymphocytes. Over the course of HIV disease, CD4 counts are used to measure the degree of immune suppression, or how effectively the body is protecting itself from the virus. Values in healthy nonpregnant adults are generally above 500 cells/mm^3. The results of this test are usually reported both as an absolute value and as a percentage of lymphocytes. The lower level of normal is about 32%. Factors other than HIV infection can cause drops in this value, including pregnancy, drug abuse, steroid use, and other illnesses; diurnal variation is also a factor. For this reason, the CD4 count is not a test used in diagnosing HIV. When the CD4 count falls below an absolute level of 200 cells/mm^3, a diagnosis of AIDS is made based on decreased immune competence.

Several genetically based tests to measure the amount of virus present in the blood are available. All of them have a lower limit, below which virus is present but not in measurable amounts and an upper limit, although greater quantities of virus may well be present. The one most frequently reported is the HIV-RNA PCR. One commonly used version of this test measures values down to 20 copies/milliliter. The same version of the test should be used consistently, because each reports slightly different values. From the standpoint of clinical care, it is essential to understand that these tests measure the level of virus only in the bloodstream. Other tissue reservoirs may persistently maintain a latent source of virus. In addition, the amount of virus in cervical secretions may vary from that in the blood.[177]

Over time, HIV mutates in the body and can become resistant to various medications, or even classes of medication. An individual may be newly infected with virus that is already resistant to medications. Phenotype and genotype assays can be performed to determine whether a rising viral load is due to resistance or to some other factor, such as not taking medication that has been prescribed. These tests should be ordered only by the person who is responsible for the long-term management of the woman's care, because the effectiveness of future medication regimens depends on careful selection among available choices.

TREATMENT OPTIONS

Treatment has become more complex as more classes of antiretroviral drugs have become available. Currently, 7 categories of medications are available, with at least 25 individual drugs currently available and nearly as many in development. The CDC publishes and regularly updates guidelines for the management of HIV disease. These guidelines discuss such issues as when to begin therapy, appropriate drug combinations for initial and continuing therapy, adherence to therapy, and evaluation of drug resistance. Current recommendations for treatment of HIV-positive individuals include beginning treatment while the immune system is intact—with a CD4 of 500 or higher.[178] Initiating therapy at higher CD4 levels serves to decrease inflammatory damage and direct viral injury to end organs, preserving general health.

With early diagnosis and treatment, life expectancies exceeding 40 years after diagnosis are not unreasonable; women tend to survive longer than men.[179] Early initiation of therapy requires commitment to adherence, and women should be counseled about the risks of nonadherence in terms of long-term survival and morbidity.

GYNECOLOGIC CARE

Women with HIV need regular gynecologic care and active management of any abnormalities found during care. On diagnosis, all women should have 6-month interval visits for 1 year. Young women with an HIV diagnosis should be offered the HPV vaccine. While women remain immunocompetent, with CD4 counts greater than 500, annual visits are acceptable for women with normal Pap test results. HIV is associated with persistent and rapid progression of Pap abnormalities, although effective management limits development of cervical cancer.[180,181] There is also an increase in vaginal, vulvar, and perianal lesions; these areas also require careful evaluation during the pelvic examination.[182]

Counseling for STI prevention and family planning is similar to that provided to any other patient. Emphasis is placed on disclosure of the HIV diagnosis to sexual partners and the importance of correct use of contraceptive measures. The increasing complexity of antiretroviral therapy (ART) has effects on contraceptive choices. The effectiveness of combined hormonal contraception is decreased by some protease inhibitors and non-nucleoside reverse transcriptase inhibitors that share a metabolic pathway in the liver.[183,184] Failure of the contraceptive implant has also been documented.[185] IUDs are safe and effective,[186-188] as is depot medroxyprogesterone acetate.[189-190] The CDC clearly states that all contraceptives are acceptable for use in HIV-infected women; the key is to be aware of the need to reinforce condom use at all times, when a method has an increased risk of failure. No woman should be denied her preferred contraceptive solely on the basis of HIV status.[191] Reinforcing the importance of condom use is essential to effective counseling in the younger population, who may feel that safer sex is no longer an issue with improved viral control.

According to the CDC Sexually Transmitted Diseases Treatment Guidelines, treatment regimens are essentially the same for all STIs in HIV-positive women.[20] The treatment of any STI and PID requires attention to duration of therapy and the possibility of inadequate treatment effect. Test of cure or follow-up visits should not be omitted in this population.

PREGNANCY-RELATED CONCERNS

During pregnancy, all HIV-positive women need to be on combination ART, in order to prevent mother-to-child transmission. For this reason, the CDC recommendation is for first trimester screening of every woman and repeat third trimester screening for women in high-incidence areas or who have personal risk factors. A woman who appears for childbirth without documentation of testing should be evaluated at that time with a rapid test. In the absence of diagnosis or treatment, the risk of maternal-to-child transmission is approximately 25%. Effective ART beginning before pregnancy or immediately following organogenesis is associated with a risk of 1% or less.[191]

HIV and Older Women

About 10% of AIDS cases are found in adults over 50, many of whom know little about HIV risks and transmission. In addition, this is not a population group that regularly considers condom use for prevention of infection,[192] nor do women in this age group need protection against unplanned pregnancy. However, the physiologic thinning of vaginal mucosa and decreased lubrication following menopause actually increase risk of HIV transmission. One study found that older women are only half as likely as men to be tested for HIV,[193] although more than half of women over 60 are sexually active.[194] Another study of older adults found that active sexual lives and multiple partners were not uncommon; less than 40% of those sexually active were using condoms. A majority of men, and 80% of women, did not see themselves at risk in this study.[195] Counseling messages about safer sex cannot be limited to the young.

Safer Sex and Prevention of STI Transmission

There is good evidence that consistent use of male condoms or another adequate barrier, such as the female condom, can reduce the transmission of STIs. Condoms are not a perfect barrier. Breakage and slippage are both possible. Oil-based lubricants or medications (e.g., clindamycin cream) can degrade latex and cause it to tear.

For those infections that are easily transmitted, such as chlamydia or gonorrhea, consistent use with every sexual act is essential for effective prevention. For some infections, such as genital herpes, the inability of condoms to cover all potentially infectious tissue decreases the benefit. It has been demonstrated that even intermittent use should lower the risk of transmission for HIV.[196] Although both male and female condoms are recommended as barriers to exposure to semen, and thus infection, the male condom is a more effective barrier. According to Galvao and colleagues, patient education decreased the number of problems reported with use.[197]

For midwives and other women's health practitioners, teaching about safer sex is not the only route to prevention of genital infections. Primary prevention begins with education about delaying the onset of sexual activity, limiting numbers of partners, and maintaining a monogamous relationship. Decreasing barriers to care—cost, accessibility, stigma—makes asking for information and obtaining treatment easier. The Institute of Medicine published *The Hidden Epidemic: Confronting Sexually Transmitted Diseases* in 1997.[198] Two decades later, the disease burden is still high, and millions of women are affected. Openly addressing these issues is an essential part of providing care to women.

After all is said and done, the other barrier to reduction of the STI burden in society may be the unwillingness of providers to adhere to CDC guidelines and standard diagnostic procedures. A number of studies have documented inadequate data collection for accurate diagnoses, failure to comply with CDC recommendations for screening and treatment, and failure to provide follow-up care such as management of partners.[199-201] Landers and colleagues evaluated the predictive value of clinical diagnosis of lower genital tract disease and found that diagnosis by symptoms led to a significant number of misdiagnoses and underdiagnosis.[199] Clinical testing improved the predictive value but still did not identify all cases correctly. Trichomoniasis and BV were more accurately diagnosed in the office than yeast. Accuracy in diagnosing gonorrhea and chlamydia required laboratory testing.[199] An evaluation of emergency department care found that fewer than 10% of cases reviewed complied with all aspects of the CDC recommendations for diagnosis and management of urethritis, cervicitis, and PID.[200] Nor is switching away from public health settings the route to improved quality of care. A quality review of the transitional period from health department to private office care in one county in Washington state found that significant variations in treatment for PID existed, Gram stains were not available, and medical records were incomplete.[201]

The message for women's health practitioners is clear. Symptomatic diagnosis is an inadequate technique. Where clinical testing can be provided in the office, it must be. When the result is unclear, or a laboratory test is demonstrated to be superior, then the best techniques available should be used. Before a diagnosis of refractory or recurrent disease is made, laboratory confirmation is required. The health and quality of life for women will be improved by staying with this level of evidence in making diagnoses, and knowing and following sound recommendations for care.

Online Resources

1. CDC, "2015 Sexually Transmitted Diseases Treatment Guidelines": http://www.cdc.gov/std/tg2015/default.htm
2. CDC, *A Guide to Taking a Sexual History*: http://www.cdc.gov/std/treatment/sexualhistory.pdf
3. American Sexual Health Association: http://www.ashasexualhealth.org
4. CDC "HIV/AIDS: Guidelines and Recommendations": http://www.cdc.gov/hiv/guidelines/index.html

References

1. Petrova M, Lievens E, Malik S, Imholz N, Lebeer S. *Lactobacillus* species as biomarkers and agents that can promote various aspects of vaginal health. *Front Physiol.* 2015;6:81.
2. Ravel J, Gajer P, Abdo Z, Schneider GM, Koenig SS, McCulle SL, et al. Vaginal microbiome of reproductive-age women. *Proc Natl Acad Sci U S A.* 2011;108(Suppl 1):4680-4687.
3. Ma B, Forney LJ, Ravel J. The vaginal microbiome: rethinking health and diseases. *Annu Rev Microbiol.* 2012;66:371-389.
4. Forney LJ, Foster JA, Ledger W. The vaginal flora of healthy women is not always dominated by *Lactobacillus* species. *J Infect Dis.* 2006;194(10):1468-1469.
5. Foxman B, Wen A, Srinivasan U, Goldberg D, Marrs CF, Owen J, et al. *Mycoplasma*, bacterial vaginosis-associated bacteria BVAB3, race, and risk of preterm birth in a high-risk cohort. *Am J Obstet Gynecol.* 2014;210(3):226.e1-7.
6. Brotman RM, Klebanoff MA, Nansel TR, Yu KF, Andrews WW, Zhang J, et al. Bacterial vaginosis assessed by Gram stain and diminished colonization resistance to incident gonococcal, chlamydial, and trichomonal genital infection. *J Infect Dis.* 2010;202:1907-1915.
7. Nelson DB, Hanlon A, Nachamkin I, Haggerty C, Mastrogiannis DS, Liu C, et al. Early pregnancy changes in bacterial vaginosis-associated bacteria and preterm delivery. *Paediatr Perinat Epidemiol.* 2014;28(2):88-96.
8. Zhou X, Bent SJ, Schneider MG, Davis CC, Islam MR, Forney LJ. Characterization of vaginal microbial communities in adult healthy women using cultivation independent methods. *Microbiology.* 2004;150:2566-2573.
9. Larsen B, Monif GRG. Understanding the bacterial flora of the female genital tract. *Clin Infect Dis.* 2001;32:e69-e77.
10. Caillouette JC, Sharp CF, Zimmerman GJ, Roy S. Vaginal pH as a marker for bacterial pathogens and menopausal status. *Am J Obstet Gynecol.* 1997;176:1270-1277.

11. Pabich WL, Fihn SD, Stamm WE, Scholes D, Boyko EJ, Gupta K. Prevalence and determinants of vaginal flora in postmenopausal women. *J Infect Dis.* 2003;188:1054-1058.

12. Chappell CA, Rohan LC, Moncla BJ, Wang L, Meyn LA, Bunge K, et al. The effects of reproductive hormones on the physical properties of cervicovaginal fluid. *Am J Obstet Gynecol.* 2014;211(3):226.e1-e7.

13. Hickey RJ, Zhou X, Settles ML, Erb J, Malone K, Hansmann MA, et al. Vaginal microbiota of adolescent girls prior to the onset of menarche resemble those of reproductive-age women. *MBio.* 2015;6(2):ii, e00097-15.

14. Hillier Sl, Lau RJ. Vaginal microflora in postmenopausal women who have not received estrogen replacement therapy. *Clin Infect Dis.* 1997;25(Suppl 2):S123-S126.

15. Hoffmann JN, You HM, Hedberg EC, Jordan JA, McClintock MK. Prevalence of bacterial vaginosis and *Candida* among postmenopausal women in the United States. *J Gerontol B Psychol Sci Soc Sci.* 2014;69(Suppl 2):S205-S214.

16. Hillier SL, Krohn MA, Klebanoff SJ, Eschenbach DA. The relationship of hydrogen peroxide producing lactobacilli to bacterial vaginosis and genital microflora in pregnant women. *Obstet Gynecol.* 1992;79:369-373.

17. US Preventive Services Task Force. Final Recommendation Statement: Sexually Transmitted Infections: Behavioral Counseling. 2014. Available at: http://www.uspreventiveservicestaskforce.org/Page/Document/UpdateSummaryFinal/sexually-transmitted-infections-behavioral-counseling. Accessed May 24, 2016.

18. Haley N, Maheux B, Rivard M, Gervais A. Sexual health risk assessment and counseling in primary care: how involved are general practitioners and obstetrician-gynecologists. *Am J Public Health.* 1999;89:899-902.

19. Whiteside JL, Katz T, Anthes T, Boardman L, Peipert JF. Risks and adverse outcomes of sexually transmitted diseases: patients' attitudes and beliefs. *J Reprod Med.* 2001;46:34-38.

20. Centers for Disease Control and Prevention. Sexually transmitted diseases treatment guidelines, 2015. *MMWR Recomm Rep.* 2015;64(No. RR-3):1-137. Available at: http://www.cdc.gov/STI/tg2015/clinical.htm. Accessed May 24, 2016.

21. Clark LR, Brasseux C, Richmond D, Getson P, D'Angelo LJ. Are adolescents accurate in self-report of frequencies of sexually transmitted diseases and pregnancies? *J Adolesc Health.* 1997;21:91-96.

22. STD/HIV Risk Assessment: A Quick Reference Guide. Seattle STD/HIV Prevention Training Center. Seattle: University of Washington Center for Health Education and Research.

23. Anderson JR. *A Guide to the Clinical Care of Women with HIV.* Rockville, MD: US Department of Health and Human Services, Health Resources and Services Administration; 2001.

24. Diamant AL, Schuster MA, McGuigan K, Lever J. Lesbians' sexual history with men: implications for taking a sexual history. *Arch Intern Med.* 1999;159:2730-2736.

25. Marrazzo JM, Coffey P, Bingham A. Sexual practices, risk perception and knowledge of sexually transmitted disease risk among lesbian and bisexual women. *Perspect Sex Reprod Health.* 2005;37(1):6-12.

26. Bostwick WB, Hughes TL, Everett B. Health behavior, status, and outcomes among a community-based sample of lesbian and bisexual women. *LGBT Health.* 2015;2(2):121-126.

27. Brown JD, Melchiono MW. Health concerns of sexual minority adolescent girls. *Curr Opin Pediatr.* 2006;18(4):359-364.

28. Oshri A, Handley ED, Sutton TE, Wortel S, Burnette ML. Developmental trajectories of substance use among sexual minority girls: associations with sexual victimization and sexual health risk. *J Adolesc Health.* 2014;55(1):100-106.

29. Gorgos LM, Marrazzo JM. Sexually transmitted infections among women who have sex with women. *Clin Infect Dis.* 2011;53(Suppl 3):S84-S91.

30. Hobbs MC, Seña AC. Modern diagnosis of *Trichomonas vaginalis* infection. *Sex Transm Infect.* 2013;89:434-438.

31. Centers for Disease Control and Prevention. Recommendations for the laboratory-based detection of *Chlamydia trachomatis* and *Neisseria gonorrhoeae*—2014. *MMWR Recomm Rep.* 2014;63(RR02);1-19.

32. Falk L, Coble BI, Mjörnberg PA, Fredlund H. Sampling for *Chlamydia trachomatis* infection—a comparison of vaginal, first-catch urine, combined vaginal and first-catch urine and endocervical sampling. *Int J STD AIDS.* 2010;21:283-287.

33. Centers for Disease Control. CLIA provider performed (PPM) procedures. Atlanta, GA: US Department of Health and Human Services. Available at: https://www.cms.gov/regulations-and-guidance/legislation/clia/downloads/ppmplist.pdf. Accessed June 1, 2016.

34. Giraldo P, Von Nowaskonski A, Gomes FAM, Linhares I, Neves NA, Witkin SS. Vaginal colonization by *Candida* in asymptomatic women with and

without a history of recurrent vulvovaginal candidiasis. *Obstet Gynecol*. 2000;95:413-416.

35. Beigi RH, Meyn LA, Moore DM, Krohn MA, Hillier SL. Vaginal yeast colonization in nonpregnant women: a longitudinal study. *Obstet Gynecol*. 2004;104:926-930.

36. Anderson MR, Klink K, Cohressen A. Evaluation of vaginal complaints. *JAMA*. 2004;291:1368-1379.

37. Spinillo A, Capuzzo E, Gulminetti R, Marone P, Colonna L, Piazzi G. Prevalence of and risk factors for fungal vaginitis caused by non-albicans species. *Am J Obstet Gynecol*. 1997;176:138-141.

38. Sobel JD, Faro S, Force RW, Foxman B, Ledger WJ, Nyirjesy PR, et al. Vulvovaginal candidiasis: epidemiologic, diagnostic, and therapeutic considerations. *Am J Obstet Gynecol*. 1998;178: 203-211.

39. Wiesenfeld HC, Macio I. The infrequent use of office based diagnostic tests for vaginitis. *Am J Obstet Gynecol*. 1999;181:39-41.

40. Ferris DG, Dekle C, Litaker MS. Women's use of over-the-counter antifungal pharmaceutical products for gynecologic symptoms. *J Fam Pract*. 1996;42:595-600.

41. Allen-Davis JT, Beck A, Parker R, Ellis JL, Polley D. Assessment of vulvovaginal complaints: accuracy of telephone triage and in-office diagnosis. *Obstet Gynecol*. 2002;99:18-22.

42. Foxman B. The epidemiology of vulvovaginal candidiasis: risk factors. *Am J Public Health*. 1990;80:329-331.

43. Spinillo A, Capuzzo E, Acciano S, de Santolo A, Zara F. Effect of antibiotic use on the prevalence of symptomatic vulvovaginal candidiasis. *Am J Obstet Gynecol*. 1999;180:14-17.

44. Eckert LO, Hawes SE, Stevens CE, Koutsky LA, Eschenbach DA, Holmes KK. Vulvovaginal candidiasis: clinical manifestations, risk factors, management algorithm. *Obstet Gynecol*. 1998;92:757-765.

45. Watson MC, Grimshaw JM, Bond CM, Mollison J, Ludbrook A. Oral versus intra-vaginal imidazole and triazole anti-fungal agents for the treatment of uncomplicated vulvovaginal candidiasis (thrush): a systematic review. *BJOG Int J Obstet Gynaecol*. 2002;109:85-95.

46. Marchaim D, Lemanek L, Bheemreddy S, Kaye KS, Sobel JD. Fluconazole-resistant *Candida albicans* vulvovaginitis. *Obstet Gynecol*. 2012;120(6): 1407-1414.

47. Sobel JD, Chaim W. Treatment of *Torulopsis glabrata* vaginitis: retrospective review of boric acid therapy. *Clin Infect Dis*. 1997;24:649-652.

48. Falagas ME, Betsi G, Athanasiou S. Probiotics for prevention of recurrent vulvovaginal candidiasis: a review. *J Antimicrob Chemother*. 2006;58(2):266-272.

49. Vicariotto F, Del Piano M, Mogna L, Mogna G. Effectiveness of the association of 2 probiotic strains formulated in a slow release vaginal product, in women affected by vulvovaginal candidiasis: a pilot study. *J Clin Gastroenterol*. 2012;46(Suppl):S73-80.

50. Cherpes TL, Hillier SL, Meyn LA, Busch JL, Krohn MA. A delicate balance: risk factors for acquisition of bacterial vaginosis include sexual activity, absence of hydrogen peroxide-producing lactobacilli, black race, and positive herpes simplex virus type 2 serology. *Sex Transm Dis*. 2008;35(1):78-83.

51. Marrazzo JM, Koutsky LA, Eschenbach DA, Agnew K, Stine K, Hillier SL. Characterization of vaginal flora and bacterial vaginosis in women who have sex with women. *J Infect Dis*. 2002;185(9):1307-1313.

52. Marrazzo JM. Interpreting the epidemiology and natural history of bacterial vaginosis: are we still confused? *Anaerobe*. 2011;17(4):186-190.

53. Koumans EH, Sternberg M, Bruce C, McQuillan G, Kendrick J, Sutton M, et al. The prevalence of bacterial vaginosis in the United States, 2001–2004: associations with symptoms, sexual behaviors, and reproductive health. *Sex Transm Dis*. 2007;34:864-869.

54. Beigi RH, Wiesenfeld HC, Hillier SL, Straw T, Krohn MA. Factors associated with absence of H2O2 producing *Lactobacillus* among women with bacterial vaginosis. *J Infect Dis*. 2005;191:924-929.

55. Mirmonsef P, Krass L, Landay A, Spear GT. The role of bacterial vaginosis and trichomonas in HIV transmission across the female genital tract. *Curr HIV Res*. 2012;10(3):202-210.

56. Wiesenfeld HC, Hillier SL, Krohn MA, Landers DV, Sweet RL. Bacterial vaginosis is a strong predictor of *Neisseria gonorrhea* and *Chlamydia trachomatis* infection. *Clin Infect Dis*. 2003;36:663-668.

57. Borgdorff H, Tsivtsivadze E, Verhelst R, Marzorati M, Jurriaans S, Ndayisaba GF, et al. *Lactobacillus*-dominated cervicovaginal microbiota associated with reduced HIV/STI prevalence and genital HIV viral load in African women. *ISME J*. 2014;8(9): 1781-1793.

58. Nelson DB, Hanlon A, Nachamkin I, Haggerty C, Mastrogiannis DS, Liu C, et al. Early pregnancy changes in bacterial vaginosis-associated bacteria and preterm delivery. *Paediatr Perinat Epidemiol*. 2014;28(2):88-96.

59. Nugent RP, Krohn MA, Hillier SL. Reliability of diagnosing bacterial vaginosis is improved by a

standardized method of Gram stain interpretation. *J Clin Microbiol.* 1991;29:297-301.

60. Schwebke JR, Hillier SL, Dobel JD, McGregor JA, Sweet RL. Validity of the vaginal Gram stain for the diagnosis of bacterial vaginosis. *Obstet Gynecol.* 1996; 88:573-576.

61. Gutman RE, Peipert JF, Weitzen S, Blume J. Evaluation of clinical methods for diagnosing bacterial vaginosis. *Obstet Gynecol.* 2005;105:551-556.

62. Thomason JL, Gelbart SM, Anderson RJ, Walt AK, Osypowski PJ, Broekhuizen FF. Statistical evaluation of diagnostic criteria for bacterial vaginosis. *Am J Obstet Gynecol.* 1990;162:15-60.

63. Geisler WM, Yu S, Venglarik M, Schwebke JR. Vaginal leukocyte counts in women with bacterial vaginosis: relation to vaginal and cervical infections. *Sex Transm Infect.* 2004;80:401-405.

64. Austin MN, Beigi RH, Meyn LA, Hillier SL. Microbiologic response to treatment of bacterial vaginosis with topical clindamycin or metronidazole. *J Clin Microbiol.* 2005;43(9):4492-4497.

65. Reid G, Bocking A. The potential for probiotics to prevent bacterial vaginosis and preterm labor. *Am J Obstet Gynecol.* 2003;189:1202-1208.

66. Ya W, Reifer C, Miller LE. Efficacy of vaginal probiotic capsules for recurrent bacterial vaginosis: a double-blind, randomized, placebo-controlled study. *Am J Obstet Gynecol.* 2010;203(2):120.e1-6.

67. Brocklehurst P, Gordon A, Heatley E, Milan SJ. Antibiotics for treating bacterial vaginosis in pregnancy. *Cochrane Database Syst Rev.* 2013;1: CD000262.

68. Shennan A, Crawshaw S, Briley A, Hawken J, Seed P, Jones G, et al. A randomised controlled trial of metronidazole for the prevention of preterm birth in women positive for cervicovaginal fetal fibronectin: the PREMET study. *BJOG.* 2006;113:65-74.

69. Okun N, Gronau KA, Hannah ME. Antibiotics for bacterial vaginosis or *Trichomonas vaginalis* in pregnancy: a systematic review. *Obstet Gynecol.* 2005;105:857-868.

70. Sutton M, Sternberg M, Koumans EH, McQuillan G, Berman S, Markowitz L. The prevalence of *Trichomonas vaginalis* infection among reproductive-age women in the United States, 2001–2004. *Clin Infect Dis.* 2007;45(10):1319-1326.

71. Krieger JN. Trichomoniasis in men: old issues and new data. *Sex Transm Dis.* 1995;22:83-96.

72. Coleman JS, Gaydos CA, Witter F. *Trichomonas vaginalis* vaginitis in obstetrics and gynecology practice: new concepts and controversies. *Obstet Gynecol Surv.* 2013;68(1):43-50.

73. McClelland RS, Sangare L, Hassan WM, Lavreys L, Mandaliya K, Kiarie J, et al. Infection with *Trichomonas vaginalis* increases the risk of HIV-1 acquisition. *J Infect Dis.* 2007;195:698-702.

74. Silver BJ, Guy RJ, Kaldor JM, Jamil MS, Rumbold AR. *Trichomonas vaginalis* as a cause of perinatal morbidity: a systematic review and meta-analysis. *Sex Transm Dis.* 2014;41(6):369-376.

75. Krieger JN, Tam MR, Stevens CE, Nielsen IO, Hale J, Kiviat NB, et al. Diagnosis of trichomoniasis: comparison of conventional wet mount examination with cytologic studies, cultures, and monoclonal antibody staining of direct specimens. *JAMA.* 1988;259:1223-1227.

76. Wiese W, Patel SR, Patel SC, Ohl CA, Estrada CA. A meta-analysis of the Papanicolaou smear and wet mount for the diagnosis of vaginal trichomoniasis. *Am J Med.* 2000;108:301-308.

77. Nicollai LM, Kopicko JJ, Kassie A, Petros H, Clark RA, Kissinger P. Incidence and predictors of reinfection with *Trichomonas vaginalis* in HIV infected women. *Sex Transm Dis.* 2000;27:284-288.

78. Klebanoff MA, Carey JC, Hauth JC, Hillier SL, Nugent RP, Thom EA, et al. Failure of metronidazole to prevent preterm delivery among pregnant women with asymptomatic *Trichomonas vaginalis* infection. *N Engl J Med.* 2001;345:487-493.

79. Manhart LE, Critchlow CW, Holmes KK, Dutro SM, Eschenbach DA, Stevens CE, et al. Mucopurulent cervicitis and *Mycoplasma genitalium.* *J Infect Dis.* 2003;187:650-657.

80. Schwebke JR, Weiss HL. Interrelationships of bacterial vaginosis and cervical inflammation. *Sex Transm Dis.* 2002;29:59-64.

81. Centers for Disease Control and Prevention. 2013 Sexually Transmitted Disease Surveillance: Gonorrhea. Atlanta, GA: US Department of Health and Human Services; 2014. Available at: http://www .cdc.gov/std/stats13/gonorrhea.htm. Accessed May 24, 2016.

82. Ram S, Rice P. Gonococcal infections. In: Faro S, Soper DE, eds. *Infectious Diseases in Women.* Philadelphia, PA: WB Saunders Company; 2001.

83. Steinhandler L, Peipert JF, Heber W, Montagno A, Cruikshank C. Combination of bacterial vaginosis and leucorrhea as a predictor of cervical chlamydial or gonococcal infection. *Obstet Gynecol.* 2002;99: 603-607.

84. Centers for Disease Control and Prevention. 2013 Sexually Transmitted Disease Surveillance: Chlamydia. Atlanta, GA: US Department of Health and Human Services; 2014. Available at: http://www.cdc .gov/std/stats13/chlamydia.htm. Accessed May 24, 2016.

85. Haggerty CL, Gottlieb SL, Taylor BD, Low N, Xu F, Ness RB. Risk of sequelae after *Chlamydia*

trachomatis genital infection in women. *J Infect Dis.* 2010;201(Suppl 2):S134-S155.

86. Sellors JW, Walter SD, Howard M. A new visual indicator of chlamydial cervicitis? *Sex Transm Infect.* 2000;76:46-48.

87. LeFevre ML. USPSTF: screening for chlamydia and gonorrhea. *Ann Intern Med.* 2014;161:902-910.

88. Renault CA, Israelski DM, Levy V, Fujikawa BK, Kellogg TA, Klausner JD. Time to clearance of *Chlamydia trachomatis* ribosomal RNA in women treated for chlamydial infection. *Sex Health.* 2011;8:69-73.

89. Ryan GM Jr, Abdella TN, McNeeley SG, Baselski VS, Drummond DE. *Chlamydia trachomatis* infection in pregnancy and the effect of treatment on outcome. *Am J Obstet Gynecol.* 1990;162:34-39.

90. Centers for Disease Control and Prevention. STD 2013 Sexually Transmitted Diseases Surveillance: Syphilis. Available at: http://www.cdc.gov/std/stats13/syphilis.htm. Accessed May 24, 2016.

91. Singh AE, Romanowski B. Syphilis: review with emphasis on clinical, epidemiologic, and some biologic features. *Clin Microbiol Rev.* 1999;12(2):187-209.

92. Centers for Disease Control and Prevention, Association of Public Health Laboratories. Laboratory diagnostic testing for *Treponema pallidum*, Expert Consultation Meeting Summary Report, January 13-15, 2009, Atlanta, GA. Available at: http://www.aphl.org/aphlprograms/infectious/std/Documents/ID_2009Jan_Laboratory-Guidelines-Treponema-pallidum-Meeting-Report.pdf. Accessed May 24, 2016.

93. Nandwani R, Evans DT. Are you sure it's syphilis? A review of false positive serology. *Int J STD AIDS.* 1995;6:241-248.

94. Centers for Disease Control and Prevention. STD2013 Sexually Transmitted Diseases Surveillance: Other Sexually Transmitted Diseases. http://www.cdc.gov/std/stats13/other.htm. Accessed May 24, 2016.

95. Lewis DA. Chancroid: clinical manifestations, diagnosis, and management. *Sex Transm Infect.* 2003;79:68-71.

96. Bradley H, Markowitz L, Gibson T, McQuillan G. Seroprevalence of herpes simplex virus types 1 and 2—United States, 1999–2010. *J Infect Dis.* 209(3):325-333.

97. Xu F, Sternberg MR, Kottiri BJ, McQuillan GM, Lee FK, Nahmias AJ, et al. Trends in herpes simplex virus type 1 and type 2 seroprevalence in the United States. *JAMA.* 2006;296(8):964-973.

98. Fanfair RN, Zaidi A, Taylor LD, Xu F, Gottlieb S, Markowitz L. Trends in seroprevalence of herpes simplex virus type 2 among non-Hispanic blacks and non-Hispanic whites aged 14 to 49 years—United States, 1988 to 2010. *Sex Transm Dis.* 2013;40(11):860-864.

99. Cowan FM, Copas A, Johnson AM, Ashley R, Corey L, Mindel A. Herpes simplex virus type 1 infection: a sexually transmitted infection of adolescence? *Sex Transm Infect.* 2002;78:346-348.

100. Satterwhite CL, Torrone E, Meites E, Dunne EF, Mahajan R, Ocfemia MC, et al. Sexually transmitted infections among US women and men: prevalence and incidence estimates, 2008. *Sex Transm Dis.* 2013;40(30):187-193.

101. Bernstein DI, Bellamy AR, Hook EW 3rd, Levin MJ, Wald A, Ewell MG, et al. Epidemiology, clinical presentation, and antibody response to primary infection with herpes simplex virus type 1 and type 2 in young women. *Clin Infect Dis.* 2013;56(3):344-351.

102. Cherpes TL, Meyn LA, Krohn MA, Hillier SL. Risk factors for infection with herpes simplex virus type 2. *Sex Transm Dis.* 2003;30:405-410.

103. Gottlieb SL, Douglas JM, Schmid DS, Bolan G, Iatesta M, Malotte CK, et al. Seroprevalence and correlates of herpes simplex virus type 2 infection in five sexually transmitted disease clinics. *J Infect Dis.* 2002;186:1381-1389.

104. Centers for Disease Control and Prevention. Seroprevalence of herpes simplex virus type 2 among persons aged 14–49 years—United States, 2005–2008. *MMWR.* 2010;59(15):456-459.

105. Wald A, Zeh J, Selke S, Ashley RL, Corey L. Virologic characteristics of subclinical and symptomatic genital herpes infections. *N Engl J Med.* 1995;333:770-775.

106. Wald A, Zeh J, Selke S, Warren T, Ryncarz AJ, Ashley R, et al. Reactivation of genital herpes simplex virus type 2 infection in asymptomatic seropositive persons. *N Engl J Med.* 2000;342:844-850.

107. Mertz GJ, Benedetti J, Ashley R, Selke SA, Corey L. Risk factors for the sexual transmission of genital herpes. *Ann Intern Med.* 1992;116:197-202.

108. Wald A, Langenberg AG, Link K, Izu AE, Ashley R, Warren T, et al. Effect of condoms on reducing the transmission of herpes simplex virus type 2 from men to women. *JAMA.* 2001;285:3100-3106.

109. Corey L, Wald A, Patel R, Sacks S, Tyring SK, Warren T, et al. Once-daily valacyclovir to reduce the risk of transmission of genital herpes. *N Engl J Med.* 2004:350:11-20.

110. American College of Obstetricians and Gynecologists. Gynecologic herpes simplex infections. ACOG Practice Bulletin No. 57. *Obstet Gynecol.* 2004;104:1111-1117.

111. Lautenschlager S, Eichmsnn A. The heterogeneous clinical spectrum of genital herpes. *Dermatology.* 2001;202:211-219.

112. Ross K, Johnston C, Wald A. Herpes simplex virus type 2 serological testing and psychosocial harm: a systematic review. *Sex Transm Infect.* 2011;87:594-600.

113. Patrick DM, Rosenthal SL, Stanberry LR, Hurst C, Ebel C. Patient satisfaction with care for genital herpes: insights from a global survey. *Sex Transm Infect.* 2004;80:192-197.

114. Hanson D, Diven DG. Molluscum contagiosum. *Dermatol Online J.* 9(2):2. Available at: http://dermatology.cdlib.org/92/reviews/molluscum/diven.html. Accessed May 24, 2016.

115. Centers for Disease Control and Prevention. Molluscum Contagiosum. http://www.cdc.gov/poxvirus/molluscum-contagiosum/. Accessed May 24, 2016.

116. de Villiers EM, Fauquet C, Broker TR, Bernard HU, zur Hausen H. Classification of papillomaviruses. *Virology.* 2004;324:17-27.

117. Petrosky E, Bocchini JA, Hariri S, Chesson H, Curtis CR, Saraiya M, et al. Use of 9-valent human papillomavirus (HPV) vaccine: updated HPV vaccination recommendations of the Advisory Committee on Immunization Practices. *MMWR.* 2015;64(11);300-304.

118. Edwards L, Ferenczy A, Eron L, Baker D, Owens ML, Fox TL, et al. Self-administered topical 5% imiquimod cream for external anogenital warts. *Arch Dermatol.* 1998;134:25-30.

119. Wiesenfeld HC, Sweet RL, Ness RB, Krohn MA, Amortegui AJ, Hillier SL. Comparison of acute and subclinical pelvic inflammatory disease. *Sex Transm Dis.* 2005;32:400-405.

120. Jossens MO, Schachter J, Sweet RL. Risk factors associated with pelvic inflammatory disease of differing microbial etiologies. *Obstet Gynecol.* 1994;83:989-997.

121. Jossens MO, Eskenazi B, Schachter J, Sweet RL. Risk factors for pelvic inflammatory disease: a case control study. *Sex Transm Dis.* 1996;23:239-247.

122. Miller HG, Cain VS, Rogers SM, Gribble JN, Turner CF. Correlates of sexually transmitted bacterial infections among U.S. women in 1995. *Fam Plan Perspect.* 1999;31:4-9, 23.

123. Walsh T, Grimes D, Frezieres R, Nelson A, Bernstein L, Coulson A, et al. Randomised controlled trial of prophylactic antibiotics before insertion of intra-uterine devices: IUD Study Group. *Lancet.* 1998; 351:1005-1008.

124. Beckmann KR, Melzer-Lang MD, Gorelick MH. Emergency department management of sexually transmitted infections in U.S. adolescents: results from the National Hospital Ambulatory Medical Care Survey. *Ann Emerg Med.* 2004;43:333-338.

125. Walker CK, Wiesenfeld HC. Antibiotic therapy for acute pelvic inflammatory disease: the 2006 CDC sexually transmitted diseases treatment guidelines. *Clin Infect Dis.* 2007;28(Supp 1):S29-S36.

126. Centers for Disease Control and Prevention. U.S. selected practice recommendations for contraceptive use, 2013: adapted from the World Health Organization selected practice recommendations for contraceptive use, 2nd ed. *MMWR Recomm Rep.* 2013;62(RR-05):1-46.

127. Tepper NK, Steenland MW, Gaffield ME, Marchbanks PA, Curtis KM. Retention of intrauterine devices in women who acquire pelvic inflammatory disease: a systematic review. *Contraception.* 2013;87:655-660.

128. Centers for Disease Control and Prevention. Surveillance for Viral Hepatitis—United States, 2013. Available at: http://www.cdc.gov/hepatitis/statistics/2013surveillance/commentary.htm. Accessed May 24, 2016.

129. Centers for Disease Control and Prevention. Viral Hepatitis—Hepatitis D Information. Available at: http://www.cdc.gov/hepatitis/HDV/index.htm. Accessed May 24, 2016.

130. World Health Organization. Hepatitis D. Available at: http://www.who.int/csr/disease/hepatitis/whocdscsrncs20011/en/. Accessed May 24, 2016.

131. Centers for Disease Control and Prevention. Viral Hepatitis—Hepatitis E Information. Available at: http://www.cdc.gov/hepatitis/HEV/index.htm. Accessed May 24, 2016.

132. Kunholm MH, Purcell RH, McQuillan GM, Engle RE, Wasley A, Nelson KE. Epidemiology of hepatitis E virus in the United States: results from the Third National Health and Nutrition Examination Survey, 1988–1994. *J Infect Dis.* 2009;200(1): 48-56.

133. Centers for Disease Control and Prevention. Hepatitis A. Available at: http://www.cdc.gov/hepatitis/hav/havfaq.htm#general. Accessed May 24, 2016.

134. Fiore AE. Hepatitis A transmitted by food. *Clin Infect Dis.* 2004;38:705-715.

135. Klevens RM, Miller JT, Iqbal K, Thomas A, Rizzo EM, Hanson H, et al. The evolving epidemiology of hepatitis A in the United States: incidence and molecular epidemiology from population-based surveillance, 2005–2007. *Arch Intern Med.* 2010; 170(20):1811-1818.

136. Bower WA, Nainan OV, Han X, Margolis HS. Duration of viremia in hepatitis A virus infection. *J Infect Dis.* 2000;182:12-7.

137. Centers for Disease Control and Prevention. Hepatitis A. In: *The Pink Book: Epidemiology & Prevention*

of Vaccine-Preventable Diseases. 13th ed. 2015. Available at: http://www.cdc.gov/vaccines/pubs/pinkbook/downloads/hepa.pdf. Accessed May 24, 2016.

138. Fiore AE, Wasley A, Bell BP. Prevention of hepatitis A through active or passive immunization: recommendations of the Advisory Committee on Immunization Practices (ACIP). *MMWR.* 2006;55(RR07):1-23.

139. Kyrlagkitis I, Cramp ME, Smith H, Portmann B, O'Grady J. Acute hepatitis A virus infection: a review of prognostic factors from 25 years experience in a tertiary referral center. *Hepatogastroenterology.* 2002;49:524-528.

140. Brown GR, Persley K. Hepatitis A epidemic in the elderly. *South Med J.* 2002;95:826-833.

141. Koff RS. Seroepidemiology of HAV in the United States. *J Infect Dis.* 1995;171(Suppl 1):s19-s23.

142. Lawrence ML, Lawrence RA. The evidence for breastfeeding: given the benefits of breastfeeding, what contraindications exist? *Pediatr Clin North Am.* 2001;48:1.

143. Centers for Disease Control and Prevention. Viral Hepatitis—Hepatitis B Information. Available at: http://www.cdc.gov/hepatitis/hbv/. Accessed May 24, 2016.

144. Centers for Disease Control and Prevention. Hepatitis B. Available at: http://www.cdc.gov/hepatitis/statistics/2013surveillance/commentary.htm#hepatitisB. Accessed May 24, 2016.

145. Kim WR. Epidemiology of hepatitis B in the United States. *Hepatology.* 2009;49(5 Suppl):S28-S34.

146. Wasley AM, Kruszon-Moran D, Kuhnert WL, Simard EP, Finelli L, McQuillan G, et al. The prevalence of hepatitis B virus infection in the United States in the era of vaccination. *J Infect Dis.* 2010;202(2):192-201.

147. Ioannou GN. Hepatitis B virus in the United States: infection, exposure, and immunity rates in a nationally representative survey. *Ann Intern Med.* 2011;154(5):319-328.

148. Chan HLY, Lok ASF. Hepatitis B in adults: a clinical perspective. *Clin Liver Dis.* 1999;3(2):291-307.

149. Centers for Disease Control and Prevention. A comprehensive immunization strategy to eliminate transmission of hepatitis B virus infection in the United States. Recommendations of the Advisory Committee on Immunization Practices (ACIP). Part 1: Immunization of Infants, Children, and Adolescents. *MMWR Recomm Rep.* 2005;54(RR16):1-23.

150. Centers for Disease Control and Prevention. A comprehensive immunization strategy to eliminate transmission of hepatitis B virus infection in the United States. Recommendations of the Advisory Committee on Immunization Practices (ACIP). Part 2: Immunization of Adults. *MMWR Recomm Rep.* 2006;55(RR-16):1-33.

151. Lok ASF, McMahon BJ. Chronic hepatitis B: update 2009. *Hepatology.* 2009;50(3):1-35.

152. World Health Organization. Guidelines for the Prevention, Care and Treatment of Persons with Chronic Hepatitis B Infection. Geneva, Switzerland: World Health Organization; 2015. Available at: http://www.ncbi.nlm.nih.gov/books/NBK305553/. Accessed May 24, 2016.

153. Centers for Disease Control and Prevention. Viral Hepatitis—Hepatitis C Information. Available at: http://www.cdc.gov/hepatitis/HCV/index.htm. Accessed May 24, 2016.

154. Williams IT, Bell BP, Kuhnert W, Alter MJ. Incidence and transmission patterns of acute hepatitis C in the United States, 1982–2006. *Arch Intern Med.* 2011;171(3):242-248.

155. Ghany MG, Strader DB, Thomas DL, Seeff LB. Diagnosis, management, and treatment of hepatitis C: an update. *Hepatology.* 2009;49(4):1335-1374.

156. Terrault NA, Dodge JL, Murphy EL, Tavis JE, Kiss A, Levin TR, et al. Sexual transmission of hepatitis C virus among monogamous heterosexual couples: the HCV Partners Study. *Hepatology.* 2013;57(3):881-889.

157. Carney K, Dhalla S, Aytaman A, Tenner CT, Francois F. Association of tattooing and hepatitis C virus infection: a multicenter case-control study. *Hepatology.* 2013;57(6):2117-2123. doi:10.1002/hep.26245.

158. Missiha SB, Ostrowski M, Heathcote EJ. Disease progression in chronic hepatitis C: modifiable and nonmodifiable factors. *Gastroenterology.* 2008;134(6):1699-1714.

159. Sabatino G, Ramenghi LA, di Marzio M, Pizzigallo E. Vertical transmission of hepatitis C virus: an epidemiological study on 2,980 pregnant women in Italy. *Eur J Epidemiol.* 1996;12:443-447.

160. Centers for Disease Control and Prevention. HIV Surveillance of Women. Available at: http://www.cdc.gov/HIV/library/slidesets/index.html. Accessed June 1, 2016.

161. Beck EJ, Mandalia S, Leonard K, Griffith RJ, Harris JRW, Miller DL. Case-control study of sexually transmitted diseases as cofactors for HIV-1 transmission. *Int J STD AIDS.* 1996;7:34-38.

162. Martin HL, Richardson BA, Nyange PM, Lavreys L, Hillier SL, Chohan B, et al. Vaginal lactobacilli, microbial flora, and risk of human immunodeficiency virus type 1 and sexually transmitted disease acquisition. *J Infect Dis.* 1999;180:1863-1868.

163. Rotchford K, Strum AW, Wilkinson D. Effect of co-infection with STDs and STD treatment on HIV shedding in genital-tract secretions. *Sex Transm Dis.* 2000;27:243-248.

164. Branson BM, Handsfield HH, Lampe MA, Janssen RS, Taylor AW, Lyss SB, et al. Revised Recommendations for HIV Testing of Adults, Adolescents, and Pregnant Women in Health-Care Settings. Available at: http://www.cdc.gov/mmwr/preview/mmwrhtml/rr5514a1.htm. Accessed May 24, 2016.

165. Centers for Disease Control and Prevention. HIV among women. Available at: http://www.cdc.gov/hiv/group/gender/women/index.html. Accessed May 24, 2016.

166. Shacker TW, Hughes JP, Shea T, Coombs RW, Corey L. Biologic and virologic characteristics of primary HIV infection. *Ann Intern Med.* 1998;128(8):313-320.

167. Schneider E, Whitmore S, Glynn MK, Dominguez K, Mitsch A, McKenna MT. Revised surveillance case definitions for HIV infection among adults, adolescents, and children aged <18 months and for HIV infection and AIDS among children aged 18 months to <13 years—United States, 2008. *MMWR.* 2008;57(RR10):1-8.

168. Centers for Disease Control and Prevention. WHO and HHS/CDC Prevention of Mother-to-Child Transmission of HIV (PMTCT) Generic Training Package Components - Presentation Module 1. Available at: http://www.cdc.gov/globalaids/Resources/pmtct-care/pmtct-who-hhs-cmpntsM1.html. Accessed May 24, 2016.

169. Farzadegan H, Hoover DR, Astemborski J, Lyles CM, Margolick JB, Markham RB, et al. Sex differences in HIV-1 viral load and progression to AIDS. *Lancet.* 1998;352:510-514.

170. Marks G, Crepaz N, Janssen RS. Estimating sexual transmission of HIV from persons aware and unaware that they are infected with the virus in the USA. *AIDS.* 2006;20:1447-1450.

171. Cohen MS, Chen YQ, McCauley M, Gamble T, Hosseinipour MC, Kumarasamy N, et al. Prevention of HIV-1 infection with early antiretroviral therapy. *N Engl J Med.* 2011;365(6):493-505.

172. Donnell D, Baeten JM, Kiarie J, Thomas KK, Stevens W, Cohen CR, et al. Heterosexual HIV-1 transmission after initiation of antiretroviral therapy: a prospective cohort analysis. *Lancet.* 2010;375:2092-2098.

173. Attia S, Egger M, Müller M, Zwahlen M, Low N. Sexual transmission of HIV according to viral load and antiretroviral therapy: systematic review and meta-analysis. *AIDS.* 2009;23(11):1307-1404.

174. US Public Health Service. Preexposure Prophylaxis for the Prevention of HIV Infection in the United States—2014: A Clinical Practice Guideline. Available at: http://www.cdc.gov/hiv/pdf/PrEPguidelines2014.pdf. Accessed May 24, 2016.

175. O'Brien ME, Richardson-Alston G, Ayoub M, Magnus M, Peterman TA, Kissinger P. Prevalence and correlates of HIV serostatus disclosure. *Sex Transm Dis.* 2003;30:731-735.

176. Ciccarone DH, Kanouse DE, Collins RL, Miu A, Chen JL, Morton SC, et al. Sex without disclosure if positive HIV serostatus in a U.S. probability sample of persons receiving care for HIV infection. *Am J Public Health.* 2003;93:949-954.

177. Uvin SC, Caliendo AM. Cervico-vaginal human immunodeficiency virus secretion and plasma viral load in human immunodeficiency virus-seropositive women. *Obstet Gynecol.* 1997;90(5):739-743.

178. Panel on Antiretroviral Guidelines for Adults and Adolescents. Guidelines for the use of antiretroviral agents in HIV-1-infected adults and adolescents. US Department of Health and Human Services. Available at: http://aidsinfo.nih.gov/contentfiles/lvguidelines/AdultandAdolescentGL.pdf. Accessed May 24, 2016.

179. The Antiretroviral Therapy Cohort Collaboration. Life expectancy of individuals on combination antiretroviral therapy in high-income countries: a collaborative analysis of 14 cohort studies. *Lancet.* 2008;372(9635):293-299.

180. Schuman P, Ohmit SE, Klein RS, Duerr A, Cu-Uvin S, Jamieson DJ, et al. Longitudinal study of cervical squamous intraepithelial lesions in human immunodeficiency virus (HIV)-seropositive and at-risk HIV-seronegative women. HIV Epidemiology Research Study (HERS) Group. *J Infect Dis.* 2003;188:128-136.

181. Massad LS, Evans CT, Minkoff H, Watts DH, Strickler HD, Darragh T, et al. Natural history of grade 1 cervical intraepithelial neoplasia in women with human immunodeficiency virus. *Obstet Gynecol.* 2004;104:1077-1085.

182. Conley LJ, Ellerbrock TV, Bush TJ, Chiasson MA, Sawo D, Wright TC. HIV-1 infection and risk of vulvovaginal and perianal condylomata acuminata and intraepithelial neoplasia: a prospective cohort study. *Lancet.* 2002;359:108-113.

183. El-Ibiary SY, Cocohoba JM. Effects of HIV antiretrovirals on the pharmacokinetics of hormonal contraceptives. *Eur J Contracept Reprod Health Care.* 2008;13:123-132.

184. Vogler MA, Patterson K, Kamemoto L, Park JG, Watts H, Aweeka F, et al. Contraceptive efficacy of

oral and transdermal hormones when coadministered with protease inhibitors in HIV-1-infected women: pharmacokinetic results of ACTG trial A5188. *J Acquir Immune Defic Syndr*. 2010;55(4): 473-482.

185. Leticee N, Viard JP, Yamgnane A, Karmochkine M, Benachi A. Contraceptive failure of etonogestrel implant in patients treated with antiretrovirals including efavirenz. *Contraception*. 2012;85(4):425-427.

186. Heikinheimo O, Lehtovirta P, Aho I, Ristola M, Paavonen J. The levonorgestrel-releasing intrauterine system in human immunodeficiency virus-infected women: a 5-year follow-up study. *Am J Obstet Gynecol*. 2011;204(2):126.e1-e4.

187. Curtis KM, Nanda K, Kapp N. Safety of hormonal and intrauterine methods of contraception for women with HIV/AIDS: a systematic review. *AIDS*. 2009;23(Suppl 1):S55-S67.

188. Lehtovirta P, Paavonen J, Heikinheimo O. Experience with the levonorgestrel-releasing intrauterine system among HIV infected women. *Contraception*. 2007;75(1):37-39.

189. Cohn SE, Park JG, Watts DH, Stek A, Hitti J, Clax PA, et al. Depo-medroxyprogesterone in women on antiretroviral therapy: effective contraception and lack of clinically significant interactions. *Clin Pharmacol Ther*. 2007;81(2):222-227.

190. Watts DH, Park JG, Cohn SE, Yu S, Hitti J, Stek A, et al. Safety and tolerability of depot medroxyprogesterone acetate among HIV-infected women on antiretroviral therapy: ACTG A5093. *Contraception*. 2008;77(2):84-90.

191. Centers for Disease Control and Prevention. Recommendations for Use of Antiretroviral Drugs in Pregnant HIV-1-Infected Women for Maternal Health and Interventions to Reduce Perinatal HIV Transmission in the United States. Available at: https://aidsinfo.nih.gov/contentfiles/lvguidelines/perinatalgl.pdf. Accessed May 24, 2016.

192. Schick V, Herbenick D, Reece M, Sanders SA, Dodge B, Middlestadt SE, et al. Sexual behaviors, condom use, and sexual health of Americans over 50: implications for sexual health promotion for older adults. *J Sex Med*. 2010;7(Suppl 5):315-329.

193. Mack KA, Bland SD. HIV testing behaviors and attitudes regarding HIV/AIDS of adults aged 50-64. *Gerontologist*. 1999;39(6):687-694.

194. Zablotsky D, Kennedy M. Risk factors and HIV transmission to midlife and older women: knowledge, options, and the initiation of safer sexual practices. *J Acquir Immune Defic Syndr*. 2003;33(Suppl 2): S122-S130.

195. Allison-Ottley S, Weston C, Hennawi G, Nichols M, Eldred L, Ferguson RP. Sexual practices of older adults in a high HIV prevalence environment. *Md Med J*. 1999;48(6):287-291.

196. Pinkerton SD, Abramson PR. Occasional condom use and HIV risk reduction. *J AIDS Hum Retrovirol*. 1996;13:456-460.

197. Galvao LW, Oliviera LC, Diaz J, Kim D, Marchi N, van Dam J, et al. Effectiveness of female and male condoms in preventing exposure to semen during vaginal intercourse: a randomized trial. *Contraception*. 2005;71:130-136.

198. Committee on Prevention and Control of Sexually Transmitted Diseases. *The Hidden Epidemic: Confronting Sexually Transmitted Diseases*. Washington, DC: National Academy Press; 1997.

199. Landers, DV, Wiesenfeld HC, Heine RP, Krohn MA, Hillier SL. Predictive value of the clinical diagnosis of lower genital tract infection in women. *Am J Obstet Gynecol*. 2004;190:1004-1008.

200. Kane BG, Degutis LC, Sayward HK, D'Onofrio G. Compliance with the Centers for Disease Control and Prevention recommendations for the diagnosis and treatment of sexually transmitted diseases. *Acad Emerg Med*. 2004;11:371-377.

201. Eubanks C, Lafferty WE, Kimball AM, MacCornack R, Kassler WJ. Privatization of STD services in Tacoma Washington: a quality review. *Sex Transm Dis*. 1999;26:537-542.

CHAPTER 22

THE REPRODUCTIVE SYSTEM

Penny Wortman | Susan M. Yount | Jan M. Kriebs

Caring for women, whether in primary care-or in a position dedicated to women's health, involves an appreciation of those normal and abnormal conditions that occur only in women. Gender differences in language use, social and economic barriers to seeking care, and a host of other personal factors can make it challenging to elicit what actually is concerning the woman who comes into your office. She may present for routine care with unexpressed concerns. Sometimes she will be troubled by a normal physiologic change or a minor problem; other times, she will be concerned about a serious infection, abnormal bleeding, or possible malignancy. This chapter is limited to gynecologic topics and cancer screening that can arise in the primary care office. Pregnancy after the first trimester and contraception are not discussed.

Essential History, Physical Examination, and Testing

The female reproductive organs are sheltered within the pelvis except during pregnancy. These consist of paired ovaries and fallopian tubes, the uterus, cervix, and vagina. Externally, the visible portions of the female anatomy include the clitoris, labia majora and minora, and vaginal introitus. **Figure 22-1** depicts the normal position of the pelvic organs. **Figure 22-2** depicts the internal reproductive organs and external genitalia.

History

A woman's health history extends beyond the general medical history in several aspects. Many clinicians will discover that forms created to document medical history will need to be adapted to capture this information in ways that will be easy to access at future visits. The medical history expands to include a comprehensive menstrual and reproductive history. Components of this history are shown in **Table 22-1**. The menstrual cycle is typically recorded in women of reproductive age as: age of menarche/length of cycle/number of bleeding days during menses (e.g., 12/28/4). Pain associated with or preceding the menses is documented along with any other symptoms, the estimated amount of bleeding (e.g., light,

Figure 22-1 Placement of pelvic organs.

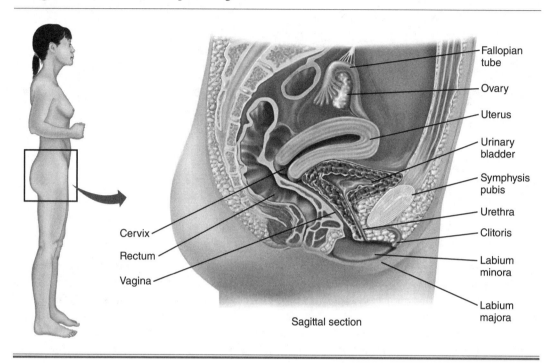

Fallopian tube

Ovary

Uterus

Urinary bladder

Symphysis pubis

Urethra

Clitoris

Labium minora

Labium majora

Cervix

Rectum

Vagina

Sagittal section

heavy), and any intermenstrual bleeding or spotting. Responses to these questions can help to identify intrauterine or ectopic pregnancies, ovarian cysts, fibroids, and endometriosis. The pregnancy history includes details of all pregnancies and births, and is summarized in **Table 22-2**.

The social history provides an opportunity to determine whether the woman is in a partnered relationship, the gender of her partner, and how many people are in the home. Employment, exercise and activity level, nutrition, and use of substances (tobacco, alcohol, marijuana where legal, illicit drugs, and use of others' prescriptions) are included in the social history. A sexual history is collected, including onset of sexual activity and number of partners. Specific family history

should inquire about cancers, endocrine disorders, and bleeding disorders.

Taking a comprehensive history will provide many clues to assess the causes of current complaints, but this is also the opportunity to gather information that will inform many other aspects of care. For example, family composition and history of postpartum depression may lead to evaluation of stress or mental health problems that are impacting her lived experience of midlife. Failure to plan for contraception may lead to an unintended pregnancy. Seeing the woman holistically gives clinicians the opportunity to provide exemplary care.

The review of systems that follows the history allows the clinician to explore in more depth the current complaint and history of present

Figure 22-2 The reproductive system. A. Anterior view of the uterus. B. Female reproductive organs, rectal.

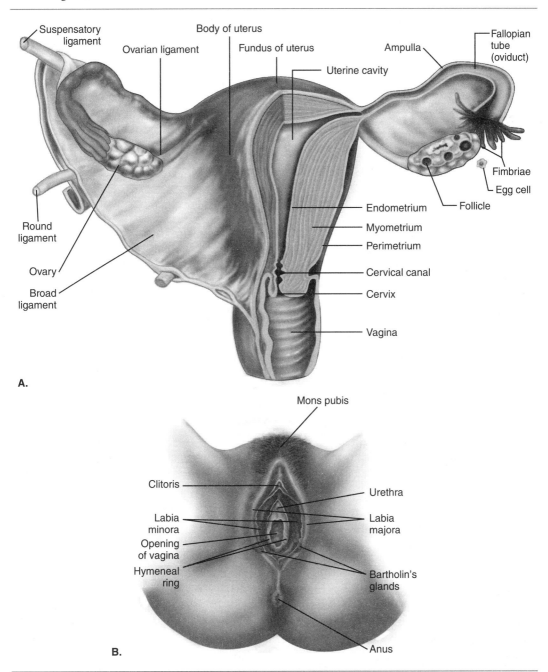

Table 22-1 Components of the Reproductive History

Gynecologic

Menstrual:
- Onset of menarche
- Last menses date and normalcy
- Length of menstrual cycle and number of bleeding days
- Symptoms associated with menstrual cycle
- Intermenstrual bleeding

Menopausal (as appropriate):
- Perimenopause symptoms
- Date of menopause
- Surgical or natural
- Hormone therapy

Contraceptive/procreative:
- Current method
- Former methods and reason for discontinuation
- Use of condom or barrier
- Childbearing plans

Cervical cancer screening:
- Last screen
- Abnormal results
- Colposcopy
- Cervical treatment/surgery

Infectious:
- Sexually transmitted diseases
- Benign vaginal infections

Pregnancy
- Number and outcome of all pregnancies
- Ectopic or molar pregnancy outcomes
- Complications of pregnancy or birth
- Medical problems (e.g., postpartum depression, gestational diabetes, hypertension)
- Genetic testing

Table 22-2 Documenting Pregnancy

Gravida: total number of pregnancies

Parity: number of births after 20 weeks' gestation

Term: births after 37 completed weeks' gestation

Preterm: births between 20 and 37 weeks' gestation

Abortion: includes spontaneous miscarriage and elective terminations before 20 completed weeks of pregnancy

Living: currently living children

This may be written in various ways. The simplest is G/P (i.e., number of pregnancies, number of viable births). The more useful method is G/TPAL.

Physical Examination

A minimum standard for the women's health examination includes evaluation of the breasts, abdomen, and pelvis. Examination of the thyroid gland, the upper body lymphatics, and lower extremities, as well as assessment of costovertebral angle tenderness, is often included, or a general screening physical may be performed. The choice of components for the examination is made based on purpose of the visit, current concerns, and the history and review of systems. The general physical examination and abdominal examination are addressed elsewhere. Examination of the pelvis includes inspection, speculum, and bimanual evaluation. Observation may reveal discharge, erythema or irritation, alterations in skin color or texture, or lesions of the external genitalia. Speculum examination provides not only an opportunity to collect specimens but an observation of cervical changes, any lesions or masses in the vagina or at the cervix, and bleeding sources. The bimanual examination allows an assessment of changes in the cervix; the size, shape, regularity, and position of the uterus and ovaries; localization of pain; and any associated masses. Checking lymph nodes that drain from the pelvis is also

condition that are the stated reason for the visit. It also permits assessment of symptoms in other body systems that may help with a differential diagnosis. This is the opportunity to put the past and present together before performing an examination.

necessary. When appropriate, rectal examination is done to identify masses, nodularity, the size and shape of an extroverted uterus, and any bowel abnormalities. **Table 22-3** provides information on the purpose and contents of the examination.

Laboratory and Imaging

Pregnancy testing—either urine or blood—is often the first test ordered in women's health. It is relevant to the management of any pain or

---

Table 22-3 The Reproductive System Examination

Constitutional:
- Vital signs
- Body hair distribution: thinning or unusual distribution
- Body fat distribution: central, even, or hip areas
- Skin: pallor, texture, petechiae, acanthosis nigricans (neck, axilla, and groin)
- Signs of possible androgen excess: acne, alopecia, and hirsutism
- Signs of anemia: pale mucous membranes, delayed capillary refill

Thyroid:
- Size, shape, mobility, and symmetry
- Palpate for enlargement, mobility, nodules, or tumors

Breast
- Visualization of size, shape, surface vascularity, skin changes, lesions
- Systematic palpation for masses and their characterization

Abdominal examination:
- Visualization of masses, striae, skin changes
- Palpation light and deep: guarding, rebound tenderness, masses, lymphadenopathy
- Note if masses are mobile, tender, or nontender
- Costovertebral angle tenderness if appropriate to history

External pelvic examination:
- Visual: atrophy, excoriation, discoloration, discharge, lesions, or trauma; hair pattern
- Palpation: groin lymphadenopathy, Bartholin's urethra and Skene's assessment for discharge
- Note if masses are mobile, tender, or nontender

Speculum exam:
- Visual: vaginal shape, color, tissue integrity, rugae, discharge, polyps, nodules
- Visual: cervical shape, color, vascularity, erosion, lesions, friability, discharge, polyps
- Assess for trauma or foreign body in vault

Bimanual exam:
- Vagina: tenderness, vaginismus, pliability, length, presence of cystocele or rectocele
- Cervix: tenderness, shape, mobility, closed or open
- Uterus: shape, size, position, masses or irregularity, asymmetry
- Adnexa: ovaries palpable or not, masses, pain or tenderness, asymmetry
- Note if masses are mobile, tender, or nontender

Rectovaginal:
- Sphincter tone, tissue integrity, presence of hemorrhoids or fissures, pain or tenderness
- Presence of rectocele
- Palpation of posterior wall of retroverted or retroflexed uterus

menstrual abnormality in women who are of reproductive age. Pregnancy status impacts which imaging studies will be ordered, which procedures can be performed, and which medications can be prescribed. Regardless of the woman's reported sexual activity, the test should be ordered. This may require tact, but the data are vital. A courteous and careful explanation can be offered if necessary, clarifying that ruling out pregnancy is standard practice. It is better to perform an unnecessary, inexpensive urine pregnancy test than to miss a concealed or unrecognized pregnancy.

Blood work ordered during gynecologic visits may include a complete blood count (CBC) to screen for anemia, evaluation for thyroid disorders with thyroid-stimulating hormone (TSH) and free T4, assessment of insulin and glucose metabolism with an insulin level, fasting blood

sugar or formal diabetes panel, or screening for infections such as human immunodeficiency virus (HIV), syphilis, hepatitis, or herpes. Studies for specific conditions are discussed in the sections that follow. Urine specimens may be collected to screen for infection or stones.

Samples for the Papanicolaou (Pap) test and human papillomavirus (HPV) co-testing are collected according to current recommendations. The technique is described in **Table 22-4**. Timing of the tests and interpretation of results are discussed in the section on cervical cancer screening. Screening for cervical cancer is one of the most successful programs for eradication of a malignancy ever created.

The most common imaging study in gynecology is a pelvic ultrasound, which may be performed transabdominally or transvaginally, depending on the information sought. Transvaginal scans are

Table 22-4 Performance of a Papanicolaou Test

Liquid-based specimen collection, in which the specimen is collected at the cervix, has become the standard where available, due to improved ability to interpret abnormalities. This material can also be used for human papillomavirus (HPV) testing (step 6). In a conventional Pap smear, a slide is made directly from the specimen collected at the cervix. An extended-tip spatula plus endocervical brush technique or broom plus endocervical brush has been shown to provide the most accurate results and should be used whenever available (steps 7 and 8).

1. Insert a moistened speculum into the vagina and visualize the cervix.
2. If only a Pap test is being performed, a small amount of water-based gel can be used to lubricate the speculum.
3. Using a spatula or broom, sweep the cervix, rotating the spatula or broom 360° to cover the entire ectocervix. An extended-tip spatula is the preferred device. If the squamocolumnar junction is visible, it should be included.
4. Remove the device without touching the vaginal sidewalls; rotate it gently in liquid medium to dislodge the cells, or roll across a clean slide, depending on whether a liquid or dry collection method is used.
5. For dry specimens only: Place one flat side on the top half of the slide and stroke once to the end of the slide. Then turn the spatula or brush over and place the other flat side on the bottom half of the slide and stroke once to the end of the slide. If the specimen is too thick, take the edge of the device and, with a single light stroke down the slide, remove the excess.
6. Insert a cervical brush into the endocervix approximately 2 cm and rotate through 90°–180°.
7. Repeat the procedure for processing as in steps 4 and 5.
8. If a dry technique is used, the specimen should immediately be fixed before transport to preserve cellular integrity.

sometimes perceived as invasive, as, indeed, are speculum examinations. However, they provide information that cannot be seen abdominally in many cases.

The Menstrual Cycle and Symptomatic Conditions

The normal menstrual cycle requires both anatomic integrity and effective hormonal control along the *hypothalamic-pituitary-ovarian (HPO) axis*. Hypothalamic release of gonadotropin-releasing hormone (GnRH) factors, composed of follicle-stimulating factor and luteinizing hormone–releasing factor, stimulates the anterior pituitary to release luteinizing hormone (LH) and follicle-stimulating hormone (FSH) as well as prolactin into the circulation. FSH and LH provoke ovarian release of estrogen and progesterone in a complex cycle of positive and negative feedback loops. The interaction of estrogen and progesterone stimulates the development and shedding of the endometrial lining of the uterus and the ovarian development and release of a mature follicle as an oocyte. Under the influence of estrogen secreted by the ovary, the scant lining (1–2 mm at the end of menses) thickens to 12 mm by the time of the LH surge that triggers ovulation. Progesterone secreted by the corpus luteum controls the second, secretory phase of endometrial development in a normal cycle. **Figure 22-3** depicts the interaction of pituitary and ovarian stimulation of the uterus and ovary during a healthy cycle. Note that the menstrual cycle is always counted from the first day of the menses.

Figure 22-3 Phases of the menstrual cycle.

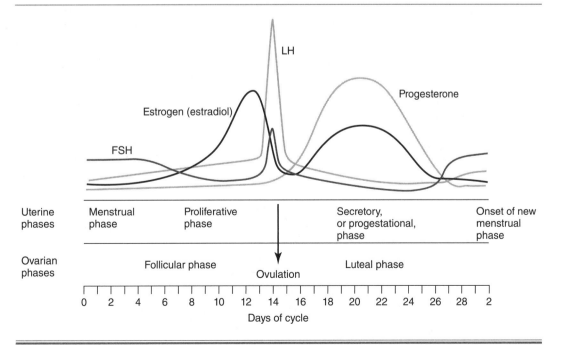

Menarche

As a girl matures, the development of breast buds and body hair signals the approach of menarche. The average age at *menarche* in the United States has remained between 12 and 13 years of age for many years.[1] Ninety percent of girls will not menstruate before the age of 11; 98% will menstruate by age 15.[2] African American girls and those with childhood obesity are prone to earlier age at menarche.[1-4] Exposure to environmental toxins may also play a role in early development of puberty.

In the first 2 years after menarche, anovulatory cycles caused by immature development of the HPO axis cause some irregularity in the length of cycles and degree of bleeding. While the average for this time is 21–45 days, with up to 7 bleeding days, much longer periods without bleeding may occur.[5] The American College of Obstetricians and Gynecologists (ACOG) recommends evaluation for possible menstrual abnormalities if any of the following occur in adolescents: no menses within 3 years of *thelarche* (onset of breast development); no menses by age 15; no menses by age 14 with a history of hirsutism, excessive exercise, or signs of an eating disorder; no menses for 90 days; menses are frequently fewer than 21 or greater than 45 days apart; menses last more than 7 days or are heavy enough to soak through a pad in 1–2 hours; or there is a personal or family history of easy bruising or a bleeding disorder.[6]

Premenstrual Syndrome

Premenstrual syndrome (PMS) has been defined as symptoms that occur only during the luteal phase, are not an exacerbation of another disorder, are severe enough to interfere with daily function, and cause significant distress.[7] There is a broad spectrum of possible complaints and how they are expressed. The symptoms may be either somatic (e.g., bloating, cramping, breast tenderness) or affective (e.g., moodiness, irritability, anger). For 5–8% of women, the symptoms are severe;[8] many of these women meet criteria for premenstrual dysphoric disorder (PMDD), which affects 2–5% of women and requires an affective symptom for diagnosis.[9] Obesity, smoking, history of abuse, and, less clearly, alcohol use have been linked to increased risks of PMS.[10-13]

Rather than abnormal levels of sex hormones as the underlying cause of PMS, acute sensitivity to the normal fluctuation of those hormones, timing of hormone excretion for thyroid or circadian hormones such as melatonin and cortisol, or neurotransmitters such as serotonin have been proposed as mediators for the affective symptoms of PMS.[8]

The diagnosis of PMS is based on having a woman track her symptoms for at least two cycles. This allows a pattern to emerge. A daily calendar of symptoms and the timing of menses are used for this purpose. Women who are experiencing the same symptoms at other times of their cycle need to be evaluated for other causes. For example, depression or another mental health issue may be the cause of the psychologic complaints; gastrointestinal disease may produce bloating or crampy pain. Note that this does not mean her symptoms are not real, only that there is another explanation that must be sought.

Treatment of mild PMS may be achieved with lifestyle changes, including increasing the proportion of complex carbohydrates, increasing exercise, and decreasing the use of sodium, simple sugars, alcohol, caffeine, and tobacco. Combined hormonal contraceptives have been tried, although the evidence is not clear regarding benefits; however, extended cycles may, by decreasing the frequency of cycles, also decrease occurrence of symptoms.[14] Hormonal contraception is more likely to relieve physical symptoms than psychological ones; drospirenone is the progestin component most likely to provide overall relief.[15]

Selective serotonin reuptake inhibitors (SSRIs) are the first-line therapy for severe PMS, and can be used either continuously or only during the luteal phase of the menstrual cycle.[16] Continuous use has been reported to yield greater benefit than intermittent dosing.[17] No particular SSRI has been shown to be preferable for this indication.[17] Other approaches may be combined with these methods. Nonsteroidal anti-inflammatory drugs (NSAIDs) and diuretics can be used for short-term relief of physical symptoms.[16] Vitamin B_6 in moderate doses—50 to 100 mg per day—may be recommended.[18] Calcium supplementation has been shown to reduce both affective and physical symptoms.[19] See **Table 22-5** for use of these and other complementary treatments for PMS. The evidence for other possible herbal remedies such as evening primrose oil, St. John's wart, Gingko biloba, and crocus sativa is insufficient to recommend their use.

Dysmenorrhea

Both a complaint in otherwise healthy women and a marker for underlying conditions, menstrual cramping can be a disruptive factor in women's lives. The problem affects between 16% and 93% of menstruating women in different reviews.[20-23] *Primary dysmenorrhea* is the term used for menstrual pain where no pathology exists. Secondary causes can include fibroids, endometriosis, uterine cancer, pelvic inflammatory disease, and placement of nonhormonal intrauterine devices (IUDs). Ju and colleagues reported that 2–29% of women are severely affected. Advancing age, parity, and use of oral contraceptives were inversely associated with dysmenorrhea in this review. Family history and stress increased the likelihood that a woman would experience dysmenorrhea.[23] Other factors associated with increased pain or duration of menstrual cramping may include either low body mass index (BMI) or obesity, smoking, low socioeconomic status, sexual abuse, PMS, early menarche, and long cycle duration or heavy flow.[21,22,24]

In adolescents, primary dysmenorrhea arises with the onset of ovulatory cycles, usually within a year of menarche.[25] Onset in adulthood suggests the possibility of secondary causes. Symptoms include spasmodic cramping, originating centrally in the lower abdomen and radiating into the groin and thighs. Cramping begins immediately within a few hours prior to menstrual onset and lasts up to 36 hours, during the time when

Table 22-5 Complementary and Alternative Medicine for Premenstrual Syndrome

	Dose	Symptoms Relieved
Supplement		
Vitamin B_6 (pyridoxine)	50–100 mg/day	Mastalgia, swollen breasts, bloating, depression
Calcium carbonate	1200–1600 mg/day	Mood, water retention, food cravings
Magnesium	200–500 mg/day	Bloating during luteal phase
Herbal		
Chasteberry (*Vitex agnus-castus*)	20–40 mg/day	Breast engorgement, core symptoms

prostaglandin F2-alpha (PGF2α) release from the endometrium is highest. Elevated PGF2α produces enhanced uterine contractions, leading to hypoxia-associated pain. Low back pain, nausea, and diarrhea may be present.[25]

Treatment for dysmenorrhea includes the use of NSAIDs and, for women who desire contraception, either long-acting progesterone contraceptives or combined hormonal contraceptives. Table 22-6 lists appropriate drugs and their length of action. Menstrual pain unrelieved with these therapies should be referred for further evaluation.

Menopausal Symptoms

Menopause is a retrospective definition—only after 12 months without menstrual bleeding can the date of the last menses be stated. Average age for cessation of menses in the United States is 51. Primary ovarian insufficiency may cause amenorrhea before age 40 in 1% of women; when the

Table 22-6 NSAIDs for Management of Dysmenorrhea

Drug Name: Generic (Brand)	Dose/Route	Frequency	Onset/Peak	Duration
Acetylsalicylic acid (aspirin)	325–650 mg PO Do not exceed 4 g/day.	q 3–4 h	15–20 min/1–3 h	3–6 hours
Diclofenac potassium (Cataflam)	50 mg PO *Or* 100 mg loading dose followed by 50 mg q 8 h	3 times daily	30 minutes/1 h 2–3 h	8 hours
Ibuprofen (Advil, Motrin, Midol IB)			Varies/30 minutes/ 1 to 2 h	4–6 h
Ketoprofen (Orudis, Orudis KT)	25–50 mg PO	q 6–8 hours Maximum dose 300 mg/daily	30 minute/2 h 2–3 h/6–7 h	Up to 6 h Unknown
Naproxen (Naprosyn)	500 mg PO, then 250 mg PO	250–500 mg PO q 6–8 h up to 1000 mg to 1.25 g/daily	30–60 minutes/ 1 h/2–4 h	6–8 h
Naproxen sodium (Aleve)	550 mg PO, then 275 mg	275 mg PO q 6–8 h up to 1375 mg/ daily	1 h/1–4 h	7 h
Naproxen sodium (Naprelan)	Sustained-release formulation 375-mg or 500-mg tablets. Dose is 1000 mg PO.	Once daily	30–60 minutes/ 4–6 h with empty stomach; 12 h with food Peak unknown	Unknown

h = hours, PO = per os (by mouth), q = every

last menses occurs before age 40 due to surgical or natural causes, the term *premature menopause* is used. Early menopause, between ages 40 and 45, affects approximately 5% of women.[26] The term *menopause transition* can be used to describe the period between the first alteration in menstrual cycles and the final menses. The Stages of Reproductive Aging Workshop (STRAW) criteria for describing this transition from reproductive to post-reproductive life recognize a two-phase *perimenopause*.[27] In the first phase, menstrual cycles increasingly vary in length and amount, but ovulation and pregnancy may still occur. During this time, there is variability in FSH levels. In the 1 to 3 years immediately prior to menopause, intervals of amenorrhea commonly increase and may last more than 60 days, and vasomotor symptoms (flushing, hot flashes) increase. FSH level stabilizes above 25 international units/L. The early post-menopause phase, including the first year without menses, is the time when vasomotor symptoms are most likely.

During this transition, many physical, hormonal, and psychological changes begin. The North American Menopause Society (NAMS) recommendations for clinical care describe changes in every body system with aging.[26] The physical changes associated with aging are discussed elsewhere in this text. Here, the focus is on management of the symptoms experienced by many women during menopause. Loss of concentration and associated disruption of cognition, lack of sleep, and increased stress are common complaints during this time. Some women find that the vaginal atrophy and loss of lubrication associated with hormonal change decrease sexual satisfaction and libido; other women find liberation in knowing that pregnancy is no longer a concern.[27] Sexual activity continues long beyond menopause for more than 50% of all women.[28] Among women 65–74 years of age, two-thirds still believe sexual activity to be an important part of life, even as they report decreasing frequency and ability.[27]

Vasomotor symptoms are the most troubling part of this transition for many women. Hormonal instability triggers vasomotor changes that cause hot flashes and disrupt sleep. As estradiol decreases and estrone (a weaker estrogen) increases, norepinephrine production is stimulated. This leads to a narrower "thermo-neutral zone" and increased experience of both sweating and chills.[29] Up to 80% of women experience hot flashes.[30] Incidence is highest among African American women and lowest among Asians. Avis and colleagues reported that the average duration of significant vasomotor symptoms was greater than 7 years, with 4.5 years of symptoms occurring after the last menses. Early onset of symptoms during perimenopause and African American race were linked to longer duration in this study.[31] Moderate to severe vasomotor symptoms have been documented in women in their 60s.[32] Smoking and increased BMI are related to symptom severity.[33]

Atrophic changes and loss of pelvic support contribute to the condition previously referred to as vulvovaginal atrophy. The term *genitourinary syndrome of menopause* is currently preferred as being both more accurate and more acceptable. The NAMS definition includes changes to the labia, clitoris, vestibule, introitus, vagina, urethra, and bladder associated with decreased sex steroid production. Associated symptoms include genital dryness, burning, or irritation; decreased lubrication, pain, or discomfort associated with sexual activity; urinary symptoms such as urgency or dysuria; and recurrent urinary tract infections.[34]

Whether depression is caused by the menopausal transition is an open question. While most women do not meet criteria for depressive disorders, they may experience decreased sense of well-being or depressed mood. Certainly, the stressors of family and professional life are significant for women, many of whom will still be caring for children as their older relatives begin to need support. Physiologic changes, including vasomotor symptoms and insomnia may disrupt the sense of wellbeing. Some women find the physical and visible signs of aging to be distressing. Women with a history of depression are particularly at risk during this transition.

Specific care of the woman during menopause and beyond can include nonhormonal and complementary and alternative therapies for vasomotor and genitourinary symptoms, use of hormone-replacement therapy, and recommendations for counseling or treatment if depression, anxiety, or stress are affecting her ability to cope. Some of the choices for nonhormonal management of vasomotor symptoms are shown in **Table 22-7**. Herbal remedies are often sought by women who do not wish to take hormone therapy. Those most often used, regardless of their effectiveness, are listed in **Table 22-8**. Note that not all of these actually have a beneficial effect; while herbs are indeed medications, evidence of safety and efficacy is not universally available. This list is provided to assist in advising women about whether their preferred choice is safe and effective.

Women may also ask about bioidentical hormones as a way to treat menopause symptoms more naturally. Bioidentical hormones are plant compounds that contain hormonal equivalents of the prescriptive therapies, including any of the following: estriol, estrone, estradiol, testosterone, micronized progesterone, or dehydroepiandrosterone (DHEA).[35,36] These products are not regulated by the US Food and Drug Administration (FDA). As with many of the herbal products, there is little scientific evidence for safety and efficacy with these drugs. By one estimate, more than 2.5 million women choose to use these annually.[36] Prescribers should consider whether an FDA-approved product is available and suitable for women asking about herbal or compounded products and discuss the risks and benefits of various options.

Hormonal therapy for management of vasomotor symptoms, vaginal atrophy, and other problems associated with reproductive aging is a complex topic. Options include continuous cyclic combinations of estrogen and progestin or estrogen-only and progestin-only pills. Any women with a uterus should have both progestin and a systemic estrogen to help prevent endometrial hyperplasia.[37] The use of a progestin is not required when only vaginal estrogen is used, although some experts advocate for sonographic evaluation of endometrial lining when these are used for an extended duration. Recently, DHEA vaginal suppositories have been reported to be an additional therapy for pain and vaginal dryness and atrophy following menopause.[38]

Basic principles include starting as soon as symptoms are concerning to the woman with the lowest dose and for the shortest time appropriate to manage symptoms, switching to a vaginal formula if only genital symptoms are being treated, and counseling women accurately about the risks and benefits of extended therapy.[39] According to NAMS, "To maximize safety, the initiation of [hormone therapy] HT should be considered for healthy symptomatic women who are within 10 years of menopause or aged younger

Table 22-7 Nonhormonal Choices to Treat Vasomotor Symptoms

	Starting Dose
SSRI/SNRI	
Fluoxetine (Prozac)	20 mg/day
Paroxetine (Paxil)	12.5–25 mg/day
Venlafaxine (Effexor)	37.5–75 mg/day
Desvenlafaxine (Pristiq)	50–100 mg/day
Anticonvulsant	
Gabapentin (Neurontin)	300 mg/day at bedtime

SNRI = serotonin-norepinephrine reuptake inhibitor,
SSRI = selective serotonin reuptake inhibitor

Table 22-8 Herbal Remedies Used Most Often for Relief of Menopausal Symptoms

Herb	Proposed Effects on Menopausal Symptoms	Provision of Therapy	Clinical Summary
Black cohosh (*Cimicifuga racemosa*)	Diminishes hot flashes	20 mg twice/day of proprietary standardized extract; recommended dose of Remifemin supplement is 40–80 mg/day	Possible evidence of benefit for hot-flash relief. Most widely studied herb for menopausal symptoms, but recent studies have many methodological limitations. Much variation in brands and preparations.
Chasteberry (*Vitex agnus-castus*)	Diminishes PMS symptoms; regulates menses	250 mg of crude herb or 20 mg/day of 12:1 ratio of standardized extract	Evidence of benefit for PMS symptoms. Possible benefits for regulating irregular perimenopausal bleeding. Popular in Europe and approved therapy in Germany for PMS, mastalgia, and menopause symptoms.
Dong quai (*Angelica sinensis*)	Treats various gynecologic conditions; diminishes hot flashes	2 capsules 2–3 times/day	No data indicating effectiveness. Usually used in conjunction with other herbs. Can trigger heavy uterine bleeding; avoid in women with fibroids or coagulation problems.
Evening primrose oil (*Oenothera biennis*)	Diminishes hot flashes and breast tenderness	1500–4000 mg/day in divided doses	No data indicating effectiveness.
Gingko (*Gingko biloba*)	Promotes good memory	40–80 mg of standardized extract taken 3 times/day	No data indicating effectiveness. Potential safety concerns regarding increased bleeding, including subdural hematoma.
Ginseng (*Panax ginseng*)	Improves mood, minimizes fatigue	100–600 mg/day of standardized extract in divided doses	No data indicating effectiveness for hot flashes. Possible effectiveness for overall feelings of wellbeing. Significant problems with purity of preparations.
Kava (*Piper methysticum*)	Minimizes irritability, promotes sleep	150–300 mg of root extract per day in divided doses	Effective for treating anxiety, but effect is small. Possible hepatotoxicity; some experts recommend avoiding completely.

(continues)

Table 22-8 Herbal Remedies Used Most Often for Relief of Menopausal Symptoms (*continued*)

Herb	Proposed Effects on Menopausal Symptoms	Provision of Therapy	Clinical Summary
Licorice root (*Glycyrrhiza glabra*)	Diminishes hot flashes	5–15 mg/day of root equivalent in divided doses	No data indicating effectiveness. High doses or long-term use can cause HTN and kidney, liver, or cardiac dysfunction.
St. John's wort (*Hypericum perforatum*)	Diminishes hot flashes, decreases irritability, treats depression	300 mg of standardized extract taken 3 times/day	Evidence of benefit for mood stabilization. Mixed evidence for hot-flash relief. Sometimes used in conjunction with black cohosh. Do not use with SSRIs and certain other medications.
Valerian (*Valeriana officinalis*)	Promotes sleep; decreases anxiety	Insomnia: 300–600 mg aqueous extract 30–60 min before bed. Anxiety: 150–300 mg aqueous extract each morning and 300–400 mg each evening	Evidence of benefit for insomnia and anxiety. Few side effects at recommended dosages and with relatively short-term use.
Wild yam (*Dioscorea villosa*)	Diminishes hot flashes	Unknown	No demonstrated benefits. Wild yam cream does not convert to progesterone in the body as product manufacturers claim.

HTN = hypertension, PMS = premenstrual syndrome, SSRI = selective serotonin reuptake inhibitor.

Data from North American Menopause Society. *Menopause Practice: A Clinician's Guide.* 4th ed. Mayfield Heights, OH: North American Menopause Society; 2010; Guttuso T. Effective and clinically meaningful non-hormonal hot flash therapies. *Maturitas.* 2012;72:6-12; Andrews JC. Vasomotor symptoms: an evidence-based approach to medical management. *J Clin Outcome Manage.* 2011;18:112-118; Borrelli F, Ernst E. Alternative and complementary therapies for the menopause. *Maturitas.* 2010;66:333-343; Hall E, Frey BN, Soares CN. Non-hormonal treatment strategies for vasomotor symptoms: a critical review. *Drugs.* 2011;71:287-304; Panay N. Taking an integrated approach: managing women with phytoestrogens. *Climacteric.* 2011;14:2-7; Geller SE, Shulman LP, van Breemen RB, et al. Safety and efficacy of black cohosh and red clover for the management of vasomotor symptoms: a randomized controlled trial. *Menopause.* 2009;16:1156-1166; Darsareh F, Taavoni S, Joolaee S, Haghani H. Effect of aromatherapy massage on menopausal symptoms: a randomized placebo-controlled clinical trial. *Menopause.* 2012;19:995-9; Regestein QR. Is there anything special about valerian? *Menopause.* 2011;18:937-939; Taavoni S, Ekbatani N, Kashaniayn M, Haghani H. Effect of valerian on sleep quality in postmenopausal women: a randomized, placebo-controlled clinical trial. *Menopause.* 2011;18:951-955; Leach MJ, Moore V. Black cohosh (*Cimicifuga* spp.) for menopausal symptoms. *Cochrane Database Syst Rev.* 2012;9:CD007244. doi:10.1002/14651858.CD007244.pub2.

than 60 years and who do not have contraindications to use of HT."[40] Contraindications to estrogen-containing therapy include: undiagnosed abnormal bleeding (whether before or after menopause); history of, known, or suspected breast cancer; known or suspected estrogen-dependent malignancy; current or history of deep vein thrombosis or pulmonary embolism; current or recent stroke or heart attack; liver disease; or possible pregnancy. Smoking is not a contraindication.[37] Use of vaginal preparations containing estrogen does not carry the same level of risk. Women with risk factors who wish to use a topical or vaginal preparation should discuss this with a clinician experienced in management of menopause. Similarly, given that many women will still be symptomatic into their 60s, treatment should not be discontinued simply because of age.[41] Women wishing to continue systemic therapy should discuss this with an experienced clinician.[40,41]

Bleeding Disorders

Amenorrhea

Primary amenorrhea is defined as the absence of menarche by 15 years of age in a girl with normal growth and secondary sexual characteristics. *Secondary amenorrhea* is the absence of regular menses, once established, for more than 90 days or of irregularly cycling menses for 6 months. Although a 28-day cycle is average, significant variation can exist with a normally functioning HPO axis. Missing a single menses is part of normal variation, as is variable length of cycles (21–45 days in adolescents, 21–35 days in adult women). Very few women have clockwork cycles that never vary.

Many factors can precipitate amenorrhea, not the least of which are pregnancy and hormonal contraception. Amenorrhea not related to pregnancy, lactation, or menopause occurs in 3–4% of the reproductive-aged population.[42,43]

Anatomic abnormalities, ovarian failure, and anovulation resulting from endocrine disorders are the major categories identified.[44]

The history for a woman who complains of irregular or absent cycles includes age at menarche, her normal pattern, including whether any cyclic irregularity is present, and the length of her cycles (3–5 days is average, 2–7 days is normal). The history assesses for possible associations including family history of delayed menses; chemotherapy or radiation therapy; pituitary, hypothalamic, or adrenal disorders; chronic illness; sudden weight loss, eating disorders, or extremes of weight; exercise pattern; sexual activity; vasomotor symptoms; stress; and substance use.

Primary amenorrhea may be caused by hypothalamic disorders, hypothyroidism, androgen insensitivity, outflow tract anomalies such as imperforate hymen, transverse vaginal septum, or Mullerian agenesis/dysgenesis.[44] About 15% of women with primary amenorrhea will have an abnormal genital examination.[45]

Causes of secondary amenorrhea include eating disorders, stress, obesity, chronic or acute illness, rapid weight loss, drug use, thyroid or adrenal disease, prolactinomas and other pituitary tumors, ovarian tumors, premature menopause, and polycystic ovarian syndrome (PCOS). Eating disorders and the female athlete triad (low energy intake/disordered eating, amenorrhea, and osteoporosis) are common causes in otherwise normal young women. Even when young athletes do not have an eating disorder, increased exercise and low food intake can lead to development of this disorder.[46]

The initial evaluation for secondary amenorrhea includes a physical examination, but focuses on the laboratory results. On examination, the thyroid is palpated, and signs of hirsutism or acne (related to PCOS, adrenal disorders, and androgen excess), striae, and fat distribution (associated with Cushing's syndrome) are noted. A pregnancy test is always performed. TSH, FSH, and prolactin levels identify the most common causes.

In most cases, other symptoms of thyroid disease precede amenorrhea. A patient with elevated prolactin levels (especially if over 100 ng/mL), galactorrhea, headaches, or visual disturbances should receive magnetic resonance imaging (MRI) to rule out a pituitary tumor.[45,47,48] Pharmacologic causes of hyperprolactinemia include estrogens, opiates, some antipsychotics, antidepressants, and antihypertensives, among others.[49] FSH abnormalities can lead to diagnoses of premature ovarian failure or PCOS.

Reproductive-aged women with episodes of amenorrhea, who have been ruled out for pregnancy and have normal thyroid and pituitary function, can be given a progesterone challenge. Medroxyprogesterone acetate (Provera) 5–10 mg daily for 5–10 days or progesterone (Prometrium) 400 mg daily at bedtime for 10 days may be prescribed. The medication is taken only until menstrual bleeding begins. Resetting the hormonal cycle may resolve the problem. Recurrences should be evaluated for the underlying diagnosis. If there are no results, then further evaluation is necessary, and the woman should be referred for care.

Polycystic Ovarian Syndrome

PCOS is the most common endocrine disorder among reproductive-aged women, and the menstrual cycle abnormality most often linked to infertility.[50] The reported prevalence varies widely, depending on the choice of criteria, ranging from 6% to as high as 18% in some populations.[51] It is heterogeneous in severity and presentation and may display different phenotypes in different ethnic groups.[52] This heterogeneity may contribute to the frequent failure to assign a diagnosis, reported as being as high as 68% in one study comparing criteria for diagnosis.[51]

Characteristics of the condition include hyperandrogenism, ovulatory dysfunction, and/or polycystic ovaries seen on ultrasound.[53] At least two of the three must be present for the diagnosis to be made, and other conditions causing menstrual irregularity should be excluded. When considering PCOS as a diagnosis in adolescents, irregular or absent menses and laboratory evidence of hyperandrogenic state are required.[54] Multiple ovarian cysts may occur as a normal maturational finding.

Women may present with complaints of any or all of the following: amenorrhea or irregular menses, infertility, hirsutism, acne, oily skin, dandruff, obesity, and thinning hair.[55,56] Family history should be elicited, because PCOS tends to cluster in families; infertility, diabetes, and cardiac disease are all relevant. On examination, multiple skin tags and acanthosis nigricans may be noted. BMI and blood pressure are assessed. Waist circumference is obtained as part of the consideration of metabolic syndrome. As many as 80% of women with PCOS are obese, but this is not a requirement for diagnosis. Laboratory evaluation when PCOS is suspected includes FSH, TSH, prolactin, testosterone, dehydroepiandrosterone-sulfate, and 17-hydroxyprogesterone (17-OHP). Metabolic screening with a 2-hour glucose tolerance test and fasting insulin level may be considered.[56,57]

Some women go undiagnosed until infertility becomes a concern. Although the majority of women with PCOS are fertile, it is the single dominant cause of anovulatory infertility. Long-term consequences include psychological concerns affecting quality of life, such as anxiety, depression, or decreased self-esteem.[58,59] Metabolic manifestations include impaired glucose tolerance, insulin resistance, hyperinsulinemia, type 2 diabetes, dyslipidemia, metabolic syndrome, and obesity.[55] The rate of cardiovascular disease is increased among women with PCOS compared to women without the condition who have similar metabolic profiles.[60] Rates of spontaneous abortion, preeclampsia, preterm birth, and gestational diabetes are all increased among women with PCOS, even after controlling for the influence of obesity on pregnancy outcomes.[61,62] Time to conception and rates of preterm birth are increased among overweight versus normal-weight women with the condition.[63]

Women suspected of PCOS who do not desire pregnancy can consider combined hormonal contraception (CHC) for control of daily symptoms and menstrual regulation. Weight loss may help to regulate cycles and improve insulin resistance. It is possibly the single most useful strategy among obese women with PCOS. Metformin has been used to reduce insulin resistance, which can offer long-term health benefits and possibly assist with weight loss and return of normal ovulation. It is most effective when combined with a program of weight loss and increased physical activity.[64] If these methods are not effective, women should be referred for reproductive endocrine evaluation or be cared for by a clinician experienced in managing PCOS.

Abnormal Uterine Bleeding

Abnormal uterine bleeding (AUB) has been described in terms of the amount and irregularity of the menstrual flow. The historical terms are being replaced with plain English, as shown in **Table 22-9**.

Prevalence of bleeding abnormalities among reproductive-aged women has been estimated at 11–13% in the general population and increases with age, peaking around 24% in those ages 36–40 years.[65] The causes are varied. The definitive description of abnormal bleeding uses the consensus documents developed by the International Federation of Gynecology and Obstetrics (FIGO) and endorsed by ACOG.[66,67] This methodology, which distinguishes between structural and nonstructural causes, is shown in **Table 22-10**. AUB can also be described in terms of ovulatory and anovulatory causes. Ovulatory abnormalities are more common and may be endocrine or structural in nature; cycles are generally regular but heavy or prolonged.[67] Anovulatory causes are associated with bleeding that is irregular in amount, frequency, and duration.

Because the underlying causes of chronic AUB are so diverse—ranging from hypo- or hyperthyroid conditions to structural problems, to

---

Table 22-9 Terminology to Describe Abnormal Uterine Bleeding (AUB)

- *Irregular menstrual bleeding*: variation > 20 days during a 1-year period
- *Absent menstrual bleeding (amenorrhea)*: no bleeding for > 90 days
- *Infrequent menstrual bleeding*: < 3 episodes within 90 days
- *Frequent menstrual bleeding*: > 4 episodes within 90 days
- *Heavy menstrual bleeding*: excessive menstrual blood loss that interferes with any aspect of a woman's quality of life; may occur alone or in combination with other symptoms
- *Prolonged menstrual bleeding*: menses lasting more than 8 days on a regular basis
- *Acute AUB*: an episode of bleeding in a non-pregnant woman of reproductive age sufficient to require immediate intervention
- *Chronic AUB*: uterine bleeding that is abnormal in duration, volume, and/or frequency that has been present for most of the last 6 months

Data from Munro MG, Critchley HO, Broder MS, Fraser IS, FIGO Working Group on Menstrual Disorders. FIGO classification system (PALM-COEIN) for causes of abnormal uterine bleeding in nongravid women of reproductive age. *Int J Gynaecol Obstet*. 2011;113(1):3-13; Fraser IS, Critchley HOD, Broder M, Munro MG. The FIGO recommendations on terminologies and definitions for normal and abnormal uterine bleeding. *Semin Reprod Med*. 2011;29:383-390.

Table 22-10 PALM-COEIN

PALM (structural)	**P**olyp
	Adenomyosis
	Leiomyoma
	Malignancy/hyperplasia
COEIN (nonstructural)	**C**oagulopathy (medication, genetic, or acquired)
	Ovulatory dysfunction
	Endometrial
	Iatrogenic
	Not yet classified

Data from Munro MG, Critchley HO, Broder MS, Fraser IS; FIGO Working Group on Menstrual Disorders. FIGO classification system (PALM-COEIN) for causes of abnormal uterine bleeding in nongravid women of reproductive age. *Int J Gynaecol Obstet.* 2011;113(1):3-13.

disruption of the HPO axis, to coagulation disorders, to endometrial cancer—the initial evaluation must address a broad differential. Evaluation for AUB begins with a history that elicits not only the current symptoms but seeks for historical associations. A complete menstrual, sexual, and gynecologic history is obtained. Family menstrual information is requested, particularly age at menarche and menopause for first-degree relatives, as well as any reproductive system problems or diagnoses. The medical history seeks clues to possible medical conditions affecting the HPO axis or blood clotting. Details of the abnormal bleeding include onset, pattern, amount, hemorrhagic events, whether clots or tissue were passed, any accidents where pads or tampons overflowed, and any premenstrual or menstrual symptoms including back pain or pelvic fullness. Symptoms of anemia and those of chronic illness should be assessed during the review of systems. Headaches, changes in mood or libido, blurred vision, changes in head or facial/body hair, skin changes or acne lesions, vocal changes, difficulty in swallowing or neck pain, sudden weight changes, temperature intolerance, and bowel or bladder function are questioned. Medication or alternative therapies are determined.[68,69] A complete gynecologic examination as described earlier in this chapter is performed. The evaluation for AUB including laboratory and imaging studies is outlined in **Table 22-11** and discussed in the paragraphs that follow.

The laboratory tests are ordered based on a differential created from the history, examination, and initial blood work. All women with a new complaint of AUB should have a pregnancy test, CBC, and thyroid screen. Other tests that can be considered based on the amount and timing of menstrual flow include FSH, LH, prolactin, and serial progesterone levels. All adolescents and women with a history of bleeding abnormalities should be screened with thrombin and partial thromboplastin time, and for von Willebrand's factor deficiency if that test is readily available.[70,71] Liver function and ferritin may also be considered.[68] Transvaginal ultrasound (TVUS) is recommended by ACOG as the first-line study.[67] While TVUS is readily available and safe, it may miss up to 18% of lesions.[69] It is performed on days 4–6 of the menstrual cycle, when an endometrial depth of < 4 mm is considered normal.[72] Endometrial biopsy is indicated in women over 45 as a first-line test.[67] Some clinicians may choose saline-infused sonohysterography rather than TVUS in order to maximize identification of lesions in the uterine cavity.[67,69]

Menorrhagia is excessive blood flow; for research purposes, this is defined as 80 mL/cycle—not the way women evaluate menstrual flow.[73] To evaluate for menorrhagia in the nonacute setting, the following data are collected: whether this is a new event or longstanding; a description of how many days the menses last and how many have heavy flow; how often a pad or tampon is changed and which size is used; and clotting, color, and duration of heavy flow. Women should

Table 22-11 Assessment of Abnormal Uterine Bleeding

Etiologies	Investigation
Polyp Adenomyosis Leiomyoma Malignancy and hyperplasia	History: • Risk factors • Physical exam Imaging studies: • Ultrasound • MRI • Endometrial biopsy
Coagulopathy Ovulatory dysfunction Endometrial Iatrogenic Not yet classified	History: • Risk factors • Hormonal contraception (i.e., use, misusing, or discontinued) • Intrauterine contraception (history of use) Laboratory studies: • Endocrine: TSH, prolactin • Hormones: FSH, LH • Coagulation indices • Pregnancy test • Endometrial biopsy

FSH = follicle-stimulating hormone, LH = luteinizing hormone, MRI = magnetic resonance imaging, TSH = thyroid-stimulating hormone.

Data from Munro MG, Critchley HO, Broder MS, Fraser IS; FIGO Working Group on Menstrual Disorders. FIGO classification system (PALM-COEIN) for causes of abnormal uterine bleeding in nongravid women of reproductive age. *Int J Gynaecol Obstet.* 2011;113(1):3-13.

be asked about how the bleeding affects their personal life, work, or school. As many as 13% of women with heavy menstrual bleeding have von Willebrand disease, while 17–20% may have an underlying coagulation disorder.[69,74] In contrast, many women who report heavy flows have a few hours or single day in which bleeding is symptomatic. In the absence of anemia or acute blood loss, menstrual control with hormonal contraceptives may be all that is needed.

In the first 2 years following menarche, most adolescents will not have achieved regular ovulation, and up to 50% of cycles in the first year will be anovulatory.[75] Thus, most heavy bleeding in the early years following menarche is essentially normal unless heavy enough to cause

symptomatic anemia.[72] When an adolescent has had persistently heavy menses since menarche and is having regular, ovulatory cycles, 65% will have a bleeding disorder.[76] Either contraceptive medication for control of menstruation or NSAIDs can be offered.

New-onset bleeding, especially if intermenstrual, in a woman with established regular cycles may represent early pregnancy or an infection such as cervicitis, salpingitis, or endometritis. A pregnancy test and screening for *Chlamydia trachomatis, Neisseria gonorrhoeae,* and *Trichomonas* are indicated.

If acute-onset bleeding is sufficient to cause severe anemia or hypovolemia, the initial evaluation is directed toward fluid resuscitation and blood product replacement, while the history, examination, and laboratory testing are used to assess for alternative sources of bleeding and for the causes of chronic AUB.[77] Women with a positive pregnancy test and vaginal bleeding should immediately be referred to an obstetric provider. When pain is also present, the referral is made on an emergent basis, because an evaluation for ectopic pregnancy is essential and required immediately.

Medications, whether prescriptive or herbal, can lead to bleeding abnormalities. Hormonal contraceptives, anticoagulants, SSRIs, antipsychotics, tamoxifen, and herbals (e.g., ginseng) have all been implicated.

Once the evaluation is complete, management of idiopathic heavy menstrual bleeding can include use of long-acting progesterone contraceptives (IUD, implant), combined hormonal contraceptives, or progesterone, with or without estrogen or NSAIDs.[68,69] If the heavy flow is limited to the first days of otherwise normal menses and the woman does not desire contraception, NSAIDs taken during the first 3 days of the menses may help. If these do not resolve the problem, the woman should be referred for further evaluation.

Bleeding that occurs more than 12 months following cessation of menses is always abnormal. It can represent transient scant bleeding as the endometrium atrophies, but the greater risk is for premalignant endometrial hyperplasia and uterine cancer. Up to 14% of postmenopausal bleeding is associated with cancer diagnoses. TVUS evaluation for hyperplasia of the endometrium is the initial screen.[78] Endometrial thickness of 4 mm or less effectively excludes malignancy.[79]

Evaluation of Pelvic Pain

Pelvic pain is a common complaint among reproductive-aged and elder women. Acute pain may be associated with an early pregnancy, in which case normal corpus luteum development, ectopic pregnancy, or spontaneous loss may be the cause. In the second and early third trimesters, stretching of the round ligaments as the uterus enlarges also may produce discomfort. Acute pain may also herald pelvic inflammatory disease, endometritis, or ovarian torsion. Nongynecologic causes of acute pain such as appendicitis and bladder infection are discussed elsewhere in this text.

In contrast, chronic pelvic pain is experienced by between 5.7% and 26.6% of women.[80] Vulvodynia, adenomyosis, and endometriosis are common causes of chronic pain, as are pelvic adhesions after surgery or infection and uterine or ovarian masses.[81] Pain may be cyclic or constant; sharp, dull, or cramping; and unilateral, central, or diffuse. Dyspareunia, pain with intercourse, is multifactorial and overlaps with diagnoses such as endometriosis and vulvodynia. Reproductive and nonreproductive causes of pelvic pain are listed in **Tables 22-12, 22-13**, and **22-14**.

The essential history and examination for pelvic pain include the standard questions for evaluating symptoms:

- Onset
- Location and extent
- Timing and duration
- Character
- Aggravating factors
- Associated symptoms
- How relief is obtained
- Impact on daily life

An abdominal and a pelvic examination are required. A pregnancy test is always performed unless the woman is more than 12 months post menopause. Additional laboratory and imaging studies address the suspected diagnosis. Testing for urinary tract infections and sexually transmitted infections (STIs) is often appropriate and should be performed when the suspicion of an infectious cause arises. Transvaginal and abdominal ultrasound are the first-line imaging studies for pelvic pain when a gynecologic or obstetric cause is suspected, because the reproductive organs can be readily seen.[82] MRI and computerized tomography (CT) are used when initial results are unclear or a gastrointestinal or urologic source of pain is suspected. CT is preferred except during pregnancy, when MRI is preferred due to lack of radiation exposure.[82]

Table 22-12 Reproductive System Causes of Pelvic Pain

Diagnosis	Presenting/Clinical Features
Gynecologic	
Dysmenorrhea	Pain just prior to and during menstrual period
Endometriosis	Dysmenorrhea, irregular menses
Endometritis	Febrile, tender uterus, usually post-procedure or postpartum
Functional ovarian cyst	Aching or sharp, intermittent pain
Leiomyoma	Menorrhagia, solid uterus mass seen on ultrasound
Mittelschmerz	Sharp unilateral pain around time of ovulation
Ovarian torsion	Sudden onset of extreme pain in lower abdomen that radiates to back, side, and thigh
Physiologic/functional cyst	Premenopausal, fluid-filled unilocular cyst without solid component seen on ultrasound
Ruptured ovarian cyst	Sudden, intense unilateral pain
Pelvic inflammatory disease	Acute pain on examination, purulent cervical discharge
Tubo-ovarian abscess	Abdominal or pelvic pain, fever, elevated white blood cell count, complex mass seen on ultrasound
Primary ovarian malignancy	Ascites, solid or complex ovarian mass seen on ultrasound
Obstetric	
Corpus luteum of pregnancy	Dull or sharp one-sided pain in the first trimester of pregnancy
Ectopic pregnancy	Missed period, positive hCG, empty uterus, complex mass on ultrasound, vaginal bleeding
Round ligament pain	Sharp or pulling pain, unilateral or bilateral, associated with uterine enlargement
Spontaneous abortion	Crampy or severe central pain, associated with bleeding
Theca lutein cyst	Very high hCG, multiple gestation, or trophoblastic disease

hCG = human chorionic gonadotropin

Data from Kriebs JM. Common conditions in primary care. In: King TL, Brucker MC, Kriebs JM, Fahey JO, Gegor CL, Varney H. *Varney's Midwifery.* 5th ed. Burlington, MA: Jones & Bartlett Learning; 2015:219-263; Raughley, MJ. Abdominal pain and masses in pregnancy. In: Angelini DJ, LaFontaine D, eds. *Obstetric Triage and Emergency Protocols.* New York, NY: Springer Publishing Company; 2012.

Table 22-13 Causes of Painful Intercourse

Lack of libido or arousal

Decreased vaginal lubrication due to decreased estrogen (e.g., with age, breastfeeding)

Vaginismus

Partner factors (rushed or rough intercourse)

History of sexual abuse or trauma

Vaginal or vulvar infections, especially *Candida* and herpes simplex virus

Vulvar dermatoses

Allergy to latex, vaginal hygiene preparation, or other substance

Fear of pregnancy or contraceptive failure

History of infertility

Uterine prolapse

Anatomic malformation (e.g., vaginal septum)

Vaginal scarring, as with episiotomy or laceration during childbirth

History of hysterectomy (vaginal shortening or narrowing)

Endometriosis

Fibroid uterus

Ovarian cysts

Retroflexed uterus

Pelvic adhesions

Medications, including some antidepressants, antihypertensives, antihistamines, and oral contraceptives

Radiation therapy

Table 22-14 Nonreproductive Causes of Abdominal Pain

Aortic dissection

Appendicitis

Ulcer

Diverticulosis

Irritable bowel syndrome

Inflammatory bowel disease

Bowel obstruction

Constipation

Cystitis

Cholecystitis

Pancreatitis

Pyelonephritis

Renal stones

Gastroenteritis

Strangulated hernia

Data from Kriebs JM. Common conditions in primary care. In: King TL, Brucker MC, Kriebs JM, Fahey JO, Gegor CL, Varney H. *Varney's Midwifery.* 5th ed. Burlington, MA: Jones & Bartlett Learning; 2015:219-263; Flasar MH, Goldberg E. Acute abdominal pain. *Med Clin North Am.* 2006;90(3):481-503.

Ovarian Torsion

In ovarian torsion, the ovary, the fallopian tube, or both twist on the vascular pedicle resulting in arterial, venous, or lymphatic obstruction; ischemia and ovarian infarction; and massive ovarian edema. It is a surgical emergency requiring prompt intervention to preserve fertility.

Ovarian torsion has been estimated to represent between 2.5% and 7.4% of all acute gynecologic emergencies, although the true incidence may be even higher.[83] Ovarian torsion is often associated with ovarian cysts, primarily dermoid cysts.[84] Additional predisposing factors include an enlarged ovary, such as with PCOS; excess length of fallopian tube or utero-ovarian ligaments; ovarian hyperstimulation; pelvic inflammatory disease; and a history of pelvic surgery, such as a tubal ligation or laparoscopic hysterectomy.[83-85] The most common age for diagnosis is before 30 years; 70–80% of torsions occur during the reproductive years.[86] However, prepubescent girls and postmenopausal women may also experience torsion. Approximately 12–25% of ovarian torsions occur during pregnancy.[86] Torsion during pregnancy is most common before the third trimester; occurrence decreases when abdominal space is more compressed.[85]

The most common symptom of ovarian torsion is the abrupt onset of extreme sharp or colicky pain in the lower abdomen radiating to the side of the affected tube. About two-thirds of torsion events are located at the right adnexa. The pain may radiate to the flank, back, thigh, or groin and increases in severity over time. Nausea, diarrhea, constipation, and vomiting may occur along with urinary frequency and urgency.

Physical examination reveals rigidity of the abdomen and rebound tenderness. A tender, palpable mass and cervical motion tenderness may be noted on vaginal exam. Laboratory findings may reveal leukocytosis. The use of color Doppler during TVUS is the most reliable technique for diagnosis, but is limited by the fact that blood flow to the ovary may persist in more than 50% of cases. Laparoscopy both confirms the diagnosis and allows the surgeon to untwist the adnexa in an effort to preserve fertility. Viability of the ovary is determined by the absence of ischemia. A resection or excision is performed when ischemia is present or a lesion is present.

Vulvodynia

Vulvodynia is vulvar discomfort, usually a burning pain, lasting at least 3 months, when neither visible lesions nor a neurologic diagnosis can be found.[87] Pain may be generalized or localized to a single area, be persistent (unprovoked), occur in response to stimuli (provoked), or may be mixed in type.[87] Lifetime prevalence is at least 8%.[88] Other estimates reported range from 10% to 28% for any occurrence of pain consistent with

vulvodynia.[89] The condition is more prevalent among Hispanics than white women and less prevalent among African American women.[90,91] Provoked vulvodynia is reported to be the most common cause of sexual pain in women under 30 years of age.[92] In one study, urogenital symptoms, other comorbid pain conditions, posttraumatic stress disorder, and sleep disturbances were found to be risk factors. Associated symptoms include pain after intercourse, current pain with intercourse, or history of vulvar pain and urinary burning.[91] Remaining sexually active despite symptoms is common, although frequency may be decreased, as is pleasure. Alternatives to vaginal intercourse, such as receptive oral sex or masturbation, may be less likely to elicit pain.[93]

The derivation of the condition is unclear and may involve local or central sensitization of the nerves. Alternatively, it may be a somatization syndrome without obvious neurologic injury or deficit.[94] Potential influences or predisposing factors include inflammatory or immunologic responses, infections, levels of sex hormones, genetics, psychological factors, and pelvic floor abnormalities. An association with sexual abuse as a child or adult has been debated.[94] Because many women with vulvodynia have other urogenital conditions and may have been treated for vulvovaginal candidiasis repeatedly without benefit, vulvodynia becomes a diagnosis of exclusion.[90]

Evaluation includes screening for bladder, vaginal, and vulvar infections; vulvar dermatoses; prior injury or abuse; and neurologic disease. Eliciting specific point pain can assist the diagnosis. A soft cotton swab is used to press gently along the labia majora, interlabial sulcus, perineum, prepuce, labia minora, and clitoris, followed by the vulvar vestibule at the 2:00, 4:00, 6:00, 8:00, and 10:00 positions.[94] Abnormal sensation along the labia minora with normal sensation elsewhere suggests vulvodynia.[94] A pediatric speculum inserted without contact with the vestibule is used to inspect the vagina and cervix. Bimanual examination may also require use of a single finger to avoid triggering pain.

One subset of vulvodynia, *vestibulodynia* (also called vulvar vestibulitis or vestibular adenitis) is provoked by pain associated with entry into the vagina, such as by tampons, speculum, or sexual activity, and limited to the vestibule. Inflammation and tenderness to palpation of the vestibule are characteristic.

Management of vulvodynia can require multiple trials to determine the most effective relief. Educating the woman and her partner and providing reassurance that this is not "all in her head" are essential, as is offering sexual or personal counseling to help her cope with the stress and depression that often accompany chronic pain. Multiple trials may be necessary to identify what works best. Lifestyle modifications to avoid possible chemical or mechanical irritants can be recommended, such as choosing loose clothing, unscented mild soaps, and showering rather than bathing. Biofeedback, cognitive behavioral therapy, and pelvic floor physical therapy all may be of benefit. Use of topical lidocaine (5% ointment or 2% gel) or EMLA (lidocaine 2.5% and prilocaine 2.5%) cream may make sexual activity less unpleasant, although women may experience side effects including burning or numbness, as may their partners. Overnight use of lidocaine 5% applied to the vulva and inserted into the vestibule on a cotton swab has also been shown to provide some relief. Acupuncture and hypnosis have also been studied and are low-risk adjuncts to therapy.[93,94]

Antidepressants have been used in treating vulvodynia and other neuropathic pain syndromes.[94] The tricyclics amitriptyline, nortriptyline, and desipramine have been used, as well as venlafaxine and duloxetine. If none of these has proven beneficial, referral to a provider skilled in gynecologic pain management should be made. It has been pointed out that overall success in treating vulvodynia hovers around 50%, suggesting that continued exploration of multidisciplinary approaches to this complicated gynecologic problem is needed.[95]

Dyspareunia

Pain during intercourse has many causes, ranging from latex allergies and vaginal *Candida* infections to a history of sexual trauma, decreased libido, or a loss of lubrication after menopause. *Dyspareunia* is the general term for pain that occurs as part of the act of intercourse—before, during, or after penetration. Prevalence estimates are between 10% and 20% of all US women.[96,97] The history of when and how pain occurs should be collected privately unless the woman indicates, when she is alone with her clinician, that she would like to have her partner present. No clinician should ever make assumptions about the factors affecting a woman's experience of sexual intercourse or imply in any way that it is not a real physical symptom. This is a topic that is often stigmatizing and painful to discuss. Gentle questioning and an assurance that a solution will be found eventually are important.

The history of this complaint includes specifics of when the pain begins during the sex act; where it is located; and whether it is cramping, burning, itchy, or sharp. Further, it is important to ask if this is a new problem or a persistent one, whether it happens with all partners and in all situations, and whether the physical position affects the pain. The physical examination should begin with careful inspection of the external genitalia and progress with the use of a small speculum to visualize the vagina and cervix. If the woman is tense or experiencing vaginismus, use of a pediatric or vaginal speculum may be necessary for her to tolerate the examination.

The bimanual should be performed initially with a single digit, again to reduce pressure and pain during the examination. This can be followed with the usual bimanual examination to more fully assess the pelvic organs, if she is able to tolerate the examination.

Vaginismus has been described as physical, involuntary contraction of the pelvic floor muscles that restricts penetration of the vagina.[98] The *Diagnostic and Statistical Manual of Mental Disorders* (DSM-5) links vaginismus, dyspareunia, and provoked vestibulodynia under a single diagnosis, genito-pelvic pain/penetration disorder.[99] Diagnosis requires persistence for 6 months and 75–100% occurrence. Women with a diagnosis of vaginismus experience more fear and pelvic muscle tension than those with the other diagnoses, although there is not a clear dividing line.[100] This makes clinical diagnosis of vaginismus based on examination difficult. One possible discriminator during history taking is to assess whether women complaining of long-standing pain with intercourse persist in (i.e., continue to voluntarily participate in) or avoid intercourse due to fear. The former is more likely to be dyspareunia; the latter, vaginismus.[101] While this does not resolve the problem, it may provide clues to next steps in counseling and care. It is also important to realize that these diagnoses are part of the *mental* health system and do not address the gynecologic causes of sexual pain or discomfort.

A partial list of causes of vulvar and vaginal pain associated with intercourse is provided in **Table 22-15**. Not all are dyspareunia, but the differential should consider a broad range of possibilities. Treatment depends on the underlying issue. If the experience of sex is painful and no physical or historical reason can be found, referral to an experienced practitioner, whether in gynecologic pain management or sexual health, is appropriate.

Table 22-15 Causes of Pain During Intercourse

Herpes genitalis

Candidal vulvovaginitis

Genital warts

Lichen sclerosus

Lichen planus

Pelvic inflammatory disease

Vulvodynia

Vaginal injury from trauma, childbirth, or surgery

Fear of pregnancy

History of infertility

History of sexual assault or abuse

Lack of vaginal lubrication (lack of arousal)

Vaginal atrophy

Allergy to latex or spermicide

Advancing pregnancy

Pelvic organ prolapse

Uterine Abnormalities

Congenital Uterine Abnormalities (CUA)

The reproductive organs form from the Müllerian ducts during the embryologic period. Disruptions of this process lead to a variety of abnormalities in the shape of the uterus, cervix, and vagina. The American Fertility Society describes seven categories of congenital abnormalities: hypoplasia/agenesis (absent development), unicornuate uterine cavity, uterine didelphys (complete duplication of cervix, uterus, and tube), bicornuate uterus with division above the cervix, and septate, arcuate, or T-shaped uterine cavities.[102] **Figure 22-4** depicts common malformations of the uterus.

Figure 22-4 Common uterine abnormalities.

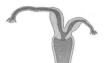

Communicating unicornuate: rudimentary horn with an endometrial cavity that communicates with the single-horned uterus. The chances of infertility, endometriosis, and dysmenorrhea are increased with this anatomic condition.

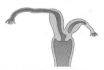

Noncommunicating unicornuate: rudimentary horn with an endometrial cavity that does not communicate with the single-horned uterus.

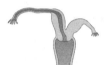

Unicornuate: Rudimentary horn with no endometrial cavity.

Unicornuate: no rudimentary horn.

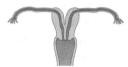

Didelphus: two separate cavities, each with its own cervix.

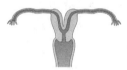

Complete bicornuate uterus: two separate uterine cavities separated by myometrial tissue and one cervix. It is estimated that 60% of women with a bicornuate uterus can maintain a pregnancy, although prior reconstructive surgery may be required to do so, and the risks of a spontaneous abortion or a preterm delivery are higher than those in women without this anatomic condition.

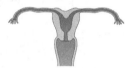

Partial bicornuate uterus: the septum is confined to the fundus.

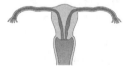

Complete septate: The septum extends into the internal cervical os. The septate uterus has two cavities separated by avascular tissue and one cervix. While individuals with a septate uterus can become pregnant, the outcome is often a spontaneous abortion or a fetus with growth malformations.

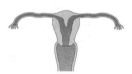

Partial septate: The septum does not reach the internal os.

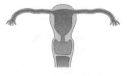

Transverse vaginal septa:

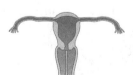

Vertical vaginal septa:

Data from American Fertility Society. The American Fertility Society classifications of adnexal adhesions, distal tubal occlusion, tubal occlusion secondary to tubal ligation, tubal pregnancies, Müllerian anomalies and intrauterine adhesions. *Fertil Steril.* 1988;49:944-955.

One systematic review including 94 observational studies put the cumulative prevalence of CUA at 5.5% in an unselected population, rising to 24.5% among women experiencing both infertility and recurrent miscarriage.[103] In another series of women recruited at random to be evaluated for CUA, the overall rate was 9.8%.[104]

History may suggest a uterine structural abnormality. Examples include absence of menarche in the presence of sexual maturity (e.g., absent cervix) or when pain occurs with menses (noncommunicating uterine horn). In most cases, women will not display symptoms. These structural issues can complicate the gynecologic examination and contribute to obstetric complications. For example, an infection in one side of a duplicate cervix might not be picked up if the examiner only noted and evaluated one side. Infertility and obstetric outcomes can be affected by uterine shape and patency. When speculum and bimanual examination suggest a structural concern, imaging should be ordered to further evaluate the anatomy.

Initial imaging for CUA includes ultrasound, which is readily available but limited in women with high BMI or overlying bowel gas, and may have limited ability to visualize the shape of the uterus. Three-dimensional ultrasound improves the assessment of structure.[105] Hysterosalpingoscopy permits evaluation of the uterine cavity and tubal patency.[106] MRI has high clinical correlation and excellent ability to characterize uterine structure. It is the standard diagnostic imaging modality.[107,108]

The nature of the structural problem dictates next steps. For asymptomatic women who do not desire pregnancy in the near future, a discussion with an experienced gynecologic specialist may suffice to discuss possible risks and complications. Women with pain from outflow tract abnormalities require surgical intervention. If pregnancy is in a woman's plans, then consultation with an obstetrician to discuss possible

complications is essential. CUAs have been associated with a decreased pregnancy rate; increased risk of spontaneous abortion; increased rates of preterm delivery, low birth weight, and perinatal mortality; and increased rate of malpresentation at delivery.[109,110]

Uterine Fibroids

Leiomyomas, or fibroids, are benign smooth-muscle neoplasms. The uterus is a common location, along with the small bowel and esophagus. In the uterus they may be termed *myomas* or *fibromyomas*. Incidence increases with age until menopause. Estimated prevalence among women over 30 years is 20–50%. An ultrasound study has reported cumulative incidence of myomas by age 50 years to be > 80% for black women and nearly 70% for white women.[111] Both estrogen and progesterone stimulate fibroid growth, explaining their rarity before menarche and regression post menopause. African American women have a significantly greater incidence of fibroids, higher numbers of fibroids, and greater total uterine weight, compared to white women.[112,113] Other risk factors include high BMI and factors that increase exposure to estrogen such as nulliparity and early menarche.[114,115] Parity is protective in the same way that CHC may be, by reducing overall estrogen stimulus.[114,116] Other research has not reported a reduction in incidence with CHC but found a significant reduction in risk associated with the use of progestin-only contraception, specifically Norplant.[117] The data on the influence of smoking are contradictory, but smoking may decrease the incidence of fibroids.[111,114]

The majority of fibroids remain asymptomatic and are an incidental finding on routine examination, either in the office or on ultrasound. The most common symptom of fibroids is heavy or prolonged menstrual bleeding, which may be sufficient to lead to symptomatic anemia. They are the "L" (for leiomyoma) in the PALM-COEIN system for describing AUB. "Bulk" symptoms caused by large fibroids include difficulty with urination (either frequency or difficulty with voiding) or with bowel function, and a swollen abdomen that may give the appearance of pregnancy. Some women complain of dysmenorrhea, often persisting throughout the menses, or of persistent pelvic or lower abdominal pain. An increased risk of miscarriage or difficulty conceiving may be seen.[118] Pregnancy outcomes may be adversely affected by large fibroids; increased rates of cesarean birth, malpresentation, and preterm births have been reported.[119,120] In one large international survey, more than 50% of women with diagnosed fibroids reported negative effects on their personal relationships or professional lives.[121]

Fibroid location within the uterus varies. *Subserosal* fibroids are located in the external layer of uterine tissue, the serosa or perimetrium, and may develop outward from a central stalk, in which case they are called pedunculated fibroids. *Intramural* fibroids are located within the muscle wall (myometrium) of the uterus, while *submucosal* fibroids lie next to the uterine cavity, just under the mucosal (endometrial) layer. (See **Figure 22-5**.)

When the history suggests fibroids, abdominal palpation for uterine enlargement is documented. The pelvic examination includes careful delineation of uterine shape and size, as well as recto-vaginal assessment of the posterior wall of the uterus for masses. Ultrasound is the initial imaging strategy, because it will distinguish between pregnancy, fibroids, and ovarian masses as potential causes of an enlarged uterus. Laboratory assessment includes a CBC, and, if indicated, a pregnancy test. Thyroid function testing and evaluation for bleeding disorders may be warranted in select cases.[118] Endometrial biopsy is indicated when the woman is 45 or older, has irregular bleeding, or when the risk of hyperplasia is increased as with obesity or anovulation. Prior to discussing treatments, saline hysterography or

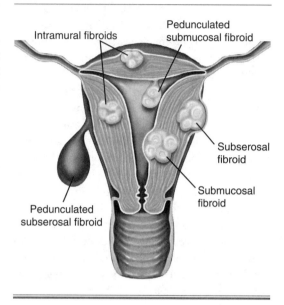

Figure 22-5 Uterine fibroid types.

MRI may be indicated to evaluate the placement, size, and vascularity of fibroids.[121]

The treatment of fibroids is dependent on the degree of symptoms and the woman's preference for maintaining fertility; asymptomatic fibroids do not require therapy although their growth should be monitored over time with clinical and ultrasound evaluation. Women whose only complaint is heavy or prolonged menstrual bleeding may opt for progestin-containing IUDs or combined contraceptives. If an IUD is chosen, she should be counseled about an increased expulsion rate (12% in one study) among women with submucosal fibroids,[122] and the potential need for future surgery. Hysterectomy is the definitive procedure and prevents recurrence and is reported to improve quality of life, although the rates of reported complications are high.[121] Some women will be given GnRH agonists prior to surgery to induce amenorrhea, shrink tumor size, and decrease risk of adverse events. The procedure can be performed either abdominally or vaginally and as an open or laparoscopic procedure.[121] For women who wish to retain fertility, myomectomy and uterine artery embolization are alternatives.[123] These and other techniques require medical participation in care. With the exception of women with small fibroids whose only complaints are related to heavy menstrual bleeding, women with symptomatic fibroids should be offered consultation with a gynecologic surgeon to discuss surgical and medical approaches to fibroid management.

Leiomyosarcoma

Sarcomas are soft tissue cancers, and uterine leiomyosarcomas are a rare but significant finding following surgery for uterine fibroids. In one recent series, the reported rate of all uterine sarcomas among women with surgical removal of fibroids was 0.29% (an incidence of 1 out of 335 women);[124] in another, the rate specifically for leiomyosarcoma diagnosed on pathology when benign fibroids were anticipated was 0.54% (1 out of 183 women).[125]

Abnormalities of the Endometrium

Growth of endometrial tissue beyond the uterine lining may present as adenomyosis or endometriosis. *Hyperplasia* is the overgrowth of endometrial tissue within the uterine cavity. Among the structural causes of AUB, adenomyosis is the "A" in PALM-COEIN and endometrial hyperplasia is, as part of the spectrum leading to endometrial cancer, included in the "M." Endometriosis falls within the nonstructural causes as part of the endometrial "E."

Adenomyosis

Adenomyosis is defined as growth of endometrial tissue into the myometrium. The invasion by endometrial glands and stroma may lead to hypertrophy of the myometrium. It may be diffuse—evenly distributed throughout—or focal—occurring in nodular lesions or adenomyomas. It is most commonly diagnosed among women in their 40s. Estimates of prevalence have been as low as 1% and as high as 70%, although the reported range based on hysterectomy specimens is between 20% and 30%.[126,127] Risk factors include early menarche, higher parity, short menstrual cycles, use of combined oral contraceptives, prior uterine surgery, and overweight and obesity.[127,128]

In the reproductive history, infertility may be reported. Symptoms include heavy menstrual bleeding, dysmenorrhea, painful intercourse, and chronic pelvic pain; uterine enlargement or tenderness may be found on examination. The uterus is generally described as being globular and is rarely larger than 12 weeks size.[129] Diagnosis is complicated, because similar signs and symptoms may be produced by endometriosis, uterine fibroids, endometrial cancer, and ovarian masses.[130]

When adenomyosis is suspected, TVUS is the first-line diagnostic method. MRI provides more detail, but is too costly to be an ideal first-line tool. A systematic review found both to be reliable diagnostic methods, with MRI having greater specificity.[131]

Therapy for adenomyosis includes CHC, depot medroxyprogesterone (Depo-Provera), and the levonorgestrel intrauterine system (LNG-IUS; Mirena). Of these, the LNG-IUS is considered most effective.[132,133] Other fertility-sparing treatments include NSAIDs, tranexamic acid (a fibrinolytic agent used to promote normal clotting), and GnRH agonists. Tranexamic acid cannot be used in women on estrogen-containing contraception or who have a history of thrombosis. The GnRH agonists produce menopausal symptoms, are costly, and are commonly used presurgically to reduce uterine bulk or improve anemia. The definitive treatment for persistent symptoms is hysterectomy, which will also confirm the diagnosis. At least one study has found LNG-IUS to be equally effective in treating symptoms and improving quality of life when compared to hysterectomy.[134] Clinicians should consider when and whether to refer, and discuss the risks and benefits of various management strategies before beginning treatment for presumed adenomyosis.

ENDOMETRIOSIS

Endometriosis is the displacement of endometrial tissue outside the uterine cavity, causing an inflammatory response. **Figure 22-6** shows potential locations for extrauterine implantation of endometrial tissue. Additionally, endometrial lesions may be found distant from the uterus in the thorax, upper abdomen, and diaphragm. A number of causes have been proposed, ranging from menstrual blood flow out the fallopian tubes carrying endometrial cells (retrograde menstruation) to genetic predisposition, alterations in cell physiology, immunologic function, lymphatic drainage or hormonal function, and exposure to endocrine disruptors such as dioxin.[135,136] Prevalence is 6–10% among reproductive-aged women.[137] However, among women with pelvic pain or infertility, the prevalence is as high as 35–50%.[138]

The symptoms of endometriosis are variable, with many women experiencing minor complaints or being asymptomatic. Common complaints include severe pain during the menses, chronic pelvic pain, and deep dyspareunia. Other symptoms may include menorrhagia, low back pain, abdominal-pelvic pain, cystitis, or irritable bowel syndrome including pain on defection.[139] Hematuria and hematochezia may be noted with

Figure 22-6 Locations of endometriosis lesions.

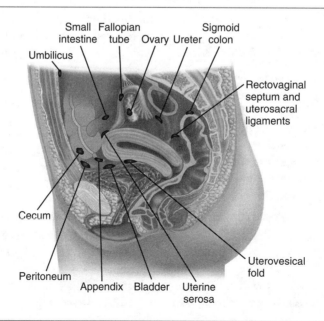

lesions in the bladder or bowel. The degree of pain is not correlated with severity of disease, and the symptoms overlap broadly with other conditions, including symptoms of appendicitis and other nongynecologic conditions.

Physical examination may be negative or include findings associated with advancing lesions. These include a retroflexed, fixed uterus; palpable nodules along the ligaments; or cervical motion tenderness. Alternative causes of pain must be excluded with appropriate testing.

The combination of nonspecific symptoms and difficulty in visualizing lesions leads to delay in diagnosis up to 10 or more years.[140] Ultrasound or MRI may pick up progressive disease with larger plaques, but the absence of endometrial lesions on imaging does not preclude the eventual diagnosis. The only definitive diagnostic technique is laparoscopic or open surgery during which lesions are observed and biopsied.

Treatment may address symptom management, controlling symptoms by decreasing the frequency or amount of menstrual bleeding. Medications commonly used include NSAIDs, hormonal contraception (including extended-cycle methods of combined estrogen-progestin methods and progestogen-only methods), danazol (Danocrine), or GnRH agonists. Danazol was previously the preferred regimen, but it has many androgenic side effects. A Cochrane review reported that menstrual suppression with the LNG-IUS, GnRH agonists, and danazol was effective for pain reduction.[141] Infertile women with endometriosis may benefit from surgical removal of lesions or the use of GnRH agonists in preparation for assisted reproduction. Hysterectomy, with or without preservation of the ovaries, is the definitive therapy. A small percentage of women have persistent symptoms even with bilateral salpingo-oophorectomy. However, ACOG does not recommend deferring estrogen-replacement therapy following removal of the ovaries.[142] Because the definitive therapies are surgical, early referral of infertile women with suspected endometriosis and women with persistent pain after a trial of contraceptive therapy is an essential part of management.

ENDOMETRIAL HYPERPLASIA

Overgrowth of the endometrial lining of the uterus is termed *hyperplasia*. The potential for malignant transformation is a major concern. Among premenopausal women, the incidence of endometrial hyperplasia is highest among those with PCOS and oligomenorrhea at 20%, and among those with AUB at 10%.[143,144] Following menopause, vaginal bleeding is more likely to be associated with endometrial carcinoma; according to one study, women with thickened endometrium had a 24% risk of cancer compared to a 6% risk among those with thinner uterine lining.[145] Risk factors for endometrial hyperplasia are the same as for endometrial cancer and include unopposed estrogen (early menarche, chronic anovulation, late menopause), nulliparity, obesity, and diabetes, as well as tamoxifen use.[146,147]

Of the two currently used methods for describing the condition, one, the World Health Organization (WHO) criteria, is purely descriptive. This methodology characterizes hyperplasia by histology based on glandular complexity and nuclear atypia: 1) simple hyperplasia, 2) complex hyperplasia, 3) simple hyperplasia with atypia, and 4) complex hyperplasia with atypia. The other, *endometrial intraepithelial neoplasia terminology*, classifies disease based on pathology. Categories include: 1) benign (benign endometrial hyperplasia), 2) premalignant (endometrial intraepithelial neoplasia), and 3) malignant (endometrial adenocarcinoma, endometrioid type, well differentiated).[148]

For women who are still menstruating, ultrasound is less helpful than endometrial biopsy or dilation and curettage in the assessment of menorrhagia. Among postmenopausal women, an endometrial stripe on ultrasound should be

< 1 mm; values of 5 mm or greater identify 95% of endometrial cancers.[147] Total hysterectomy is the standard recommended therapy for postmenopausal hyperplasia or endometrial intraepithelial neoplasia. For women of reproductive age who desire to maintain fertility, medical treatments may be used first. Progestins are the first-line option.[147] Women with a diagnosis of endometrial hyperplasia should be seen by a gynecologist to discuss their options.

Screening for Endometrial Cancer

Endometrial cancer is the most common reproductive cancer in women. Slightly less than 3% of American women will be diagnosed with endometrial cancer in their lifetime.[149] The average age at diagnosis is 61, and 90% of cases are diagnosed in women over 50 years of age.[150] Historically, the risk was highest for Caucasian women, but since 2010 that gap has decreased for African Americans and American Indian/Alaska native groups. Mortality, however, remains higher among African American women than for any other ethnic group.[151] Overall, more than 80% of women diagnosed with endometrial cancer will survive more than 5 years.

Risk of endometrial cancer increases with exposure to estrogen. This can result from endogenous factors—early menarche, late menopause, chronic anovulation, nulliparity—or from exogenous sources such as estrogen-only hormone therapy, environmental sources, or tamoxifen. Other risk factors for endometrial cancer include obesity, cirrhosis, diabetes, and genetic predisposition (e.g., Lynch syndrome). Protective factors include being physically active, pregnancy, breastfeeding, and the use of progestin-only or combined hormonal contraceptives.[150,151]

The most common presenting symptom is AUB or postmenopausal bleeding. TVUS or endometrial sampling is the preferred initial assessment for postmenopausal bleeding; in premenopausal women TVUS has not been shown to be an effective tool so endometrial sampling is the standard for initial screening.[152] Atypical glandular cells seen on Pap testing should be followed with endometrial biopsy or dilation and curettage in any woman over 35 or with risk factors for endometrial cancer.[150] Women in whom endometrial cancer is suspected should be referred to a gynecologic oncology center or to an experienced gynecologic surgeon if no specialist is available.

Pelvic Organ Prolapse

Pelvic organ prolapse (POP) is caused by weakening of the musculature that supports the bladder, bowel, and uterus. It is defined by location and degree of distortion of normal anatomy. Overall rates of pelvic floor weakness approximate 50% of the older female population,[153] although rates vary widely by ethnicity and risk factors. Hispanic women have the highest risk by ethnicity, while African American women have the lowest.[154] In the Women's Health Initiative study, rates of POP among women with an intact uterus were 14.2% for uterine prolapse, 34.3% for cystocele, and 18.6% for rectocele.[153] Rates of cystocele and rectocele were similar among women who had undergone hysterectomy.[153] Enterocele is the descent of bowel into the vaginal vault behind a pelvic floor weakness and is most commonly seen after hysterectomy. Factors associated with POP include parity, obesity, injury from surgery or trauma, chronic straining to defecate, and advancing age. Less common associations are sacral nerve damage, connective tissue disorders, increased abdominal pressure, and congenital disorders.[154-156] Although overweight and obesity are associated with POP, weight loss does not appear to remedy the problem.[155]

The history for pelvic floor disorders includes a complete reproductive history and surgical history. Review of systems includes problems with voiding, such as difficulty with initiation or any incontinence, constipation or straining, abdominal-pelvic or low back pain, and sense of pressure or of "things falling out."

Rectocele

Patient complaints specific to rectocele include pelvic or low back pain, a sensation of fullness along the back wall of the rectum causing constipation, and a need to strain or manually support the perineum and vaginal wall during defecation. Some women may note discomfort or pain during sex. Alternatively, with the woman in lithotomy position, a single speculum blade can be used to lift the anterior vaginal wall and she can be asked to bear down. A soft, reducible bulge should be seen on the lower two-thirds of the posterior wall. Bulging high up on the posterior wall is from an enterocele. During the bimanual examination, the rectocele may be palpable if the lower bowel is full of stool. The bulge may also be felt when she bears down.

Cystocele

If the weakened area involves the upper part of the urethra and the bladder, the term used is *cystourethrocele*, or *urethrocele* if only the urethra is involved. Stress incontinence frequently accompanies the disorder; when sacral nerves are damaged, overflow or urgency may also occur.[156] Examination to identify the problem includes using the posterior speculum blade to retract the posterior wall of the vagina and having the woman Valsalva or bear down to bring the bulge into view.[156] Urethroceles are seen low down on the anterior wall, while cystoceles are seen in the upper two-thirds. Even if the woman has not reported incontinence, the presence of a cystocele warrants re-questioning about specific urinary symptoms.

Figure 22-7 shows the location and appearance of cystoceles and rectoceles.

Uterine Prolapse

Prolapse of the uterus is described based on the amount of descent through the vagina. **Figure** 22-8 shows the degrees of uterine prolapse. History specific to uterine prolapse includes pelvic pressure, sensation of her uterus falling out, pain or discomfort with intercourse, and, with severe prolapse, bladder or bowel abnormalities that have developed due to the pressure of the uterus

Figure 22-7 Cystocele, rectocele, enterocele.

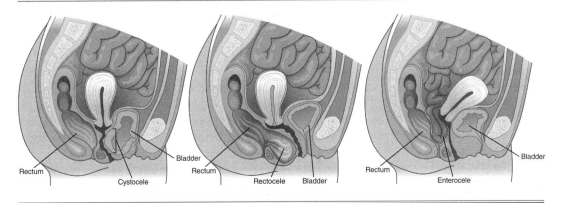

Figure 22-8 Degrees of uterine prolapse.

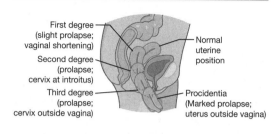

against the bladder, urethra, and rectum. Identification is by visualization of the vagina and cervix and assessment of the degree of descent.[157]

Management of Pelvic Organ Prolapse

For mild degrees of pelvic floor relaxation, Kegel exercises, more generically known as pelvic floor muscle training, should be the first intervention.[158,159] See **Box 22-1** for patient instructions for pelvic floor exercises. These can be demonstrated during the pelvic examination; women experiencing difficulty in mastering the technique can be referred for assistance through physical therapy.

Pessary fitting may improve comfort and reduce symptoms. Depending on the degree of descent, either a supportive pessary such as a ring or Hodge pessary or a space-occupying pessary such as a doughnut or Gellhorn may be used. It is recommended that clinicians be trained in the various types and their use before beginning this practice. Women will need instruction regarding positioning, cleaning, and possible complications of pessary use. Among complications of pessary use, a change in vaginal discharge is most common. Serious problems may include a malodorous discharge, erosion, spotty bleeding, necrosis, or fistula.[160] Women with severe symptoms should be referred for surgical management.

Adnexal Masses

Ovarian masses include various benign cysts, ectopic pregnancy, hydrosalpinx, tubo-ovarian abcess, and ovarian cancers. Only benign and malignant masses of the ovary are discussed here. Evaluation of pain or fullness on pelvic examination includes pregnancy testing, screening for possible infectious causes, and pelvic ultrasound, which will help to identify and eliminate from the differential diagnosis ectopic pregnancy, hydrosalpinx, and tubo-ovarian abscess. Ectopic pregnancy is a life-threatening emergency. When an adnexal mass is palpated on clinical examination and the pregnancy test is positive, a quantitative beta-human chorionic gonadotropin (hCG) is drawn, and the woman is immediately referred for ultrasound evaluation to discriminate a benign corpus luteum of pregnancy from an ectopic

---

Box 22-1 Pelvic Floor Exercise Instructions

1. Identify the pelvic floor muscles by trying to stop the flow of urine when on the toilet. The muscle that contracts to stop urine flow also surrounds the vagina. Do not continue to perform the exercise during voiding, to avoid bladder problems.
2. The exercise can be done standing, sitting or lying down.
3. Tighten the muscle slowly, hold and relax slowly. The goal is to hold for 10 seconds and relax for 10 seconds before repeating.
4. The goal is 10 repetitions, 3 times a day.

implantation. *Hydrosalpinx* is a fluid-filled block-age of one or both fallopian tubes as a result of ad-hesions, infection, or endometriosis. It is seen on ultrasound and should be referred to a gynecolo-gist, particularly if the woman is experiencing in-fertility. *Tubo-ovarian abscess* is the result of pelvic inflammatory disease causing infection within the fallopian tube. Immediate antibiotic therapy is required, possibly with drainage of the pus-filled blockage. The finding mandates immediate refer-ral for further evaluation by a gynecologist.

Benign Ovarian Cysts

The incidence of an ovarian cyst is approximately 8% among premenopausal women and 14% or higher among postmenopausal women.[161,162] The risk of malignancy increases with age, but most adnexal masses found in menopausal women are benign. Various types of cysts and cystic masses occur around the adnexa. The most common are functional cysts and dermoid cysts. Other types not discussed include cystadenomas, peritoneal cysts, and fibromas.

The term *functional cyst* describes a cyst formed as part of the ovulatory cycle that may resolve spon-taneously or rupture, causing pain. Multiple fol-licles develop within the ovary in each menstrual cycle. At ovulation the dominant follicle ruptures to release an oocyte. Simple functional cysts are described as *follicular* (in which the egg is not re-leased and the fluid-filled sac remains) or as a *corpus luteum* (the follicle does not resolve after ovula-tion but continues to grow and retain fluid). If the woman conceives, the corpus luteum may persist throughout the first trimester. A *hemorrhagic cyst* is one in which there is bleeding into a functional cyst. Simple cysts < 10 cm in diameter are almost always benign. Fewer than 1% will become malignant.[163]

Dermoid cysts, also called benign cystic teratomas, are formed when residual embryonic cells form into a mass contained within a sac-like membrane. They may contain mature hair, tooth or bone fragments,

skin, muscle, or fat tissue.[163] The median age at diagnosis is 32 years, with a wide range—from 5 to 85 years of age in one retrospective series.[164] Children and adolescents are more likely to pres-ent with abdominal pain and to have larger tu-mors.[164] Dermoids are the most common germ cell neoplasm, accounting for up to 20% of all ovarian masses; malignant transformation occurs in 1–2% of cases. When a malignancy results, most cases are squamous cell carcinomas. This diagnosis is usu-ally made among women over 45 years of age.[165] When dermoid cysts enlarge, they have a high risk for ovarian torsion. Unlike simple fluid-filled cysts, dermoid cysts can reach sizes of 35 cm or more.[164]

Most benign cysts are asymptomatic and are incidental findings on examination. Pain from a rupturing functional cyst or bleeding within a cyst may bring a woman in with an urgent complaint. Pelvic fullness or pressure may be associated with an enlarging cyst. Acute-onset pain may be asso-ciated with torsion of an ovary enlarged by a cyst.

Ovarian Cancer

According to the National Cancer Institute, ovar-ian cancers make up 3% of cancer diagnoses among women, but have a poor overall prognosis, being the fifth leading cause of cancer deaths.[166] While 22,000 women were diagnosed with ovarian can-cer in 2014, 14,000 died from the disease.[166] Risk factors for ovarian cancer include family history of the disease; genetic mutations including BRCA1, BRCA2, and Lynch syndrome (hereditary non-polyposis colorectal cancer); use of estrogen-only hormone therapy or of fertility drugs; exposure to talc; obesity; and tall stature.[167] Compared to a general population risk of 1.6%, women with BRCA1 mutation have a 35–60% risk, and those with BRCA2 a lifetime risk of up to 25%.[162] While families positive for Lynch syndrome have lower ovarian cancer risks (~10%), this and other more recently identified genetic risks contribute significantly to the burden of disease.[167]

Ovarian cancers are difficult to diagnose at an early stage. The symptoms are often vague and include feelings of fullness or bloating, diffuse abdominal discomfort, irregular vaginal bleeding, or an abnormal discharge. The lack of an effective screening test, such as mammography or Pap testing, contributes to the difficulty of diagnosis. Symptoms are often present for months or years before a diagnosis is made. Ascites, shortness of breath, weight gain, and abdominal distension are late signs associated with advanced disease.

Diagnosis and Management of Adnexal Masses

A family history of reproductive cancer, advancing age, and a reproductive and medical history suggestive of PCOS all increase the likelihood of finding an adnexal mass. Specific additional risk

factors for ovarian cancer are noted in the previous section. Specific questions about abdominal symptoms, vaginal bleeding or discharge, and prior medication use should be incorporated into the history and review of systems for adnexal masses. On examination, enlargement of the adnexa and tenderness to palpation may be noted. TVUS is the next step in identification, and Doppler blood flow assessment should be incorporated into these studies. MRI or CT may be needed to confirm or exclude specific causes. ACOG recommends quantitative hCG, CBC, and TVUS for premenopausal women as an initial workup.[168] Ultrasound identification of a simple cyst < 10 cm in diameter is almost always benign. Thickened or irregular tumor walls, solid components of the mass, and nodular components of the wall are associated with increased cancer risk. Classification of follow up for benign-appearing cysts is provided in **Table 22-16**.

Table 22-16 Follow Up for Benign-Appearing Cysts

Simple cysts, premenopausal women	≤ 3 cm, physiologic, no follow up < 5 cm, benign, no follow up < 7 cm, yearly follow up ≥ 7 cm, refer for further imaging with MRI or surgical excision
Simple cysts, postmenopausal women	≤ 1 cm, physiologic < 7 cm, yearly follow up > 7 cm, refer for further imaging with MRI or surgical excision
Dermoid tumors	MRI, refer for evaluation
Hemorrhagic cysts, premenopausal women	≤ 5 cm, no follow up > 5 cm, 6- to 12-week follow up
Hemorrhagic cysts, early postmenopausal women	Regardless of size, 6- to 12-week follow up
Hemorrhagic cysts, postmenopausal women	Refer for surgical evaluation

MRI = magnetic resonance imaging

Data from Levine D, Brown DL, Andreotti RF, Benacerraf B, Benson CB, Brewster WR, et al. Management of asymptomatic ovarian and other adnexal cysts imaged at US: Society of Radiologists in Ultrasound consensus conference statement. *Radiology.* 2010;256:943-954; Ackerman S, Irshad A, Lewis M, Anis M. Ovarian cystic lesions. *Radiol Clin North Am.* 2013;51:1067-1085.

The International Ovarian Tumor Analysis (IOTA) group proposed guidelines for interpreting the malignancy risk of adnexal masses seen on ultrasound. Benign characteristics include unilocular cyst, no solid component greater than 7 mm, presence of acoustic shadows (indicates fluid), smooth multilocular tumor < 10 cm, and no blood flow on Doppler. Characteristics that help predict malignancy include irregular solid tumor, ascites, 4 or more papillary structures, irregular multilocular-solid mass ≥ 10 cm, and strong blood flow to the mass.[169] New research has shown that the Simple Rules from the International Ovarian Tumor Analysis group can be used to predict risk and simply to sort adnexal masses into benign, malignant, and inconclusive categories.[170]

CA-125 is elevated in most cases of ovarian cancer. Levels may be normal in early-stage disease and in some less common types of ovarian malignancy. It is not effective as a screen, because many women with benign abdominal or gynecologic conditions ranging from pancreatitis, diverticulitis, inflammatory bowel disease, liver disease, pelvic inflammatory disease, fibroids, endometriosis, or a ruptured cyst to recent surgery can have elevated CA-125 levels. There is some evidence that in postmenopausal women the predictive value of CA-125 is higher. Thus, ACOG recommends collecting CA-125 and obtaining a TVUS in the evaluation of adnexal masses after menopause.[168] A large randomized controlled trial of combined TVUS and CA-125 screening did not reduce cancer mortality, compared with usual care.[171]

As a general rule, any clinician who is not experienced in the management of ovarian masses should consider consultation at an early stage, at least to review ultrasound findings. Possible ectopic pregnancy, tubo-ovarian abscesses, and solid or multiseptated ovarian masses should always have high-priority referrals. In the case of possible ectopic pregnancy, the referral is to an emergency setting. If there is any suspicion of ovarian malignancy, referral is to a gynecologic oncologist.

Vulvar Dermatoses and Vulvar Cancers

Irritation and itching on the vulva can be the result of numerous problems, from infections such as *Candida* to allergies and contact dermatitis. Three of the more common presentations, lichen simplex chronicus (LSC), lichen planus (LP), and lichen sclerosus (LS), are each histologically distinctive diseases, although they have similar names. The name "lichen" is intended to evoke the image of rough-surfaced lichen heaped on a smooth-surfaced rock. A list of differential diagnoses is provided in **Table 22-17**.

Table 22-17 Differential Diagnosis for Vulvar Dermatitis

Infectious:
- *Candida*
- Aerobic vaginitis
- Bacterial vaginosis
- Herpes simplex virus
- Human papillomavirus
- *Trichomonas vaginalis*
- *Chlamydia trachomatis*
- Molluscum contagiosum

Infestation:
- Scabies
- Pubic lice (*Phthirus pubis*)

Allergic dermatitis

Contact dermatitis

Psoriasis

Hydradenitis

Vulvar neoplasia

Evaluation of Dermatoses

The diagnosis of vulvar conditions requires evaluation of symptoms, with attention to the degree and type of pain (e.g., itch versus burn), its onset, persistence, and associated factors. The history and review of symptoms related to vulvovaginal symptoms are extensive. The family and medical history should look for allergic, autoimmune, neurologic, or endocrine disorders that might affect tissue integrity and sensation; gastrointestinal or urinary conditions that could expose tissue to irritation (e.g., urinary incontinence, diarrhea); reproductive and gynecologic history for menstrual status, pregnancy outcomes, infections, or injury; sexual history for contraception and practices; possible history of assault or abuse; and assessment of hygiene, including what cleaning and menstrual products are used.

On examination, inspection of the entire genital area is essential, from the mons to the anus. Changes in the appearance of the tissue such as discoloration, rash, lesions, or textural changes are noted. Palpation for masses, inflamed Skene's or Bartholin's glands, and urethral irritation is performed prior to a complete pelvic examination. The color, volume, and odor of any vaginal discharge is noted. Testing for STIs and benign vaginal infections is performed.

Contact Dermatitis— Allergic and Irritant

Contact dermatitis may occur as a result of chafing against fabric, prolonged exposure to warm, moist clothing (e.g., exercise or swimwear), exposure to an irritating substance (e.g., scented cleansers), or an allergic response (e.g., latex). Exposure to allergens and irritants is the cause of 50% of chronic itching[172] and all vulvar complaints. The appearance of the labia is reddened and scaly with increased rugosity (wrinkling). Contact dermatitis may occur acutely, within minutes of exposure to a powerful irritant or as a result of repeated exposure to a milder irritant that nevertheless damages the skin.[173]

Management for allergic or irritant vulvar dermatitis includes collecting a scrupulous history of all exposures (tampons, pads, hygiene products, laundry, etc.) eliminating all potential irritants and allergens including synthetic clothing worn tight to the skin, and the use of medium- to high-potency topical steroid ointments. If symptoms do not clear, allergy patch testing may be in order.[172]

Lichen Simplex Chronicus

LSC, one of the most common causes of vulvar itching, is often the result of a contact dermatitis, chafing, or other irritation. It is considered to be part of the spectrum of atopic reactions that includes eczema and neurodermatitis. It can occur on normal-appearing skin or as a reaction to an underlying skin condition. In addition, LSC is more common among women with anxiety disorders or emotional stress. The primary symptom is a chronic, itch-scratch-itch cycle leading to thickening and toughening of skin. The itching may be intermittent or continuous. It is worsened by heat, humidity, exposure to body fluids (urine, stool, vaginal discharge), and by medications or hygiene products. Because it has an atopic component, the itch may persist even in the absence of the original stimulus. Some women awaken from sleep to find themselves scratching or are in too much discomfort to sleep well.

On examination, the skin is thickened with increased wrinkling and a leathery texture. Excoriation from scratching, fissures, or erosions may be present. The skin may be reddened or have areas of discoloration. The labia may be swollen in response to constant rubbing.[174]

Healing requires time for tissue to repair itself and a reduction in inflammation to resolve the itch-scratch cycle. Treatment requires combination therapy with a potent topical corticosteroid, symptomatic treatment with topical anesthetics to block itching, nighttime sedation if required, treatment of secondary bacterial and fungal infections, identification and treatment of underlying conditions, and elimination of irritants.[173]

Lichen Sclerosus

LS a chronic inflammatory skin disease, usually confined to the perineal and perianal areas. It is believed to have an autoimmune component,[174] with other proposed predisposing factors including a low-estrogen environment and genetics.[175] Prevalence has been estimated over a range of 0.1% to as high as 1.7%. LS occurs more frequently in women than in men and has a bimodal onset with peaks around puberty and menopause.[176]

Women with LS experience intense pruritus so serious that it may interfere with sleep, and they may complain of pain with intercourse, when voiding, or around the anus. The initial signs are sharply outlined erythematous areas, often initially around the clitoris. Pale, shiny, or crinkled plaques develop. Eventually, the skin loses its pigmentation and becomes thin and fragile. Petechiae, excoriation, or fissures may be present as a result of scratching.[177] Secondary infections may occur and contribute to progression of the symptoms. Over time, the vulvar architecture is lost as the labia majora and minora fuse. The clitoris may be entirely covered by the fused tissue atrophy, and scarring can result. The disfigurement can be extreme with almost total closure of the introitus. In about 60% of cases, the perianal area will also be involved.[178]

Evaluation includes careful pelvic examination. Because several conditions result in the formation of white plaques, a biopsy is recommended to establish a definite diagnosis. The differential diagnoses for leukoplakia (white plaques) include HPV, LP, LSC, vitiligo, and vulvar intraepithelial neoplasia. Testing for autoimmune diseases including thyroid disease should be considered due to increased prevalence in women with LS.

Management strategies for LS include evaluation for secondary yeast or bacterial infections, avoidance of irritants, and treatment with a high-potency topical steroid. Initially, the steroid is applied daily for 8–12 weeks before transitioning to weekly lifetime maintenance with a mid- to high-potency steroid.[175] Alternatively, some women with mild cases may be able to use an emollient, rather than steroids, for maintenance.[176] Symptoms should clear in the majority of women within 3 months; scarring will not regress. Older women are less likely to experience improvement.[175] Women whose symptoms do not resolve with this treatment should be referred for evaluation. Other medical therapies including the calcineurin inhibitors may be considered; however, they carry a warning related to the potential increase in malignancy when they are applied and should not be used as first-line therapy or by an inexperienced provider. There is a 3% or greater risk of developing squamous cell carcinoma in lesions of LS.[175,179]

Lichen Planus

LP is an inflammatory disorder of the mucous membranes that impacts the vulva and vagina in about half of all cases in women. Other tissues involved include the ear, mouth and esophagus, and skin. It is believed to have an autoimmune component.[174] The prevalence of LP is not well defined, but is believed to be < 2%.[180] The disease is seen most commonly among postmenopausal women but may arise at any age.[179] The most common variant is erosive LP, which produces erosions into tissue from the clitoris back along the labia and around the introitus. The spread of lesions into the vagina helps to distinguish LP from LS.

The initial complaint is itching, burning, or pain in the vulva. Women may complain of dyspareunia and of abnormal vaginal bleeding or discharge. On inspection, patches of bright-red, shiny tissue are seen (glazed erythema). The classic early lesions are small, purple, polygonal papules with a lacy reticulate white overlay. As the disease progresses, scarring and adhesions may be seen to narrow the introitus, and vulvar architecture may be lost.

Diagnostic criteria have been proposed for LP. The presence of three out of nine characteristics is necessary to make the diagnosis. The criteria include symptoms of pain or burning, involvement of other mucosal tissue with similar lesions, vaginal inflammation, erosions or glazed erythema at the vaginal opening, reddened or eroded areas surrounded by a reticulated pattern (Wickham's striae) and a hyperkeratotic border, scarring and loss of vulvovaginal architecture, and three histologic characteristics determined on biopsy.[181]

Comfort care for management of pain can be offered. Because LP is strongly associated with lesions in multiple parts of the body and is a more severe presentation than LS, referral for management is wise. A dermatologic consult may also be required. First-line therapy of LP is with superpotent topical or oral steroids. Systemic medications may be needed if touching the affected area is too painful or if the disease is extensive or severe.[175,179] Lifetime management is necessary for the disease. Unlike LS, the relationship of LP to vulvar cancers is not clear; however, the potential for increased risk is suggested by a review of the several small reports available.[182]

Vulvar Cancer

Cancers of the vulva and vagina are rare, with a lifetime prevalence for vulvar cancer of 0.3% of women. Together, vulvar and vaginal cancers are only 6–7 % of all reproductive cancers. More than 70% of women diagnosed with vulvar cancer will survive more than 5 years.[183] Risk factors include HPV infection, smoking, prior diagnosis of cervical cancer or precancer, HIV, and other causes of immune suppression.[184] Seventy percent of vaginal and vulvar cancers are caused by HPV. Prior diagnosis of LS or LP may increase risks.

Squamous cell carcinoma accounts for more than 95% of all cases, followed by melanoma and other rare types. There are two main etiologies of vulvar cancer. HPV-related cancer occurs most often in women 35–75 years of age, while vulvar nonneoplastic epithelial disorders, including LS, which lead to cancer occur primarily among postmenopausal women.[185]

Common symptoms include vulvar pain, irritation or bleeding, skin discoloration or lesions, masses or erosive lesions, and pain associated with voiding or sex. Vulvar intraepithelial neoplasia, a form of carcinoma in situ, may closely resemble the appearance of vulvar dermatoses. Changes in vulvar appearance should always spur consideration of risk factors and evaluation with vulvar biopsy. There is no effective screening test for vulvar and vaginal cancers. Prevention is the most effective approach. Vaccination with an HPV vaccine, for both girls and boys, prior to the onset of sexual activity is the best tool for eradication of vulvar carcinoma.

While surgery, radiation, and chemotherapy are standard treatments for vulvar cancers, the use of biologics such as imiquimod cream have shown promise in treatment. As with other perineal lesions, early referral in the face of unclear diagnosis is the most prudent course.

Cervical Cancer Screening

Sexually transmitted HPV includes about 40 of the 100 or more identified strains. The pervasiveness of risk can be seen in the fact that more than half of sexually active adults are infected with one

Table 22-18 Vaccines to Prevent HPV Infection

Vaccine	Date Available	Strains Covered	Approved for
Gardasil (quadrivalent)	2006	6, 11, 16, 18	Females and males
Cervarix (bivalent)	2009	16, 18	Females
Gardasil 9 (9-valent)	2014	6, 11, 16, 18, 31, 33, 45, 52, and 58	Females and males

or more strains of HPV. Of these, some are responsible for genital warts, while others, the high-risk or oncogenic types, are responsible for almost all cervical cancer. HPV is found in 90.6% of cervical cancer specimens and 98.8% of carcinoma in situ of the cervix.[186]

Transmission is through exposure to infected skin, mucous membranes, or bodily fluids via any type of sexual contact. More than 79 million adults are infected with HPV; most new infections occur among those under 25 years old, and many will clear spontaneously within 2 years. The identification of HPV on testing in women over 30 indicates a higher likelihood of persistent infection. HPV prevalence is highest among Hispanic and African American women.[187]

Two types of HPV, 16 and 18, are the cause of 70% of cervical cancers in the United States.[187] Smoking, an impaired immune response, and HIV are known to increase the risk of progressive disease. The prevention of cervical cancer is achieved through a combination of vaccination against HPV and regularly scheduled screening. In 2015, an estimated 13,000 American women were expected to be diagnosed with cervical cancer, and 4,000 or so were expected to die.[188] Reduction in cervical cancer rates by more than 50% is directly attributable to widespread screening with the Pap smear and, more recently, HPV testing.[188] Disparities in screening

are narrowing between younger black and white women, although they remain high among older blacks.[190,191]

Vaccination against HPV to prevent cervical cancer and genital warts has been available in the United States since 2006. Three vaccines are available, as shown in **Table 22-18**. All are recommended to be given between ages 9 and 26, with recommended start date for the 3 injection series at age 11 or 12 years. The bivalent vaccine is estimated to cover 66% of potential cervical cancer cases; adding the additional strains that make up the 9-valent vaccine covers an additional 4.2% to 18.3%.[186] Although the *Healthy People 2020* goal is that 80% of eligible adolescents will be vaccinated, rates are significantly lower.[192] In 2014, 39.7% of girls had received all 3 doses by age 17; only 21.6% of boys had completed the series. Rates vary widely by state. Hispanic and African American girls are more likely to receive all or part of the series than white girls. Children living below the poverty level were more likely to be vaccinated.[193] Multiple factors contribute to the poor rates of vaccination including provider attitudes, attitudes of families toward a vaccine directed against an STI, and, prior to the passage of the Patient Protection and Affordable Care Act, access to insurance coverage.[192]

While women's health practitioners can and should recommend HPV vaccine to all eligible women, the burden of timely vaccination (i.e., before the onset of sexual activity) falls primarily on pediatricians and family doctors, many of whom are reluctant to discuss the vaccine or do not store it in their offices.[192] Inquiring about vaccination history is a key part of the history taken at the time of a first visit and updated regularly.

Secondary prevention of cervical cancer occurs with scheduled screening. National guidelines have changed in recent years as our understanding of HPV and precancerous cervical changes has grown. The addition of direct testing for HPV has also contributed to the revisions. Current recommendations are to begin testing for cervical cancer no earlier than age 21, regardless of age at first sexual activity, except for women living with HIV. The high rate of clearance of HPV in young women, the recognition that a cervical intraepithelial neoplasia (CIN) grade 1 report probably indicates acute HPV infection, the slow progress of cervical changes, and the potential for cervical injury with aggressive treatment in healthy women all contribute to these recommendations.[194] In this population, education about HPV vaccination, contraception, and STIs is the most valuable strategy for preventing cancer.[195]

In general, for women ages 21–29, cytology testing every 3 years without HPV screening is indicated. After age 30 and continuing until at least age 65, women with negative prior results should have cytology testing with HPV co-testing every 5 years or cytology every 3 years.[196] Women who have co-testing that is HPV negative have a minimal risk of developing cervical cancer within the next 6 years.[197] After age 65, women with persistently negative screening may cease screening for cervical cancer.[198] These are women who have never had CIN-2 or higher reported as an abnormality and who have had three screens with cytology alone or two screens with cytology and HPV testing within 10 years, and for whom the last test was within 5 years. Women with history of significant abnormalities should continue for 20 years after spontaneous or treatment-based resolution of HPV.[196] It is possible, although not yet standard, to test with HPV screening alone.[197] When this route is chosen, 3 years is an appropriate interval for retesting.[198] Management for HPV 16– or 18–positive results is direct referral to colposcopy; women with other high-risk HPV types should have cytology testing and be reevaluated in 12 months.[197]

The Bethesda System for reporting of cervical cytology describes the standard terminology for interpreting cervical cytology. The categories are shown in **Table 22-19**. Management of test results incorporates information from HPV co-testing when available. For example, when the Pap test is negative, but the HPV is positive, repeat co-testing in 12 months is indicated, or, if types 16 or 18 are present, refer for colposcopy. Conversely, if the cytology is atypical cells of undetermined significance (ASCUS) but HPV is negative, a 3-year interval is appropriate.[196] Of note, women with insufficient specimens should have the test repeated within 2–4 months unless HPV co-testing shows HPV types 16 or 18, in which case colposcopy is indicated.[197]

Management of abnormal cervical cytology can be kept current in clinical practice by following guidelines published by the American Society for Colposcopy and Cervical Pathology (ASCCP). These are readily available on their website (www.asccp.org/guidelines) and can be downloaded to mobile devices.[199] Changes occur with advancing knowledge of disease. For example, in the most recent update, a change was made regarding the management of women under 25 with ASCUS or low-grade squamous intraepithelial results. The current recommendation is to avoid colposcopy, but repeat the cytology screening in 1 year, with further testing based on the persistence of abnormal results.[199]

Table 22-19 The 2014 Bethesda System for the Interpretation of Cervical Cytology

SPECIMEN TYPE:
Indicate conventional smear (Pap smear) vs. liquid-based preparation vs. other

SPECIMEN ADEQUACY
- Satisfactory for evaluation (*describe presence or absence of endocervical/transformation zone component and any other quality indicators, e.g., partially obscuring blood, inflammation, etc.*)
- Unsatisfactory for evaluation . . . (*specify reason*)
  - Specimen rejected/not processed (*specify reason*)
  - Specimen processed and examined, but unsatisfactory for evaluation of epithelial abnormality because of (*specify reason*)

GENERAL CATEGORIZATION (*optional*)
- Negative for Intraepithelial Lesion or Malignancy
- Other: See Interpretation/Result (*e.g., endometrial cells in a woman ≥45 years of age*)
- Epithelial Cell Abnormality: See Interpretation/Result (*speci al 'squamous' or 'glandular' as appropriate*)

INTERPRETATION/RESULT
NEGATIVE FOR INTRAEPITHELIAL LESION OR MALIGNANCY
(*When there is no cellular evidence of neoplasia, state this in the General Categorization above and/or in the Interpretation/Result section of the report--whether or not there are organisms or other non-neoplastic findings*)

*Non-Neoplastic Findings (**optional to report**)*
- Non-neoplastic cellular variations
  - Squamous metaplasia
  - Keratotic changes
  - Tubal metaplasia.
  - Atrophy
  - Pregnancy-associated changes
- Reactive cellular changes associated with:
  - Inflammation (includes typical repair)
  - Lymphocytic (follicular) cervicitis
  - Radiation
  - Intrauterine contraceptive device (IUD)
- Glandular cells status post hysterectomy

Organisms
- *Trichomonas vaginalis*
- Fungal organisms morphologically consistent with *Candida* spp.
- Shift in flora suggestive of bacterial vaginosis
- Bacteria morphologically consistent with *Actinomyces* spp.
- Cellular changes consistent with herpes simplex virus
- Cellular changes consistent with cytomegalovirus

OTHER
- Endometrial cells (*in a woman ≥45 years of age*)
(*Specify if "negative for squamous intraepithelial lesion"*)

(continues)

Table 22-19 The 2014 Bethesda System for the Interpretation of Cervical Cytology (*continued*)

EPITHELIAL CELL ABNORMALITIES

SQUAMOUS CELL
- Atypical squamous cells
  - of undetermined significance (ASC-US)
  - cannot exclude HSIL (ASC-H)
- Low-grade squamous intraepithelial lesion (LSIL)
  (*encompassing: HPV/mild dysplasia/CIN 1*).
- High-grade squamous intraepithelial lesion (HSIL)
  (*encompassing: moderate and severe dysplasia, CIS; CIN 2 and CIN 3*)
  - with features suspicious for invasion (*if invasion is suspected*)
- Squamous cell carcinoma

GLANDULAR CELL
- Atypical
  - endocervical cells (NOS *or specify in comments*)
  - endometrial cells (NOS *or specify in comments*)
  - glandular cells (NOS *or specify in comments*)
- Atypical
  - endocervical cells, favor neoplastic
  - glandular cells, favor neoplastic
- Endocervical adenocarcinoma in situ
- Adenocarcinoma
  - endocervical
  - endometrial
  - extrauterine
  - not otherwise specified (NOS)

OTHER MALIGNANT NEOPLASMS: (*specify*)

ADJUNCTIVE TESTING
Provide a brief description of the test method(s) and report the result so that it is easily understood by the clinician.

COMPUTER-ASSISTED INTERPRETATION OF CERVICAL CYTOLOGY
If case examined by an automated device, sped), device and result.

EDUCATIONAL NOTES AND COMMENTS APPENDED TO CYTOLOGY REPORTS (*optional*)
Suggestions should be concise and consistent with clinical follow-up guidelines published by professional organizations (references to relevant publications may be included).

Conclusion

Reproductive concerns regarding health and sexuality are common among women, but many women will not raise these issues unless asked. Incorporating a comprehensive history and careful gynecologic examination into women's health leads to improvements that may range from increased vaccination rates to more effective contraceptive use. Addressing women's concerns improves overall health and wellbeing.

It is essential that primary care providers have access to resources that include current guidelines and to reliable consultation and referral providers. While many of the topics addressed in this chapter can be managed in primary women's health, others require specialists to provide best care.

References

1. Chumlea WC, Schubert CM, Roche AF, Kulin HE, Lee PA, Himes JH, et al. Age at menarche and racial comparisons in US girls. *Pediatrics*. 2003;111(1):110-113.
2. Finer LB, Philbin JM. Trends in ages at key reproductive transitions in the United States, 1951-2010. *Womens Health Issues*. 2014;24(3):e271-9. doi:10.1016/j.whi.2014.02.002.
3. Anderson S, Dallal G, Must A. Relative weight and race influence average age at menarche: results from two nationally representative surveys of US girls studied 25 years apart. *Pediatrics*. 2003;111(4):844-850.
4. Currie C, Ahluwalia N, Godeau E, Nic Gabhainn S, Due P, Currie DB. Is obesity at individual and national level associated with lower age at menarche? Evidence from 34 countries in the Health Behaviour in School-aged Children Study. *J Adolesc Health*. 2012;50(6):621-626. doi:10.1016/j.jadohealth.2011.10.254.
5. World Health Organization Task Force on Adolescent Reproductive Health. World Health Organization multicenter study on menstrual and ovulatory patterns in adolescent girls. II. Longitudinal study of menstrual patterns in the early postmenarcheal period, duration of bleeding episodes and menstrual cycles. *Adolesc Health Care*. 1986;7(4):236-244.
6. American College of Obstetricians and Gynecologists Committee on Adolescent Health. Menstruation in girls and adolescents: using the menstrual cycle as a vital sign. *Obstet Gynecol*. 2015;126(6):e143-e146. doi:10.1097/AOG.0000000000001215.
7. O'Brien PMS, Bäckström T, Brown C, Dennerstein L, Endicott J, Epperson CN, et al. Towards a consensus on diagnostic criteria, measurement and trial design of the premenstrual disorders: the ISPMD Montreal consensus. *Arch Womens Ment Health*. 2011;14(1):13-21. doi:10.1007/s00737-010-0201-3.
8. Yonkers KA, O'Brien PMS, Eriksson E. Premenstrual syndrome. *Lancet*. 2008;371(9619):1200-1210. doi:10.1016/S0140-6736(08)60527-9.
9. Epperson CN, Steiner M, Hartlage SA, Eriksson E, Schmidt PJ, Jones I, et al. Premenstrual dysphoric disorder: evidence for a new category for DSM-5. *Am J Psychiatry*. 2012;169(5):465.
10. Bertone-Johnson ER, Hankinson SE, Johnson SR, Manson JE. Cigarette smoking and the development of premenstrual syndrome. *Am J Epidemiol*. 2008;168(8):938-945. doi:10.1093/aje/kwn194.
11. Bertone-Johnson ER, Hankinson SE, Willett WC, Johnson SR, Manson JE. Adiposity and the development of premenstrual syndrome. *J Womens Health*. 2010;19(11):1955-1962. doi:10.1089/jwh.2010.2128.
12. Bertone-Johnson ER, Hankinson SE, Johnson SR, Manson JE. Timing of alcohol use and the incidence of premenstrual syndrome and probable premenstrual dysphoric disorder. *J Womens Health*. 2009;18(12):1945-1953. doi:10.1089/jwh.2009.1468.
13. Bertone-Johnson ER, Whitcomb BW, Missmer SA, Manson JE, Hankinson SE, Rich-Edwards JW. Early life emotional, physical, and sexual abuse and the development of premenstrual syndrome: a longitudinal study. *J Womens Health*. 2014;23(9):729-739. doi:10.1089/jwh.2013.4674.
14. Freeman EW, Halbreich U, Grubb GS, Rapkin AJ, Skouby SO, Smith L, et al. An overview of four studies of a continuous oral contraceptive (levonorgestrel 90 mcg/ethinyl estradiol 20 mcg) on premenstrual dysphoric disorder and premenstrual syndrome. *Contraception*. 2012;85(5):437-445. doi:10.1016/j.contraception.2011.09.010.
15. Coffee AL, Kuehl TJ, Willis S, Sulak PJ. Oral contraceptives and premenstrual symptoms: comparison of a 21/7 and extended regimen. *Am J Obstet Gynecol*. 2006;195(5):1311-1319.

16. Jarvis CI, Lynch AM, Morin AK. Management strategies for premenstrual syndrome/premenstrual dysphoric disorder. *Ann Pharmacother.* 2008;42: 967-968. doi:10.1345/aph.1K673.

17. Shah NR, Jones JB, Aperi J, Shemtov R, Karne A, Borenstein J. Selective serotonin reuptake inhibitors for premenstrual syndrome and premenstrual dysphoric disorder: a meta-analysis. *Obstet Gynecol.* 2008;111(5): 1175-1182. doi:10.1097/AOG.0b013e31816fd73b.

18. Wyatt KM, Dimmock PW, Jones PW, Shaughn O'Brien PM. Efficacy of vitamin B-6 in the treatment of premenstrual syndrome: systematic review. *BMJ.* 1999;318(7195):1375-1381.

19. Thys-Jacobs S, Starkey P, Bernstein D, Tian J. Calcium carbonate and the premenstrual syndrome: effects on premenstrual and menstrual symptoms. Premenstrual Syndrome Study Group. *Am J Obstet Gynecol.* 1998;179(2):444-452.

20. Jamieson DJ, Steege JF. The prevalence of dysmenorrhea, dyspareunia, pelvic pain, and irritable bowel syndrome in primary care practices. *Obstet Gynecol.* 1996;87(1):55-58.

21. Harlow SD, Park M. A longitudinal study of risk factors for the occurrence, duration and severity of menstrual cramps in a cohort of college women. *Br J Obstet Gynaecol.* 1996;103(11):1134-1142.

22. Parker MA, Sneddon AE, Arbon P. The menstrual disorder of teenagers (MDOT) study: determining typical menstrual patterns and menstrual disturbance in a large population-based study of Australian teenagers. *BJOG.* 2010;117(2):185-192.

23. Ju H, Mark Jones M, Mishra G. The prevalence and risk factors of dysmenorrhea. *Epidemiol Rev.* 2014;36(1):104-13. doi:10.1093/epirev/mxt009.

24. Latthe P, Mignini L, Gray R, Hills R, Khan K. Factors predisposing women to chronic pelvic pain: systematic review. *BMJ.* 2006;332(7544):749.

25. Dawood MY. Primary dysmenorrhea: advances in pathogenesis and management. *Obstet Gynecol.* 2006;108:428-441.

26. Shifren JL, Gass ML; NAMS Recommendations for Clinical Care of Midlife Women Working Group. The North American Menopause Society recommendations for clinical care of midlife women. *Menopause.* 2014;21(10):1038-1062. doi:10.1097/ GME.0000000000000319.

27. Harlow SD, Gass M, Hall JE, Lobo R, Maki P, Rebar RW, et al. Executive summary of the Stages of Reproductive Aging Workshop + 10: addressing the unfinished agenda of staging reproductive aging. *Menopause.* 2012;19(4):387-395. doi:10.1097/ gme.0b013e31824d8f40.

28. Lonnèe-Hoffmann RAM, Dennerstein L, Lehert P, Szoeke C. Sexual function in the late postmenopause:

a decade of follow-up in a population-based cohort of Australian women. *J Sex Med.* 2014;11:2029-2038.

29. Krause MS, Nakajima ST. Hormonal and nonhormonal treatment of vasomotor symptoms. *Obstet Gynecol Clin North Am.* 2015;42:163-179.

30. Thurston RC, Joffe H. Vasomotor symptoms and menopause: findings from the study of Women's Health Across the Nation. *Obstet Gynecol Clin North Am.* 2011;38(3):489-501. doi:10.1016/j.ogc .2011.05.006.

31. Avis NE, Crawford SL, Greendale G, Bromberger JT, Everson-Rose SA, Gold EB, et al. Duration of menopausal vasomotor symptoms over the menopause transition. *JAMA Intern Med.* 2015;175(4):531-539. doi:10.1001/jamainternmed.2014.8063.

32. Gartoulla P, Worsley R, Bell RJ, Davis SR. Moderate to severe vasomotor and sexual symptoms remain problematic for women aged 60 to 65 years. *Menopause.* 2015;22(7):694-701. doi:10.1097/ GME.0000000000000383.

33. Gold EB, Block G, Crawford S, Lachance L, FitzGerald G, Miracle H, et al. Lifestyle and demographic factors in relation to vasomotor symptoms: baseline results from the Study of Women's Health Across the Nation. *Am J Epidemiol.* 2004;159(12): 1189-1199.

34. Portman DJ, Gass ML; Vulvovaginal Atrophy Terminology Consensus Conference Panel. Genitourinary syndrome of menopause: new terminology for vulvovaginal atrophy from the International Society for the Study of Women's Sexual Health and the North American Menopause Society. *Maturitas.* 2014;79(3): 349-354. doi:10.1016/j.maturitas.2014.07.013.

35. American College of Obstetricians and Gynecologists Committee on Gynecologic Practice, American Society for Reproductive Medicine Practice Committee. Compounded bioidentical menopausal hormone therapy. *Fertil Steril.* 2012;98(2):308-312.

36. Pinkerton JV, Santoro N. Compounded bioidentical hormone therapy: identifying use trends and knowledge gaps among US women. *Menopause.* 2015;22(9): 926-936. doi:10.1097/GME.0000000000000420.

37. Roberts H, Hickey M. Managing the menopause: an update. *Maturitas.* 2016;86:53-58. doi:10.1016/j. maturitas.2016.01.007.

38. Labrie F, Archer DF, Koltun W, Vachon A, Young D, Frenette L, et al. Efficacy of intravaginal dehydroepiandrosterone (DHEA) on moderate to severe dyspareunia and vaginal dryness, symptoms of vulvovaginal atrophy, and of the genitourinary syndrome of menopause. *Menopause.* 2016;23(3):243-256. doi: 10.1097/ GME.0000000000000571.

39. Schmidt P. The 2012 hormone therapy position statement of the North American Menopause Society.

Menopause. 2012;19(3):257-271. doi:10.1097/gme.0b013e31824b970a.

40. The North American Menopause Society. The North American Menopause Society statement on continuing use of systemic hormone therapy after age 65. *Menopause.* 2015;22(7):1.

41. American College of Obstetricians and Gynecologists. Practice Bulletin No. 141: management of menopausal symptoms. *Obstet Gynecol.* 2014;123: 202-216.

42. Pettersson F, Fries H, Nillius SJ. Epidemiology of secondary amenorrhea. I. Incidence and prevalence rates. *Am J Obstet Gynecol.* 1973;117:80-86.

43. Bachmann GA, Kemmann E. Prevalence of oligomenorrhea and amenorrhea in a college population. *Am J Obstet Gynecol.* 1982;144:98-102.

44. Marsh CA, Grimstead FW. Primary amenorrhea: diagnosis and management. *Obstet Gynecol Surv.* 2014; 69:603-612. doi:10.1097/OGX.0000000000000111.

45. Rebar R. Evaluation of amenorrhea, anovulation, and abnormal bleeding. In: De Groot LJ, Beck-Peccoz P, Chrousos G, et al., eds. *Endotext.* South Dartmouth, MA: MDText.com, Inc.

46. Javed A, Tebben PJ, Fischer PR, Lteif AN. Female athlete triad and its components: toward improved screening and management. *Mayo Clin Proc.* 2013;88(9):996-1009.

47. Practice Committee of the American Society for Reproductive Medicine. Current evaluation of amenorrhea. *Fertil Steril.* 2008;90:S219-S225.

48. Klein DA, Poth MA. Amenorrhea: an approach to diagnosis and management. *Am Fam Physician.* 2013;87(11):781-788.

49. Torre DL, Falorni A. Pharmacological causes of hyperprolactinemia. *Ther Clin Risk Manag.* 2007; 3(5):929-951.

50. Azziz R, Woods KS, Reyna R, Key TJ, Knochenhauer ES, Yildiz BO. The prevalence and features of the polycystic ovary syndrome in an unselected population. *J Clin Endocrinol Metab.* 2004;89:2745-2749.

51. March WA, Moore VM, Willson KJ, Phillips DIW, Norman RJ, Davies MJ. The prevalence of polycystic ovary syndrome in a community sample assessed under contrasting diagnostic criteria. *Hum Reprod.* 2010;25(2):544-551.

52. Wang S, Alvero R. Racial and ethnic differences in physiology and clinical symptoms of polycystic ovary syndrome. *Semin Reprod Med.* 2013;31(5):365-369. doi:10.1055/s-0033-1348895.

53. Rotterdam ESHRE/ASRM-Sponsored PCOS Consensus Workshop Group. Revised 2003 consensus on diagnostic criteria and long-term health risks related to polycystic ovary syndrome (PCOS). *Hum Reprod.* 2004;19(1):41.

54. Rosenfield RL. The diagnosis of polycystic ovary syndrome in adolescents. *Pediatrics.* 2015;136(6):1154-1165. doi:10.1542/peds.2015-1430.

55. Teede H, Deeks A, Moran L. Polycystic ovary syndrome: a complex condition with psychological, reproductive and metabolic manifestations that impacts on health across the lifespan. *BMC Med.* 2010; 8:41. doi:10.1186/1741-7015-8-41.

56. Sheehan MT. Polycystic ovarian syndrome: diagnosis and management. *Clin Med Res.* 2004;2(1):13-27.

57. ACOG Committee on Practice Bulletins—Gynecology. ACOG Practice Bulletin No. 108: Polycystic ovary syndrome. *Obstet Gynecol.* 2009;114(4): 936-949. doi:10.1097/AOG.0b013e3181bd12cb.

58. Deeks AA, Gibson-Helm ME, Teede HJ. Anxiety and depression in polycystic ovary syndrome: a comprehensive investigation. *Fertil Steril.* 2010;93(7): 2421-2423. doi:10.1016/j.fertnstert.2009.09.018.

59. Himelein MJ, Thatcher SS. Polycystic ovary syndrome and mental health: a review. *Obstet Gynecol Surv.* 2006;61:723-732. doi:10.1097/01.ogx.0000243772.33357.84.

60. Shaw LJ, Bairey Merz CN, Azziz R, Stanczyk FZ, Sopko G, Braunstein GD, et al. Postmenopausal women with a history of irregular menses and elevated androgen measurements at high risk for worsening cardiovascular event-free survival: results from the National Institutes of Health-National Heart, Lung, and Blood Institute sponsored Women's Ischemia Syndrome Evaluation. *J Clin Endocrinol Metab.* 2008;93:1276-1284. doi:10.1210/jc.2007-0425.

61. Rees DA, Jenkins-Jones S, Morgan CL. Contemporary reproductive outcomes for patients with polycystic ovary syndrome: a retrospective observational study. *J Clin Endocrinol Metab.* 2016;101(4):1664-1672.

62. Boomsma CM, Eijkemans MJ, Hughes EG, Visser GH, Fauser BC, Macklon NS. A meta-analysis of pregnancy outcomes in women with polycystic ovary syndrome. *Hum Reprod Update.* 2006;12(6):673-683.

63. De Frène V, Vansteelandt S, T'Sjoen G, Gerris J, Somers S, Vercruysse L, et al. A retrospective study of the pregnancy, delivery and neonatal outcome in overweight versus normal weight women with polycystic ovary syndrome. *Hum Reprod.* 2014;29(10): 2333-2338. doi:10.1093/humrep/deu154.

64. Naderpoor N, Shorakae S, de Courten B, Misso ML, Moran LJ, Teede HJ. Metformin and lifestyle modification in polycystic ovary syndrome: systematic review and meta-analysis. *Hum Reprod Update.* 2015;21(5):560-574. doi:10.1093/humupd/dmv025.

65. Marret H, Fauconnier A, Chabbert-Buffet N, Cravello L, Golfier F, Gondry J, et al. Clinical practice guidelines on menorrhagia: management of

abnormal uterine bleeding before menopause. *Eur J Obstet Gynecol Reprod Biol.* 2010;152(2):133-137. doi: 10.1016/j.ejogrb.2010.07.016.

66. Munro MG, Critchley HO, Broder MS, Fraser IS; FIGO Working Group on Menstrual Disorders. FIGO classification system (PALM-COEIN) for causes of abnormal uterine bleeding in nongravid women of reproductive age. *Int J Gynaecol Obstet.* 2011;113(1):3-13. doi:10.1016/j.ijgo.2010.11.011.

67. American College of Obstetricians and Gynecologists Committee on Practice Bulletins—Gynecology. Practice bulletin no. 128: diagnosis of abnormal uterine bleeding in reproductive-aged women. *Obstet Gynecol.* 2012;120(1):197-206. doi:10.1097/AOG.0b013e318262e320.

68. Twiss JJ. A new look at abnormal uterine bleeding. *Nurse Pract.* 2013;38(12):22-30; quiz 31. doi:10.1097/01.NPR.0000437574.76024.ef.

69. Bradley LD, Gueye NA. The medical management of abnormal uterine bleeding in reproductive-aged women. *Am J Obstet Gynecol.* 2016;214(1):31-44. doi:10.1016/j.ajog.2015.07.044.

70. Shankar M, Lee CA, Sabin CA, Economides DL, Kadir RA. von Willebrand disease in women with menorrhagia: a systematic review. *BJOG.* 2004;111(7):734-740.

71. Minjarez DA, Bradshaw KD. Abnormal uterine bleeding in adolescents. *Obstet Gynecol Clin North Am.* 2000;27(1):63-78.

72. Davidson BR, DiPiero CM, Govoni KD, Littleton SS, Neal JL. Abnormal uterine bleeding during the reproductive years. *J Midwifery Womens Health.* 2012;57(3):248-254.

73. Fraser IS, Critchley HO, Munro MG, Broder M; Writing Group for this Menstrual Agreement Process. A process designed to lead to international agreement on terminologies and definitions used to describe abnormalities of menstrual bleeding. *Fertil Steril.* 2007;87(3):466-476.

74. Kadir RA, Economides DL, Sabin CA, Owens D, Lee CA. Frequency of inherited bleeding disorders in women with menorrhagia. *Lancet.* 1998;351(9101)485-489.

75. Hickey M, Balen A. Menstrual disorders in adolescence: investigation and management. *Hum Reprod Update.* 2003;9(5):493-504.

76. Wilkinson JP, Kadir RA. Management of abnormal uterine bleeding in adolescents. *J Pediatr Adolesc Gynecol.* 2010;23(6):S22-S30.

77. American College of Obstetricians and Gynecologists. Committee Opinion No. 557. Management of acute abnormal uterine bleeding in nonpregnant reproductive-aged women. *Obstet Gynecol.* 2013; 121:891-896.

78. American College of Obstetricians and Gynecologists. The role of transvaginal ultrasonography in the evaluation of postmenopausal bleeding. ACOG Committee Opinion No. 440. *Obstet Gynecol.* 2009; 114:409-411.

79. Gull B, Karlsson B, Milsom I, Granberg S. Can ultrasound replace dilation and curettage? A longitudinal evaluation of postmenopausal bleeding and transvaginal sonographic measurement of the endometrium as predictors of endometrial cancer. *Am J Obstet Gynecol.* 2003;188:401-408.

80. Ahangari A. Prevalence of chronic pelvic pain among women: an updated review. *Pain Physician.* 2014; 17(2):E141-E147.

81. Speer LM, Mushkbar S, Erbele T. Chronic pelvic pain in women. *Am Fam Physician.* 2016;93(5):380-387.

82. Bhosale PR, Javitt MC, Atri M, Harris RD, Kang SK, Meyer BJ, et al. ACR Appropriateness Criteria® Acute Pelvic Pain in the Reproductive Age Group. *Ultrasound Q.* 2015 Nov 19. [Epub ahead of print]

83. Huchon C, Fauconnier A. Adnexal torsion: a literature review. *Eur J Obstet Gynecol Reprod Biol.* 2010;150(1): 8-12. doi:10.1016/j.ejogrb.2010.02.006.

84. Melcer Y, Sarig-Meth T, Maymon R, Pansky M, Vaknin Z, Smorgick N. Similar but different: a comparison of adnexal torsion in pediatric, adolescent, and pregnant and reproductive-age women. *J Womens Health (Larchmt).* 2015;25(4):391-396.

85. Sasaki KJ, Miller CE. Adnexal torsion: review of the literature. *J Minim Invasive Gynecol.* 2014;21(2):196-202. doi:10.1016/j.jmig.2013.09.010.

86. Hasson J, Tsafrir Z, Azem F, Bar-On S, Almog B, Mashiach R, et al. Comparison of adnexal torsion between pregnant and nonpregnant women. *Am J Obstet Gynecol.* 2010;202(6):536.e1-6. doi: 10.1016/j.ajog.2009.11.028.

87. Haefner HK. Report of the International Society for the Study of Vulvovaginal Disease: terminology and classification of vulvodynia. *J Low Genit Tract Dis.* 2007;11:48-49.

88. Harlow B, Kunitz C, Nguyen R, Rydell SA, Turner RM, MacLehose RF. Prevalence of symptoms consistent with a diagnosis of vulvodynia: population-based estimates from 2 geographic regions. *Am J Obstet Gynecol.* 2014;210:40.e1.

89. Pukall CF, Goldstein AT, Bergeron S, Foster D, Stein A, Kellogg-Spadt S, et al. Vulvodynia: definition, prevalence, impact, and pathophysiological factors. *J Sex Med.* 2016;13(3):291-304. doi: 0.1016/j.jsxm.2015.12.021.

90. Harlow BL, Stewart EG. A population-based assessment of chronic unexplained vulvar pain: have we underestimated the prevalence of vulvodynia? *J Am Med Womens Assoc.* 2003;58:82.

91. Reed BD, Legocki LJ, Plegue MA, Sen A, Haefner HK, Harlow SD. Factors associated with vulvodynia incidence. *Obstet Gynecol.* 2014;123(201):225-231. doi:10.1097/AOG.0000000000000066.

92. Sadownik LA. Etiology, diagnosis, and clinical management of vulvodynia. *Int J Womens Health.* 2014;6:437-449. doi:10.2147/IJWH.S37660.

93. Reed BD, Advincula AP, Fonde KR, Gorenflo DW, Haefner HK. Sexual activities and attitudes of women with vulvar dysesthesia. *Obstet Gynecol.* 2003; 102:325-331.

94. Cox KJ, Neville CE. Assessment and management options for women with vulvodynia. *J Midwifery Womens Health.* 2012;57:231-240. doi: 10.1111/j.1542-2011.2012.00162.x.

95. Gunter J. Vulvodynia: new thoughts on a devastating condition. *Obstet Gynecol Surv.* 2007;62(12): 812-819.

96. Laumann EO, Paik A, Rosen RC. Sexual dysfunction in the United States: prevalence and predictors [published correction appears in *JAMA.* 1999;281(13):1174]. *JAMA.* 1999;281(6):537-544.

97. Simons JS, Carey MP. Prevalence of sexual dysfunctions: results from a decade of research. *Arch Sex Behav.* 2001;30(2):177-219.

98. Seehusen DA, Baird DC, Bode DV. Dyspareunia in women. *Am Fam Physician.* 2014;90(7):465-470.

99. American Psychiatric Association. *Diagnostic and Statistical Manual of Mental Disorders, 5th Edition: DSM-5.* Arlington, VA: American Psychiatric Publishing; 2013.

100. Lahaie MA, Amsel R, Khalifé S, Boyer S, Faaborg-Andersen M, Binik YM. Can fear, pain, and muscle tension discriminate vaginismus from dyspareunia/provoked vestibulodynia? implications for the new DSM-5 diagnosis of genito-pelvic pain/penetration disorder. *Arch Sex Behav.* 2015;44(6):1537-1550. doi:10.1007/s10508-014-0430-z.

101. Brauer M, Lakeman M, van Lunsen R, Laan E. Predictors of task-persistent and fear-avoiding behaviors in women with sexual pain disorders. *J Sex Med.* 2014;11:3051-3063.

102. Buttram VC, Jr, Gomel V, Siegler A, DeCherney A, Gibbons W, March C. The American Fertility Society classifications of adnexal adhesions, distal tubal occlusion, tubal occlusion secondary to tubal ligation, tubal pregnancies, Müllerian anomalies and intrauterine adhesions. *Fertil Steril.* 1988;49:944-955.

103. Chan YY, Jayaprakasan K, Zamora J, Thornton JG, Raine-Fenning N, Coomarasamy A. The prevalence of congenital uterine anomalies in unselected and high-risk populations: a systematic review. *Hum Reprod Update.* 2011;17(6):761-771. doi:10.1093/humupd/dmr028.

104. Dreisler E, Stampe Sørensen S. Müllerian duct anomalies diagnosed by saline contrast sonohysterography: prevalence in a general population. *Fertil Steril.* 2014;102(2):525-529. doi:10.1016/j.fertnstert.2014.04.043.

105. Chandler TM, Machan LS, Cooperberg PL, Harris AC, Chang SD. Müllerian duct anomalies: from diagnosis to intervention. *Br J Radiol.* 2009;82(984): 1034-1042. doi:10.1259/bjr/99354802.

106. Behr SC, Courtier JL, Qayyum A. Imaging of müllerian duct anomalies. *Radiographics.* 2012;(6): E233-E250.

107. Mueller GC, Hussain HK, Smith YR, Quint EH, Carlos RC, Johnson TD, et al. Müllerian duct anomalies: comparison of MRI diagnosis and clinical diagnosis. *AJR Am J Roentgenol.* 2007;189: 1294-1302.

108. Marcal L, Nothaft MA, Coelho F, Volpato R, Iyer R. Mullerian duct anomalies: MR imaging. *Abdom Imaging.* 2011;36(6):756-764.

109. Chan YY, Jayaprakasan K, Tan A, Thornton JG, Coomarasamy A, Raine-Fenning NJ. Reproductive outcomes in women with congenital uterine anomalies: a systematic review. *Ultrasound Obstet Gynecol.* 2011;38:371-382. doi:10.1002/uog.10056 (2011B).

110. Venetis CA, Papadopoulos SP, Campo R, Gordts S, Tarlatzis BC, Grimbizis GF. Clinical implications of congenital uterine anomalies: a meta-analysis of comparative studies. *Reprod Biomed Online.* 2014;29(6): 665-683. doi:10.1016/j.rbmo.2014.09.006.

111. Baird DD, Dunson DB, Hill MC, Cousins D, Schectman JM. High cumulative incidence of uterine leiomyoma in black and white women: ultrasound evidence. *Am J Obstet Gynecol.* 2003;188(1): 100-107.

112. Moorman PG, Leppert P, Myers ER, Wang F. Comparison of characteristics of fibroids in African American and white women undergoing pre-menopausal hysterectomy. *Fertil Steril.* 2013;99(3):768-776.e1. doi:10.1016/j.fertnstert.2012.10.039.

113. Marshall LM, Spiegelman D, Barbieri RL, Goldman MB, Manson JE, Colditz GA, et al. Variation in the incidence of uterine leiomyoma among premenopausal women by age and race. *Obstet Gynecol.* 1997;90(6):967-973.

114. Faerstein E, Szklo M, Rosenshein N. Risk factors for uterine leiomyoma: a practice-based case-control study. I. African-American heritage, reproductive history, body size, and smoking. *Am J Epidemiol.* 2001;153(1):1-10. doi:10.1093/aje/153.1.1.

115. Chen CR, Buck GM, Courey NG, Perez KM, Wactawski-Wende J. Risk factors for uterine fibroids among women undergoing tubal sterilization. *Am J Epidemiol.* 2001;153(1):20-26.

116. Parazzini F. Risk factors for clinically diagnosed uterine fibroids in women around menopause. *Maturitas.* 2006;55(2):174-179.

117. Wise LA, Palmer JR, Harlow BL, Spiegelman D, Stewart EA, Adams-Campbell LL, et al. Reproductive factors, hormonal contraception, and risk of uterine leiomyomata in African-American women: a prospective study. *Am J Epidemiol.* 2004;159:113-123.

118. Stewart EA. Uterine fibroids. *N Engl J Med.* 2015; 372:1646-1655. doi:10.1056/NEJMcp1411029.

119. Klatsky PC, Tran ND, Caughey AB, Fujimoto VY. Fibroids and reproductive outcomes: a systematic literature review from conception to delivery. *Am J Obstet Gynecol.* 2008;198:357-366.

120. Michels KA, Edwards DRV, Baird DD, Savitz DA, Hartmann KE. Uterine leiomyomata and cesarean birth risk: a prospective cohort with standardized imaging. *Ann Epidemiol.* 2014;24(2):122-126. doi:10.1016/j.annepidem.2013.10.017.

121. Zimmermann A, Bernuit D, Gerlinger C, Schaefers M, Geppert K. Prevalence, symptoms and management of uterine fibroids: an international internet-based survey of 21,746 women. *BMC Womens Health.* 2012;12:6.

122. Mercorio F, De Simone R, Di Spiezio Sardo A, Cerrota G, Bifulco G, Vanacore F, et al. The effect of a levonorgestrel-releasing intrauterine device in the treatment of myoma-related menorrhagia. *Contraception.* 2003;67:277-280.

123. American College of Obstetricians and Gynecologists. Alternatives to hysterectomy in the management of leiomyomas. ACOG Practice Bulletin No. 96. *Obstet Gynecol.* 2008;112:201-207.

124. Paul PG, Rengaraj V, Das T, Garg R, Thomas M, Khurd AS. Uterine sarcomas in patients undergoing surgery for presumed leiomyomas: 10 years' experience. *J Minim Invasive Gynecol.* 2016;23(3):384-389. doi:10.1016/j.jmig.2015.11.012.

125. Lieng M, Berner E, Busund B. Risk of morcellation of uterine leiomyosarcomas in laparoscopic supracervical hysterectomy and laparoscopic myomectomy, a retrospective trial including 4791 women. *J Minim Invasive Gynecol.* 2015;22(3):410-414. doi: 10.1016/j.jmig.2014.10.022.

126. Struble J, Reid S, Bedaiwy MA. Adenomyosis: a clinical review of a challenging gynecologic condition. *J Minim Invasive Gynecol.* 2016;23(2):164-185. doi: 10.1016/j.jmig.2015.09.018.

127. Vercellini P, Viganò P, Somigliana E, Daguati R, Abbiati A, Fedele L. Adenomyosis: epidemiological factors. *Best Pract Res Clin Obstet Gynecol.* 2006; 20(4):465-477.

128. Templeman C, Marshall SF, Ursin G, Horn-Ross PL, Clarke CA, Allen M, et al. Adenomyosis and endometriosis in the California Teachers Study. *Fertil Steril.* 2008;90:415-424.

129. Levgur M. Diagnosis of adenomyosis: a review. *J Reprod Med.* 2007;52:177-193.

130. Cockerham AZ. Adenomyosis: a challenge in clinical gynecology. *J Midwifery Womens Health.* 2012;57: 212-220. doi:10.1111/j.1542-2011.2011.00117.x.

131. Champaneria R, Abedin P, Daniels J, Balogun M, Khan KS. Ultrasound scan and magnetic resonance imaging for the diagnosis of adenomyosis: systematic review comparing test accuracy. *Acta Obstet Gynecol Scand.* 2010;89:1374-1384.

132. Cho S, Nam A, Kim H, Chay D, Park K, Cho DJ, et al. Clinical effects of the levonorgestrel-releasing intrauterine device in patients with adenomyosis. *Am J Obstet Gynecol.* 2008;198:373.e1-e7.

133. Fedele L, Bianchi S, Raffaelli R, Portuese A, Dorta M. Treatment of adenomyosis-associated menorrhagia with a levonorgestrel-releasing intrauterine device. *Fertil Steril.* 1997;68:426-429.

134. Ozdegirmenci O, Kayikcioglu F, Akgul MA, Kaplan M, Karcaaltincaba M, Haberal A, et al. Comparison of levonorgestrel intrauterine system versus hysterectomy on efficacy and quality of life in patients with adenomyosis. *Fertil Steril.* 2011;95(2):497-502.

135. Burney RO, Giudice LC. Pathogenesis and pathophysiology of endometriosis. *Fertil Steril.* 2012;98(3): 511-519. doi:10.1016/j.fertnstert.2012.06.029.

136. McCool WF, Durain DC. Gynecologic disorders. In: King TL, Brucker MC, Kriebs JM, Fahey JO, Gegor CL, Varney H, eds. *Varney's Midwifery.* 5th ed. Burlington, MA: Jones & Bartlett Learning.

137. Eskenazi B, Warner ML. Epidemiology of endometriosis. *Obstet Gynecol Clin North Am.* 1997;24:235-258.

138. Meuleman C, Vandenabeele B, Fieuws S, Spiessens C, Timmerman D, D'Hooghe T. High prevalence of endometriosis in infertile women with normal ovulation and normospermic partners. *Fertil Steril.* 2009; 92:68-74.

139. Ballard K, Seaman H, De Vries C, Wright J. Can symptomatology help in the diagnosis of endometriosis? Findings from a national case–control study—Part 1. *BJOG.* 2008;115:1382-1391. doi: 10.1111/j.1471-0528.2008.01878.x.

140. Dunselman GAJ, Vermuelen N, Becker C. ESHRE guideline: management of women with endometriosis. *Hum Reprod.* 2014;29:400-412. doi:10.1093/humrep/det457.

141. Brown J, Farquhar C. Endometriosis: an overview of Cochrane Reviews. *Cochrane Database Syst*

Rev. 2014;3:CD009590. doi:10.1002/14651858. CD009590.pub2.

142. American College of Obstetricians and Gynecologists. Management of endometriosis. Practice Bulletin No. 113. *Obstet Gynecol.* 2010;116:223-236.

143. Park JC, Lim SY, Jang TK, Bae JG, Kim JI, Rhee JH. Endometrial histology and predictable clinical factors for endometrial disease in women with polycystic ovary syndrome. *Clin Exp Reprod Med.* 2011;38: 42-46.

144. Ash SJ, Farrell SA, Flowerden G. Endometrial biopsy in DUB. *J Reprod Med.* 1996;41:892-896.

145. Opolskiene G, Sladkevicius P, Valentin L. Prediction of endometrial malignancy in women with postmenopausal bleeding and sonographic endometrial thickness ≥4.5 mm. *Ultrasound Obstet Gynecol.* 2011;37:232-240.

146. Armstrong AJ, Hurd WW, Elguero S, Barker NM, Zanotti KM. Diagnosis and management of endometrial hyperplasia. *J Minim Invasive Gynecol.* 2012; 19(5):562-571. doi:10.1016/j.jmig.2012.05.009.

147. Trimble CL, Method M, Leitao M, Lu K, Ioffe O, Hampton M, et al. Management of endometrial precancers. *Obstet Gynecol.* 2012;120(5):1160-1175.

148. Baak JPA, Mutter GL. EIN and WHO94. *J Clin Pathol.* 2005;58:11-6. doi:10.1136/jcp.2004.021071.

149. National Cancer Institute. SEER Stat Fact Sheets: Endometrial Cancer. Available at: http://seer.cancer.gov/statfacts/html/corp.html. Accessed May 25, 2016.

150. Sorosky JI. Endometrial cancer. *Obstet Gynecol.* 2012;120(2 Pt 1):383-397. doi:10.1097/AOG.0b013e3182605bf1.

151. National Cancer Institute. A snapshot of endometrial cancer: Incidence and mortality. Available at: http://www.cancer.gov/research/progress/snapshots/endometrial. Accessed May 25, 2016.

152. American College of Obstetricians and Gynecologists. Endometrial cancer. Practice Bulletin No. 149. *Obstet Gynecol.* 2015;125:1006-1026.

153. Maher C, Feiner B, Baessler K, Schmid C. Surgical management of pelvic organ prolapse in women. *Cochrane Database Syst Rev.* 2013;4:CD004014. doi:10.1002/14651858.CD004014.pub5.

154. Hendrix SL, Clark A, Nygaard I, Aragaki A, Barnabei V, McTiernan A. Pelvic organ prolapse in the Women's Health Initiative: gravity and gravidity. *Am J Obstet Gynecol.* 2002;186(6):1160-1166.

155. Kudish BI, Iglesia CB, Sokol RJ, Cochrane B, Richter HE, Larson J, et al. Effect of weight change on natural history of pelvic organ prolapse. *Obstet Gynecol.* 2009;113(1):81-88. doi:10.1097/AOG.0b013e318190a0dd.

156. McNeeley SG. Cystoceles, Urethroceles, Enteroceles, and Rectoceles. *Merck Manual.* Available at: http://www.merckmanuals.com/professional/gynecology-and-obstetrics/pelvic-relaxation-syndromes/cystoceles,-urethroceles,-enteroceles,-and-rectoceles. Accessed May 25, 2016.

157. McNeeley SG. Uterine and Vaginal Prolapse. *Merck Manual.* Available at: http://www.merckmanuals.com/professional/gynecology-and-obstetrics/pelvic-relaxation-syndromes/uterine-and-vaginal-prolapse. Accessed May 25, 2016.

158. Hagen S, Stark D. Conservative prevention and management of pelvic organ prolapse in women. *Cochrane Database Syst Rev.* 2011;12:CD003882. doi:10.1002/14651858.CD003882.pub4.

159. Braekken IH, Majida M, Engh ME, Bø K. Can pelvic floor muscle training reverse pelvic organ prolapse and reduce prolapse symptoms? An assessor-blinded, randomized, controlled trial. *Am J Obstet Gynecol.* 2010;203(2):170.e1-7. doi: 10.1016/j.ajog.2010.02.037.

160. Abdulaziz M, Stothers L, Lazare D, Macnab A. An integrative review and severity classification of complications related to pessary use in the treatment of female pelvic organ prolapse. *Can Urol Assoc J.* 2015;9(5-6):E400-6. doi:10.5489/cuaj.2783.

161. Borgfeldt C, Andolf E. Transvaginal sonographic ovarian findings in a random sample of women 25-40 years old. *Ultrasound Obstet Gynecol.* 1999;13: 345-350.

162. Greenlee RT, Kessel B, Williams CR, Riley TL, Ragard LR, Hartge P, et al. Prevalence, incidence, and natural history of simple ovarian cysts among women > 55 years old in a large cancer screening trial. *Am J Obstet Gynecol.* 2010;202:373.e1-E9.

163. Ackerman S, Irshad A, Lewis M, Anis M. Ovarian cystic lesions. *Radiol Clin North Am.* 2013;51: 1067-1085.

164. Kim MJ, Kim NY, Lee DY, Yoon BK, Choi D. Clinical characteristics of ovarian teratoma: age-focused retrospective analysis of 580 cases. *Am J Obstet Gynecol.* 2011;205(1):32.e1-4. doi:10.1016/j.ajog.2011.02.044.

165. Dos Santos L, Mok E, Iasonos A, Park K, Soslow RA, Aghajanian C, et al. Squamous cell carcinoma arising in mature cystic teratoma of the ovary: a case series and review of the literature. *Gynecol Oncol.* 2007;105(2):321-324.

166. National Cancer Institute. Ovarian, Fallopian Tube, and Primary Peritoneal Cancer—Health Professional Version. Available at: http://www.cancer.gov/types/ovarian/hp. Accessed June 2, 2016.

167. Pennington KP, Swisher EM. Hereditary ovarian cancer: beyond the usual suspects. *Gynecol Oncol.* 2012;124(2):347-353. doi:10.1016/j.ygyno.2011.12.415.

168. American College of Obstetricians and Gynecologists. Management of adnexal masses. ACOG Practice Bulletin No. 83. *Obstet Gynecol.* 2007; 110:201-214. Reaffirmed 2015.

169. Timmerman D, Testa AC, Bourne T, Ameye L, Jurkovic D, Van Holsbeke C, et al. Simple ultrasound-based rules for the diagnosis of ovarian cancer. *Ultrasound Obstet Gynecol.* 2008;31:681-690. doi:10.1002/uog.5365.

170. Timmerman D, Van Calster B, Testa A, Savelli L, Fischerova D, Froyman W, et al. Predicting the risk of malignancy in adnexal masses based on the Simple Rules from the International Ovarian Tumor Analysis group. *Am J Obstet Gynecol.* 2016;214(4):424-437. doi:10.1016/j.ajog.2016.01.007.

171. Buys SS, Partridge E, Black A, Johnson CC, Lamerato L, Isaacs C, et al. Effect of screening on ovarian cancer mortality: the Prostate, Lung, Colorectal and Ovarian (PLCO) cancer screening randomized controlled trial. *JAMA.* 2011;305(22):2295-2303. doi:10.1001/jama.2011.766.

172. Lambert J. Pruritus in female patients. *Biomed Res Int.* 2014;2014:541867. doi:10.1155/2014/541867.

173. Stewart KA. Clinical care of vulvar pruritus, with emphasis on one common cause, lichen simplex chronicus. *Dermatol Clin.* 2010;28:669-680.

174. Cooper SM, Ali I, Baldo M, Wojnarowska F. The association of lichen sclerosus and erosive lichen planus of the vulva with autoimmune disease: a case-control study. *Arch Dermatol.* 2008;144(11): 1432-1435.

175. Thorstensen KA, Birenbaum DL. Recognition and management of vulvar dermatologic conditions: lichen sclerosus, lichen planus, and lichen simplex chronicus. *J Midwifery Womens Health.* 2012;57:260-275. doi:10.1111/j.1542-2011.2012.00175.x.

176. Fistarol SK, Itin PH. Diagnosis and treatment of lichen sclerosus: an update. *Am J Clin Dermatol.* 2013;14(1):27-47. doi:10.1007/s40257-012-0006-4.

177. McPherson T, Cooper S. Vulval lichen sclerosus and lichen planus. *Dermatol Ther.* 2010;23(5):529-532.

178. Smith YR, Haefner HK. Vulvar lichen sclerosus: pathophysiology and treatment. *Am J Clin Dermatol.* 2004;5(2):105-125.

179. Piplin C. Erosive diseases of the vulva. *Dermatol Clin.* 2010;28:737-751.

180. Schlosser BJ. Lichen planus and lichenoid reactions of the oral mucosa. *Dermatol Ther.* 2010;23(3):251-267.

181. Simpson R, Thomas K, Leighton P, Murphy R. Diagnostic criteria for erosive lichen planus affecting the vulva: an international electronic-Delphi consensus exercise. *Br J Dermatol.* 2013;169(2):337-343. doi:10.1111/bjd.12334.

182. Simpson RC, Murphy R. Is vulval erosive lichen planus a premalignant condition? *Arch Dermatol.* 2012;148(11):1314-1316. doi:10.1001/2013.jamadermatol.84.

183. National Cancer Institute. SEER Stat Fact Sheets: Vulvar Cancer. Available at: http://seer.cancer.gov/statfacts/html/vulva.html. Accessed May 25, 2016.

184. Centers for Disease Control and Prevention. Vaginal and Vulvar Cancers. Available at: http://www.cdc.gov/cancer/vagvulv/index.htm. Accessed May 25, 2016.

185. Alkatout I, Schubert M, Garbrecht N, Weigel MT, Jonat W, Mundhenke C, et al. Vulvar cancer: epidemiology, clinical presentation, and management options. *Int J Womens Health.* 2015;7:305-313. doi:10.2147/IJWH.S68979.

186. Saraiya M, Unger ER, Thompson TD, Lynch CF, Hernandez BY, Lyu CW, et al. US Assessment of HPV types in cancers: implications for current and 9-valent HPV vaccines. *J Natl Cancer Inst.* 2015;107:djv086. doi:10.1093/jnci/djv086.

187. Jemal A, Simard EP, Dorell C, Noone AM, Markowitz LE, Kohler B, et al. Annual report to the nation on the status of cancer, 1975-2009, featuring the burden and trends in human papillomavirus (HPV)–associated cancers and HPV vaccination coverage levels. *J Natl Cancer Inst.* 2013;105(3):175-201. doi:10.1093/jnci/djs491.

188. Siegel RL, Miller KD, Jemal A. Cancer statistics, 2015. *CA Cancer J Clin.* 2015;65(1):5-29. doi:10.3322/caac.21254.

189. Howlader N, Noone AM, Krapcho M, Garshell J, Miller D, Altekruse SF, et al. SEER Cancer Statistics Review, 1975-2012. Bethesda, MD National Cancer Institute. Available at: http://seer.cancer.gov/csr/1975_2012/. Accessed May 25, 2016.

190. Simard EP, Naishadham D, Saslow D, Jemal A. Age-specific trends in black-white disparities in cervical cancer incidence in the United States: 1975-2009. *Gynecol Oncol.* 2012;127(3):611-615. doi:10.1016/j.ygyno.2012.08.021.

191. Beavis AL, Levinson KL. Preventing cervical cancer in the United States: barriers and resolutions for HPV vaccination. *Front Oncol.* 2016;6:19. doi:10.3389/fonc.2016.00019.

192. Healthy People 2020. Immunization and Infectious Diseases. 2015. Available at: http://www.healthypeople.gov/2020/topics-objectives/

topic/immunization-and-infectious-diseases/objectives?topicId=23. Accessed May 25, 2016.

193. Centers for Disease Control and Prevention. Teen Vaccination Coverage. Available at: http://www.cdc.gov/vaccines/parents/vacc-coverage-teens.html. Accessed May 25, 2016.

194. Moscicki A-B, Cox JT. Practice improvement in cervical screening and management (PICSM): symposium on management of cervical abnormalities in adolescents and young women. *J Low Genit Tract Dis*. 2010;14(1):73-80.

195. American College of Obstetricians and Gynecologists. Practice Bulletin No. 157: cervical cancer screening and prevention. *Obstet Gynecol*. 2016;127(1):e1-20. doi:10.1097/AOG.0000000000001263.

196. Saslow D, Solomon D, Lawson HW, Killackey M, Kulasingam SL, Cain J, et al. American Cancer Society, American Society for Colposcopy and Cervical Pathology, and American Society for Clinical Pathology Screening Guidelines for the Prevention and Early Detection of Cervical Cancer. *CA Cancer J Clin*. 2012;62(3):147-172. doi:10.3322/caac.21139.

197. Dillner J, Rebolj M, Birembaut P, Petry K-U, Szarewski A, Munk C, et al. Long term predictive values of cytology and human papillomavirus testing in cervical cancer screening: joint European cohort study. *BMJ*. 2008;337:a1754.

198. Huh WK, Ault KA, Chelmow D, Davey DD, Goulart RA, Garcia FA, et al. Use of primary high-risk human papillomavirus testing for cervical cancer screening: interim clinical guidance. *Obstet Gynecol*. 2015;125(2):330-337. doi:10.1097/AOG.0000000000000669.

199. American Society of Colposcopy and Cervical Pathology. Guidelines. Available at: http://www.asccp.org/guidelines. Accessed May 24, 2016.

CHAPTER 23

MUSCULOSKELETAL CONDITIONS

Deborah L. Schofield

Patients frequently present with musculoskeletal complaints in primary care women's health practice. Orthopedic conditions cannot be diagnosed or managed without knowledge of skeletal and muscular anatomy and the nervous system, because symptoms may arise from any of these components. Providers should be able to assess whether care is within their competence, or whether referral to an orthopedist (or subspecialist) is required.

Structures of the Musculoskeletal System

Bones, muscles, joints, tendons, ligaments, cartilage, and bursae compose the musculoskeletal system (MS), which functions to support and permit movement of the body. If any component of the system is compromised by injury or trauma, quality of life can be impacted. Disability from pain and immobility affect the woman's ability to perform her daily activities.

The framework of the MS is composed of the 206 bones that provide skeletal support to the associated soft tissue structures of the body. The bones are classified into four types: long bones, such as the humerus and femur; short bones, such as the metacarpals and phalanges; irregular bones, such as the carpal bones of the hand; and flat bones, such as the ribs.

Joints, the functional units of the MS, permit mobility. Joints connect all elements of the MS and are classified into two distinct types: non-synovial joints, which are composed of fibrous tissue or cartilage and are immovable or slightly movable, like those of intervertebral joints, and synovial joints, which are freely movable joints enclosed in a lubricant-filled cavity. The synovial fluid reduces friction between the component parts of the joint. Bursae are sacs surrounding the synovial joints to contain this fluid.

Cartilage is the fibrous tissue that covers the surface of opposing bones, such as in the knee or shoulder joints. Ligaments are fibrous bands running directly from one bone to another to strengthen the joint. They help prevent movement in undesirable directions. Lastly, tendons are strong fibrous cords that attach skeletal muscle to bone and permit the contraction of these muscles to produce movement.

Assessment

History

When a woman mentions problems related to the MS as the chief complaint, an appropriately focused history includes the following items. First, it must be determined whether the complaint is acute in nature, due to an injury, or whether the complaint is related to a chronic problem with an acute exacerbation. The characteristics of the complaint must then be elicited. (See **Box 23-1**.)

The examiner also needs a current list of any medications or allergies the client may have and history of any previous illness or surgery. Questions regarding the patient's family, occupational, and social history provide information about any genetic predisposition, living or work conditions that may cause or exacerbate the condition, and the woman's ability to access resources to assist with daily needs.

Physical Examination

The initial approach to the focused MS physical examination begins with an assessment of the client's gait, balance, and posture. The provider can begin this assessment as the woman enters the exam room and while she is seated during the initial history, noting any gait abnormalities, movement difficulties, or abnormal posturing. Gait should be assessed by noting the base of support, stride, and stance. Posture is assessed by the woman's ability to sit or stand erect, with the head midline, noting any deviation. Grimacing or guarding of particular areas of the body is noted, as are the woman's overall appearance and demeanor.

A full musculoskeletal assessment incorporates an evaluation of the spinal column, thorough palpation of all muscles and joints, active and passive range of motion, and determination of muscle strength of all joints, comparing each side of the body bilaterally. Size, symmetry, and alignment of bilateral structures are assessed. If the woman presents with a unilateral complaint, care should be taken to evaluate the unaffected side prior to the affected side. Importantly, the provider must note any swelling, deformity, increased curvature, crepitus, laxity, immobility, tremors or muscle spasm, muscle weakness, or complaint of pain. The examination of a particular area is not continued past the point where motion or pressure becomes painful.

Several validated pain scales are in common use, among them the Visual Analogue Scale, the Numerical Rating Scale, the Verbal Rating Scale, and the Faces Pain Scale-Revised. In a recent study, the Numerical Rating Pain Scale has been shown to be best able to detect differences in gender-specific ratings of pain intensity.[1]

Box 23-1 History for MS Complaint

Time and mechanism of injury or onset of chronic problem
The length of time the complaint has been present
The area(s) of the body affected by the problem
Location, duration, and quality of any pain
Any weakness, stiffness, or difficulty with balance or coordination
Spasm or immobility
Skin breakdown or alteration
Aggravating and alleviating factors (i.e., activity or rest)

A neurovascular assessment is also an essential component of the examination when there is an MS complaint; this rules out any compromise of the nerves and vascular structures related to the affected areas. Each cranial nerve is assessed, as are muscle strength, peripheral pulses, and the color, turgor, and sensation of the overlying skin and associated soft tissues.

Laboratory testing and diagnostic procedures are specific to the diagnoses being considered and are discussed in the appropriate sections that follow.

Low Back Pain

The most common musculoskeletal complaint seen in primary care is low back pain, with close to 90% of adults having one or more episodes of back pain at some point during their lifetime. About 97% of adults with low back pain have a mechanical injury (strain, sprain, disc injury, or trauma); 85% of these will not have

a specific pathologic diagnosis.[2] Descriptions of various symptoms can be used to help identify the cause of pain, such as areas of local tenderness, loss of lower extremity sensation, and loss of motor control. The evaluation of a low back complaint includes ruling out underlying medical disorders such as infection, metastatic cancers, inflammatory bowel disease, pyelonephritis, or referred pain from another abdominal or pelvic disorder. Psychogenic pain secondary to depression must also be considered. Other conditions affecting the back include scoliosis and osteoporosis, which may or may not be associated with pain; these are discussed later in this chapter. The common musculoskeletal causes of low back pain are shown in **Table 23-1**.

Low back pain can occur as a result of injury to the spinal muscles or lumbar strain, compression of a nerve root that arises from the vertebral column due to degenerative disc disease, herniated nucleus pulposus, inflammation, or vertebral fracture. In the most common presentation, the patient

Table 23-1 Common Causes of Low Back Pain

Disorder	Type of Pain	Location	Clinical Signs	Average Age of Onset
Lumbosacral strain	Spasmodic Aching Worsens with movement	Low back area Buttocks	Point tenderness Decreased ROM	20–45
Herniated nucleus pulposa	Shooting pain Lower extremity numbness Increases with bending	Buttocks Lower extremity Calf	Lower extremity weakness Decreased lower extremity reflexes Straight leg raises – positive	30–55
Osteoarthritis	Aching/shooting pain Pinching quality Increases with activity	Low back Lower extremity	Asymmetric LE reflexes Weakness of LE	>50

Abbreviations: ROM, range of motion; LE, lower extremity.

presents with a complaint of pain in the low back, buttock, and posterior thigh, which is described as aching or having a "spasm"-like quality. There is often local tenderness and decreased spinal motion. Loss of sensation secondary to nerve damage can cause weakness or numbness in the buttocks and lower extremity along the affected dermatome (area of spinal nerve distribution).

Diagnosis of Low Back Pain

Recent literature offers guidelines on the diagnosis and management of the patient presenting with low back pain. Specifically, "red flags" to alert providers to more serious underlying conditions include unexplained weight loss, trauma, and focal or diffuse neurologic findings.[3] In addition, being older than 50 years of age, elevated temperature > 100.4°F/38°C, loss of bowel or bladder function, and bilateral (as opposed to central or unilateral) pain may signal more complex problems.

A thorough medical history, inclusive of any previous injury or trauma, medications, surgeries, and chronic illnesses, provides a basis for the examination and eventual diagnosis of low back pain. Psychosocial factors to be considered include employment, hobbies, sports, and potential stressors in the home or work environment. Specific history questions related to back pain include time of onset, duration, location, and type of pain (shooting, burning, etc.). It is also important for the clinician to establish any potential aggravating or alleviating factors, such as lifting, movement, heat, or massage. The presence or absence of sciatica should be determined, because this is a major contributor to the differential diagnosis.

The examination of a patient presenting with back pain includes gait evaluation, assessment of active and passive range of motion, and a neurologic examination that assesses sensation, peripheral motor function, and deep tendon reflexes. The symmetry of the spine and muscle tone and mass are evaluated. An abdominal, pelvic, and rectal examination may be necessary to rule out gastro-intestinal (GI) involvement, uterine and ovarian causes, and cauda equina syndrome, respectively. Finally, clues to possible systemic causes of pain such as malignancy should be sought.

Straight leg raises (SLR) are performed as part of the musculoskeletal exam for low back pain. During SLR, reported pain in the low back or buttock is considered a positive finding and indicates nerve root involvement. The examiner checks to be sure that the pain is reproducible when the patient is distracted from the exercise. Sciatic pain is differentiated from tightness on the posterior leg.[4]

If a clear diagnosis of muscle and ligament strain exists, further diagnostic studies are not indicated. Plain-film x-rays in the acute phase of low back pain management, without the finding of red flags on physical exam, have not been found to improve clinical outcomes as compared with usual clinical care.[5,6] For patients with low back pain, imaging (x-rays, magnetic resonance imaging [MRI], or computed tomography [CT]) should only be considered when a patient exhibits a "red flag" physical finding or exhibits no improvement at the 4 to 6 week follow-up visit. Consideration should also be given to refer the patient to a provider skilled in the management of musculoskeletal problems.[7] **Table 23-2** indicates reasons to consider imaging modalities.

Lumbosacral Strain

Low back pain that presents with a sharp pain in the low back region as lumbosacral strain prevents the woman from walking or enjoying her normal activities. Lumbosacral strain is common in women 16 to 40 years of age and is among the 10 most common diagnoses in the primary care office.[8] Immediate pain may be associated with the movement that initiates the strain, but pain often develops or worsens 12 to 36 hours after an injury, as associated soft tissues become swollen.

Table 23-2 Indications for Radiographs in Patients with Acute Low Back Pain

History of trauma

Neurologic deficit

Symptoms of systemic illness

Temperature >100.4°F/38°C

History of:

    Cancer

    Glucocorticoid use

    Substance abuse (drugs or alcohol)

Symptoms are usually confined to the low back, buttocks, and thighs. Common descriptors are spasm, burning, or "twinging." Standing and bending are aggravating factors for pain caused by lumbosacral strain; lumbosacral strain also may worsen on inspiration or with sudden movement. Rest and reclining tend to provide relief. For pain relief, nonsteroidal anti-inflammatory drugs (NSAIDs) are commonly used and are now available in oral and topical formulations. The lowest effective dose and short-term use (2–3 weeks) of an NSAID is optimal, to avoid potential GI and cardiovascular toxicity.[8] Common NSAIDs used in musculoskeletal injury are shown in **Table 23-3**. Muscle relaxants and benzodiazepines have not been shown to be more effective than NSAIDs but can be considered as adjunctive therapy with caution due to their increased effects of sedation.[9] Narcotics may also be beneficial for relief of acute pain for a short period of time, not greater than 72 hours' duration. However, caution should be taken when using narcotics for acute lumbar strain, due to the potential for dependence with long-term use.[9] Additionally, intermittent application of ice packs during the first 48 to 72 hours may be beneficial,

Table 23-3 Nonsteroidal Anti-Inflammatory Drugs for Management of Musculoskeletal Injury

Ibuprofen (Motrin, Advil)	Rx 600–800 mg po every 6–8 hours OTC 200–400 mg po every 4–6 hours, package labeling specifies not more than 6 tablets/day
Celecoxib (Celebrex)	400 mg po, then 200 mg po every 12 hours
Diclofenac potassium (Cataflam)*	50 mg po tid
Diflunisal (Dolobid)	1000 mg po then 500 mg po every 8–12 hours
Naproxen sodium** (Anaprox 275 mg)	550 mg po then 275 mg po every 6–8 hours or 550 mg every 12 hours
(Anaprox DS)	550 mg po every 12 hours
(Aleve) OTC	220 mg po every 6–8 hours

*Diclofenac sodium (Voltaren, Voltaren XR) is used primarily for symptoms of arthritis, rather than musculoskeletal injury.

**Naproxen (Naprosen, EC-Naprosen) has a slower onset of action and is not generally used for this purpose.

Comment: Use of nonsteroidal anti-inflammatory drugs increases the incidence of gastrointestinal disorders and may also increase the risk of cardiovascular events. Medications used for long-term therapy should be carefully monitored for adverse effects.

Abbreviations: OTC, over the counter; DS, double strength.

with heat application if necessary after 72 hours. The cold reduces swelling and bleeding into the tissues, while heat relaxes the muscles and promotes blood flow.

Activity should be encouraged, because bedrest may worsen lumbosacral strain.[10-11] Stretching and strengthening exercises have been demonstrated to be most effective, regardless of whether the pain is from an acute incident or a chronic condition. Exercises with a focus on strengthening both lumbar spine extensors and core muscles, along with an individualized approach, should be considered to increase individual adherence.[11,12] Low-impact aerobic exercise is a good adjunct to therapy after 2 weeks, including activities such as walking, swimming, and light biking. Participation in structured exercise programs appears to have long-term benefits, including decreased work absence and decreased pain scores.[13] When combined with education and exercise programs, massage therapy has been demonstrated to be beneficial and long lasting for chronic and subacute pain.[14] Trials regarding the benefit of acupuncture for this purpose are unclear.[15] Counseling should also be directed to patient lifestyle, because maintaining normal weight and increasing regular exercise activities may assist in limiting recurrence.

Lumbosacral strain usually resolves without further treatment; however, follow up to assess recovery is recommended 1 month following the initial visit.

Other Conditions Presenting as Low Back Pain

In clients presenting with a herniated disc (herniated nucleus pulposus), pain is felt in the buttock or radiating down into the lower extremity as opposed to localizing in the low back area. This condition is related to compression of the nerve root as it emanates from the spinal column, most often at the L4–L5 level, with the possibility of

the L5–S1 level being affected either alone or with other vertebrae.

Sciatica is the term used for this irritation of the nerve root. The pain is sharp and radiates down the posterior or lateral portion of the leg to the foot. Numbness and tingling are common. If the compression is progressive, weakness, decreased muscle tone, and diminished reflexes of the affected lower extremity will develop.[4] Clients with these symptoms should be referred to orthopedics or physical medicine for further evaluation and treatment. Herniation at the thoracic level is rare; however, it should be considered as part of the differential diagnosis of chest and upper extremity complaints. When suspected, a referral for care should be obtained promptly.

Compression fractures are most commonly seen in association with osteoporosis, glucocorticoid use, and metastatic cancer. The onset of pain is sharp. Typically, the distribution of the pain is lateral rather than extending into the lower extremities. As with herniation of a lumbar disc, patients in whom compression fracture is suspected should be promptly referred to an orthopedic specialist. Any condition that presents with loss of bowel and bladder function (cauda equina syndrome) and those involving paralysis or suspected aneurysm should be considered emergent and be referred to an emergency department or surgeon immediately.

Some patients suffering from depression will present with somatic symptoms as their primary complaint. In general, these patients will have symptoms that are more severe than the history and examination suggest. Thorough evaluation is still required to ensure that the medical diagnosis is not obscured by the psychologic one.

Malingering must be considered as a possibility in patients presenting with low back pain. Maneuvers such as axial loading, where the examiner places downward pressure on the top of the head, that elicit pain and inappropriate complaints of pain on palpation to the areas of the low back that are not involved are clues for the examiner to consider malingering as a potential diagnosis.

Clinicians also must be aware that patients with drug-seeking behaviors will feign back pain to garner opioid medications. In the absence of a secure diagnosis, it is not advisable for the provider to prescribe controlled substances for pain relief. In addition, if the patient has a clinician who is managing a chronic condition such as low back pain, all prescriptions for controlled substances are deferred to that clinician.

Sprain Injuries

Unlike a strain, in which there is injury to a segment of a muscle related to excessive forcible stretch, a sprain is an injury to the ligamentous structures of the body. Sprains occur near a joint, whereas strains present within the muscle body, which often helps to differentiate between the two forms of injury. Common sites of sprain injury are the wrist, elbow, knee, and ankle.

Loss of continuity when the ligaments are overstretched may result in one of three types of sprains:

- First degree: mildly stretched
- Second degree: moderately stretched with some tearing of the ligament
- Third degree: severely stretched with complete tear (avulsion) of the ligament

The most common sprain is that of the ankle, and these injuries typically occur when someone is walking or running on an uneven surface. Inversion injury to the lateral area of the ankle is the most common presentation. Cardinal signs of ankle sprain include immediate pain, immediate inability to bear weight, the sensation of a "pop" or "snap" and locking of the ankle, and joint swelling within 1 hour of injury.

Diagnosis of sprain requires a thorough examination of both ankles, beginning with the unaffected side. **Figure 23-1** illustrates the parts of the ankle. All structures of the ankle joint are observed and palpated, looking for inflammation, swelling, deformity, hematoma or pallor, intact pulses, crepitation, and decreased active and/or passive range of motion. The inability to bear weight and joint instability are also assessed, using Talar tilt and anterior drawer tests (**Figure 23-2**).

Ankle sprains do not require radiography unless criteria suggestive of fracture are met. The Ottawa ankle criteria, a set of highly useful criteria for the management of ankle injuries, recommend radiologic studies if there is pain at either the lateral or medial malleolus with bone tenderness at the posterior edge or tip, or an inability to bear weight both immediately after the injury and in the emergency department.[16]

Management of sprain is a two-step process. The therapeutic plan for the first 48 hours includes avoidance of weight-bearing activity, using crutches or splints as necessary, NSAIDs for pain relief, and (P)RICE(S) therapy—(protection), rest, ice, compression, elevation (and support) (**Table 23-4**).[17] An air compression support may be more useful than elastic bandages.

After the first 2 days, soaking the affected joint alternately in warm and cold water, dorsiflexion/plantarflexion exercises, and isometric resistance exercises can be started. Use of compression bandages can be continued to reduce swelling and stabilize the joint. Plastic braces also may be used to stabilize the ankle during recovery. For first- and second-degree sprains, these measures will usually suffice. However, third-degree sprains with complete ligament tear often require surgery.[17] Conservative management of even third-degree sprains may be sufficient; physical therapy focusing on balance, increasing muscle strength and flexibility surrounding the joint.

Figure 23-1 Lateral view of the ankle.

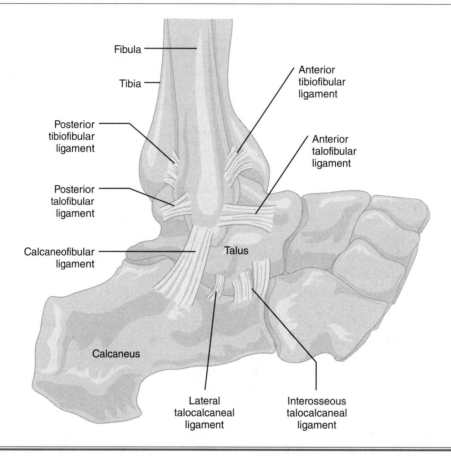

Fibula

Tibia

Anterior tibiofibular ligament

Posterior tibiofibular ligament

Anterior talofibular ligament

Posterior talofibular ligament

Calcaneofibular ligament

Talus

Calcaneus

Lateral talocalcaneal ligament

Interosseous talocalcaneal ligament

Four to 6 weeks is an average time for recovery from pain and obvious disability. During that time, the clinician should continue to monitor for a possible fracture and for neurovascular compromise. Ankle fractures are rare and involve the malleoli either unilaterally or bilaterally.

Although sprains often are regarded as minor injuries, severe sprains require orthopedic evaluation and joint immobilization during healing. If the degree of injury is unclear or the examination suggests the need for radiology, referral to an orthopedic provider is indicated. Finally, patients need to understand that resolution of pain does not indicate complete recovery of ligament strength, which may take several months, depending on the severity of the injury.

Figure 23-2 Talar tilt and anterior drawer tests to assess ankle sprain.

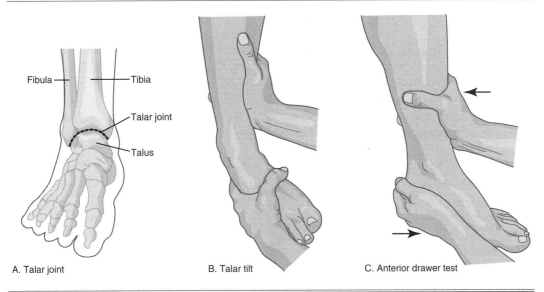

A. Talar joint   B. Talar tilt   C. Anterior drawer test

Table 23-4 Management of Pain from a Sprain Using the RICE Mnemonic

- Rest – Use a cane on the opposite side from the injury, crutches as necessary, and reduce activity to the minimum necessary.
- Ice – Applied for 20 minutes 4 to 8 times a day.
- Compression – Elastic bandages, an air cast, or splints may be applied for support.
- Elevation – Above the level of the heart if possible.

Data from Wolfe MW, Uhl TL, Mattacola CG, McCluskey LC. Management of ankle sprains. *Am Fam Physician*. 2001;63: 93-104.

Costochondritis

Costochondritis is an inflammation in the interface between the bony and cartilaginous area of the thoracic cage, the costochondral junction, which causes chest pain. Often, more than one area may be involved, and edema may be associated with the affected joints. Women are more affected, accounting for 70% of all cases of costochondritis.[18] The woman with costochondritis usually presents with unilateral pain and can point to the location of maximum discomfort. Pain may be sharp or dull, and duration varies. The pain is increased on movement and with deep inspiration and expiration, and is usually relieved with rest, change of position, and quiet breathing.

The patient may report trauma due to repetitive movements or moving heavy objects. However, in some cases, women may not be aware of the condition until the affected area is palpated, such as during breast exam or chest percussion. On examination, pain is elicited by palpating the involved costochondral joint(s).

A chest x-ray may be ordered to rule out more serious conditions such as pneumonia and to assess the possibility of any rib fractures. Anyone presenting with chest pain should be evaluated for a potential cardiac or respiratory condition such as myocardial infarction, pericarditis, or pleurisy before a diagnosis of costochondritis is finalized.

Management of costochondritis includes NSAIDs, cold and heat applications, and light exercise to stretch the chest wall muscles. Narcotic analgesics are usually not indicated. The course of the condition is self-limiting, with complete resolution in 4 to 6 weeks. Education should include advisement to avoid activities that overuse chest muscles and reassurance that the findings are not dangerous.[19]

Carpal Tunnel Syndrome

Carpal tunnel syndrome (CTS) is a frequent cause of pain and numbness in the hands and a major contributor to work absences. Estimates of lifetime risk are as high as 10%.[20] Women have an increased incidence relative to men, with the majority of the reported difference occurring between 20 and 40 years of age. Work-related CTS is most common in women and non-work-related incidence peaks after age 50.[21]

Atroshi and colleagues' survey reported that close to 15% of individuals in their sample had symptoms of pain, numbness, or tingling along the median nerve. After clinical examination and electrophysiological testing, about 20% of those who were symptomatic met the criteria for diagnosis.[21]

Women who engage in occupations that involve repetitive wrist movements, whether in an office or manual labor settings, are most likely to be affected. Hobbies that require frequent repetitive movements, such as knitting, can also increase risk, and medical conditions such as hypothyroidism, diabetes mellitus, and rheumatoid arthritis may play a role. Excessive computer use is frequently cited as likely to increase risk of CTS. At least 1 large survey found a minimal effect other than with use of a computer mouse for more than 30 hours a week.[22]

Women are also prone to injury when their estrogen levels are lower than usual, including during pregnancy, lactation, and menopause. Pregnancy-related CTS presents most often in the third trimester as a transient problem and is associated with edema of the hands and wrists.[23]

CTS is an entrapment neuropathy caused by compression of the median nerve and hand tendons as they pass through the carpal tunnel, a narrow ligamentous passage between the small bones of the wrists. The pressure results in inflammation and swelling of the soft tissue structures, with the presenting complaints of pain in the wrists and numbness in the hands and fingers. Occasionally, pain will radiate up the affected arm. The pain is related to ischemia of the median nerve more often than actual nerve damage. Discomfort is often first noticed at night.

Numbness of the hand occurs mainly in the thumb, index, and middle fingers, with the most significant loss of sensation centrally. A protracted course of carpal tunnel pain can involve the fourth digit and the distal portion of the fifth digit. Grip may be decreased as nerve innervation of the hand muscles is impaired.

Examination of the patient reveals decreased sensation of the palm in the distribution of the median nerve as well as the fingers. **Figure 23-3** shows the area of the hand innervated by the median nerve. In persistent conditions, thumb weakness and thenar atrophy (decreased muscle mass

Figure 23-3 Distribution of sensation by the radial (R), median (M), and ulnar (U) nerves.

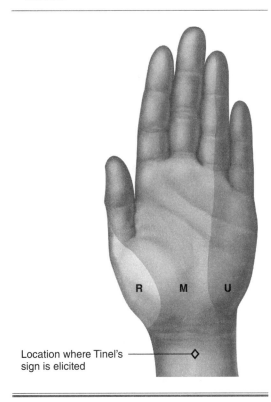

Location where Tinel's sign is elicited

of the wrist. Tinel sign is positive when tapping over the median nerve on the volar aspect of the wrist elicits paresthesia. Both are standard parts of the evaluation when CTS is suspected. Positive results indicate the need for further evaluation.

Electromyelogram (EMG; nerve conduction) studies are necessary for a definitive diagnosis; the EMG also provides information about the severity of median nerve compromise. In terms of imaging for the detection of CTS, x-rays have little value in making a diagnosis. A study employing the combination of ultrasound and MRI to diagnose CTS indicated its usefulness, but the technique requires further study for approval in the United States.[24]

Mild CTS is managed with NSAIDs, wrist rests, and assistive devices that prevent the injured area from being subjected to the repetitive trauma of certain activities. The use of wrist splints when at rest can maintain the wrist and hand in a neutral position to promote relief. Inexpensive wrist splints are available at medical supply houses. For most effective use, splints should be fitted by a physical therapist or orthopedic clinician. Corticosteroid injections may be necessary and should be considered based on the severity of nerve involvement. Surgery is the definitive treatment for severe CTS, although it does not lead to complete resolution in all cases.

Except for the transient syndrome of late pregnancy, women with CTS should be referred to an orthopedist if the relief measures discussed here do not provide prompt relief. Options for treatment are limited during the course of pregnancy. Early onset in pregnancy is associated with poorer outcomes.[25]

at the base of the thumb) can be found. Attention should be given to other conditions that may produce similar symptoms, testing for diabetes or arthritis and looking for indication of strains or fractures.[23] Assessment of other possible neurologic causes is also necessary. While CTS and related symptoms are the most common cause of hand pain, cervical spine injury and other nerve entrapments can exist.

Two easy tests for in-office screening involve Phalen and Tinel signs (**Figure 23-4**). A positive Phalen sign results in numbness and paresthesia in the affected area after 60 seconds of hyperflexion

Scoliosis

Scoliosis is a progressive disorder usually identified in childhood, which has been found to progress more in girls and affects young women

Figure 23-4 A. Phalen's test. B. Tinel's sign.

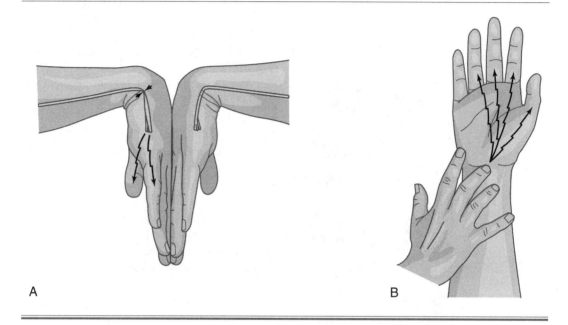

A

B

twice as often as young men.[26] The overall incidence is about 3 to 5 per 1000 children. Most commonly, it is an idiopathic disease that develops after age 10, although other conditions may underlie its development, such as cerebral palsy or polio. It also appears as part of some congenital syndromes. There is lateral curvature of the spinal column with vertebral rotation. Pain rarely accompanies this condition; however, pain may be present in clients with adjunct clinical conditions of the spine such as spondylolisthesis (forward subluxation of a vertebra) or spinal tumor. Figure 23-5 depicts the spine curvatures attributable to scoliosis.[27]

Idiopathic scoliosis has been studied over a 50-year period by Weinstein and colleagues. Their findings included a generally high standard of function and productive adult life. The incidence of back pain and shortness of breath were higher than in the comparison group. No other significant difficulties were reported.[28] Increased risk of osteoporosis related to bracing for treatment of scoliosis has been posited. Snyder and colleagues studied adolescent females and found increases in spinal bone density appropriate for age and menstrual status.[29]

Unlevel shoulders and protruding scapulae are cues for the examiner to evaluate the client for scoliosis. A right thoracic curvature is most common and presents with the right shoulder deviating in a forward rotation and the medial border of the scapula deviating posteriorly. Physical examination to evaluate for scoliosis includes a baseline assessment of client posture and body contour. An abnormal rib cage shape or an asymmetric waist also should trigger

Figure 23-5 Curve patterns of the spine.

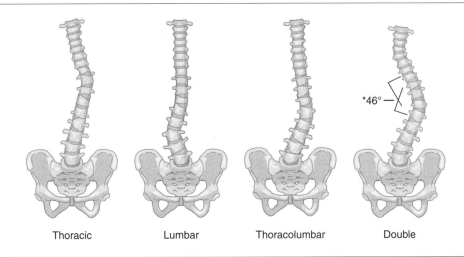

Thoracic	Lumbar	Thoracolumbar	Double

National Institute of Arthritis and Musculoskeletal and Skin Diseases, National Institutes of Health. Scoliosis. http://niams.nih.gov/Health_Info/Scoliosis/default.asp#curved. 2015. Accessed May 27, 2016.

consideration of scoliosis. A forward-bend test is used to assess the potential extent of spinal curvature. The patient is asked to bend forward from the waist, presenting the spine to identify any curvature. Whenever a forward-bend test is positive (i.e., the spine is not aligned normally), the patient should be referred for orthopedic evaluation.

The plan of management is based on degree of spinal deformity and bone maturity. Although girls are more likely to progress, as are those with > 50° of curvature at the end of bone growth, idiopathic scoliosis often becomes stable after bone growth is complete.[30] Common management for milder forms of scoliosis include observation with follow-up x-rays at regular intervals. More severe forms are treated with mechanical bracing and surgery. Exercise, chiropractic, transcutaneous electrical stimulation,

and nutritional interventions have not been shown to help.[30] The women's healthcare provider's participation in management is limited to encouraging the patient to follow through with orthopedic visits.

During pregnancy, uncorrected scoliosis may be problematic for the mother because of the increased stress placed on the spine by the enlarging uterus. At delivery, women who have had surgery to repair the spinal curve may be unable to have regional anesthesia. When the provider is aware of a history of scoliosis repair or, indeed, any spinal surgery, an anesthesia consult should be scheduled prior to the onset of labor. This holds true even when the management plan for labor does not include regional anesthesia. In the event of an emergency, the mother and her fetus will be best served by a well informed anesthesia team.

Arthritic Conditions

There are more than 100 causes of arthritic pain. The etiologies are diverse, and management of arthropathies is beyond the scope of this text or of women's health care. Including the rheumatoid diseases, they range from infections such as Lyme disease to lupus to fibromyalgia. Four of the most common conditions are presented here, because all primary care clinicians should be able to recognize and refer appropriately women with these joint diseases. Osteoarthritis is the most common of these, affecting as many as 27 million Americans; incidence increases with age.[31] It is a degenerative disease of the cartilage, with associated bone overgrowth. In contrast, rheumatoid arthritis is a chronic inflammatory process with an immunologic basis that affects about 1.3 million adults.[32] Gout, with about 6 million self-reports of diagnoses,[32] is the result of uric acid deposits in tendons and joints and is uncommon in premenopausal women. Fibromyalgia, a syndrome classed with the rheumatic diseases, is a condition found predominantly in women, estimated to have an occurrence of as much as 4.9% over the lifetime, with the incidence increasing as women age.[31] Symptoms common to many of the arthritic and rheumatoid diseases are shown in **Box 23-2**.

Relevant history for arthritic and rheumatoid conditions includes the onset, persistence, and quality of pain; effect of activity and rest; number of joints affected; recent illnesses or injuries; current medications; and whether family members have a history of these conditions. Often, patients are asked to maintain a daily journal of symptoms. The examination includes assessment of the joints for erythema, warmth, pain, and range of motion. A number of laboratory tests and procedures may be ordered, depending on the differential diagnosis for each patient.

As with other health problems considered in this chapter, NSAIDs are often considered as a treatment option for arthritic conditions. All NSAIDs

---

Box 23-2 Common Symptoms of Arthritis

- Swelling in one or more joints
- Stiffness around the joints that lasts for at least one hour in the early morning
- Constant or recurring pain or tenderness in a joint
- Difficulty using or moving a joint normally
- Warmth and redness in a joint

Data from National Institute of Arthritis, Musculoskeletal and Skin Diseases. Rheumatoid Arthritis. Health Information. http://www.niams.nih.gov/health%5Finfo/rheumatic%5Fdisease/. 2016. Accessed June 6, 2016.

---

share an increased risk of gastric toxicity, which can limit their utility. The adverse effects can range from stomach discomfort to bleeding or perforation.[33] The cyclooxygenase-2 (COX-2)-specific inhibitors were developed to offer similar pain relief with reduced GI effects. However, at least two of the drugs in this class (valdecoxib [Bextra] and rofecoxib [Vioxx]) have been withdrawn from the market based on increased risk of cardiovascular events such as myocardial infarction and ischemic stroke, and other drugs in this class also have a demonstrated increase in cardiovascular risk.[34,35] Providers using these medications should be aware of these and other risks associated with NSAID and COX-2 use and advise patients carefully. There is some evidence that patients may neither receive adequate information regarding medication options, nor be followed with appropriate monitoring to reduce risks of medication use.[36,37]

Osteoarthritis

Osteoarthritis is primarily a chronic hypertrophic arthropathy in which there is degeneration of the articular cartilage and reactive osteophyte formation in a joint space, leading to degenerative joint disease. Osteoarthritis has a peak incidence at age 65, with women being affected more than men at a rate of 2:1. The joints most commonly involved are the knees, hips, hands, cervical spine, and lumbar spine. Osteoarthritis usually affects joints unilaterally and asymmetrically.[38]

Development of osteoarthritis is associated with overuse, physical stressors, obesity, and joint laxity. Secondary forms of osteoarthritis also may develop following autoimmune diseases, avascular necrosis, chronic illness, and infection.

There is a strong genetic component for hand and hip osteoarthritis, but less so for knee problems. The role of estrogen in the prevention or development of osteoarthritis is unclear, but it may have a mild protective benefit related to increased bone mass.[39] However, the most recent US Preventive Services Task Force statement recommends against the use of combined estrogen/progestin preparations in postmenopausal women for chronic conditions.[40] Maintaining a normal weight throughout life can be important in reducing the risk of osteoarthritis.[41] Particularly for older women, obesity is strongly linked to osteoarthritis in the knees, and weight-reduction programs can reduce risk by more than 50%.[42,43]

Bony sclerosis, loss of cartilage, and osteophyte formation all lead to joint space narrowing. The narrowed joint space causes symptoms that include pain that is aggravated by weight-bearing pressure and morning stiffness. Acute inflammatory flares due to overuse and environmental temperature change are common to osteoarthritis. Over time, progressive deformation of the joints leads to increasing disability, pain, limitation in range of motion, and joint instability.

Diagnosis is made with a combination of history, examination, and radiography. When suspected in a women's health setting, osteoarthritis should be referred to a clinician with skills in orthopedic diagnosis and management.

Treatment options for osteoarthritis include acetaminophen and ibuprofen, tramadol (a synthetic opioid agonist), rest, weight reduction, intraarticular corticosteroid injection, and physiotherapy. A newer class of intraarticular medications, the hyaluronans (macromolecule supplementation), has been found to be effective at pain relief when compared to NSAID therapy and intraarticular placebo therapy.[44] Capsaicin creams have demonstrated some benefit. End-stage osteoarthritis may require surgery. Although a number of complementary therapies have been suggested, none have demonstrated long-term benefits. In several cases, a strong placebo effect has been noted.[45]

Rheumatoid Arthritis

Rheumatoid arthritis is a chronic inflammatory arthropathy that occurs bilaterally in joints of the hands, hips, and knees. The condition usually begins in 1 to 2 joints and often will progress to 20 or more, initially affecting the proximal interphalangeal, metacarpophalangeal, and metatarsophalangeal joints. It affects small joints primarily, but any peripheral joint may be affected. There is often synovial proliferation (pannus), inflammation synovitis, and erosion of the articular surfaces of the bones in affected joints.

Rheumatoid arthritis is characterized clinically by inflammation of a joint, tenderness to palpation of the affected joints, limited joint function, and morning stiffness that lasts longer than an hour. There may also be associated fever, fatigue, and inflammatory vascular conditions accompanying this autoimmune disorder. The disease exists in remitting-relapsing and progressive forms.

Young age at onset and female sex have been identified in some studies as being related to poorer outcomes. Level of joint erosion at diagnosis may also provide clues as to eventual disability, although clinical markers are most predictive of the likelihood of remissions (**Table 23-5**).[46]

Because of the possibility of multisystem involvement, rheumatoid arthritis is best evaluated and managed by a rheumatologist. Diagnostic laboratory testing includes rheumatoid arthritis factor and erythrocyte sedimentation rate. A positive

Table 23-5 Features of Rheumatoid Arthritis

- Tender, warm, swollen joints
- Symmetrical pattern of affected joints
- Joint inflammation often affecting the wrist and finger joints closest to the hand
- Joint inflammation sometimes affecting other joints, including the neck, shoulders, elbows, hips, knees, ankles, and feet
- Fatigue, occasional fevers, a general sense of not feeling well
- Pain and stiffness lasting for more than 30 minutes in the morning or after a long rest
- Symptoms that last for many years
- Variability of symptoms among people with the disease

Data from National Institute of Arthritis, Musculoskeletal and Skin Diseases. Rheumatoid Arthritis. Health Information. http://www.niams.nih.gov/health%5Finfo/rheumatic%5Fdisease/. 2016. Accessed June 6, 2016; Gossec L, Dougados M, Goupille P, Cantarel A, Sibilia J, Meyer O, et al. Prognostic factors for remission in early rheumatoid arthritis: a multiparameter prospective study. *Ann Rheum Dis.* 2004;63:675-680.

rheumatoid arthritis factor result and increased erythrocyte sedimentation rate support the diagnosis of rheumatoid arthritis.

Women in whom rheumatoid arthritis is suspected should be told that early diagnosis and management improve the likelihood of maintaining functional capacity. Management can include pain control with NSAIDs; corticosteroids for symptomatic relief on a short-term basis; medications to delay or prevent disease progression, known as disease-modifying antirheumatic drugs (DMARDs); and regular monitoring of symptoms to achieve remission.[47] Surgery can be used to replace destroyed joints. Prevention of osteoporosis, to which rheumatoid arthritis patients are prone, secondary to inactivity and steroid treatment, is an additional concern.

Gout

Gout is an erosive arthritis that results from the deposition of sodium urate crystals in connective tissue or in one or more joints, with the first occurrence often being in the big toes. Gout is most common in males over 40; women most frequently develop gout after menopause. The incidence range is 5.0 to 6.6 per 1000 in men and 1.0 to 3.0 per 1000 in women, although self-reported cases are approximately twice those levels.[31] A condition that resembles gout in clinical findings is called pseudogout, or chondrocalcinosis; it is caused by calcium phosphate deposits.

The pathologic basis of gout is either overproduction or underexcretion of uric acid. Many cases are idiopathic. Among the associated factors for increased risk are genetic predisposition, obesity, excessive alcohol intake, high-purine diet (e.g., liver, dried beans), lead exposure, and medications including diuretics, salicylates, and niacin.[48]

Prevention of gout includes dietary changes, specifically the avoidance of dietary fats and purine-rich foods such as organ meats and aged cheeses. Rapid-weight-loss diets can stimulate new attacks and should be avoided. Avoidance of alcohol, particularly of excessive drinking, is essential to prevent recurrences.[48]

The classic presentation of gout is unilateral pain in the first metatarsophalangeal joint (podagra). In the first episode, sudden onset of pain, worsening over several hours, is followed by complete recovery within days or weeks. On examination there is pain to palpation, swelling, decreased mobility, and inflammation of the affected joint. Intermittent periods without any symptoms occur, although these become shorter over time. As the disease advances, multiple joints can be involved, and healing is slowed.[49] Intermittent hyperuricemia is found in gout but is not pathognomonic. Diagnosis is made by aspiration of synovial fluid for evaluation of monosodium urate crystals (MSU); these can accumulate in joints as crystals and are called tophi. Ultrasound and dual-energy CT have proved useful in clarifying diagnoses.[50]

Initial plain films of joints affected by gout are negative, because involvement is confined to the soft tissues and there is asymmetric inflammation in affected joints. Later stages of chronic gout show notable changes, and "punched-out" lesions appear in the bony structures on x-ray. After several years of chronic gout, large tophi are a hallmark sign and can be seen on x-ray along with joint space narrowing.

Treatment of acute gout is accomplished with NSAIDs, particularly indomethacin (Indocin), and rest of the affected joint. Injectable corticosteroids may also be used to provide local pain relief. Long-term treatment of gout includes allopurinol, probenecid, and colchicine. Allopurinol is not used during an acute attack, because it may aggravate symptoms. As with the other arthritic conditions, referral to a clinician skilled in gout management is most appropriate.

Fibromyalgia

Fibromyalgia is a chronic disorder characterized by diffuse muscle pain, fatigue, sleep disturbance, and multiple tender points on various areas of the body. It affects as many as 1 in 50 Americans; women are 6 times more likely to be diagnosed with fibromyalgia as compared to men.[51] Persons with other rheumatic diseases (i.e., lupus and rheumatoid arthritis) are also prone to fibromyalgia. The differential diagnosis includes hypothyroidism, rheumatoid arthritis, adrenal dysfunction, myeloma, and depressive conditions.[51]

Fibromyalgia is considered a rheumatic disorder; however, it is not a true arthritis. There is no inflammation of the joints, nor is there any destruction of the associated tissues such as cartilage or muscle. Pain and fatigue, headache, sleep disturbances, morning stiffness, increased sensitivity to heat or cold, and extremity numbness and tingling are common symptoms. By virtue of the potentially myriad symptoms, it is considered a syndrome rather than a disease. The actual cause of fibromyalgia is unknown. Musculoskeletal, neurologic, genetic, and psychologic factors may contribute to the development of this disorder.[53] Recent research suggests that fibromyalgia demonstrates a familial pattern, and it may be linked to strong family or personal history of mood disorders.[52]

According to the original American College of Rheumatology guidelines, for a diagnosis of fibromyalgia to be considered, the examiner must elicit > 10 of 18 tender points on various areas of the body (**Figure 23-6**), while applying at least 4 kg of pressure to the site. Complaints of widespread pain lasting 3 months or longer and affecting all 4 quadrants of the body (above and below the waist and bilaterally) are other criteria required for a diagnosis.[53] This diagnosis is often not correctly made in primary care.[54] In an update published in 2010, reliance on clinician elicited trigger points was recommended to be replaced by the following three criteria, all of which must be met: specific combinations of high scores on the Widespread Pain Index and symptom severity scales; persistent symptoms at that level for at least 3 months; no other disorder that explains the pain. There are 19 possible pain areas identified in the widespread pain index. The symptom severity scale asks about degree of problems with fatigue, waking unrefreshed, and cognitive problems within the last week; and about overall severity of somatic symptoms such as gastrointestinal symptoms, dizziness, shortness of breath or wheezing, and tinnitus.[54]

Figure 23-6 Tender points of the body.

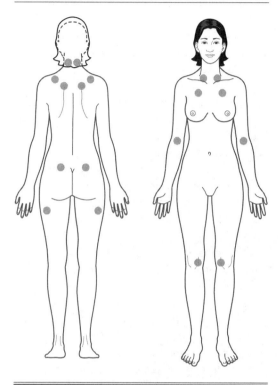

Data from National Institute of Arthritis, Musculoskeletal and Skin Diseases. Health Topics. Fibromyalgia. http://www.nih.gov/hi/topics/fibromyalgia/fibrofs.htm; American College of Rheumatology. The American College of Rheumatology 1990 criteria for the classification of fibromyalgia. *Arthritis Rheum.* 1990; 33(2):160-172.

A team treatment approach has been proven to be most effective, with primary care, physical medicine, and psychotherapy professionals lending clinical expertise to provide a well-rounded treatment plan. Women's health practitioners need to be aware of the diagnosis and management for fibromyalgia, but should not offer primary care for women with a suspected diagnosis outside of such a team setting.

Ample data demonstrate that structured exercise programs are a major contributor to improved health and quality of life.[55-57] Counseling or other interventions to deal with comorbid mood disorders can benefit women for whom these are affecting fibromyalgia management.[58,59] Combinations of exercise, patient education, provision of behavioral therapy, and medication are most frequently effective.[55,60]

Milnacipran (Savella), a serotonin and norepinephrine reuptake inhibitor, is approved for the treatment of fibromyalgia. Other medications often used in management of symptoms include tricyclic antidepressants to deal with depressive symptoms, pain, and fatigue; cyclobenzaprine (Flexeril); pregabalin (Lyrica); and gabapentin (Neurontin).[51,61] Tramadol is the only opioid with demonstrated effectiveness. Acetaminophen is more effective than NSAIDs.[61]

Complementary therapies that have been explored include massage, chiropractic, acupuncture, and a variety of dietary supplements, but no solid evidence supports their effectiveness at this time.[51] However, given the interrelationship of mental status and pain in fibromyalgia, patients should discuss these therapies with their primary provider.

Osteoporosis

Osteoporosis affects 25% of American women over 65, and osteopenia occurs in more than 50%.[62] As many as 40% of Caucasian women over 50 will have an osteoporosis-related fracture during the remainder of their lives.[63] Rates of osteoporosis are highest among Hispanic and Caucasian women.[62] Although rates are lower among African-American women, once diagnosed, the fracture risk is identical. As the population ages, dramatic increases are predicted for rates of fracture and the resultant morbidity.

According to the Centers for Disease Control and Prevention, 250,000 elder adults are hospitalized for hip fractures annually; three out of four of them are women.[64]

Osteoporosis is a diffuse skeletal disease with increased bone fragility and fracture risk.[64] The condition is characterized by the deterioration of bone mass, with osteoclast (bone resorbing) activity exceeding osteoblast (bone forming) cell activity. Primary osteoporosis is seen in both males and females at all ages. Secondary osteoporosis can be the result of medications, disease states, or genetic predisposition. Medications can induce osteoporosis by causing hypogonadism or interfering with vitamin D metabolism. **Table 23-6** lists risk factors for primary and secondary osteoporosis.

Peak bone mass is attained in 95% of women by age 16, although further small increases are possible before age 30.[67,68] Genetic factors account for about 75% of the variation in peak bone mass.[69] Until menopause, there is little further alteration in a woman's bone mass and structure. Following the decrease in circulating estrogens that accompanies the cessation of

Table 23-6 Risk Factors for Primary and Secondary Osteoporosis

Primary	Methotrexate
Older age	Cholestyramine
Low body weight	Diseases include:
Low BMI	Malnutrition (e.g., anorexia nervosa)
Sedentary lifestyle	Vitamin B_{12} deficiency
Fair skin	Diabetes mellitus
Female gender	Hyperthyroidism
Postmenopausal status (without current HRT)	Hyperparathyroidism
	Hyperprolactinemia
Hypogonadic states	Cushing's disease
Low calcium intake	Rheumatoid arthritia
Family history	Organ transplant survivors
Tobacco use	Gastrectomy patients
Excess alcohol use	Inflammatory bowel disease
Secondary	Genetic risks include:
Medications include:	Marfan syndrome
Medroxyprogesterone	Thalassemia
Corticosteroids	Celiac disease
Antiepileptics	Hemochromatosis
SSRI antidepressants	Osteogenesis imperfecta
Excess thyroid hormone	Homocystinuria
Chronic heparin, coumadin treatment	Ehlers Danlos syndrome

Data from Osteoporosis prevention, diagnosis, and therapy. *NIH Consens Statement.* 2000;17(1):1-36; International Osteoporosis Foundation. Who's at risk. https://www.iofbonehealth.org/whos-risk. n.d. Accessed June 11, 2016; Cosman F, de Beur SJ, LeBoff MS, et al. Clinician's guide to prevention and treatment of osteoporosis. *Osteoporos Int.* 2014;25(10): 2359-2381. doi:10.1007/s00198-014-2794-2.

menses, bone density drops dramatically over several years. Women using hormonal therapy delay but do not prevent this change.

Screening

Clinically, osteoporosis is defined as decreased bone mineral density (BMD) that is more than 2.5 standard deviations below that of a healthy 25-year-old individual of the same sex, as evaluated by dual-energy x-ray absorption (DEXA) scan of the lumbar vertebrae and hip. *Osteopenia* is the term used when bone density is decreased to 1 to 2.5 standard deviations below the mean. The term used to describe these scores is *T score*. The *Z score* is a measurement of BMD in relation to age- and sex-adjusted norms; a normal Z score does not rule out osteoporotic changes in adults, because bone loss is common in older individuals. While a Z score provides a comparative assessment of age-matched bone density levels, it is not used to indicate whether treatment is needed. Treatment is based on the T score. The complete World Health Organization criteria for diagnosis are shown in **Table 23-7**.[70]

The US Preventive Services Task Force recommends BMD screening in all women age 65 and older, regardless of risk factors and in women under 65 whose personal risk is equivalent to that of a 65-year-old woman.[71] Other methods of screening for osteoporosis include peripheral dual x-ray absorptiometry (pDXA) and single-energy x-ray absorptiometry (SXA), which measure bone density in the forearm, finger, or heel; quantitative CT, which measures trabecular and cortical bone density at various sites; and ultrasound densitometry. Ultrasound measurements are generally not as precise as pDXA or SXA, but appear to predict fracture risk as well as other measures of bone density. Serum or urine biochemical markers can identify changes in bone turnover but are not used in lieu of BMD evaluation.

Several screening tools are available for provider use; none are specific enough to use instead of BMD, although they can be used to screen for additional women who are at risk and require evaluation. One of these tools, the online fracture risk assessment tool (FRAX), developed by the World Health Organization, is available as an app or at multiple websites. It estimates the fracture risk within 10 years for the following at-risk populations: postmenopausal women and men aged 50 years and older, those diagnosed with osteopenia, and persons who have not taken medications for osteoporosis.[72]

Table 23-7 WHO Criteria for Diagnosis of Osteoporosis

DEXA Score for Women after Menopause	T Score
Normal	−1.0 to 0+
Osteopenia	−2.5 to −1.0
Osteoporosis	< −2.5
Severe Osteoporosis	< −2.5 with fragility fracture

Data from World Health Organization. *Assessment of fracture risk and its application to screening for postmenopausal osteoporosis: report of a WHO study group.* Geneva, Switzerland: World Health Organization; 1994.

Osteoporosis Prevention

The most effective preventive measures for osteoporosis are those that increase peak bone mass in the young adult years and promote adequate calcium and vitamin D intake. Thus, counseling to increase exercise, promote healthy dietary habits, and decrease tobacco and alcohol use are core parts of health maintenance visits for all women of reproductive age, beginning in adolescence. Assessments of dietary intake of calcium and sun exposure for stimulation of vitamin D production are also valuable. All women whose diets are deficient should be encouraged to supplement appropriately. Screening with serum 25-hydroxyvitamin D levels should be considered

Calcium supplementation as needed to reach an intake of 1200 mg per day is recommended for women over 50 years of age.[72] However, levels higher than 1500 mg per day may increase the risk of kidney stones; dietary intake should be evaluated when recommending supplementation. At least one author has identified the necessary vitamin D intake for those without sun exposure to be 1000 international units per day.[73] The National Osteoporosis Foundation Guidelines recommends 800–100 IU for those over 50.[72] Many women who are postmenopausal, even those on osteoporosis therapy, remain vitamin D deficient, which directly impacts the body's ability to maintain bone mass.[75] Medications to prevent osteoporosis are listed in **Table 23-8.**

Fall-prevention strategies should be discussed. Although the use of hormonal therapy has decreased in the wake of evidence that risks of cardiovascular disease and cancer are increased, they remain available and can be considered in the context of individual risks and benefits; however, they are not the first choice to consider.

Although medroxyprogesterone acetate (Depo-Provera) has been shown to have at least a short-term negative effect on BMD in young women,[74] some recent evidence indicates that inadequate levels of vitamin D among women receiving medroxyprogesterone and adolescents with a low calcium intake and greater alcohol use were associated with a higher bone density loss.[75] Therefore, a discussion of risks of bone loss should be part of contraceptive counseling for this product in addition to counseling on the adequate intake of vitamin D and screening for alcohol use. Additionally, in recommending medroxyprogesterone, the clinician should consider whether additional risk factors for decreased bone mass exist, remembering that young women can also develop osteoporosis. Studies indicate that bone density increases to normal levels following discontinuation of

Table 23-8 Medications Used in the Prevention or Treatment of Osteoporosis

Bisphosphonates

   Alendronate (Fosamax)

      Prevention: 5 mg daily or 35 mg once per week

      Treatment: 10 mg daily or 70 mg once per week

      Risendronate (Actonel)

      Prevention/Treatment: 5 mg daily or 35 mg once per week

Selective Estrogen Receptor Modulators

   Raloxifene (Evista)

      Prevention/Treatment: 60 mg daily

Hormone Therapies

   Estrogens (such as Climara, Estrace, Estraderm, Estratab, Menostar, Ogen, Ortho-Est, Premarin, Vivelle)

      Prevention: dosage varies

   Estrogens and Progestins (such as Activella, FemHrt, Premphase, Prempro)

      Prevention: dosage varies

Calcitonin (Miacalcin)

Treatment: 100 Units IM or SC, every other day, or three times a week

Calcium Supplements

   1200–1500 mg elemental calcium daily

Vitamin D Supplements

   800 IU daily

Abbreviations: IM, intramuscular; SC, subcutaneous; IU, international units.

medroxyprogesterone.[76] Combined hormonal contraception, in contrast, does not have a significant effect on bone density.[77]

Pregnancy and lactation have been shown to produce a short-term decrease in BMD in some women, but this effect does not increase osteoporosis risk in later life.[78–81]

Presentation

Osteoporosis can present silently or with minimal symptoms, reinforcing the importance of screening and attention to risk factors presented in the history. Loss of height and changes in spinal curvature suggest its presence. A decrease in height is an indicator of loss of height of the vertebrae. For this reason, it is necessary to monitor a woman's height at each preventive visit. On examination, an increased thoracic kyphosis or decreased curvature of the lumbar lordosis is commonly seen when the woman is in a standing position.

Localized spinal tenderness may be present, with spinal flexion increasing pain more than extension. When the vertebrae are involved in osteoporosis, the woman may present with neck or back pain. Osteoporosis of the spinal column causes weakening and pathologic wedge-fracture of the vertebrae, which, in turn, may sublux and exert pressure on spinal peripheral nerve roots.

Fracture is a late presentation in osteoporosis. Most commonly, the wrist, lumbar vertebrae, and hip are at risk. Relative risk of fracture increases 2 to 3 times with each 1.0 decrease in T score. However, there is significant overlap between T scores of those with and without fracture.[82] Increasing age also independently increases fracture risk due to factors including bone changes such as decreased flexibility and increased brittleness, decreasing weight with age, decreased visual acuity, mental confusion, and loss of stability.

Hip fracture has been demonstrated to be the most likely injury to reduce survival, resulting in excess mortality between 8% and 36%. A 20% with hip fracture as a result of osteoporosis will require nursing home care; only 40% will recover full function.[72]

Management of Osteoporosis

Management of osteoporosis incorporates tobacco cessation, limiting alcohol intake, adequate dietary or supplemental calcium and vitamin D, nonpharmacologic therapy including calcium supplementation and vitamin D supplements, and weight-bearing exercise. The National Osteoporosis Foundation recommends beginning medical therapy to reduce fracture risk in postmenopausal women with BMD T scores below 2.5 in the absence of risk factors and in women with T scores between −1.0 and −2.5 if there is an increased 10 year risk of hip fracture.[72]

Current pharmacologic options for osteoporosis prevention and treatment are shown in Table 23-8. Each has side effects and risks; women should be advised regarding these effects for safety and to prevent nonadherence. Estrogen and estrogen/progesterone combined hormone therapy can be used with caution for osteoporosis prevention. They may be particularly useful in young women with premature menopause or surgical removal of the ovaries who are in their 30s and 40s.

Counseling includes the importance of adequate calcium and vitamin D supplementation, increasing activity by adding weight-bearing and muscle-strengthening exercises, and fall prevention. A 30-minute walk at least 3 times a week is effective exercise.

Conclusion

This chapter has presented a range of MS conditions that primary care providers, including midwives and other women's health practitioners, can expect to see in practice. Not all are appropriate for management in the women's health setting. Others, such as osteoporosis, are central to the care of older women. In making decisions about when to treat and when to refer, each provider should always be aware of both her or his own skill set and the resources available.

References

1. Ferreira-Valente MA, Pais-Ribeiro JL, Jensen MP. Validity of four pain intensity rating scales. *Pain.* 2011;152:2399-2404.

2. Deyo RA, Weinstein JN. Low back pain. *NEJM.* 2001;344:363-370.

3. Koes, BW, van Tulder M, Lin, CW, Macedo, LG, McAuley, J, Maher, C. An updated overview of clinical guidelines for the management of non-specific low back pain in primary care. *Eur Spine J.* 2011;19;2075-2094.

4. Goroll AH, Mulley AG. Evaluation of low back pain. In: Goroll AH, Mulley AG, eds. *Primary Care Medicine.* 6th ed. Philadelphia, PA: Lippincott Williams & Wilkins; 2009.

5. Kendrick D, Fielding K, Bentley E, Miller P, Kerslake R, Pringle M. The role of radiography in primary care patients with low back pain of at least 6 weeks duration: a randomized (unblended) controlled trial. *Health Technol Assess.* 2001;5:1-69.

6. Chou, R, Qaseem, A, Owens, DK, Shekelle PC. Diagnostic imaging for low back pain: advice for high-value health care from the American College of Physicians. *Ann Intern Med.* 2011;154:181-189.

7. Toward Optimized Practice. Guideline for the evidence-informed primary care management of low back pain. Edmonton, AB: Toward Optimized Practice; 2011: 37. Available at: https://www.guideline.gov/content.aspx?id=37954. Accessed May 27, 2016.

8. Kuritzky L, Samraj G. Nonsteroidal anti-inflammatory drugs in the treatment of low back pain. *J Pain Res.* 2012;5:579-590.

9. Chou, R. Pharmacologic management of low back pain. *Drugs.* 2010;70:387-402.

10. Adams T. Conservative Treatment of Low Back Pain in the Older Adult: A Literature Review. [A senior research project submitted in partial requirement for the degree of Doctor of Chiropractic]; 2012. Available at: http://www.logan.edu/mm/files/LRC/Senior-Research/2012-Apr-01.pdf. Accessed May 27, 2016.

11. Hayden JA, van Tulder MW, Tomlinson G. Systematic review: strategies for using exercise therapy to improve outcomes in chronic low back pain. *Ann Intern Med.* 2005;142:776-785.

12. Hayden JA, van Tulder MW, Malmivaara AAV, Koes BW. Meta-analysis: exercise therapy for non-specific back pain. *Ann Intern Med.* 2005;142:765-775.

13. Moffett JK, Torgerson D, Bell-Syer S, Jackson D, Llewelyn-Phillips H, Farrin A, Barber J. Randomised controlled trial of exercise for low back pain: clinical outcomes, costs, and preferences. *BMJ.* 1999;319:279-283.

14. Furlan, AD, Imamura M, Dryden T, Irvin E. Massage for low back pain: an updated systematic review within the framework of the Cochrane Back Review Group. *Spine.* 2009;34:1669-1684.

15. Cherkin D, Sherman K, Avins A, Erro J, Ichikawa L, Barlow W, et al. A randomized trial comparing acupuncture, simulated acupuncture, and usual care for chronic low back pain. *Arch Intern Med.* 2009; 169:858-866.

16. Jenkins M, Sitler M, Kelly J. Clinical usefulness of the Ottawa ankle rules for detecting fractures of the ankle and midfoot. *J Athl Train.* 2010;45:480-482.

17. Wolfe MW, Uhl TL, Mattacola CG, McCluskey LC. Management of ankle sprains. *Am Fam Physician.* 2001;63:93-104.

18. McGarr, K, Tong I. *The Five Minute Clinical Companion to Women's Health.* 2nd ed. Philadelphia, PA: Lippincott, Williams & Wilkins; 2013.

19. Proulx, AM, Zyrd, TW. Costochondritis: diagnosis and treatment. *Am Fam Physician.* 2009;80:617-620.

20. Franzblau A, Werner RA. What is carpal tunnel syndrome? *JAMA.* 1999;282:186-187.

21. Atroshi I, Gummesson C, Johnsson R, Omstein E, Ranstam J, Rosen I. Prevalence of carpal tunnel syndrome in a general population. *JAMA.* 1999;282: 153-158.

22. Andersen JR. Computer use and the carpal tunnel syndrome. *JAMA.* 2003;289:2963-2969.

23. LeBlanc KE, Cestia W. Carpal tunnel syndrome. *Am Fam Physician.* 2011;83:952-8.

24. Keberle M, Kenn W, Reiners K, Peter M, Haerten R, Hahn D. Technical advances in ultrasound and MR imaging of carpal tunnel syndrome. *Eur Radiol.* 2000;10:1043-1050.

25. Padua L, Aprile I, Caliandro P, Mondelli M, Pasqualetti P, Tonali PA; for the Italian Carpal Tunnel Syndrome Study Group. Carpal tunnel syndrome in pregnancy: multiperspective follow up of untreated cases. *Neurology.* 2002;59:1643-1646.

26. Bunnell, WP. Selective screening for scoliosis. *Clin Orthop Res.* 2005;434:40-45.

27. National Institute of Arthritis and Musculoskeletal and Skin Diseases, National Institutes of Health. Scoliosis. Available at: http://niams.nih.gov/Health_Info/Scoliosis/default.asp#curved. Accessed May 27, 2016.

28. Weinstein SL, Dolan LA, Spratt KF, Peterson KK, Spoonamore MJ, Ponsetti IV. Health and function of patients with untreated idiopathic scoliosis: a 50-year natural history study. *JAMA.* 2003;289: 559-567.

29. Snyder BD, Katz DA, Myers ER, Breitenbach MA, Emans JB. Bone density accumulation is not affected by brace treatment of idiopathic scoliosis in adolescent girls. *J Pediatr Orthop.* 2005;25:423-428.

30. Hresko, MT. Idiopathic scoliosis in adolescents. *NEJM.* 2013;368:834-881.

31. Lawrence R, Felson D, Helmick C, Arnold L, Choi H, Deyo R, et al. Estimates of the prevalence of arthritis and other rheumatic conditions in the United States, Part II. *Arthritis Rheum.* 2008;58:26-35.

32. Helmick CG, Felson DT, Lawrence RC, Gabriel S, Hirsch R, Kwoh CK, et al. Estimates of the prevalence of arthritis and other rheumatic conditions in the United States. Part I. *Arthritis Rheum.* 2008;58(1):15-25.

33. Laine L. The gastrointestinal side effects of nonselective NSAIDs and COX-2-selective inhibitors. *Semin Arthritis Rheum.* 2002;32(3 Suppl 1):25-32.

34. Mukherjee D, Nissen SE, Topol EJ. Risk of cardiovascular events associated with selective COX-2 inhibitors. *JAMA.* 2001;286:954-959.

35. Solomon SD, McMurray JJV, Pfeffer MA, Wittes J, Fowler R, Finn P, et al. Cardiovascular risk associated with celecoxib in a clinical trial for colorectal adenoma prevention. *N Engl J Med.* 2005;352:1071-1080.

36. Fraenkel L, Wittink DR, Concato J, Fried T. Informed choice and the widespread use of anti-inflammatory drugs. *Arthritis Rheum.* 2004;51:210-214.

37. Patino FG, Olivieri J, Allison JJ, Mikuls TR, Moreland L, Kovac SH, et al. Nonsteroidal anti-inflammatory drug toxicity monitoring and safety practices. *J Rheumatol.* 2003;30:2680-2688.

38. Sinusas K. Osteoarthritis: diagnosis and treatment. *Am Fam Physician.* 2012;85(1):49-56.

39. Felson DT. Osteoarthritis: new insights. Part 1: the disease and its risk factors. *Ann Intern Med.* 2000; 133:635-646.

40. Moyer VA. Menopausal hormone therapy for the primary prevention of chronic conditions: US Preventive Services Task Force recommendation statement. *Ann Intern Med.* 2013;158:47-54.

41. Gelber AC, Hochberg MC, Mead LA, Wang NY, Wigley FM, Klag MJ. Body mass index in young men and the risk of subsequent knee and hip osteoarthritis. *Am J Med.* 1999;107:542-548.

42. Felson DT, Anderson JJ, Naimark A, Walker AM, Meenan RF. Obesity and knee osteoarthritis: The Framingham Study. *Ann Intern Med.* 1988;109:18-24.

43. Felson DT, Shang Y, Anthony JM, Naimark A, Anderson JJ. Weight loss reduces the risk for symptomatic knee arthritis in women: The Framingham study. *Ann Intern Med.* 1992;116:535-539.

44. Neustadt DH. Intra-articular injections for osteoarthritis of the knee. *Cleve Clin J Med.* 2006;10:897-8, 901-4, 906-911.

45. Felson DT. Osteoarthritis: new insights. Part 2: treatment approaches. *Ann Intern Med.* 2000;133: 726-737.

46. Gossec L, Dougados M, Goupille P, Cantarel A, Sibilia J, Meyer O, et al. Prognostic factors for remission in early rheumatoid arthritis: a multiparameter prospective study. *Ann Rheum Dis.* 2004;63: 675-680.

47. Kim SY, Schneeweiss S, Liu J, Solomon D. Effects of disease-modifying anti-rheumatic drugs on nonvertebral fracture risk in rheumatoid arthritis: a population-based cohort study. *J Bone Miner Res.* 2012;27:789-796.

48. National Institutes of Arthritis and Musculoskeletal Diseases. Questions and answers about gout. National Institutes of Health; 2015. Available at: http://www.niams.nih.gov/health_info/gout/. Accessed May 27, 2016.

49. Burns, C, Wortmann, R. Latest evidence on gout management: what the clinician needs to know. *Ther Adv Chronic Dis.* 2012;3:271-286.

50. Sivera F, Andrés M, Carmona L, Kydd AS, Moi J, Seth R, et al. Multinational evidence-based recommendations for the diagnosis and management of gout: integrating systematic literature review and expert opinion of a broad panel of rheumatologists in the 3e initiative. *Ann Rheum Dis.* 2014; 73(2):328-335.

51. Wierwille L. Fibromyalgia: diagnosing and managing a complex syndrome. *J Am Acad Nurse Pract.* 2012;24:184-192.

52. Raphael KG, Janal MN, Nayak S, Schwartz JE, Gallagher RM. Familial aggregation of depression in fibromyalgia: a community-based test of alternate hypotheses. *Pain.* 2004;110(1-2):449-460.

53. Wolfe F, Smythe HA, Yunus MB, Bennett RM, Bombardier C, Goldenberg DL, et al. The American College of Rheumatology 1990 criteria for the classification of fibromyalgia. Report of the multicenter criteria committee. *Arthritis Rheum.* 1990. 33:160-172.

54. Wolfe F, Clauw DJ, Fitzcharles MA, Goldenberg DL, Katz RS, Mease P, et al. The American College of Rheumatology preliminary diagnostic criteria for fibromyalgia and measurement of symptom severity. *Arthritis Care Res* (Hoboken). 2010 May; 62(5): 600-610. doi: 10.1002/acr.20140.

55. Gowans SE, Dehueck A, Voss S, Silaj A, Abbey SE. Six-month and one-year followup of 23 weeks of aerobic exercise for individuals with fibromyalgia. *Arthritis Rheum.* 2004;51:890-898.

56. Lemstra M, Olszynski WP. The effectiveness of multidisciplinary rehabilitation in the treatment of fibromyalgia. *Clin J Pain.* 2005;21:166-174.

57. Mannerkorpi K. Exercise in fibromyalgia. *Curr Opin Rheumatol.* 2005;17:190-194.

58. Thieme K, Turk DC, Flor H. Comorbid depression and anxiety in fibromyalgia syndrome: relationship to somatic and psychosocial variables. *Psychosom Med.* 2004;66:837-844.

59. Turk DC, Robinson JP, Burwinkle T. Prevalence of fear of pain and activity in patients with fibromyalgia syndrome. *J Pain.* 2004;5:483-490.

60. Goldenberg DL, Burckhardt C, Crofford L. Management of fibromyalgia syndrome. *JAMA.* 2004;292:2388-2395.

61. Skaer TL. Fibromyalgia: disease synopsis, medication cost effectiveness and economic burden. *Pharmacoeconomics.* 2014;32(5):457-466.

62. Looker AC, Frenk SM. Percentage of Adults Aged 65 and Over With Osteoporosis or Low Bone Mass at the Femur Neck or Lumbar Spine: United States, 2005–2010. Available at: http://www.cdc.gov/nchs/data/hestat/osteoporsis/osteoporosis2005_2010.htm. Accessed June 12, 2016.

63. Cummings SR, Melton LJ, III. Epidemiology and outcomes of osteoporotic fractures. *Lancet.* 2002;359(9319):1761-1767.

64. National Hospital Discharge Survey (NHDS), National Center for Health Statistics. Health Data Interactive, Health Care Use and Expenditures. Available at: www.cdc.gov/nchs/hdi.htm. Accessed June 11, 2016.

65. Osteoporosis prevention, diagnosis, and therapy. *NIH Consens Statement.* 2000;17(1):1-36.

66. International Osteoporosis Foundation. Who's at Risk? Available at: https://www.iofbonehealth.org/whos-risk. Accessed June 11, 2016.

67. Theintz B, Ruchs R, Rizzoli R, Slosman D, Clavien H, Sizonenko C, Bonjour J. Longitudinal monitoring of bone mass accumulation in healthy adolescents: evidence for a marked reduction after 16 years of age at the levels of lumbar spine and femoral neck in female subjects. *J Clin Endo Metab.* 1992;75:1060-1065.

68. Recker RR, Davies KM, Hinders SM, Heaney RP, Stegman MR, Kimmel DB. Bone gain in young adult women. *JAMA.* 1992;268:2403-2408.

69. Matcovic V, Fontana D, Tominac C, Goel P, Chestnut CH, III. Factors that influence peak bone mass formation: A study of calcium balance and the inheritance of bone mass adolescent females. *Am J Clin Nutr.* 1990;52:878-888.

70. World Health Organization. *Assessment of Fracture Risk and Its Application to Screening for Osteoporosis: Report of a WHO Study Group.* Geneva, Switzerland: World Health Organization; 1994.

71. US Preventive Services Task Force. Osteoporosis: Screening. 2011. Available at: http://www.uspreventiveservicestaskforce.org/Page/Document/UpdateSummaryFinal/osteoporosis-screening. Accessed May 27, 2016.

72. Cosman F, de Beur SJ, LeBoff MS, et al. Clinician's Guide to Prevention and Treatment of Osteoporosis. Osteoporosis International. 2014;25(10):2359-2381. doi:10.1007/s00198-014-2794-2.

73. Holick MF, Siris ES, Binkley N, Beard MK, Khan A, Katzer JT, et al. Prevalence of vitamin D inadequacy among postmenopausal North American women receiving osteoporosis therapy. *J Clin Endocrinol Metab.* 2005;90(6):3215-3224.

74. Clark MK, Sowers MR, Nichols S, Levy B. Bone mineral density changes over two years in first time users of depot medroxyprogesterone acetate. Fertil Steril. 2004;82:1580-1586.

75. Harel Z, Wolter K, Gold MA, Cromer B, Stager M, Johnson CC, et al. Biopsychosocial variables associated with substantial bone mineral density loss during the use of depot medroxyprogesterone acetate in adolescents: adolescents who lost 5% or more from baseline vs. those who lost less than 5%. *Contraception.* 2010;82:503-512.

76. Scholes D, La Croix AZ, Ichiwara LE, Barlow WE, Ott SM. Change in bone mineral density among adolescent women using and discontinuing depot medroxyprogesterone acetate contraception. *Arch Pediatr Adolesc Med.* 2005;159:139-144.

77. Berenson AB, Breitkopf CR, Grady JJ, Rickert VI, Thomas A. Effects of hormonal contraception on bone mineral density after 24 months of use. *Obstet Gynecol.* 2004;103(5 Pt 1):899-906.

78. Kalkwarf HJ, Specker BL. Bone mineral changes during pregnancy and lactation. *Endocrine.* 2002;17:49-53.

79. Ritchie LD, Fung EB, Halloran BP, Turnlund JR, Van Loan MD, Cann CE, et al. A longitudinal study of calcium homeostasis during human pregnancy and lactation and after resumption of menses. *Am J Clin Nutr.* 1998;67:693-701.

80. Kalkwarf HJ. Lactation and maternal bone health. *Adv Exp Med Biol.* 2004;554:101-14.

81. Kalkwarf HJ, Specker BL, Ho M. Effects of calcium supplementation on calcium homeostasis and bone turnover in lactating women. *J Clin Endocrinol Metab.* 1999;84:464-470.

82. Wainwright SA, Marshall LM, Ensrud KE, Cauley JA, Black DM, Hillier T, et al. Study of Osteoporotic Fractures Research Group. Hip fracture in women without osteoporosis. *J Clin Endocrinol Metab.* 2005;90:2787-2793.

CHAPTER 24

DERMATOLOGY

Barbara K. Hackley | Jan M. Kriebs

Women often seek the advice of their women's health provider on common skin-related problems. While many skin conditions are benign, others can herald systemic diseases or cancer, and some are specific to pregnancy. Thus, women's health providers play a pivotal role in the recognition and management of common skin problems, but also help women access appropriate and timely care for serious conditions. This chapter provides an overview of some of the more commonly seen conditions and is not intended to provide comprehensive therapeutic recommendations.

The Skin

The skin consists of three layers: the epidermis, dermis, and hypodermis (subcutaneous layer) (**Figure 24-1**). The *epidermis* is a continually renewing, stratified, squamous epithelium. Its primary function is protective. *Keratinocytes*, the main constituent, are formed in the basal cell layer of the epidermis. The basal cell layer also contains melanocytes, which produce *melanin*

and transfer it to neighboring keratinocytes.[1] Melanin helps to filter out ultraviolet (UV) sunrays and protect the skin. Half of the keratinocytes remain in place, while the other half migrate upward through the other upper three layers of the epidermis, first through the stratum spinosum, then the stratum granulosum, and finally into the outermost layer of the skin, the stratum corneum. Langerhans cells, which have immunologic functions, are found in the stratum spinosum. The keratinocytes become flatter and lose their nuclei in the granular layer. In the outermost layer, the stratum corneum, the skin is composed of overlapping cornified cells with no nuclei that are stuck together with lipid glue, forming a durable waterproof barrier.[1] When the outer layer of the skin becomes thickened or horny, the term *keratosis* is used.

The *dermis* is the middle layer of the skin. It is intimately connected to the epidermis above and is a supportive matrix of connective tissue, although it also contains hair follicles and sebaceous and sweat glands. More than 70% of the dermis is made up of collagen, giving it strength. It also contains elastin, which provides elasticity

Figure 24-1 The skin.

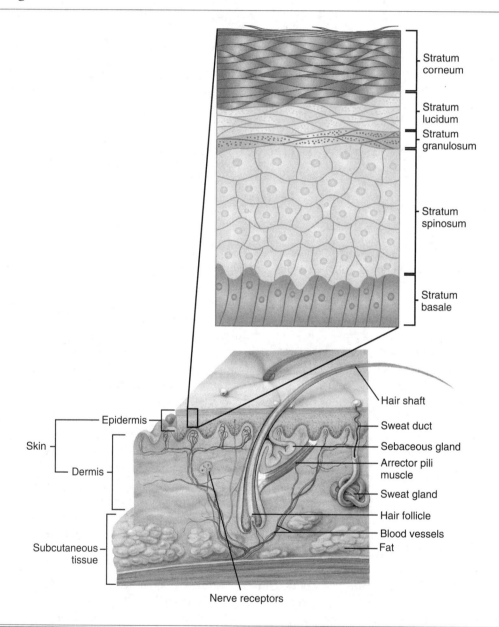

to the skin. Other cells found in the dermis include fibroblasts (which synthesize collagen, elastin, and connective tissue), dermal dendric cells, mast cells, macrophages, and lymphocytes.[1] Nerves course through the dermal layer and sense pain, touch, pressure, and temperature. Blood vessels bring nutrients and by dilating and contracting help regulate body temperature.

The *hypodermis* or *subcutaneous layer* is the deepest layer and is composed of fat, connective tissue that separates the fat into lobules, nerves, and blood vessels; the fatty tissue is biologically active and subject to inflammatory responses. This layer insulates the body and helps regulate body temperature. Fat in the hypodermis also serves as an energy store that can be utilized in times of energy deficit.

Burden of Skin Diseases

Many skin diseases are minor and transient in nature; others are persistent and may cause permanent scarring or skin changes. Some dermatologic disorders involving sensitive areas of the body such as the face, hands, and genitals can cause significant distress for women; however, the distress experienced not always correlate with the seriousness or extent of the disease. For example, teens who are dealing with core developmental issues related to body image and sexuality can have a significant psychosocial reaction to even mild disfigurement from acne. Depression, suicidal ideation, and sexual dysfunction can coexist with skin diseases that affect sensitive areas or those that involve disfigurement, so consideration of psychiatric and psychosocial factors must be addressed when assessing patients with dermatologic problems. It is important to recognize the patient who may be at high risk of developing psychosocial and psychiatric comorbidity. Major life events have been reported to exacerbate some

skin disorders, and, conversely, psychosocial stress may result from the impact of the skin disorder upon the quality of life of the patient.[2,3] Management of the distressed patient with skin conditions requires aggressive treatment; this patient is likely to be best served by immediate referral to a dermatologist. The patient may also benefit from referral to a psychiatric provider for assessment and treatment of any mental health comorbidity.

Essential History, Physical, and Laboratory Evaluation

History

History taking includes all the essential components of any medical history including menstrual, gynecologic, obstetric, sexual, medical, surgical, and family histories. In collecting the complete history, hormonal changes, potential exposures, and other risk factors may appear. The general condition of the woman's health is assessed; family history of atopy is determined. *Atopy* is an immune response to common, naturally occurring allergens with the continual production of immunoglobin E (IgE) antibodies. It commonly presents as atopic dermatitis, although allergic rhinitis and allergic asthma, which are related disorders, occur even more frequently. These conditions likely have a shared genetic basis, because they are often clustered in families. A family history of any of these conditions increases the chance that a woman may present with an atopy-related condition.

Further details of the condition in question should be ascertained as part of the history of present condition—in particular, recent exposures to chemicals, temperature extremes such as heat or cold, and drug ingestion. Other questions should elicit information about timing (onset and duration), initial appearance and change over time, whether this is an isolated or recurrent problem, and, if recurrent, a description of prior episodes. Inquiries should also be made regarding previous treatments, including the use of over-the-counter (OTC) medications, prescription drugs, or complementary therapies. During a review of systems, additional questions should be addressed to specifics of the current problem.

Physical Examination

Looking is the most important skill in diagnosing and treating skin diseases and is one that can be learned by primary care providers. Because diseases have locations of predilection, the clinician must know where to look as well as how to look. Not looking is more serious than not knowing exactly what is observed (**Figure 24-2**).

Figure 24-2 Location of common skin conditions.

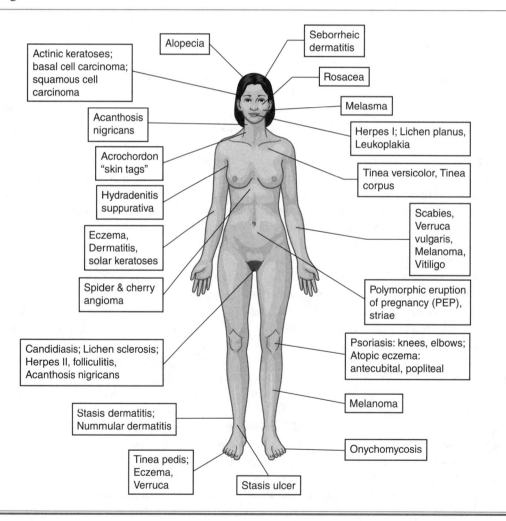

What is seen may be a primary lesion or the result of secondary irritation. Scratching or previous treatment with OTC preparations may alter the look of the lesion. When observing a skin lesion, looking and palpation are required. The lesion must be viewed with good lighting from various angles and may need to be touched, stretched, pinched, or moistened in order to appreciate the characteristics of the lesion.

Full-body examination provides the opportunity for identifying serious skin problems. Because 82% of the US population sees a health provider at least once a year,[4] it is possible to incorporate individual screening and education on skin health into routine care, including periodic gynecologic examinations, which may improve outcomes. Melanomas are more likely to be smaller when detected by primary care providers than those detected by a woman or her family.[5] Because women are often fully undressed at the gynecology visit, it is the perfect opportunity for detection. Hair, nails, and mucous membranes are all ectodermal structures closely related to skin and so should be included in the examination. This is an opportunity to observe for atypical nevi, in particular. These are discussed in the section on melanoma.

The initial examination of the lesion or rash allows the provider to focus the history in a productive manner. The history of this occurrence should be obtained while doing the physical examination. Knowledge about various dermatologic conditions allows the clinician to focus on suspected areas of probable involvement. For example, psoriasis is often found on elbows and knees but can also involve the nails. Some conditions can affect similar types of skin. For example, lichen planus (LP) often affects the mucous membranes of both the genital area and the oral cavity.

Skin inspection requires good lighting. Dim lighting reduces color and increases shadows, but too much light interferes with observation of skin surfaces. Daylight is the optimal light source for viewing lesions. The next best choice is a blue incandescent light. Skin diseases assume unusual hues when observed under white fluorescent lighting; such lighting is too strong. Examining with a 5–10× magnifying glass is also helpful.[6]

To define the differential diagnoses, a description of the lesion is essential. The main descriptors of skin lesions include morphology, color, arrangement, and distribution. Morphology characterizes the size, texture, and elevation of the individual lesion. Lesions can also be described by shape from round or oval to more complex appearances. Noting color can also be helpful, including whether the color changes when the lesion is compressed. The margins can be well defined or not. **Table 24-1** lists terms and descriptions of various skin manifestations.

Lesions may be singular or multiple. If multiple, they can be described by their arrangement and distribution. Grouped arrangements are described as linear, circular, arciform, herpetiform, or reticulated. Disseminated lesions can be described as scattered or diffuse. Distribution includes the extent of the involvement: isolated, localized, and regional. Patterns can be described as characteristic of specific conditions, such as those seen in Lyme disease, candidiasis, or acne; described using more general terms, such as symmetrical; or described by location, such as present in exposed or intertriginous areas.

Simple office-based tests can be done to help determine the diagnosis. One is to stroke the flexor surface of the forearm or upper back with a wooden tongue depressor. In certain conditions, a red linear wheal called *dermographism* will occur. However, in women with atopic dermatitis, stroking will cause a white line without urtication to form where the skin was stroked. Diascopy is the use of a glass slide to dehematize a lesion by applying pressure. If pressure on the glass slide causes a red lesion to blanch, the lesion is caused by vascular dilation. Extravascular lesions such as hemorrhages, pigmentations, and cellular infiltrates will

Table 24-1 Descriptors for Skin Lesions

Term	Description
Type	
Blister	Fluid-filled superficial lesion, ≤ 1 cm
Bulla	Fluid-filled lesion, > 1 cm
Carbuncle	Clustered furuncules
Furuncules	Boil, skin abcess
Macule	Flat, well circumscribed change in skin color
Nodule	Solid lesion involving dermis/subcutaneous tissue, > 1 cm
Papule	Solid superficial raised lesion, < 1 cm
Petechiae	Small blood deposits under the skin, < 0.5 cm
Plaque	Solid superficial raised lesion, ≥ 1 cm
Pupura	Extravasion of blood under the skin in a rash
Pustule	Superficial lesion containing purulent matter
Striae	Linear atrophic lesions
Vesicle	Fluid-filled lesion at surface of epidermis, < 0.5 cm
Wheal	Raised edematous tissue; irregular in size, shape, and color; may involve dermis
Color	
Brown	Hypermelanosis
Red	Erythema, violaceous, purpureus (does not blanch)
White	Leukoderma, hypomelanosis, leukoplakia
Other colors	Vary with disease process (e.g., black or gray with skin cancers)
Appearance	
Crust	Dried serum, blood, or pus; also used to describe thickened epidermis with psoriasis or eczema
Desquamation/Scaling	Loss of epidermal tissue in large flakes
Ecchymosis	Bruising
Erosion	Slight depression of skin caused by loss of epidermis
Excoriation	Skin torn, abraded, or irritated by scratching
Fissure	Linear tear
Lichenification	Epidermal hypertrophy, thickened, leathery texture
Ulcer	Open round or oval lesion in epidermis and dermis
Shape	
Annular	Raised lesion surrounding a cleared center
Arciform	Shaped in an arc
Herpetiform	Clustered blisters
Reticulated	Lacy, weblike
Serpiginous	Curving, snakelike, serpentine
Umbilicated	Having a central depression

not blanch under pressure. If it is unclear whether a small lesion is fluid filled (vesicle or pustule) or solid (papule), puncture with a fine sterile needle will demonstrate the difference if exudate is expressed. Dermatologists use a Wood's light (UV light at 360 nm) to diagnose certain types of

Table 24-2 KOH Wet Mount for Cutaneous Fungal Infections

1. Hold a # 15 surgical blade perpendicular to the skin surface and smoothly but firmly draw the blade against the scale of the lesion with several short strokes. If a border is present, the blade should be held at right angles to the fringe of the scale.
2. The scale is separated and placed on the slide and covered with the cover slip. KOH 10–20% is applied by a toothpick or eyedropper to the edge of cover slip and allowed to seep beneath the cover slip by capillary action.
3. The slide is gently heated under a low flame and pressed to separate the epithelial cells from the fungal hyphae.
4. Lower the condenser of the microscope and dim the light to enhance the contrast, making identification of the hyphae easier.

fungal infections. Potassium hydroxide (KOH) preparation of scales is diagnostic for fungal organisms of the skin and can be done in the office setting of the primary care provider (**Table 24-2**).

Laboratory Evaluation

Although visualization of the skin is the most important component of diagnosis for most lesions in a gynecology practice, at times laboratory examination may contribute to the diagnosis. Examples of tests to consider include cultures for bacteria and virology, microscopy for wet mounts including yeast, laboratory evaluation of blood for signs of diabetes or polycystic ovarian syndrome, and serology for syphilis. Although biopsies of the skin, especially of the vulva, are done in a gynecology practice, referral to a dermatologist is commonly done if a biopsy is warranted for lesions at other locations of the body.

Common Signs and Symptoms

Management of specific skin diseases is discussed in detail in this section; however, the same treatments are often used to manage the same symptoms irrespective of the underlying etiology. This section discusses supportive care used to treat dry skin, urticaria, pruritis, and intertrigo.

Dry Skin (Xerosis)

Most soap is alkaline in pH, while the skin has a pH of 4 to 5.5. Use of soap can damage, irritate, and dry the skin. Individuals with dry, itchy skin can use nonsoap cleansers that are neutral in pH, hypoallergenic, and fragrance free. Other tips to reduce skin dryness include showering with warm rather than hot water, showering for no more than 5 to 10 minutes, and applying moisturizer immediately after bathing.[7]

Preserving the integrity of normal skin is the first requirement for healthy skin, particularly if it is dry. This can be managed with a variety of moisturizers that restore water and lipids to the epidermis. These products include lotions, creams, ointments, and pastes that should be applied after bathing and then patted dry. *Lotions* are liquid (either alcohol or water) solutions and are used to treat inflammation and for rehydration. They absorb quickly and, unless they contain alcohol, are not drying. Because they are thinner and easy to apply over large areas, they are best for areas that are hairy, prone to folliculitis, or intertriginous. *Creams* are an emulsion of water and oil, either of which may predominate; when oil predominates, they are greasier but also have greater emollient effect. *Ointments* are a semisolid compound containing a hydrocarbon. They can both rehydrate and occlude, preventing further water loss, but they are difficult to remove and therefore less acceptable to some women. Unlike creams, they do not require a preservative, and thus may be less allergenic in susceptible individuals. *Pastes* are a mixture of powder and ointment; they are best for skin conditions that require hydration but affect defined areas such as psoriasis. The addition of powder makes them more adherent. No matter what vehicle is chosen, repeated applications are important, especially for women who wash frequently. Gel products are not used for hydration; they are nonfluid colloids that become liquid when applied to the skin. Although used as a transport mechanism for skin medications, they are not emollient.

There is no need for expensive preparations if the main aim is rehydration, because ingredients are very similar despite wide differences in price. Petroleum jelly and mineral oil are inexpensive and effective choices and are often recommended as first-line agents for rehydration.

Additives can increase the effectiveness of products. Products containing urea 5% to 10% (Aquacare, Carmol) or lactic acid 5% to 12% (Lac Hydrin) are particularly useful in helping hydrate skin that has a thick epidermal layer. These substances can penetrate the thicker epidermis and act as a chemical exfoliant. Other products use microsphere delivery systems, where the active ingredient is incorporated into a polymeric matrix. This allows a higher concentration of the drug to be delivered, increasing diffusion and availability of the active ingredient while decreasing irritation. Acne treatments using benzoyl peroxide and tretinoin have employed this approach to create more tolerable products.

Urticaria

Urticaria is a common, distinctive, and variably pruritic reaction to a variety of stimuli. The transient wheals are edematous papules and plaques and larger edematous areas that involve the dermis. The lesions are surrounded by a reflex erythema. Urticaria usually resolves quickly, within 1 to 24 hours. When the deep dermis, subcutaneous,

or submucosal tissue is involved, it is called *angioedema*. Angioedema is more often described as being painful rather than itchy and takes longer to resolve than wheals, up to 72 hours. Angioedema accompanied by difficulty breathing is a precursor of anaphylaxis and warrants immediate transfer to a higher level of care. These symptoms may be spontaneous and self-limited, but they also may be indicative of the presence of other medical conditions.[8]

Previous classification systems divided the various types of urticaria into groups based on their underlying cause. These categories included IgE-mediated causes (atopy, allergens, parasites), physical triggers (cold, sun, exercise, vibration), and autoimmune and hereditary causes, among others.[9] However, a 2013 international consensus guideline, released by the World Allergy Organization, the European Dermatology Forum, and representatives from 21 national and international societies, suggested a more practical approach.[8] They first suggest classifying urticaria as acute or chronic (< vs. ≥ 6 weeks' duration). Next, urticaria can be classified as being spontaneous or induced by external stimuli. These classifications can be used to determine if only supportive care is needed or if further diagnostic testing is needed (see **Table 24-3**).

A directed history can help focus the differential list. If a woman reports fever, malaise, and/or joint/bone pain, then an autoinflammatory disease should be suspected. Wheals that last more than 24 hours might indicate vasculitis, which can be confirmed by biopsy. If a woman reports that her wheals are in response to certain exposures such as heat, cold, or sunlight, then a dermatologist can order specific provocation tests. A medication and family history should be obtained, because certain medications such as angiotensin-convertin enzyme (ACE) inhibitors and nonsteroidal anti-inflammatory drugs (NSAIDs) and hereditary conditions are associated with angioedema.[8]

Women's health providers generally do not manage any of the serious forms of urticaria, but

Table 24-3 Urticaria

Type	Subtype	Laboratory	Possible Entities
Spontaneous	Acute	None	Unknown
	Chronic	Differential blood count ESR or CRP Possibly: thyroid function tests, liver enzymes	Infections (*H. pylori*, hepatitis B or C, EBV) Allergy Thyroid disorder Dietary triggers Parasites
Inducible	Cold	Confirm with cold provocation test (ice cube, cold water, cold wind)	Infections
	Delayed pressure	Confirm with pressure test	
	Heat	Confirm with heat provocation test	
	Solar	UV and visible light of different wavelengths	Rule out other light-induced dermatoses
	Contact dermatitis	Skin tests	
	Drug	Stop use of suspected product	

CRP = C-reactive protein, EBV = Epstein-Barr virus, ESR = erythrocyte sedimentation rate, UV = ultraviolet.

Data from Zuberbier T, Aberer W, Asero R, Bindslev-Jensen C, Brzoza Z, Canonica GW, et al. The EAACI/GA2LEN/EDF/WAO guideline for the definition, classification, diagnosis, and management of urticaria: the 2013 revision and update. *Allergy*. 2014;69(7):868-887; Bernstein JA, Lang DM, Khan DA, Craig T, Dreyfus D, Hsieh F, et al. The diagnosis and management of acute and chronic urticaria: 2014 update. *J Allergy Clin Immunol*. 2014;133(5):1270-1277.e66.

women with spontaneous acute symptoms may seek care from their women's health provider. Cool baths are soothing, but hot showers are contraindicated to prevent worsening pruritus and urticaria. Topical steroids are not effective. All suspected triggers should be stopped (e.g., food, aspirin) and second-generation antihistamines prescribed; doses may need to be high to afford relief. Suggested products include nondrowsy H1 blockers, including loratadine (Claritin), cetirizine (Zyrtec), and fexofenadine (Allegra). Women who do not get complete relief from second-generation antihistamines should be referred to a dermatologist for evaluation and adjunctive therapy. Other treatment modalities include prescribing high-dose antihistamines, combining several antihistamine products together, and use of omalizumab or montelukast. Very rarely, a 10-day course of corticosteroids may be needed.[8,10]

Children and adults with serious known allergies in which urticaria occurs should carry epinephrine (i.e., EpiPen) to use in case of an emergency. If exposure to an allergen occurs and the woman experiences difficulty breathing or swelling in the throat or tongue, 9-1-1 should be called immediately and epinephrine administered. Women should also always carry an oral antihistamine to take in addition to intramuscular epinephrine if serious symptoms develop.

Pruritus

Itching, or *pruritis*, is the major symptom of many skin conditions, especially inflammatory ones,

Table 24-4 Chronic Pruritus

Type	Conditions	Diagnostic Clues
Dermatologic	Atopic eczema	Often the first symptom at the beginning of a flare. Can be provoked by allergens, emotional stress, contact with irritants, or overheating.
	Contact dermatitis	Acute exposure can lead to blisters, oozing, or erythema. Chronic exposure is associated with scaling, erythema, hyperkeratosis, lichenification, and fissures. Commonly affects hands, fingers, and face.
	Insect bite	Localized itchiness.
	Psoriasis	Experienced by 85%; worsened by stress, heat, and xerosis. Can also experience crawling and burning sensations.
	Scabies	Itching commences within 3 to 6 weeks in primary infestation, within a few days in secondary ones.
	Urticaria	Intense itchiness, stinging, or prickling sensation.
	Xerosis	Dry skin, worse in the winter and as individuals age.
Systemic	Cholestasis	Generalized, migratory pruritus not relieved with scratching. Worse at night. Often worse on hands and feet.
	Chronic kidney disease	Localized or generalized pruritus. Waxes just before and during dialysis and wanes the day after dialysis. Pattern repeats.
	HIV infection	Can be due to a number of causes: folliculitis, seborrheic dermatitis, scabies, xerosis, and drug eruptions, among others.
	Hodgkin's lymphoma	Severe persistent generalized pruritus.
	Hyperthyroidism	Severe generalized pruritus.
	Polycythemia vera	Pruritus worse after contact with water.
Neuropathic	Neuropathy	Generally localized pruritus. Can be due to tumors of the central nervous system, stroke, or multiple sclerosis.
	Postherpetic itch	Severe pruritus that persists after resolution of infection.
Psychogenic	Obsessive-compulsive disorder	Sleep generally not interrupted.
	Substance abuse	

Data from Weisshaar E, Fleischer AB, Bernhard JD, Cropley TG. Pruritus and dysesthesia. In: Bolognia JL, Jorizzo JL, Schaffer JV, eds. *Dermatology*. 3rd ed. Philadelphia, PA: Elsevier Saunders; 2012; Yosipovitch G, Bernhard JD. Chronic pruritus. *N Engl J Med*. 2013;368:1625-1634.

and systematic diseases (**Table 24-4**).[11,12] Whatever the underlying cause, itch evokes scratching, which increases inflammation and stimulates nerve fibers, leading to a vicious cycle called the "itch-scratch cycle." This cycle can alter the integrity of the skin, leading to barrier damage.

Incessant rubbing and scratching can result in *lichenification*, which is a well developed plaque with marked accentuation of the skin creases. Lichenification can occur secondarily to a primary skin lesion, but it can also occur in the absence of a primary skin lesion. The need to scratch can be triggered by emotional or systemic conditions and does not always represent a primary skin disorder.[12] The common sites for lichenification are in locations easily reached, such as the nape of the neck, below the elbow, the ankle, the buttock, and the genitals. Postinflammatory hyperpigmentation or hypopigmentation is common.

Treatment is directed by the underlying etiology. Supportive options during therapy include:[12]

- Topical
  - Emollients to treat *xerosis* or lichenification
  - Anesthetics such as capsaicin or a mixture of lidocaine/prilocaine to desensitize local peripheral nerve fibers
  - Coolants such as topical menthol
  - Topical corticosteroids to reduce inflammation
- Systemic therapies
  - Oral antihistamines to reduce itch and induce drowsiness, allowing affected individuals to sleep through the night
  - Gabapentin for neuropathic pain and itch
  - Antidepressants such as paroxetine, mirtazapine, and amitriptyline for generalized pruritus or neuropathic itch
  - UV light for atopic dermatitis, psoriasis, or pruritus from kidney disease

See specific conditions described in the sections that follow for further details on management of skin diseases involving irritation.

Intertrigo

Intertrigo is any inflammatory dermatosis involving body folds and results from chafing and moisture. Obese individuals, athletes, and those with immunosuppression from diabetes or human immunodeficiency virus (HIV) may be prone to intertrigo.[13] Moisture in the skin folds increases the risk for developing a secondary bacterial (erythrasma) or fungal infection. Common sites for intertrigo include beneath the breasts and in the axillae, antecubital fossae, inguinal folds, and abdominal folds (panniculus) above the symphysis pubis. In intertrigo, red plaques are seen opposite each other on either side of the skin fold, creating a mirror image. Heat is thought to aggravate the condition. Poor hygiene may contribute to the incidence.

There is general agreement that the best prevention is to keep the affected areas clean and dry by minimizing skin-on-skin friction, heat, and moisture in and around skin folds. These goals can be achieved by using techniques to promote dryness (e.g., separating the skin folds with absorbent cotton or other materials or disrobing and exposing affected areas to low heat from a hair dryer or electric light bulb), minimize friction (e.g., the use of skin protectants such as petroleum jelly or zinc oxide), and encourage healing (e.g., the application of wet tea bags, Domeboro soaks, hydrocolloid dressings, Burrow's solution, or witch hazel compresses). Women with intertrigo should be advised to wear light, nonconstrictive, absorbent clothing.[13]

Secondary bacterial and/or fungal infections require treatment. Multiple organisms, including *Staphylococcus aureus* or group A beta-hemolytic *Streptococcus* can cause bacterial infection. Treatment with topical therapies (e.g., mupirocin, erythromycin) is usually sufficient. Rarely, oral antibiotics (e.g., penicillin, first-generation cephalosporins) may be needed. Topical antifungal agents are preferred, with oral fluconazole reserved for use in resistant cases. Low-potency topical steroids (e.g., hydrocortisone 1% cream) can be used if the underlying cause is thought to be due to atopic dermatitis.[13]

Therapeutic Approaches

Use of Topical Corticosteroids

Topical corticosteroids are commonly used to treat pruritus and inflammation and are an integral component of the management of almost all skin conditions. This section reviews the principles governing their use and will help the clinician choose the correct dose and vehicle of topical corticosteroids. It also discusses management strategies that will result in the safe use of these products.

Topical corticosteroids are grouped by strength from I to VII (strongest to weakest; **Table 24-5**). When choosing a product, the group to which it belongs is the indicator of the strength, not the percentage as noted on the package. The percentage noted on the package refers to the concentration of the active ingredient in the vehicle (cream, ointment, etc.). Because the different vehicles have characteristics that affect absorption rates, it is important to choose both active ingredient and carrier correctly. It is essential that the product chosen be the correct strength for the specific condition being treated and be used for an appropriate amount of time. It is of little value to prescribe a product from the weaker categories when it is not of sufficient strength to be therapeutic. Weaker, supposedly "safer" strengths can fail to provide adequate activity and control.

The super-potent topical steroids from Class I are the strongest agents available and are used for difficult-to-treat conditions such as psoriasis and hand eczema. They have the potential to cause serious side effects. Hypothalamic-pituitary-adrenal

Table 24-5 Topical Steroids: From Least to Most Potent by Class

Potency (I Is Most Potent)	Generic Name	Brand Names/Percent Active Ingredient/Vehicle
VII	Hydrocortisone widely available as generic	LactiCare/1.0-AC/lotion LactiCare/2.5-AC/lotion
		Hytone/2.5/cream, lotion, ointment
	Hydrocortisone acetate	Epifoam/1.0/foam spray
VI	Desonide	DesOwen/0.05/cream, lotion
	Flurandrenolide	Cordran SP/0.025/cream
	Fluocinolone acetonide	Capex/0.01/shampoo Derma-Smoothe/0.01/oil
	Prednicarbate	Aclovate/0.05/cream, ointment
	Triamcinolone acetonide	Aristocort A/0.025/cream
V	Betamethasone valerate cream	Betatrex/0.1/cream
	Clocortolone pivalate	Cloderm/0.1/cream
	Desonide	DesOwen/0.05/ointment Tridesilon/0.05/ointment
	Fluocinolone acetonide	Synalar/0.025/cream Synemol/0.025/cream
	Flurandrenolide	Cordran SP/0.05/cream Cordran/0.5/ lotion Cordran/0.025/ointment
	Hydrocortisone butyrate	Locoid/0.1/cream Locoid Lipocream/0.1/ointment, solution
	Hydrocortisone valerate	Westcort/0.2/cream
	Triamcinolone acetamide	Aristocort/0.1/cream Kenalog/0.1/cream, lotion

Table 24-5 Topical Steroids: From Least to Most Potent by Class

Potency (I Is Most Potent)	Generic Name	Brand Names/Percent Active Ingredient/Vehicle
IV	Amcinonide	Cyclocort/0.1/cream
	Betamethasone valerate	Luxiq/0.12/foam
	Fluocinolone acetonide	Synalar/0.025/ointment
	Flurandrenolide	Cordran/0.05/ointment
	Mometasone furoate	Elocon/0.1/cream, lotion
	Prednicarbate	Dermatop-E/0.1/ointment
	Triamcinolone acetonide	Aristocort A/0.1/ointment Kenalog/0.1/ointment
III	Amcinonide	Cyclocort/0.1/cream, lotion
	Betamethasone dipropionate	Alphatrex/0.05/cream, ointment Diprosone/0.05/cream, lotion
	Betamethasone valerate	Betatrex/0.1/ointment
	Fluticasone propionate	Cutivate/0.005/ointment
	Mometasone furoate	Elocon/0.1/ointment
	Triamcinolone acetonide	Aristocort A/0.5/cream Kenalog/0.5/cream
II	Amcinonide	Cyclocort/0.1/ointment
	Augmented betamethasone dipropionate	Diprolene AF/0.05/cream
	Betamethasone dipropionate	Diprosone/0.1/aerosol Diprosone/0.05/ointment
	Desoximetasone	Topicort/0.25/cream
	Diflorasone diacetate	Psorcon-E/0.05/cream, ointment
	Fluocinonide	Lidex-E/0.05/cream Lidex/0.05/cream, gel, ointment, solution
	Halcinonide	Halog/0.1/cream, ointment, solution Halog-E/0.1/cream
	Mometasone furoate	Elocon/0.1/ointment
I	Augmented betamethasone dipropionate	Diprolene/0.05/gel, lotion, ointment
	Clobetasol propionate	Cormax/0.05/cream, ointment, scalp solution Olux/0.05/foam Temovate-E/0.05/cream Temovate/0.05/gel, ointment
	Diflorasone diacetate	Psorcon/0.05/ointment
	Flurandrenolide	Cordran/0.05/tape
	Halobetasol propionate	Ultravate/0.05/cream, ointment

axis suppression, hyperglycemia, and glycosuria occur rarely with the use of topical corticosteroids, but have been reported if the area being treated is large, occlusive dressings are used, or treatment is prolonged. Adverse dermatologic reactions are more common. These include thinning of the epidermis, striae, purpura, and maceration. Side effects are more likely to occur with higher potency products, with continuous use, in the elderly, and in those with thinner skin.[7]

In general, Class I and II corticosteroids are best prescribed under the direction of a dermatologist. Classes III through VII are prescribed more commonly in primary care practice. While adverse reactions are less common with use of mid- to low-potency steroids, following certain guidelines will minimize the risk. They should be applied no more than twice a day and be limited to 2 to 6 weeks' duration. If no improvement is seen, then a referral to a dermatologist is necessary. Steroid atrophy and other dermatologic reactions can develop in the areas being treated if an individual is treated for too long a time or with too strong a product.

Particular care should be used in treating skin conditions found on the face or in intertriginous areas. Use of lower potency corticosteroids in these areas is more likely to result in side effects than if same-strength products are used on other parts of the body. Therefore, using the lowest potency products available (Class VI or VII) for the shortest period of time is recommended for treating skin conditions in more vulnerable areas.

Using occlusive dressings can also increase the potency of corticosteroids. While they can markedly improve the response to treatment in more severe presentations, they also increase the risk of developing serious side effects related to corticosteroid use.

Topical corticosteroids are mixed in various bases: creams, lotions, gels, or ointments. Ointments allow greater penetration than creams or lotions and, therefore, are more potent. The type of vehicle can affect potency to such an extent that it can change the classification of a corticosteroid. For example, hydrocortisone valerate (Westcort) ointment 0.2% is classified as a Class IV steroid; however, it is categorized as a Class V corticosteroid if prescribed as a cream. Ointments are also usually preservative free, whereas creams are more likely to contain preservatives that may cause irritation. However, many patients prefer the feel of a cream or lotion to gels or ointments and may discontinue use of products that feel "greasy."

Steroids may be mixed with antimicrobial agents. Lotrisone cream, which contains an antifungal agent and the corticosteroid betamethasone diproprionate, is expensive and indicated only when there is a fungal diagnosis. Another combined product is Mycolog II, which is an antifungal agent with triamcinolone (Class VI).

Referral to a dermatologist is warranted if prompt improvement is not seen with low- to medium-dose corticosteroid therapy, if the diagnosis is in doubt, or if the use of high-dose corticosteroids or the use of an adjunctive treatment, such as occlusive dressings, is needed.

Management of Common Conditions

Eczematous Disorders

Eczema derives from the Greek word *ekzein*, meaning to erupt, ferment, or boil. Acute eczema is an inflammation of the skin characterized by erythema, edema, and vesiculation with weeping of acute lesions. Pruritus is severe. Subacute eczema is more organized and often associated with excoriation, scaling, and erythematous papules or plaques, grouped or scattered over erythematous skin. In chronic eczema, thickened, lichenified skin is seen. The mainstay of treatment is avoiding irritants and keeping the skin moisturized. In acute flares, cool wet compresses and topical steroid creams allow vasoconstriction and suppress inflammation and itching. Oral corticosteroids are used only for severe or generalized or acute eczema.

ATOPIC ECZEMA

Atopy (atopic dermatitis, AD) is now thought to be a result of interactions between genetics and environmental factors. Individuals with eczema often have an inherited tendency toward hypersensitivity and may present with asthma and allergic rhinitis in addition to eczema. Women with atopy tend to have inherently dry skin that makes them vulnerable to environmental irritants. They also have a lower itch threshold that is triggered by seasonal changes or contact with substances such as sweat, occlusive clothing, or wool. Emotional stress may also be a trigger. Adult manifestations include flexural involvement, hand manifestations, and upper eyelid dermatitis.

Treatment includes regular use of moisturizers and episodic use of topical corticosteroids during a flare. Generally, twice-daily use of topical corticosteroids is sufficient to induce remission. Use of high-potency topical steroids is limited to 1 to 2 weeks if possible. Remission can be maintained by twice-weekly application of lower potency products in eczema-prone areas.[14] Aggravating factors should be avoided. Up to one-third of patients with refractory eczema are thought to have food allergies. Avoiding problematic foods and other environmental irritants may be helpful. Clothing should be soft and light; cotton is an excellent choice. Stress-reduction techniques may be helpful.[14]

Referral to a dermatologist, who can offer other treatment modalities, should be obtained in persistent cases. Topical calcineurin is an anti-inflammatory agent that is thought to be equivalent to mid-potency corticosteroids in effectiveness and is less likely to cause local skin atopy. Thus, it may be recommended for use for facial or eyelid eczema despite the rare risk of lymphoma associated with its use.[14] Oral antihistamines with a sedating effect such as diphenhydramine (Benadryl) or hydroxyzine (Atarax) do little to control pruritus but may allow individuals with atopy to sleep better at night and control allergies, which are a common trigger for eczema. Oral vitamin D supplementation may be helpful, because it has been found to reduce eczematous flares by up to 80% (compared to 17% in the control group) in some trials.[14]

S. aureus can cause secondary infections of eczematous lesions, but even colonization is problematic as it is thought to trigger flares. Twice-weekly baths with diluted bleach equivalent to the concentration in a swimming pool (¼ to ½ cup household bleach in a 40-gallon bath tub) can result in marked clinical improvements in some patients. Refractory cases may benefit from wet wraps with concomitant topical corticosteroids.[14]

CONTACT DERMATITIS

Contact dermatitis is a generic term applied to acute or chronic inflammatory reactions to substances that come in contact with the skin. Eighty percent of contact dermatitis cases are due to contact with local irritants, and 20% are due to a type IV hypersensitivity reaction to allergens.[15] The problem is closely linked to occupation because of irritants encountered on the job. The response may be immediate or delayed, and symptoms include pruritus and inflammation. Common triggers are nickel; occupational exposure to chromate (found in cement and other industrial processes); contact with poison ivy, oak, or sumac; chronic exposure to water (hairdressers, bakers, pastry cooks) or friction (poorly fitting clothes or prosthetic limbs); and contact with chemicals or solvents, rubber or neoprene, topical anesthetics, or topical antibiotics such as bacitracin and neomycin.[15]

The causes of contact dermatitis can be differentiated by a careful history, and sometimes by the appearance and location of the lesions. Contact with irritants often results in red, fissured, painful, mildly pruritic lesions, typically with indistinct borders, localized to the region of contact.[15] Exposure to allergens will result in the same symptoms experienced after prior exposures and often presents with redness, edema, and vesicles. The rash may spread locally or become disseminated. Treatment consists of avoidance of the offending irritant or allergen, cool compresses, use of nonsoap cleansers to reduce dryness, use of emollients for rehydration, and topical corticosteroids to treat inflammation.[15]

Nummular Eczema

Nummular eczema is a chronic, pruritic, round, coin-shaped plaque composed of grouped small papules and vesicles on an erythematous base, scale, and crust. The margins are often more pronounced than the central portion. Lesions are more common in the winter months due to lack of humidity and increased use of hot water and soap. It is most commonly confused with tinea corporis, but can be differentiated from tinea corporis by distinctive characteristics: location (dorsa of the hands, extensor surfaces of the forearms, upper arms, legs, thighs, and feet), appearance (crusting and scaling surface and lack of central clearing), and past history of eczema. The differential diagnosis should include psoriasis, Bowen's disease, mycosis fungoides, and tinea corporis.[16] Treatment consists of removal of any triggering agents and use of mild corticosteroids and emollients. Higher potency II or III topical steroids are used in resistant cases. Rarely, other therapies, such as topical tacrolimus or pimecrolimus, coal tar preparations, or UV light therapy are needed.[16,17]

Stasis Dermatitis

Stasis dermatitis, the result of chronic venous insufficiency, may be seen in older women. It is associated with varicose and dilated veins. It is a progressive disease, often starting with edema, which resolves at night. The skin becomes dry and itchy. Over time, the edema becomes more extensive and persistent and is accompanied by inflammation. The skin, subcutaneous adipose tissue, and deep fascia become adherent and form a firm circular cuff in the distal calf. The skin may show hemosiderin pigmentation. Venous ulcers can develop spontaneously or as a result of scratching or trauma. Lichenification is also common. Differential diagnoses include contact dermatitis and cellulitis. Treatment is directed at the underlying pathology: compression stockings to improve venous return, lifestyle changes, exercise of the calf muscles, and surgery if needed. Topical treatment is the same as for other types of eczemas: topical corticosteroids and emollients.[16]

Seborrheic Dermatitis

Seborrheic dermatitis occurs in areas of the skin where active sebaceous glands are found and is thought to be partially due to sebum overproduction. In adults, greasy scales and yellow–red coalescing macules, patches, and papules may be found on the scalp, face, or ears, and less commonly in the central chest or skin folds.[16] The mildest form is dandruff, a dry scaling rash of the scalp. More extensive involvement of the scalp can occur. Other affected sites include the eyebrows, glabella, nasolabial folds, and the cheeks. There may be associated blepharitis or otitis externa.[18] Differential diagnosis for suspected seborrheic dermatitis on the scalp included psoriasis, pediculosis, fungal infections, and eczema. For facial presentations, other possibilities should be considered, including eczema, lupus, rosacea, and contact dermatitis.[18]

Seborrheic dermatitis in adults tends to be chronic with periods of remission and exacerbation. Treatment focuses on control of symptoms. Dandruff is best treated with medicated shampoos that include selenium sulfide, ketoconazole, tar, or salicylic acid.[19] Facial lesions are treated with antifungal and sometimes topical corticosteroids.[18] Of these agents, the strongest evidence supports the use of antifungal agents, which are considered first-line agents. Topical selenium sulfide has been found to be slightly less effective and associated with more local irritation than 2% ketoconazole.[18,19]

Psoriasis

Psoriasis is a chronic, immune-mediated disorder that encompasses genetic predisposition and environmental triggers. The world prevalence is approximately 1–3%.[20] It is a hereditary disorder; if 1 parent has the disease, the offspring have an 14% chance of having the disease, but if both parents have psoriasis, the child has a 41% chance.[21] Flares can be triggered by stress, trauma, infections, or medications. Psoriasis is a papulosquamous disease; that is, it is manifested as scaling with papules and plaques. Most frequently, it affects the elbows, knees, and scalp but can affect any portion of the skin, nails, and joints. The lesions are sharply marginated with a silvery-white scale. It is associated with increased risk of arthritis, cardiovascular disease, and cancer in those with severe presentations. The differential list is broad and includes seborrheic dermatitis, squamous cell carcinoma, mycosis fungoides variant of cutaneous T cell lymphoma, hypertrophic lichen planus, drug eruptions, and pityriasis rosea, among other possibilities.[21]

Most patients will already have a diagnosis of psoriasis when they present to a gynecologic visit and should be referred to a dermatologist if a new diagnosis is suspected. The expression, "the heartbreak of psoriasis," is not a joke. The name literally means "humiliation." It can be disfiguring and very difficult to treat. It is lifelong and characterized by recurrent exacerbations and remissions. Psoriasis is not managed in the primary care women's health setting. Treatment is usually multimodal and often includes a combination of topical vitamin D_3 analogues and corticosteroids. Other treatment options include topical anthralin, topical tazarotene, phototherapy, and oral methotrexate among other therapies.[21]

Diseases of the Sebaceous and Apocrine Glands

ACNE

Acne is an inflammation of the pilosebaceous unit (pustular eruption) of the face and trunk that occurs in adolescence and may persist into adulthood. It may manifest itself as papules, papulopustules, or nodules plus cysts. Pitted, depressed, or hypertrophic scarring may occur with all types, but this happens more frequently with nodulocystic acne. Women may have premenstrual flares. Controversy remains about whether diet influences acne.[22,23] A 2009 review found that Western diets with a high intake of dairy, fat, and high-glycemic-index foods may worsen the course.[22]

Comedones result from abnormalities in the proliferation and differentiation of ductal keratinocytes in the skin. Retention of hyperproliferating keratinocytes and corneocytes in the duct cause a plug of sebaceous and keratin material to form. It may be that abnormalities in the sebaceous lipid composition, androgens, local cytokine production, and colonization by particular bacteria encourage comedo formation. Comedo formation may be primarily an inflammatory process. This would explain why antibacterial agents (benzoyl peroxide) and antimicrobial therapy (oral and topical antibiotics) work so well. *Propionibacterium acnes* has been implicated in the pathogenesis of acne for more than 100 years.

Acne lesions are divided into noninflammatory and inflammatory lesions. The former (comedones) consist of open papular lesions (blackheads) and closed papular lesions (whiteheads). Inflammatory acne is characterized by the presence of papules, pustules, and nodules (cysts). The pustules have a visible central core of purulent exudates. Nodules become suppurative or hemorrhagic. Recurring rupture and re-epithelialization of cysts lead to epithelial-lined tracts, often accompanied by severe scarring.

Tretinoins are prescribed as initial therapy in almost all cases. They prevent the formation of comedones, help clear existing comedones, have anti-inflammatory properties, and can help maintain control after systemic drugs are discontinued. Their most common side effects are burning, stinging, dryness, and scaling.[24] Adapalene appears to be one of the better tolerated products.[25] Topical retinoids are thought to normalize keratinization and reduce follicular plugging. Ongoing use prevents formation of microcomedones, which are precursor lesions to all forms of acne.

Treatment approaches vary according to the severity of the presentation (**Table 24-6**). Monotherapy with a tretinoin is used for the initial treatment of noninflammatory acne. If no response is seen in 4 to 8 weeks, topical benzoyl peroxide agents are added. Individuals with mild inflammatory acne are commonly started with two products, a tretinoin and a benzoyl peroxide agent. Benzoyl peroxide has antibacterial properties and is most effective if combined with a tretinoin. If the combination of these two products is inadequate, topical antibiotics can be added. Individuals with moderate inflammatory acne are usually started on a three-drug regimen (tretinoin, benzoyl peroxide, and topical antibiotics). It is important to add on benzoyl peroxide first, because it can help prevent antibiotic resistance to topical (and oral) antibiotics. Patience is required, because it takes up to 2 months for most topical regimens to show their full effect.[25]

Individuals with moderate to severe acne need more aggressive treatment. Moderate acne responds best to oral antibiotics.[25] Preferred first-line agents, if tolerated, are doxycycline or minocycline.[25] Erythromycin is becoming increasingly resistant to *P. acnes*.[24] Control, defined as a marked reduction in the formation of new inflammatory lesion, can take 3 to 6 months.[24] Once control is achieved, antibiotics are stopped and maintenance is generally achieved with ongoing use of tretinoin.[24,25] Oral contraceptives can also be used as adjunctive therapy in women and may be particularly useful in long-term control. A recent meta-analysis found that oral antibiotics outperformed oral contraceptives at 3 months, but by 6 months results were equivalent. Women on a 6-month course of antibiotics had a 52% reduction in the number of total acne lesions compared to a 55% reduction for those on oral contraceptives and a 29% reduction for those on placebo.[26]

Isotretinoin is reserved for use with severe cystic acne, with acne that causes scarring, and for persistent cases unresponsive to less aggressive therapy. Potential adverse effects include increases in liver enzymes and triglycerides and possibly a negative impact on bone health and increased risk for inflammatory bowel disease and depression.[24] However, the greatest concern is prenatal exposure. Isotretinoin use is contraindicated in pregnancy. Fetal exposure to isotretinoin during pregnancy can cause severe craniofacial, cardiac, and central nervous system anomalies. Women taking it should have monthly pregnancy tests and use two forms of contraception. Dermatologists register any women taking the drug, and the patient must sign a consent form.

Other agents are sometimes used. Dapsone 5% gel is thought to be particularly effective

Table 24-6 Treatment of Acne

Type	Treatment	
Clinical Presentation	Therapy	Products

Comedones	Topical retinoid	Adapalene
		    Cream, lotion (0.1%)
		    Gel (0.1%, 0.3%)
		Tazarotene
		    Cream, gel (0.05%, 0.1%)
		Tretinoin
		    Cream (0.025%, 0.05%, 0.1%)
		    Gel (0.01%, 0.025%, 0.05%)
		    Microsphere gel (0.04%, 0.1%)

Mild inflammatory with papules and pustules	Topical retinoid
	Benzoyl peroxide
		Single agents:
		• See above for topical retinoid
		• Benzoyl peroxide
		    Formulations: cream, gel, lotion, pad,
		        wash (2.5% to 10%)
		Combination products:
		• Adapalene/benzoyl peroxide
		Gel (0.1%/2.5%)

Moderate inflammatory with papules and pustules	Topical retinoid
	Benzoyl peroxide
	Topical antibiotic
		Single agents:
		• See above for retinoids
		• See above for benzoyl
		• Clindamycin
		    Foam, gel, lotion, solution (1.0%)
		• Erythromycin
		    Gel, ointment, solution (2%)
		Combination products:
		• Clindamycin/tretinoin
		    Gel (1.2%/0.025%)
		• Erythromycin/benzoyl peroxide
		• Gel 3%/5%

Moderate inflammatory with papules, pustules, and nodules Severe inflammatory with papules and pustules	Topical retinoid Benzoyl peroxide Oral antibiotic	See above: retinoids and benzoyl peroxide Oral antibiotics: • Doxycycline • Minocycline • Erythromycin • Trimethoprim-sulfamethoxazole
Severe inflammatory with papules, pustules, and nodules	Oral isotretinoin	Claravis Sotret Myorisan Amnesteem Absorica

against inflammatory lesions, especially if it is combined with a tretinoin.[24] Salicylic acid is an active ingredient in many OTC anti-acne products, but appears to be less efficacious than benzoyl peroxide.[24]

Acne is a chronic condition. Therapy is usually continuous and prolonged, so referral to a dermatologist is indicated for moderate to severe cases. Women with milder presentations who respond well to topical agents or hormonal contraception do not require a referral. Women over the age of 25 with acne usually have long-term, low-grade acne. A workup for polycystic ovarian syndrome (PCOS) is indicated if the woman has irregular cycles, hirsutism, or obesity.

Alternative therapies for acne have been explored. According to a recent Cochrane review, a low-glycemic-load diet, tea tree oil, and bee venom may reduce total lesions, but the studies are weak. No other alternative therapies have been shown to have a positive effect.[27]

Rosacea (Rosacea Acne)

Rosacea is a common, chronic facial disorder of the pilosebaceous unit. The hallmark sign is diffuse centrofacial erythema, which intensifies during a flare. Inflammatory papulopustular lesions may or may not be present, but if present are most commonly found on the central face. Rosacea can also affect the nose (phymatous rosacea) and eyes (ocular rosacea).[28] With phymatous rosacea, the nose appears red and swollen; less commonly the forehead or chin is affected. Ocular rosacea should be suspected if a woman reports sensitivity to light; gritty, scratchy, itchy, red, or bloodshot eyes; blurred vision; eye allergies; or foreign body sensation.[28] Triggers vary by individual and include heat, stress, sunlight, alcohol, and certain foods and medications.[29,30]

Rosacea more commonly affects women than men, adults compared to children, and individuals of Northern European descent with fair skin.

It is rare in darker skinned persons. With rosacea, there is often a long history of flushing with hot fluids, spicy foods, or alcohol. It may follow acne but usually arises de novo. The differential diagnosis should include chronic sun damage, contact dermatitis, seborrheic dermatitis, lupus, and alcohol or niacin ingestion.[28]

Treatment includes avoidance of triggers through lifestyle modifications. Medication options are determined by symptoms. Topical metronidazole (twice-daily application of 0.75% gel, cream, or lotion; once-daily application of 1% gel or cream) and azelaic acid (15% gel twice-daily application) are US Food and Drug Administration (FDA)–approved for the treatment of inflammatory lesions. Topical sodium sulfacetamide 10%/sulfur 5% formulations have also long been used for the treatment of rosacea but are less commonly used today due to their strong smell and the availability of other effective products.[29]

Unfortunately, while first-line topical agents effectively treat inflammatory lesions, they are not effective at minimizing background erythema due to fixed dilation and enlargement of the underlying facial vasculature. A newer product, an alpha-adrenergic receptor agonist (brimonidine tartrate), has been approved to treat background flushing. It increases vasomotor tone and shunts blood flow into deeper tissue.[29] Other topical agents not expressly approved for treatment of rosacea are also sometimes used and/or are under investigation for the treatment of rosacea. These include tretinoin, topical clindamycin, benzoyl peroxide, and permethrin.[30] No topical agents improve telangiectasia, the permanent dilation of superficial blood vessels. It is treated with laser therapy.[29]

Oral antibiotics, ideally given for a limited amount of time, are used to treat more extensive inflammatory lesions (i.e., papules, pustules, nodules) if topical agents are insufficient. Oral isotretinoin is used if severe inflammatory lesions are present and is also sometimes used in the treatment of phymatous rosacea.

Relapse of rosacea occurs in 25% of patients. Therefore, maintenance topical therapy for 6 months is recommended once control is achieved.

HIDRADENITIS SUPPURATIVA (ACNE INVERSA)

Hidradenitis suppurativa (HS) is a chronic, relapsing disease of the skin areas containing apocrine glands (axillae, breasts, groin, genital, buttocks). The prevalence has been reported to be as high as 4%; the incidence is 3 times higher in women than in men.[31] Symptoms often first occur around the time of puberty.[32] Smoking, obesity, and family history have all been associated with the development of HS.[31] The associated pain and disfiguring lesions may bring women to see their women's health provider, as this is both a socially distressing condition and one in which the chronic pain significantly affects quality of life.

Because the initial nodule forms in the pilosebaceous follicular ducts, the similarity to acne pathogenesis has led to a proposal to change the name to acne inversa. The inflammatory nodule may resolve or may form a channel to the surface and drain purulent or seropurulent material from the abscess. Eventually, sinus tracts form with fibrosis and ropy scarring; hypertrophic and keloidal scars and contractures may ensue. In the early stages, differential diagnoses include boils, granuloma inguinale, lymphogranuloma venereum, pilonidal cysts, and dermal cysts, but as the woman's symptoms worsen the diagnosis becomes more evident.[33]

Treatment for mild cases includes management of personal hygiene with loose clothing, no shaving of the affected area, warm compresses, avoidance of heat and humidity, and topical antiseptics or antibacterials.[33] Topical clindamycin and resorcinol cream have demonstrated benefit.[34] First-line oral antibiotics include clindamycin plus rifampin. Other antibiotics used include dicloxacillin, minocycline, and tetracycline. Long-term antibiotics are best managed by a dermatologist, who is better placed to evaluate disease progression or remission.

If lesions are painful, severe, or persist after initial therapy, referral to a dermatologist is warranted. Long-term antibiotics, intermittent steroids, and surgery or cryotherapy have been the primary therapies, and more recently tumor necrosis factor-alfa inhibitors have been tried.[32] New biologics, including adalimumab and infliximab, are effective and coming into use for severe cases.[34]

Disorders of Hair Follicles

ALOPECIA

Hair loss in women is often very disturbing. Androgenetic alopecia is a physiologic reaction to androgens in genetically predisposed individuals of both sexes. In women, there is diffuse hair thinning that begins between puberty and 40 years of age. The hair thins first in the frontal and parietal regions.[35] Androgenetic alopecia is polygenic and can be inherited from either side of the family.[36] Many women show no evidence of hyperandrogenism, suggesting that there is a multifactorial cause for the hair loss.

Most women with alopecia do not require laboratory hormonal evaluation. If, however, the woman has irregular menstrual cycles, severe acne, infertility, or galactorrhea, then dehydroepiandrosterone sulfate (DHEAS), serum-free or total testosterone, and prolactin levels may help to point to a diagnosis of PCOS, pituitary adenoma (galactorrhea), or other constitutional disease. Other common causes of hair loss are ruled out by measurement of thyroid hormones, serum iron and ferritin, complete blood count, and rapid plasma reagin.[35]

Treatment includes use of 2% topical minoxidil solution, applied twice a day; a 5% solution is used on men. Use of the stronger solution by women may result in increased hair growth on the forehead and face. Finasteride has not been demonstrated to be as effective in women as in men;[37] further, it is not recommended for use in women due to fetal risks if pregnancy occurs.

If hormonal contraception is desired, a product low in androgenic activity (i.e., Yasmin or Ortho Tri-Cyclen Lo) should be considered.

HIRSUTISM

Hirsutism is excessive hair growth in androgen-dependent hair patterns: the face, chest, areola, linea nigra, inner thighs, and external genitalia. Defining this condition is difficult because there is considerable individual and ethnic variation in the degree and pattern of body hair.[38] In the extreme on this spectrum, however, there may be an association with hyperandrogenism. This is the case with PCOS, the most common pathologic cause of hirsutism, and with idiopathic hirsutism, when no endocrine abnormalities are noted.

According to the Endocrine Society, androgen-level testing is required when hirsutism is severe, or is associated with rapid onset or progression or with any of the following: menstrual irregularity, infertility, central obesity, acanthosis nigricans, or clitoromegaly.[39] Additional testing should include a pregnancy test if amenorrhea is present, DHEAS, thyroid studies, prolactin, pelvic ultrasound, and other evaluation as warranted by additional symptoms (e.g., for Cushing's syndrome).[39]

For most women, reassurance that they have no masculinizing or other serious disease is all that is needed. Some women will ask about cosmetic treatments, and laser hair removal can be recommended if shaving or depilation is not acceptable. Oral contraceptives with a low androgenic profile should be chosen for women who require contraception. If this has limited effect, an antiandrogen medication such as spironolactone can be added after 6 months.[39] Referral to a dermatologist or endocrinologist is indicated at this point.

Bacterial Skin Infections

Bacterial skin infections are most often caused by S. aureus, with which more than one-third of Americans are colonized at any time.[40,41] Surface infections associated with S. aureus range from folliculitis to more complex boils and cellulitis. The rise of methicillin-resistant S. aureus (MRSA) as a cause of skin and soft-tissue infections has paralleled the rise of antibiotic resistance generally in the United States. About 2% of adults are colonized.[40]

Infectious *folliculitis* presents with a nodule or pustule surrounding a hair follicle, generally with complaints of itching or mild pain. In addition to staphylococcal infections, *Pseudomonas* or other bacteria may be involved; other less common causes include viral or fungal infections and ingrown hairs. Predisposing factors include shaving or waxing hairy regions such as the axillae and the pubic area, previous skin damage, and immune suppression. Investigation of causative factors should include use of hot tubs, swimming pools, exposure to chemicals, and the possibility of other causes of dermatitis. Folliculitis is responsive to antibiotic and hygienic measures. Heat and friction should be minimized. Warm or cold compresses offer some relief for the pain and itching. Topical clindamycin 1% cream and mupirocin are acceptable first-line therapies.

Furuncules (boils) develop as a result of the spread of a bacterial infection in the epidermis. The furuncle begins as a small, painful, inflammatory follicular nodule that becomes pustular, develops central necrosis within a few days, and heals after a discharge of necrotic material, often leaving a scar. Predisposing conditions for development of furuncles include chronic staphylococcal carrier state, diabetes mellitus, malnutrition, and HIV infection.[42] *Carbuncles,* a cluster of boils that have enlarged and penetrated the subcutaneous tissue, indicate a more significant infection.

S. aureus is the most common infecting organism. Although Gram stain can be performed, the Infectious Diseases Society of America states that except in severe disease, empiric treatment is appropriate.[43] Inspection of scrapings from the lesion under the microscope with KOH can be done if a fungal cause is suspected.

Incision and drainage (I&D) of purulent lesions is the first-line of therapy for uncomplicated furuncles or carbuncles that do not open and drain spontaneously. MRSA should be considered if local incidence is high or lesions are widespread, recurrent, or resistant to treatment. Oral anti-staphylococcal antibiotics such as clindamycin, dicloxacillin, cephalexin, or trimethoprim-sulfamethoxazole (TMP-SMX) should be used as initial therapy along with I&D if systemic inflammatory response syndrome (SIRS), temperature > 38ºC, tachypnea, tachycardia, or elevated white blood cell count is present.[43] Antibiotics should also be considered for women with immunosuppression. Consultation is warranted at this point. Recurrent lesions warrant I&D, culture, and consideration of mupirocin nasal decolonization.

Cellulitis, a deeper infection with erythema, swelling, and tender, poorly demarcated edges, is associated with poor circulation and conditions that predispose to poor healing. Cellulitis also develops frequently near surgical wounds or trauma sites. Other dermatoses, such as athlete's foot or stasis dermatitis, may provide the entry for infection.

The lower extremities are most at risk. If the leg is affected, elevation improves circulation to the area. Pain can be alleviated somewhat with Burrow's solution compresses. Cellulitis is managed based on presence or absence of SIRS, but in every case involves infectious disease consultation. When no additional symptoms are present, oral antibiotics effective against both *Staphylococcus* and *Streptococcus* species are appropriate. Otherwise, hospital evaluation for parenteral therapy is indicated.[43] Skin sloughing, tissue anesthesia, bullae, or any other additional symptoms also warrant emergent referral.

Impetigo

Impetigo occurs most commonly in small children; in adults, it is often a secondary infection. *S. aureus* and *Streptococcus pyogenes* are the most common infectious agents. Predisposing factors include warm ambient temperature; humidity; presence of another skin disease, especially atopic dermatitis; prior antibiotic therapy; poor hygiene; crowded living conditions; and neglected minor skin trauma. Transient superficial small vesicles or pustules rupture and result in erosions, which in turn become crusted.

The disease is self-limiting, but if not treated may be of long duration. Topical therapy with mupirocin or fusidic acid is equally or more effective than oral antibiotics.[44] Oral antibiotics are administered for widespread infection. TMP-SMX, amoxicillin-clavulanic acid, dicloxacillin, cephalexin, minocycline, and tetracycline are among the antibiotics used for 7-day therapy.[45]

Erythrasma Intertrigo

Obese women, those with pendulous breasts, serious athletes, and others may have chronic chafing and inflammation in intertriginous areas. Deep body folds are less able to dry out with perspiration. Erythrasma intertrigo is a chronic bacterial infection caused by *Corynebacterium minutissimum* that can happen when intertrigo (inflammation of the tissue folds) is present. This microbe is part of the normal skin flora that can cause superficial infection under circumstances such as diabetes, increased humidity, and prolonged periods of occlusion or maceration. In appearance, brownish macules spread and run together.[46] It is often mistaken for a widespread fungal infection, but the KOH prep will be negative.

Treatment is with topical or oral antibiotics. When group A beta-hemolytic *Streptococcus* is implicated, topical or oral therapy can be combined with a low-potency topical steroid.[46] Of note, there is no good evidence for preventive or treatment measures for the underlying chafing, beyond hygiene measures and weight loss.[47]

Fungal Infections

TINEA CORPORIS

Tinea corporis (ringworm) is a superficial dermatophyte that appears on the body other than the palms and soles, genital area, and scalp, favoring intertriginous areas. Fungal genera that cause tinea corporis include *Trichophyton, Microsporum,* and *Epidermophyton;* the most common source is *T. rubrum.* The incubation period can be from days to months.

Initial presentation is as a scaling, erythematous plaque. Central clearing follows as the plaque enlarges, causing annular lesions. At the margins, papules, pustules, and vesicular lesions may be noted in a generally raised edge. Lesions range widely in size and are sharply marginated. Pruritus is common in early infection. Individuals may contract the infection from other people, animal or environmental sources, or may self-inoculate from a distant lesion.

The differential includes other dermatoses such as tinea versicolor and candidiasis, psoriasis, pityriasis rosea, eczema, seborrhea, and other rashes. Diagnosis may be made on the basis of appearance and confirmed by scraping and KOH preparation on a slide. If the appearance is atypical or KOH is negative but the appearance suggests tinea infection, a fungal culture can be sent.[48]

Superficial lesions respond to antifungal creams (terbinafine [Lamisil] and butenafine [Lotrimin Ultra]) applied twice daily for a minimum of 2 weeks, and at least 1 week following resolution of the lesions. Tinea pedis (athlete's foot) is caused by the same organisms and is treated in the same way. Extensive lesions or those resistant to therapy require oral therapy including terbinafine or griseofulvin and should be treated by a dermatologist.[48]

PITYRIASIS VERSICOLOR

Pityriasis versicolor (PV) is a chronic benign dermatosis caused by the lipophilic yeasts *Malassezia* species. The organism is part of the normal skin flora but is opportunistic in the right circumstances. Excess heat and humidity, perspiration, and oily skin can be predisposing factors. It is often seen in adolescence or young adulthood, a time with high sebaceous activity, but persists into adulthood for many susceptible individuals. It is particularly common in individuals exposed to high humidity, such as those residing in subtropical or tropical zones. Circumstances that may lower the skin's resistance to this organism and allow for its overgrowth include pregnancy, malnutrition, corticosteroid therapy, immunosuppression, and hormonal contraception.

The lesions present as small, circular patches on the upper trunk, often in the intertriginous area below or between the breasts. They may be hypo- or hyperpigmented depending on the underlying skin tone (see **Color Plate 1**). Clinical findings can be confirmed by positive KOH preparation.

The greatest concern for women who have PV is cosmetic, because of the blotchy pigmentation. Tissue with resolved PV lesions will not tan until the superficial cells are replaced. Topical agents used in treatment include selenium sulfide (2.5%) lotion or shampoo applied daily for 10 to 15 minutes, followed by a shower, for 1 week. Alternately, azole creams (ketoconazole, econazole, miconazole, clotrimazole) can be applied twice a day for 2 weeks, and at least 1 week following resolution. Systemic agents such as oral ketoconazole are off label for use for PV, so if topical agents are not successful, referral to a

Table 24-7 Antifungal Agents

Generic Name	Brand Name	Uses
Miconazole	Monistat, Monistat-Derm	*Candida*
Clotrimazole	Lotrimin, Mycelex	*Candida*
Fluconazole	Diflucan	*Candida*
Griseofulvin	Grisfulvin V; Gris-PEG	Tinea
Ketoconazole	Nizoral	Tinea, *Candida*; drink citrus or cranberry juice for better absorption
Terbinafine	Lamisil	Onychomycosis
Nystatin	Nilstat	*Candida*
Itraconazole	Sporanox	Onychomycosis
Clotrimazole and betamethasone dipropionate	Lotrisone	Antifungal with potent topical steroid for inflamed fungal infections (short duration only)
Nystatin and Triamcinolone topical	Mycolog II	Antifungal with medium potency steroid (short duration only)

dermatologist is recommended. **Table 24-7** lists antifungal agents.

ONYCHOMYCOSIS

Onchyomycosis is a fungal infection of the nail that occurs in about 10% of young adults, rising to a prevalence of 50% among the elderly.[49] It is a dominant cause of nail damage and discoloration. The primary pathogens are dermatophytes from genus *Trichophyton*. Candidal species may also cause onychomycosis, although in these cases it is usually found on the fingernails rather than toenails in immunocompetent persons.

Damage can range from cracking along the edge or superficial flaking to total disruption and destruction of the nail.[50] Separation of the nail from the underlying nail bed, debris under the nail, thickening, flaking, and changes in color are indicative of onychomycosis. The differential

diagnosis for onychomycosis includes chronic nail trauma, dermatitis, lichen planus, psoriasis of the nails, melanoma, and other less common conditions.[51]

Diagnosis is made by clinical evaluation, microscopic KOH preparation, and examination for hyphae, and it is confirmed by culture or polymerase chain reaction. Because microscopic evaluation for onychomycosis requires multiple specimens that are often obtained by drilling into the nail, this procedure may best be performed by an experienced clinician.

Onychomycosis will not resolve spontaneously. The nail is formed from keratin, which is avascular and absorbs topical agents poorly. Treatment will last for weeks or months, and a clinical cure (80–100% improvement in appearance) may take up to a year, depending on the extent of damage. Medications include ciclopirox (nail lacquer applied daily, left in place without washing for 8 hours, removed weekly, with the nails kept trimmed), oral fluconazole (Diflucan), itraconazole (Sporanox), and terbinafine (Lamisil). Nail debridement may also be required on a regular basis during treatment. None of these medications is guaranteed to produce a complete mycotic cure; the success rate for the most effective medication (terbinafine) is only 76%.[50] Other therapies, including laser treatment, have been tried with varying success.

Because of the possibility of misdiagnosis on clinical examination and the need for prolonged treatment, as well as the possibility of significant side effects including liver damage, gastrointestinal distress, rash, prolonged QT interval, and Stevens-Johnson syndrome,[50] treatment by an experienced clinician is recommended.

Viral Infections

CUTANEOUS HUMAN PAPILLOMAVIRUS

More than 100 strains of human papillomavirus (HPV) exist, each with its preferred tissue location for development of disease. Common warts, flat warts, and deep plantar warts each develop from multiple different strains. Transmission can be by autoinoculation, transmission between individuals, or through environmental exposure. Viral particles penetrate and infect the basal skin layer and rise to the surface as keratinocytes mature. Viral multiplication in the surface lesion and subsequent shedding facilitate transmission to new hosts.

The prevalence of cutaneous warts rises through childhood, peaking at around 8% at age 10 and plateauing at around 4% during adolescence. Non-Hispanic whites have higher rates of cutaneous HPV, as do those with higher educational levels and household incomes. There is no gender difference in prevalence.[52]

Common warts make up about 70% of cutaneous warts.[53] Common warts appear most frequently on the extremities, especially hands and knees, but can be found anywhere on the body. They are hyperkeratotic lesions that can grow to sizes larger than 1 cm in diameter. Flat (plane) warts occur in 4% of patients with warts.[54] They are either flat or slightly raised, often smooth or only minimally hyperkeratotic. Although individually smaller than 1 cm, they may cluster or grow together to form a larger mass, usually on the hands, face, or lower leg. Deep plantar warts (Myrmecia) form from a small papule and develop into a hyperkeratotic nodule. They penetrate deep into the skin layers, causing pain, because they are commonly found on weight-bearing surfaces of the foot or under the nails.

Diagnosis is generally clinical, based on appearance and location. If the appearance is atypical, consideration should be given to alternative causes of skin lesions. The differential diagnoses for warts include actinic keratosis (a premalignant condition), skin cancers, lichen planus, molluscum contagiosum, and other skin diseases.

Many warts resolve spontaneously. It is possible to simply advise women to wait for resolution, without harmful effect.[55] None of the therapies available provides a complete and permanent cure. The choice should be based on location, size, number, patient comorbidities, and age.[56] Personal discomfort with the appearance or physical pain or irritation based on location may also indicate the need to treat. Salicylic acid is a fairly effective OTC keratinolytic treatment that is safe for home use.[57] It can be applied to the affected area after soaking and filing down the hypertrophied tissue every day, or every other day if a patch is used, for up to 12 weeks. Common side effects include redness, irritation, and pain.[55] Cryotherapy can be used in office, but may cause scarring. Both of these modalities have 50–70% success at treating warts. Numerous other treatment are available upon referral to the dermatologist, although improved outcomes cannot be guaranteed.[55,57]

HERPES ZOSTER

Herpes zoster (shingles) is the reactivation of latent varicella zoster virus, which has lain dormant along basal root ganglia. Only those who have had wild-type varicella (chickenpox infection) are at risk; however, this includes more than 95% of those over 40 in the United States, one-third of whom will have an outbreak.[58] Childhood vaccination programs probably protect those who were vaccinated from future shingles, but do not appear to affect incidence among older adults who were not vaccinated as children.[59] About 68% of zoster cases occur in persons aged 50 years or older, affecting 1% of those older than 60 annually, at a rate of 1 million cases per year.[57,60] According to the Centers for Disease Control and Prevention (CDC), some data suggest that herpes zoster is more common among women and Caucasians; anyone who is immunocompromised has increased risk.[58, 61]

Most individuals have only one occurrence, although multiple recurrences are possible.[58] The lesions appear along a single dermatome or may cluster along 2 or more in fewer than 20% of cases. However, in every case they are limited to the pattern of those dermatomes, and they do not usually cross the midline, which can be used in making the diagnosis. Disseminated zoster, with three or more dermatomes affected, occurs primarily in individuals who are immunosuppressed.[58] At this point, it may be difficult to distinguish from an initial varicella infection.

Pre-eruptive tenderness, hyperesthesia, pain, itching, or burning in only one dermatome may appear as a prodrome; constitutional symptoms including fever, malaise, and headache may also occur prior to the rash. When lesions occur, small red papules will resolve into clusters of clear vesicles (see **Color Plate 2**). As with the initial chickenpox episode, these will continue to develop over several days, crust, and dry over a 2- to 4-week period. During the period when vesicles are present, before drying occurs, the patient is infectious. Individuals who have never had chickenpox or have not been vaccinated are at risk of developing a primary varicella infection upon exposure to the lesions.[58]

Postherpetic neuralgia (PHN), which affects 10–18% of persons with shingles, is a disabling pain syndrome that can last months or even years; there is no consistently effective treatment for PHN.[60] Symptoms include intractable pain, sensitivity to touch, and itching. Administration of corticosteroids during the acute event may help reduce the incidence of PHN.[62] Home treatment with topical analgesics or anesthetics or capsaicin cream may help with pain management. More intensive therapy should be directed by a clinician with experience in pain management.

Perhaps the most effective intervention is prevention. The Advisory Committee on Immunization Practices (ACIP) recommendation is to administer the Zostavax vaccine at or after age 60.[63] The vaccine is FDA approved for those over 50. However, the long-term efficacy of the vaccine is unknown, given that immunity wanes over time. For that reason, the ACIP has not lowered the recommended age.

PITYRIASIS ROSEA

Pityriasis rosea is a benign, self-limited *exanthem* (a widespread rash) of unknown etiology that is suspected to be the result of reactivation of one of the human herpes viruses.[64] It has a distinctive morphology and runs a characteristic course. The first clinical manifestation is a herald patch, a solitary annular lesion from 2 to 10 cm across that appears anywhere on the body, but usually on the trunk or upper arms. Within 10 to 14 days, a papulosquamous rash spreads across the trunk and extremities. Apart from the herald patch, the eruption is symmetrically oriented along lines of skin cleavage. The rash lasts for 2 to 12 weeks, and post-inflammatory hyper- or hypopigmentation may last for many months. As many as half of those affected experience moderate to severe itching.[65]

The diagnosis of pityriasis rosea is made clinically. The differential diagnosis includes tinea corporis, nummular eczema—when only the herald patch is present, and secondary syphilis. Treatment is symptomatic: Patients who are pruritic may benefit from emollients, mild topical corticosteroids, and antipruritic medications. A Cochrane review reported that no treatments had adequately demonstrated efficacy.[65] Women with suspected pityriasis should also be tested for syphilis.

Other Skin Infections

PHTHIRUS PUBIS

Phthirus pubis (crab lice) is an insect infestation of hair-bearing regions. The crab louse is found only in humans and is transmitted sexually. The lifecycle from nit (egg) to nymph (immature louse) to adult lasts 3 to 4 weeks. Adult lice can survive for less than 48 hours without feeding on human blood, so transmission from objects (e.g., clothing, bed linens) is uncommon. Most commonly found in the genital area, the lice and their eggs can be found on other coarse hairs including leg and axillary hair, eyebrows, and eyelashes.[66] One summary of world data gives an incidence of approximately 2% of the adult population.[67]

On physical examination, the nits are firmly attached to the hair in the pubic or anal regions, and the small (< 0.2 cm) adult lice can be seen (**Figure 24-3**). Use of a magnifying glass and direct light may be required to confirm diagnosis. The adult insects have a pronounced crab-like appearance, giving them their common name.

The recommended treatment includes permethrin 1% cream rinse applied to affected areas and washed off after 10 minutes, or pyrethrins with piperonyl butoxide applied to the affected area and washed off after 10 minutes. Both of these are safe for pregnancy and lactation. The CDC's sexually transmitted disease (STD) treatment

Figure 24-3 Crab louse.

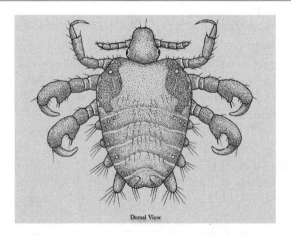

Dorsal View

guidelines should be accessed for the most current treatment recommendations.[68] Treatment can be repeated in 1 week. All bed linens, clothing, and fabric furniture should be decontaminated. All sexual partners for the last month also require treatment.[68]

Because phthisis pubis has a preference for the genital area and is spread almost exclusively through sexual content, the presence of pubic lice on the eyelashes or eyebrows of children should initiate an evaluation for possible sexual abuse.[66]

SCABIES

Scabies is an infestation by the mite *Sarcoptes scabiei*. The lifecycle is 1 to 2 months in 4 stages from egg to larva to nymph to adult. Adult female mites burrow into the skin, often between fingers and toes or along contact lines for clothing (e.g., bra lines or belt area) and lay eggs there. Transmission is typically sexual among adults. Prolonged skin-to-skin contact is generally required. Fomite transmission is unusual, but nonsexual contact in crowded homes or communities can provide the needed conditions for transmission.[69]

On first infection, initial symptoms, caused by allergic response to the mites and waste products, may take 2 to 6 weeks to develop. Recurrent infection produces symptoms within the first week, as the body is already sensitized. It is manifested by severe, intractable pruritus and a red papular rash. Itching is commonly worst at night. The burrows may be seen as a serpiginous track that is grayish white or skin colored. Commonly found in the webbing between the fingers, on the wrists, or sides of hands or feet, it can also be found in skin folds, the genital area, and in warm intertriginous regions. Scabies should be considered whenever any generalized pruritic eruption does not respond to topical corticosteroids or oral prednisone.

Scabies is usually treated topically with permethrin cream 5% (Elimite, Acticin) applied overnight for 8 to 14 hours. It is applied to the entire skin surface below the neck, including under the fingernails, toenails, and in the umbilicus. Treatment should be repeated in 1 week. Oral ivermectin is an alternative treatment. The CDC STD guidelines should be accessed for the most current treatment recommendations.[68] Ivermectin is probably safe for use in pregnancy and lactation, but permethrin 5% is preferred.[68]

All sexual partners need evaluation for infestation, as do any others in the home environment. The home and the examining room need to be cleaned thoroughly, and all clothing and bedding should be washed and dried by machine. Stuffed animals or other unwashable material should be kept away from contact with humans for 72 hours; storage in a sealed black garbage bag is suitable. Insecticides, fumigation, and extermination are not necessary.[68]

Crusted, or Norwegian, scabies is a severe, aggressive form of the infection, found most commonly in immunocompromised individuals. Crusting occurs because the mites multiply rapidly in the absence of a strong immune response. The infection is more easily transmitted due to the high parasite load and flaking off of the crusted material. Immediate treatment with a combination of topical and oral agents and referral for further evaluation of the woman's health are essential.[69]

LYME DISEASE

Lyme disease is caused by the spirochete *Borrelia burgdorferi*, a bacterial parasite of the black-legged tick (often called deer tick). Within the United States, the infection is most prevalent in the Northeast, upper Midwest, and Mid-Atlantic, with 14 states having 95% of the disease burden. The range is slowly spreading west and south; some cases have been identified along the Pacific coast.[70] More than 30,000 confirmed and probable cases were reported in 2014.[71] In its initial phase, Lyme disease is a localized skin eruption. Incubation lasts 3–30 days, followed by an initial localized stage with a small red papule expanding to an annular or erythematous patch in up to 80% of affected individuals, lymphadenopathy, and possible flulike symptoms (see **Color Plate 4**). The appearance of the erythema migrans patch is significantly associated with diagnosis of Lyme, but is not required. When it is seen, diagnosis may be made by clinical inspection, but antibody titers are not reliably positive until 4–6 weeks after exposure.[72] The disease becomes disseminated, initially with symptoms that include multiple secondary annular rashes, flulike symptoms, and lymphadenopathy as well as transient arthritis and mild hepatitis. Left untreated, the progress of disseminated Lyme includes rheumatologic, cardiac, and neurologic complications. Post-treatment, some individuals continue to experience symptoms such as fatigue, memory loss, myalgia, or arthritis.[70]

Laboratory findings include elevated transaminase levels and erythrocyte sedimentation rate, microscopic hematuria, and proteinuria. Diagnosis is by antibody testing; the CDC recommends two-stage testing with an enzyme immunoassay (EIA) or indirect immunofluorescence assay (IFA) followed by IgG/IgM Western blot.[70]

Adults with early Lyme disease who do not have cardiac or neurologic symptoms should be treated with 14–21 days of doxycycline 100 mg twice a day, amoxicillin 500 mg 3 times a day, or cefuroxime axetil (Ceftin) 500 mg twice a day.[73] IgG may persist for years if a strong immune response was initially developed; this is not evidence of persistent infection. Although retreatment may occasionally be required, prolonged antibiotic therapy carries greater risks than benefits when Lyme disease is diagnosed during the localized or early disseminated phases.[70]

Prophylaxis of Lyme disease may be offered only when *all* of the following can be verified:

- An *Ixodes scapularis* tick is found that is reliably estimated to have been attached for > 36 hours.
- Prophylaxis can be started within 72 hours of removing the tick.

- The local rate of *I. scapularis* infection with *B. burgdorferi* is ≥ 20%.
- Doxycycline treatment is not contraindicated.[73]

There is disagreement in the literature as to the existence, prevalence, and appropriate management of a chronic Lyme syndrome in treated individuals, separate from the possible damage caused by untreated infection.[70,72,74] A physician experienced in infectious disease should manage the treatment of Lyme disease.

Disorders of Blood Vessels

CHERRY ANGIOMA

These are common, asymptomatic, benign vascular lesions. Bright red to violaceous in color, these domed lesions form from capillaries and post-capillary venules that are dilated. They are non-bleaching lesions (i.e., they do not turn pale when compressed). They develop in up to 50% of adults, increase in number with age, and are most commonly found on the trunk, although they may develop at any location. They may first appear in pregnancy and in patients with elevated prolactin levels or as a result of exposure to chemicals.[75,76] Sudden occurrence of these lesions may be associated with occult malignancy; in this situation, the woman should be referred to dermatology.

ANGIOKERATOMA

Angiokeratomas appear as asymptomatic, deep red to maroon or blue to black sharply defined, 0.5- to 1.0-cm papules. Over time they darken and develop a rough or scaly surface. They will bleed if they are abraded. Although they are more common in men than in women, lesions may occur on the vulva in middle and later life and persist indefinitely.[77] They may occur in younger women on oral contraceptives or during pregnancy, possibly because of increased venous pressure. Because they may overlap with malignant lesions in appearance, biopsy may be needed to make the diagnosis.

SPIDER ANGIOMA

These lesions are common, asymptomatic arteriolar papules with a distinct clinical appearance. They result from dilation of a previously existing blood vessel, and most commonly are found on the face, neck, and upper trunk. They are found in 10% to 15% of adults and are also common in young children.[78] They often increase in number in pregnancy and during oral contraceptive use, in which case they may resolve or decrease in prominence after childbirth or cessation of contraception. Thyrotoxicosis and chronic liver disease are also associated with development of spider angiomas.[78] They are regarded as a clinical symptom of hepatitis C[79] and are linked to cirrhosis and liver failure. For this reason, even when pregnancy or oral contraception is the most likely explanation, a careful history for alcohol abuse and evaluation of liver function are warranted when new spider nevi are found on clinical examination.

Pigment Disorders

VITILIGO

Vitiligo is a progressive depigmentation of the skin from loss of melanocytes. It occurs in less than 1% of the world population. All races and both sexes are equally affected, although those with darker skin have more noticeable effects. Average age of onset is in the 20s.[80] Patches can appear anywhere on the body, including on mucous tissue, and may be associated with graying hair in the affected area.

Vitiligo has a genetic predisposition and is considered to have features of autoimmune disease, although whether the pigment loss is cytokine mediated or from direct destruction of melanocytes is unknown. When older women develop new-onset vitiligo, consideration should be given to the presence of other comorbidities, such as thyroid dysfunction, rheumatoid arthritis, diabetes mellitus, and alopecia areata.[81] Other conditions that have been associated include adrenocortical insufficiency and pernicious anemia.[80]

The umbrella descriptors are segmental (limited to one side of the body) and non-segmental (including a variety of patterns that are bilateral), also called simply vitiligo. When vitiligo appears as a localized focus, it typically will progress to 1 of the primary categories over 1 to 2 years, after which if there is no change it is classified as focal vitiligo.[82] Mixed types may appear. The classification matters, because true segmental vitiligo progresses rapidly in the first 2 years and then usually remains stable; it also has increased hair follicle involvement.[82]

Diagnosis is made by clinical examination of white tissue patches that may appear in many patterns. Biopsy can confirm the diagnosis.

Treatment focuses on decreasing the distinction between normal and depigmented skin. The best evidence for short-term efficacy, according to a Cochrane review, is for corticosteroids plus UV light therapy.[83]

In early-stage vitiligo, topical corticosteroids may promote repigmentation, but their use is best for small lesions and is limited to short-term use, due to the risk of striae and skin atrophy with chronic use. Sunscreens with a sun protection factor (SPF) of 30 or higher can be recommended to protect the macules and to prevent tanning of the normal skin. This limits the contrast between normal skin and depigmented skin. Cosmetics can be used to mask the discrepancy in skin color.

An additional consideration is the psychological burden of changed appearance. Vitiligo is associated with psychiatric comorbidities and diminished quality of life.[81] Counseling should be recommended to women who express distress or concern about how they will deal with the change in their appearance.

A variety of other light therapies and chemical depigmentation of normal skin are recommended, as may surgical procedures. These are managed by an experienced clinician, with consideration of patient tolerance and preference.

SOLAR LENTIGO

Solar lintingnes are < 3 cm, yellow to brown hyperpigmented, well circumscribed lesions on sun-exposed surfaces of the skin. Whites and Asians with skin types that freckle (see section on skin types later in this chapter) are more likely to develop lentigines.[84] These lesions do not darken in response to sun exposure as freckles do. They develop in response to actinic damage and increase in number with age.

Prevention is the easiest treatment. Use of sunscreens and avoidance of sunburn can prevent or diminish the development of these lesions. Therapies for those who want to reduce the appearance of lentigines include topical hydroquinone, mequinol/tretinoin, and retinoids such as tazarotene and adapalene. All of these may produce side effects. Skin discoloration and sensitivity are associated with hydroquinone; inflammation, skin dryness, and sensitivity are associated with tretinoin and the retinoids. Other therapies include chemical peels, cryotherapy, and laser therapy.[84,85] None of these give ideal results. Women should discuss how to manage solar lentigines with an experienced clinician before deciding whether to treat for cosmetic improvement.

When lentigines display rapid growth, have associated pain or itching, bleed when abraded, are atypical in appearance, or have a keratotic surface, they should be biopsied to distinguish these lesions from skin cancers.[84]

ACANTHOSIS NIGRICANS

Acanthosis nigricans is a skin condition characterized by thick, darkened velvety patches found most commonly in skin folds and around the neck. Prevalence is highest among Native Americans and African Americans.[86] The strongest associations are insulin resistance, diabetes, and obesity.[87]

A large, multisite study found higher rates among minorities in a population where the condition was common across the lifespan and highly associated with risk factors for diabetes.[88] In gynecologic practice, acanthosis nigricans is important because it can be a marker for PCOS, hyperinsulinemia, and insulin resistance in women with obesity.[87] When observed, women should receive dietary and exercise education to support weight loss and be screened for metabolic syndrome and diabetes. Women who wish to explore potential medical therapy can be referred; topical retinoids may offer some benefit.[86]

Benign Skin Tumors and Conditions

ACROCHORDON

Skin tags are common, benign pedunculated lesions that are either skin colored or hyperpigmented. Skin tags occur in about 25% of the population, increasing in incidence with age and obesity.[75,89] They vary in size from 1 mm to 10 mm and occasionally become several centimeters in diameter. Most common locations include the neck and intertriginous areas. Friction against clothing may promote their development. When multiple tags are present, they may represent an increased risk of diabetes, abnormal lipid metabolism, liver abnormalities, and hypertension.[90,91]

Skin tags may be removed for cosmetic reasons, or because they are causing further irritation. Small lesions can be ligated or trimmed with scissors in the office, using a topical anesthetic for excision. Smaller lesions can be removed with cryotherapy or shave excision.[75] If the diagnosis is unclear based on an atypical appearance, the acrochordon should be seen by a dermatologist before being removed.

DERMATOFIBROMA

Dermatofibromas are small (usually < 1 cm), button-like nodules most commonly found on the legs. They are now considered to represent true neoplasms, but have previously been thought of as sequelae of minor trauma such as shaving or insect bites. They are important in that they can be misdiagnosed instead of a malignancy. Dermatofibromas vary widely in color. Dermatofibromas are fixed in the skin but can be moved over the underlying subcutaneous fat. One characteristic that helps to confirm a diagnosis is Fitzpatrick's sign—retraction and dimpling when compressed. The lesions may remain stable for many years, and some regress. No intervention is indicated, unless there is a suspicion of malignancy, in which case a punch or excisional biopsy is required.[75]

Melanocytic Nevus (Mole)

Benign moles are persistent, sharply circumcised lesions. Their appearance varies with the tissue type from which they arise. Melanocytic moles are macular or papular, soft, tan to black lesions, typically less than 5 mm in diameter. Most are seen at birth or develop during childhood and adolescence. Having multiple moles is not uncommon; many individuals will develop up to 40 nevi. Most moles are found on the upper body. Large moles, those with mottled or unusual coloration, and those that are rapidly growing may indicate a risk for melanoma and should be evaluated promptly.[92]

Syringoma

Syringomas are benign adenomas (a benign epithelial structure usually arranged like a gland) of the intraepidermal eccrine ducts. There may be a familial tendency. Syringomas occur most frequently in women, beginning at puberty. They are 1- to 2-mm, firm, skin-colored or yellow papules; most often they appear as multiple papules around the eyes but are also found on the labia. The papules are asymptomatic, stable in size, and persistent. If the lesions are considered disfiguring, they can be removed with electrosurgery.

Seborrheic Keratosis

Seborrheic keratoses (SK) are persistent, benign lesions of variable appearance (See **Color Plate 5**). There is no gender or racial preference; the incidence increases with age. These are among the most common skin tumors seen by dermatologists, affecting about 83 million individuals in the United States. Lesions may be found anywhere on the body, most commonly in the presternal area, and can be single or multiple.

Initially, the appearance is of a small, hyperkeratotic macule. Over time, SK lesions enlarge, thicken, and become hyperpigmented.[93] The surface is typically waxy in texture and roughened or wartlike in appearance. They appear to be "stuck" onto the skin, rather than contiguous with surrounding tissue. Most are less than 3 cm in size when fully developed. The color of the lesions varies, but most are tan to black. *Dermatosis papulosa nigra* describes seborrheic dermatoses most commonly found in individuals with darker skin tones. These lesions are 1- to 2-mm, dark-brown keratotic papules concentrated around the eyes and on the cheeks.[75]

Treatment with cryotherapy, curettage, or excision is usually for cosmetic reasons or because of irritation, such as when the lesion is abraded by clothing.[93] SK can be confused with melanoma. Both vary in color and size and may be irregular in shape. For this reason, if the diagnosis is not clear, an excisional biopsy should be performed.[75] When in doubt, the woman's health clinician can always refer the woman to a dermatologist for evaluation.

Keloids

Keloids are hypertrophic scars that extend beyond the initial incision or wound. They form as a result of abnormal collagen production and breakdown of the healing process. Unlike typically hypertrophic scars, they tend to develop more slowly and over a longer time, are more common on the upper body, do not regress with healing, and persist after removal or revision.[94] They are more common in Africans, Asians, and Hispanics. Development is most common between the ages of 10 and 30 years.[95] In appearance, keloids have a smooth or ropy surface and are of irregular shape. Apart from the cosmetic concerns, complaints may include pruritus, pain, and sensitivity to touch.[94]

Prevention requires that the individual prone to developing keloids avoid skin trauma from piercing or tattoos; vaccination, acne, burns, injuries, and surgical procedures all may promote keloid growth. When skin trauma occurs, promoting wound healing and decreasing tension on the site, while avoiding stretching, may help reduce keloid development.

When surgery is planned, women should discuss with their surgeon what precautions can be taken to reduce risk. Therapies for keloid are best applied before the development of scar tissue. These may include silicone gel sheeting applied after the procedure to reduce traction, intralesional injections of corticosteroids or fluorouracil, or application of imiquimod. Pulsed dye laser may be used. Therapies used to reduce keloid size later include excision or cryotherapy with injected corticosteroids. Unfortunately, all methods have significant side effects, and surgical removal can lead to regrowth in more than 50% of cases.[94-96]

EPIDERMOID (INCLUSION) CYSTS

An epidermoid cyst is a firm, mobile, subcutaneous cyst originating from true epidermis, most often from a hair follicle. They are most common on the head and upper body. These lesions are formed by a cystic enclosure of epithelium within the dermis that becomes filled with keratin and lipid-rich debris. They grow slowly and may persist indefinitely; they may be subject to external trauma and rupture because of their thin walls. Inflammation after rupture of an epidermal cyst can be misdiagnosed as an infection. Symptomatic or recurrent cysts can be removed.

Asymptomatic cysts occurring anywhere other than the face need no attention.[75]

Brittle Nails

Nail disorders, ranging from infections to brittle or cracking nails, make up 10% of dermatologic complaints.[97] The most common cause of brittle nails is dehydration of the nail plate, usually from exposure to damaging agents. Common causes include acetone, alkaline liquids, organic solvents, and frequent hand washing.[98] Direct trauma to the nail plate, nail biting, typing, playing a musical instrument, or using the nail as a tool to pry or scrape can lead to trauma, which can lead to dehydration. Frequent hand washing causes the nail plate to expand and contract repeatedly as the nail absorbs and loses water, which places a strain on the protein structures and onychocyte bridges, and results in weakening and destruction of the protein links between the cells that comprise the nail.[98] As a consequence, the nail loses its ability to retain water and becomes brittle and susceptible to splitting, cracking, and peeling. Brittleness occurs because of a loss of flexibility.

Poor nutrition can cause brittle nails, so eating disorders should be considered along with vitamin deficiencies when evaluating this condition.[96] Brittle nails are also associated with aging. Atherosclerosis of small arteries decreases blood flow to the nail matrix and can reduce growth and flexibility.[99] The nails thicken and develop longitudinal ridges that contribute to brittleness.

Proper nail care helps to maintain nail health.[97] Suggestions to help with brittle nails include regular trimming to avoid direct trauma. This should be done after bathing when the nails are soft. Filing after trimming keeps the edges smooth, and buffing gently keeps the surfaces smooth. Wearing gloves to avoid precipitating factors such as exposure to chemicals and soaps will help. Avoiding all contact with water is impossible, but the nails and the periungual skin should be moisturized several times a day and after each hand washing.

For extreme problems, a nightly routine may be suggested. Soaking the hands (or feet) for 20 minutes in lukewarm water, followed by application of a moisturizer and covering with white cotton gloves is effective in treating brittle and splitting nails.[98] Applying nail enamel that does not contain formaldehyde and toluene may improve nails, but the polish should not be removed more frequently than once weekly. There is no evidence that vitamin supplementation with vitamins A, C, or E; retinoids; retinol; silicon; zinc; iron; copper; selenium; calcium; or vitamin B_{12} (cyanocobalamin) will improve nail quality, absent a specific dietary deficiency, nor will they resolve the effects of underlying disease.[98,100,101] Brittle nail syndrome appears to abate with supplementation with a 2.5-mg dose of biotin daily or a 10-mg dose of silicon daily.[101]

The Skin and Aging

Many of the visible signs of aging occur in the skin. Eighty percent of aging appearance is caused by UV exposure. Other contributors are smoking, nutrition, stress, and illness.[102] Changes due to sun exposure are termed *dermatoheliosis* or *photoaging*. Photoaging caused by UV light is apparent by the age of 40 and produces coarse and fine wrinkles, uneven and blotchy skin pigmentation, freckles, and distinct solar lentigines.[103] Telangiectasias may also be attributed to sun damage. Dilated sebaceous glands may produce persistent lesions known as solar comedones that are primarily on the upper cheek and nose. Seborrheic dermatosis and actinic keratosis are also effects of UV exposure over time. Drying skin, thinning of the epidermis, and *ptosis* (sagging, inelastic skin) caused by loss of collagen and elastin in the skin are related to age rather than sun exposure.[104] *Poikiloderma* describes the combination of epidermal atrophy, hyperpigmentation and hypopigmentation, and telangiectasia.

Skin changes are most notable in persons with fair skin. Fitzpatrick Skin photo types are shown in **Table 24-8**. Persons with all skin types can suffer sun-related damage, although it may not be as evident with darker skin tones. Persons of color

Table 24-8 Skin Photo Type (SPT)

SPT Class	Tanning	Descriptors	Constitutive Color	Other Factors
I	Never	Melanocompromised	White	Regardless of hair and eye color, always burns within 30 minutes of exposure
II	Rarely	Melanocompromised	White	Sunburns easily; tans with difficulty
III	Over time	Melanocompetent	White	Some sunburn with short exposures, but over time develop deep tanning
IV	Easily	Melanocompetent	White	Tans easily and never sunburns with short exposures
V	Always—rare burn	Melanocompetent	Brown	Can sunburn with long exposures
VI	Always tans	Melanocompetent	Black	Can sunburn with long exposures

are more likely to have slow-to-develop, deep folds rather than finer wrinkles, and are less at risk for skin cancers.[20]

Sunscreen that has an SPF of 15 blocks 93% of UVB, and an SPF of 45 blocks 97% consistently when properly applied. There is evidence that use of an adequate (SPF 30) sunscreen will prevent skin damage.[103] However, most people use too little sunscreen and reapply too rarely.[105] Individuals may also use products that do not effectively block UVA radiation, since not all commercial sunscreens block both UVB and UVA radiation. Therefore, women should be encouraged to read product labels to ensure that they are purchasing a broad-spectrum sunscreen.

Treatment with topical retinoids reverses some photoaging, causing skin pigmentation to become lighter and more uniform. New collagen and new blood vessels form within the papillary dermis. However, treatment must be continued for effects to remain. Peeling agents can also improve skin texture and appearance. Alpha-hydroxy acids reduce hyperkeratosis and promote epidermal hyperplasia. Laser resurfacing damages the papillary dermis, which causes a thin zone of scar formation (new collagen), effectively reducing wrinkles. These and other therapies should be prescribed by an experienced provider.

Premalignant and Malignant Skin Tumors

Skin cancers are the most common malignancy group in the United States and one of the most easily preventable.[106,107] The incidence is higher than for all other cancers combined.[108] More than 5 million US adults visit a health provider each year for treatment of a skin cancer.[109] The non-melanoma skin cancers (squamous cell carcinoma [SCC] and basal cell carcinoma [BCC]) are both more prevalent than melanoma and less deadly. The American Cancer Society estimate for 2015 was 3.5 million new cases of non-melanoma skin cancer (NMSC) and about 73,000 cases of melanoma.[110] In 2012, there were more than 68,000 cases of melanoma, among which were 28,080 women. Of the 13,000-plus deaths from skin cancer each year, melanoma accounts for more than 75%. Melanoma accounted for more than 3200 deaths in women in 2012.[111]

The primary risk factor for skin cancer is unprotected exposure to UV rays. In addition to sunlight, indoor tanning increases risk. Some worksites further increase risk because of reflected sunlight from light-colored surfaces. Examples include lifeguards, construction workers, and agricultural workers.[112] Fair skin tones, living at high altitude, older age, personal history of blistering sunburns, moles, decreased immunocompetence, family history of skin cancer, and exposure to certain substances or medications increase risk. Toxic substance exposures include arsenic, coal tar, and paraffin. Medications that increase sun sensitivity include thiazides, diuretics, tetracyclines, sulfa antibiotics, and NSAIDs. Use of tanning beds or UV phototherapy treatment also increases risk.

Recurrence rates are high; 50% of those with a NMSC will have a second cancer within 5 years, usually of the same type (BCC or SCC).[113] Risk factors for recurrence of both BCC and SCC include larger size, higher risk location, poorly defined borders, subtype, and other historical factors. High-risk locations include the face, genitals, hands, and feet.[114]

Suspicion of any skin cancer is an indication for prompt referral to a dermatologist. Women with large numbers of nevi (> 50) or enlarging, bleeding, or irregularly colored moles should be referred for a visual full-body scan.

Actinic Keratosis

Actinic keratosis (AK) is a carcinoma in situ precursor to squamous cell carcinoma. In the

Rotterdam Study, a large European cohort, prevalence of AK among women was 26–31%, reflecting the primarily fair-skinned European population.[115] The study's authors noted that data on AK incidence are widely variable, with rates as high as 40–60% reported in some white populations, and much lower rates elsewhere. Extensive areas of sun-damaged skin, advancing age, light pigmentation status, immunosuppression, severe baldness, skin wrinkling, and high tendency for sunburn are significantly associated with extensive actinic damage and risk for progression.[115,116]

AK presents as rough, scaly, ill-defined reddish to reddish-brown macules or papules, often on an erythematous base.[117] The lesions develop on chronically sun-exposed areas such as the face, forearms and hands, and scalp (see **Color Plate 6**). The key to clinical diagnosis is the gritty, sandpaper-like sensation felt when palpating these lesions.[118] Lesions may follow 1 of 3 paths: Some regress spontaneously, some remain stable, and some transform further into squamous cell carcinoma.[119] A Veterans Affairs study reported a 70% regression rate over 4 years and a 2.5% progression to SCC.[120] The same study noted that about two-thirds of all new SCCs and one-third of all new BCCs were found at the site of AK lesions.[120] These lesions are considered to have undergone invasive malignant transformation when they become enlarged and indurated or ulcerated or bleed.

Referral to a dermatologist is indicated when AK is suspected. Diagnosis is made by biopsy or evaluation under fluorescence. Surgical removal, cryotherapy, or topical application of 5-fluorouracil (5-FU), imiquimod cream, ingenol mebutate gel, or diclofenac gel can be used to treat AK.[118]

Basal Cell Carcinoma

BCC is the most common type of skin cancer, accounting for 80–90% of NMSC in women.[109] The association of BCC with UV damage is weaker than for SCC, although childhood exposure is an important risk factor. The tumor may occur at any age, and the incidence of BCC increases markedly after the age of 40.[121]

BCCs are usually slow-growing tumors. Although they rarely metastasize, they may penetrate to muscle or bone underlying the lesion and cause extensive damage.

Lesions are most common on the head, particularly on the nose. About one-third occur in areas of skin with little or no sun exposure.[114,122] Early BCCs are commonly small, translucent, or pearly, and telangiectasia is often present.[114] Pinching or stretching a BCC to blanch it may highlight the pearly quality (see **Color Plate 7**). As the lesion progresses, a smooth, skin-colored indurated (hardened) nodule with a rolled edge will develop. A pigmented BCC may be confused with melanoma, but the BCC usually has a pink or reddish component with a suggestion of waxiness.

Therapy is by surgical excision, Mohs surgery in high-risk lesions, or use of imiquimod, cryotherapy, or 5-fluorouracil; radiotherapy and electrodessication with curettage are also used in select populations. Vismodegib, a Hedgehog-signaling pathway inhibitor that affects cellular signal pathways activated in BCC, is being used in advanced disease.[123,124]

Squamous Cell Carcinoma

SCC accounts for up to 20% of NMSC in women, but is considered more deadly than BCC.[107] Apart from the presence of AK, risk factors include chronic skin injury such as ulcers or sinus tracts, exposure to radiation, immunosuppression, and xeroderma pigmentosa.[125]

SCC lesions are often tender, with an elevated, often scaly pink base peripheral to an overlying crust. Induration may be present (see **Color Plate 8**). They sometimes occur as an indurated keratotic nodule or scale within long-standing scars. Enlargement, thickening, location on or behind the ear, poor histologic differentiation, and development of fibrosis indicate increased risk of metastasis, which occurs in about 1.9–2.6% of cases.[126,127]

Treatment options include surgical excision with margin evaluation, Mohs surgery, radiation, curettage and electrodesiccation, and cryosurgery. Adjuvant therapy may be offered after surgery, but there is little evidence comparing any of the treatment options.[128,129]

Melanoma

More than 28,000 cases of melanoma occurred in US women in 2012; more than 3200 deaths occurred, making this the 7th leading cause of death among women.[111] In 2011, there was an incidence rate in the United States of 15.7 per 100,000 women (20.1 for white women).[111] The estimates continue to climb; over the lifespan, slightly more than 2% of the US population will be diagnosed with melanoma.[130] Those most at risk are fair-skinned individuals with sun or other UV exposure, those with a large number of nevi, and those with dysplastic nevi. Family history increases risk twofold.[131] Overall, men have higher incidence rates, as do whites, although among those under 40 rates in women are almost twice those in men.[132] Invasive melanoma is the 3rd leading cancer of young adults.[132] The surge in melanoma among young women has been linked to indoor tanning.[133,134]

Melanoma is characterized by the uncontrolled growth of melanocytes and can spread to lymph nodes and, by extension, to internal organs.[132] Although there is a 91% 5-year survival rate, early detection is essential; metastatic disease has a 5-year survival rate of 15%.[130,132] Melanoma comprises only 5–6% of all skin cancers, but it accounts for 75% of skin cancer deaths.[135]

Universal screening for skin cancer has been controversial, with the US Preventive Services Task Force finding inadequate evidence for universal screening in 2009.[136] Recently, Weinstock and others have called for a reevaluation of the benefits and risks of screening, based on current evidence that screening specifically for melanoma can reduce mortality.[137]

Dysplastic nevi that may be melanoma precursor lesions are larger and rougher than common moles, irregular in outline, and irregularly pigmented.[131,138] The typical nodular form of melanoma is an elevated brown-black papule or nodule. The superficial spreading form, which has a higher incidence in younger individuals, is a flat, irregularly pigmented macule, patch, or plaque (see **Color Plate 9**). While many lesions are found on the lower legs, the incidence of truncal lesions is becoming more common in young women.[139] The acral-lentiginous melanoma is a flat, spreading lesion found on the soles, palm, or fingers/toes as a variably pigmented tan to brown to black patch or plaques.

While the ABCDE guidelines for recognizing melanoma (**Table 24-9**) are a useful reminder for identifying potential dangerous lesions, there is

Table 24-9 Mnemonic for Malignant Melanoma

A	Asymmetry
B	Border is irregular with irregularly scalloped edges
C	Color is mottled, haphazard colors in various shades of brown, black, blue, gray, red, and white
D	Diameter is large, greater than the tip of a pencil eraser; enlargement in size may be the most important sign
E	Elevation is almost always present with surface distortion; in situ and acral (foot) lesions may be flat

no single criterion that is absolutely indicative of whether a lesion is benign or malignant. A high index of suspicion should be maintained for any pigmented lesion, particularly those that are new or have changed. As women's health exam offers more opportunities than most primary care visits to see large areas of the skin, given the nature of the examination. All clinicians should be not only familiar with the lesion characteristics that are most concerning for melanoma, but also the history and current findings that suggest a changing lesion.

Prevention and Education

Prevention is the most important aspect of primary care for melanoma and NMSC. The annual gynecology exam and obstetric visits are opportunities for teaching women ways to minimize their, and their families', risks. Simple measures such as avoiding UV rays, especially in childhood and adolescence, and between the hours of 10:00 am and 4:00 pm at any age, and wearing tightly woven clothing and hats can be protective. Such points should be made to young women in their childbearing years and are just as important as other health messages, such as the benefit of avoiding exposure to smoke for young children, the need for all children to use car seats and seat belts, and similar topics.

Physiologic Changes of Pregnancy

Skin, hair, and nail changes are common in pregnancy. Sebaceous gland secretions increase, as does sweat gland function. Vascular dilation occurs as fluid circulation increases, making blood vessels more visible. Small vascular lesions such as spider angiomas or cherry angiomas may increase in number and become more prominent. Varicosities of the vulva and legs may develop or be exacerbated by the pressure exerted on venous return by the growing uterus. Mucous membranes become more vascularized in pregnancy. Gingivitis, nosebleeds, and postcoital spotting are common as a result of these changes.

Localized or generalized hyperpigmentation occurs to some extent in 90% of pregnant women. Such lesions are apt to be more pronounced in darker skinned individuals but are noticeable in light-skinned women as well.[140] The most commonly seen change is darkening of the line between the umbilicus and the symphysis pubis, the *linea nigra*. It often occurs several months into the first pregnancy and earlier in subsequent pregnancies. Darkening of the nipples, areolas, the external genitalia, and the axillae are usual. *Melasma gravidarum*, formerly called chloasma, or mask of pregnancy, occurs on the face in many women and will persist in up to 30% of those affected.

Other than acrochordon, skin lesions should not grow during pregnancy. Moles may appear to enlarge as the underlying tissue is stretched, but nevi that are growing should be biopsied to eliminate the possibility of skin cancer. There is no difference in the prognosis for skin malignancies, including melanoma, when diagnosed during pregnancy unless definitive treatment is delayed out of concern for the fetus.

Striae gravidarum (stretch marks) occur in nearly all women by the end of the pregnancy. They are commonly seen on the abdomen but may be observed on the breasts, hips, and thighs. They are pink to purple atrophic lines that develop at right angles to the skin tension lines. After the birth of the baby, they typically become more flesh colored or pale and thinner. Risk factors include young age, family history, extremes of skin type (fairest and darkest), excess weight, and high weight gain.[141] There is little evidence that topical preparations prevent or decrease the appearance of stretch marks, although Indian pennywort (*Centella asiatica*) and bitter almond oil have shown some promise.[142,143]

Hair and nails also undergo changes in pregnancy. Increased hair growth is seen, particularly in dark-skinned women or women who already have abundant hair. After birth, the hair follicles resume the normal pattern of growth and loss. *Telogen effluvium* results in the loss of terminal scalp hairs about 1 to 5 months postpartum. Women often need reassurance that it is a self-limiting process and that baldness will not occur. Nails can become brittle and soft in the early months of pregnancy. In some women nails grow faster during the pregnancy.

Specific Dermatoses of Pregnancy

Dermatologic findings in pregnancy include both physiologic changes and specific dermatoses. All of the common dermatoses are pruritic. The dermatoses are differentiated on appearance, timing in pregnancy, and laboratory findings when indicated. Neither polymorphic eruption of pregnancy nor atopic eruption of pregnancy carries fetal risk; pemphigoid gestationis and intrahepatic cholestasis of pregnancy are more serious conditions both for mother and fetus.

POLYMORPHIC ERUPTION OF PREGNANCY

Polymorphic eruption of pregnancy (PEP), formerly called pruritic urticarial papules and plaques of pregnancy (PUPPP), is a benign, self-limiting inflammatory condition.[144] It occurs in about 1 in 160 pregnant women.[145] Although the older term accurately described the itching and appearance of most cases, as many as 50% of women develop additional lesions including vesicles, wheals or even bullae, erythema, or eczematous lesions. It is most often seen in fair-skinned primigravidas, developing in late pregnancy or immediately postpartum.[146] The rash is commonly confined to the abdomen and thighs, sparing the periumbilical area. The rash often occurs first within striae. The avoidance of the umbilicus and the presence of rash crossing striae are clues to clinical diagnosis. In some cases, the hips and back are involved, but a whole-body rash is rare.

Because PEP is self-limiting and without serious sequelae, reassurance and symptomatic treatment are usually all that is necessary. Cool wet compresses, oatmeal baths, antipruritic lotions, and topical steroids can be used. Medium-potency steroids such as clobetasone butyrate 0.05% (Class V) are generally needed to control itch, but milder presentations may respond to lower potency steroids such as hydrocortisone 0.01%. Prednisone in a tapering dose of 30 to 40 mg may be used daily for 7 to 10 days in extreme cases. Antihistamines are not as effective as topical corticosteroids in controlling itch, but may be a helpful adjunctive measure. Because the itchiness associated with PEP can be especially bothersome at night, antihistamines may be particularly useful if taken in the evening.

ATOPIC ERUPTION OF PREGNANCY

Several formerly described syndromes, such as prurigo, are now classified together as atopic eruption of pregnancy (AEP). Women prone to atopy (allergies, asthma, eczema) may develop a pruritic rash that is papular and may form eczematous plaques. The rash tends to be wider spread than in PEP and to start on the neck or chest rather than in striae. The diagnosis is made based on timing in pregnancy (75% before the third trimester), history of atopy, and absence of other possible conditions. Elevated IgE and eosinophilia may be found. It is now thought to represent half of all dermatoses of pregnancy.[147] Treatment with mild topical steroids and antihistamines should resolve the rash and itching. Oral corticosteroids can be given in severe cases. This condition is likely to recur in future pregnancies.

Pemphigoid Gestationis

Pemphigoid gestationis (PG) is a rare autoimmune bullous disease that occurs during pregnancy and the postpartum period. The initial lesions are small urticarial papules, which develop into vesicles and eventually, large, tense bullae on an inflamed background.[144] Unlike PEP, lesions are usually seen around the umbilicus before spreading widely across the body. PG most commonly presents during the second or third trimester, but may occur earlier or immediately postpartum. The course of the disease often remits and recurs with a flare, or worsening, near term.[147]

Maternal risks include erosion or scarring at the site of lesions and concomitant autoimmune disorders including thyroiditis or Graves' disease. Women should be aware that the disease may recur with the use of combined hormonal contraception or with a future pregnancy.[147] Fetal risks associated with PG include preterm birth, growth restriction, and the development of a vesicular rash on the newborn.

Therapy includes relief of pruritus, suppression of blister formation, and prevention of erosions. Use of topical or systemic corticosteroids combined with emollients and systemic antihistamines is usual. The patient with PG should be referred to a maternal–fetal medicine specialist.

Intrahepatic Cholestasis of Pregnancy

Intrahepatic cholestasis of pregnancy (ICP) has a worldwide prevalence of 1% with wide population variance.[144] The disease develops late in the third trimester and presents with severe itching. The rash is secondary and appears as a result of scratching. Often, the initial pruritus occurs on the palms and soles of the feet, before rapidly spreading. Excoriation, papules, and nodules develop as the condition progresses. There is a genetic component to susceptibility to ICP, and recurrence is likely in future pregnancies.[144]

The spreading pattern of the rash, elevated transaminase levels, and elevated bile salt levels are diagnostic. Treatment should be started immediately with ursodeoxycholic acid,[148,149] which has been shown to decrease fetal loss and preterm delivery, to reduce maternal pruritus, and improve laboratory values. Early delivery may be indicated to protect the fetus.

Conclusion

As primary care providers, midwives and women's health providers have innumerable opportunities to observe skin lesions, become familiar with characteristics of various diseases, treat simpler and more straightforward problems, and refer in a timely matter to the dermatologist for management of more persistent or severe presentations.

References

1. Gawkrodger DJ, Ardern-Jones MR. Microanatomy of the skin. In: Gawkrodger DJ, Ardern-Jones MR, eds. *Dermatology: An Illustrated Colour Text*. 5th ed. Philadelphia, PA: Elsevier; 2012.
2. Hong J, Koo B, Koo J. The psychosocial and occupational impact of chronic skin disease. *Dermatol Ther*. 2008;21(1):54-59.
3. Dunn L, O'Neill J, Feldman S. Acne in adolescents: quality of life, self-esteem, mood, and psychological disorders. *Dermatol Online J*. 2011;17(1):1.
4. Blackwell D, Lucas J, Clarke T. Summary health statistics for US adults: National Health Interview Survey, 2012. National Center for Health Statistics; 2014. Available at: http://www.cdc.gov/nchs/data/series/sr_10/sr10_260.pdf. Accessed June 2, 2016.
5. Mayer JE, Swetter SM, Fu T, Geller AC. Screening, early detection, education, and trends for melanoma: current status (2007–2013) and future directions: Part II. Screening, education, and future directions. *J Am Acad Dermatol*. 2014;71(4):611.e1-e10.

6. Gawkrodger DJ, Ardern-Jones MR. Practical clinic procedures. In: Gawkrodger DJ, Ardern-Jones MR, eds. *Dermatology: An Illustrated Colour Text*. 5th ed. Philadelphia, PA: Elsevier Ltd; 2012.

7. Eichenfield L, Tom W, Berger T, Krol A, Paller AS, Schwarzenberger K, et al. Guidelines of care for the management of atopic dermatitis: section 2: Management and treatment of atopic dermatitis with topical therapies. *J Am Acad Dermatol.* 2014;71(1):116-132.

8. Zuberbier T, Aberer W, Asero R, Bindslev-Jensen C, Brzoza Z, Canonica GW, et al. The EAACI/GA2LEN/EDF/WAO guideline for the definition, classification, diagnosis, and management of urticaria: the 2013 revision and update. *Allergy.* 2014;69(7):868-887.

9. Grattan CE. Urticaria and Angioedema. In: Bolognia JL, Jorizzo JL, Schaffer JV, eds. *Dermatology.* 3rd ed. Philadelphia, PA: Elsevier Saunders; 2012.

10. Bernstein JA, Lang DM, Khan DA, Craig T, Dreyfus D, Hsieh F, et al. The diagnosis and management of acute and chronic urticaria: 2014 update. *J Allergy Clin Immunol.* 2014;133(5):1270-1277.

11. Weisshaar E, Fleischer AB, Bernhard JD, Cropley TG. Pruritus and dysesthesia. In: Bolognia JL, Jorizzo JL, Schaffer JV, eds. *Dermatology.* 3rd ed. Philadelphia, PA: Elsevier Saunders; 2012.

12. Yosipovitch G, Bernhard JD. Chronic pruritus. *N Engl J Med.* 2013;368:1625-1634.

13. Kalra MG, Higgins KE, Kinney BS. Intertrigo and secondary skin infections. *Am Fam Physician.* 2014;89(7):569-573.

14. Lio PA, Lee M, LeBovidge J, Timmons KG, Schneider L. Clinical management of atopic dermatitis: practical highlights and updates from the atopic dermatitis practice parameter 2012. *J Allergy Clin Immunol Pract.* 2014;2(4):361-336.

15. Anderson BE. Contact dermatitis. In: Ferri FF, ed. *Ferri's Clinical Advisor 2016*. Philadelphia, PA: Elsevier; 2016.

16. Reider N, O Fritsch P. Other eczematous eruptions. In: Bolognia JL, Jorizzo JL, Schaffer JV, eds. *Dermatology.* 3rd ed. Philadelphia, PA: Elsevier Saunders; 2012.

17. Halberg M. Nummular eczema. *J Emerg Med.* 2012;43(5):e327-e328.

18. Zaidi Z, Lanigan S. Eczema. In: *Dermatology in Clinical Practice*. New York, NY: Springer-Verlag London Limited; 2010:151-162.

19. Naldi L, Rebora A. Seborrheic dermatitis. *N Engl J Med.* 2009;360:387-396.

20. Kimball AB. Skin differences, needs, and disorders across global populations. *J Investig Dermatol Symp Proc.* 2008;13(1):2-5.

21. van de Kerkhof PC, O Nestlé F. Psoriasis. In: Bolognia JL, Jorizzo JL, Schaffer JV, eds. *Dermatology.* 3rd ed. Philadelphia, PA: Elsevier Saunders; 2012.

22. Spencer EH, Ferdowsian HR, Barnard ND. Diet and acne: a review of the evidence. *Int J Dermatol.* 2009;48:339-347

23. Bowe, Whitney P, Joshi SS, Shalita AR. Diet and acne. *J Am Acad Dermatol.* 2010;63(1):124-141.

24. Eichenfield LF, Krakowski AC, Piggott C, Del Rosso J, Baldwin H, Fallon Friedlander S, et al. Evidence-based recommendations for the diagnosis and treatment of pediatric acne. *Pediatrics.* 2013;131(Suppl 3):163-186.

25. Titus S, Hodge J. Diagnosis and treatment of acne. *Am Fam Physician.* 2012;86(8):734-740.

26. Koo EB, Petersen TD, Kimball AB. Meta-analysis comparing efficacy of antibiotics versus oral contraceptives in acne vulgaris. *J Am Acad Dermatol.* 2014;71(3):450-459.

27. Cao H, Yang G, Wang Y, Liu JP, Smith CA, Luo H, et al. Complementary therapies for acne vulgaris. *Cochrane Database Syst Rev.* 2015;1:CD009436. doi:10.1002/14651858.CD009436.pub2.

28. Del Rosso J, Thiboutot D, Gallo R, Webster G, Tanghetti E, Eichenfield L, et al. Consensus recommendations from the American Acne & Rosacea Society on the management of rosacea, part 1: a status report on the disease state, general measures, and adjunctive skin care. *Cutis.* 2013;92(5):234-240.

29. Del Rosso J, Thiboutot D, Gallo R, Webster G, Tanghetti E, Eichenfield L, et al. Consensus recommendations from the American Acne & Rosacea Society on the management of rosacea, part 2: a status report on topical agents. *Cutis.* 2013;92(6):277-284.

30. Elewski BE, Draelos Z, Dréno B, Jansen T, Layton A, Picardo M. Rosacea—global diversity and optimized outcome: proposed international consensus from the Rosacea International Expert Group. *J Eur Acad Dermatol Venereol.* 2011;25(2):188-200.

31. Dufour DN, Emtestam L, Jemec GB. Hidradenitis suppurativa: a common and burdensome, yet under-recognised, inflammatory skin disease. *Postgrad Med J.* 2014;90(1062):216-221.

32. Alikhan A, Lynch PJ, Eisen DB. Hidradenitis suppurativa: a comprehensive review. *Am Acad Dermatol.* 2009;60(4):539-61; quiz 562-3. doi:10.1016/j.jaad.2008.11.911.

33. Shah N. Hidradenitis suppurativa: a treatment challenge. *Am Fam Physician.* 2005;72(8):1547-1552.

34. Deckers IE, Prens EP. An update on medical treatment options for hidradenitis suppurativa. *Drugs.* 2016;76(2):215-229.

35. Price, Vera H. Androgenetic alopecia in women. *J Investig Dermatol Symp Proc*. 2003;8:24-27.

36. Ellis JA, Harrap SB. The genetics of androgenetic alopecia. *Clin Dermatol*. 2001;19(2):149-154.

37. Price VH, Roberts JL, Hordinsky M, Olsen EA, Savin R, Bergfeld W, et al. Lack of efficacy of finasteride in postmenopausal women with androgenetic alopecia. *J Am Acad Dermatol*. 2000;43:768-776.

38. Dawber RP, Sinclair RD. Hirsuties. *Clin Dermatol*. 2001;19:189-199.

39. Martin KA, Chang RJ, Ehrmann DA, Ibanez L, Lobo RA, Rosenfield RL, et al. Evaluation and treatment of hirsutism in premenopausal women: an Endocrine Society clinical practice guideline. *J Clin Endocrinol Metab*. 2008;93(4):1105-1120.

40. Centers for Disease Control and Prevention. Methicillin-resistant *Staphylococcus aureus* (MRSA) Infections. Available at: http://www.cdc.gov/mrsa /tracking/. Accessed June 7, 2016.

41. Wertheim HFL, Melles DC, Vos MC, van Leeuwen W, van Belkum A, Verbrugh HA, et al. The role of nasal carriage in *Staphylococcus aureus* infections. *Lancet Infect Dis*. 2005;5:751-762.

42. Lulemo-Aguilar J, Sabat-Santandreu M. Folliculitis: recognition and management. *Am J Clin Dermatol*. 2004;5(5):301-310.

43. Stevens DL, Bisno AL, Chambers HF, Dellinger EP, Goldstein EJ, Gorbach SL, et al. Practice guidelines for the diagnosis and management of skin and soft tissue infections: 2014 update by the Infectious Diseases Society of America. *Clin Infect Dis*. 2014;59(2): e10-e52.

44. Bangert S, Levy M, Hebert AA. Bacterial resistance and impetigo treatment trends: a review. *Pediatr Dermatol*. 2012;29(3):243-248.

45. Hartman-Adams H, Banvard C, Juckett G. Impetigo: diagnosis and treatment. *Am Fam Physician*. 2014;90(4):229-235.

46. Janniger CK, Schwartz RA, Szepietowski JC, Reich A. Intertrigo and common secondary skin infections. *Am Fam Physician*. 2005;72(5):833-838.

47. Mistiaen P, van Halm-Walters M. Prevention and treatment of intertrigo in large skin folds of adults: a systematic review. *BMC Nursing*. 2010;9:12. doi:10.1186/1472-6955-9-12.

48. Ely JW, Rosenfeld S, Seabury Stone M. Diagnosis and management of tinea infections. *Am Fam Physician*. 2014;90(10):702-710.

49. Thomas J, Jacobson GA, Narkowicz CK, Peterson GM, Burnet H, Sharpe C. Toenail onychomycosis: an important global disease burden. *J Clin Pharm Ther*. 2010;35(5):497-519.

50. Westerberg DP, Voyack MJ. Onychomycosis: current trends in diagnosis and treatment. *Am Fam Physician*. 2013;88(11):762-770.

51. Allevato MA. Diseases mimicking onychomycosis. *Clin Dermatol*. 2010;28(2):164-177.

52. Silverberg JI, Silverberg NB. The US prevalence of common warts in childhood: a population-based study. *J Investig Dermatol*. 2013;133:2788-2790. doi:10.1038/jid.2013.226.

53. Plasencia JM. Cutaneous warts. *Dermatology*. 2000;27(2):423-434.

54. Micali G, Dall'Oglio F, Nasca MR, Tedeschi A. Management of cutaneous warts: an evidence-based approach. *Am J Clin Dermatol*. 2004;5(5):311-317.

55. Mulhem E, Pinelis S. Treatment of nongenital cutaneous warts. *Am Fam Physician*. 2011;84(3):288-293.

56. Kollipara R, Ekhlassi E, Downing C, Guidry J, Lee M, Tyring SK. Advancements in pharmacotherapy for noncancerous manifestations of HPV. *J Clin Med*. 2015;4(5):832-846. doi:10.3390/jcm4050832.

57. Kwok CS, Gibbs S, Bennett C, Holland R, Abbott R. Topical treatments for cutaneous warts. *Cochrane Database Syst Rev*. 2012;9:CD001781. doi:10.1002/ 14651858.CD001781.pub3.

58. Centers for Disease Control and Prevention. Shingles (Herpes Zoster). Available at: http://www.cdc .gov/shingles/hcp/. Accessed June 7, 2016.

59. Yawn BP, Saddier P, Wollan PC, St Sauver JL, Kurland MJ, Sy LS. A population-based study of the incidence and complication rates of herpes zoster before zoster vaccine introduction. *Mayo Clin Proc*. 2007;82:1341-1349.

60. Leung J, Harpaz R, Molinar N-Ai, Jumaan A, Zhou F. Herpes zoster incidence among insured persons in the United States, 1993–2006: evaluation of impact of varicella vaccination. *Clin Infect Dis*. 2011;52(3):332-340. doi:10.1093/cid/ciq077.

61. Thomas SL, Hall AJ. What does epidemiology tell us about risk factors for herpes zoster? *Lancet Infect Dis*. 2004;4(1):26-33.

62. Han Y, Zhang J, Chen N, He L, Zhou M, Zhu C. Corticosteroids for preventing postherpetic neuralgia. *Cochrane Database Syst Rev*. 2013;3:CD005582. doi:10.1002/14651858.CD005582.pub4.

63. Centers for Disease Control and Prevention. Update on recommendations for use of herpes zoster vaccine. *MMWR*. 2014;63(33);729-731.

64. Broccolo F, Drago F, Careddu AM, Foglieni C, Turbino L, Cocuzza CE, et al. Additional evidence that pityriasis rosea is associated with reactivation of human herpesvirus-6 and -7. *J Invest Dermatol*. 2005;124(6):1234-1240.

65. Chuh AAT, Dofitas BL, Comisel G, Reveiz L, Sharma V, Garner SE, et al. Interventions for pityriasis rosea. *Cochrane Database Syst Rev.* 2007;2:CD005068. doi:10.1002/14651858.CD005068.pub2.
66. Centers for Disease Control and Prevention. Parasites—Lice. Available at: http://www.cdc.gov/parasites/lice/index.html. Accessed June 7, 2016.
67. Anderson AL, Chaney E. Pubic lice (*Pthirus pubis*): history, biology, and treatment versus knowledge and beliefs of US college students. *Int J Environ Res Public Health.* 2009;6(2):592-600. doi:10.3390/ijerph6020592.
68. Centers for Disease Control and Prevention. Sexually transmitted diseases treatment guidelines, 2015. *MMWR Recomm Rep.* 2015;64(RR-3):1-137.
69. Centers for Disease Control and Prevention. Parasites—Scabies. Available at: http://www.cdc.gov/parasites/scabies/index.html. Accessed June 7, 2016.
70. Centers for Disease Control and Prevention. Lyme Disease. Available at: http://www.cdc.gov/lyme/index.html. Accessed June 7, 2016.
71. Centers for Disease Control and Prevention. *Tickborne Diseases of the United States: A Reference Manual for Health Care Providers.* 3rd ed. 2015. Available at: https://www.cdc.gov/lyme/resources/tickborne-diseases.pdf. Accessed June 7, 2016.
72. Halperin JJ, Baker P, Wormser GP. Common misconceptions about Lyme disease. *Am J Med.* 2013;126:264.e1-e7.
73. Wormser GP, Dattwyler RJ, Shapiro ED, Halperin JJ, Steere AC, Klempner MS, et al. The clinical assessment, treatment, and prevention of Lyme disease, human granulocytic anaplasmosis, and babesiosis: clinical practice guidelines by the Infectious Diseases Society of America. *Clin Infect Dis.* 2007;43:1089-134.
74. Delong AK, Blossom B, Maloney EL, Phillips SE. Antibiotic retreatment of Lyme disease in patients with persistent symptoms: a biostatistical review of randomized, placebo-controlled, clinical trials. *Contemp Clin Trials.* 2012;33(6):1132-1142. doi:10.1016/j.cct.2012.08.009.
75. Luba MC, Bangs SA, Mohler AM, Stulberg DL. Common benign skin tumors. *Am Fam Physician.* 2003;67(4):729-738.
76. Kim J-H, Park H, Ahn SK. Cherry angiomas on the scalp. *Case Rep Dermatol.* 2009;1(1):82-86. doi:10.1159/000251395.
77. Kudur MH, Hulmani M. Giant angiokeratoma of Fordyce over the vulva in a middle-aged woman: case report and review of literature. *Indian J Dermatol.* 2013;58(3):242. doi:10.4103/0019-5154.110856.
78. Khasnis A, Gokula R M. Spider nevus. *J Postgrad Med.* 2002;48:307.
79. Romagnuolo J, Jhangri GS, Jewell LD, Bain VG. Predicting the liver histology in chronic hepatitis C: how good is the clinician? *Am J Gastroenterol.* 2001;96:3165-3174.
80. National Institute of Arthritis and Musculoskeletal and Skin Diseases. Vitiligo. Available at: http://www.niams.nih.gov/Health_Info/Vitiligo/#7. Accessed June 7, 2016.
81. Alikhan A, Felsten LM, Daly M, Petronic-Rosic V. Vitiligo: a comprehensive overview Part I. Introduction, epidemiology, quality of life, diagnosis, differential diagnosis, associations, histopathology, etiology, and work-up. *J Am Acad Dermatol.* 2011;65(3):473-491. doi:10.1016/j.jaad.2010.11.061.
82. Ezzedine K, Lim HW, Suzuki T, Katayama I, Hamzavi I, Lan CC, et al. Revised classification/nomenclature of vitiligo and related issues: the Vitiligo Global Issues Consensus Conference. *Pigment Cell Melanoma Res.* 2012;25(3):E1-E13. doi:10.1111/j.1755-148X.2012.00997.x.
83. Whitton ME, Pinart M, Batchelor J, Lushey C, Leonardi-Bee J, González U. Interventions for vitiligo. *Cochrane Database Syst Rev.* 2015;2:CD003263. doi:10.1002/14651858.CD003263.pub5.
84. Plensdorf S, Martinez J. Common pigmentation disorders. *Am Fam Physician.* 2009;79(2):109-116.
85. Ortonne JP, Pandya AG, Lui H, Hexsel D. Treatment of solar lentigines. *J Am Acad Dermatol.* 2006;54(5 Suppl 2):S262-S271.
86. Higgins SP, Freemark M, Prose NS. Acanthosis nigricans: a practical approach to evaluation and management. *Dermatol Online J.* 2008;14(9):2.
87. Hermanns-Le T, Scheen A, Pierard GE. Acanthosis nigricans associated with insulin resistance. *Am J Clin Dermatol.* 2004;5(3):199-203.
88. Kong AS, Williams RL, Rhyne R, Urias-Sandoval V, Cardinali G, Weller NF, et al. Acanthosis nigricans: high prevalence and association with diabetes in a practice-based research network consortium—a PRImary care Multi-Ethnic network (PRIME Net) study. *J Am Board Fam Medicine.* 2010;23(4):476-485. doi:10.3122/jabfm.2010.04.090221.
89. Boza JC, Trindade EN, Peruzzo J, Sachett L, Rech L, Cestari TF. Skin manifestations of obesity: a comparative study. *J Eur Acad Dermatol Venereol.* 2012;26(10):1220-1223.
90. Senel E, Salmanoglu M, Solmazgül E, Berçik Inal B. Acrochordons as a cutaneous sign of impaired carbohydrate metabolism, hyperlipidemia, liver enzyme abnormalities and hypertension: a case-control

study. *J Eur Acad Dermatol Venereol.* 2011 Dec 21. doi:10.1111/j.1468-3083.2011.04396.x. [Epub ahead of print]

91. Akpnar F, Dervs E. Association between acrochordons and the components of metabolic syndrome. *Eur J Dermatol.* 2012;22(1):106-110.

92. National Cancer Institute. Common Moles, Dysplastic Nevi, and Risk of Melanoma. Available at: http://www.cancer.gov/types/skin/moles-factsheet. Accessed June 7, 2016.

93. Jackson JM, Alexis A, Berman B, Berson DS, Taylor S, Weiss JS. Current understanding of seborrheic keratosis: prevalence, etiology, clinical presentation, diagnosis, and management. *J Drugs Dermatol.* 2015;14(10):1119-1125.

94. Juckett G, Hartman-Adams H. Management of keloids and hypertrophic scars. *Am Fam Physician.* 2009;80(3):253-260.

95. Kundu RV, Patterson S. Dermatologic conditions in skin of color: part II. Disorders occurring predominately in skin of color. *Am Fam Physician.* 2013;87(12):859-865.

96. Ogawa R. The most current algorithms for the treatment and prevention of hypertrophic scars and keloids. *Plast Reconstr Surg.* 2010;125(2):557-568. doi:10.1097/PRS.0b013e3181c82dd5.

97. Cashman MW, Sloan SB. Nutrition and nail disease. *Clin Dermatol.* 2010;28(4):420-425. doi:10.1016/j.clindermatol.2010.03.037.

98. Scher RK, Fleckman P, Tulumbas B, McCollam L, Enfanto P. Brittle nail syndrome: treatment options and the role of the nurse. *Dermatol Nurs.* 2003; 15(1):15-23.

99. Kechijian P. Brittle fingernails. *Dermatol Clin.* 1985;3(3):421-429.

100. Reid IR. Calcium supplements and nail quality. *N Engl J Med.* 2000;343(24):1817.

101. Scheinfeld N, Dahdah MJ, Scher R. Vitamins and minerals: their role in nail health and disease. *J Drugs Dermatol.* 2007;6(8):782-787.

102. Flament F, Bazin R, Laquieze S, Rubert V, Simonpietri E, Piot B. Effect of the sun on visible clinical signs of aging in Caucasian skin. *Clin Cosmet Investig Dermatol.* 2013;6:221-232.

103. Stern RS, Treatment of photoaging. *N Engl J Med.* 2004:350:1526-1534.

104. Jackson R. Elderly and sun-affected skin. Distinguishing between changes caused by aging and changes caused by habitual exposure to sun. *Can Fam Physician.* 2001;47:1236-1243.

105. Boyd AS, Naylor M, Cameron GS, Pearse AD, Gaskell SA, Neldner KH. The effects of chronic sunscreen use on the histologic changes of dermatoheliosis. *J Am Acad Dermatol.* 1995;33:941-946.

106. Lomas A, Leonardi-Bee J, Bath-Hextall F. A systematic review of worldwide incidence of nonmelanoma skin cancer. *Br J Dermatol.* 2012;166(5):1069-1080.

107. US Department of Health and Human Services. *The Surgeon General's Call to Action to Prevent Skin Cancer.* Washington, DC: US Department of Health and Human Services, Office of the Surgeon General; 2014.

108. Stern RS. Prevalence of a history of skin cancer in 2007: results of an incidence-based model. *Arch Dermatol.* 2010;146(3):279-282.

109. Agency for Healthcare Research and Quality. Medical Expenditure Panel Survey. Rockville, MD:. US Department of Health and Human Services. Available at: http://meps.ahrq.gov/mepsweb/. Accessed June 7, 2016.

110. American Cancer Society. Skin Cancer Facts. Available at: http://www.cancer.org/cancer/cancercauses/sunanduvexposure/skin-cancer-facts.

111. Centers for Disease Control and Prevention. Skin Cancer Statistics. Available at: http://www.cdc.gov/cancer/skin/statistics/. Accessed June 7, 2016.

112. National Institute for Occupational Safety and Health. Sun Exposure. Available at: http://www.cdc.gov/niosh/topics/sunexposure/. Accessed June 7, 2016.

113. Karagas MR, Stukel TA, Greenberg ER, Baron JA, Mott LA, Stern RS. Risk of subsequent basal cell carcinoma and squamous cell carcinoma of the skin among patients with prior skin cancer. *JAMA.* 1992;267(24):3305.

114. Firnhaber JM. Diagnosis and treatment of basal cell and squamous cell carcinoma. *Am Fam Physician.* 2012;86(2):161-168.

115. Flohil SC, van der Leest RJ, Dowlatshahi EA, Hofman A, de Vries E, Nijsten T. Prevalence of actinic keratosis and its risk factors in the general population: the Rotterdam Study. *J Invest Dermatol.* 2013;133(8):1971-8. doi:10.1038/jid.2013.134.

116. Berman B, Cockerell CJ. Pathobiology of actinic keratosis: ultraviolet-dependent keratinocyte proliferation. *J Am Acad Dermatol.* 2013;68(1):S10-S19.

117. Roewert-Huber J, Stockfleth E, Kerl H. Pathology and pathobiology of actinic (solar) keratosis—an update. *Br J Dermatol.* 2007;157(Suppl 2):18-20.

118. Rigel DS, Stein Gold LF. The importance of early diagnosis and treatment of actinic keratosis. *J Am Acad Dermatol.* 2013;68(1):S20-S27.

119. Anwar J, Wrone D, Kimyai-Asadi A, Alam M. The development of actinic keratosis into invasive

squamous cell carcinoma: evidence and evolving classification schemes. *Clin Dermatol.* 2004;22(3): 189-196.

120. Criscione VD, Weinstock MA, Naylor MF, Luque C, Eide MJ, Bingham SF. Actinic keratoses: natural history and risk of malignant transformation in the Veterans Affairs topical tretinoin chemoprevention trial. *Cancer.* 2009;115:2523-2530. doi:10.1002/cncr.24284.

121. Marcil I, Stern RS. Risk of developing a subsequent nonmelanoma skin cancer in patients with a history of nonmelanoma skin cancer: a critical review of the literature and meta-analysis. *Arch Dermatol.* 2000;136(12):1524-1530.

122. Bath-Hextall F, Bong J, Perkins W, Williams H. Interventions for basal cell carcinoma of the skin: systematic review. *BMJ.* 2004;329(7468):705.

123. Clark CM, Furniss M, Mackay-Wiggan JM. Basal cell carcinoma: an evidence-based treatment update. *Am J Clin Dermatol.* 2014;15(3):197-216. doi:10.1007/s40257-014-0070-z.

124. Proctor AE, Thompson LA, O'Bryant CL. Vismodegib: an inhibitor of the Hedgehog signaling pathway in the treatment of basal cell carcinoma. *Ann Pharmacother.* 2014;48(1):99-106. doi:10.1177/1060028013506696.

125. Alam M, Ratner D. Cutaneous squamous-cell carcinoma. *N Engl J Med.* 2001;344(13):975-983.

126. Brantsch KD, Meisner C, Schönfisch B, Trilling B, Wehner-Caroli J, Röcken M, et al. Analysis of risk factors determining prognosis of cutaneous squamous-cell carcinoma: a prospective study. *Lancet Oncol.* 2008;9:713.

127. Brougham ND, Dennett ER, Cameron R, Tan ST. The incidence of metastasis from cutaneous squamous cell carcinoma and the impact of its risk factors. *J Surg Oncol.* 2012;106:811.

128. National Cancer Institute. Squamous Cell Carcinoma of the Skin Treatment. Available at: http://www.cancer.gov/types/skin/hp/skin-treatment-pdq#link/_383_toc. Accessed June 7, 2016.

129. Lansbury L, Bath-Hextall F, Perkins W, Stanton W, Leonardi-Bee J. Interventions for non-metastatic squamous cell carcinoma of the skin: systematic review and pooled analysis of observational studies. *BMJ.* 2013;347:f6153. doi:10.1136/bmj.f6153.

130. Howlader N, Noone AM, Krapcho M, Garshell J, Miller D, Altekruse SF, et al. (eds). *SEER Cancer Statistics Review, 1975–2012.* Bethesda, MD: National Cancer Institute. Available at: http://seer.cancer.gov/csr/1975_2012/. Accessed June 7, 2016.

131. Tucker MA. Melanoma epidemiology. *Hematol Oncol Clin North Am.* 2009;23(3):383-395, vii. doi:10.1016/j.hoc.2009.03.010.

132. Weir HK, Marrett LD, Cokkinides V, Barnholtz-Sloan J, Patel P, Tai E, et al. Melanoma in adolescents and young adults (ages 15–39 years): United States, 1999–2006. *Am Acad Dermatol.* 2011;65 (5 suppl 1):S38-S49.

133. Little EG, Eide MJ. Update on the current state of melanoma incidence. *Dermatol Clin.* 2012; 30(3):355-361.

134. Boniol M, Autier P, Boyle P, Gandini S. Cutaneous melanoma attributable to sunbed use: systematic review and meta-analysis. *BMJ.* 2012;345: e4757.

135. Wolff TA, Tai E, Miller T. Screening for skin cancer: update of the evidence. *Ann Intern Med.* 2008; 150:194-198.

136. US Preventive Services Task Force. Screening for skin cancer: US Preventive Services Task Force recommendation statement. *Ann Intern Med.* 2009; 150:188-193.

137. Weinstock MA. Reducing death from melanoma and standards of evidence. *J Investig Dermatol.* 2012;132:1311-1312. doi:10.1038/jid.2012.57.

138. Friedman RJ, Farber MJ, Warycha MA, Papathasis N, Miller MK, Heilman ER. The "dysplastic" nevus. *Clin Dermatol.* 2009;27(1):103-115.

139. Bradford PT, Anderson WF, Purdue MP, Goldstein AM, Tucker MA. Rising melanoma incidence rates of the trunk among younger women in the United States. *Cancer Epidemiol Biomarkers Prev.* 2010;19(9):2401-2406.

140. Beard MP, Millington GW. Recent developments in the specific dermatoses of pregnancy. *Clin Exp Dermatol.* 2012;37:1-4.

141. Picard D, Sellier S, Houivet E, Marpeau L, Fournet P, Thobois B, et al. Incidence and risk factors for striae gravidarum. *J Am Acad Dermatol.* 2015; 73(4):699-700. doi:10.1016/j.jaad.2015.06.037.

142. Brennan M, Young G, Devane D. Topical preparations for preventing stretch marks in pregnancy. *Cochrane Database Syst Rev.* 2012;11:CD000066. doi:10.1002/14651858.CD000066.pub2.

143. Korgavkar K, Wang F. Stretch marks during pregnancy: a review of topical prevention. *Br J Dermatol.* 2015;172(3):606-615. doi:10.1111/bjd.13426.

144. Sävervall C, Sand FL, Thomsen SF. Dermatological diseases associated with pregnancy: pemphigoid gestationis, polymorphic eruption of pregnancy, intrahepatic cholestasis of pregnancy, and atopic eruption of pregnancy. *Dermatol Res Pract.* 2015; 2015:979635. doi:10.1155/2015/979635.

145. Ambros-Rudolph CM. Dermatoses of pregnancy—clues to diagnosis, fetal risk, and therapy. *Ann Dermatol.* 2011;23(3):265-275. doi:10.5021/ad.2011.23.3.265.

146. Rudolph CM, Al-Fares S, Vaughan-Jones SA, Müllegger RR, Kerl H, Black MM. Polymorphic eruption of pregnancy: clinicopathology and potential trigger factors in 181 patients. *Br J Dermatol*. 2006;154(1):54-60.

147. Ambros-Rudolph CM, Müllegger RR, Vaughan-Jones SA, Kerl H, Black MM. The specific dermatoses of pregnancy revisited and reclassified: results of a retrospective two-center study on 505 pregnant patients. *J Am Acad Dermatol*. 2006;54(3):395-404.

148. Gurung V, Middleton P, Milan SJ, Hague W, Thornton JG. Interventions for treating cholestasis in pregnancy. *Cochrane Database Syst Rev*. 2013;6: CD000493. doi:10.1002/14651858.CD000493. pub2.

149. Bacq Y, Sentilhes L, Reyes HB, Glantz A, Kondrack-iene J, Binder T, et al. Efficacy of ursodeoxycholic acid in treating intrahepatic cholestasis of pregnancy: a meta-analysis. *Gastroenterology*. 2012;143(6): 1492-501. doi:10.1053/j.gastro.2012.08.004.

CHAPTER 25

ANTIMICROBIALS

Kathryn Niemeyer

Antimicrobial is the global term for any medication that kills or inhibits the growth of a micro-organism. These medications are among the most widely prescribed in primary healthcare settings.[1,2] Based on a 2010 sample of 70% of the prescriptions in the United States, it was estimated that 50% of antibiotic prescriptions were unnecessary.[3] Responsible prescribing practices depend on knowledge of microbiology, pharmacology, host factors affecting infectious disease processes, potential responses to pharmacotherapy, toxicity risks, and local and global patterns of resistance.[2] Likewise, responsible prescribing is informed by knowledge of the consequences of overprescribing and includes the judicious application of professional judgment to discern when it is appropriate to prescribe antimicrobial medications or when other interventions should be recommended.

The *microbiome*, or normal flora, residing within and on the human body is diverse and exists in delicate balance. This balanced diversity of our resident bacteria supports and protects human health and normal physiologic functioning.[4] Initiation of antimicrobial therapy may upset that balance, offering the opportunity for superimposed infection and the elimination of essential bacterial species.[4] The consequences from antimicrobial therapies may potentially be life threatening. Both the frequency of antibiotic prescriptions and how early in life antibiotics are prescribed may correlate to the increased frequency and severity of chronic diseases such as obesity, allergies, celiac disease, and inflammatory bowel diseases.[4]

By adhering to appropriate evidence-based prescribing practices and practicing antibiotic stewardship, the primary care provider combats the crisis of emerging antimicrobial resistance and disease causation. Guidelines for appropriate antibiotic prescribing include differentiating viral from bacterial infections, encouraging palliative therapy for viral infections, recommending appropriate immunizations, and educating women and their families regarding the judicious use of antibiotics and simple infection control measures like handwashing.[5,6]

There may be additional health benefits associated with cautious prescribing habits and educating individuals regarding the appropriate use of antibiotics. For example, in 2004, a case-control study performed by Velicer and colleagues identified a relationship between antibiotic use and breast cancer.[7] Researchers compared the computerized pharmacy records of 2266 women with primary, invasive breast cancer to the records of 7953 randomly selected women without breast cancer and found that increased antibiotic exposure was associated with an increase in the incidence of and mortality from breast cancer. Two measures of antibiotic exposure (cumulative use in number of days and total number of antibiotic prescriptions) were utilized based on data from the health plan pharmacy. The relative risk of breast cancer increased in all categories of antibiotic use with each increment in days of use or number of prescriptions.[7] Furthermore, it is theorized that increases in the early development of breast cancer in BRCA-positive women born after 1940, in contrast to BRCA-positive women born before 1940, is likely due to environmental changes rather than changes in genes. The role of bacteria in estrogen metabolism is speculated to be a causative factor.[4] Fuhrman and colleagues provided initial research to demonstrate that gut microbiome diversity influences endogenous estrogen metabolism.[8] Research is beginning to evaluate the complex relationship between microbiome diversity and estrogen metabolism that may explain the relationship between breast cancer and antibiotic use. This emerging knowledge, while not evidence of a causal relationship between antibiotic use and the risk of breast cancer, is an example of a rationale for prudent prescribing habits.

The term *antimicrobial* refers to natural or synthetic agents or drugs used in the treatment of infections caused by microorganisms such as bacteria, viruses, fungi, or protozoa.[2] While including brief sections on antiviral and antifungal medications, this chapter focuses on antibacterial therapy and is designed to clarify the relationship between pathogen and antibacterial medication, identify simple rules to follow when prescribing, and foster a level of confidence in initiating antibacterial therapy based on best practices. Specific pharmacotherapeutic guidelines for common health conditions encountered in the primary care setting, as well as pharmacotherapy for viral, fungal, and protozoal infections, are discussed in greater detail in related chapters.

Microbiology

A fundamental understanding of microbiology is essential to understanding how antibacterial medications work. The most clinically useful antibacterials are selectively toxic chemicals that exploit the cellular and biochemical differences between pathogen and host in order to eradicate infection with the fewest host side effects. These differences in structure and function between bacterial cells and human cells provide a mechanism for antibacterials to interfere with the replication and growth of microorganisms (*bacteriostatic* agents) or kill invading pathogens (*bactericidal* agents). This distinction is important, because the bacteriostatic agents rely on an intact immune system for maximum therapeutic benefit.

Bacteria are prokaryotes—single cells or groups of cells without nuclei. Single-stranded deoxyribonucleic acid (DNA) lies in the cytoplasm. The genetic material in a human eukaryote is contained within the cell nucleus, encased in the nuclear membrane. Unlike eukaryotes, the plasma cell membrane of bacteria is surrounded by a cell wall composed primarily of peptidoglycan, a protein unique to bacteria. This bacterial cell wall is necessary to maintain the osmotic pressure of the cellular contents, essentially preventing the cell from exploding. Interfering with cell wall synthesis is lethal to bacterial cells.

Differing biochemical functions within the host and bacterial invader also provide potential for interference with the growth and development of pathogenic colonization. For example, both bacteria and human cells require folate for DNA synthesis. Although humans rely on dietary folate, bacteria must synthesize folate in order to reproduce. Blocking bacterial folate synthesis effectively inhibits DNA replication.

Bacteria are classified as Gram-positive or Gram-negative depending on their color reaction to a staining technique developed by Hans Gram in 1884. The principal difference between Gram-positive and Gram-negative organisms is the composition of the cell wall. The cell wall of Gram-positive organisms is simple in structure. The complexity of the composition of the cell wall of Gram-negative organisms, in which the peptidoglycan layer is surrounded by lipopolysaccharides and encased in an outer lipid membrane, creates a more significant barrier to penetration by an antibacterial agent.

The shape of individual bacteria may be spherical (cocci), rod-shaped (bacilli), or curved and spiral (spirochetes). Diplococci refer to cocci in pairs (*Neisseria gonorrhoeae*), streptococci refer to cocci in chains (*Streptococcus pyogenes*), and staphylococci refer to clusters of cocci (*Staphylococcus aureus*). Bacteria are also classified as aerobic or anaerobic depending on their need for oxygen to grow and reproduce.

Some tiny Gram-negative bacteria, such as *Chlamydia* and *Mycoplasma*, do not share the common characteristics of other bacteria and were initially believed to be viruses. *Chlamydia*, the most primitive of bacteria, is an obligate intracellular parasite. Like viruses, *Chlamydia* depends on the host cell to perform essential metabolic processes; unlike viruses, these microbes contain both DNA and ribonucleic acid (RNA). *Mycoplasmas* are the tiniest cellular microbes. Because they do not have a cell wall, their shape is amorphous and they are resistant to antimicrobials that interfere with cell wall synthesis.

The integrity of host immunity, including biological barriers and innate and adaptive immune systems, affects the ability of the individual to actively fight infection. Other host factors may contribute to particular susceptibility to infections. For example, *Chlamydia trachomatis* invades the columnar epithelium of the cervix. The adolescent female is more likely than the adult female to have a cervical ectropion, with columnar epithelium on the ectocervix. This makes the adolescent cervix more vulnerable to invasion by *Chlamydia*. The cervical ectropion associated with the use of combined oral contraceptives creates a similar situation and a similarly increased risk.

Many bacterial infections are due to the overgrowth of bacteria that are part of the normal microbiome in or on a particular site. For example, *S. aureus* can be found on the skin of a healthy individual. These bacteria are opportunistic pathogens. In small numbers they are relatively harmless to the host; however, under certain host conditions, such as a break in the skin or a reduced immune response, *S. aureus* may proliferate, causing carbuncles, furuncles, mastitis, impetigo, or cellulitis. A viral or fungal infection may also provide the right conditions for opportunistic pathogens such as *S. aureus* to multiply and cause a secondary infection. Tinea pedis causes breaks in the skin between the toes that may, with the right combination of conditions, become secondarily infected with *S. aureus* or *S. pyogenes*, another bacterium frequently found on the skin. The vesicles and ulcers of herpes simplex virus also provide these bacteria with a portal of entry into soft tissue.

Bacterial infections also occur as an organism migrates and proliferates from one anatomical site to another site not usually colonized by that organism. *Escherichia coli*, for example, is part of the normal microbiome of the colon. When the urogenital tract is contaminated by *E. coli* (or when *E. coli* is transported to the urogenital tract), it easily multiplies in the sterile environment of the bladder, causing cystitis.

Some bacterial infections are the result of exposure to microbes that are not part of the normal

Table 25-1 Common Pathogens: Gram-positive Aerobes

Organism	Common Anatomical Sites of Colonization	Common Infections Caused by Opportunistic Pathogens
Cocci		
Streptococcus Group A	Respiratory	Strep pharyngitis, scarlet fever, rheumatic fever
S. pyogenes	Skin	Impetigo, cellulitis, toxic shock syndrome
Streptococcus Group B *S. agalactiae*	Genitourinary	Neonatal sepsis
S. pneumoniae	Respiratory	Pneumonia, meningitis, sinusitis
Staphylococcus		
S. aureus	Skin and soft tissue	Mastitis, carbuncles, furuncles, folliculitis, impetigo, cellulitis,
	Respiratory Gastrointestinal	Sinusitis
S. saprophyticus	Gastrointestinal tract	Urinary tract infection
Enterococcus species	Gastrointestinal tract	Urinary tract infection
	Genitourinary	Nosocomial infections
Rods		
Bacillus anthracis	Not part of normal flora: Spores enter through skin, respiratory, gastrointestinal routes	Anthrax
Listeria species	Not part of normal flora: Ingested in contaminated food (cheese)	Listeriosis, meningitis, septicemia, abscess, encephalitis
Corynebacterium C. diphtheriae	Genitourinary	Diptheria
Mobiluncus species	Genitourinary	Bacterial vaginosis
Lactobacillus species	Genitourinary Gastrointestinal Skin	Nonpathogenic
Spirochetes		
Treponema pallidum	Not part of normal flora	Syphilis

flora, such as *Bacillus anthracis* or *C. trachomatis.* Tables 25-1, 25-2, and 25-3 summarize the characteristics, common anatomical sites of colonization, and associated primary care conditions of some common human pathogens.

Antibiotic Classifications

The term *antibiotic* refers to the earliest antibacterials that were produced by microbes, which were isolated and harvested from culture and able to

Table 25-2 Common Pathogens: Gram-negative Aerobes

Organism	Common Anatomical Sites of Colonization	Common Infections Caused by Opportunistic Pathogens
Cocci		
Neisseria	Not part of normal flora:	
N. gonorrhoeae	Sexually transmitted	Gonorrhea of the urogenital tract, pharynx, arthritis
N. meningitidis	Respiratory	Meningitis
Rods		
Escherichia coli	Gastrointestinal tract (colon)	Urinary tract infection
Klebsiella species	Gastrointestinal tract (colon)	Urinary tract infection Pneumonia
Proteus species	Gastrointestinal tract (colon)	Urinary tract infection
Moraxella		
M. catarrhalis	Respiratory	Pneumonia, sinusitis
Haemophilus influenzae	Respiratory	Meningitis, pneumonia, sinusitis, conjunctivitis, otitis media
Pseudomonas species *P. aeruginosa*	Skin	Otitis externa, skin and soft tissue infections
Helicobacter pylori	Gastrointestinal tract	Bacterial gastritis, duodenal ulcers
Primitive Species		
Chlamydia	Not part of normal flora	
C. pneumoniae		Pneumonia
C. trachomatis		Chlamydial cervicitis, pelvic inflammatory disease, urethritis, newborn pneumonia, conjunctivitis/trachoma (neonatal and adult eye disease)
Mycoplasma pneumoniae	Respiratory	Atypical pneumonia

harm other microbes.[2] Drugs produced in a laboratory, either natural derivatives or synthetic, that are capable of killing or suppressing microorganisms are considered antimicrobial. Quinolones are an example of synthetic chemical compounds. Today, the terms *antibiotic* and *antimicrobial* are often used interchangeably.[2]

Antibiotics may have a narrow spectrum of activity effective against a select group of microbes or a broad spectrum effective against a number of types of bacteria. Antibiotics are classified according to similarities in chemical structure, mechanism of action, and antibacterial activity. Pharmaceuticals are also labeled by the US Food and Drug Administration (FDA) according to real and potential perinatal and neonatal effects when prescribed in pregnancy.

The FDA pregnancy categories were initiated to simplify provider selection of medications,

Table 25-3 Common Pathogens: Anaerobic Bacteria

Organism	Common Anatomical Sites of Colonization	Common Infections Caused by Opportunistic Pathogens
	Gram-Positive Anaerobic Rods	
Clostridium		
C. difficile	Gastrointestinal tract	*C. difficile*–associated disease
C. tetani	Genitourinary	Tetanus
Propionibacterium		
P. acnes	Skin (pilosebaceous glands)	Acne
	Gram-Negative Anaerobic Rods	
Bacteroides	Gastrointestinal tract	Wound infection, peritonitis
Prevotella species	Gastrointestinal tract, vagina	Abscesses
Fusobacterium species	Gastrointestinal tract Respiratory	Oral and respiratory infections

but were confusing and misleading when choosing pharmacotherapy. Categories delineating safe drug use in pregnancy are difficult to ascribe primarily because conducting randomized controlled trials in pregnant women is unethical. Scientific data are often not available, particularly for new drugs. Pregnancy drug registries and meta-analyses of retrospective studies provide the most reliable information regarding drug use in pregnancy.

In 2014, the FDA issued a "final rule" regarding regulations governing drug and biological product labeling in pregnancy, labor and delivery, and nursing mothers. This rule eliminates over time the previously used categories A, B, C, D, and X. Drug and biological product information will include a summary of the risks associated with use during pregnancy, birth, and lactation with a discussion of the data and relevant information supporting the summary. Labeling will also include relevant information on pregnancy testing, contraception, and infertility for both males and females with reproductive potential.[9] The new labeling regulation was designed to provide a consistent format for information on drug benefits compared to risks in order to assist healthcare providers in making prescribing decisions and with counseling women on drug use in pregnancy and lactation.[9]

The American Academy of Pediatrics (AAP) and the World Health Organization (WHO) publish recommendations regarding the use of medications during lactation. These organizations review the clinical literature to determine the amount of drug found in breast milk after maternal ingestion, serum levels of the drug in infants following exposure in breast milk, and reported and possible adverse effects on the breast-feeding infant. While the AAP asserts that the degree of caution typically imposed on nursing mothers may be overstated, it is often not based on evidence. In actuality, only a small number of medications are contraindicated. The AAP acknowledges the need for more information on drug excretion in breast milk.[10] When making medication decisions with lactating mothers, the need for the drug is weighed along with the potential breast milk excretion amounts, effects on milk production, infant age and absorption, and potential adverse effects on the infant.[10] The AAP recommends prescribers utilize the most up-to-date information source on lactation when prescribing. The online database LactMed is part of the National Library of Medicine's Toxicology Data Network site and includes the most up-to-date information on medications and lactation.[10]

Classifications of drugs and potential adverse effects cited in this text are limited to commonly reported effects and those serious or toxic effects that are less frequent but warrant precaution or are associated with morbidity and mortality. The antibiotic classes and specific antibiotics discussed in detail in this chapter are those most likely to be used in the primary care setting and include the following:

- Beta-lactams
  - Penicillins
  - Cephalosporins
- Macrolides
- Lincosamides
- Quinolones
- Tetracyclines
- Metronidazole
- Sulfonamides and trimethoprim
- Aminoglycosides
- Nitrofurantoin
- Oxazolidinone

Beta-Lactams (β-Lactams)

The β-lactams include the penicillins and the cephalosporins, which share a common core chemical structure, the four-membered β-lactam ring. Beta-lactams are bactericidal agents that interfere with the synthesis of peptidoglycan, the principal component of the bacterial cell wall, resulting in cell lysis. The β-lactams have little effect on the metabolic and biochemical functioning of human cells, because human cells are eukaryotes and have no cell wall. As a result, there

are few toxic effects associated with the β-lactams; however, the broad-spectrum drugs in this group may disturb the balance of microbiota in the gut, causing gastrointestinal (GI) disturbance.

The most common adverse effects are nausea, vomiting, diarrhea, and headache. Urticaria and skin rash are less common, as are true hypersensitivity reactions, characterized by life-threatening anaphylaxis and respiratory distress. Approximately 1–5 per 10,000 individuals treated with penicillin will have a true anaphylactic response; severe reactions are even less common with the use of cephalosporins.[11] When evaluating hypersensitivity reactions, the clinician should obtain a careful history to distinguish hypersensitivity from common adverse effects. Skin testing may be warranted in clinical situations when the β-lactams are the preferred therapeutic option in order to document a true allergic response. Cross-hypersensitivity between the penicillins and cephalosporins occurs in fewer than 10% of cases and is more common with earlier generation cephalosporins such as cephalexin and ceftriaxone.[11,12] When alternatives are viable, selection of another class of medications is prudent when there is a history of hypersensitivity to one or the other.

The natural penicillins were the first antimicrobial agents to be used in a wide variety of clinical situations. In 1928, Alexander Fleming discovered that a mold of the genus *Penicillium* growing on a culture medium with staphylococci produced an antibacterial substance. It was not until 1940 that Chain and Florey successfully harvested the first natural penicillins from cultures of *Penicillium notatum* and a year later demonstrated their effectiveness in combating bacterial infections in a human subject. Penicillin G became widely available by 1950 and continues to be an effective agent in the treatment of infections caused by many Gram-positive and Gram-negative cocci, anaerobes, and spirochetes such as *Treponema pallidum*. After more than 50 years of clinical use, penicillin remains the drug of choice for infections caused by group A and group B β-hemolytic *Streptococcus* as well as all stages of syphilis.[13] Penicillin G is given parenterally due to its poor absorption from the GI tract. Penicillin VK is available as an oral preparation.

The effectiveness of the β-lactams depends on the presence of actively growing and dividing bacterial cells; their effectiveness is compromised when used in combination with bacteriostatic agents such as erythromycin or the tetracyclines. The mechanism of resistance to this class of drugs is the evolution of β-lactamase-producing bacteria, particularly in Gram-positive organisms such as *Staphylococcus* and *N. gonorrhoeae*, as well as Gram-negative enteric bacilli such as *E. coli*, *Klebsiella* species, and *Proteus* species. Both of the β-lactamases, penicillinase and cephalosporinase, produced by resistant bacteria cleave the β-lactam ring, inactivating the antimicrobial properties of the drug.

The emergence of β-lactamase-producing bacteria led to the development of penicillinase-resistant penicillins, semisynthetic compounds that include cloxacillin, dicloxacillin, oxacillin, methicillin, and nafcillin. These drugs have a narrow spectrum specific to the treatment of infections due to penicillinase-producing *Staphylococcus* such as *S. aureus*.

The aminopenicillins, ampicillin (Omnipen) and amoxicillin (Amoxil), are also semisynthetic derivatives of natural penicillin that have a broader spectrum of activity than the natural penicillins with better coverage of Gram-negative organisms including *E. coli*, *Haemophilus influenzae*, and *Proteus mirabilis*. Amoxicillin has higher bioavailability following oral administration, allowing for a less frequent dosing schedule (three times daily) than ampicillin or penicillin VK (four times daily). The half-life of the aminopenicillins and penicillin VK is 1 hour compared to the 30-minute half-life of penicillin G. Because it is better absorbed than ampicillin, amoxicillin is

less likely to interfere with the balance of intestinal microbiota; therefore, it is less likely to cause the watery diarrhea associated with pseudomembranous colitis.

β-lactamase inhibitors such as clavulanic acid and sulbactam have weak antibacterial activity alone, but when combined with the aminopenicillins extend the spectrum of activity of these drugs to include penicillinase-producing bacteria. Clavulanic acid and sulbactam each contains a β-lactam ring that binds to and inactivates β-lactamase. Augmentin is the combination of 125 milligrams (mg) of clavulanic acid with 250 mg, 500 mg, or 875 mg of amoxicillin. Note that the dose of clavulanic acid is constant in all these preparations; therefore, two 250-mg tablets may not be substituted for one 500-mg tablet. Ampicillin is combined with sulbactam to form the parenteral drug Unasyn.

While β-lactams in combination with aminoglycosides are the antibiotics of choice for *Pseudomonas* infections, many resistant strains are emerging. Antibiotic selection should be determined by the infection site, extent and severity of infection, and community resistance patterns. Selection of appropriate antibiotics may include combination or secondary antibiotics such as a third-generation cephalosporin or ciprofloxacin.[14] Extended-spectrum penicillins, including ticarcillin (Ticar), mezlocillin (Mezlin), and piperacillin (Pipracil), may be useful in combination with the β-lactamase inhibitors to provide broader coverage of β-lactamase-producing organisms.

The cephalosporins are defined in terms of "generation." The first-generation cephalosporins, the earliest developed, are rarely employed as first-line therapy with a few exceptions. First-generation cephalosporins are most active against Gram-positive aerobic cocci and are resistant to the β-lactamases produced by staphylococci. They are effective in treating skin and soft tissue infections caused by staphylococci and streptococci such as impetigo.[2,15] Impetigo may manifest as a primary lesion or a secondary dermatological lesion. For example, the ulcers in a severe primary episode of herpes simplex virus may become impetiginized—secondarily infected with group A β-hemolytic streptococci.

The first-generation parenteral cephalosporin, cefazolin (Ancef, Kefzol), is frequently employed as prophylactic therapy in surgical procedures. Lamont and colleagues explain that antibiotic treatment for cesarean birth is optimized,[16] theoretically and according to earlier research,[17] with the use of cefazolin or ampicillin as single agents. Second- or third-generation cephalosporins or combination drug regimens offer no additional benefit. While the Cochrane Database of Systematic Reviews, the American College of Obstetricians and Gynecologists, and the Centers for Disease Control and Prevention (CDC) make recommendations for the prophylactic use of first-generation cephalosporins with cesarean births,[16] a recent Cochrane review notes that different antibiotic regimens used with cesarean birth had similar infection rate reductions when compared to no antibiotic treatment.[18]

Moving from first to third generation, the cephalosporins exhibit greater Gram-negative coverage at the expense of Gram-positive coverage. Second-generation cephalosporins such as cefaclor (Ceclor), because of their activity against both Gram-positive *Streptococcus* and Gram-negative *Moraxella* and *H. influenzae,* are effective in treating both otitis media and community-acquired pneumonia. The third-generation cephalosporin parenteral ceftriaxone (Rocephin) is an effective single-dose therapy for *N. gonorrhoeae,* given in conjunction with a single dose of azithromycin. As a result of increasing antimicrobial resistance, gonorrhea must be treated with a two-drug regimen; oral cefixime is only recommended for use with azithromycin when ceftriaxone is unavailable, as a result of increasing resistance.[13] Ceftriaxone crosses the blood–brain barrier, making it

an effective therapy for meningitis. In addition to renal excretion, ceftriaxone is 40% eliminated in bile, and unlike other cephalosporins does not require dose adjustment in individuals with renal impairment. Of the cephalosporins, the third-generation cephalosporin ceftazidime (Fortaz, Tazidime) offers the best coverage of *Pseudomonas.*

The β-lactams have variable absorption depending on the specific drug and route of administration. All are widely distributed following oral or parenteral administration. With the exception of some of the third-generation cephalosporins, β-lactams do not cross the blood–brain barrier. Elimination is primarily via the kidneys by tubular secretion. The β-lactams are generally considered to be pregnancy category B and are compatible with breastfeeding according to the AAP.[19] Limited evidence suggests that exposure to amoxicillin or ampicillin, but not the cephalosporins or other penicillins, may be associated with oral clefts in the first trimester and necrotizing enterocolitis in the third trimester. These findings, however, are preliminary and need to be confirmed in future studies.[19] **Table 25-4** lists the β-lactams and their antibacterial activity.

Macrolides

The basic chemical structure of the macrolides, including the antibiotics erythromycin, clarithromycin, and azithromycin, is a lactone ring. The macrolides inhibit protein synthesis and are classified as bacteriostatic agents; however, in some concentrations and in some circumstances, they may be bactericidal. Erythromycin has been in clinical use since the 1950s and is available in several different salts (erythromycin base, erythromycin estolate, erythromycin stearate, and erythromycin ethylsuccinate). Clarithromycin (Biaxin) and azithromycin (Zithromax), the newer macrolides, have longer serum half-lives than erythromycin, permitting a more convenient oral dosing

Table 25-4 Beta-Lactams

Bactericidal Agents	
Penicillins	**Antimicrobial Activity**
Natural penicillins	**Narrow-spectrum:** Gram-positive cocci Gram-negative cocci Some anaerobes Spirochetes
Penicillinase-resistant penicillins: • Cloxacillin, dicloxacillin, oxacillin, methicillin, nafcillin	Penicillinase-producing *Staphylococcus*
Aminopenicillins: • Ampicillin, amoxicillin	**Broad-spectrum:** Gram-positive cocci Better Gram-negative cocci coverage Some anaerobes
Aminopenicillins + β-lactamase inhibitors: • Augmentin (amoxicillin + clavulanic acid) • Unasyn (ampicillin + sulbactam)	Extends the spectrum of the aminopenicillins to include penicillinase-producing bacteria
Extended-spectrum penicillins: • Ticarcillin, mezlocillin, piperacillin	Pseudomonal infections
Cephalosporins	**Antimicrobial Activity**
First generation: • Cephalexin, cefazolin, cefadroxil Second generation: • Cefaclor, cefotetan, cefoxitin, cefprozil, cefuroxime Third generation: • Ceftriaxone, cefixime, ceftazidime, cefdinir, cefditoren, cefotaxime, cefpodoxime, ceftibuten, ceftizoxime	Similar to the penicillins Moving from first to third generation, the cephalosporins exhibit greater Gram-negative coverage and less Gram-positive coverage Ceftazidime covers *Pseudomonas aeruginosa*

schedule. Clarithromycin requires twice-daily dosing, azithromycin is given once daily, and erythromycin is given four times daily. Azithromycin is designed to produce fewer GI symptoms and better absorption than erythromycin, thereby achieving and maintaining higher tissue levels for longer periods.

Macrolides are commonly used in clinical practice and are usually well tolerated. However, side effects and adverse reactions can occur. These drugs are metabolized in the liver, primarily eliminated in bile, and should be used with caution in patients with altered liver function. The macrolides can be prescribed during pregnancy and lactation with the exception of erythromycin estolate,[19] which is more likely to be associated with hepatotoxicity than the other formulations. The most severe and frequent side effects of the macrolides are GI upset. Nausea, vomiting, diarrhea, abdominal cramping, and anorexia are common. Erythromycin interacts with many drugs and may be synergistic or antagonistic. Synergistic interactions cause increased blood levels and toxicity, as with theophylline and lovastatin. Antagonistic interactions occur when administered in conjunction with the penicillins. A thorough history of current medications should be obtained prior to the initiation of any antimicrobial therapy, because all of these agents have the potential to interact with other drugs.

In the primary care setting, the macrolides are most frequently prescribed for upper and lower respiratory tract infections caused by *S. pyogenes, Streptococcus pneumoniae, H. influenzae,* and *Mycoplasma pneumoniae.* Azithromycin in a single one-gram dose is a CDC-recommended treatment for *Chlamydia* in the nonpregnant woman and is used with ceftriaxone for the treatment of gonorrhea.[13] Single-dose azithromycin is the primary recommended treatment for *C. trachomatis* during pregnancy. Amoxicillin and erythromycin base are alternatives, with the caveat that frequent GI side effects may interfere with completing the course of therapy with erythromycin base.[13]

Approved in 2007 and similar to macrolide antibiotics, ketolide antibiotics inhibit bacterial protein synthesis. In contrast to macrolides, ketolides are active against macrolide-resistant bacteria. Telithromycin is the only FDA-approved ketolide antibiotic and has only one indication, community-acquired pneumonia caused by *S. pneumoniae* that is penicillin and macrolide

resistant. This single indication is due to the high risk of severe adverse effects including GI disturbances and liver damage.[2] **Table 25-5** lists the macrolides and their antibacterial activity.

Lincosamides

Lincomycin, the first lincosamide, was isolated from the mold *Streptomyces lincolnensis.* Clindamycin, a derivative of lincomycin, is formed by the replacement of a hydroxyl group with a chlorine atom. Due to its superior antibacterial activity and better oral bioavailability, clindamycin has essentially replaced lincomycin in clinical use.[20]

Like the macrolides, clindamycin is bacteriostatic and inhibits bacterial protein synthesis. It has a broad spectrum of activity that includes streptococci, staphylococci, and *Mycoplasma hominis.* Clindamycin does not cover Gram-positive enterococci or the aerobic Gram-negative bacilli such as *E. coli, Klebsiella, Proteus,* or *H. influenzae.*

Clindamycin is often employed in treating mixed anaerobic infections. It is effective against most anaerobes with the exception of *Clostridium difficile.* Among the broad-spectrum antibiotics, clindamycin poses the most significant risk of *C. difficile*-associated disease (CDAD) or what was formerly called pseudomembranous colitis.[2] Clindamycin effectively destroys

Table 25-5 Macrolides

Bacteriostatic Agents	
Macrolide	**Antimicrobial Activity**
First generation: • Erythromycin base, erythromycin ethyl succinate	Spectrum similar to the penicillins: Gram-positive and Gram-negative aerobic bacteria *Chlamydia trachomatis*
Second generation: • Azithromycin, clarithromycin, fidaxomicin	Spectrum similar to the penicillins: Gram-positive and Gram-negative aerobic bacteria Azithromycin active against chlamydia and gonorrhea Fidaxomicin used for treatment of *C. difficile*

competing microorganisms, allowing *C. difficile* to proliferate, leading to profuse watery diarrhea. *C. difficile*–associated disease (CDAD) is a life-threatening condition and should be suspected when an individual presents with profuse watery diarrhea up to 6 weeks following a clindamycin regimen or while taking any broad-spectrum antibiotic.[2] While CDAD is related to antibiotic use and caused by the destruction of good gut bacteria, infection results from external contamination. Contamination is more likely in hospitals or long-term care settings. Treatment consists of discontinuing current antibiotic therapy and initiating treatment with fidaxomicin (a narrow-spectrum macrolide approved in 2011 for *C. difficile* diarrhea), vancomycin, or metronidazole (discussed later). Likewise, fecal transplants may be indicated as treatment.[2] While the cure rate with fidaxomicin is higher, vancomycin and metronidazole drugs are effective in CDAD.[2] Metronidazole and fidaxomicin are the first-line therapies to reduce the risk of encouraging the development of vancomycin-resistant organisms. Additionally, metronidazole is less expensive than vancomycin. Fluid and electrolyte replacement should be initiated, and the individual observed for improvement of symptoms.

Clindamycin is available in oral, topical, and parenteral preparations. Following oral or parenteral administration, clindamycin is rapidly distributed in tissue and bone, which makes it particularly useful in treating staphylococcal infections of the bones and joints. The half-life of clindamycin is 21 hours; it is partially metabolized in the liver and excreted in urine and bile. Like the macrolides, oral or topical preparations of clindamycin are considered to be safe in pregnancy.[13,19] Topical clindamycin cream and oral clindamycin, in addition to metronidazole, are effective in the treatment of bacterial vaginosis in pregnant and nonpregnant women.[13] LactMed considers clindamycin to have the potential to cause adverse effects on the breastfed infant's GI flora and recommends using an alternative medicine when breastfeeding.[21] However, the AAP classifies clindamycin as being compatible with breastfeeding, because bloody stools were noted only in one small case series of two breastfeeding infants whose mothers were taking clindamycin. In both cases, symptoms resolved completely and rapidly with cessation of breastfeeding.[19]

Fluoroquinolones

The fluoroquinolones (also referred to as quinolones) are bactericidal. They impair synthesis and repair of bacterial DNA by inhibiting DNA gyrase. They can be categorized by generations. The first-generation quinolone, nalidixic acid, was introduced in 1963 for the treatment of urinary tract infection (UTI). Due to rapid absorption and renal elimination following oral administration, this drug does not exhibit systemic effects. It is no longer used due to the prevalence of resistant organisms.

Second-generation (ciprofloxacin, ofloxacin) and third-generation (levofloxacin) fluoroquinolones are synthetic fluorinated analogs of nalidixic acid. Following oral administration, they are well absorbed from the gut with high bioavailability. Ciprofloxacin (Cipro) and ofloxacin (Floxin) are active against most Gram-negative aerobic rods, including drug-resistant *Pseudomonas* and *Enterobacter* species. They do not have effective anaerobic activity and have poor Gram-positive coverage with the exceptions of *Bacillus anthracis* and the Gram-positive aerobic rod, *Chlamydia* species. Common urinary pathogens including *E. coli* and *Klebsiella* are sensitive to ciprofloxacin; likewise, most bacteria-causing enteritis such as *Salmonella*, *Shigella*, *Campylobacter jejuni*, and *E. coli* are sensitive to ciprofloxacin.[2] Quinolones are no longer recommended for *Neisseria gonorrhoeae* due to resistance.[13]

The third-generation quinolone, levofloxacin (Levaquin), has broad Gram-positive and

Gram-negative coverage with better absorption, bioavailability (99%), and longer half-life than the second-generation drugs. It is given once daily and is excreted unchanged in urine. Levofloxacin is useful in treating upper and lower respiratory infections (sinusitis, pneumonia, infections of the skin and skin structures, UTIs, and bacterial prostatitis). Due to its expense and the propensity for resistance to develop in the quinolones, it is best reserved for infections that are resistant to other drug therapies or when an agent with its broad spectrum of activity is clearly indicated. Levofloxacin is a good choice for highly resistant strains of *S. pneumoniae*.[2]

Absorption of the quinolones is impaired in the presence of divalent or trivalent cations (magnesium, calcium, aluminum, zinc). Antacids, vitamins, and dairy products containing these substances should be avoided for several hours before and after administration. While ofloxacin is excreted almost entirely via the kidney, ciprofloxacin is metabolized in the liver and partially excreted via the biliary route.

The most common side effects of the quinolones are mild GI upset, including nausea, vomiting, and diarrhea (with potential for *C. difficile*); dizziness; headache; rash; photosensitivity; and exacerbation of the effects of caffeine. Quinolones have been associated with prolonged QT interval, exacerbation of myasthenia gravis, and spontaneous tendinopathies like ruptures of the Achilles tendon.[2] In 2013, the FDA issued a safety warning for fluoroquinolones as a class regarding the risk of permanent peripheral neuropathy as a result of oral or injected medication use.[22] Persons who report tingling or loss of sensation in their extremities should stop their medication immediately and not be rechallenged with another quinolone. Further, many of the newer quinolones have been withdrawn from the market due to severe side effects, ranging from liver and cardiac damage to hypoglycemia.[23]

In May 2016, the FDA advised against the use of fluoroquinolones as the first-line drug for acute respiratory infections such as sinusitis and bronchitis and for acute urinary tract infections, when another drug is available for use. The safety report noted that use is associated with increased risks of "disabling and potentially permanent serious side effects that can occur together. . . . [involving] the tendons, muscles, joints, nerves, and central nervous system."[24] For this reason, despite their effectiveness, these medications should only be used when there is not another effective medication available, whether as a result of resistance or individual intolerance of other medications.[24]

Studies in young animals have shown damage to growing cartilage. Because of the potential for irreversible arthropathies in children and effects on juvenile cartilage and joint development from exposure to the fluoroquinolones, fluoroquinolones historically have not been recommended in individuals younger than 18 years.[25,26] In 2004, ciprofloxacin and levofloxacin were approved for use in children for postexposure management of inhalation anthrax. Likewise, in 2004, ciprofloxacin was approved for use in children (1–17 years of age) for complicated UTI and pyelonephritis. As use of fluoroquinolones increases in children, the controversy continues and more research is needed.[25,26]

Fluoroquinolones are currently classified as pregnancy category C antibiotics; adverse effects have been seen in animal studies, but the evidence in human studies is difficult to interpret.[19] In 2009, Crider and colleagues, in a National Birth Defects Prevention Study, demonstrated a link between quinolone exposures and tetralogy of Fallot defect in 42 case mothers compared to 14 control mothers.[27] However, no discernable pattern could be identified between specific birth defects and quinolone use in most studies reporting an association between quinolones and birth defects. Further, the overall risk appears to be small, because the majority of studies have not reported a link between quinolone use and birth defects.[19,28] However, given the controversy surrounding their safety, authoritative recommendations vary. Some authorities recommend cautious use only in the first trimester and others recommend the avoidance of the quinolones in pregnancy and the use of other safer products if possible.[19] When a fluoroquinolone is the best choice for treatment, their use is reasonable. As an example of such an indication, the FDA identifies ciprofloxacin use as appropriate in pregnant women exposed to anthrax.[29] Fluoroquinolones are considered compatible with breastfeeding according to LactMed. It is theorized that the calcium in the milk may block quinolone absorption in the newborn; however, there is little evidence to support this premise.[21] Table 25-6 lists the quinolones and their antibacterial activity.

Glycopeptide

Vancomycin (Vancocin), a glycopeptide in a class of its own, is highly effective against Gram-positive bacteria. It is used intravenously for the treatment of C. difficile; methicillin-resistant Staphylococcus aureus (MRSA); serious skin, blood, or bone infections; endocarditis; and resistant pneumococci infections. Due to its efficacy against many resistant microbes and the need to decrease the risk that bacteria will develop resistance, its use is reserved for circumstances in which there is no alternative.[2] Vancomycin is not absorbed from the GI tract and, as a result, is not useful in the primary care setting except as a therapeutic alternative to metronidazole in the treatment of C. difficile infections. Vancomycin effectively covers C. difficile in the gut; cost and the potential for resistance mean that it is not a first-line therapy. Vancomycin is bactericidal, inhibiting cell wall synthesis and associated with the adverse reactions of angioedema, hypotension, and red neck syndrome. Although vancomycin has been associated with ototoxicity and nephrotoxicity, in its newer more purified forms toxicity is rarely seen. It is considered compatible with pregnancy and lactation; however, only limited human data are available on its safety in breastfeeding.[19]

Table 25-6 Fluoroquinolones

Bactericidal Agents	
Quinolone	Antimicrobial Activity
First generation: • Nalidixic acid, others	Gram-negative organisms associated with urinary tract infection
Second generation: • Ciprofloxacin, ofloxacin	Gram-negative aerobic rods: Pseudomonas species Enterobacter species Chlamydia trachomatis Neisseria gonorrhoeae Bacillus anthracis
Third generation: • Levofloxacin	Gram-positive and Gram-negative aerobes
Fourth generation: • Moxifloxacin	S. pneumoniae (including multidrug-resistant strains), Haemophilus influenzae, Moraxella catarrhalis, Mycoplasma pneumoniae, Chlamydia pneumoniae, or Klebsiella pneumoniae

Tetracyclines

The tetracyclines are broad-spectrum bacteriostatic agents that inhibit bacterial protein synthesis. Four fused cyclic rings form the common chemical structure of tetracycline, doxycycline, and minocycline. Doxycycline and minocycline have several advantages over tetracycline. The longer half-life of both allows a less frequent dosing schedule than tetracycline, and food, milk, and antacids do not impair absorption. Unlike tetracycline, doxycycline and minocycline are excreted in bile and are good choices for individuals with impaired renal function.

Common adverse effects of the tetracyclines include GI disturbance and photosensitivity. Minocycline has been associated with dizziness and vertigo. The tetracyclines are not recommended in pregnancy and not recommended for children younger than 8 years of age.[19] They chelate (bind to) calcium ions in the tissues that are calcifying at the time of administration. Tetracyclines have the potential to cause permanent discoloration of the teeth and can inhibit bone growth, causing deformities. Because tetracyclines are inactivated by calcium, concurrent administration with calcium-containing food is not recommended. Because they are excreted in breast milk in low concentrations and serum levels in breastfeeding infants exposed to these medications are undetectable, the tetracyclines are considered compatible with breastfeeding.[30]

Tetracyclines were introduced in 1948. Their spectrum of activity includes many Gram-positive aerobes including spirochetes, Gram-negative aerobes including *Mycoplasma* and *Chlamydia*, and some anaerobes such as bacteroides species. Increasing resistance and the availability of alternative drugs have undermined their clinical usefulness. They do remain an effective alternative for some conditions in individuals with penicillin allergy. Doxycycline is an alternative treatment for syphilis in nonpregnant persons,

Table 25-7 Tetracyclines

Bacteriostatic Agents	
Tetracycline	**Antimicrobial Activity**
Tetracycline	Many Gram-positive aerobic bacteria including spirochetes
Doxycycline	Many Gram-negative aerobic bacteria including *Mycoplasma* and *Chlamydia*
Minocycline	Some anaerobes including *Bacteroides* species

penicillin-allergic individuals, and for chlamydial infections, but is no longer a viable treatment option for gonorrheal infections due to resistance.[13] Minocycline is an effective treatment for acne and rosacea.[2] **Table 25-7** lists the tetracyclines and their scope of activity.

Nitroimidazoles

Metronidazole and tinidazole are the only drugs in this class currently available in the United States. The spectrum of activity includes most anaerobic bacteria, including *C. difficile* and some protozoa, notably *Trichomonas*. Either metronidazole or tinidazole is recommended for *Trichomoniasis vaginalis* infections. While tinidazole is more expensive, it has a longer half-life and fewer GI side effects, and evidence suggests it is equivalent or superior to metronidazole for *Trichomonas* therapy.[13] If persons are unable to tolerate or are allergic to tinidazole or metronidazole, they must be desensitized prior to initiation of treatment. There have been reported cases of *Trichomonas* resistance to metronidazole. Because *Trichomonas* can persist in the bladder and gut, systemic treatment and partner therapy are required.[13]

Tinidazole is only available for oral use; oral, parenteral, topical, and vaginal preparations of metronidazole are available. Topical metronidazole

is a treatment for rosacea (cystic acne). Oral
metronidazole has almost 100% bioavailability
and is the treatment of choice for *C. difficile* diarrhea. Metronidazole given either vaginally or
orally is effective treatment for the mixed anaerobic vaginal colonization associated with bacterial
vaginosis.

Even though there are no data demonstrating mutagenic effects in humans, metronidazole
and tinidazole are not recommended to be used
in the first trimester of pregnancy.[19] Of the two,
metronidazole is preferred later in pregnancy
because of the paucity of safety data on tinidazole in pregnancy.[19] Vaginal preparations may be
used without concern during breastfeeding, but
oral nitroimidazoles should be avoided. The AAP
classifies these products as having potential toxicity during breastfeeding based on limited human data. Women taking metronidazole should
pump and discard breast milk for 24 hours
post-administration.[19]

The nitroimidazoles have no activity against
aerobic bacteria, which increases their advantage
in treating bacterial vaginosis.[2] Gram-positive
rods, hydrogen peroxide–producing *Lactobacillus*
species are largely responsible for maintaining
the vaginal ecosystem by promoting an acidic
environment. Bacterial vaginosis occurs when
colonization by lactobacilli is disrupted, the
vaginal pH rises, and anaerobic bacteria thrive.
Lactobacilli-sparing treatment with metronidazole may allow for recolonization and a return to
the natural balance of flora in the genital tract.
Table 25-8 lists the nitroimidazoles and their
scope of activity.

Sulfonamides and Trimethoprim

The first antimicrobial agents available for treatment of systemic bacterial infections were the
sulfonamides.[2] These synthetic agents, first formulated in 1932, are no longer employed as
single agents due to the evolution of resistant

Table 25-8 Nitroimidazoles

Bacteriostatic Agents	
Nitroimidazole	**Antimicrobial Activity**
Metronidazole Tinidazole	Most anaerobic bacteria including *Clostridium*

microbes, the prevalence of hypersensitivity reactions, and the availability of alternative drugs
with a similar spectrum of activity and fewer
potential side effects. When sulfamethoxazole is
combined with trimethoprim (TMP-SMX), the
result is a drug with enhanced Gram-positive and
Gram-negative coverage and less risk of resistance
than when either drug is used alone.[2]

Sulfamethoxazole and trimethoprim are bacteriostatic agents alone and bactericidal in combination. Because each drug interferes with folate
synthesis in a different metabolic step, the combination has a synergistic effect. Common side
effects of the sulfonamides include nausea, vomiting, headache, and allergic reactions. Hypersensitivity to the sulfonamides may be severe and life
threatening. Therapy should be discontinued with
the onset of skin rash, sore throat, fever, cough,
shortness of breath, or any signs of adverse reaction. Increasing fluid intake during the course of
therapy is recommended to prevent crystalluria.
The sulfonamides along with quinolones, nitrofurantoin, and cotrimoxazole have been associated with hemolytic anemia in individuals with
glucose-6-phosphate dehydrogenase (G6PD) deficiency, including the term fetus.[31]

TMP-SMX is rapidly absorbed following
oral administration with peak blood levels at
1–4 hours. Elimination is primarily through the
kidney. Due to this drug's potential to interfere
with folic acid metabolism, it should be avoided
in individuals with folate deficiency (megaloblastic anemia). In a large case-control study

(N = 13,155), Crider and colleagues reported that the sulfonamides were associated with increased risk of a number of birth defects including anencephaly (adjusted odds ration [AOR] = 3.4; 95% confidence interval [CI], 1.3–8.8), hypoplastic left heart syndrome (AOR = 3.2; 95% CI, 1.3–7.6), coarctation of the aorta (AOR = 2.7; 95% CI, 1.3–5.6), choanal atresia (AOR = 8.0; 95% CI, 2.7–23.5), transverse limb deficiency (AOR = 2.5; 95% CI, 1.0–5.9), and diaphragmatic hernia (AOR = 2.4; 95% CI, 1.1–5.4).[27] However, in their analysis of the totality of the evidence, Briggs and Freeman conclude that other factors, in particular the combination with trimethoprim, may account for these associations. They suggest that TMP-SMX should be avoided in the last trimester of pregnancy.[19] TMP-SMX has low concentrations in breast milk. While rare toxicities have been reported in nursing infants, it is considered compatible with breastfeeding by the AAP.[19] Other authorities suggest it is safer to use after the newborn period.[32] TMP-SMX should be avoided while breastfeeding G6PD-deficient infants.[32]

Aminoglycosides

Rarely employed in the primary care setting, the parenteral aminoglycosides, gentamicin, amikacin, streptomycin, and tobramycin are reserved for severe systemic infections due to Gram-negative aerobes resistant to other medications. The aminoglycosides carry a black box warning related to the potential for an associated high risk of neurotoxicity, ototoxicity, nephrotoxicity, and neuromuscular blockade.[2] Toxicity is related to serum levels and duration of therapy. The narrow therapeutic window for aminoglycosides requires monitoring of blood levels. The aminoglycosides are bactericidal agents that inhibit bacterial protein synthesis. Gentamicin is frequently used in conjunction with penicillin or vancomycin, a combination that has a synergistic effect and increases the efficacy of gentamicin. Elimination is via the kidney. The use of gentamycin in pregnancy is classified as being low risk based on human data.[19] Due to poor drug-to-breast milk transference and poor newborn absorption, the aminoglycosides are considered compatible with breastfeeding. Infant monitoring for diarrhea or candidiasis is recommended.[21]

Oral preparations of neomycin and puromycin are poorly absorbed, so their use is limited to a few specific intestinal infections. Neomycin is used in conjunction with erythromycin to reduce bowel microbiota prior to elective colorectal surgery, and puromycin is useful for a local effect against some intestinal protozoa.[2] Neomycin is also available as topical treatment for infections of the skin, eyes, and ears (Neosporin, Cortisporin). **Table 25-9** lists aminoglycosides and their scope of activity.

Table 25-9 Aminoglycosides

Bactericidal Agents	
Aminoglycoside	**Antimicrobial Activity**
Gentamicin, amikacin, streptomycin, tobramycin, neomycin	Penicillin/methicillin-resistant strains of *Staphylococcus* Gram-negative aerobic bacteria including *Enterobacter*, *E. coli*, *Klebsiella*, *Proteus*, *Pseudomonas*
Puromycin	Intestinal protozoa

Nitrofurantoin

Nitrofurantoin, available as microcrystals (Furadantin), macrocrystals (Macrodantin), or monohydrate/macrocrystals (Macrobid), is a broad-spectrum urinary antiseptic active against most organisms responsible for UTIs with the exception of *Proteus* species. *Proteus* species create alkaline urine that inhibits the activity of nitrofurantoin, a drug that works best in an acid environment. The absorption, metabolism, and renal excretion of nitrofurantoin are so efficient that there are no systemic antimicrobial effects and few host side effects other than mild GI upset; occasionally, severe pulmonary toxicity is seen in some individuals.[33] While magnesium interferes with the absorption of all forms of nitrofurantoin and macrocrystal forms have fewer gastric side effects due to slower absorption, all forms are equally effective.[2] Nitrofurantoin in low concentrations has bacteriostatic effects and at high concentrations is bactericidal. Bacteria DNA is damaged by the enzymatic conversion of nitrofurantoin to a reactive form.[2]

As with the sulfonamides, cotrimoxazole, and quinolones, nitrofurantoin is associated with hemolytic anemia in individuals with G6PD deficiency, including neonates exposed in utero.[31] An estimated 400 million individuals worldwide are affected by G6PD deficiency, the most common enzyme deficiency.[34] Hemolytic anemia and prolonged neonatal jaundice are the most serious associated conditions with G6PD deficiency.[35] Nitrofurantoin should be avoided after 36 weeks' gestation due to potential fetal risks of hemolytic anemia, which can occur in both healthy fetuses and those with G6PD deficiency.[19] It is actively transported into breast milk and has been rarely associated with adverse events in breastfeeding infants.[19] The AAP considers breastfeeding to be compatible with nitrofurantoin.[19] Nitrofurantoin should be avoided in newborns affected by G6PD deficiency or who have prolonged, unexplained

Table 25-10 Nitrofurantoin

Urinary Antiseptic	
Nitrofurantoin	Antimicrobial Activity
Microcrystals (Furadantin) Macrocrystals (Macrodantin) Monohydrate/ macrocrystals (Macrobid)	Most organisms responsible for urinary tract infection including *E. coli*, *Klebsiella*, *Enterococcus*, and *Enterobacter*, except *Proteus* species

jaundice.[35] **Table 25-10** lists nitrofurantoins and their scope of activity.

Oxazolidinone

Linezolid was developed in the 1990s and is the first in a class of oxazolidinone antibiotics active with aerobic Gram-positive bacteria. Pathogens receptive to linezolid include *Enterococcus faecium* (vancomycin-sensitive and -resistant strains) and *Enterococcus faecalis* (vancomycin-resistant strains), *S. aureus* (methicillin-sensitive and -resistant strains), *Staphylococcus epidermis* (methicillin-resistant strains), and *Staphylococcus pneumoniae* (penicillin-sensitive and -resistant strains). Linezolid is bacteriostatic and uniquely inhibits protein synthesis. The mechanism for inhibiting protein synthesis assures no cross-resistance with other agents. Resistance to linezolid is rare and if it occurs is secondary to prolonged treatment for vancomycin-resistant enterococci (VRE). Uses are reserved for severe pneumonias and skin and skin structure infections resistant to other antibiotics.[2]

Linezolid is available in oral tablets, powder for suspension, and intravenous solution and is tolerated well. It should be used with caution in pregnancy. There is no information to estimate risk or safety during pregnancy or breastfeeding, and should be avoided pending further study.[19] The most frequent side effects are gastric disturbances, and the most severe is myelosuppression. Rare side effects are optic and peripheral neuropathies. Severity of side effect risk is correlated to duration of treatment. Persons with phenylketonuria should not take linezolid, and caution should be used with persons on selective serotonin reuptake inhibitors.[2]

Antiviral Medications

Viruses are obligate parasites employing the biochemistry of the host cells in order to live, grow, and replicate. Because of this cellular "hijacking" by viruses, it is difficult to develop safe and effective antiviral drugs without potential risks to the host. Antiviral medications biochemically interfere with viral reproduction and may act at any of several points in the replication cycle. These include at entry of the viral particle into the host cell, replication of the RNA or DNA, attachment to the cellular genetic structure, protein synthesis, or detachment from the host cell (**Figure 25-1**).

When compared to the advances made in the treatment of bacterial infections, treatment of viral infections is limited.[2] Antiviral drugs are available for the treatment of influenza and respiratory syncytial virus, hepatitis B and C, varicella zoster

Figure 25-1 Viral lifecycle.

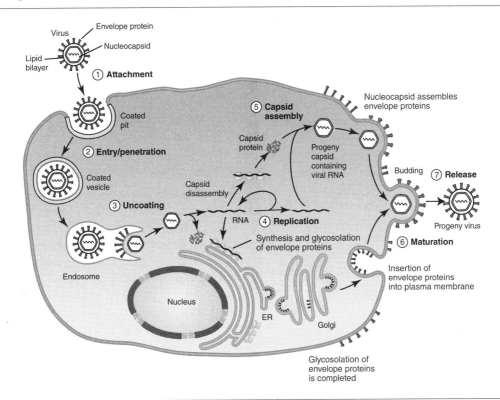

virus (VZV), herpes simplex virus (HSV), and human immunodeficiency virus (HIV). Most are addressed elsewhere in this text; the treatment of herpes viruses causing chickenpox, shingles, and orolabial or genital herpes simplex is discussed here.

Infections from HSV can manifest on the mouth, skin, or genitalia; VZV is responsible for herpes zoster (shingles) and varicella (chickenpox). Acyclovir, valacyclovir, and famciclovir are used systemically and topically to treat viruses from the herpes virus group. Acyclovir is less bioavailable than either of the other, newer medications, which are prodrugs—they are metabolized into an active form once absorbed into the body. However, it is also the least expensive and often used as the first-line treatment, as long as the patient can tolerate the more frequent dosing schedule. Acyclovir is also the only one available for intravenous use.

Use of these drugs is most common in HSV. Oral herpes lesions can be treated during both primary and secondary infections with acyclovir, valacyclovir, or famciclovir. Childhood varicella in healthy children does not generally require treatment; adult infection is more likely to be severe and has increased risk for varicella pneumonia. Because treatment will reduce risk of complications and shorten the acute course, use of acyclovir is recommended.[36]

Acyclovir has few side effects—primarily nausea, diarrhea, or headache. Long-term or high-dose use can produce more severe effects. When used intravenously, nephrotoxicity can occur, as can neurologic symptoms.[2] Acyclovir is considered safe to use in pregnancy, lactation, and with neonates. Approximately 1% of the typical infant acyclovir dose transfers to breast milk and is not associated with adverse effects.[37]

Ganciclovir is a synthetic antiviral drug approved for use with the herpes virus, cytomegalovirus (CMV). It is used only in immunocompromised persons for the prevention and treatment of CMV and is associated with severe adverse reactions including thrombocytopenia and granulocytopenia. Ganciclovir is teratogenic and embryotoxic in laboratory studies and potentially in humans. Bioavailability is low but increased by 4–5% if taken with food. Even though the prodrug valganciclovir has greater bioavailability, it retains the same risks as ganciclovir for mutagenesis. Neither drug is recommended in pregnancy.[2] However, other authorities suggest it can be used to treat life-threatening illness or to prevent fetal infection, because CMV infection significantly increases the risk of malformations in exposed fetuses.[19] Pregnancy should be avoided until 90 days after ganciclovir use is discontinued.[2]

Antifungal Medications

Infections that are mycotic in origin can be systemic or superficial and opportunistic or nonopportunistic. Antifungal agents used to treat symptomatic mycotic infections include polyene antibiotics, azoles, echinocandins, and flucytosine, a pyrimidine analog used in combination with amphotericin B. Nystatin and amphotericin B are polyene antibiotics considered to be broad-spectrum antifungals useful in common systemic fungal infections.

Polyene Antibiotics

Nystatin and amphotericin B, the oldest antifungal drugs, are broad-spectrum polyenes. Binding to fungal cell membranes, polyenes cause transmembrane ionic leakage and fungal death.[38] Amphotericin B continues to be a potent systemic antifungal used for serious infections. Nystatin is commonly used for treatment of topical *Candida* infections, although it is less efficacious against other fungal types.

Azoles

Itraconazole, fluconazole, voriconazole, and ketoconazole are broad-spectrum antifungal drugs that provide a less toxic oral systemic fungal treatment alternative to amphotericin B. The azoles, exemplified by the prototype itraconazole, disrupt the fungal cell wall causing increased permeability and loss of cellular integrity. Consequently, while inhibiting fungal cytochrome P450–dependent enzymes, the azoles also inhibit host cytochrome P450 enzymes, resulting in the potential to increase serum levels of various other drugs.[2] For superficial mycotic infections, clotrimazole; ketoconazole; miconazole; the newer econazole, oxiconazole; and sertaconazole may be employed.

Itraconazole treats blastomycosis, histoplasmosis, paracoccidioidomycosis, and sporotrichosis and is an acceptable alternative to amphotericin B for aspergillosis, candidiasis, and coccidioidomycosis. Itraconazole is also useful for superficial mycotic infections. Fluconazole can be used as a single-dose oral regimen following topical therapy for vulvovaginal candidiasis and is likewise recommended prophylactically on a weekly basis for recurrent vulvovaginal candidiasis. Topically, oral candidiasis is treated with nystatin, clotrimazole, or miconazole. In addition to GI symptoms, rash, headache, and edema, azoles can cause hepatic injury, have multiple drug interactions, and have a negative cardiac inotropic effect leading to reductions in cardiac ejection fraction. Ketoconazole may occasionally cause severe and fatal hepatic necrosis.[2]

The choice of antifungal agents is altered in pregnancy and lactation. Amphotericin B remains the medication of choice for systemic fungal infections during pregnancy due to the teratogenic and embryotoxic effects of azoles in both human and animal data.[38] It is the safest systemic antifungal drug and is FDA category B.[38] Although amphotericin B is theoretically considered acceptable with breastfeeding, no information exists on milk excretion levels.[38] Of the systemic antifungals, fluconazole is one of the most frequently used agents in nonpregnant women. It is considered safe to use for treatment of systemic candidiasis in infants and in lower doses for children, but is a category D for pregnancy at > 300 mg total dose. It may also be used during lactation, because only low amounts are excreted into breast milk.[39]

Topical agents are preferred for treatment of vaginitis and fungal skin infections. Topical azoles and terbinafine are considered safe in pregnancy. Nystatin, used topically and orally for candidiasis, is considered pregnancy category A because of poor absorption. Emerging data suggest that nystatin be avoided during 8–14 weeks' gestation based on possible associations with hypospadias,[38] although in their analysis, Briggs and Freeman state that nystatin is safe in pregnancy.[19] Topical use of nystatin is considered safe with breastfeeding, but paraffin-based nystatin ointments on the nipples should be avoided.[40,41]

Additional Antifungal Medications

Echinocandins (caspofungin, micafungin, and anidulafungin) are the newest class of antifungals used to treat systemic mycosis. Echinocandins act by disrupting the fungal cell wall and are virtually equivalent in therapeutic potential. Echinocandins are broad-spectrum drugs that are active against *Aspergillus* and *Candida* species. Caspofungin is affected by cytochrome P450 hepatic inducers and, consequently, may need dosage adjustments. Micafungin has demonstrated some capacity for elevating liver enzymes, and anidulafungin may induce histamine reactions and liver damage.[2] In the laboratory, echinocandins are embryotoxic and teratogenic in animals. While the echinocandins are considered to be pregnancy category C, there are no available human data, and there is evidence of harm in animal studies. Therefore, the echinocandins are best avoided in pregnancy.[38]

Griseofulvin is used in superficial mycosis and disrupts fungal mitosis, affecting only actively growing fungi. Griseofulvin is used for dermatophytic infections of the skin, hair, and nails. It is not effective with *Candida* species. Absorption of griseofulvin is increased with concomitant ingestion of fat. This drug may cause hepatic toxicity and the induction of increased metabolism of drugs taken concurrently.[2] Griseofulvin should be avoided in pregnancy and lactation because of limited data on its safety in pregnancy.[19] While the limited studies to date in humans do not demonstrate harm, there is evidence of embryotoxicity and teratogenicity in animals.[38] Males are advised to wait 6 months post-administration prior to fathering a child.[42]

Antimicrobial Resistance

The WHO conducts worldwide surveillance on the extent and severity of the risks from antibiotic resistance.[5] The WHO has identified antimicrobial resistance as a current global crisis with international implications. In the United States, antibiotic resistance is considered one of the most urgent public health problems with an associated economic burden of $60 billion per year.[1] Each year in the United States, approximately 2 million people are impacted by antibiotic resistance, with at least 23,000 related deaths.[43] In response to this growing concern, many nations have implemented programs to combat the threat of emerging microbes or new "superbugs" that are impervious to even the most powerful drugs.

Antimicrobial resistance refers to the natural evolutionary process of genetic mutation that results in microbes becoming immune to the effects of antimicrobial drugs. Genetic mutation results in survival of microbes resistant to antibiotics. Microbes have acquired the capacity to share that resistance vertically and horizontally with other microbes. Vertical movement of resistance is transference of resistance when microbes meet in the human GI tract or in biofilms, which are thick, gelatin-like layers that surround bacteria to

protect them. Resistance is spread horizontally with gene sharing in a process likened to microbial sexual activity. Natural selection favors the propagation of resistant gene strains.[4,5] The process of resistance is accelerated with widespread use of antibiotics. The more antibiotics are used, the quicker resistance will develop. Likewise, the lifespan of each antibiotic will decrease. The broader the spectrum of the antibiotic, the broader the scope is for resistance.[4]

Contributing Factors

Microbial resistance is the natural outcome of overexposure to antibiotics in humans and food-producing animals.[4,5] It represents extensive antibiotic overuse, oftentimes due to the lack of discretionary prescribing by clinicians. This is compounded by unreasonable expectations for antibiotics by the public. Since the advent of antibiotics in the 1940s, antibiotics have been considered wonder drugs and frequently viewed as a panacea for infections.[4,5] Population-based data from 2000–2010 have shown that overall antibiotic prescribing has remained stable or has decreased for children, adolescents, and adults, but has increased 30% for those over 65 years of age and doubled for those over 80 years.[1] Persons visiting their primary care providers in 2010 were more likely to receive an antibiotic than they would have in 2000.[1,44] Prescriptions of broad-spectrum antibiotics have increased across all age groups,[1] with azithromycin being the most frequently prescribed antibiotic.[3] While it is well known that the overuse of broad-spectrum antibiotics contributes to resistance, prescriptions of broad-spectrum antibiotics have more than doubled from 2000 to 2010. In 2010, broad-spectrum prescriptions represented 46% of antibiotics prescribed.[1] Overprescribing results in the inappropriate use of antibiotics by the public and is related, to a great extent, to the treatment of viral upper respiratory, sinus, and ear infections and uncomplicated cystitis in both children and adults.

Selecting the wrong drug in the treatment of infection is another common error favoring the development of antibiotic resistance. As best practices change with emerging research, healthcare providers need to be aware of and incorporate these changes in prescribing patterns. For example, while current recommendations for acute sinusitis have changed from amoxicillin to amoxicillin-clavulanate, prescribing patterns show that prescribing broader-spectrum quinolones and macrolides as first-line treatments is common.[44]

Healthcare providers often prescribe antibiotics because it is a stated or implied wish of the patient. Indiscriminate use of antibiotics comes, in part, from a lack of knowledge. In a systematic review and meta-analysis of 26 and 24 studies, respectively, on public perceptions of antibiotics, Gualano and colleagues found that more than half of those surveyed did not know antibiotics were not useful for viruses, and only 59% expressed awareness of antibiotic resistance.[45] Almost half of those surveyed reported stopping antibiotics once they felt better. This is consistent with earlier studies and reports from Europe concluding that misguided beliefs and expectations are associated with a lack of awareness of the danger of antibiotic overuse.[46,47]

Humans do not consume the majority of antibiotics sold in the United States. Most of the antibiotics sold are for farm feedlot use for industrial food animals such as chickens, turkeys, pigs, dairy and beef cattle, and farmed fish. Of all antibiotics sold in the United States, 70–80% are for optimizing feed efficiency in animals for food. Antibiotics are used subtherapeutically for growth promotion of animals in order to fatten them up and increase production.[4,48,49] Animal and human use of antibiotics has resulted in antibiotic residues in the US food and water supplies.[4,50]

Microbial resistance is amplified in humans due to antibiotic residue in animal-related food products. There is a growing body of evidence relating the uses of antibiotics in animals, therapeutically, prophylactically, and as growth enhancers, to the progression of antibiotic resistance in humans.[4,5,51] WHO recognizes the relationship between the applications of antibiotics in animals as a contributing factor in global antibiotic resistance in humans.[5] In response, the European Union has banned certain antibiotic growth promoters in animals. The CDC acknowledged that the use of antibiotics as growth promoters in animals is unnecessary. However, even though the FDA has outlined a path to eliminate the use of antibiotics for growth promotion in food animals, no restrictive measures and minimal compliance monitoring are in place at this time.[43]

Another causal factor associated with antibiotic resistance is the failure to develop and discover new antibiotics with novel mechanisms of action.[49] No completely new classes of antimicrobial drugs have been developed or discovered since the 1990s. This lack of discovery and development compounds antibiotic resistance and creates an acute need. There are infections that are now untreatable; as we use more broad-spectrum antibiotics, more resistance will develop. Considering that the broader the antibiotic coverage the greater the sales, broad-spectrum antibiotics are more profitable for pharmaceutical companies.[4] The primary factor interfering with antibiotic research and development is cost. Reportedly, the time spent on development is not profitable when compared to sales costs and short treatment periods. As further resistance develops, the duration of time that an antibiotic will be effective is limited.

Outcomes Associated with Microbial Resistance

What are the outcomes likely to result from microbial resistance? When 70 international experts met in 2011 to discuss the challenge of antibiotic resistance, they outlined the known and expected health implications of antibiotic resistance.[49] Antibiotic resistance increases the human and economic burden of infectious diseases. Infections will become untreatable and will be associated with rising rates of morbidity and mortality. Microbial resistance is anticipated to spread aggressively. Microbes are also expected to develop new mechanisms of resistance. Finally, the increasing threat of multidrug resistance, the reuse of old drugs with poor safety profiles, and community-wide cross-contamination are likely to lead to "resistance globalization."[49] In summary, antimicrobial resistance is expected to have serious and negative consequences to humanity from the inability to effectively treat infectious diseases.

Blaser posited a novel and compelling theory in his book *Missing Microbes*.[4] What if the overuse of antibiotics has destroyed essential microbes and microbial diversity that exist in useful and crucial compatibility with humans? Blaser argues that the elimination of essential microbes and reduction in the diversity of resident microbial populations from the overuse of antibiotics in our food and clinical medicine may play a causal role in disease. Obesity, asthma and allergies, food allergies, inflammatory bowel diseases, celiac disease, autism, diabetes mellitus type 1, precocious puberty, and breast cancer may be wholly or in part due to the overuse of antibiotics.[4] Antibiotics are responsible for ecological disturbances in the microbiota. With a renewed focus on the study of the human microbiome, emphasis is being placed on the persistent and perhaps permanent changes in the microbiome from ongoing exposure to antibiotics. Antibiotics target pathogenic bacteria and affect commensal inhabitants of the host as well. The extent to which this exposure affects the microbiome depends on host gut microbiota characteristics, antibiotic properties, and patterns of resistance. Changes in the microbiota

may prove to have significant long-term impacts on health.[52]

Actions Needed to Prevent Microbial Resistance

The 3rd World Healthcare-Associated Infections (HAI) Forum, held in June 2011, recommended a platform of change to help protect against the globalization of antibiotic resistance.[49] Recommendations included the use of infection-control practices designed to limit the transmission of resistant bacteria, a worldwide antibiotic stewardship strategy and the development and use of diagnostic techniques to reduce inappropriate antibiotic use, mechanisms to fast-track the development of new antibiotics and vaccines, and the development and implementation of education programs directed toward healthcare providers and consumers. These steps will require changes in consumer and provider behavior, as well as policy and legislative support on national and international levels to provide the infrastructure and funding needed to implement these suggestions.[49]

Antibiotic stewardship requires changes in prescribing patterns and the modification of farming practices. It involves the prescriber and the patient, as well as the community. For the prescriber, antibiotic stewardship begins with correct diagnosis of bacterial infections. This includes differentiating bacterial infections from viral infections. Where possible, the responsible pathogen should be identified before treatment is instituted. Identification of the pathogenic organism is essential in that it directs prescription of an agent with the narrowest spectrum of activity needed to target that specific pathogen. The site of the infection, clinical symptoms, epidemiological data, and culture results, when indicated and available, all contribute to identifying an organism or group of probable organisms for a particular infection. Selecting a drug with a narrow spectrum reduces the risk of interfering with the host's normal microbiota in addition to reducing the risk of encouraging resistance.

There are occasions when the clinician can make a diagnosis based on clinical symptoms alone. For example, when a client presents with dysuria, frequency of urination, and suprapubic pain in the absence of evidence suggestive of complicated cystitis or pyelonephritis, there is ample clinical evidence to support the diagnosis of acute uncomplicated cystitis (AUC). The diagnosis can be confirmed with a midstream urine dipstick positive for leukocyte esterase and nitrites.[53]

Initiating empiric therapy for a presumptive diagnosis requires knowledge regarding the most common pathogens for the identified infection, as well as susceptibility and resistance patterns in the community. In the case of AUC in women, *E. coli* is the most frequent uropathogen, accounting for 75% to 95% of infections. *Klebsiella* or *Proteus mirabilis* and *Staphylococcus saprophyticus* infections account for an additional 5% to 10% of infections.[54] Because of increasing antibiotic resistance, the β-lactams and the aminopenicillins have limited usefulness in treating UTIs. The prevalence of aminopenicillin-resistant bacteria may be as high as 30%. Therefore, careful selection of an antimicrobial must be based on current knowledge of the profile of common pathogens in the surrounding community.

Prescribing patterns also suggest that healthcare professionals are affected by pharmaceutical marketing practices when selecting an antimicrobial agent. Although a 3-day course of therapy of TMP-SMX (Bactrim) is recommended as a first-line empiric treatment for AUC, one study reviewing the prescriptive histories in a cohort of more than 13,000 individuals with a diagnosis of AUC found that only 37% of physicians prescribed TMP-SMX, and that it was frequently prescribed for a longer duration than the recommended 3-day course.[55] Fluoroquinolones, heavily marketed by pharmaceutical companies for

the treatment of cystitis and more expensive than Bactrim, were given in 32% of cases. Other drugs prescribed in the study included erythromycin, amoxicillin, azithromycin, and other β-lactams, none of which are appropriate therapies for cystitis. In their discussion, the researchers suggested that using fluoroquinolones as first-line treatment for acute, sporadic cystitis would accelerate resistance rates, result in more treatment failures, and ultimately lead to the use of less effective and safe alternatives.[55] Further, they called for better and more widespread education for providers on the appropriate selection of an antibiotic, as well as the appropriate dose and duration of treatment, as an important strategy in preventing antibiotic resistance.[55] Shorter courses of therapy are often, as in the case of AUC, as effective as longer courses with less risk of contributing to the emergence of resistant organisms.

There are other instances when empiric therapy is warranted: when delaying treatment may cause serious morbidity or even death or when there is a significant risk of transmitting the infection to others. When the invading microbe has not been identified, broad-spectrum antimicrobials or combinations of drugs may be employed that cover the greatest number of possible microorganisms. The clinician should change to an antibiotic with a narrower spectrum if indicated, once the results of culture and sensitivity are available.

In addition to following appropriate prescribing practices, providers can promote appropriate antibiotic use by educating patients, addressing their concerns, and recommending appropriate nonantibiotic therapies for symptomatic relief. Effective treatment is based on shared decision making between providers and patients.[6,43] Table 25-11 outlines the guidelines for improved therapeutic effect and reduced risk of resistance in initiating antimicrobial therapy.

While widely used, the risks of antibacterial soaps and cleaning agents may outweigh their

Table 25-11 Initiating Antibacterial Therapy

Guideline	Rationale
Document a bacterial (as opposed to viral) infection, and identify a suspected pathogen based on the site of infection, clinical evidence, epidemiological patterns, and culture when indicated.	• Antibiotics are not effective in treating viral infections. • Targeting a specific microbe is less likely to disturb the balance of the microbiome, reducing the risk of superimposed infection. • Therapy directed at a specific organism reduces the risk of encouraging resistance.
Identify host factors that may influence pharmacodynamics and pharmacokinetics: age, weight, health, allergies, integrity of the immune system, impaired liver or kidney function, medications, pregnancy, lactation.	• Absorption, distribution, and elimination of drugs are host dependent. • Side effects and adverse reactions can be minimized when therapy is tailored to the individual.
Review patterns of antimicrobial resistance in the community, and select an agent with the narrowest spectrum and best efficacy against the suspected pathogen.	• Selecting an agent with a narrow spectrum reduces the risk of encouraging drug resistance in the individual and the community.
Consider route, dosing schedule, and duration of therapy.	• Shorter courses of therapy are frequently as effective as longer courses and reduce the risk of emerging resistance. • Individualizing route, dosing schedule, and duration of therapy promotes adherence to the drug regimen.
Consider cost and availability.	• Newer, more expensive drugs do not necessarily offer advantages over tried and true therapies.
Educate patient regarding healthy drug use and alternatives to antibiotics when appropriate.	• Resistance is exacerbated when individuals "share" antibiotics with friends, self-medicate with incomplete or inappropriate therapies, or fail to take medication correctly. • Public education on appropriate antibiotic use and overuse promotes antibiotic-saving, resistance-reducing decision making.
Educate patient regarding the natural history of the infection, emphasizing palliative therapies and infection control measures.	• Changing attitudes, beliefs, and behaviors of the public regarding antibiotic use and infection control helps avoid overuse and misuse of antibiotics.

benefits. Antibacterial soaps and cleaning agents are related in some laboratory studies to antibiotic resistance, yet they are no more effective in preventing infection or reducing bacterial levels on the hands than plain soap.[56] Further, up to 76% of adults and children using commercial soap brands excrete triclosan, the active ingredient in many products, in their urine.[57] Consequently, in 2013, the FDA proposed a rule change to require that manufacturers of antibacterial soaps demonstrate that their products are safe for daily use and more effective than hand soap in preventing infection.[58] As of this writing, the rule is not yet final. The American Medical Association advocates regulation by the FDA of antibacterial agents in home products because of a potential link of the use of these products to antibiotic resistance and the lack of proven benefit. They further suggest the products, which promote antibiotic resistance, should be removed from the market.[59]

Summary

The core of primary health care is health promotion and disease prevention. The holistic philosophy of health care engages people as participants in their own health and wellness. Prescribing healthy lifestyle choices that promote healthy immunity such as balanced nutrition, exercise, smoking cessation, healthy weight, and stress

reduction are important infection-prevention techniques. Clinicians should take a cautious approach to intervention, utilizing antimicrobial therapy only when indicated, carefully choosing an evidence-based course of therapy, and educating patients about infections in relation to the rationale, risks, and benefits of drug therapy. Completing a course of medication, avoiding sharing or self-initiating drug therapy, and recommending pharmacologic and nonpharmacologic palliative therapies are included in the plan. By following a few simple rules, clinicians can effectively manage common bacterial infections without promoting microbial resistance.

Resources

Burton GRW, Engelkirk PG. *Microbiology for the Health Sciences*. 9th ed. Philadelphia, PA: Lippincott Williams & Wilkins, 2011.
LactMed: http://toxnet.nlm.nih.gov/newtoxnet/lactmed .htm
Reprotox: https://reprotox.org/

References

1. Lee GC, Reveles KR, Attridge RT, Lawson KA, Mansi I A, Lewis II J S, et al. Outpatient antibiotic prescribing in the United States: 2000–2010. *BMC Med.* 2014;12:96.
2. Burchaum JR, Rosenthal LD. *Lehne's Pharmacology for Nursing Care.* 9th ed. Philadelphia, PA: Saunders Elsevier; 2016.
3. Hicks LA, Taylor TH, Hunkler RJ. US outpatient antibiotic prescribing, 2010. *N Engl J Med.* 2013;368(15):1461-1462.
4. Blaser MJ. *Missing Microbes.* New York, NY: Picador, Henry Holt and Co.; 2014.
5. World Health Organization. *Antimicrobial Resistance: Global Report on Surveillane.* Geneva, Switzerland: WHO Press; 2014.
6. World Health Organization. WHO Factsheet, Antimicrobial Resistance. 2015. Available at: http://www.who.int/mediacentre/factsheets/fs194/en/. Accessed June 3, 2016.
7. Velicer CM, Heckbert SR, Lampe JW, Potter JD, Robertson CA, Taplin SH. Antibiotic use in relation to the risk of breast cancer. *JAMA.* 2004; 291(7):827-835.
8. Fuhrman BJ, Feigelson HS, Flores R, Gail MH, Xu X, Ravel J, et al. Associations of the fecal microbiome with urinary estrogens and estrogen metabolites in postmenopausal women. *J Clin Endocrinol Metab.* 2014;99(12):4632-4640.
9. US Food and Drug Administration. Content and Format of Labeling for Human Prescription Drug and Biological Products; Requirements for Pregnancy and Lactation Labeling. Available at: https://www.federalregister.gov/articles/2014/12/04/2014-28241/content-and-format-of-labeling-for-human-prescription-drug-and-biological-products-requirements-for#h-20 10. Accessed June 3, 2016.
10. Sachs HC, Committee on Drugs. The transfer of drugs and therapeutics into human breast milk: an update on selected topics. *Pediatrics* 2013;132(3):e796-e809.
11. Bhattacharya S. The facts about penicillin allergy: a review. *J Adv Pharm Technol Res.* 2010;1(1):11-17.

12. Campagna JD, Bond MC, Schabelman E, Hayes BD.The use of cephalosporins in penicillin-allergic patients: a literature review. *J Emerg Med.* 2012;42(5): 612-620.

13. Centers for Disease Control and Prevention. Sexually transmitted diseases treatment guidelines, 2015. *MMWR Recomm Rep.* 2015;64(RR-3):1-137.

14. Gianarellou H. Prescribing guidelines for severe *Pseudomonas* infections. *J Antimicrob Chemother.* 2002;49(2):229-233.

15. Turkoski BB, Lance BR, Bonfiglio MF. *Drug Information Handbook for Advanced Practice Nursing.* 15th ed. Cleveland, OH: Lexi-Comp; 2014.

16. Lamont RF, Sobel J, Kusanovic JP, Vaisbuch E, Mazaki-Tovi S, Kim SK, et al. Current debate on the use of antibiotic prophylaxis for cesarean section. *BJOG.* 2011;118(2):193-201.

17. Hopkins L, Smaill F. Antibiotic prophylaxis regimens and drugs for cesarean section. *Cochrane Database Syst Rev.* 2000;2:CD001136.

18. Smaill FM, Grivell RM. Antibiotic prophylaxis versus no prophyaxis for preventing infection after cesarean section. *Cochrane Database Syst Rev.* 2014;10:CD007482.

19. Briggs GG, Freeman RK. *Drugs in Pregnancy and Lactation.* 10th ed. Philadelphia, PA: Wolters Kluwer; 2015.

20. Page C, Curtis M, Sutter M, Walker M, Hoffman B. *Integrated Pharmacology.* 3rd ed. Edinburgh, Scotland: Mosby; 2006.

21. US National Library of Medicine. LactMed: Clindamycin. National Institutes of Health; 2014. Available at: http://toxnet.nlm.nih.gov/cgi-bin/sis/search2/r?dbs+lactmed:@term+@DOCNO+343. Accessed June 3, 2016.

22. Food and Drug Administration. FDA Drug Safety Communication: FDA requires label changes to warn of risk for possibly permanent nerve damage from antibacterial fluoroquinolone drugs taken by mouth or by injection. Available at: http://www.fda.gov/Drugs/DrugSafety/ucm365050.htm. Accessed June 3, 2016.

23. Schlecht HP, Bruno C. Fluoroquinolones. In: *Merck Manual: Professional version.* 2015. Available at: http://www.merckmanuals.com/professional/infectious-diseases/bacteria-and-antibacterial-drugs/fluoroquinolones. Accessed June 3, 2016.

24. Food and Drug Administration. FDA Drug Safety Communication: FDA advises restricting fluoroquinolone antibiotic use for certain uncomplicated infections; warns about disabling side effects that can occur together. Available at: http://www.fda.gov/Drugs/DrugSafety/ucm500143.htm. Accessed June 14, 2016.

25. Kline JM, Wietholter JP, Kline VT, Confer J. Pediatric antibiotic use: a focused review of fluoroquinolones and tetracyclines. *US Pharm.* 2012;37(8):56-69.

26. Choi SH, Kim EY, Kim YJ. Systemic use of fluoroquinolone in children. Korean J of Pediatr. 2013;56(5):196-201.

27. Crider KS, Cleves MA, Reefhus J, Berry RJ, Hobbs CA, Hu DJ. Antibacterial medication use during pregnancy and risk of birth defects. *Arch Pediatr Adolesc Med.* 2009;163(11):978-985.

28. Yefet ERS, Chazam B, Akel H, Romano SZN. The safety of quinolones in pregnancy. *Obstet Gynecol Surv.* 2014;69(11):681-694.

29. Food and Drug Administration. CIPRO (Ciprofloxacin) Use by Pregnant and Lactating Women. Available at: http://www.fda.gov/Drugs/EmergencyPreparedness/BioterrorismandDrugPreparedness/ucm130712.htm. Accessed June 3, 2016.

30. US National Library of Medicine. LactMed: Tetracycline. National Institutes of Health; 2014. Available at: http://toxnet.nlm.nih.gov/cgi-bin/sis/search2/r?dbs+lactmed:@term+@DOCNO+252. Accessed June 3, 2016.

31. Luzzatto L, Seneca E. G6PD deficiency: a classic example of pharmacogenetics with ongoing clinical implications. Br J Haematol. 2014;164:469-480.

32. US National Library of Medicine. LactMed: Trimethoprim-sulfamethoxazole. National Institutes of Health; 2014. Available at: http://toxnet.nlm.nih.gov/cgi-bin/sis/search2/r?dbs+lactmed:@term+@DOCNO+417. Accessed June 3, 2016.

33. Chudnofsky CR, Otten EJ. Acute pulmonary toxicity to nitrofurantoin. *J Emerg Med.* 1989;7:15-19.

34. Nkhoma ET, Poole C, Vannappagari V, Hall SA, Beutler E. The global prevalence of glucose-6-phosphate dehydrogenase deficiency: a systematic review and meta-analysis. *Blood Cells Mol Dis.* 2009;42(3):276-278.

35. Watchko JF. Common hematologic problems in the newborn nursery. *Pediatric Clin N Am.* 2015; 62:509-524.

36. Gnann JW. Antiviral therapy of varicella-zoster virus infections. In: Arvin A, Campadelli-Fiume G, Mocarski E, Moore PS, Roizman B, Whitley R, et al., eds. *Human Herpesviruses: Biology, Therapy, and Immunoprophylaxis.* Cambridge, UK: Cambridge University Press; 2007.

37. US National Library of Medicine. LactMed: Acyclovir. National Institutes of Health; 2015. Available at: http://toxnet.nlm.nih.gov/cgi-bin/sis/search2/r?dbs+lactmed:@term+@DOCNO+331. Accessed June 3, 2016.

38. Pilmis B, Jullien V, Sobel J, Lecuit M, Lortholary O, Charlier C. Antifungal drugs during pregnancy:

an updated review. *J Antimicrob Chemother.* 2015; 70:14-22.

39. US National Library of Medicine. LactMed: Amphotericin B. National Institutes of Health; 2013. http://toxnet.nlm.nih.gov/cgi-bin/sis/search2/r?dbs+lactmed:@term+@DOCNO+446. Accessed June 3, 2016.

40. US National Library of Medicine. LactMed; Fluconazole. National Institutes of Health; 2013. Available at: http://toxnet.nlm.nih.gov/cgi-bin/sis/search2/r?dbs+lactmed:@term+@DOCNO+357. Accessed June 3, 2016.

41. US National Library of Medicine. LactMed: Nystatin. National Institutes of Health; 2013. Available at: http://toxnet.nlm.nih.gov/cgi-bin/sis/search2/r?dbs+lactmed:@term+@DOCNO+374. Accessed June 3, 2016.

42. US Food and Drug Administration. Griseofulvin. Full prescribing information. Available at: http://www.accessdata.fda.gov/drugsatfda_docs/label/2014/062279s022lbl.pdf. Accessed June 3, 2016.

43. Centers for Disease Control and Prevention. Antibiotic resistance threats in the United States, 2013. Available at: http://www.cdc.gov/drugresistance/threat-report-2013. Accessed June 3, 2016.

44. Fairlie T, Shapiro DJ, Hersh A, Hicks LA. Research letters: national trends in visit rates and antibiotic prescribing for adults with acute sinusitis. *Arch Intern Med.* 2012;172(19):1513-1514.

45. Gualano MR, Gili R, Scaioli G, Bert F, Siliquini R. General population's knowledge and attitudes about antibiotics: a systematic review and meta-analysis. *Pharmacoepidemiol Drug Safety.* 2015;24:2-10.

46. Vanden Eng J, Marcus R, Hadler JL, Imhoff B, Vugia DJ, Cieslak PR, et al. Consumer attitudes and use of antibiotics. *Emerg Infect Dis.* 2003;9(9):1128-1135.

47. Read RC, Cornaglia G, Kahlmeter G. European Society of Clinical Microbiology and Infectious Diseases Professional Affairs Workshop Group: professional challenges and opportunities in clinical microbiology and infectious diseases in Europe. *Lancet Infect Dis.* 2011;11:408-415.

48. Cabello F, Godfrey H, Tomova A, Ivanova L, Dolz H, Millanao A, et al. Antimicrobial use in aquaculture re-examined: its relevance to antimicrobial resistance and to animal and human health. *Environ Microbiol.* 2013;15(7):1917-1942.

49. Carlet J, Jarlier V, Harbarth S, Voss A, Gossens H, Pittet D. Ready for a world without antibiotics? The Pensieres antibiotic resistance call to action. *Antimicrob Resist Infect Control.* 2012;111:1-13.

50. Consumers Union. The Overuse of Antibiotics in Food Animals Threatens Public Health. Available at: https://consumersunion.org/wp-content/uploads/2013/02/Overuse_of_Antibiotics_On_Farms.pdf. Accessed June 3, 2016.

51. Singer RS, Finch R, Wegener HC, Bywater R, Waters J, Iipsitch M. Antibiotic resistance—the interplay between antibiotic use in animals and human beings. *Lancet.* 2003;3:47-51.

52. Jernberg C, Lofmark S, Edlund C, Jansson JK. Long-term impacts of antibiotic exposure on the human intestinal microbiota. *Microbiology.* 2010;156:3216-3223.

53. Colgan R, Williams M. Diagnosis and treatment of acute uncomplicated cystitis. *Am Fam Physician.* 2011;84(7):771-776.

54. Imam TH. Bacterial Urinary Tract Infections. *Merck Manual.* 2015. Available at: http://www.merckmanuals.com/professional/genitourinary-disorders/urinary-tract-infection. Accessed June 3, 2016.

55. McEwen LN, Farjo R, Foxman B. Antibiotic prescribing for cystitis: how well does it match published guidelines? *Ann Epidemiol.* 2003;13(6):482.

56. Aiello AE, Larson EL, Levy SB. Consumer antibacterial soaps: effective or just risky? *Clin Infect Dis.* 2007;45:S137-S147.

57. Bergstrom KG. Update on antibacterial soaps: the FDA takes a second look at triclosans. J Drugs Dermatol. 2014;13(4):501-503.

58. US Food and Drug Administration. FDA issues proposed rule to determine safety and effectiveness of antibacterial soaps. 2013. Available at: http://www.fda.gov/NewsEvents/Newsroom/PressAnnouncements/ucm378542.htm. Accessed June 3, 2016.

59. Tan L, Nielsen N, Young D, Trizna Z. Use of antimicrobial agents in consumer products. *Arch Dermatol.* 2002;138(8):1082-1086.

CHAPTER 26

COMPLEMENTARY AND INTEGRATIVE HEALTH CARE IN PRIMARY CARE

Kathryn Niemeyer

Complementary and alternative medicine (CAM) is a consumer-driven healthcare phenomenon. In 2007, a National Health Interview Survey showed that approximately 38.3% of adults and 11.8 % of children in the United States used some form of CAM in the last year.[1,2] Patient expectations, healthcare systems concerns, the rising incidence of chronic disease, and costs of disease-centered health care are some of the reasons for the scientific community's interest in CAM.[3] Even when the patient has to pay out of pocket for CAM therapies due to a lack of insurance coverage, CAM use has increased steadily since 2006.[2]

The purpose of this chapter is to introduce women's health providers to CAM and integrative health care. This chapter discusses various definitions of CAM and integrative health care and the state of research and issues surrounding research in integrative health care with CAM systems and therapies. Commonly used CAM therapies, as reported by the National

Center for Complementary and Integrative Health (NCCIH; formerly the National Center for Complementary and Alternative Medicine [NCCAM]), and the role of the women's healthcare provider in the application of integrative health in primary care are also explored.

Complementary and Alternative Health Care

CAM refers to "whole systems" of medicine and to treatment therapies or modalities that have developed separate from, but on a spectrum with, conventional health care.[4,5] CAM is an inclusive descriptor referring to medical, nursing, or healthcare therapies that are complementary or alternative to conventional allopathic health care.[6] These systems of care and therapies are holistic and complex in nature and address whole-person health and wellbeing, disease prevention, and symptom presentations.[5,7,8] Systems of CAM include homeopathy, naturopathy, chiropractic, and culturally embedded systems of medicine such as Western herbal medicine, Ayurveda (also called Ayurvedic medicine), and traditional Chinese medicine (TCM). CAM modalities refer to therapies such as aromatherapy, nutritional and botanical supplementation, movement therapies such as tai chi and yoga, bodywork (i.e., massage therapy, cranial-sacral manipulation, or acupressure), body–mind modalities (i.e., biofeedback, mindfulness meditation, hypnosis, and prayer), and energy work such as therapeutic touch (see Table 26-1).

Integrative Health Care

Integrative health care is a relatively new concept and refers to the inclusion of CAM in personalized, relationship- and evidence-based models

of health care centering on whole-person care or treatment.[5,7,9] While CAM terminology is widely understood and recognized, it is being replaced by or subsumed in the term *integrative medicine* or *integrative health* (see **Box 26-1**). Integrative medicine as a model of care has the potential to shift evidence-based CAM into the conventional healthcare arena. This allows for third-party reimbursement, a broader audience, and more comprehensive and inclusive models of care. While CAM can be integrated into practice at multiple levels, women's health providers are in a unique position to engage in integrative health care in primary care depending on their level of expertise. Some women's health providers may have the training needed to offer select CAM modalities, while others will be more comfortable partnering with expert CAM practitioners.

Consistent with integrative health, nursing and other disciplines are rooted in the belief that

Table 26-1 Categories of Complementary Health Modalities and Systems

Category of Practice	Specific Practice
Natural products	Dietary supplements including vitamins, minerals, probiotics, botanical products, enzymes, hormones or hormone-like products, amino acids, essential fatty acids, other biologics
Mind–body practices	Meditation; relaxation; deep breathing; hypnotherapy; biofeedback; guided imagery; prayer; arts and music; humor; aromatherapy; nutrition; bodywork including acupuncture, acupressure, massage therapies, shiatsu, movement therapies (Feldenkrais, Alexander, Pilates, Rolfing, structural integration, Trager psychophysical integration); spinal and osteo- manipulation (including chiropractic and osteopathic medicines); reflexology; tai chi; qigong; yoga
Energy medicine	Therapeutic touch, healing touch, Reiki, and energy therapies; earthing; biophysical devices including magnetism, electricity, light
Whole systems	Traditional healers; Ayurvedic medicine; traditional Chinese medicine; homeopathy; naturopathy; Western herbal medicine; other indigenous healing systems including Southern African, Sufism, Kampo, Native American healing

Data from National Center for Complementary and Integrative Health. Complementary, alternative, or integrative health: what's in a name? Available at: https://nccih.nih.gov/health/integrative-health#integrative. 2016. Accessed June 6, 2016; Micozzi MS. *Fundamentals of Complementary and Alternative Medicine.* 4th ed. Philadelphia, PA: Saunders Elsevier; 2011.

Box 26-1 Integrative Health Care Defined

Integrative nursing is finding "meaning and purpose in relationships . . . [providing] opportunities for healing within a co-created relationship based on mutuality and participatory engagement" and:

> collaborative interprofessional relationships built on trust and mutual respect. . . . integrative nursing invites each of us to embrace the moral commitment of healthcare to be in right relationship with the earth, the people we care for, our communities, and ourselves, creating a system that is responsive, compassionate, and caring. . . . Integrative nurses use a full complement of therapies to support and augment the healing process in a manner that first considers the least invasive and intensive therapy. (p. 542)*

Integrative medicine is a newly emerging form of health care: "It is patient-centered, healing-oriented, and embraces conventional and complementary therapies . . . focus[ing] on the whole person and life-style . . . and a willingness to use all appropriate therapeutic approaches." (p. 3)**

Integrative healthcare "is focused on whole person/whole system care that is grounded in relationships and prevention, and is delivered by interprofessional teams that include conventional (allopathic) as well as complementary/alternative therapies." (p. 6)† "When guided by the principle that people have innate healing capacity, the healthcare system becomes supportive rather than directive; providers become partners rather than prescribers; and consumers become active rather than passive." (p. 542)§

* Data from Koithan M. Gazing with soft eyes. In: Kreitzer MJ, Koithan M, eds. *Integrative Nursing*. Oxford, UK: Oxford University Press; 2014.

** Maizes V, Rakel D, Niemiec C. Integrative medicine and patient-centered care. *Explore (NY)*. 2009;5(5):277-289.

† Koithan M. Concepts and principles of integrative nursing. In: Kreitzer MJ, Koithan M, eds. *Integrative Nursing*. Oxford, UK: University Press; 2014.

§ Koithan M. Gazing with soft eyes. In: Kreitzer MJ, Koithan, M, eds. *Integrative Nursing*. Oxford, UK: University Press; 2014.

---

the whole person demonstrates complexity and is an irreducible integrated bio-psycho-social-spiritual being with adaptive organization at multiple levels or dimensions. While flexible and dynamic, the whole person is embedded in and inseparable from internal environmental relationships and relationships extending out to the external environment.[7,10] Healing has been described as "the emergence of right relationship at one or more levels of the human experience."[11,12] *Right relationship* is further defined as order and coherence at multiple levels of the whole person, where the whole is greater than the sum of the parts.[12-14] Therefore, extending the goal beyond curing the person and reducing symptoms, women's health providers engaging in integrative health care are interested in whole-person healing and strive for mutually determined

patient-centered outcomes such as "wellbeing, energy, happiness, clarity, and purpose."[7]

State of Research in CAM

One reason inconsistencies in health care exist is the lack of clinically relevant research methods.[15] Among all the research designs, the randomized controlled trial (RCT) has been held to provide the highest quality evidence. RCTs are considered to be the "gold standard" in research designs, because potential intervening and confabulating variables can be controlled, reduced, or eliminated in order to ascribe causation between the dependent and independent variables. However, RCTs most commonly include young, white healthy males with a normal body mass index (BMI) and measure short-term outcomes. The ideal subject is studied in ideal conditions. This provides greater confidence of a linear cause and effect but limits the generalizability of RCTs to the broader population. The lack of applicability of the results of RCTs to real life circumstances has prompted a call for more clinically relevant research methods.[16] While often venerated as providing the strongest level of evidence and therefore proof, RCTs are in actuality only one potential source of evidence and may offer inconclusive proof.

Emerging research on CAM consists of mixed and multiple levels evidence. Understanding the "state of the science" in a particular field is based partly on meta-analysis methodology, where data from several studies are pooled and analyzed. However, meta-analyses or systematic reviews can only be done if there is a substantial body of research already existing that permits summative evaluation. Different CAM modalities and systems have varying degrees of evidence supporting their use. For example, mindfulness meditation, the use of probiotics, and tai chi all have multiple strong, high-quality studies supporting their use in various healthcare situations. There is a plethora of emerging research on other aspects of TCM, especially acupuncture and Chinese herbal medicines, for use with multiple health problems or medical diagnoses. Less human research exists on the energy therapies. Researchers have been unable to consistently demonstrate positive outcomes from intact whole systems of CAM that concurrently implement multiple healthcare modalities, such as Ayurveda or Western herbal medicine.

CAM modalities can be considered to be under researched because of the relative deficiency of quality RCTs. This relative lack of research may be due to several reasons. First, commonly used research designs such as RCTs are inappropriate for use with many CAM modalities; an RCT does not provide a broad enough lens to look at whole systems of medicine.[17] Golden makes the case that RCTs are often not suitable for evaluating CAM therapies that produce global or nonspecific outcomes or have multilayered treatments.[18] Because of homogeneity, RCTs are not relevant to real-life situations and lack generalizability. Further, RCTs fail to account for several factors that may affect the effectiveness of various CAM modalities: 1) the clinical experience of the practitioner, 2) the synergism that can occur with multiple dimensions of CAM therapies, and 3) contextual factors. Therefore, RCTs by their design may not be the best approach for evaluating the effectiveness of CAM.

Herbal medicine offers an example of the difficulty in studying CAM methodologies. Herbal therapy using whole crude plant parts is a system of medicine that selects herbs for an individual patient and works synergistically with the body to promote healing and health. Currently, research on herbal medicines can be divided into two types. The first looks at herbs as they would be studied in conventional pharmaceutical research, as single, static chemical agents. The second examines herbs as complex multichemical living organisms as they are used in Western herbal medicine: close to their natural state (as crude plant teas and tinctures), in combination with other herbs, and matched to the needs of a particular individual. The majority of herb research conducted to date, including laboratory and human studies, is conducted from a pharmaceutical perspective on single herbal agents, extracted chemical parts of herbs, or synthetic or amplified components of whole plants. This pharmaceutical model of research looks at herbs using a reductionist framework. Because of the lack of standardization from one product to another, preparations and dosing vary and results are product specific. These factors make it difficult to interpret results.

Unfortunately, little research has been conducted using a broader framework to evaluate the impact of herbal therapy. Studies looking at herbal medicine as a whole system of medicine where complex crude plant materials are used in personalized formulations are few, primarily because science lacks a research vehicle or model to measure outcomes in complex beings using complex therapies.[19,20] Therefore, research findings may not be generalizable to real-life herb use, especially if multiple whole crude plants are used together. Consequently, the pharmaceutical model of research often fails to capture outcomes reported in whole systems of CAM.

The state of the science for herbal medicine is comparable to that for nutrition, because many of the same methodological issues affect both fields. As with herbal medicine, the validity and generalization of findings from RCTs evaluating the impact of food and nutrition on health and wellbeing are being questioned.[21] Like medicinal herbs, foods are not eaten in isolation.

The second major factor inhibiting the quality and quantity of research on CAM is the lack of funding. Until CAM therapeutics are considered as financially viable complements or alternatives to well funded medical interventions (pharmaceuticals) or until a shift to whole-person care occurs, CAM research will not be broadly funded. Research is frequently driven by potential economic profit, and until CAM therapies demonstrate the potential for economic profit, limited resources will be directed to research on CAM. Despite the lack of funding, two forces are driving increased research in this area—public interest in CAM and the push to create integrative health care.

A more effective research approach may be one that is multimodeled and based on new, more inclusive research attitudes and a shift away from a mono-research culture where every study is judged in relationship to the RCT. Several alternatives have been proposed. One suggestion is the utilization and valuing of multiple different qualitative, quantitative, and population-based studies with each research design contributing to the evidence base. Instead of a research hierarchy, evidence would be built using a mixed-methods approach to research.[22] Walach and colleagues suggest a similar model of evidence, with the circle as a structure to define what constitutes evidence.[23] The circle is composed of large, well-conducted studies using multiple designs to provide large, relevant data sets.

Increasingly, studies using new models of research are being reported in the literature. Some of these models are closely aligned with clinical research, while others are more pragmatic. These models include quasi-experimental designs, applied clinical research, population-based observational studies, and research where CAM is added onto conventional therapies. In addition, new outcome tools and measures are being applied in research, which address CAM's long-term, global, and nonspecific outcomes. An example would be an outcome tool that measures changes in symptom presentation along with functional changes and changes in overall experience of wellbeing, which may include emotion, sensation, and energy level. Appropriate research models and measures assuring validity, credibility, and rigor are emerging specific to integrative health care and CAM research needs.

Lastly, the evidence base on CAM, as well as in conventional medicine, should integrate knowledge gleaned from practice and research, as suggested by the Institute of Medicine (IOM). According to the IOM, evidence-based practice is the *application of systematically generated knowledge* in the decision-making process for the provision of "best care." It integrates "individual clinical expertise with the best available external evidence."[16] In this model, evidence building values the results of high-quality studies, as well as clinical expertise. Clinical expertise is what emerges from multiple ways of knowing. This includes, along with scientific empirical knowing,

knowing that comes from personal experience (ethical and intuitive knowing), practice knowledge (praxis), traditional knowing, and knowing that has origins in the narrative or aesthetic.[24-26] Traditional knowing refers to the accumulation of knowledge over time by a group of people living in close contact with nature. It is built through the narrative story, observation, and experience and is adaptive to changing environments.[27] While research in CAM is not as prolific as in other fields, clinical wisdom—derived from the expertise of seasoned practitioners of CAM—is available to guide practice and research in CAM.

In summary, when evaluating CAM research, it is essential to be knowledgeable about current research issues in the field, to understand the limitations of the linear causal model, and to appreciate that RCTs may not be the most appropriate research approach to evaluating complex systems of CAM or CAM therapeutic modalities. Further, it is important to investigate how the patient is using the CAM modality, what her values and preferences are, and to search for and evaluate research that reflects those specific usages. Evidence-based practice reflects a personalized approach that emerges from the assimilation of science, experiential wisdom, and patient preference.

Insufficient funding, lack of agreement on how to research whole systems of CAM, and the inability to agree on what outcomes to measure have slowed the development of a comprehensive evidence base for CAM. New research models are emerging from efforts to capture the complexity, context, and reality of interventions in whole systems of CAM. CAM has been used throughout history and is widely used today. Thus, it has social value and deserves better evidence of its effectiveness and safety.

Use of CAM in the General Population

CAM modalities are widely used as self-medication, often without the support, guidance, or advice of healthcare providers or experts in CAM. CAM therapies that are readily available to the general

public include over-the-counter products and home remedies. In 2007, the National Health Interview Survey was used to collect CAM usage data on 23,393 US adults and 9417 children. It was found that of the nearly 40% of adults who used CAM, the most frequently used therapies were natural products other than vitamins and minerals, which were categorized in the survey as non-practitioner-based therapies. The nonvitamin, nonmineral natural products, in order of frequency of use, included fish oil or omega-3, glucosamine, echinacea, flaxseed oil or pills, ginseng, combination herb pills, ginkgo biloba, chondroitin, garlic, and coenzyme Q10 (CoQ10 or ubiquinone). The four top reasons provided for use of CAM modalities were back pain, neck pain, joint pain, and arthritis.[1,2] Unfortunately, this report provided no information on why persons were using the particular nutritional supplements, nor did the report provide information on which particular CAM therapies were being used for back, neck, joint pain, and arthritis. **Table 26-2** provides a brief overview of the natural products most commonly used. The level of evidence to support their use varies; some have clear support, while others are indeterminate or lack support for use.[2,28] The presence of an accessible resource indicates only that research exists, not that it supports a recommendation for use. The reader should investigate products with which they are unfamiliar before making recommendations.

Integrative Health Care in the Primary Care Setting

Role of Women's Health Providers in Integrative Practice

Integrative health care represents a shift from the dominant medical paradigm of traditional healthcare models. However, nursing and other health disciplines have meta-theoretical perspectives and theories that align with whole-person, relationship-based care, which forms the foundation of CAM. These perspectives are consistent with values inherent in integrative health care. The paradigm shift moves health care from a disease-centered reductionist perspective to a health and wellbeing perspective grounded in multiplicity and complexity science. Integrative health care addresses symptom presentations and the root cause of those symptoms, the variables and life factors that support that root

Table 26-2 Most Common Natural Products Used in the United States: Historical Use and Potential Uses Studied

Natural Supplement	Type of Product	Traditional Indications	Accessible Resources
Echinacea	Herb extract	*Echinacea* species are used for infections (respiratory, gastric, dermatological, urinary) and venomous bites.	Cochrane review: • Common cold
Ginseng	Herb extract	Panax ginsengs have been used to support visceral organs and calm nerves and for loss of stamina, chronic immune deficiency, chronic conditions, and recovery from depletion.	Cochrane reviews: • Cognition • Heart failure • Protocol for cancer Additional human studies: • Diabetes, endurance athletes, cancer, radiation injury and cancer-related fatigue, erectile dysfunction, COPD, night duty work, quality of life
Ginkgo biloba	Leaf extract	No history of use of ginkgo leaf (the plant part used in research and processed ginkgo products).	Cochrane reviews: • Macular degeneration • Cognitive impairment and dementia • Acute ischemic stroke • Intermittent claudication • Tinnitus • Cognitive improvement in healthy individuals Systematic review: • Alzheimer's disease
Garlic	Herb and food extract	Has been ingested as food. This use has been culturally determined.	Cochrane reviews: • Common cold • Cardiovascular mortality in hypertension • Preeclampsia prevention • Peripheral arterial occlusive disease • Diabetes mellitus (protocol) • Adjunct for pulmonary infection in cystic fibrosis

(continues)

Table 26-2 Most Common Natural Products Used in the United States: Historical Use and Potential Uses Studied (*continued*)

Natural Supplement	Type of Product	Traditional Indications	Accessible Resources
Fish oil/ omega-3	Food extract: essential fatty acids	No history of use as extract from food.	Cochrane reviews: • Kidney transplant • Asthma • Ulcerative colitis • Crohn's remission • Retinitis pigmentosa • Atopic eczema • IgA nephropathy • Cancer cachexia • Pregnancy • Rheumatoid arthritis (protocol) • Hypertension (protocol) • Schizophrenia • Preterm infants • Cognitive decline and dementia • Diabetes mellitus type 2 • Postnatal depression • Patency of arteriovenous fistulae and grafts • Allergies in children • Intermittent claudication • Breastfeeding for increasing growth and development • Dysmenorrhea • Dyslipidemia in HIV • Cystic fibrosis • Liver transplant Additional human studies: • Stress, hostility in young adults, self-report health status, cancer risk, Alzheimer's disease, depression Systematic reviews: • Heart disease mortality, cardiovascular disease risk
Flaxseed oil/pills	Food extract: essential fatty acids	No history of use as extract from food.	Controlled trials: • Dry eye • Diabetes mellitus • Cardioprotection • Skin • Dyslipidemia • Platelets • Blood pressure • Hemodialysis • PCOS • Rheumatoid arthritis

Natural Supplement	Type of Product	Traditional Indications	Accessible Resources
Glucosamine	Monosaccharide Usual source: extraction from exoskeletons of crustaceans or fermented grain	No history of use as extract from food.	Cochrane reviews: • Osteoarthritis • TMJ osteoarthritis • Diabetes mellitus type 2 • Patellofemoral pain syndrome
Chondroitin	Nutritional extract Polysaccharide	No history of use as extract from food.	Cochrane reviews: • Nail psoriasis • Diabetic kidney disease • Osteoarthritis
Coenzyme Q10	Vitamin-like nutrient benzoquinone Biologically, exists in mitochondria of human cells, and foods. Human production is endogenous synthesis. Supplement source: synthesis	No history or tradition of use.	Cochrane reviews: • Heart failure • Parkinson's disease • Hypertension • Mitochondrial disorders • Huntington's disease • Childhood cancer • Adult cancer • ALS • MS Additional human studies: • Persons treated with statin drugs, migraine prevention, periodontal disease

ALS = amyotrophic lateral sclerosis, COPD = chronic obstructive pulmonary disease, HIV = human immunodeficiency virus, IgA = immunoglobulin A, MS = multiple sclerosis, PCOS = polycystic ovarian syndrome, TMJ = temporomandibular joint.

Data from National Center for Complementary and Integrative Health. The use of complementary and alternative medicine in the United States. Bethesda, MD: US Department of Health and Human Services, National Institutes of Health; 2008. https://nccih.nih.gov/research/statistics/2007/camsurvey_fs1.htm. Accessed June 6, 2016; Yance DR. *Adaptogens in Medical Herbalism.* Rochester, VT: Healing Arts Press; 2013.

cause, and a person's global sense of wellness and wellbeing.[7,10,24,29,30] The overarching beliefs of integrative health care include the belief in the person's innate self-healing capabilities and self-determination. Thus, every person is an active participant in her own health and wellbeing.[31] By working together, women, integrative healthcare practitioners, and women's healthcare providers less skilled in CAM can create healing environments that support and enable personal healing (see **Box 26-2**).[32,33] This occurs through tolerance, acceptance, and the practice of other ways of being and doing. Integrative medicine is rooted in the premise that health and health care are responsive to the whole person, dynamic, and constantly evolving as new knowledge emerges.[7,31]

Operationalizing integrative health care occurs on a spectrum, at multiple levels, and varies by each individual practitioner. There is no

---

Box 26-2 Principles Foundational to Integrative Health Care

- Humans coexist with and are inseparable from their environments.
- Humans have innate capacities for health and healing.
- Nature offers restoration and healing for the human.
- Integrative care is whole-person centered and relationship based.
- Integrative care is informed by evidence and uses a full range of therapies to support and augment healing, moving from the least invasive/intensive to more, depending on the individual context.
  - Providers facilitate the best conditions for healing.
- Integrative care focuses on the health and wellbeing of the caregiver in addition to those served.
- Healing is an emergent (time-intensive) and subjective experience and includes movement toward greater complexity, order, coherence, and creativity in the whole person.

Data from Ringdahl D. Integrative nursing and symptom management. In: Kreitzer MJ, Koithan M, eds. *Integrative Nursing.* Oxford, UK: Oxford University Press; 2014:187-199; Niemeyer K, Koithan M, Bell I. Traditional knowledge of Western herbal medicine and complex systems science. *J Herb Med.* 2013;3:112-119.

---

established model of practice for integrative health care that fits all environments. Clinicians integrate CAM systems and modalities in different ways. Some women's health providers offer no CAM modalities, others have sufficient expertise in some modalities to offer CAM-specific care, and a few are integrative practitioners with extensive expertise in multiple CAM systems and modalities. For example, some clinicians may make herbal supplement recommendations or refer patients to traditional practitioners for CAM, while others may have the knowledge and skill to offer specific CAM systems or therapies, such as massage therapy, therapeutic touch, or herbal medicine, based on education and experience. More advanced integrative practitioners have knowledge and skills in counseling broadly on healthy lifestyle practices that extend beyond the boundaries of conventional health care. This additional knowledge and skill, along with the extra time allotted to visits by integrative practitioners, and the knowledge and judgment on how to integrate CAM with conventional medical therapies, are all essential components in providing integrative care at an expert level.

The skills that many integrative practitioners bring to health care include knowledge and experience with person-centered change theories, processes to generate new patterns and habits, and motivational strategies. Likewise, knowledge of nutrition for wellness, including nutritional and herbal supplements, movement and exercise, interventions for healthy sleep, and the role of spirituality, community, attitude, and emotions in wellbeing form the foundation of integrative health care.[34] For example, nutritional counseling in integrative health care includes strategies to change from a dietary pattern that promotes disease and inflammation to a plant-based, food additive–free diet.[35,36] Besides recommending vitamin D3, fish oil, and magnesium supplements, women's health providers practicing expert integrative health care may encourage patients to take healthy probiotic mixes or an individually tailored dietary supplement of protein fractions (i.e., L-lysine or L-carnitine), extracted concentrated nutrients or nutritional cofactors (e.g., para-aminobenzoic acid [PABA], spirulina), phytohormones (i.e., melatonin or wild yam–based products), or basic herbal medicines. Patient coaching may include schedules or plans for movement and exercise-based lifestyle changes or sleep-promoting protocols. Integrative practitioners may address attitude and emotional and spiritual wellbeing by promoting mediation practices such as mindfulness and community engagement or by altering personal relationships. Less experienced women's health providers can partner with CAM practitioners within their community to expand their skills or be able to refer to their patients to experts in the field. To do this, clinicians need a broad understanding of CAM systems and practices, need to develop linkages with CAM experts in their local practice area, and should have a working knowledge of nonpractitioner-provided CAM modalities.

Qualifications for CAM Practitioners

What constitutes a credible CAM practitioner and with whom should women's health providers be partnering? Clinicians should look for training, credibility, and experience with safe practices. While experience in a field yields a degree of expertise and potential credibility, there is no uniform licensing, educational, or regulatory criteria or credentialing for CAM practitioners. Credentials or qualifications vary according to the therapy and may further vary within the body of practitioners. Credentials include certifications, informal educational course work or apprentice programs, formal degree programs, and degree programs with licensing. Licensing exists for practitioners of acupuncture, chiropractic, naturopathy, massage therapy, and TCM, but licensing is limited on a state-to-state basis.

Each CAM field or system of medicine has its own markers for acceptable practitioners; unless practitioners are licensed, there is little professional accountability or regulation of practice. These markers may be certifications of completion of educational programs (massage therapist, naturopathic certifications). Certifications may be stand-alone criteria, or they may be added on to degrees or practice licenses. Educational programs vary and can range from online programs to years-long apprenticeship programs or person-to-person classroom instruction. Many CAM therapies have degree programs with or without state or national licensure (e.g., a master's of science in herbal medicine has no licensing associated with it, but doctors of TCM are licensed). Titling from professional organizations can also indicate that uniform practitioner standards are met (e.g., RH is the "registered herbalist" designation from the American Herbalists Guild).

To complicate the issue of qualifications and credentialing, several CAM systems and modalities have different levels of practitioners. Homeopathic or naturopathic practitioners may have either completed certification programs or hold clinical doctorate degrees and be licensed as professionals in their system of medicine. In some states where licensing is not accepted, there has been a rise in certification programs. For example, naturopathic doctors (NDs) are licensed in 17 states. Licensure indicates graduation from an accredited naturopathic medical school and successful completion of a national licensing exam. In states that do not recognize ND licensure, there are certification programs with practitioners potentially using the ND credential without the license. It would be fair to say the public is to a great degree unaware of these differences. Credentialing and practitioner experience are fraught with inconsistencies and personal variations. The minimal acceptable credential or standard for a practitioner would be completion of a credible and reliable educational program.

Like physicians and nurses, CAM practitioners may have different levels of expertise in the evaluation of research in their field, but should have a thorough understanding of the theoretical base and application of their therapeutic practice to be credible. Women's health providers have the responsibility to explore the expertise and credibility of the CAM practitioners in their geographic location, have knowledge of the appropriate application of the therapies, and have an understanding of the theoretical basis and research supporting the practice.

Integrative Healthcare Practice Models

The foundation of integrative health care is understanding the state of the science in the various therapies and their safety and effectiveness, as well as awareness that knowledge is generated from multiple ways of knowing. Oftentimes, blending the practice of conventional health care with CAM therapies depends on developing mutual trust and respect, communication, and collaboration. These processes are essential to be able to provide synergistic treatment that results in health promotion, disease prevention, and enhanced wellbeing.[32,37]

Practice models for integrative health care are evolving. By definition, integrative health care includes many modalities and blends evidence-based complementary systems and modalities of health care with conventional medical therapeutics.[6] Women's health providers may have additional education in a CAM system or therapeutic modality or they may practice conventional health care within an integrative practice environment where other practitioners offer CAM. There are various forms of integrative practice models. Some models offer some, but not all, CAM systems or modalities. Others may be led by a CAM practitioner, while in other models the women's health provider may act as gatekeeper or care coordinator.[37] Each model is relationship based and results in the blending of conventional with complementary health care. Theoretically, integrative health care utilizes the best (both biomedical and experiential evidence) of both conventional and CAM therapies to provide personalized, patient-driven, and empowered care when appropriate. Integrative health care involves fostering interdisciplinary partners with openness, receptivity to the subjective experience, shared visions of health, and communication. Integrative practices promote a softer

environment where practitioners spend more time and have a deeper level of communication with patients, appreciating the subjective experience.[38-40]

Integrative Healthcare Outcomes

The effectiveness of integrative healthcare practices is often difficult to measure because of the synergy resulting from using multiple whole-person therapies in different contexts. In evaluating the outcomes associated with integrative healthcare practices, the focus is most often on the particular therapy or CAM modality in question and on the qualifications and experience of the practitioner. However, what is often not appreciated is the influence of the recipient or patient on the success of integrative health care. The characteristics of the patient, her experiences with CAM, the quality and depth of her social networks, her underlying health beliefs, and economic resources can potentially mediate or moderate healing outcomes from integrative health care. As with conventional medicine, which addresses outcomes in terms of patient compliance, integrative health care relies on patient engagement, participation, motivation, self-efficacy, and readiness to change and persevere. In addition, the healing environment contextualizes success. The healing environment is composed of multiple contributing or distracting variables including interface factors such as time constraints, characteristics of the physical space, personalities involved, the quality of the therapeutic relationship, and the value ascribed to integrative health care.[24]

Applications of Integrative Medicine: Herbal Medicine

While it is beyond the scope of this chapter to review all the research findings on any of the CAM modalities or systems, it is important for women's health providers to have a basic comprehension of common herbal medicines that are available over the counter (**Table 26-3** provides an overview of the historical uses of common herbs). Similarly, it is valuable to know about basic patient education in nutrition and lifestyle that is offered by the provider engaging in integrative practices and how it is different from what conventional providers may offer.

Bone and Mills state that out of all CAM therapies, herbal medicine or phytotherapy has "the most scientific support."[41] Even though there is still a "paucity" of human studies on whole crude herbs, there are reports of consistent therapeutic performance and clinical effects of crude plant medicines by herbal practitioners. As of 2010, clinical trials existed for 156 plants; the 9 plants with the most clinical trial data included:[42]

- *Althaea officinalis* or marshmallow root
- *Calendula officinalis* or calendula
- *Centella asiatica* or Gotu kola
- *Echinacea purpurea* or purple coneflower
- *Passiflora incarnata* or passion flower
- *Punica granatum* or pomegranate
- *Vaccinium macrocarpon* or cranberry
- *Vaccinium myrtillus* or bilberry (similar to the US wild blueberry)
- *Valeriana officinalis* or valerian

At the same time, 12% of the commercially available herbal plants had only minimal evidence. Bone and Mills suggest that in the absence of data to support efficacy of herbal use, evidence of well established use over time can be considered clinical data.[41] See Table 26-3 for a review of common herbs.[43,44]

When investigating or gathering information on herbal medicine it is important to consider the following:

- *The system of medicine in which the use of an herb originated.* The herbal use within that system may be significantly different from the research-supported herb in dose, indications,

or the form the patient obtains from the health food store or pharmacy. Whether the patient is taking a nutritional supplement derived from part of the plant or the whole plant may result in significant differences in indications and outcomes and has implications for the generalizability of study findings. The whole plant in a crude form (like tincture or tea) is different from the extracted, augmented, or synthesized ingredients typically found in capsule or tablet forms. When taken close to their natural state, medicinal plants may be similar to foods but still considered medicine (consider cranberry and bilberry as food then processed as medicine).

- *Whether the patient is self-medicating with herbal medicine or has received an herbal medication after consultation with an herbalist.* Registered herbalists in the United States often have a thorough understanding and working knowledge of 100–300 herbs. They are more likely to be able to make effective recommendations for use.
- *Whether the patient is using an herb in isolation or as combined therapy.* If the patient is using a product composed of an isolated herb fraction or singular active ingredient, taking an extract of the whole medicinal plant along with the supplement may result in synergistic effects and better outcomes.
- *Using sources to investigate herbs that provide both the binomial botanical name and common name of the plant.*
- *Using multiple sources of knowledge, including current publications originating from experts or herbalists from the particular tradition or system under consideration, along with sources discussing the science and research of herbal medicines.* Typically, sources written by practitioners provide a practice context, the history and traditions of use, dose, and form along with a review of current research. Herbs are complex matrices of chemical components and as such are different from pharmaceuticals.[19,20]

Table 26-3 Common Herbs and Historical Uses and Uses Supported by Clinical Trials

Common Name	Binomial	Therapeutic Parts	Key Therapeutic Actions	Key Indications	Clinical Trial Evidence for Use
Aloe vera	*Aloe barbadensis*	Leaf (resin and gel)	Resin: laxative Gel or juice: alterative, anti-inflammatory, antimicrobial	Resin: constipation, hemorrhoids, anal fissure Gel or juice: irritable bowel Topical for skin	Clinical trials support: Dried latex of leaves: constipation Gel: topically for burns, erythema, genital herpes virus, seborrheic dermatitis
Black cohosh	*Actaea racemosa*	Root	Estrogen modulation, anti-inflammation, uterine tonic, spasmolytic	Menstruation disorders, arthritis, myalgia, tinnitus, whooping cough, asthma	Clinical trials support: menopause symptoms
Calendula	*Calendula officinalis*	Flower	Vulnerary, cholagogue, lymphatic, antimicrobial	External wounds, cysts, and inflammation; oral, GI, GU, eye infections; ulcers; swollen glands	Clinical trials support: upper respiratory inflammation; topically for skin inflammation, wounds, and rashes
Chamomile (German)	*Matricaria recutita* or *Chamomilla recutita*	Flower	Anti-inflammatory, spasmolytic, mild sedative, carminative, vulnerary	Nervous dyspepsia or diarrhea, flatulence, dysmenorrhea, catarrh, anxiety	Clinical trials support: anxiety, GI complaints, diarrhea (in combination with pectin), menopause (in combination with dong quai) infantile colic (in combination), topical for wounds and eczema
Echinacea	*Echinacea angustifolia* or *Echinacea purpurea*	Root, whole plant	Alterative, anti-inflammatory, antiseptic (respiratory, GI, GU, topical), immunomodulator, lymphatic, antimicrobial	Acute or chronic bacterial, viral, and protozoal infections (respiratory, GI, GU, skin); inflammation	Clinical trials support: upper respiratory tract infections and infection prophylaxis

Elder	*Sambucus nigra*	Berry, flower	Berries: immune enhancing, antiviral, antioxidant. Flowers: diaphoretic, anticatarrhal	Berries: acute viral respiratory infections. Flowers: respiratory infection, asthma, fever	Clinical trials support: influenza
Fennel	*Foeniculum vulgare*	Fruit	Carminative, galactagogue, spasmolytic, antimicrobial	Intestinal colic, flatulence, dyspepsia, anorexia, nausea, vomiting, suppressed lactation, catarrh, eye wash for conjunctivitis	Clinical trials support: IBS, in combination with other herbs, dyspepsia, flatulence, chronic constipation, infantile colic, cough, topically for hirsutism. Essential oil: dysmenorrhea, infantile colic
Feverfew	*Tanacetum parthenium*	Leaf	Anti-allergic, respiratory spasmolytic, anti-inflammatory	Cough, debility, fever, dyspepsia	Clinical trials support: migraine and tension headache prevention
Ginger	*Zingiber officinale*	Root	Bitter tonic, cholagogue	Digestive weakness, abdominal bloating, flatulence, nausea, colic, constipation, cachexia, debility, fever, colds, asthma, arthritis	Clinical trials support: dyspepsia, motion sickness nausea, pregnancy nausea, osteoarthritis, dysmenorrhea, and gastroparesis
Ginkgo	*Ginkgo biloba*	Leaf	Antiplatelet activating factor, circulatory stimulant, neuroprotective, cognition enhancing	No well documented historical use of ginkgo leaf	Clinical trials support: disorders and symptoms of restricted cerebral blood flow, vertigo, tinnitus, peripheral arterial disease, cardiovascular risks, early stages of Alzheimer-type degenerative dementia, multi-infarct dementia, reduced retinal blood flow, diabetic retinopathy and neuropathy, congestive dysmenorrhea and PMS, altitude sickness, asthma, radiation damage prophylaxis, anxiety

(continues)

Table 26-3 Common Herbs and Historical Uses and Uses Supported by Clinical Trials *(continued)*

Common Name	Binomial	Therapeutic Parts	Key Therapeutic Actions	Key Indications	Clinical Trial Evidence for Use
Ginseng (American or Korean)	*Panax ginseng*	Root	Adaptogen, tonic, immunomodulator, cardiotonic, male tonic, cancer protectant, cognitive enhancing	Aging, heart failure, digestive complaints, hypothermia, palpitations, exhaustion, debilitation and weakness, anxiety, immune deficiency, diminished memory and focus, depression, cancer, chronic disease, DM2, erectile dysfunction, menopausal symptoms	Clinical trials support: improvements of performance and well-being, cardiovascular deficits, CHF, performance with stress, cognitive performance, DM2, erectile dysfunction, lipid panels, risks of certain cancer
Hawthorne	*Crataegus* spp.	Leaf, flower, berry	Peripheral vasodilator, cardiotonic, antiarrhythmic, antioxidant, collagen stabilizing	Mild heart conditions such as hypertension, angina pectoris, and tachycardia; arteriosclerosis	Clinical trials support: stages I and II CHF, mild hypertension, anxiety in combination, topically for acne
Lemon balm	*Melissa officinalis*	Leaf	Sedative, carminative, spasmolytic, antiviral, diaphoretic, cholinergic	Restlessness, anxiety, depression, insomnia, neuralgia, dyspepsia, flatulence, topically for HSV	Clinical trials support: insomnia, anxiety, restlessness, functional GI complaints
Licorice	*Glycyrrhiza glabra*	Root	Adaptogen, adrenal tonic, antitussive, anti-inflammatory, mild laxative	Bronchitis, cough, peptic ulcers, gastritis, adrenal insufficiency, urinary inflammation, physical stress, constipation; topically for mouth ulcers, dermatitis, acne	Clinical trials support: In combination for: GI ulceration, PCOS, hyperprolactinemia. Glycyrrhizin or deglycyrrhizinated forms for: gastric and duodenal ulcers, functional dyspepsia, insulin resistance. IV: viral hepatitis, oral lichen planus

Common name	Latin name	Part used	Actions	Uses/Indications	Clinical trials support
Milk thistle or St. Mary's thistle	*Silybum marianum*	Seed	Digestive tonic, hepatotonic, antioxidant, cholagogue	Gallbladder disorders; alcoholism; liver toxicity or fatty liver; hepatitis A, B, C; jaundice; hyperlipidemia; gastric bloating	Clinical trials support: dyspepsia, supportive for chronic inflammatory and cirrhotic liver disease (nonalcoholic or alcoholic), Child-Pugh grade A cirrhosis, cirrhosis complications, xenobiotic exposure
Nettles	*Urtica dioica*	Leaf Root	Leaf: antiallergic, antirheumatic, diuretic, alterative, styptic; Root: anti-prostatic	Leaf: allergic rhinitis, diarrhea, internal bleeding, bladder irritation; Topically: burns, wounds, inflammation, dermatitis, urticaria, arthritis	Clinical trials support: Allergic rhinitis; Topically: osteoarthritis; Root: BPH, chronic prostatitis
Peppermint	*Mentha piperita*	Leaf	Spasmolytic, carminative, cholagogue, antiemetic, antitussive, antimicrobial, mild sedative, antipruritic topically	Dyspepsia, intestinal colic, flatulence, cramps, gastritis, nausea, catarrh, colds	Clinical trials support: spasmodic complaints of the GI tract, IBS (oil of peppermint), postoperative nausea, inhalation for asthma, topically for headaches, in combination for dyspepsia
Saw palmetto	*Serenoa repens*	Fruit	Anti-inflammatory, male tonic, anti-prostatic, spasmolytic	Inflammation of the respiratory tract, GU tract, atrophy of the sexual tissue, aphrodisiac	Clinical trials support: mild to moderate BPH (in combination), male-pattern baldness
St. John's wort	*Hypericum perforatum*	Aerial parts	Nervine tonic, antiviral, vulnerary, anxiolytic	Neuralgias, rheumatism, mild psychological disorders, menopausal anxiety, nervousness; topically in oil for wounds, bruises, dermatitis	Clinical trials support: mild to moderate depression, HSV, premature ejaculation, menopausal psychological symptoms, PMS, OCD, IBS, social phobia; topically for wound healing, dermatitis, and scar reduction
Thyme	*Thymus vulgaris*	Leaf Flower	Expectorant, spasmolytic, antibacterial, antifungal, rubefacient (topically)	Cough, bronchitis, catarrh, asthma, pharyngitis (topically), gastritis, dyspepsia, colic, and diarrhea	Clinical trials support: productive cough, in combination for acute bronchitis

(continues)

Table 26-3 Common Herbs and Historical Uses and Uses Supported by Clinical Trials *(continued)*

Common Name	Binomial	Therapeutic Parts	Key Therapeutic Actions	Key Indications	Clinical Trial Evidence for Use
Turmeric	*Curcuma longa*	Rhizome	Anti-inflammatory, antiplatelet, cholagogue, hepatoprotective, antioxidant	Poor digestion and liver function, topically for skin disorders	Clinical trials support: Curcuma: rheumatoid arthritis, osteoarthritis, postoperative inflammation, inflammatory bowel disease, HIV-associated diarrhea, orbital inflammatory syndrome, uveitis, topically for psoriasis Turmeric: osteoarthritis, hyperlipidemia, IBS, topically for precancerous lesions
Valerian	*Valeriana officinalis*	Root Rhizome	Mild sedative, hypnotic, anxiolytic, antispasmodic, nervine tonic	To promote sleep, nervous unrest, stress, neuralgia, epilepsy; to relieve spasm of smooth muscles	Clinical trials support: nervous tension, restlessness, insomnia, in combination for depression or anxiety

BPH = benign prostatic hyperplasia, CHF = congestive heart failure, DM2 = diabetes mellitus type 2, GI = gastrointestinal, GU = genitourinary, HIV = human immunodeficiency virus, HSV = herpes simplex virus, IBS = irritable bowel syndrome, IV = intravenous, OCD = obsessive-compulsive disorder, PCOS = polycystic ovarian syndrome, PMS = premenstrual syndrome.

Data from Bone K. *The Ultimate Herbal Compendium.* Warwick, Australia: Phytotherapy Press; 2007; Bone K, Mills S. *Principles and Practice of Phytotherapy.* 2nd ed. Edinburgh, Scotland: Churchill Livingstone, Elsevier; 2013; Thomsen M. *Phytotherapy Desk Reference.* 4th ed. Hobart, TAS, Australia; Global Natural Medicine; 2009.

Box 26-3 Glossary of Traditional Herbal Actions

Adaptogen: increases overall nonspecific resistance or adaptation to physical, environmental, emotional, or biological stressors and promotes normal biological function

Alterative: improves detoxification processes

Anticatarrhal: relieves excessive mucus

Carminative: soothes the stomach and intestines; relieves gas, pain, and spasms

Cholagogue: increases the release of bile from the gallbladder

Galactagogue: increases the flow of breast milk

Nervine: improves the tone, vigor, and function of the nervous system

Tonic: strengthens and improves the tone and vigor of the whole; improves general health and wellbeing

Vulnerary: provides wound healing with local application

Bone K, Mills S. *Principles and Practice of Phytotherapy.* Edinburgh, Scotland: Churchill Livingstone, Elsevier; 2013; Libster MM. *The Nurse Herbalist: Integrative Insights for Holistic Practice.* Naperville, IL: Golden Apple Publications; 2012.

Therefore, they should not be likened to drugs or described primarily by using pharmaceutical terminology in isolation from the traditional descriptions. Herbs are different from pharmaceuticals, act differently, and are described differently by herbal practitioners (see **Box 26-3**).[41,45] Books written by non-herbalists about herbs may potentially be incomplete and fail to differentiate between plant species or to provide the context and value in traditional knowledge or traditional descriptive terminology by reducing herb descriptions to pharmaceutical descriptions. Similarly, precautions may be overstated and based on conjecture and theory rather than actual risk from quality reports of incidents where there is credible causation linking an herb to an adverse event.[46] Reporting of adverse events should distinguish between those adverse events correlated with use of the actual herb and those associated with use of a contaminated or adulterated product.[41]

- *Creating or adapting a personal-use database on herbal medicines for quick reference.*
- *Remembering that no herb or herb combination is a "cure all" and outcomes are likely time intensive.*

Caution should be taken with the following herbs:[41]

- *Hypericum perforatum* (St. John's wort) impacts drug metabolism at the level of the cytochrome P450 system in the liver and may speed up the breakdown of particular drugs such as oral contraceptives and statin drugs.
- Pyrrolizidine alkaloids are cumulative and toxic to the liver. They are found in herbs like *Symphytum officinale* (comfrey root), *Tussilago farfara* (coltsfoot), and *Senecio* species and should be limited to external use only.
- Hepatotoxicity has been associated with *Teucrium chamaedrys* (germander), *Larrea tridentate* (Chaparral), *Kava kava,* and *Actaea racemosa* (black cohosh). However, the causal association between hepatotoxicity and both kava and black cohosh continues to be unclear.
- "Chinese herb nephropathy" has been reported with herb combinations used in Chinese medicines containing or contaminated with aristolochic acid (*Aristolochia* spp.).
- Symptoms of toxicity have been associated with the use of *Caulophyllum thalictroides* (blue cohosh) and *Mentha pulegium* (pennyroyal).

- Thujone-containing herbs (*Thuja occidentalis* or thuja, *Salvia officinalis* or sage, *Tanacetum vulgare* or tansy, *Artemisia absinthium* or wormwood, *Achillea millefolium* or yarrow) may initiate headaches or result in a decreased seizure threshold in epileptics.
- Common adverse reactions include the following:
  - *Glycyrrhiza glabra* (licorice) may contribute to hypertension with sodium and fluid retention with prolonged high-dose usage (more than 3 g per day).
  - Tannin-containing herbs may inhibit absorption of trace elements, iron, and B vitamins.
  - Echinacea, kava, and prickly ash (*Zanthoxylum* spp.) may cause tingling in the mouth and promote saliva production.
  - St. John's wort may cause allergic skin reactions in some cases. Photosensitivity is unlikely.
  - Kava or any sedative herbs may cause rebound mild lethargy in some individuals.
  - Valerian use may result in an increase in dreams in some individuals, and some individuals may respond idiosyncratically with alertness and wakefulness.
  - Laxative herbs can result in electrolyte loss or abdominal pain with abuse.
  - Misuse of adaptogens may result in overstimulation in some individuals.
  - Echinacea use in autoimmune disease is controversial.
- Caution should always be taken with drugs that have a narrow therapeutic window, such as warfarin and immunomodulators used with organ transplants. Concurrent usage with herbs is not recommended unless expressly recommended by a registered herbalist after a thorough consultation.
- Caution should be taken with pregnancy, breastfeeding, and very young children. The guideline of avoiding all medicines to the extent possible in pregnancy also applies to herbal medicines. Herbs should also be used sparingly, if at all, in children. Pregnant and breastfeeding women and children should consult a registered herbalist and an integrative practitioner prior to using any herbs.
- Allergic reactions are possible, but uncommon, with the use of herbs.
- Herbs considered to be "low dose," such as *Atropa belladonna* (belladonna), *Chelidonium majus* (greater celandine), *Convallaria majalis* (lily of the valley), *Datura stramonium* (Jimson weed), *Ephedra sinica* (ephedra), *Gelsemium sempervirens* (gelsemium), *Hyoscyamus niger* (stinking nightshade or black henbane), and *Lobelia inflate* (Indian tobacco or puke weed), are potentially toxic and should only be prescribed by professional or registered herbalists or herbalists with experience in prescribing these herbs. Additional herbs with dose-related precautions include *Adonis vernalis* (false hellebore or pheasant's eye), *Bryonia dioica* (red and white bryony), *Sanguinaria canadensis* (bloodroot), *Phytolacca decandra* (poke root or pokeweed), and potentially (depending on source and level of supervision) *Piper methysticum* (*Kava kava*).
- See selected resources on herb precautions and herb–drug interactions at the end of this chapter.

Integrative Medicine: Food and Nutrition

Food and eating-related health problems are rapidly becoming central issues in American health care.[35] Obesity is common and increases the risk of diseases such as diabetes mellitus type 2, cardiovascular disease, and cancer.[36] In addition, there have been increases in allergies and food intolerances. Consequently, it is critical that all healthcare providers understand the role food plays in disease, the culture of food, how personal food choices are made, and the factors that lead to different eating patterns.

Akin to having "health food stores" in contrast to supermarkets, integrative health care's approach to diet and nutrition stands in contrast to conventional approaches to diet and nutrition. Food quality and production practices prevalent in the US industrialized food supply are seen in relation to the fact that the "standard American diet" is emerging as a major contributor to disease. Instead of contributing to disease, the food people eat can be foundational to health promotion, disease prevention, and wellness. Food provides fuel for daily living and is the basic substrate of health.[47] In short, the food we eat is directly related to the health of the organism and quality of living.[48]

Food, eating habits, and eating patterns are deeply connected to rituals associated with home, nurturing, and often religious cultures. Food can represent comfort, substance, fulfillment, belonging, wellbeing, or medicine, but also inflammation and disease. For some people, specific food choices may be part of the diet, because certain foods make them feel good emotionally or may be avoided because they create fear. Additionally, food choices are often a matter of the knowledge one enters the supermarket with, the immediate monetary costs of the food, and what is available and appealing at the supermarket. Considering the emotional connections we have with food and the value we give to food selections, it is often a challenge for the integrative practitioner to redefine the meanings associated with food, to shift food values, and to promote new habits and patterns of eating.

Integrative health providers promote a healthful relationship with food among patients in their care. Having a healthy relationship with food is manifested by food choices that reflect quality and variety, as well as eating patterns that are conducive to energy distribution, activity, and emotional fulfillment. Dietary coaching should include a thorough dietary assessment of food content, habits, and patterns along with personal resources, interest in and motivation to change, and barriers to healthful eating. Women's health providers can function as a resource when promoting changes in food selections and eating patterns, and can become expert in nutritional counseling.

Integrative health practitioners focus on the importance of food quality in promoting health in their counseling. This approach is in contrast to the one recommended by the US Department of Agriculture, *MyPlate,* which recommends educating individuals solely on defined amounts and proportions of various foods. Humans have co-evolved with plants and have a history of eating lean wild meats and plants, and later cultivated plants. Never before in history had humans, to the extent they do today, consumed foods that have been genetically modified; exposed to pesticides and herbicides; prepared in or augmented in laboratories; or contained fillers, preservatives, flavor enhancers, or artificial colorants; or bathed in sugar, salt, and fat.[35] Never before had humans eaten meat from contained (as opposed to free-range or grazed) and medicated animals in the proportion that they are being consumed today.

Our foods have become increasingly industrialized, processed, manipulated, and monocultured over time. These processes have an adverse impact on public health and the global environment. Integrative health care acts to deter the negative effects of the standard American food culture on the health of individuals and the environment by promoting plant-based eating and the consumption of real food.

Food Recommendations

Healthy eating recommendations promoted by integrative healthcare practitioners include the following:

- Strive to eat a plant-based diet composed of whole, real foods. Strive to eat less. Individuals should consume high-quality omega-3, -6, and -9 fats; whole grains; fresh vegetables and fruits of multiple colors and varieties; beans and legumes; nuts and seeds; and lean meats and wild fish.

- If animal products are consumed, quality should guide the selection. Animal products, in moderation, are considered a side dish rather than the center of the meal. Animal products should be from animals raised and kept in a manner that is congruent with conditions they are biologically compatible with and healthful for the animal. For dairy and beef cattle, healthy living conditions include grazing and ruminating on grass as a way of life; for poultry, this includes being able to be free range with the opportunity to eat grubs and work the dirt. Likewise, animals should not be stressed by caging or given hormones or antibiotics to increase production. Processing should result in rendered products that promote the health of the animal and add health value to the consumer. Following these principles is not only ethical but affects the taste and nutrient content of the food product. Livestock that graze on grasses as opposed to being confined in a contained space, are fed primarily non-genetically modified grains, and are given minimal (or no) antibiotics and hormones produce meat and dairy products with a greater proportion of good fats to saturated or bad fats. Thus, the quality of life for animals raised for human consumption directly impacts the health-related quality of the food yield from these animals. Dietary intake of saturated fats is reduced when eating livestock that has been grazed or eggs from free-range chickens.

- Eat organic to the extent possible (e.g., when affordable and available). This assures a reduction in the consumption of genetically modified foods, pesticides, herbicides, and food additives, which are contained in various degrees in food products and likely transfer to humans. While organic foods cost more up-front, the payback is in taste and potentially improved health outcomes.

- Eat real foods and foods as close to their wild form as possible. Minimize the intake of food containing food additives (e.g., additives used for color, flavor, preservation, enhancement) or those that are highly processed (see **Table 26-4**). Real foods replace processed food and food products. Processed food products tend to be cheap and high calorie, and have minimal nutritional value. Processed foods including restaurant foods that use preprepared foods products are high in salt, sugar, and poor-quality fats. "Natural flavorings" are typically artificial, chemically derived substances that smell and perhaps taste like real food; these are added to enhance flavor and thus manipulate the consumer into buying more of the product based on the enhanced taste value.

Integrative healthcare providers also address food for diagnostic purposes with short-term elimination diets or detoxification diet protocols. In both instances, specific foods are restricted (usually 2–4 weeks in duration) to evaluate tolerance or to assist with the natural physiologic detoxification processes to counteract the effects of environmental toxins. Likewise, practitioners may feel an affinity for and ease of instruction in certain established diets, such as the Mediterranean diet, Dean Ornish's low-fat heart diet, or a no-added-sugar diet.

Food as an intervention or vehicle for health and wellbeing should be personalized, and a plan should be developed that promotes healthy, stress-free eating specific to the individual. Over time, food selection and eating become intentional and a time of mindfulness. Enabling success with new foods and new eating patterns may require learning where and how to shop, how to read labels and identify food additives, how to prepare foods or menus, and how to structure calorie or protein

Table 26-4 Foods and Food Additives to Avoid and Healthy Substitutes

Foods to Avoid	Substitutes
Trans fats and excessive saturated fats	Organic olive oil, grape seed oil, coconut oil
White sugar, sugar substitutes, and white flour Additives: corn syrup, glucose, fructose, high fructose corn syrup, maltodextrin, sorbitol, mannitol, xanthan gum, modified and unmodified starches, dextrins, citric acid, lactic acid, monosodium glutamate (MSG), ethanol, maltose, polyols, caramel color, ascorbic acid, sugar alcohols, natural flavors, nitrates (often added to meats), "any ingredient you can't read or pronounce"	Organic Stevia, Sucanat, rice syrup, honey, maple syrup, molasses in moderate amounts
Industrialized, refined, and processed foods (process of removing) or real-food substitutes	Eat real foods, less of them, and mostly plants and organic to the extent possible

Data from Pollan M. *The Omnivore's Dilema*. London, UK: Penguin; 2006.

intake throughout the day. More than just giving generic dietary advice, the integrative practitioner coaches, teaches, and enables change with food selection and eating patterns and helps individuals create a better food environment; these changes set the stage for health and wellbeing.

Nutritional Supplements

The relationship between food and health is difficult to research.[21] As with herbal medicines, each food is complex, with multiple macro- and micronutrients and chemicals existing together and acting synergistically to yield nutritional value of the whole. The effect of the whole food is potentially greater than if the parts are extracted and separated from the whole. Research, in the quest to study nutrition, has taken a reductionist approach and focused on extracted parts and their effects outside the context of the whole food (see **Box 26-4**).[49] We now know that extracted parts do not always have the same beneficial effect as when the part is nested in the whole food. Because of this, it is more beneficial to get nutrition

Box 26-4 Natural Product Defined

Natural products refer to those substances found in nature, produced by living systems, including secondary metabolites. Natural substances may be biologically native to or derived from humans, animals, plants, minerals, and organic chemicals.

Natural products on the market often in actuality are synthetic analogs of natural products, chemical derivatives, or isolated and purified parts extracted from natural substances. Natural products or nutritional supplements are developed in laboratories.

Modified from Nicolaou KC, Vourloumis D, Winssinger N, Baran PS. The art and science of total synthesis at the dawn of the twenty-first century. *Angew Chem Int Ed Engl.* 2000;39:44-120.

from food rather than supplements for prevention of health problems.

Nutritional research provides a body of information on nutritional supplements and functional foods. *Functional foods* refer to foods that have nutritional factors added that potentially increase their nutrient value. This artificially pumps up the reported nutritional value in processed food products. Nutritional supplements are parts of food—substances that are extracted, synthesized, and/or augmented to provide a dose of the nutritional component, which is not accessible when consuming a less-than-optimal diet. While nutritional supplementation is based on the sentiment that "if a little is good, then more is better," little consistent evidence from human studies exists to support broad claims of effectiveness and clinical value for mega-doses of vitamins and minerals, antioxidants in supplement form, or many of the concentrated doses of synthesized biologics (e.g., amino acids, alpha-lipoic acid, S-adenosyl methionine). While the use of nutritional supplements is supported by case reports and holds promise for research, basic questions are still unanswered. It is yet unknown whether many of the available nutritional supplements are beneficial and, if so, who might best benefit from their use. Nutritional supplements that have research supporting their use include vitamin D3, B-complex vitamins, probiotics, lutein, glucosamine, omega-3, and CoQ10.

By being on the forefront of food awareness, integrative healthcare practitioners negotiate new understandings of food and new relationships with food. The origins and relationship of health and wellbeing to food quality and health are fostered with intelligent, mindful, and intentional food selection and eating.

Integrative Health Care: Healthy Lifestyle

In addition to making referrals to partners in integrative health care, women's health providers can offer integrative interventions from their own skill sets, help guide women in the selection of healthy food and the use of herbal medicine, and empower women to be involved in their health and healing processes. Along with this, guidance should be given on how to make therapeutic

lifestyle changes that are personalized and can advance health and prevent disease. Therapeutic lifestyle modifications include exercise and activity, optimal sleep, spirituality or religious practices, emotional wellbeing and attitudinal positivity, and engagement in fulfilling community and personal relationships.

General guidelines for exercise include becoming active whenever possible. An active lifestyle, as opposed to a sedentary one, is one in which individuals take every opportunity to be upright and moving. The type, amount, and frequency of recommended physical activity should be adapted to the individual, well balanced, occur on most days of the week, and be strenuous enough to cause the person to get out of breath and break a sweat. Whole-body exercise routines include upper and lower body involvement, flexibility, weight resistance, and aerobic heart-healthy exercising. Each person's activity and exercise level should promote healthy weight. The minimal recommendation of 150 minutes a week of moderate-intensity aerobic exercise can be difficult to achieve; however, people who walk are more likely to meet this guideline than nonwalkers.[50] Walking is adaptive to each person's environment and circumstances. It is an opportunity for persons to be outside in nature; it is also simple to do and free. Tai chi is an excellent option for older adults and has multiple health benefits. Yoga is beneficial for any age group. Women should know that exercise is not a 1:1 relationship between calories consumed and those burned at the time of exercise; rather, additional benefit comes from the prolonged increase in metabolism and resultant efficiency in using calories induced by regular exercise.

Optimal sleep is integral to preventing functional impairment during the day. Often, a sleep hygiene protocol along with relaxing herbal teas and a mild over-the-counter product such as melatonin, a homeopathic calming pill, or herbal sedative combinations and management of nighttime hypoglycemia are helpful for sleep if the person does not desire pharmaceuticals.[51,52]

Whole-person health and wellbeing include recognition and integration of many aspects of health, including physical-biological health, mental-emotional health, having a positive attitude and purpose in life, spirituality, engagement in social and community relationships, and fulfillment. Health and wellbeing for whole systems are reflected by adaptability, flexibility, and complexity, as well as "fitness" to an ever-changing landscape.[10] Health emerges from the lived experience of right relationships, balancing all of the bio-psycho-socio-spiritual dimensions, and congruence within and without the environment of the human organism.[11] It is the integration and interactions of the whole that manifests in right relationships. While it is easy for the integrative practitioner to compartmentalize health promotion and disease prevention by applying multiple additive interventions, basic lifestyle changes are complicated and involve intangible elements such as experience and consciousness of purpose that both move a person toward or hold them back or apart from the dynamics of wellbeing. Attention to these contextual elements should not be overlooked or underestimated.

Most women's health providers develop strong and enduring relationships with the women in their care. Clinicians can facilitate healing by using these relationships and their knowledge of a woman's strengths and resources to promote healthy changes. Through the astute use of theories of change and the integration of CAM systems or therapies into clinical practice, women's health providers can make it possible for women to make and sustain healthy changes in their lives. However, this requires an in-depth knowledge of and referral to community resources, as well as consultation as needed and desired with expert integrative healthcare partners.

Conclusion

Integrative health care represents a shift in focus from a one-size-fits-all, disease-centered approach to participative personalized health promotion and disease prevention. Along with offering conventional interventions, integrative healthcare providers support personal choices to use nonconventional therapies, natural earth-centered therapies, and the least aggressive and least invasive therapies for disease prevention and health promotion. Appreciation is given for the knowledge and wisdom that emerge from different ways of knowing—from the expertise gleaned through repeated use through history and from research. Women's health providers engaging in integrative health care bring an understanding of whole systems, CAM interventions or therapeutics, and personal expertise in CAM systems or modalities into the healthcare environment. While additional education in integrative health care is requisite for expert practice, women's health providers can work collaboratively with integrative healthcare practitioners to promote the health and wellbeing of women in their care.

Selected Resources for Herbal Medicine

Traditional Western herbalism:
> Grieve M. (1931/1936). *A Modern Herbal.* New York, NY: Courier.
> Hoffmann, D. (2003). Medical Herbalism. Rochester: Healing Arts Press.

Traditional Western herbalism and nursing:
> Libster MM. *The Nurse Herbalist.* Naperville, IL: Golden Apple Publications; 2012.

Traditional Western herbalism with a review of current research:
> Bone K, Mills S. *Principles and Practice of Phytotherapy.* 2nd ed. Edinburgh, Scotland: Churchill Livingstone, Elsevier; 2014.
> Yance DR. *Adaptogens in Medical Herbalism.* Rochester, VT: Healing Arts Press; 2013.

Safety and interactions of herbal medicine:
> Stargrove M, Treasure J, McKee DL. *Herb, Nutrient and Drug Interactions: Clinical Implications and Therapeutic Strategies.* St. Louis, MO: Mosby, Elsevier; 2007.
> Brinker F. *Herbal Contraindications and Drug Interactions: Plus Herbal Adjuncts with Medicines.* 4th ed. Sandy: Eclectic Medical Publications; 2010.

Online Resources

National Center for Complementary and Integrative Health: https://nccih.nih.gov/
- Dietary and Herbal Supplements: https://nccih.nih.gov/health/supplements

- Herbs at a glance: https://nccih.nih.gov/health/herbsataglance.htm

National Institutes of Health Office of Dietary Supplements: https://ods.od.nih.gov/factsheets/BotanicalBackground-HealthProfessional/

References

1. Barnes PM, Bloom B, Nahin RL. Complementary and alternative medicine use among adults and children: United States, 2007. *Natl Health Stat Rep.* 2008;10(12):1-23.
2. National Center for Complementary and Integrative Health. The use of complementary and alternative medicine in the United States. Bethesda, MD: US Department of Health and Human Services, National Institutes of Health. 2008. Available at: https://nccih.nih.gov/research/statistics/2007/camsurvey_fs1.htm. Accessed June 6, 2016.
3. Stumpf SH, Shapiro SJ, Hardy ML. Divining integrative medicine. *eCAM.* 2008;5(4):409-413.
4. National Center for Complementary and Integrative Health. Complementary, Alternative, or Integrative Health: What's in a Name? Bethesda, MD: US Department of Health and Human Services. National Institutes of Health; 2015. Available at: https://nccih.nih.gov/health/integrative-health. Accessed June 7, 2016.
5. Maizes V, Rakel D, Niemiec C. Integrative medicine and patient-centered care. Institute of Medicine Summit on Integrative Medicine and the Health of the Public, 2009. Available at: http://www.canyonranchinstitute.org/storage/documents/Integrative_Medicine_and_Patient_Centered_Care.pdf. Accessed June 7, 2016.
6. National Center for Complementary and Integrative Health. Integrative Medicine. Available at: https://nccih.nih.gov/health/integrative-health#integrative. Accessed June 7, 2016.
7. Koithan M. Concepts and principles of integrative nursing. In: Kreitzer MJ, Koithan M, eds. *Integrative Nursing.* Oxford, UK: Oxford University Press; 2014.
8. Micozzi MS. *Fundamentals of Complementary and Alternative Medicine.* 4th ed. Philadelphia, PA: Saunders Elsevier; 2011.
9. Weil A. Dr. Andrew Weil's vision for the future of integrative medicine. YouTube; 2012. Available at: https://www.youtube.com/watch?v=FDQmgpBVOMY. Accessed June 7, 2016.
10. Koithan M, Bell I, Niemeyer K, Pincus D. A complex systems science perspective for whole systems of complementary and alternative medicine research. *Forsch Komplementarmed.* 2012;19(suppl 1):7-14.
11. Quinn J. Transpersonal human caring and healing. In: Dossey BM, Keegan L, eds. *Holistic Nursing: A Handbook for Practice.* 6th ed. Burlington, MA: Jones & Bartlett Learning; 2013.
12. Quinn J. The integrated nurse: wholeness, self-discovery, and self-care. In: Kreitzer MJ, Koithan M, eds. *Integrative Nursing.* Oxford, UK: Oxford University Press; 2014.
13. Bar-Yam Y. The dynamics of complex systems: examples, questions, methods, and concepts. In: *Dynamics of Complex Systems.* Boulder, CO: Westview Press; 2003.
14. Zimmerman B, Lindberg C, Plesk P. A complexity science primer: what is complexity science and how should I learn about it? In: Zimmerman B, Lindberg C, Plesk P, eds. *Edgeware: Insights from Complexity Science for Health Care Leaders.* 2nd ed. Irving, TX: VHA Inc.; 2001.
15. Koithan M. Gazing with soft eyes. In: Kreitzer MJ, Koithan M, eds. *Integrative Nursing.* Oxford, UK: Oxford University Press, 2014.
16. McCellan MB, MCGinnis MJ, Nabel EG, Olsen LM. *Evidence-Based Medicine and the Changing Nature of Healthcare: 2007 IOM Annual Meeting Summary.* Washington, DC: The National Academies Press; 2008. Available at: http://www.nap.edu/openbook.php?record_id=12041. Accessed June 7, 2016.
17. Aickin M. Innovative designs and analysis. In: Lewith GT, Jonas WB, Walach H, eds. *Clinical Research in Complementary Therapies Principles, Problems and Solutions.* Edinburgh, Scotland: Churchill Livingstone, Elsevier; 2011.
18. Golden I. Beyond randomized controlled trials: evidence in complementary medicine. *J Evidence-Based Complement Altern Med.* 2012;17(1):72-75.
19. Niemeyer K, Bell I, Koithan M. Complex systems science and traditional knowledge of Western herbal

medicine. *J Herb Med*. 2013;3(3):112-119. doi: 10.1016/j.hermed.2013.03.001.

20. Spelman K. Ecological pharmacy: from Gaia to pharmacology. In: Micozzi MS, ed. *Fundamentals of Complementary and Alternative Medicine*. Philadelphia, PA: Saunders Elsevier; 2011.

21. Challem J. The blind leading the blind: common problems with the nature of clinical trials. *Altern Complement Ther*. 2011;17(5):279-283.

22. Jonas WB, Lewith GT. Towards standards of evidence for CAM research and practice. In: Lewith GT, Jonas WB, Walach H, eds. *Clinical Research in Complementary Therapies Principles Problems and Solutions*. Edinburgh, Scotland: Churchill Livingstone, Elsevier; 2011.

23. Walach H, Falkenberg T, Fonnebo V, Lewith G, Jonas W. Circular instead of hierarchical: methodological principles for evaluation of complex interventions. *BMC Med Res Methodol*. 2006;6(29):1-9.

24. Niemeyer K. Personalizing Western Herbal Medicine: Weaving a Tapestry of Right Relationships: A Grounded Theory Study [Dissertation]. Ann Arbor, MI: ProQuest, University of Arizona; 2013.

25. Carper BA. Fundamental patterns of knowing in nursing. In: Reed PG, Shearer NBC, eds. *Perspectives on Nursing Theory*. 5th ed. Philadelphia, PA: Lippincott Williams & Wilkins; 1978.

26. Chinn PL, Kramer MK. *Integrated Theory and Knowledge Development*. 7th ed. St. Louis, MO: Mosby Elsevier; 2008.

27. Dutfield G. Protecting traditional knowledge and folklore: A review or progress in diplomacy and policy formation. Geneva, Switzerland International Centre for Trade and Sustainable Development (ICTSD), United Nations Conference on Trade and Development (UNCTAD); 2003. Available at: http://www.ictsd.org/downloads/2008/06/cs_dutfield.pdf. Accessed June 7, 2016.

28. Yance DR. *Adaptogens in Medical Herbalism*. Rochester, VT: Healing Arts Press; 2013.

29. Koithan M, Verhoef M, Bell I, White M, Mulkins A, Ritenbaugh C. The process of whole person healing: unstuckness and beyond. *J Altern Complement Med*. 2007;13(6):659-668.

30. Rioux J. A complex, nonlinear dynamic systems perspective on Ayruveda and Ayurvedic research. *J Altern Complement Med*. 2012;18(7):709-718.

31. Quinn J. The integrated nurse: way of the healer. In: Kreitzer MJ, Koithan M, eds. *Integrative Nursing*. Oxford, UK: Oxford University Press; 2014.

32. Ringdahl D. Integrative nursing and symptom management. In: Kreitzer MJ Koithan M, eds. *Integrative*

Nursing. New York, NY: Oxford University Press; 2014:187-199.

33. Niemeyer K, Koithan M, Bell I. Traditional knowledge of Western herbal medicine and complex systems science. *J Herb Med*. 2013;3:112-119.

34. Kreitzer MJ, DeLagran L, Uptmor A. Advancing wellbeing in people, organizations, and communities. In: Kreitzer MJ, Koithan M, eds. *Integrative Nursing*. Oxford, UK: Oxford University Press; 2014.

35. Pollan M. *Omnivore's Dilema*. London, UK: Penguin; 2006.

36. Centers for Disease Control and Prevention. The Health Effects of Overweight and Obesity. Available at: http://www.cdc.gov/healthyweight/effects/. Accessed June 7, 2016.

37. Templeman K, Robinson A. Integrative medicine models in contemporary primary health care. *Complement Ther Med*. 2011;19:84-92.

38. Boon H, Verhoef M, O'Hara D, Findlay B. From parallel practice to integrative health care: a conceptual framework. *BMC Health Serv Res*. 2004;4(15):1-5.

39. Rhead JC. The deeper signifcance of integrative medicine. *J Altern Complement Med*. 2014;20(5):329.

40. Gray B, OstMed M, Orrock P. Investigation into factors influencing roles, relationships, and referrals in integrative medicine. *J Altern Complement Med*. 2014;20(5):342-346.

41. Bone K, Mills S. *Principles and Practice of Phytotherapy*. 2nd ed. Edinburgh, Scotland: Churchill Livingstone, Elsevier; 2013.

42. Cravotto G, Boffa L, Genzini L, Garella D. Phytotherapeutics: an evaluation of the potential of 1000 plants. *J Clin Pharm Ther*. 2010;35:11-48.

43. Bone. K. *The Ultimate Herbal Compendium*. Warwick, Australia: Phytotherapy Press; 2007.

44. Thomsen, M. *Phytotherapy Desk Reference*. 4th ed. Hobart, TAS, Australia; Global Natural Medicine; 2009.

45. Libster MM. *The Nurse-Herbalist: Integrative Insights for Holistic Practice*. Naperville, IL: Golden Apple Publications; 2012.

46. Briggs J. Natural Product Research at NIH. Where are we now? Where next? National Center for Complementary and Integrative Health; 2015. Available for fee at: https://apha.confex.com/apha/143am/webprogram/Paper331400.html.

47. Bland JS. Environmental inputs. In: Jones DS, ed. *Textbook of Functional Medicine*. Gig Harbor, WA: Institute for Functional Medicine; 2010.

48. Gaby AR. *Nutritional Medicine*. Concord, NH: Fritz Perlberg Publishing; 2011.

49. Nicolaou KC, Vourloumis D, Winssinger N, Baran PS. The art and science of total synthesis at the dawn

of the twenty-first century. *Angew Chem Int Ed Engl.* 2000;39:44-120.

50. Centers for Disease Control and Prevention. Vital signs: walking among adults—United States, 2005 and 2010. *MMWR.* 2012;61(31);595-601.

51. Bove M. Addressing the many causes of insomnia. Medicines from the Earth Lecture Notes; 2014:20-33.

52. Romm, A. Insomnia. *J Am Herb Guild.* 2004; 8(2):14-22.

Index

Page numbers followed by *b*, *f*, or *t* indicate material in boxes, figures, or tables, respectively.

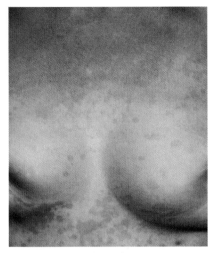

Plate 1: Pityriasis versicolor

Courtesy of CDC/Dr. Lucille K. Georg

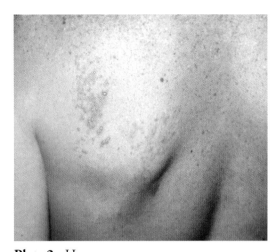

Plate 2: Herpes zoster

© Biophoto Associates/Science Source. Enhancement by: Mary Martin

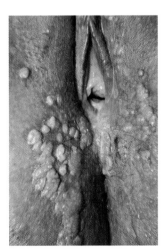

Plate 3: Condyloma lata

Courtesy of CDC/Joyce Ayers

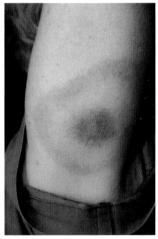

Plate 4: Erythema Migrans

Courtesy of CDC/James Gathany

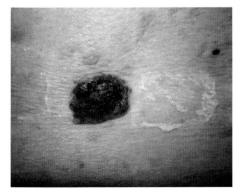

Plate 5: Seborrheic keratosis

Courtesy of CDC/ Dr. Steve Kraus

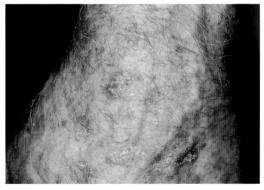

Plate 6: Actinic keratosis

Courtesy of Skin Cancer Foundation

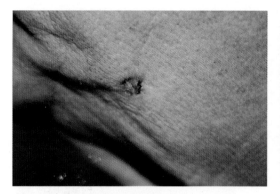

Plate 7: Basal cell carcinoma

Courtesy of National Cancer Institute/Kelly Nelson, M.D.

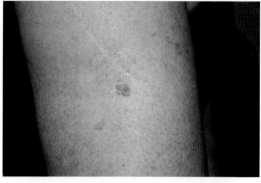

Plate 8: Squamous cell carcinoma

Courtesy of National Cancer Institute/Kelly Nelson, M.D.

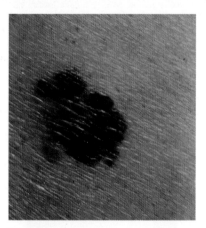

Plate 9: Melanoma

Courtesy of National Cancer Institute/Laurence Meyer, MD, PhD

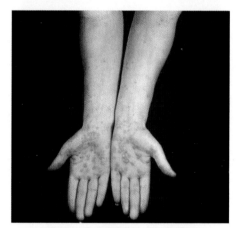

Plate 10: Rash of Secondary Syphilis

Courtesy of CDC/Robert Sumpter

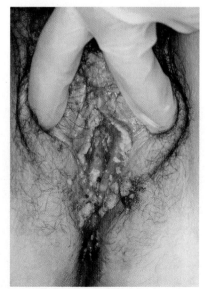

Plate 11: Condyloma accuminata (genital HPV)

Courtesy of CDC/Joe Millar

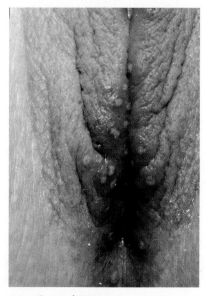

Plate 12: Genital Herpes

© Dr. Hercules Robinson/Phototake